Cooper's
FUNDAMENTALS
of HAND THERAPY

Clinical Reasoning and Treatment Guidelines for Common Diagnoses of the Upper Extremity

Third Edition

CHRISTINE M. WIETLISBACH, OTD, CHT, MPA

Hand Therapist
Eisenhower Health
Palm Springs and Rancho Mirage, CA

Adjunct Assistant Professor
Occupational Therapy Program
West Coast University
Los Angeles, CA

Lecturer and Clinical Faculty
Occupational Therapy Program
Loma Linda University
Loma Linda, CA

Adjunct Assistant Professor
Occupational Therapy Program
Rocky Mountain University of Health Professions
Provo, UT

ELSEVIER

Elsevier
3251 Riverport Lane
St. Louis, Missouri 63043

Senior Content Strategist: Lauren Willis
Senior Content Development Manager: Lisa Newton
Senior Content Development Specialist: Danielle M. Frazier
Publishing Services Manager: Shereen Jameel
Senior Project Manager: Umarani Natarajan
Design Direction: Bridget Hoette

Printed in the United States of America

Last digit is the print number: 9 8 7 6 5 4

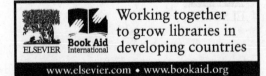

Contributors and Reviewer

Sarah Baier, BSc, BPHE, MScOT, CHT
Occupational Therapist
Roth McFarlane Hand and Upper Limb Centre
St. Joseph's Health Care London
London, Ontario, Canada

Prosper Benhaim, MD
Associate Professor and Chief of Hand Surgery
Department of Orthopaedic Surgery
UCLA Medical Center
Los Angeles, California

Andrea Bialocerkowski, PhD, BAppSc(Physio), MAppSc(Physio), GradDipPubHlth
Professor
School of Allied Health Sciences
Griffith University
Gold Coast, Queensland, Australia

Michael John Borst, OTD, MS, BA, CHT, OTR
Associate Professor
Occupational Therapy
Concordia University Wisconsin
Mequon, Wisconsin

Mark Butler, PT, DPT, OCS, Cert. MDT
Adjunct Associate Professor
School of Health Professions
Rutgers University
Blackwood, New Jersey

Lecturer
Physical Therapy
Stockton University
Galloway, New Jersey

Lecturer
Doctor of Physical Therapy Program
DeSales University
Center Valley, Pennsylvania

Center Manager
NovaCare
Select Medical
Medford, New Jersey

Angela C. Chu, BAppSc(OT)
Occupational Therapy Department
Austin Health
Heidelberg, Victoria, Australia

Cynthia Cooper, MFA, MA, OTR/L, CHT
Cooper Hand Therapy
Carlsbad, California

Lori DeMott, OTD, OTR/L, CHT
Associated Faculty
The Ohio State University
Occupational Therapy Division
College of Medicine School of Health & Rehabilitation Sciences
Columbus, Ohio

Lisa Deshaies, OTR/L, CHT
Clinical Specialist
Outpatient Therapy Services
Rancho Los Amigos National Rehabilitation Center
Downey, California

Adjunct Clinical Faculty
Division of Occupational Science and Occupational Therapy
University of Southern California
Los Angeles, California

Goldie Eder, LICSW, BCD
Lecturer
Psychiatry
Harvard Medical School
Cambridge, Massachusetts

Associate Clinical Professor
School for Social Work
Smith College
Northampton, Massachusetts

Lori Falkel, PT, MOMT, CHT, DPT
Peace Corps Community Health Volunteer
Vancouver, Washington

Sharon R. Flinn, PhD, MEd, OTR/L, CHT, FAOTA
Professor Emeritus
The Ohio State University
Columbus, Ohio

Louann Gulick Gaub, MSA, OTR/L, CHT
Hand Therapy Manager
Hand Therapy, Sawmill Location
Orthopedic ONE
Upper Arlington, Ohio

Luella Grangaard, MS, OTR/L, CHT
Manager
Occupational Therapy
Eisenhower Health
Rancho Mirage, California

Mojca Herman, MA, OTR/L, CHT
Owner/Therapist
Hand and Upper Extremity
Advanced Therapy Center
Torrance, California

Bridget Hill, PhD, Grad Dip Physio
Epworth Monash Rehabilitation Medicine Unit
Epworth HealthCare
Melbourne, Australia

Melissa J. Hirth, BOT, MSc (Hand & Upper Limb Rehab)
Occupational Therapy
Austin Health
Heidelberg, Victoria, Australia

Julianne Wright Howell, MS, PT, CHT
Self-Employed
Saint Joseph, Michigan

Kendyl Brock Hunter, OTR/L, CHT
Clinical Specialist
Hand Therapy
BenchMark Rehab Partners
Cleveland, Georgia

Cynthia Clare Ivy, MEd, OTD, CHT
Associate Clinical Professor
Occupational Therapy
Northern Arizona University
Phoenix, Arizona

Assistant Professor
Physical Medicine Rehabilitation
Mayo Clinic
Phoenix, Arizona

Certified Hand Therapist
Hand Therapy
Mayo Clinic
Phoenix, Arizona

Saba Kamal, OTR, CHT
Director
Hands-On-Care
San Jose, California

Steven Kempton, MD
Hand Surgeon
Orthopedic Surgery
UCLA Medical Center
Los Angeles, California

Linda Klein, OTR, CHT
Hand Therapy Manager
Hand to Shoulder Specialists of Wisconsin
Glendale, Wisconsin

Paige E. Kurtz, MS, OTR/L, CHT
Advanced Clinical Rehabilitation Specialist
Hand Therapy
Sentara Therapy Centers
Chesapeake and Virginia Beach, Virginia

Adjunct Faculty
School of Rehabilitation Sciences, Doctorate in Physical Therapy
Old Dominion University
Norfolk, Virginia

Renee B. Lonner, LCSW, BCD
Licensed Clinical Social Worker
Private Practice
Sherman Oaks, California

Kathryn S. McQueen, OTD, OTR/L, CHT
Occupational Therapist
Occupational Therapy, Milliken Hand Rehabilitation Center
Washington University School of Medicine
Saint Louis, Missouri

Sarah Mee, MSc Hand Therapy, PG Dip Biomechanics, DipCOT
Consultant Hand Therapist
Hand Therapy Department
Chelsea and Westminster NHS Foundation Trust
London, United Kingdom

Lecturer and Director
NES Hand Therapy Training
London, United Kingdom

Joel Moorhead, MD, PhD
Physician Advisor
Tucson Medical Center
Tucson, Arizona

Anne Michelle Moscony, OTD, OTR/L, CHT
Contributing Faculty
Occupational Therapy
University of St. Augustine
St. Augustine, Florida

Certified Hand Therapist
Occupational Therapy
Ability Rehabilitation
Orlando and Winter Park, Florida

Lisa O'Brien, PhD, MClinSci, BAppSci(OT)
Associate Professor
Occupational Therapy
Monash University
Melbourne, Victoria, Australia

Aida E. Olvera-Dyckes, MSOP, BS/OT

Occupational Therapist
Ascension Health, Outpatient Hand Therapy
Southfield, Michigan

Carol Page, PT, DPT, CHT

Program Director, Hand Therapy Fellowship
Rehabilitation
Hospital for Special Surgery
New York, New York

Senior Director
Rehabilitation
Hospital for Special Surgery
New York, New York

Julie Pal, BSOT, OTR/L, CHT

Dept of Occupational Therapy/Outpatient Rehabilitation
Saint Luke's Hospital
Kansas City, Missouri

Tim Pemberton, MSOT, OTR/L

Occupational Therapist
Occupational Therapy, Milliken Hand Rehabilitation Center
Washington University School of Medicine
St. Louis, Missouri

Gillian Porter, MA, MOT

Occupational Therapist
Occupational Therapy
SWAN Rehab
Phoenix, Arizona

Luke Steven Robinson, BOccTherapy(Hons), PhD Candidate

Lecturer
Occupational Therapy
Monash University
Melbourne, Victoria, Australia

Deborah A. Schwartz, OTD, OTR/L, CHT

Product and Educational Specialist
Physical Rehabilitation
Orfit Industries America
Leonia, New Jersey

Emily Seeley, BScOT, CHT

Occupational Therapist
Division of Hand Therapy, Roth McFarlane Hand and
Upper Limb Centre
St. Joseph's Health Care London
London, Ontario, Canada

Gary Solomon, MS, OTR/L, CHT

Director
Hand Therapy
Chicago Metro Hand Therapy, LLC
Arlington Heights, Illinois

Peggy Stein, OTD, OTR/L, CHT

Active Wellness, LLC
Corvallis, Oregon

Susan Watkins Stralka, BS, MS, DPT

Consultant /Physical Therapy
Plymouth, Massachusetts

Mike Szekeres, PhD, OT Reg(Ont.), CHT

Associate Scientist
Occupational Therapy
Lawson Health and Research Institute
London, Ontario, Canada

Director
Hand Therapy
Hand Therapy Canada
London, Ontario, Canada

Lara Taggart, EdD, OTR/L

Lecturer
Occupational Therapy Doctoral Program
Northern Arizona University
Phoenix, Arizona

Jackie Wallman, BSOT, OTR/L, CHT

Manager
Outpatient Rehabilitation Services
Saint Luke's Hospital
Kansas City, Missouri

Maura Ann Walsh, OTR/L, CHT

Senior Occupational Therapist
Certified Hand Therapist
Rehabilitation Services
Newton Wellesley Hospital-Ambulatory Care Center
Newton, Massachusetts

Susan Weiss, OTR/L, CHT

Director
Education Department
Exploring Hand Therapy
Saint Petersburg, Florida

Colleen West, MS, OTR/L

Occupational Therapist
Advanced Home Health
Mesa, Arizona

Adjunct Faculty
Occupational Therapy
A.T. Still University
Mesa, Arizona

Christine M. Wietlisbach, OTD, CHT, MPA
Hand Therapist
Eisenhower Health
Palm Springs and Rancho Mirage, California

Adjunct Assistant Professor
Occupational Therapy Program
West Coast University
Los Angeles, California

Lecturer and Clinical Faculty
Occupational Therapy Program
Loma Linda University
Loma Linda, California

Adjunct Assistant Professor
Occupational Therapy Program
Rocky Mountain University of Health Professions
Provo, Utah

REVIEWER

Rhonda Powell, OTD, OTR/L, CHT
Occupational Therapist
Occupational Therapy, Milliken Hand Rehabilitation Center
Washington University School of Medicine
Saint Louis, Missouri

To all my students: past, present, and future.
You allow me the joy of teaching in the classroom and in the clinic.
This book is for you.

Foreword

Welcome to the third edition of *Cooper's Fundamentals of Hand Therapy*! This book has long been considered one of the premiere resources for students and therapists new to hand therapy, and I am honored to have the opportunity to contribute some words about this new edition. This textbook is important and unique because it addresses the novice hand therapist in understandable language and describes specialized practice concepts in a user-friendly format. Cynthia Cooper, the editor of previous editions, did an excellent job establishing this book in a "mentor speaks to mentee" style; and Christine Wietlisbach has carried this vision forward in exemplary fashion. For example, each diagnosis-specific chapter in this edition includes sections like: "Questions to Ask the Doctor" and "What to Say to Clients" and "Tips From the Field." The inclusion of these sections along with the writing style of each chapter makes the entire text easy to read and gives the feel of having an experienced hand therapist there guiding the reader. The content of the pages within this book does more than just tell the new hand therapist *what to do*; it guides the new hand therapist in *how to think* about management of individuals with upper extremity dysfunction.

Two highlights of this text are the wide base of contributors and the variety of topics found within. Contributors from the USA, Canada, Australia, and Great Britain help provide a worldwide perspective on several topics. While practice patterns may differ geographically, the diversified contribution that these contributors have made reinforces the fact that the fundamentals of hand therapy practice and the general principles of upper extremity management transcend location. These general principles are thoroughly covered in this book, with 39 chapters on a wide variety of diagnoses commonly seen by the hand therapist.

The second chapter of this text, "Evidence-Based Practice: The Basic Tools," is a welcome addition. This chapter explores how to critically examine research and should assist new hand therapists in understanding what they are reading in publications. Therapists should always try to incorporate the best available evidence into clinical decision making. This begins with the ability to critically appraise primary research papers and understand how these papers apply to specific clinical scenarios in practice. This new chapter offers a starting place for understanding appraisal of the literature and will hopefully inspire readers to utilize appropriate evidence in daily practice as it becomes available. While the chapters in this book are written by acknowledged experts who have been encouraged to back up their information with the most current published research, the multitude of new research papers published on a daily basis makes all text books inherently out of date shortly after publication. By understanding how to be consumers of research, therapists can use this textbook as a reliable base for understanding the fundamentals of hand therapy, and then supplement this knowledge through further literature review and analysis to make evidence-based decisions in their practice.

Once again, I am honored to have been invited to write this piece on behalf of Christine Wietlisbach. I highly recommend this textbook for students and therapists who are new to hand therapy, as it is easy to read, provides valuable clinical tips and suggestions, and includes evidence-based information on a wide variety of relevant topics from expert contributors.

Mike Szekeres, PhD, OT Reg(Ont.), CHT

Preface

There are many well-written books covering a variety of hand therapy topics. Several of these books line the shelves of my personal library, and I have enjoyed reading them while enhancing my knowledge of this wonderful area of specialty practice. However, when I was searching for a new textbook to accompany my hand therapy course at Loma Linda University in southern California, I was completely enamored with Cynthia Cooper's *Fundamentals of Hand Therapy*. At the time, the textbook was in its first edition. What I found extraordinary about this textbook was that it taught students and beginning hand therapists not only about common hand therapy diagnoses but also about *how to think about* treating these diagnoses. This element of teaching clinical reasoning in a textbook sold me on *Fundamentals of Hand Therapy*, and it has been my go-to textbook ever since.

When Cynthia asked me to take over as editor for the third edition of her textbook, I was honored. As a teacher and a clinician, there are few things more important to me than grooming the next generation of hand therapists. I believe Cooper's *Fundamentals of Hand Therapy* is integral to this mission. The textbook is divided into two parts. The first half of the book focuses on foundational knowledge relative to the hand therapy practitioner, such as functional anatomy, evaluation and assessment of the upper extremity, and orthoses. This third edition includes new foundational chapters on evidence-based hand therapy practice, physical agent modalities used in hand therapy, and facilitating adherence to the hand therapy plan of care.

The second half of the book covers clinical reasoning and treatment guidelines for common diagnoses of the upper extremity. I have preserved Cynthia's organizational format in that the diagnosis-specific chapters include information about:

- Anatomy
- Diagnosis/pathology
- Timelines and healing
- Nonoperative treatment
- Operative treatment
- Questions to ask the doctor
- What to say to clients
- Evaluation tips
- Diagnosis-specific information that affects clinical reasoning
- Tips from the field
- Precautions and concerns
- Clinical pearls
- Case examples

I believe the third edition of *Fundamentals of Hand Therapy* continues Cynthia Cooper's vision of a user-friendly and understandable textbook for physical and occupational therapy students and beginning hand therapists around the globe. It is my ardent hope that whether you are a teacher or student of hand therapy, you will enjoy this textbook as much as I do.

Christine M. Wietlisbach

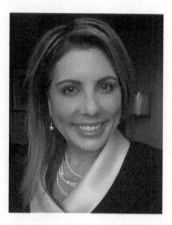

Contents

1 Fundamentals: Hand Therapy Concepts and Treatment Techniques

Cynthia Cooper

The more you know about something in detail,
the less you know about it in general.

—From *The Child in Time* by Ian McEwan,
Anchor Books, 1987

Hands are visible, expressive, and vulnerable. When clients use their hands to get dressed, eat, touch, gesture, or communicate, they are performing exquisite and complex movements. Limitations of motion or even a small scar can affect a person's life in profound ways.[1] When we touch our clients' hands, we touch their lives. Although it is very important to be knowledgeable about the details of hand anatomy and to be structure-specific in our treatment, it is equally important not to lose sight of the whole person whose extremity we are treating. We must continuously encourage clients to tell us about themselves and their needs so that their therapy can be relevant and successful. While getting to know the person we are treating, we can explain how our interventions and the client's home programs will be helpful. As a rule, I find that if I listen well, clients frequently tell me in lay terms or even show me exactly what motion or function is missing. The challenge is to identify and treat clients' specific tissues effectively while not losing sight of them as people.

Hand Therapy Concepts

The anatomy of the hand is complex. Many structures are **multiarticulate** (that is, they cross multiple joints), and little room is available for scar tissue or edema to develop without affecting function. Injury in one area of the hand can result in stiffness in other, uninjured parts. A good demonstration of this is the **quadriga effect,** which illustrates the interconnectedness of the digits. If you passively hold your ring finger extended with your other hand and then try to make a fist, you will notice how limited the whole hand can feel when just one finger is held stiff. In this example, the flexor digitorum profundus (FDP) tendons to multiple digits have a shared muscle belly. Restricting movement at one finger restricts the other fingers when they try to flex. This example reminds us that clients can be limited in motion in areas not originally injured. Therefore the therapist needs to evaluate beyond the isolated area of injury when treating clients with hand problems.

To be competent in hand therapy, therapists must be able to do more than just note decreased range of motion (ROM). They must be able to figure out what structures are restricted and how these restrictions affect function (for example, the client has decreased digital flexion due to FDP adherence, preventing him from holding the steering wheel); they then must be able to target treatment to those particular tissues. These three elements are part of all the decisions we make as hand therapists. As treatment continues, reevaluation reveals new findings with different tissues to target, and appropriate modifications and upgrades are made. This chapter addresses treatment concepts and techniques of hand therapy and concludes with some provocative thoughts to stimulate clinical reasoning.

Timelines and Healing

Tissues heal in predictable phases. However, the length of these phases varies depending on client variables, such as age and health. The three phases of healing are inflammation, fibroplasia, and maturation (also called *remodeling*). In the **inflammation phase,** vasoconstriction occurs, followed by vasodilation, with migration of white blood cells to promote **phagocytosis** in preparation for further healing. In this stage, which lasts a few days, immobilization often is advised, depending on the specifics of the diagnosis.[2] If wound contamination or delayed healing is a factor, this phase can last longer.[3]

The **fibroplasia phase** begins about 4 days after injury and lasts 2 to 6 weeks. In this phase, fibroblasts begin the formation of scar tissue. The fibroblasts lay down new collagen, on which capillary buds grow, leading to a gradual increase in the tissue's tensile strength. In this stage, active range of motion (AROM) and orthotics typically are used to promote balance in the hand and to protect the healing structures.[2]

The timeline for the **maturation (remodeling) phase** varies; this phase may even last years. In the maturation phase, the tissue's architecture changes, reflecting improved organization of the collagen fibers and a further increase in tensile strength. The tissue is more *responsive* (that is, reorganizes better) if appropriate therapy is started sooner rather than later. In this stage, gentle resistive exercises may be appropriate, and the client should be monitored for any inflammatory responses (also known as a *flare response*). Dynamic or static orthoses may also be helpful.[2]

Positioning to Counteract Deforming Forces

Predictable deforming forces act on an injured upper extremity (UE). **Edema** (swelling) routinely occurs after injury, creating tension on the tissues. The resulting predictable deformity posture is one of wrist flexion, metacarpophalangeal (MP) hyperextension, proximal interphalangeal (PIP) and distal interphalangeal (DIP) flexion, and thumb adduction.[4] This deformity position occurs as a result of tension on the extrinsic muscles caused by dorsal edema.

Use of the **antideformity (intrinsic-plus) position** (also called *safe position*) is recommended after injury unless it is contraindicated by the diagnosis (for example, it is not used after flexor tendon repair). The antideformity position consists of the wrist in neutral position or extension, the MPs in flexion, the IPs in extension (*IPs* refers to the PIP and DIP joints collectively), and the thumb in abduction with opposition (Fig. 1.1). The antideformity position maintains length in the collateral ligaments, which are vulnerable to shortening, and counteracts deforming forces.

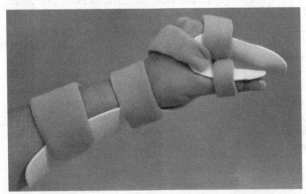

FIG. 1.1 Antideformity (intrinsic-plus) orthotic position. (From Coppard BM, Lohman H, eds. *Introduction to Splinting: A Clinical-Reasoning and Problem-Solving Approach.* 2nd ed. St Louis, MO: Mosby; 2001.)

Joint and Musculotendinous Tightness

Joint tightness is confirmed if the passive range of motion (PROM) of a joint does not change despite repositioning of proximal or distal joints. **Musculotendinous tightness** is confirmed if the PROM of a joint changes with repositioning of adjacent joints that are crossed by that particular muscle–tendon (musculotendinous) unit.[5]

Joint tightness and musculotendinous tightness can be treated with serial casting, dynamic orthoses, static progressive orthoses, or serial static orthoses (see Chapter 7 and also the Orthotics section later in this chapter). With joint tightness, splinting can focus on the stiff joint, and less consideration is needed for the position of proximal or distal joints. With musculotendinous tightness, because the tightness occurs in a structure that crosses multiple joints, the orthosis must carefully control the position of proximal (and possibly distal) joints to remodel tightness effectively along that musculotendinous unit.

The client in Fig. 1.2A had an infected PIP joint in the index finger. He was treated with hospitalization, intravenous administration of antibiotics, and joint debridement. He arrived for therapy 2 weeks later than his physician had ordered; he had no orthosis, significant edema, and a severe flexion contracture of the PIP joint. Because the stiffness was localized to the PIP joint, he needed only a digit-based extension orthosis for that joint. Fig. 1.2B shows his progress after 2 weeks of edema control and serial static digit-based orthoses.

Musculotendinous tightness can be a cause of joint tightness. Clients with tightness of the extrinsic flexors (that is, lacking passive composite digital extension with the wrist extended) are at risk of developing IP flexion contractures. Instruct these clients to passively place the MP in flexion and then to gently, passively extend the IPs to maintain PIP and DIP joint motion. In these cases, although you should consider night orthoses in composite extension to lengthen the extrinsic flexors, the better course may be to splint in a modified intrinsic-plus position with the MPs flexed as needed to support the IPs in full extension. This helps prevent IP flexion contractures.

Intrinsic or Extrinsic Extensor Muscle Tightness

Intrinsic muscles are the small muscles in the hand. **Extrinsic muscles** are longer musculotendinous units that originate proximal to the hand. Intrinsic tightness and extrinsic extensor tightness are tested by putting these muscles on stretch. This is accomplished by comparing the PROM of digital PIP and DIP flexion when the MP joint is passively extended and then passively flexed. With **interosseous muscle tightness,** passive PIP and DIP flexion is limited when the MP joint is passively extended or hyperextended (Fig. 1.3). With **extrinsic extensor tightness,** PIP and DIP flexion is limited when the MP joint is passively flexed (Fig. 1.4).[5]

To treat intrinsic tightness, perform PIP and DIP flexion with MP hyperextension. Functional orthoses are very helpful for isolating specific exercises to restore length to the intrinsics while performing daily activities (see the Orthotics section). To treat extrinsic extensor tightness, promote **composite motions** (that is, combined flexion motions of the wrist, MPs and IPs) with orthoses, gentle stretch, and exercise. Instruct the client that performing these exercises with the wrist in a variety of positions is helpful.

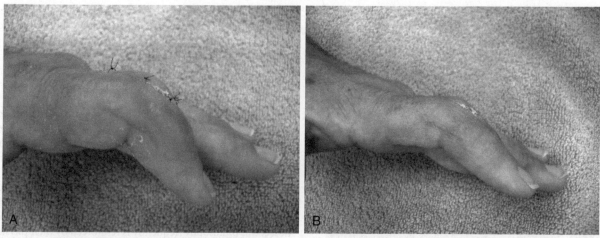

FIG. 1.2 (A) Unsplinted, infected index finger after surgery. (B) Improvement in edema and improved extension range of motion after 2 weeks.

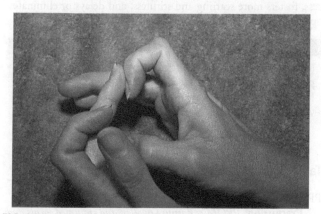

FIG. 1.3 Interosseous muscle tightness. PIP and DIP flexion is passively limited when the MP joint is passively extended or hyperextended.

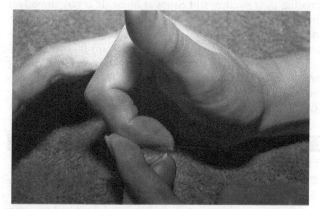

FIG. 1.4 Extrinsic extensor tightness. PIP and DIP flexion is passively limited when the MP joint is passively flexed.

Extrinsic Extensor or Flexor Tightness

Extrinsic tightness can involve the flexors or the extensors. To test for tightness, put the structure on stretch by positioning the proximal joint crossed by that structure. With extrinsic extensor tightness, passive composite digital flexion is more limited with the wrist flexed than with the wrist extended.

With extrinsic flexor tightness, passive composite digital extension is more limited with the wrist extended than with the wrist flexed.[5]

Lag or Contracture

> ◎ **Clinical Pearl**
>
> When PROM is greater than AROM at a joint, the active limitation is called lag.

A client with a PIP extensor lag is unable to actively extend the PIP joint as far as is possible passively (which may not necessarily be full extension). **Lags** may be caused by adhesions, disruption of the musculotendinous unit, or weakness.

> ◎ **Clinical Pearl**
>
> When passive limitation of joint motion exists, that limitation is called a *joint contracture*.

Joint contractures can be caused by collateral ligament tightness, adhesions, or a mechanical block. A *joint flexion contracture* is characterized by a stiff joint in a flexed position that lacks active and passive extension. A person with a joint flexion contracture whose passive extension improves may progress from having a flexion contracture to having an extensor lag. In your treatment communications and documentation, it is important to identify such changes, to use these terms correctly, and to be joint specific and motion specific. For example, you should note, "The client has full PIP passive extension but demonstrates a 30-degree PIP extensor lag."

When a lag is present (PROM exceeds AROM), treatment should focus on promoting active movement. Blocking exercises (Fig. 1.5), differential tendon gliding exercises (see Fig. 1.17), place and hold exercises (see Fig. 1.18), and dynamic or static functional orthoses can be helpful (Fig. 1.6). If a contracture is present, promote both PROM and AROM with the same exercises and with corrective orthoses, which may be the dynamic, static progressive, serial static, or casting type.

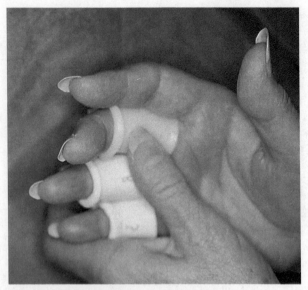

FIG. 1.5 DIP blocking exercises with the MP in various positions.

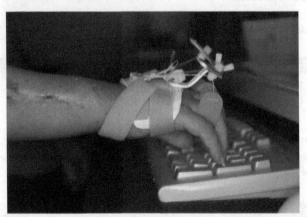

FIG. 1.6 A dynamic MP extension-assist orthosis allows the client to perform keyboard activities at the computer.

Joint End Feel

A joint with a **soft end feel** has a spongy quality at the end range. This favorable quality indicates a potential for remodeling. Orthoses for soft end feel may be the static type or the low-load, long-duration type.

A joint with a **hard end feel** has an unyielding quality at end range. This is a stiffer joint, and correcting it may require serial casting or static progressive orthoses with longer periods of splint wear.[2] Documenting the end feel and explaining the implications of your findings to the client are very important.

Nociceptive Pain Versus Neuropathic Pain[6]

Not all pain is the same physiologically or symptomatically. **Nociceptive pain** is caused by structural dysfunction, such as an arthritic wrist. Providing an orthosis to support the involved structures reduces the pain. **Neuropathic pain** is caused by some form of peripheral nerve dysfunction and is typically a sensory pain that is difficult for clients to describe in words. It may be burning or electrical. Providing sensory protection and minimizing peripheral nerve irritation reduces this type of pain.

Hand therapy clients may have nociceptive pain or neuropathic pain or a combination of the two. It is important to address this with clients so that your treatment targets their unique pain quality and can be most successful.

Preventing Pain

Precaution. *Pain with therapy is a signal that injury is occurring. Irreversible damage can result when clients or their families or, worse, therapists injure tissue by using painful force and PROM. Avoid pain in your hand therapy treatment. Being overzealous and ignoring objective signs of tissue intolerance is inexcusable.*

Teaching clients and their families that painful therapy is counterproductive can be a challenge. Often clients come to therapy with a "no pain, no gain" mentality. To make matters worse, this philosophy frequently is reinforced by their physicians and friends. Therapists have a duty to explain to their clients that imposing, prolonging, or aggravating pain slows the healing process, fosters more scarring and stiffness, and delays or eliminates opportunities to upgrade therapy.

> **Clinical Pearl**
>
> Never tell your clients, "Exercise to pain tolerance" or "Go to pain." Instead, say, "Avoid pain when you exercise. It's okay to feel a stretch that isn't painful, but it's not okay to feel pain when you exercise."

Taking Care With Passive Range of Motion

PROM of the hand should be performed gently and with care.

Precaution. *PROM can injure swollen and inflamed joints and tissues.* Colditz[5] cautions that the only joints for which manual PROM is safe are joints with a soft end feel. Nevertheless, clients may request more aggressive therapy. They may even be passively stressing their swollen, stiff hands at home. It is very important that the therapist inquire about this and put a stop to it. Explain to your client how injurious and counterproductive it is, emphasizing that delicate hand tissues are all too easily injured.

Precaution. *PROM can trigger inflammatory responses, causing additional scar production, pain, and stiffness. PROM used inappropriately or painfully can incite complex regional pain syndrome (CRPS), which is also known as reflex sympathetic dystrophy (RSD).*

> **What to Say to Clients**
>
> ### If the Doctor Orders "Aggressive Therapy"
>
> When a physician orders aggressive therapy for a client, I tell the client, "Your doctor wants you to make excellent progress. However, the reality is that tissues in the hand are delicate and can easily be injured by too much force or pressure. We will work to correct the restricted or injured tissues, and you will make the best progress by providing controlled stress to the proper structures. Painful, injurious treatment or exercise will only delay or even derail your progress. What we will do aggressively is to upgrade your program and encourage maximum results."
>
> Hopefully, physicians soon will realize the wisdom of replacing the term *aggressive* with *progressive*. Until that happens, explain to your clients that pain-free, controlled stretching and remodeling have proved to be the best course of treatment for the fragile hand tissues.

Quality of Movement and Dyscoordinate Cocontraction

Dyscoordinate cocontraction is a poor quality of movement that can result from cocontraction of antagonist muscles. Clients may demonstrate dyscoordinate cocontraction when they use excessive effort with exercise or when they fear pain with exercise or PROM, or it may be habitual. The resulting motion looks unpleasant and awkward. For example, you may feel the extensors contract as the client tries to activate the flexors. It is important not to ignore dyscoordinate cocontraction. Instead, teach the client pain-free, smooth movements that feel pleasant to perform. Replace isolated exercises with purposeful or functional activities and try proximal oscillations (small, gentle, rhythmic motions) to facilitate a more effective quality of movement. Biofeedback or electrical stimulation may also be helpful. Imagery offers additional possibilities (for example, ask your client to pretend to move the extremity through gelatin or water).[7] Do not bark at the client to "Relax!" Instead, be gentle with your voice and your verbal cues.

Adjunct Treatments

Superficial heating agents can have beneficial effects on analgesic, vascular, metabolic, and connective tissue responses. Analgesic effects are seen in diminished pain and elevated pain tolerance. Vascular effects are evidenced by reduced muscle spasms and improved pain relief. Metabolic effects are related to an increased flow of blood and oxygen to the tissues with improved provision of nutrients and removal of by-products associated with inflammation. Connective tissue effects include reduced stiffness with improved extensibility of tissues.[8]

Many clients feel that heat helps prepare the tissue for exercise and activity. The safest way to warm the tissues of hand therapy clients is aerobic exercise, unless this is contraindicated for medical reasons. Tai chi, for example, provides multijoint ROM, relaxation, and cardiac effects.

Application of external heat (for example, hot packs) is a popular method in many clinics. Although the use of heat is fine if it is not contraindicated, be mindful that heat increases edema, which acts like glue, and this may contribute to stiffness. Heat can degrade collagen and may contribute to microscopic tears in soft tissue.[9] For these reasons, be very gentle and cautious if you perform PROM after heat application. Monitor the situation to make sure that the overall benefits of heat outweigh any possible negative responses. Measuring edema is a good way to objectify these responses.

Cold therapy (also called *cryotherapy*) traditionally has been used to relieve pain and to reduce inflammation and edema after injury (and sometimes after overly aggressive therapy). Cryotherapy typically is used after acute injury to reduce bleeding by means of vasoconstriction. Cold therapy reduces postinjury edema and inflammation and raises the pain threshold. However, remember: *cold therapy can be harmful to tissues; be cautious with this modality.*

Precaution. *Do not use cryotherapy on clients with nerve injury or repair, sensory impairment, peripheral vascular disease, Raynaud's phenomenon, lupus, leukemia, multiple myeloma, neuropathy, other rheumatic disease, or cold intolerance.*

Other modalities have historically been used in hand therapy. Therapists should study these topics further. However, they also must abide by their practice acts and the regulations of their state licensing agencies regarding the use of modalities. Never use a modality for which you cannot demonstrate proper education and training.

Scar Management

Scars can take many months to heal fully. Treat scar sensitivity with desensitization. If the sensitivity causes functional limitations, provide protection, such as padding or silicone gel. Scars are mature when they are pale, supple, flatter, and no longer sensitive. Scar maturation can be facilitated by light compression (for example, with nonadherent wrap, an elastic support sleeve, or edema gloves).

Precaution. *Always check to make sure the compression on the scar is not excessive (that is, the wrap, sleeve, or glove is not too tight).*

Inserts made of padded materials or silicone gel pads also help facilitate scar maturation.[10] This padding is thought to promote neutral warmth of the area and may decrease oxygen to the collagen, thus promoting collagen maturation. Another alternative for scar management is to use paper tape applied longitudinally along the incision line once epithelialization has occurred.[11] I have found this to be very effective and cost saving for clients. In addition, paper tape helps reduce neuropathic pain.

Instruct your clients to avoid sun exposure while the scar is still immature (that is, pink or red, thick, itchy, or sensitive). Sunlight can burn the fragile scar and darken its color, affecting the cosmetic result when the scar is mature. Frequent use of sunscreen is highly recommended (see Chapter 30). Although scar massage is often performed, it is important to monitor the client's tissue response.

Precaution. *If scar massage is too aggressive, it may cause inflammation and contribute to more extensive development or thickening of scar tissue.*

Do not encourage aggressive massage; instead, teach the client to perform gentler massage that does not cause a flare of tissues. Further research on this topic is needed.

Treatment Techniques

Orthoses

Orthotic fabrication is a mainstay of therapy for UE problems. Orthoses can provide immobilization or selective mobilization. They can be used with exercise or to promote function. The topic of orthoses exceeds the scope of this chapter (see Chapter 7). I strongly advise readers to study more comprehensive resources on this subject.[2,12] In addition to learning about orthotic fabrication, readers should learn about strap placement for mechanical advantage and comfort.

Static orthoses are used to immobilize tissues, to prevent deformity, to prevent contracture of soft tissue, and to provide substitution for lost motor function. **Serial static orthoses** position the tissue for lengthening and are remolded at intervals. Static orthoses contribute to disuse, stiffness, and atrophy; therefore they should not be used more than necessary. **Static progressive orthoses** (also called *inelastic mobilization orthotics*) apply mobilizing force using nonmoving parts such as monofilament, Velcro, or screws. **Dynamic orthoses** (also called **mobilization orthoses** or **elastic mobilization orthoses**) use moving parts, such as rubber bands or spring wires, to apply a gentle force. These orthoses are used to correct deformity, to substitute for absent or impaired motor function, to provide controlled movement, and to promote wound healing or help with alignment of fractures.[12,13]

Forearm-based orthoses should cover approximately two-thirds of the forearm. Have the client bend the arm at the elbow, and note the place where the forearm meets the biceps muscle. The proximal edge of the orthosis should be one-quarter-inch distal to this so that the orthosis is not pushed distally when the client flexes the elbow. Flaring the proximal edges of the orthosis is also important to ensure that the orthotic stays in place on the arm.[14] Clearing the distal palmar crease is extremely important. If the orthosis crosses this crease, MP flexion will be impeded. When you construct a dorsal forearm-based orthosis or a forearm-based ulnar gutter, pad the area of the ulnar head because this bony prominence can become a pressure area. Always incorporate the padding into the molding of the orthosis; do not place it inside afterward as an addition. With mobilization orthosis, the best approach is to provide an orthosis your client can tolerate for long periods.

> ◎ *Clinical Pearl*
>
> Applying low tension that is tolerable and constant over prolonged periods is much more effective than applying strong forces over shorter periods.

The amount of safe force for the hand is 100 to 300 g.[15] Clients often ask that more force be used in their orthosis. These clients need repeated education that low load over a long duration is the safest and most effective way to remodel tissues and make clinical progress.

Precaution. *Painful splinting can be harmful.*

Skin blanching is a sign of high tension or incorrect orthotic mechanics.[3] The line of pull on the part being mobilized in a static progressive or dynamic orthosis must be a 90-degree angle from the **outrigger** (the structure from which the forces are directed). An outrigger can be high profile or low profile (Fig. 1.7). High-profile outriggers have certain mechanical and adjustment advantages but are bulkier and less attractive.[16]

Orthoses Used With Exercise

A dorsal dropout orthosis can be used to correct digital flexion or extrinsic extensor tightness. Mold the orthosis in a position of comfortable stretch. Use strapping as needed to keep it in place. The client should try to gently flex the digits away from the orthosis as able (Fig. 1.8). Having an object to reach for, such as a dowel in the palm, can be helpful.

Orthoses can be used to achieve various differential MP positions. The differential MP orthosis (also called a yoke) in Fig. 1.9 positions the long finger MP in greater flexion than the index and ring fingers. In this orthosis, active MP flexion of the index and ring fingers facilitates long finger flexion. Fig. 1.10 shows the opposite differential MP orthosis with the long finger MP more extended than the adjacent fingers. A yoke orthosis with the small finger MP more flexed than the ring finger might be useful for a small finger metacarpal fracture with limited MP flexion. Active PIP flexion and extension within this type of orthosis at various MP positions also promotes PIP joint ROM and tendon gliding. This orthosis can be used during a progressive gripping activity (for example, gripping a handful of dried beans, squeezing some out of the hand, and then gripping further).

A scrap of thermoplastic material can be used to create a cylinder to fit the client's available limited fist position. Sustained gripping of or holding onto this cylinder and "pumping" to flex and extend the digits around the cylinder may enhance composite digital flexion.

Chip Bags

Chip bags can be incorporated into orthotic regimens to maximize lymphatic flow and minimize the stiffness and adherence that otherwise would worsen as a result of the edema. A **chip bag** is a cotton stockinette bag filled with small foam pieces of various densities (Fig. 1.11). The foam can be cut from a variety of sources, including foam exercise blocks, padding, and soft Velcro materials. Chip bags traditionally have been used in the treatment of lymphedema; they are positioned over indurated areas of edema within external compressive garments or multilayered stretch bandages. Chip bags provide light traction on the skin, facilitate lymphatic stimulation, and promote neutral warmth. All these effects help reduce edema. The increased body heat under the chip bag and the light pressure exerted by the bag help soften thickened or fibrotic tissue.

In some cases, chip bags can be used alone without an accompanying orthosis. In such cases, they can be held in place with stockinette or a soft Velcro strap that is not applied tightly. Sometimes a less technical approach, such as using chip bags with orthosis, is a very effective option. Chip bags also can be positioned inside or in conjunction with orthoses to maximize edema control and reduce scar adherence. Clients find chip bags very comfortable. Some refer to the chip bag as their "pillow," which probably conveys the comfort they experience with it.

Soft Four-Finger Buddy Strap

A soft four-finger buddy strap can be made from Softstrap Velcro loop to provide transverse support that promotes more efficient primary function of the extrinsic flexors and extensors. This strap facilitates AROM for composite flexion and extension and for isolated extensor digitorum communis (EDC) and FDP tendon glide. It also stimulates lymphatic flow over the volar proximal phalanges, similar to chip bags. The soft four-finger buddy strap can relieve pain and promote AROM when hand stiffness is present. It also is helpful for symptom management in clients with lateral epicondylitis (tennis elbow) who have EDC involvement and pain on fisting.[17]

CASE STUDIES

CASE STUDY 1.1 ■

A client was in an altercation with a family member, and her hand was closed in a door during the argument. She was seen for malunion of a right distal radius fracture with right ulnar joint dislocation and extensor pollicis longus (EPL) rupture. She underwent open carpal tunnel release, corrective osteotomy of the distal radius fracture with internal fixation and bone grafting, and intercalary tendon grafting of the EPL tendon using the extensor indicis proprius (EIP). When the client was seen in occupational therapy, her hand was extremely swollen and stiff, and she had severe extrinsic extensor tightness that limited full fisting. She developed CRPS and was

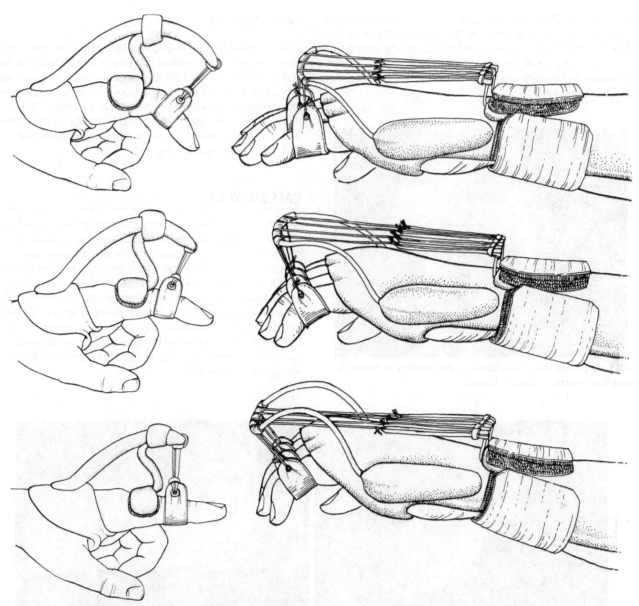

FIG. 1.7 Examples of the 90-degree angle of pull with high-profile and low-profile outriggers. (From Fess EE. Principles and methods of splinting for mobilization of joints. In: Mackin EJ, Callahan AD, Skirven TM et al. eds. *Rehabilitation of the Hand and Upper Extremity*. 5th ed. St Louis, MO: Mosby; 2002.)

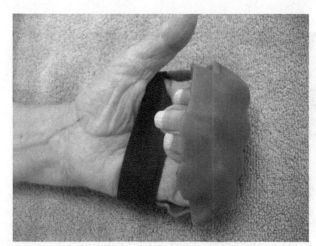

FIG. 1.8 Client performing active digital flexion in a dorsal dropout orthosis.

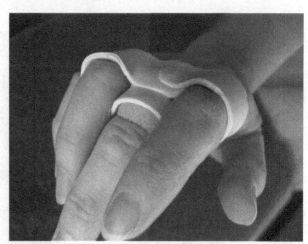

FIG. 1.9 Differential MP positioning orthosis with long finger MP more flexed than adjacent fingers.

treated successfully for this with a combination of stellate ganglion blocks and hand therapy. Note the dorsal scars and edema (Fig. 1.12A). The style of chip bag incorporated into her volar wrist orthosis is shown in Fig. 1.12B. This woman was a highly motivated client. At the time her therapy was discontinued, she had regained very good hand function.

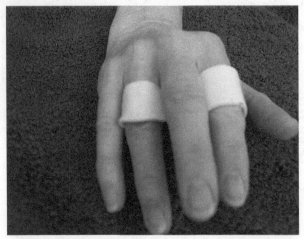

FIG. 1.10 Differential MP positioning orthosis with long finger MP more extended than adjacent fingers.

CASE STUDY 1.2 ■

A client who underwent surgery for release of a Dupuytren's contracture developed a flare reaction. Note the incisional scar and fullness of the ulnar hand (Fig. 1.13A), as well as the limitation in composite digital flexion (Fig. 1.13B). This client used a chip bag inside an exercise orthosis designed to block the MPs and promote PIP and DIP flexion exercise; the goals were to resolve intrinsic muscle tightness and promote composite digital flexion. Within 2 weeks, the client had made very good gains (Fig. 1.13C).

CASE STUDY 1.3 ■

A woman who fell while hiking sustained a displaced distal radius fracture that required external fixation and percutaneous pin fixation. More than a week passed after her fall before she went to her physician. The woman explained this by noting that she has attention deficit disorder. She came to therapy 1 day after applying an elastic bandage tightly and irregularly around her external fixator. Note the indentations left on her skin by the wrap (Fig. 1.14A). Chip bags were incorporated into the dressings and orthoses used in this case (Fig. 1.14B), and the client progressed very well in therapy. She had good composite digital extension and flexion at the time of discharge (Fig. 1.14C and D).

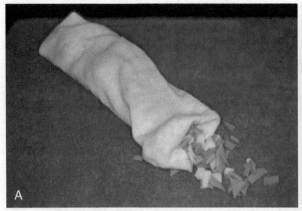
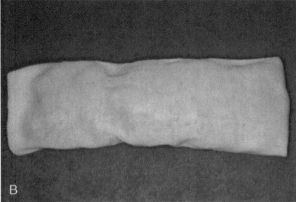

FIG. 1.11 (A) Chip bag contents consisting of small pieces of foam placed in a cotton stockinette. (B) Ends of chip bag can be folded over and taped closed.

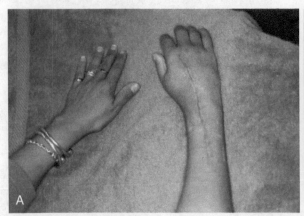
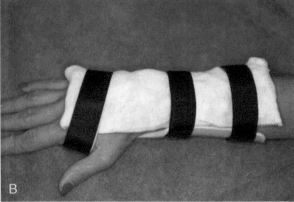

FIG. 1.12 (A) Dorsal scars and edema. (B) Style of chip bag incorporated into the client's volar wrist orthosis.

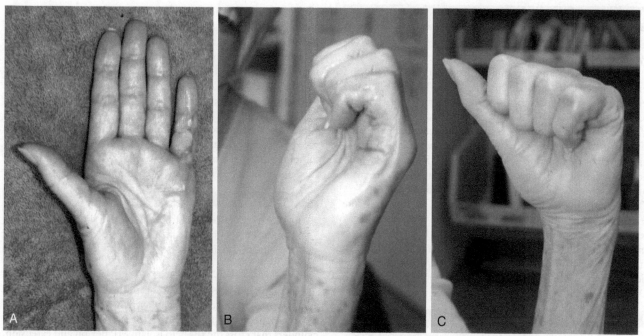

FIG. 1.13 **(A)** Flared incisional scar that developed after Dupuytren's release surgery. **(B)** Limited active composite flexion. **(C)** Full active composite flexion 2 weeks later.

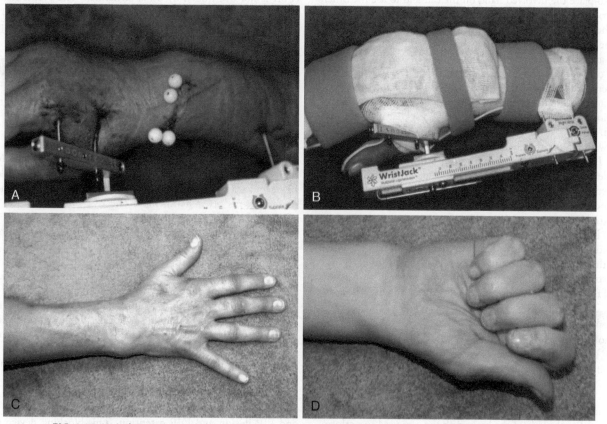

FIG. 1.14 (A) Indentations made by a tight elastic bandage applied by the client. (B) Chip bags incorporated into dressings and orthosis with external fixator hand pins. (C) and (D) Resolution of edema and active digital extension and flexion at discharge.

Exercises for Upper Extremity Therapy

Precaution. *Shoulder stiffness can develop insidiously and can be very limiting.*

Check the client's posture and proximal motion initially and then at intervals. Incorporate proximal AROM into all home exercise programs even if this is only a preventive measure (see Chapter 18).

Shorter, milder sessions of exercise performed more frequently are better than longer, intensive sessions done less often. Some clients do well at first, performing 5 repetitions 5 times a day and gradually building to 10 repetitions hourly during the day. Explain that exercises work well if the process is brief and frequent.

When working on isolated wrist extension, be sure to isolate the extensor carpi radialis brevis (ECRB), and teach clients how to extend the wrist with a soft fist that includes MP flexion. Have them hold an object so that the MPs are flexed. It is critical to retrain the ECRB to perform wrist extension. Without this isolation of motion, the client may learn to extend the wrist with EDC substitution instead of using the ECRB.

> ◎ *Clinical Pearl*
>
> Once established, the habit of extending the wrist with EDC substitution can be very hard to break.

To work on wrist active/active assistive range of motion (A/AAROM), put a towel on the table, and then place a coffee can (no bigger than the 3-lb size) on its side on the towel. Teach the client to place the involved hand on the can and to use the other hand to hold the involved hand flat on the can. The client then rolls the can using A/AAROM forward and backward. Clients like the feeling of this exercise, which also promotes proximal ROM and stimulates lymphatic flow.

In contrast to this, if extrinsic flexor tightness is a problem, the client would perform exercises involving wrist extension with simultaneous digital extension. Otherwise, exercises for wrist extension should be done primarily with a fist that includes MP flexion.

Always look at the client's wrist position when exercising the digits. Do not exercise or coax the digits into flexion with the wrist flexed unless you are deliberately trying to stretch the extrinsic extensors. It is biomechanically easier to achieve digital flexion with the wrist in extension, to achieve PIP joint flexion with the MP extended, and to achieve PIP joint extension with the MP flexed. If the client cannot sustain a position of wrist neutral or extension, use an orthosis or have the client self-support the wrist using the other hand when digital exercises are performed.

Instruct clients always to keep the upper arm locked at the side of the body when performing forearm rotation exercises.

> ◎ *Clinical Pearl*
>
> Do not perform forearm rotation exercises with the elbow on a table or even on a pillow; this prevents isolated forearm rotation and allows for substitution with humeral motions.

Teach the client that one way to do this is to keep a towel roll pressed to the side of the body with the arm used to perform forearm rotation exercises because this requires that the elbow be kept close to the body.

In some cases, AROM through functional activity and exercise may be all that is needed to enable the client to recover full UE flexibility and function. When more isolated and structure-specific exercises are needed, the exercises discussed in the following sections may be helpful.

Blocking Exercises

Blocking exercises are exercises in which proximal support is provided to promote isolated motion at a particular site. They are helpful for clients with limitation of either AROM or PROM or both. Blocking exercises exert more force than nonblocking exercises.

> ◎ *Clinical Pearl*
>
> With blocking exercises, instruct the client to hold the position at comfortable end-range for 3 to 5 seconds; this allows remodeling of the tissues.

Blocking exercises can be accomplished in a variety of ways. You can use either commercially available devices or individual devices made from scraps of orthotic materials. Digital gutters or cylinders that cross the IPs help isolate MP flexion and extension. If the cylinder is shortened to free the DIP, then DIP blocking exercises can be performed. These exercises can be done with the MP in extension or in varying degrees of flexion. Often a client exerts too strong a contraction, and the PIP tries to flex within the blocking splint. Explain to the client that isolating motion to only the DIP requires a soft quality of contraction so that the effort is not overridden by other structures. The biomechanical challenge to the FDP is greater when DIP flexion is performed with MP flexion than with MP extension. This positional progression can be used to upgrade the exercises.

> ◎ *Clinical Pearl*
>
> When a digital PIP block is used to promote MP flexion of the small finger, it is very helpful to stabilize the small finger metacarpal.

The ring and small finger metacarpals are more mobile at their carpometacarpal (CMC) joints than are the index and long finger metacarpals. If the metacarpal is supported by your hand or the client's other hand, more effective isolated motion can occur at the MP joint. This isolation and proximal support can be very helpful for clients trying to recover MP flexion after a small finger metacarpal fracture.

A blocking splint with the MPs flexed helps isolate active PIP extension (Fig. 1.15). Extending the PIP is easier biomechanically when the MP is flexed because this position promotes central slip function. This same blocking splint also promotes composite flexion exercise and can be helpful for normalizing extrinsic extensor tightness. Conversely, a blocking splint with the MPs extended (Fig. 1.16) helps to isolate active IP flexion and FDP excursion and to resolve intrinsic tightness. These types of orthoses can be used with function, or they may be used only for exercise.

A DIP cap or flexion block diverts FDP excursion to the PIP and thus promotes isolated exercise of the FDS muscle with MP and PIP flexion and DIP extension. This blocking device may also help the client exercise the flexor digitorum superficialis (FDS) fist position more easily (see the following section).

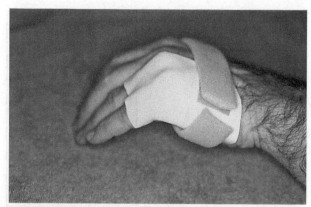

FIG. 1.15 Blocking orthosis with the MP flexed helps isolate PIP extension and promotes extrinsic extensor stretch.

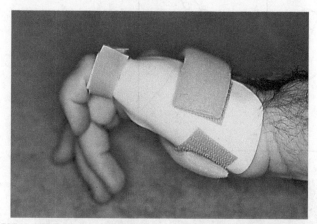

FIG. 1.16 Blocking orthosis with the MP extended helps isolate active PIP flexion and FDP excursion and also helps resolve intrinsic tightness.

Differential Tendon Gliding Exercises

Differential tendon gliding exercises are a mainstay of most home programs because they are easy to perform and they promote motion very effectively (Fig. 1.17).[18] They are a standard exercise for conservative management of carpal tunnel syndrome and are also used after carpal tunnel release. These exercises are an important option for all clients with hand or wrist stiffness. Rolling a thick highlighting pen up and down in the palm is an effective way to perform FDP gliding.

Place and Hold Exercises

Place and hold exercises can be helpful when PROM is greater than AROM (Fig. 1.18). Gently perform AAROM to position the finger (for example, in composite flexion). Then ask the client to sustain that position comfortably while releasing the assisting hand. The assisting hand may be yours or the client's other hand. Watch for co-contraction or force that is too strenuous as the client tries to sustain the exercise position. A combination of blocking exercises and place and hold exercises can be very productive. Also, you can try doing place and hold exercises with a blocking orthosis in place.

When the client releases the sustained contraction, pain sometimes may be felt in the area of a stiff joint. For instance, if the client performs place and hold exercises for composite fisting and then has PIP joint discomfort when releasing the fist, have the client relax the muscle contraction but stay in the same fisted position. While the client stays in that position, gradually provide assistance to gently begin extending the digit or digits (minimal joint distraction mobilization also can be helpful if not contraindicated). Next, ask the client to slowly actively extend the digits the rest of the way. This technique can be helpful for eliminating pain associated with end-ranges and AAROM.

Resistive Exercises

After clients have been medically cleared for them, resistive exercises are used for strengthening and to improve excursion of adherent tissue. Sometimes clients want to use a greater load than is safe for them. Teach clients that, for isolating wrist curls, they should not use as heavy a weight as they would for biceps curls.

Precaution. *Think carefully and critically about the status of your client's wrist if the person is recovering from a fracture, has had tendonitis, or is at risk for degenerative joint changes. Be very careful with wrist radial and ulnar deviation strengthening exercises because these may provoke tendonitis.*

Generally speaking, the safest course in performing resistive exercises is to use more repetitions with a lower load. This approach promotes endurance. (A more detailed discussion of resistive exercise is presented in Chapter 10.)

Resistive exercise can take many forms, including progressive resistive exercises (PREs) and exercises performed with graded grippers, rubber bands, squeeze balls, graded clothespins, and putty. For example, marbles or other objects can be embedded in putty, requiring pinch and dexterity to remove them.

Functional Activity

It is essential that the client incorporate the gains made from exercising into functional UE use at home and at work. Practicing or simulating relevant activities in the clinic can reinforce this. Examples of such activities may include tying shoes, folding clothes, manipulating coins, writing with an adapted pen, using the involved hand for handshakes, hammering, using screwdrivers, or lifting. Putty can be used to simulate activities, such as turning keys. Adding visualization to the simulation enhances the treatment. The scope of practice for either occupational therapy or physical therapy dictates some of these choices.

Ball rolling can be used for wrist AROM, composite stretching, weight bearing, and closed chain exercise. The ball can be dribbled or thrown for strengthening or sports simulation. Balloons can also be thrown or batted with the hand.

Dried beans can be used for grip and release, for progressive gripping, and for finding and removing other objects (for example, marbles) out of the beans. Instruct the client to grip the beans and then to release them with full digital extension. Wrist motions can be varied, and tenodesis can be incorporated. You also can have the client use opposition of the thumb to each finger to pick up one bean and then release it with full digital extension.

Pegs of varying sizes promote tendon gliding, sensory stimulation, and joint ROM. Fine motor activities (for example, threading beads, in-hand manipulation of marbles, and stacking blocks) can be modified with blocking orthoses to promote isolated ROM or tendon glide.

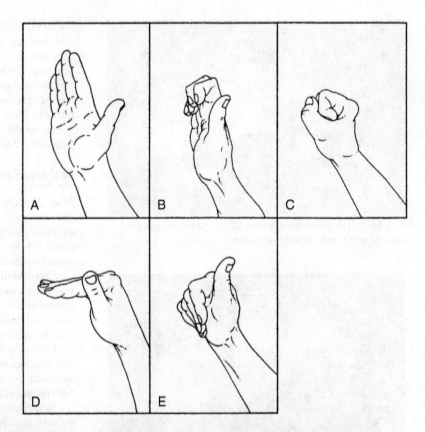

FIG. 1.17 Differential tendon gliding exercises. (A) Straight digits. (B) Hook fist. (C) Composite fist. (D) Tabletop. (E) Straight (FDS) fist. (From Rozmaryn LM, Dovelle S, Rothman ER, et al. Nerve and tendon gliding exercises and the conservative management of carpal tunnel syndrome. *J Hand Ther.* 1998; 11[3]: 171-179.)

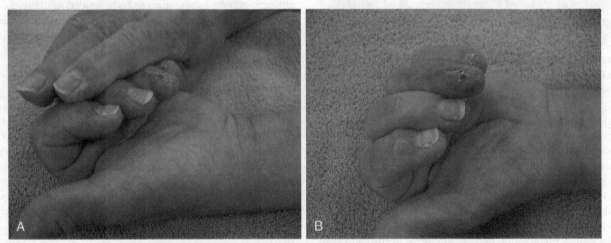

FIG. 1.18 (A) Place exercises for digital flexion. (B) Hold exercises for digital flexion.

♡ *Tips from the Field*

- Look at all your clients and their hands with interest and curiosity. For example, what do you see in Fig. 1.19?
- Be tender when you touch your clients. If your hands are cold, try to warm them up a bit before you touch the person.
- Remember that you do not have to evaluate and treat everything on the first visit.
- Never yell at or order a client to "Relax!" Instead, encourage relaxation with a calm, slow voice.
- Working on one area of stiffness sometimes can also resolve stiffness in another area.
- Example: A client who sustained a distal radius fracture had limited AROM and PROM in wrist flexion and extension and decreased ECRB excursion (that is, passive wrist extension exceeded active wrist extension). Stretching led to improved

wrist flexion. It also helped reduce ECRB adherence, which resulted in improved wrist extension.
- Example: A client had extrinsic flexor tightness after a distal radius fracture with edema and decreased wrist and hand AROM. As her extrinsic flexor tightness resolved (she recovered full passive composite extension), the active digital flexion also resolved because she had better mechanical function of the lengthened digital flexors.
- Keep the timeline open for more progress by not performing painful therapy and by avoiding a flare reaction.
- As a hand therapist, you won't be able to resolve every problem in every case. If prolonged, established stiffness is present, if the client has highly fibrotic tissue responses, or if client follow-through has been poor, residual limitations may exist that are beyond our ability to correct.

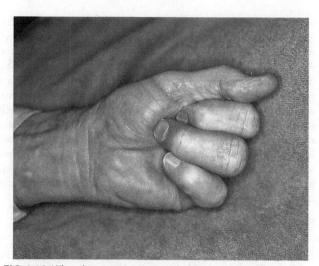

FIG. 1.19 What do you see wrong with this client's hand?

- Document explicitly if poor client follow-through is a factor. For example, a client was carrying a glass table that broke; the client received a laceration to his right-dominant forearm. Several flexor tendons and the median and ulnar nerves also were lacerated. The client missed many therapy visits and did not perform his home program (see Chapter 27). The client returned to therapy with very poor passive digital flexion, severe edema, and skin maceration. In this case, documentation would include the following: "The client had been instructed to perform hourly home program, but he reports that he did not do so. He states that he understands the need to exercise as instructed. He also states that he understands that if he does not gain passive digital flexion soon, he may lose the opportunity to make maximum clinical gains." If appropriate, the progress note to this client's physician should report that the client now agrees to increase the frequency of home exercise program (HEP) exercises, as he was previously instructed to do.
- If a client is not following through as instructed, it is important to investigate why this is happening and to work with the client to correct the situation. Clients can have a number of reasons for failing to follow their regimen. They may be uninformed about the importance of the HEP; they may think they can catch up and make progress later; they may have a secondary agenda, such as avoiding a return to work; they may be depressed; or they may need help to assimilate the HEP into their daily routine successfully.
- Help clients learn to be patient. Encourage them to continue with their home program and to celebrate small improvements. Assist them in finding meaningful ways to use their time (for example, find new interests and hobbies) if participation in an enjoyable activity has been temporarily disrupted.
- Replenish your own reserves so that you have the resources needed for complicated clinical situations. Give yourself a few moments to take some deep breaths and focus on the client as a person. Try to sense what it must be like for the client to have this injury. Carefully check for extensor habitus, which is habitual posturing in digital extension. The index finger is particularly prone to this response. Extensor habitus can occur after an injury as simple as a paper cut. It is important to identify this phenomenon and to correct it as soon as possible so

that it does not become permanent and so that joint stiffness does not occur. Buddy straps and orthoses may be helpful.
- Take one day at a time with the therapy. Do not presume that you will pick up where your last session left off. Look at your clients with fresh eyes at each visit. Ask them what is better, what they are noticing about their hands, what they are able to do functionally now, and what they are still unable to accomplish functionally.

Thinking Outside the (Treatment) Box

When to Mix and Match

Mix and match your treatment repertoire. After reading the rest of this book, try to think outside the treatment box. Be creative, and have some fun. For example, why not perform early protective motions (for example, place and hold tenodesis motions) with most of your clients?

When Less Is More

Teaching your client the benefits of a "less is more" approach to UE exercises is very important. For example, a 12-year-old girl underwent flexor tendon grafting. In therapy, when trying to isolate FDP motion at the DIP with the PIP blocked, she was co-contracting and eliciting PIP flexion instead. The therapist taught her to contract more softly to isolate the FDP more effectively. The therapist used some helpful verbal cues, such as "Don't try so hard," "Stop trying altogether," and "Stop thinking." The therapist gave these cues in a soft, gentle voice and made sure to compliment the girl and smile when her isolated motion was of better quality. This activity was followed by place and hold exercises, which progressed successfully. Even though this client was very young, she learned the quality of isolated motion well, recognizing that less is more. She also could see the improvement in her capabilities.

When to Stop Exercising for a Few Days

Another important lesson to teach clients is when to stop exercising for a short time. For example, a 53-year-old, right-dominant woman sustained a distal radius fracture when she fell while shopping. She developed significant, diffuse edema and stiffness of the shoulder, elbow, forearm, and hand. This client demonstrated objective signs of a flare response after efforts were made to upgrade her exercises gradually. She was at risk for IP flexion contractures of all digits. Her sisters came to visit her, and they all went to a spa for 4 days. During this time, the client stopped performing her assigned upper extremity exercises while she pampered herself at the spa. When she came back to therapy, she had diminished flare responses, decreased edema, and improved ROM throughout the upper extremity. It helped her immensely to stop trying so hard. She was then able to resume "trying," but with a better sense of her tissue tolerances.

When to Accept a Stiff Hand and Get On With Life

Unfortunately, hand therapists cannot fix everything. In some cases, the client's injuries may be too severe to permit a full recovery. In other cases, a family crisis may prevent therapy from continuing in a timely manner. Under circumstances such as these, the client's best course of action is to accept the residual stiffness or limitations and to resume otherwise normal living. In such cases, therapists can perform the important role of identifying and teaching compensatory techniques to maximize the client's function.[19] Also, sometimes the therapist has the responsibility to identify a clinical plateau and to help clients realize that they may have achieved all that is possible at that time.

Summary

This chapter has identified fundamental hand therapy concepts that foster clinical reasoning. It also has highlighted treatment techniques and provided guidelines to promote interventions that are safe and appropriate. Most treatment techniques are not diagnosis specific, but rather can be applied to a variety of diagnoses. As a hand therapist, the challenge you face is to be tissue specific, to be aware of clinical precautions, and to adapt the appropriate treatment from your toolbox of techniques to a given diagnosis. As you continue with this book, I encourage you to ask yourself what interventions would be most appropriate and why. I also recommend that you return to this chapter and reread it after you have read the rest of the book. Rereading this chapter at that time will help you appreciate what you have learned; that, hopefully, will be how to apply clinical reasoning in selecting safe treatment choices for clients with many different diagnoses.

References

1. Tubiana R, Thomine J-M, Mackin EJ, editors: *Examination of the hand and wrist*, ed 2, London, UK, 1996, Martin Dunitz.
2. Fess EE, Gettle KS, Philips CA, et al.: *Hand and upper extremity splinting: principles and methods*, ed 3, St Louis, MO, 2005, Elsevier.
3. Strickland JW: Biologic basis for hand and upper extremity splinting. In Fess EE, Gettle KS, Philips CA, et al.: *Hand and upper extremity splinting: principles and methods*, ed 3, St Louis, MO, 2005, Elsevier.
4. Pettengill KS: Therapist's management of the complex injury. In Skirven TM, Osterman AL, Fedorczyk JM, et al.: *Rehabilitation of the hand and upper extremity*, ed 6, Philadelphia, PA, 2011, Elsevier.
5. Colditz C: Therapist's management of the stiff hand. In Mackin EJ, Callinan N, Skirven TM, et al.: *Rehabilitation of the hand and upper extremity*, ed 6, Philadelphia, PA, 2011, Elsevier.
6. Gutierrez-Gutierrez G, Sereno M, Miralles A, et al.: Chemotherapy-induced peripheral neuropathy: clinical features, diagnosis, prevention and treatment strategies, *Clin Transl Oncol* 12(2):81–91, 2010, https://doi.org/10.1007/S12094-010-0474-z.
7. Cooper C, Liskin J, Moorhead JF: Dyscoordinate contraction: impaired quality of movement in patients with hand disorders, *OT Practice* 4:40–45, 1999.
8. Bracciano AG: Physical agent modalities. In Radomski MV, Latham C, editors: *Occupational therapy for physical dysfunction*, ed 6, Baltimore, MD, 2008, Lippincott Williams & Wilkins.
9. Chen J-J, Jin P-S, Zhao S, et al.: Effect of heat shock protein 47 on collagen synthesis of keloid in vivo, *ANZ J Surg* 81(6):425–430, 2011.
10. Anzarut A, Olson J, Singh P, et al.: The effectiveness of pressure garment therapy for the prevention of abnormal scarring after burn injury: a meta-analysis, *J Plast Reconstr Aesthet Surg* 62(1):77–84, 2009, https://doi.org/10.1016/j.bjps.2007.10.052.
11. von der Heyde RL, Evans RB: Wound classification and management. In Skirven TM, Osterman AL, Fedorczyk JM, et al.: *Rehabilitation of the hand and upper extremity*, ed 6, Philadelphia, PA, 2011, Elsevier.
12. Coppard BM, Lohman H: *Introduction to splinting: a clinical reasoning and problem-solving approach*, ed 3, St Louis, MO, 2003, Mosby.
13. Deshaies LD: Upper extremity orthoses. In Radomski MV, Latham C, editors: *Occupational therapy for physical dysfunction*, ed 6, Baltimore, MA, 2008, Lippincott Williams & Wilkins.
14. Lashgari D, Yasuda L: Orthotics. In Pendleton HM, Schultz-Krohn W, editors: *Pedretti's occupational therapy practice skills for physical dysfunction*, ed 7, St Louis, MO, 2013, Mosby.
15. Krotoski JAB, Breger-Stanton D: The forces of dynamic orthotic positioning: ten questions to ask before applying a dynamic orthosis to the hand. In Skirven TM, Osterman AL, Fedorczyk JM, et al.: *Rehabilitation of the hand and upper extremity*, ed 6, Philadelphia, PA, 2011, Elsevier.
16. Fess EE: Orthoses for mobilization of joints: principles and methods. In Skirven TM, Osterman AL, Fedorczyk JM, et al.: *Rehabilitation of the hand and upper extremity*, ed 6, Philadelphia, PA, 2011, Elsevier.
17. Cooper C, Meland NB: *Clinical implications of transverse forces on extrinsic flexors and extensors in the hand*, Seattle, WA, 2000, Unpublished paper presented at the annual meeting of the American Society of Hand Therapists, pp 5–8.
18. Bardak AN, Alp M, Erhan B, et al.: Evaluation of the clinical efficacy of conservative treatment in the management of carpal tunnel syndrome, *Adv Ther* 26(1):107–116, 2009, https://doi.org/10.1007/s12325-008-0134-7.
19. Merritt WH: Written on behalf of the stiff finger, *J Hand Ther* 11(2):74–79, 1998.

2

Evidence-Based Practice: The Basic Tools

Michael John Borst

Evidence-based practice (EBP) is an approach to client care that aims to ensure that therapists consider the highest quality and most objective information possible when making clinical decisions. It is the integration of three things: the best evidence from research, the therapist's clinical expertise, and each individual client's values and circumstances.[1] Because EBP involves the therapist's expertise as well as the client's perspective, two therapist–client teams may make two different decisions, both of them evidence based. Because EBP involves each client's situation, the same therapist may collaborate with two different clients to make two different decisions, both of them evidence based. EBP is like a three-legged stool that requires all three legs to function properly. This chapter introduces a vocabulary and framework for understanding, applying, and analyzing evidence and other resources for EBP. As you continue your EBP journey, you may wish to look at resources that are more comprehensive[1-5] or pursue further education in this area.

Five Steps to Evidence-Based Practice

Hand therapists ask many types of questions in the clinic. The most common questions typically address therapeutic interventions, but therapists also ask questions about diagnosis, prognosis, and other topics.[1,6] This chapter outlines how practitioners of EBP approach intervention and diagnosis questions using a five-step process.[1,7]

EBP Step 1: Ask an Answerable Question

Therapists ask two types of questions about clinical situations in their practice: background questions and foreground questions.[1,3] **Background questions** are general questions about the situation that therapists ask when they encounter a new diagnosis or client situation. Examples of background questions include the following:

What are the anatomical and physiological factors involved in this condition?

What do the terms in the medical record mean?

What are the possible treatment options for this condition?

What are the precautions and contraindications regarding intervention with this condition?

Textbooks, reference books, protocol manuals, and valid web-based resources can effectively answer background questions. **Foreground questions** focus on a particular choice that needs to be made about an individual client. Therapists ask foreground questions when they already have some experience working with clients with a particular condition. Textbooks and protocol manuals usually do not provide evidence-based answers to foreground questions.

Foreground intervention questions are usually phrased using the **PICO question** template:[1,3] **P**opulation, **I**ntervention, **C**omparison intervention, and **O**utcome. An example of an intervention PICO question might be:

"In middle-aged females with carpal tunnel syndrome of less than six months duration (population), how effective is a therapy program consisting of a wrist-hand orthosis with the wrist positioned at zero degrees, tendon and median nerve gliding exercises, and activity modification (intervention), compared with surgical release of the transverse carpal ligament (comparison intervention), in relieving symptoms as measured by the Boston Carpal Tunnel Questionnaire (outcome)?"

This carefully phrased question is answered by looking at the best research evidence.

EBP Step 2: Find the Best Evidence

The second step of EBP is to find the best evidence to answer the question. Research is generally categorized into two types:

Quantitative research measures and analyzes data using numbers and statistics.

Qualitative research collects data to inductively build concepts or theories and analyzes them through description.

Quantitative research is often used to describe the frequency of an event (the **prevalence** of a disease in a particular group of people), associations between events (the relationship between socioeconomic status and health care outcomes), and cause and effect (the causal relationship between smoking and lung cancer). These "events" are called variables in quantitative research. On the other hand, qualitative research is used in therapeutic settings to understand the experience of a client and how a client interprets their experiences.[8] Studies that that use both quantitative and qualitative methods are called "mixed methods." The "evidence" part of evidence-based practice often comes from quantitative research, though some advocate for using qualitative research in EBP as well.[9,10] In quantitative research the "best" evidence is often defined as research that has high internal validity and high external validity.

Internal validity is the extent to which a study was well conducted so that the results are accurate and can be trusted. An intervention study with high internal validity can confidently be used to assert a true cause and effect relationship between variables.[2] Internal validity is assessed through critical appraisal of the study (see EBP Step 3) and the **evidence hierarchy**.

The evidence hierarchy ranks study designs into levels of evidence, according to their ability to avoid systematic bias. The less bias a study has, the more likely it is that the results are valid. There are different evidence hierarchies for different types of EBP questions (intervention, diagnosis, prognosis, etc.).[2,6,7] For example, while randomized controlled trials (RCTs) work well to answer questions about intervention effectiveness, they are not useful for questions of diagnosis. Case studies and other studies without control groups are useful to identify areas needing further research but are generally inadequate evidence for clinical decision making. Various authors have proposed a variety of evidence hierarchies.[1-6,9] A simple evidence hierarchy for intervention studies[11] is in Table 2.1.

It is important to note that a particular level of evidence does not guarantee quality. It is quite possible that a poorly conducted level 1 study has less internal validity than a well-conducted level 3 study, for example. A study's statistical methods can also alter the level of evidence. For example, if a study designed to be an RCT (level 1) reports statistical differences between pre-intervention and post-intervention measures *within an intervention group* rather than post-intervention measures of differences *between* the control group and the intervention group, the study drops to a level 3 (one group, measured before and after an intervention).

External validity is the extent to which the study findings can be generalized or applied to another situation. For a study to have external validity relative to your client, the clients in the study should be similar to your client, the setting in which the study was conducted should be similar to your clinical setting, and the intervention in the study should be feasible to implement in your setting.

TABLE 2.1	Levels of Evidence for Intervention Studies
Level of Evidence	**Description**
Level 1 (lowest potential for bias)	Systematic review or metaanalysis of randomized controlled trials; randomized controlled trials (comparison of two groups with random assignment to either an intervention or control group)
Level 2	Comparison of two groups (an intervention group and a comparison group) without random assignment to groups
Level 3	One group, measured before and after an intervention, Case-control study (retrospective analysis of two groups, one that had a particular outcome and a similar group that did not)
Level 4	Case series with analysis of outcomes
Level 5 (highest potential for bias)	Case study, Expert opinion, Narrative review, Mechanism-based reasoning

(Modified from Arbesman, Scheer, and Lieberman, 2008)

EBP Step 3: Critically Appraise the Evidence

Critical appraisal refers to an assessment of how well a study was done. There are a variety of tools that therapists can use to critically appraise quantitative research studies on therapy interventions: the 7-item *Cochrane Collaboration's tool for assessing risk of bias*,[12] the 10-point *PEDro scale*,[13] CanChild's *Critical Review Form and Guidelines*,[14] and the 24-item *Evaluation of Effectiveness Study Design*,[7] among others. Evidence-based clinical practice guidelines can be helpful tools for the evidence-based practitioner and are critically appraised using the *Appraisal of Guidelines for Research & Evaluation (AGREE II) Instrument*.[15] Note that many clinical practice guidelines available online are not evidence based and therefore have little value for answering foreground questions.

Preappraised evidence is available in articles and databases that gather and appraise evidence for practitioners. Systematic reviews and metaanalyses gather all of the high-quality evidence available on a topic and combine the studies to generate conclusions. These studies should include the items described in the Preferred Reporting Items for Systematic Reviews and Meta-Analyses (PRISMA) statement,[16] available for free online. The PRISMA statement provides criteria for the structure and elements of a well-reported systematic review or meta-analysis. Review articles should be systematic reviews, not narrative reviews. A number of websites have preappraised articles or topics for the therapy practitioner:

www.pedro.org.au

www.otseeker.com

www.aota.org/Practice/Researchers/Evidence-Exchange/RDP.aspx

www.ptnow.org

www.cochranelibrary.com/cochrane-database-of-systematic-reviews/index.html

Any critical appraisal should also include a discussion of the difference between *statistically significant* differences and *clinically important* differences. In an intervention study, we often conclude that post-intervention differences between the intervention and control groups are **statistically significant** when the value of the statistic P is equal to or less than 0.05 (that is, when there is a 5% or less probability that any observed difference between groups is due to chance).[2] Sometimes 95% confidence intervals (CIs) are used for this purpose; in that case, we are 95% sure that the real difference between 2 groups falls between 2 numbers that define the lower and upper boundaries of the 95% CI. Thus if the number 0 is within a 95% CI for difference scores between groups, we conclude it is possible that no real difference exists between the two groups.

Once a study has found a statistically significant difference between interventions, we need to determine whether the difference is clinically important. It is possible that the intervention resulted in a statistically significant difference so small that it would not influence a client's ability to participate in their desired daily activities in a meaningful way. In therapy, the **minimal clinically important difference** (MCID) is the minimum difference that will result in a meaningful change in the client's abilities or outcome. This is sometimes also referred to as the "minimal clinically important change" or just the "minimal important difference."[17]

As an example, the Boston Carpal Tunnel Questionnaire Symptom Severity Scale (score range from 1 to 5) has an MCID of 1.6 for nondiabetic clients 6 months after surgery.[17] A study might find that clients who receive a certain intervention for carpal tunnel syndrome score 0.5 points better on the Symptom Severity Scale than those in a control group, and that this difference is statistically significant. However, clients will likely perceive this difference not to be "important" or "worth it" because it is far below the MCID for this scale. If an intervention study shows a result that is statistically significant but not clinically important, it may not be worth the resources required to implement it.

EBP Step 4: Make a Decision

After we have gathered and critically appraised the best available evidence, we collaborate with our client about their treatment options. We identify the client's goals for therapy and then discuss the costs, risks, and benefits of possible interventions to achieve those goals. By doing this, we use our clinical expertise to integrate the research findings with our client's values and situation to create a mutually developed client-centered plan.

EBP Step 5: Evaluate the Result

After we have chosen and implemented an evidence-based intervention or diagnostic tool with the client, it is important to reflect on what went well and what could be improved. Consider the following: (a) how well did we locate, appraise, and use the evidence? and; (b) how well did the EBP process work for the client? The answers to these questions will help improve a therapist's skills as an evidence-based practitioner.

Differential Diagnosis

Differential diagnosis is "the distinguishing between two or more diseases with similar symptoms by systematically comparing their signs and symptoms."[18] All hand therapists engage in

TABLE 2.2 Four Possible Outcomes When Using Special Tests for Differential Diagnosis

		THE TRUTH (DETERMINED BY A GOLD STANDARD TEST)	
		Condition present	Condition absent
Your test results	+	TP	FP
	–	FN	TN

TP, true positive; *FN*, False negative; *FP*, false positive; *TN*, true negative.

differential diagnosis when they seek to determine the underlying cause of a client's symptoms. Even when a physician provides a diagnosis, it is still the responsibility of the therapist to determine whether that diagnosis is the true source of the client's concerns. Understanding how to evaluate evidence and interpret diagnostic tests is important to this process.

Differential Diagnosis Step 1: Interview

Hand therapists begin the process of differential diagnosis by interviewing clients to gather details on symptom presentation and activity limitations. We ask questions about the nature, severity, and specific location of symptoms. We want to know how and when the symptoms began, how the symptoms have progressed, and what activities exacerbate the symptoms. Clients will often tell us about the most bothersome aspect of their condition but may fail to include all the details of what they are experiencing. We usually need to ask our clients a number of clarifying questions to make sure we have the complete picture. Do not assume that a symptom is not present just because your client has not mentioned it.

Once we have gathered a thorough history, we compare the client's symptom presentation to the typical clinical presentation of a variety of conditions to see which ones seem to match the best. We then create a short list of likely conditions to explore further.

Differential Diagnosis Step 2: Testing

Once we have narrowed down the possible causes of the client's symptoms to a few probable conditions, we use diagnostic tests (sometimes called special tests) to further define the symptom etiology. Special tests usually have a dichotomous outcome: a positive result (indicating that the client has the condition) or a negative result (indicating that the client does not have the condition). However, test results can be incorrect and must be interpreted using evidence that indicates how often the results are correct or incorrect, and how they tend to be incorrect. Table 2.2 illustrates the four possibilities when using special tests for differential diagnosis:

A **True Positive** (TP) is when the test result is *positive* and the client actually *has* the condition (i.e., a positive test result that is true).

A **True Negative** (TN) is when the test result is *negative* and the client actually *does not* have the condition (i.e., a negative test result that is true).

A **False Positive** (FP) is when the test result is *positive* but the client actually *does not* have the condition (i.e., a positive test result that is false).

A **False Negative** (FN) is when the test result is *negative* but the client actually *has* the condition (i.e., a negative test result that is false).

Unfortunately, no test gives only true results, but we can select tests and interpret test results based on how often and in what direction they tend to provide true or false results.

Sensitivity and Specificity: Deciding Which Test to Use

Sensitivity and specificity are measures of validity that help therapists decide which special tests to use.

Sensitivity indicates what percentage of those who actually have the condition have a positive result on the test. A highly sensitive test is good at *including* most people who *have* the condition. Therefore a negative result on a highly sensitive test can confidently rule *out* the condition for a particular individual. By itself, sensitivity does not tell us anything about a test's ability to correctly rule *in* a condition. Sensitivity = TP/(TP+FN).

Specificity indicates what percentage of those who do not have the condition have a negative result on the test. A highly specific test is good at *excluding* most people who do *not* have the condition. Therefore a positive result on a highly specific test can confidently rule *in* the condition for a particular individual. By itself, specificity does not tell us anything about a test's ability to correctly rule *out* a condition. Specificity = TN/(FP+TN).

The mnemonics **SpPin** and **SnNout** help us remember how to use sensitivity and specificity when selecting a special test[1]:

If a test has a very high degree of Specificity and the test result is Positive, then you can be fairly confident that the condition has been ruled in (SpPin).

If a test has a very high degree of Sensitivity and the test result is Negative, then you can be fairly confident that the condition has been ruled out (SnNout).

The ideal test is one that is both sensitive and specific. For example, if test A says that everyone in the world has carpal tunnel syndrome, it will have 100% sensitivity, but the specificity will be 0%, and it obviously will be of no diagnostic value. At the very least, sensitivity + specificity should be >100%. Any less than that, and the overall accuracy of the test is worse than a coin flip. It is better if a test's sensitivity and specificity are *both* >70%, as that test will generate meaningful shifts in the probability that a client has a certain condition for both positive and negative test results.

As an example, Phalen's test for carpal tunnel syndrome (in which the elbows are in 30 degrees of flexion, the forearms are supinated, and the examiner passively positions the wrists in full flexion for 60 seconds, with a positive result being the reproduction of symptoms in the distribution of the median nerve distal to the carpal tunnel) was found to have a sensitivity of 77% and specificity of 40%.[19] This study result indicates that a negative result on Phalen's test has some ability to rule out carpal tunnel syndrome, but a positive result cannot be used to rule in carpal tunnel syndrome because of the low specificity (40%). Thus we would not choose to use Phalen's test if our primary interest is confirming a diagnosis of carpal tunnel syndrome.

Sensitivity and specificity give us a general idea of whether a test is good at ruling in (because it has high specificity), ruling out (because it has high sensitivity), or both but do not help us interpret test results in a precise way for our clients. To interpret test results, we have other tools: likelihood ratios and predictive values.

Interpreting Test Results

Likelihood Ratios

Likelihood ratios (LRs) help us determine how likely it is that a client has a certain condition given a particular test result. LRs are used to interpret test results. However, before we can use likelihood ratios, we need to know how probable it is that a client has a condition based on the information we have *before* we do the test; this is called the **pretest probability**. The pretest probability of a client having a certain condition when they come to a hand therapist depends on a variety of factors: the referral source, the setting in which they are seen, the specified diagnosis, the amount and quality of diagnostic testing done previously, demographic information, and so on.

For example, in one study where physicians referred clients with either suspected carpal tunnel syndrome (CTS) or cervical radiculopathy for neurophysiological testing, only 34% of those clients actually had CTS.[19] This scenario provides a reasonable estimate of CTS prevalence at 34% in clients who are referred for evaluation of hand symptoms that could be explained by either CTS or cervical radiculopathy. Many therapists would agree that being only 34% confident of a diagnosis is not confident enough to start treatment for that condition.

LRs tell us how much the probability of a client having a particular condition increases or decreases, given a test result. If a clinical test is positive in a client, then the positive LR (LR+) for that test tells you how much the likelihood that the client has the condition *increases*. If a clinical test is negative in a client, then the negative likelihood ratio (LR−) for that test tells you how much the likelihood that the client has the condition *decreases*. Likelihood ratios are calculated from sensitivity and specificity using the following formulae[1]:

LR+ = sensitivity / (1 - specificity)

LR− = (1 - sensitivity) / specificity

Let's return to the example of a client who is referred with a diagnosis of carpal tunnel syndrome or cervical radiculopathy, but no electrophysiological testing. The pretest probability (or prevalence) of carpal tunnel syndrome in this situation is 34%. If the therapist performs a Phalen's test and obtains a positive result, the therapist can use the LR+ of 1.3[19] to calculate the posttest probability. This calculation is done using Fagan's Nomogram (Fig. 2.1A). If you draw a straight line from the pretest probability of 34% through the LR+ of 1.3, the line will intersect the posttest probability at 40% (Fig. 2.1B). Further testing can then be done with 40% as the new pretest probability.

Tests can be "chained" in sequence, with each test's posttest probability becoming the pre-test probability for the next test, but only if the tests are independent of each other (that is, if they do not test for the same condition in the same way).[1] A Phalen's test (wrists passively flexed for 60 seconds) and reverse Phalen's test (wrists passively extended for 60 seconds) are probably not independent of each other because both rely on wrist positioning increasing the pressure in the carpal tunnel. On the other hand, a Phalen's test and a Tinel's sign (Tinel's sign, not Tinel's test) (in which the median nerve is percussed with a reflex hammer) probably are independent because they test for carpal tunnel syndrome in different ways.

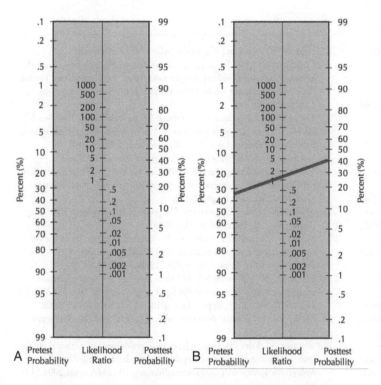

FIG. 2.1 (A) Fagan's Nomogram. (B) Calculating posttest probability, given a pretest probability of 34% and an LR+ of 1.3. *(Adapted with permission from Fagan TJ. Letter: nomogram for Bayes theorem. N Engl J Med. 1975;293:257. Copyright 2005, Massachusetts Medical Society. All rights reserved.)*

◎ *Clinical Pearl*

To use a nomogram in the clinic, print one out at https://www.cebm.net/2014/02/likelihood-ratios/ or use the interactive nomogram at http://araw.mede.uic.edu/cgi-bin/testcalc.pl

---

TABLE 2.3 Likelihood Ratios Required for a Test to be Useful[3]:

Usefulness of test	LR+	LR−
Does not change probability in a helpful way	1 to 2	1 to 0.5
Small changes in probability	2 to 5	0.5 to 0.2
Moderate changes in probability	5 to 10	0.2 to 0.1
Large and conclusive changes in probability	>10	<0.1

Table 2.3 shows the likelihood ratio values that are required to change probabilities in a helpful way.

Positive and Negative Predictive Values

Positive predictive values (PPV) and **negative predictive values** (NPV) are used after the test results have been obtained to interpret those results (the same purpose for which LRs are used). Referencing Table 2.2, the PPV = TP/(TP+FP). The PPV indicates what percent of those individuals who have a positive result on the test actually have the condition. The NPV indicates what percent of those who have a negative result on the test do not have the condition. NPV = TN/(FN+TN). You can use PPV and NPV to estimate the probability that the test result is accurate. For example, a NPV of 0.65 means that of all those clients who have a negative result on the test, 65% actually do not have the condition (and 35% do). One disadvantage of PPV and NPV is that they take the prevalence of a condition into account, and the prevalence in any particular study may differ greatly from the prevalence in your clinical setting. Before using PPVs and NPVs from a study, the practitioner must make sure that the prevalence of the condition in the study is the same as the prevalence of that condition in their own practice setting.

Finding the Evidence and Tools for Differential Diagnosis

A number of resources exist that provide sensitivity, specificity, and likelihood ratios for special tests. Two evidence-based orthopedic examination books provide a wealth of evidence regarding reliability and validity (sensitivity, specificity, and LRs) of special tests in differential diagnosis.[20,21] We can also find systematic reviews or individual studies on diagnosis through www.pubmed.gov: click on "Clinical Queries" under "PubMed Tools," type the diagnosis in the search box, then look at the articles under the "Systematic Reviews" heading, or choose the category "Diagnosis" under the "Clinical Study Categories" heading.

Perhaps the most difficult data to access is the pretest probability (or prevalence) of a condition. Ideally, this should be the prevalence in one's own clinical setting. Sometimes this can be informed by evidence (as in the carpal tunnel syndrome example presented in this chapter). Other times, we have to estimate the prevalence in our clinical population; however, we can use our clinic data to make such an estimate.

References

1. Straus SE, Glasziou P, Richardson WS, et al.: *Evidence-based medicine: how to practice and teach EBM*, ed 5, New York, NY, 2019, Elsevier.

2. Portney LG, Watkins MP: *Foundations of clinical research: applications to practice*, ed 3, Upper Saddle River, NJ, 2009, Pearson Prentice Hall.

3. Guyatt G, Rennie D, Meade MO, et al.: *Users' guides to the medical literature: a manual for evidence-based clinical practice*, ed 3, McGraw-Hill Education, 2015.

4. Fetters L, Tilson J: *Evidence-based physical therapy*, Philadelphia, PA, 2012, F. A. Davis.

5. Law M, MacDermid JC, editors: *Evidence-based rehabilitation: a guide to practice*, ed 3, Thorofare, NJ, 2014, SLACK Inc.

6. OCEBM Levels of Evidence Working Group: *The Oxford 2011 levels of evidence*, Oxford, United Kingdom, 2011, Oxford Centre for Evidence-Based Medicine. http://www.cebm.net/index.aspx?o=5653. [Accessed 20 May 2019].

7. MacDermid JC: An introduction to evidence-based practice for hand therapists, *J Hand Ther* 7(2):105–117, 2004. https://doi.org/10.1197/j.jht.2004.02.001.

8. Merriam SB, Tisdell EJ: *Qualitative research:a guide to design and implementation*, ed 4, San Fransisco, CA, 2015, Jossey-Bass.

9. Tomlin G, Borgetto B: Research pyramid: a new evidence-based practice model for occupational therapy, *Am J Occup Ther* 65(2):189–196, 2011. https://doi.org/10.5014/ajot.2011.000828.

10. Tickle-Degnen L, Bedell G: Heterarchy and hierarchy: a critical appraisal of the "levels of evidence" as a tool for clinical decision making, *Am J Occup Ther* 57(2):234–237, 2003. https://doi.org/10.5014/ajot.57.2.234.

11. Arbesman M, Scheer J, Lieberman D: Using AOTAs critically appraised topic and critically appraised paper series to link evidence to practice, *OT Practice* 13(5):18–22, 2008. https://communot.aota.org/viewdocument/05-march-31-2008.

12. Higgins JPT, Altman DG, Sterne JAC: 8.5 The Cochrane Collaboration's tool for assessing risk of bias. In Higgins JPT, Green S, editors: *Cochrane handbook for systematic reviews of interventions. Version 5.1.0*, The Cochrane Collaboration, 2011. http://handbook-5-1.cochrane.org/.

13. *Centre for Evidence-Based Physiotherapy: PEDro scale Sydney, New South Wales, Australia*, University of Sydney, 1999. https://www.pedro.org.au/english/downloads/pedro-scale/2018. [Accessed 20 May 2019].

14. Law M, Stewart D, Pollock N, et al.: *Critical Review Forms and Guidelines*, Hamilton, Ontario, 1998, Canada McMaster University. https://www.canchild.ca/en/resources/137-critical-review-forms-and-guidelines2018. [Accessed 1 April 2019].

15. AGREE Next Steps Consortium: The AGREE II Instrument 2017. https://agreetrust.org. [Accessed 20 May 2019].

16. Moher D, Liberati A, Tetzlaff J, et al.: Preferred reporting items for systematic reviews and meta-analyses: the PRISMA statement, *BMJ* 339:b2535, 2009. https://doi.org/10.1136/bmj.b2535.

17. Rodrigues JN, Mabvuure NT, Nikkhah D, et al.: Minimal important changes and differences in elective hand surgery, *J Hand Surg Eur Vol* 40(9):900–912, 2015. https://doi.org/10.1177/1753193414553908.

18. Mosby: *Mosby's medical dictionary*, ed 9, St. Louis, MO, 2013, Elsevier Mosby. 2013;533.

19. Wainner RS, Fritz JM, Irrgang JJ, et al.: Development of a clinical prediction rule for the diagnosis of carpal tunnel syndrome, *Arch Phys Med Rehabil* 86(4):609–618, 2005. https://doi.org/10.1016/j.apmr.2004.11.008.

20. Cleland JA, Koppenhaver S, Su J: *Netter's orthopedic clinical examination: an evidence-based approach*, ed 3, Philadelphia, PA, 2016, Elsevier.

21. Cook CE, Hegedus EJ: *Orthopedic physical examination tests: an evidence-based approach*, ed 2, Upper Saddle River, NJ, 2013, Pearson Education.

3

Functional Anatomy

Lori DeMott
Sharon R. Flinn

Introduction

Anatomy is the study of the physical structures within the human body. The skeleton provides a stable foundation, and muscles attach by way of bony origins and insertions that cross and influence the angle of the joints. Knowledge of the nervous system provides us with a practical understanding of muscular control both to the tendon excursion and muscle mobility. The interrelatedness of the skeleton, muscle, and nervous systems provides an understanding of how the body works during a simple task to overall performance in daily activities, simply due to the functional anatomy. Knowledge of these systems, interrelationships, and how they affect the efficacy and efficiency of movement will facilitate therapeutic interventions that lead to improved client outcomes.

The principles of functional anatomy begin with the ability to understand the components in each of the three systems. Knowledge of skeletal support, muscle orientation and location, and muscle tone influences any given action. The interaction of the neuromusculoskeletal systems is important to analyze the parts of the body systems that explain observable postures. The concept of the unconscious and compensatory mechanics of the body to overall performance is a prerequisite to the goal of improved functioning. Sound knowledge of anatomical systems and the understanding, applying, and analyzing of their interrelationship during movement is a primary directive to addressing movement dysfunction. Ultimately, in practice, the functional anatomy is an important factor in grading the success of our clients' task performance.

The focus of this chapter is to introduce a sophisticated yet understandable method of neuromusculoskeletal assessment. The recall of anatomy as an identifiable detail is mainly at the lower level of the learning hierarchy. The ability to evaluate and analyze the body systems requires looking at component anatomy and then distinguishing between limitations of the parts to the whole of functional movement. There are conditions that may appear to be limited to a single part of the body (e.g., swan neck, zigzag deformity of the wrist and fingers, rounded shoulders) yet over time this initial change may contribute to changes both proximally and distally. The sections of this chapter are divided into body parts. The local aspect of muscle balance is described in each section and then combined to the analysis of the whole in movement. Then learning progression of analysis to synthesis will be summarized in the last part of this chapter using case studies. These common clinical scenarios will illustrate abnormal deviations or faults in postural mechanics resulting from tissue imbalance that will provide examples for quick screens of the functional anatomy. The analysis of the interrelationships of systems that affect the body's ability to perform are those against-gravity movements that incorporate upper limb movements within the advanced skills of functional mobility.

Key concepts of functional anatomy are normal postural mechanics, structural components of alignment, principles of muscle function, posture and body alignment (systems interdependence), and the influences of postural deviation on body position.

Standard Postural Mechanics

There are observable muscle behaviors that influence our posture and purposeful movements, also termed functional anatomy. Essential distinctions should be made between the anatomical characteristic of body positions, both at the initial static position of a kinematic event and then the return to our neuromuscularskeletal equilibrium of balance.[1] **Static posture** is the stationary position held against gravity, whereas **dynamic posture** refers to a series of positions that continuously changes during movement and function. Both postures require equilibrium of the muscle system and are observed during relaxation, standing, sitting, or lying down.[1]

Functional anatomy, defined by postural kinematic expressions, is fundamentally based on a predictable design. The gross structure, knowledge of muscle fiber alignment, location, and the origins and insertions of human anatomy references will assist in understanding the natural tone and potential forces of a specific muscle. Standard postural mechanics work in harmony and are observed when the antagonist, agonist, and synergistic coordination of our body mechanics perform in an efficient and effective manner.

If the observed initial position of the body differs from the known standard, well-balanced posture, the therapist can assume there is potentially altered kinematics. Studies have found that there is a relationship between altered posture and musculoskeletal disorders.[2] The therapist's knowledge of the neuromusculoskeletal anatomy is paramount to identifying the specifics of the constraints and resultant soft tissue changes. Furthermore, an identified structural abnormality can be the cause or result of movement dysfunction and pain. For example, in the forward head, rounded shoulders (FHRS) position, which differs from the standard position of balanced posture, this starting position of altered anatomy can create the potential for proximal and distal disruptions in the kinematic chain of movement. During reach, the changes in joint orientation due to the core malalignment will add kinematic mechanical stress to structures, such as the acromioclavicular joint or to the muscles that originate on the lateral epicondyle.[2]

◎ *Clinical Pearl*

If the starting position of the body differs from the zero position of balance, the altered anatomy will create a disrupted kinematic chain of movement that adds stress to areas, such as the acromioclavicular joint or the muscles that originate on the lateral epicondyles.

Structural Components of Alignment

Bones, Ligaments, and Joints

Bones are responsible for the rigidity and structure of the entire foundation. The joint anatomy is designed to allow transmission of muscle force, at rest and during motion. Understanding joint structure contributes to the overall whole of functional anatomy and posture configuration. Bone-to-bone connection creates the joint. The bone segments within the joint move in relation to each other. The configuration of the bony surfaces dictates the degree of freedom of a joint and creates a type of movement hinge.

Most joints allow freedom of movement from one to three planes as the bony segments move in relationship to each other. Usually, one segment is stable while the other moves in relation to the base. As the joint moves, there can be more than one contributing articulation that influence the overall pattern of movement. For example, the shoulder girdle comprises the glenohumeral joint with scapulohumeral, sternohumeral, and clavicohumeral articulations.[3] The control and stability of the joint's axis of rotation directly relates to the articular orientation of the all of the structures. Without the rules for joint stability, the simplest movement can become weakened by the loss of mechanical advantage at any given point along the kinematic chain. This is seen in a joint dislocation, degeneration, and in segmental bone

fractures, whereby the movement is not guided, and irregular angulations are observed. Conversely, if the segments of bone are not congruent and there is altered space that changes the axis of movement, the extrinsic muscle pull can be offset, and functional movement will present with distorted mechanics that are dysfunctional and not optimal. In the occupation-based profile, the client will describe various levels of adaptation, usually not from the changes in specific movement or those of unconscious motoric compensations, but to the description of pain or loss of meaningful activity.

Throughout the body, there are many axes of rotation. In the upper limb, there are flexion–extension, abduction–adduction, internal–external, radial–ulnar, and pronation–supination axes. The wrist has two, the elbow joint has one at the ulnohumeral joint axis, and the glenohumeral joint is a ball-and-socket joint with three axes of rotation. The relationships of joint axes have a normal presentation of balance that is predictable and can be assessed at rest and during movement.

◎ *Clinical Pearl*

Joint pathologies can be observed, and should be palpated, at rest and during movements.

An altered configuration of the joint's soft tissue matrix or bony constructs lead to the joint's failure to glide and can result in various types of joint collapses and deformities.[3] With joint laxity, the axis shifts in the direction of the weakened and degraded tissue. Frequently, this is seen with attritional changes of the glenohumeral joint where the anterior capsuloligaments are weakened and attenuated. A shift in the joint axis results in tension changes in the anterior and posterior capsule and over time contributes to the formation of adhesions. Instability and adhesive phenomena are due to many types of disease manifestations. All will eventually involve the soft tissue structures of the intrinsic and extrinsic muscles that will lose the internal balance of the bony articular surface and ligamentous stability. The loss of joint stability will allow muscle to pull the articulated bone unopposed and contribute to deformity.[4]

Nervous System

The peripheral, central, and autonomic nervous systems all combine to form one internal communication system for sensing and responding to internal and external stimuli.[5] The motor and sensory functions for the upper limb come from the cervical and brachial plexus. Most nerves have an efferent motor and afferent sensory fibers arranged in bundles of axons. Layers of dense connective tissues called the epineurium, perineurium, and endoneurium protect the axons. Each layer has a unique role to support the innermost structures of the nerve, modulate compressive and tensile forces, and allow gliding between nerve fascicles and the surrounding anatomical structures.[6] Electrical impulses are rapidly conducted by way of the nodes of Ranvier along a neural pathway, which originates at the spinal cord and brainstem and terminates in the fingers and toes. Due to the continuous nature and physiology of the peripheral nervous system, motions at a distal site, such as the wrist joint, increase the strain at the cord level of the brachial plexus. Similarly, contralateral flexion of the cervical spine increases the strain in the cords of the brachial plexus and three major nerves in the arm.[5] Under tension, the neural tissue may have difficulty conducting electrical impulses, ensuring adequate blood supply, and providing adequate axonal transport, especially during movement.[6]

The complex role of the nervous system in muscular activity is to keep the body in balance. What is found in the nerve-to-muscle connections is a synchronous muscular harmony that is performed by the receptor Golgi tendon organs and the muscle spindles. These two proprioceptors are in or near muscles. Their function is to record and respond to muscle tension and changes in muscle length. They are responsible for muscle inhibition of the agonist and facilitation of the antagonist.[4] This complex feedback system from sensory receptors up to the spinal cord, to the central nervous system and back, contributes to the movement components that produce both planned and reflexive movement patterns.

The nervous system is the control center for our muscle equilibrium at rest and during motion. The complexity of the system controls muscles in isolation or in synergistic groups. Anatomical knowledge of specific locations of nerves from the spinal cord to the periphery, or at the synaptic junction of skeletal muscle, helps us understand the type of changes that occur within the musculoskeletal anatomy.

Muscles

Muscles work in groups and patterns of movement. Individual muscles have lengthening, contractile, excitable, and recoil characteristics. **Contractility** allows a muscle to shorten with force, to lengthen passively, and to move. **Excitability** allows a muscle to respond to a stimulus and to maintain chemical potentials across its cell membranes. **Extensibility** allows a muscle to be stretched, repeatedly and considerably, as needed, without being damaged. **Elasticity** allows a muscle to return to its normal length after being stretched or shortened. The result of a muscle function is an application of force. For example, a coordinated neuromuscular event occurs during the conscious decision to make a fist. The wrist extensors and flexors stabilize the wrist in approximately 35 degrees of extension, the extrinsic extensor digitorum communis (EDC) elongates into a full extensible position as the antagonist muscle, and simultaneously the extrinsic flexor digitorum profundus (FDP) and flexor digitorum superficialis (FDS) contract in their role as agonist muscles. The balanced self-selected position of 25 to 35 degrees of wrist extension and 7 degrees of ulnar deviation was found to produce optimal grip strength.[7] The coordinated muscle contractions of the wrist assist in the differentiation of tendon glide that allows terminal distal joint flexion. Simultaneously, contraction of the intrinsic lumbrical and interossei muscles increase metacarpal joint flexion, stabilize and control the joint, and allow the digits to converge into a tucked position within the palm.[4] The characteristics of the musculotendinous structures that contribute to muscle balance are located in Box 3.1. In summary, the principles of muscle function allow coordinated effort to improve both strength and flexibility of the isolated muscle and those muscles in groups.

⊚ Clinical Pearl

The wrist position is the key to changing the tension placed on the extrinsic fingers and thumb musculotendinous units.

BOX 3.1 Musculotendinous Characteristics That Contribute to Balance

1. The resting length of a muscle is the relationship and proportional stretch to the fully contracted muscle fiber.
2. At rest and even during sleep, there is a tendency of the muscle to contract and resist lengthening. This principle is influenced by the central nervous system and the intrinsic muscle structure, and by definition is our muscle tone.
3. Ordinary normal range of motion at rest or during movement is influenced by the variability of length and pull of all of our contributing anatomy due to antagonist lengthening as well as synergistic coordination.
4. Gravity and the need for skeletal stability will change the resting muscle tone and therefore change distal joint position.
5. Length and cross-section of a muscle leads to predictable excursion and levels of muscle elasticity.
6. A muscle crossing multiple joints will provide a composite excursion; a proximal joint stability is necessary for increased distal joint mobility.
7. Passive joint mobility is without influence of soft tissue elastic characteristics.
8. Muscle balance is involuntary, and over time the resting length can change or be changed by an altered axis. As the joint moves, these altered forces create imbalances and lead to deformity.

Posture: Body Alignment

Functional anatomy, defined by postural kinematic expressions, is fundamentally based on a stable, predictable design. This composite of body position is called **standard posture**. During observation, the skeletal conformation is observed and analyzed by envisioning the underlying bone positions. By knowing the preset configuration, or default design, you can visually construct the muscle anatomy and its contribution to posture. The gross structure, knowledge of muscle fiber alignment, location, and the origins and insertions of the human anatomy assist in understanding the natural tone and potential force of a specific muscle.

Skeletal alignment is observed and analyzed by envisioning the underlying interplay of the neuromusculoskeletal system. Postural configurations as a whole are the positions that are caused by changes in an isolated joint or by multiple joints. The shortened and lengthened muscle orientations are primary or secondary contributions to the observed posture. Many different conditions can cause these noted structural changes.

⊚ Clinical Pearl

Shortened muscles are not stronger muscles.

The neutral resting balance of our anatomy is the state of default or the **zero position** of the body.[3] The zero position is different from the anatomical position of the body. It represents the standard resting balance position where the upper limbs align themselves in space against gravity, where movement ceases, and where relative loads are removed. In the zero position, the upper limbs are positioned in the midrange of

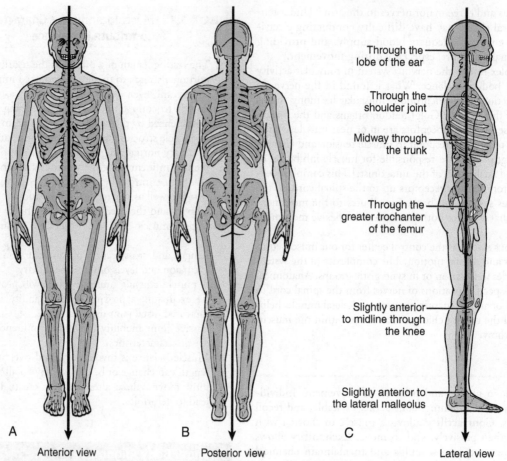

Through the
lobe of the ear

Through the
shoulder joint

Midway through
the trunk

Through the
greater trochanter
of the femur

Slightly anterior
to midline through
the knee

Slightly anterior to
the lateral malleolus

A　　　　　　　　　　B　　　　　　　　　　C

Anterior view　　　　Posterior view　　　　Lateral view

FIG. 3.1　The zero position of the body from the sagittal and coronal planes. (A) Anterior view. (B) Posterior view. (C) Lateral view. (Modified from Cameron MH, Monroe LG. *Physical Rehabilitation: Evidence-Based Examination, Evaluation, and Intervention.* St Louis, MO: Saunders Elsevier; 2007.)

glenohumeral and forearm rotation, the wrist is positioned in approximately 10 degrees of extension, and the finger joints are positioned in approximately 45 degrees of flexion. Abnormal changes in functional anatomy cannot be understood without knowledge of the standard resting balance position. Fig. 3.1 illustrates zero position.

> ### ◎ *Clinical Pearl*
> The position of the hand in relation to the zero position tells you about the functional anatomy of the scapula and suggests the orientation of the scapula and its relative position on the thorax.

The upper limb returns to this default resting position, or zero position, in most static body postures. It is an assumed position of joint alignment where the tone of muscle activity is minimal, where the origins and insertions are in a "resting" position, and where the tension of the joint is in a relaxed ligamentous balance. The residual muscle tone at rest is the muscle contraction in response to the gravitational pull. Importantly, the resting position and resultant tone of the upper limb may be different in different postures (e.g., sitting, supine, prone) due to the contributions from the base of

support and the gravitational pull and subsequent tilt of the pelvis and or scapula.

Muscle tone is defined as the continuous and passive-partial contraction of the muscle or the muscle's resistance to passive stretch during the resting state.[4] The joint angles and lines of muscle tension that are produced, as well as the whole conformation of the body, are indications as to how synergistic muscles and nervous system are performing. Typically, the points of reference are anatomical landmarks and are observed in two body planes. The **coronal plane** is vertical and divides the body into anterior and posterior halves.[3] From the coronal plane we draw a linear plumb line, or line of gravity (LOG), that forms an **axis of reference.** From the lateral view of the client, the alignment of the ear, shoulder, lateral elbow, posterior hip, anterior knee, and lateral malleolus are body landmarks that are located close to, if not directly within, the axis of reference. From the axis you can observe the flexion, extension, anterior, and posterior adaptations of the body. Similarly, the **sagittal plane** is vertical and divides the body into right and left halves.[3] Postures viewed from all sides include obvious body markers, such as head position, shoulder height and glenoid orientation, clavicle angle, scapular position, antecubital fossa (i.e., carrying angle/orientation), hand orientation, and hip height. Fig. 3.1A and B illustrates the body in the sagittal plane and provides the anterior and posterior views of the body. Fig. 3.1C illustrates the body in the coronal plane and provides a lateral view of the body with a clear view of the arm orientation.

> ### ◎ *Clinical Pearl*
>
> The scapula tilts (anteriorly, posteriorly, upwardly or downwardly). The scapular tilt changes the orientation of the limb at rest and contributes to acquired functional range of motion.

A functional anatomy screen is performed by envisioning key markers of anatomical landmarks, and bone segments, as they create altered angles in contrast to those described in the zero position. The altered angles can change the overall height or distance between parts and present with a segment line of movement from the vertical or horizontal "zero" position. The differences in these angles or projections are used to hypothesize the influence of the associated muscle function. To understand postural forces of human anatomy and to utilize these concepts in practice, we need to apply the normal orientation of the ideal skeleton and muscle alignment at rest and during movement. These "normal" default postures can then be compared to the client who has compensatory adaptation and restrictions in anatomical structures.

> ### ◎ *Clinical Pearl*
>
> An understanding of normal anatomy and the ideal positions of balance is essential to recognize the imbalances in your client's neuromusculoskeletal anatomy.

The skeletal system of the body and upper limb can be mapped to determine the standard default state of zero position. **Mapping** is a visual technique of drawing, using the design and angles of the body that creates a picture of alignment. An imaginary overlay of the skeleton on the conformation of the body creates the approximate location of the joints and bone segments. Positions of mapping are in the planes of movement. The body's coronal and sagittal planes produce the lines of reference in static and dynamic body postures. The front and back views of the body allow the best view of symmetry.

These structures assist in recognizing important landmarks. **Landmarks** are structures that identify a feature other than a joint. Examples of landmarks are the ear, forehead creases, palm and nail positions, the carry angle space, web spaces, and skin folds in the back and digital creases. An example of important landmarks as seen in Fig. 3.1 is the space between the arm and body. Fig. 3.2 identifies the mapping specific to the hand. Important landmarks for the hand are nail positions, the space between the index and thumb, the cascading flexion of the fingers, the mass of the thenar eminence, and the prominence of the ulnar head.

Once the position of the joint articulation and landmarks are identified, the **segments**, or lines drawn between articular surfaces, are identified. The design is then analyzed using the expected functional anatomy as the reference point for identifying imbalances that can contribute to pain, weakness, and restrictions in movement.

The use of the two anatomical planes, axes of reference, and mapping techniques serve as a functional anatomy screening tool that allows the therapist to compare the ideal postural alignment to that of the assumed posture of the client. The

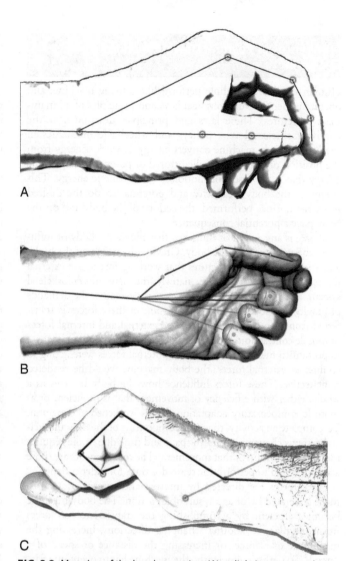

FIG. 3.2 Mapping of the hand at rest in a (A) radial view pronated position, (B) neutral forearm position, and (C) ulnar view pronated position. (From Donatelli RA. *Orthopaedic Physical Therapy.* 4th ed. St Louis, MO: Churchill Livingstone Elsevier; 2010.)

deviation from the ideal can range from slight to severe and will guide the evaluator in understanding the problems associated with joint and muscle functions. This tool can identify at a local level (joint) and global level (body posture) the differences in the contributing anatomy misalignment.[8,9] The shortened muscles (e.g., antagonist weakness, joint pain, proximal etiology) may have contributed to the observed posture or joint position that of greater deviation of flexion, extension, lateral rotation. Recognizing these postural fluctuations allows therapists to describe the contributory neuromuscular events and address the functional anatomy in their therapeutic interventions.

> ### ◎ *Clinical Pearl*
>
> With practice, the therapist performing anatomical mapping will find that this process can be envisioned, looking at the client's conformation, using the feet, knee, hip, shoulder, and ear landmarks as key visual markers and comparing them to the normal resting alignment.

Influences of Postural Deviation on the Body Position

Human systems as a whole perform like a living machine, and operate under the same physical laws and principles of all inanimate structures. These laws and principles describe how the relatively efficient levers, pulleys and wheel-axle mechanics in the human body machine convert energy to work. Energy from the position of the body is called stored or potential energy. The energy that is the result of motion is called kinetic energy. This energy is the body's capacity and potential to do the desired movement. Once performed, the actions of the body and on the body have a potential consequence.

Force is any action or influence that moves the body or influences the movement of the body. Gravity, the weight of the body, and friction on those structures that work against it, are external forces. The body's structure, namely the neuromusculoskeletal system, also generates internal forces as it overcomes the demands of gravity and loads.[10] The transmission of these forces is transferred from one part to another. The external and internal forces of muscle contraction, ligamentous restraint, and bony support are important to mention because if no internal forces were acting to counteract external forces, the body machine would be rendered noneffective. These forces influence how the body behaves as a whole, either with efficiency of movement that is proficient or as motoric compensatory adaptation that is weakened and painful. To complete an activity, the body components of the musculoskeletal systems change position in space and time due to the requirements for execution of that movement. The requirements are those actions needed to perform the desired actions for independence.

The forces are directed by internal and external demands, those generated by or as a result of an action. The body machine becomes efficient by accomplishing the transference of forces from one place to another, changing directions, increasing the magnitude of a force, or increasing the distance or speed of a force.[13] To perform efficiently, the machine has to overcome friction and the stress of loads in every action.[4] The laws of movement mechanics help in understanding the postural effect of strain and stress on the body during all body positions and actions. For the purpose of this chapter, the understanding of functional anatomy includes the interrelationships of systems, the forces that act on the body structures and the biomechanics of that motion. These are the factors contributing to our client's functional complaints.

Force is a cause (push or pull) that produces or changes the acceleration of a body.[4] The forces defined for our purposes are those that cause stress to the musculoskeletal system, which includes those of the bones, joints, and soft tissue. Body postures are attempts to move as efficiently as possible in order to successfully complete desired tasks. Importantly, the external forces of gravity continually act on all body structures. The ever-changing center of gravity is the concentrated point about which all parts balance each other and produce musculoskeletal changes down the kinematic chain. During postural changes for stability and mobility that occur with movement, the lengthening and shortening of our neuromuscular structures work against gravity to maintain the body in the best erect and stable position. The effect of internal and external forces on a body changes the mechanical balance and center of gravity. Efficient mechanical balance is based on a stable distribution of its weight throughout the entirety of the movement. In summary, proper alignment during

activity is based on the body's ability to support and adjust the weight of the gravitational pull using the functional anatomy of muscle contraction and relaxation.

Internal mechanical stresses (i.e., tensile, compressive, shearing, torsion, and bending), if they are persistent, can result in changes to the neuromusculoskeletal form. The changes in form are seen in the muscle builder or performance worker who has overdevelopment of muscle, known as chronic hypertonicity. The muscle *strain* changes the shape, volume, or both in a body as the result of excessive and/or sustained stress. Other changes to form that alter the pattern of movement are observed with the imbalance of the antagonist due to atrophy. The muscle properties change in elasticity, flexibility, and suppleness with the inability to reach the full range of motion, to return to its original shape, and to recover from distortion even when the stress has been removed.

Local changes at a joint can be observed when muscle atrophy occurs following nerve injury or complete denervation to a muscle or muscle group. The balanced equilibrium at the joint will be lost as the unopposed muscle contracts without an antagonist and alters the joint's position. A joint imbalance may be the primary contributor to a joint contracture and/or may be part of the chain of kinematic changes resulting in dysfunction. The observed deformity is accentuated when forces are applied. Functional movements that include the external forces of acceleration and gravity will generate a reaction to neuromuscular relationships. External and internal forces that create balance or imbalance subsequently result in alignment or misalignment.

A broader picture of the more global effect of skeletal changes is observed with postural variations in the normal curves of the spine. The postural variation can be seen in different combinations. The faulty posture can sit alone as a primary problem or be the contributor to secondary distal and/or proximal kinematic compensations. Faulty core postures influence distal kinematics of the upper limb and compound the internal and external stress of our movements. Thoracic flexion (kyphosis), rounded shoulder forward head (RSFH), scoliosis, and lumbar extension (lordosis) are examples of faulty postures that occur when the spine and scapular line of movement increase their distance from the line of gravity. Each of these postures presents with shortening and lengthening of corresponding muscles with elongation, weakness, shortening and/or ineffectual strengthening of the functional anatomy.[12,13]

Next, a review of the anatomical systems will be discussed in further detail including the characteristics associated with bones, joints, ligaments, muscles, tendons, and the neurovascular systems of the upper limb as well as their contribution to posture and the mechanics of movement. Each body region will be discussed with information to identify and qualify the changes that occur within the functional anatomy.

Hand, Wrist, Forearm, and Elbow

Postural deviations that are due to disease can be seen in the hands of persons with rheumatoid or osteoarthritis. The anatomical structural changes that occur over time are observed with metacarpophalangeal (MP) joint subluxation and swan neck deformities. A common MP joint change occurs when the most proximal phalanx segment tilts palmary toward the volar plate, descending and subluxing the joint. What is observed at rest is the prominent head of the metacarpal. The internal forces from muscle contractions are transmitted through the altered joint axis and changes in the moment arm of the tendon. In this example, the extensor digitorum communis tendon becomes a flexor of the finger MP joint. The change in the axis of rotation alters not only the forces applied to the MP joint but also the kinematic chain of all joints that the muscle-tendon unit controls. The anatomical redirection of the long tendon at the MP joint, in conjunction with significant joint changes, presents with a zigzag pattern of the fingers with proximal interphalangeal (PIP) joint hyperextension and distal interphalangeal (DIP) flexion joint postures. These changes in the anatomy and kinematics result in a functional loss to extend the digits for grasp. As the condition progresses, the zigzag deformity produces a locking PIP joint hyperextension posture that restricts digital flexion for all tasks.

> ### ◎ *Clinical Pearl*
>
> The kinematic chain of mobility is controlled and primarily influenced proximally.

Attritional changes at a joint may be due to ligament laxity or disease of the articular surface as found in the carpometacarpal (CMC) joint of the thumb.[14] The excessive movement during functional use causes bone surface erosions and ligament laxity. Laxity of the stabilizing deep anterior oblique ligament (DAOL), called the beak ligament, causes the joint to sublux in a radial and palmar direction. Over time, the degenerative thumb CMC joint exhibits changes in appearance as seen with a prominent ledge that extends from the radial side of the base of the thumb. The loss of joint stability changes the characteristic of the surrounding muscular anatomy. The abductor pollicis brevis weakens and the adductor pollicis muscle contracts, unopposed. The thumb CMC joint is drawn into adduction and rotational supination.[4] The imbalance of the thumb intrinsic muscles changes the axis of rotation, decreasing the transmission of flexion forces across the metacarpal joint, and moves the resting position of the MP joint from a flexed posture to extension. Over time, the metacarpal joint hyperextends as the mechanical advantage from the extensor pollicis brevis (EPB) muscle further aggravates the adductor pull on the CMC joint and the increasing severity of the contracture. The interphalangeal (IP) joint compensates for loss of metacarpal joint flexion and overly flexes to produce a functional tip pinch. The cascading events are self-perpetuating as the normal joint forces become pathological. The specific pattern of use changes the functional patterns of pinch.

The anatomy of the arthritic thumb presents with imbalances, principally at the CMC joint level, with bone erosions and capsular instability that contribute to the distal joint changes at rest and during dynamic loads.[14] Fig. 3.3 illustrates the mapping of a normal and pathological CMC joint. The dots estimate the joint location, the stars are the landmarks, and the dashes are the bone segments. The disparities between the two thumbs are clear. The line of movement has changed from a resting flexed posture to a zigzag presentation. Compared to the normal thumb, imbalances in the pathological thumb are identified by three visible landmarks; increased nail rotation, MP joint hyperextension, and a protuberance at the CMC joint caused by the subluxing metacarpal.

The function of the collateral ligaments in the human body is to provide joint stability while functional activities occur within

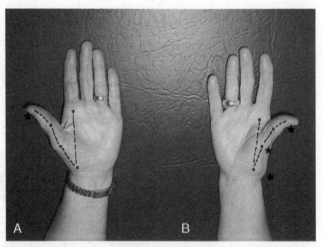

FIG. 3.3 Mapping of a (A) normal and (B) pathological carpometacarpal joint of the thumb. (Photo Lori DeMott.)

multiple planes of movement. Fig. 3.4 provides the ligamentous system of the wrist. The palmar wrist ligaments provide support between the carpal bones. The dorsal wrist ligaments provide support between the carpal bones and the radius. The palmar radioscapholunate ligament provides support for the radius, the scaphoid, and the lunate. The triangular fibrocartilage complex (TFCC) provides support between the carpal bones, the ulna, and the distal radial-ulnar joint. Each of the supporting structures is important in stabilizing the wrist in extreme ranges of wrist extension, flexion, radial deviation, and ulnar deviation.[8] Not only does stability of the joint affect mobility, but without adequate support on the ulnar border of the wrist, the amount of pinch strength on the radial side can be diminished.

Several imbalances of the wrist can occur from pathology. In the case of a displaced and angulated metacarpal fracture, the skeletal length changes and the shortened foundations can limit the ability of the extensor tendon to bring the MP joints into full extension. This is an important function in initiating grasp for large objects, placing the hand into pockets, and for the fine manipulation of using a keyboard. Injuries to the wrist ligaments themselves have stabilizing effects that redirect the pull and balance of the long extrinsic tendons. This is seen in clients with distal radioulnar joint (DRUJ) instability. During forearm pronation, the ulna migrates dorsally and a prominent ulnar styloid is observed. The CMC joint of the small finger demonstrates mild changes but an obvious collapse proximally creates a visual fovea, or depression. The extensor carpi ulnaris (ECU) tendon that inserts onto the fifth metacarpal now becomes inefficient and loses its ability to stabilize the metacarpal into extension during active grasp. The hand changes its appearance as the arch of the small metacarpal joint ascends and over time the entire hand radially deviates during grasp and pinch tasks. The ligaments by virtue of disease and overload from an altered axis will eventually cascade into instability and joint collapse. Fig. 3.5A and B, maps the expected imbalances from the same client with ligamentous instability associated with a classical malunion of a distal radius fracture. In Fig. 3.5A, shortening of the radius and carpal collapse demonstrates the radial bias of the wrist. Landmarks can be observed with increased prominence of the ulnar styloid. In Fig. 3.5B, the proximal elevation of the fifth metacarpal can be seen as a result of ulnocarpal ligament laxity. This instability results in the disruption of the distal transverse arch. Also, you will

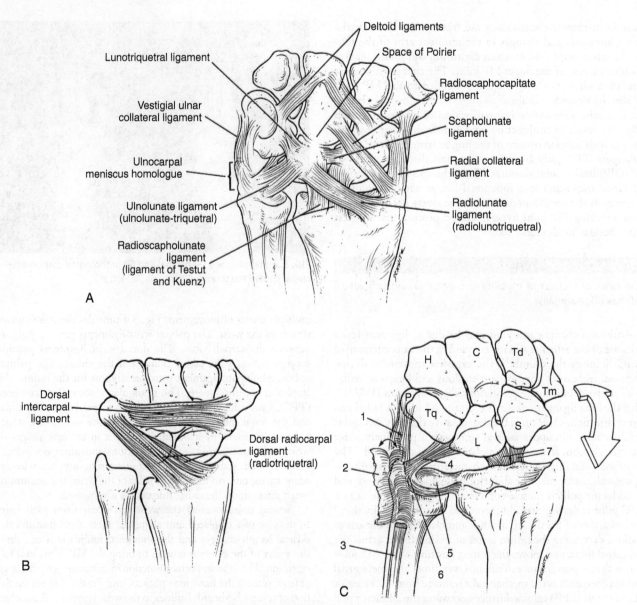

FIG. 3.4 Ligamentous anatomy of the wrist. (A) Palmar wrist ligaments. (B) Dorsal wrist ligaments. (C) Dorsal view of the flexed wrist, including the triangular fibrocartilage. 1, Ulnar collateral ligament; 2, retinacular sheath; 3, tendon of extensor carpi ulnaris; 4, ulnolunate ligament; 5, triangular fibrocartilage, 6, ulnocarpal meniscus homologue; 7, palmar radioscaphoid lunate ligament; C, capitate; H, hamate; L, lunate; P, pisiform; S, scaphoid; Td, trapezoid; Tm, trapezium; . (From Fess EE, Gettle K, Phillips C, et al. *Hand and Upper Extremity Splinting: Principles and Methods.* 3rd ed. St Louis, MO: Mosby; 2005.)

see an atrophied hypothenar eminence and a pronounced extensor digitorum minimi, which assists with wrist extension. Other landmarks can be observed with abnormal depression from the metacarpal angle and prominence of the ulnar styloid; both are indicative of possible subluxation of the wrist carpus and DRUJ imbalance.

The ligamentous structures in the fingers differ considerably from those of the wrist. Fig. 3.6 reviews the supporting structures of the finger MP and PIP joints. The design of the collateral ligament is to ensure lateral support. When the MP joint is flexed, the collateral ligament lengthens to accommodate the movement and stabilize the joint. Similarly, slack in the collateral ligament occurs when the MP joint is fully extended. In addition to the lateral support of a joint, volar reinforcement is provided

through strong membranous connections with the collateral ligament. The palmar (also called volar) plates are slack in flexion but become taut when the joint is extended, thus protecting the joint from hyperextension stresses or dislocations. Common postural changes for ligamentous instability of the fingers may include swan neck deformity of the digits. In the static and dynamic postures of the PIP joint, the palmar support attenuates over time and the lateral bands slide dorsal to the joint axis with the resulting PIP hyperextension posture.

As expected, the thumb has ligamentous supports at the IP joint, the MP joint, and the CMC joint. Of particular interest are the radial and ulnar collateral ligaments (RCLs/UCLs) of the MP joint. Fig. 3.7 illustrates the importance of this strong band of tissue in supporting pinch, especially for tip

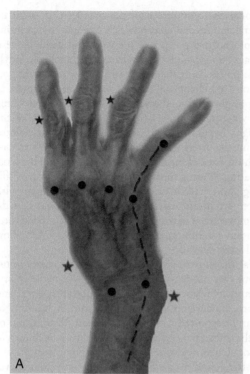

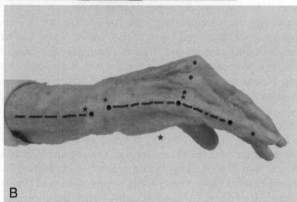

FIG. 3.5 A,B Mapping of the expected distal imbalances from liga-mentous instability of the radiocarpal, ulnocarpal, and distal radioul-nar joints. (From Sahrmann SA: *Movement system impairment syndromes of the extremities, cervical and thoracic spines: considerations for acute and long-term management,* St. Louis, 2011, Elsevier Mosby.)

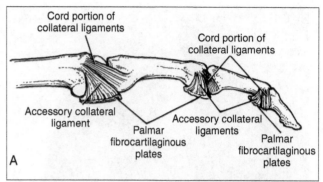

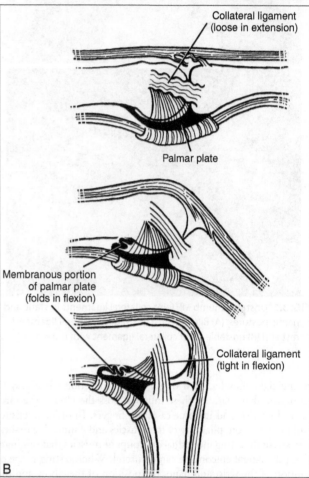

FIG. 3.6 (A) Ligamentous structures of the finger joints. (B) At the metacarpal joint level, the collateral ligaments are loose in exertion but tighten in flexion.(A, From Fess EE, Gettle K, Phillips C, et al. *Hand and Upper Extremity Splinting: Principles and Methods.* 3rd ed. St Louis, MO: Mosby; 2005; B, modified from Wynn-Parry CB. Rehabilitation of the hand. In: Fess EE, Gettle K, Phillips C, et al. *Hand and Upper Extremity Splinting: Principles and Methods.* 3rd ed. St Louis, MO: Mosby; 2005.)

and lateral pinches. Common postural imbalances can be seen with ligamentous instability when loading the joint through tip pinch. Observational mapping of unstable bilateral RCLs at rest shows increased angulation of the MP joints of the thumb, supination of the thumb nail, and loss of muscle mass in the thenar eminences (Fig. 3.7A). Similar changes can be seen with observational mapping of an unstable UCL with pinch to include radial deviation of the MP joint and rotation of the thumb nail (Fig. 3.7B).

Proper balance of the musculotendinous structures that originate from the lateral and medial epicondyles is necessary for positioning the hand in tasks away from the body. Actions of elbow extension and flexion, forearm rotation, wrist extension and flexion and some finger extension and flexion are controlled by these musculotendinous structures. Due to the length of these tissues, their actions cross as many as five joints and can influence

reaching and positioning of the hand. Static or dynamic muscle imbalances can lead to pathological joint stresses, muscle weak-ness, and ultimate limitations in functional reach and grasp patterns.

Even though all of the muscles that originate from the lateral epicondyle are innervated by the radial nerve, a different picture of function can be obtained when observing their influence on multijoint, simultaneous movements. Table 3.1 provides a listing

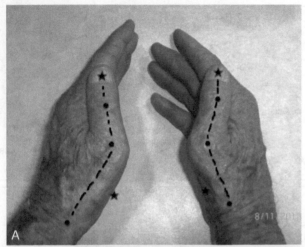

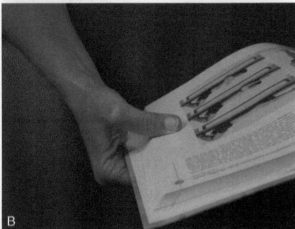

FIG. 3.7 Unstable thumb MP joint collateral ligaments in static and dynamic postures. (A) Bilateral unstable radial collateral ligaments at rest and (B) unstable ulnar collateral ligament with movement. (Martin Dunitz Ltd., 2001.)

A functional anatomy screen of the muscles that originate from the lateral and medial epicondyles is essential to determine deviations from normal posture of the wrist and hand. At rest, imbalances cause unopposed muscles from the lateral epicondyle to change the positions of the upper arm joints. In standing or sitting positions the client will present with subtle increases in the **carrying angle of the elbow**, the palm of the hand facing forward, the wrist in radial deviation, and the MP joints of the fingers in slight hyperextension. Similarly, the extrinsic flexor bias of the muscles from the medial epicondyle at rest can be observed with the back of the hand more prominent and the wrist in ulnar deviation. During movement, the client may have difficulty reaching in every plane of movement and may present with a more pronounced posture defect when carrying increased loads. Exaggerated movements of trunk flexion and glenohumeral rotation compensate for limitations in extensibility of the elbow extensors and wrist deviators.

Functional anatomy screening can be utilized to assess muscle adaptations that occur with acute and chronic nerve injury. Changes in muscle balance, and ultimately postures at rest and during movement, develop in response to pain. Symptoms of nerve pain can be reported within the cutaneous distribution or throughout the entire peripheral distribution from an injury to the nerve root. Unconsciously, the nerve response to injury is to limit the stretch and excursion that occurs with joint movement. The muscles of the upper limb limit the arc of motion by contracting the corresponding joint. An example can be seen in clients with an ulnar nerve injury. The shoulder, elbow, and wrist joints will limit tension and stress to that nerve by holding the joint in a position to limit and prevent stretch or nerve excursion. Neural tension increases with elbow flexion greater than 90 degrees and intrafascicular pressure intensifies with shoulder abduction, forearm supination, and wrist extension. The neuromuscular system will prevent this undesirable painful posture by controlling joint motion in a cohesive manner. A functional anatomy screen for the composite joints of the upper limb will find the arm bias of elbow flexion is short of 90 degrees, forearm movements range from neutral to pronation, and the wrist is flexed. If additional tension occurs, as when the client's head laterally flexes to the opposite side, the shoulder girdle and elbow may change position to accommodate proximal nerve glide without increasing neural tension. Measures are needed to decrease the pain and the neuromuscular response during intervention. Immobilization may be necessary, but overlooking the effects of pain reduction through postural modifications may lead to an undesirable response of joint and muscle adaptation.

In nerve injuries with a severe degree of conduction loss of both sensory and motor fascicules, a functional anatomy screening uses a more conventional assessment of imbalance. Frequently, manual muscle tests are performed by evaluating synergistic action of muscle groups, such as wrist extensors or finger flexors as a group. In reality, manual muscle testing can be a valuable tool in viewing muscle balance from other perspectives. Unrecognized impairments of the upper limb can be discovered due to imbalances created from a condition such as peripheral neuropathy.

The findings of a manual muscle test can be more sensitive when selecting muscles innervated by various nerve distributions. For example, Fig. 3.8A provides the distribution of the muscles associated with the radial nerve. It is important to note that more than finger and wrist extension can be involved, especially with trauma to the nerve proximal to the elbow in the midhumeral or

of the eight muscles, their origin, and their action.[3] It is easy to recognize that many of these muscles cross the elbow, the forearm, the wrist, and in some cases the fingers. In order to ensure full joint motion, pliability of the muscles and connective tissues, and strength testing individual or groups of muscles that originate from the lateral epicondyle can be useful. When testing range of motion of the wrist and hand, the position of the elbow and the forearm should be considered. For example, full passive stretch of the longest musculoskeletal structure originating on the lateral epicondyle, the EDC muscle, is obtained with elbow extension, forearm pronation, wrist flexion, and full finger flexion.

In discussing the muscles that originate from the medial epicondyle, a similar picture of function also can be obtained. Table 3.2 provides a listing of the five muscles, their origin, and their action.[3] In this case, all of the muscles are innervated by the median nerve, with the exception of one, the flexor carpi ulnaris, which is supplied by the ulnar nerve. In spite of the differences in nerve innervations, the same principles for extensibility of these muscles can apply as was suggested for the muscles originating from the lateral epicondyle. For example, full passive stretch of the longest musculoskeletal structure originating on the medial epicondyle, the FDS muscle, is obtained with elbow extension, forearm supination, wrist extension, and full finger extension.

TABLE 3.1   Muscles Originating From the Lateral Epicondyle

Muscle	Origin	Action	Position for Full Musculotendinous Flexibility
Anconeus	Lateral and posterior surfaces of proximal half of body of humerus and lateral intermuscular septum	Extends the elbow	Elbow flexion, forearm pronation
Brachioradialis	Proximal two-thirds of lateral supracondylar ridge of humerus and lateral intermuscular septum	Flexes the elbow, assists with pronating and supinating the forearm	Elbow extension, forearm pronation or supination
Supinator	Lateral epicondyle of humerus, RCL of elbow joint, annular ligament of radius, and supinator crest of ulna	Supinates the forearm	Elbow extension, forearm pronation
Extensor carpi radialis longus	Distal one-third of lateral supracondylar ridge of humerus and lateral intermuscular septum	Extends the wrist in a radial direction, assists with elbow flexion	Elbow extension, forearm pronation, wrist flexion in an ulnar direction
Extensor carpi radialis brevis	Lateral epicondyle of humerus, RCL of elbow, and deep antebrachial fossa	Extends the wrist, assists with wrist radial deviation	Elbow extension, forearm pronation, wrist flexion
Extensor carpi ulnaris	Lateral epicondyle of humerus, aponeurosis from posterior border of ulna, and deep antebrachial fossa	Extends the wrist in an ulnar direction	Elbow extension, forearm pronation, wrist flexion in a radial direction
Extensor digitorum communis	Lateral epicondyle of humerus and deep antebrachial fossa	Extends the MP joints of the second through fifth digits; in conjunction with the lumbricals and interossei, extends the PIP joints of the second through fifth digits; assists with abduction of the index, ring, and small fingers; and assists with extension of the wrist in a radial direction	Elbow extension; forearm pronation; wrist flexion; and MP, PIP, and DIP flexion of the fingers
Extensor digitorum minimi	Lateral epicondyles of humerus and deep antebrachial fossa	Extends the MP joint of the small finger; in conjunction with the lumbricals and interossei, extends the PIP joint of the small finger; assists with abduction of the small finger	Elbow extension; forearm pronation; wrist flexion; and MP, PIP, and DIP flexion of the small finger

DIP, Distal interphalangeal; *MP,* metacarpophalangeal; *PIP,* proximal interphalangeal; *RCL,* radial collateral ligament.

TABLE 3.2   Muscles Originating From the Medial Epicondyle

Muscle	Origin	Action	Position for Full Musculotendinous Flexibility
Pronator teres	Medial epicondyle of humerus, common flexor tendon, and deep antebrachial fascia	Pronates the forearm, assists with elbow flexion	Elbow extension, forearm supination
Flexor carpi radialis	Common flexor tendon of medial epicondyle of humerus and deep antebrachial fascia	Flexes the wrist in a radial direction; may assist with pronation of the forearm and elbow flexion	Elbow extension, forearm supination, wrist extension in an ulnar direction
Flexor carpi ulnaris	Common flexor tendon of medial epicondyle of humerus	Flexes the wrist in an ulnar direction; may assist with elbow flexion	Elbow extension, forearm supination, wrist extension in a radial direction
Palmaris longus	Common flexor tendon of medial epicondyle of humerus and deep antebrachial fascia	Tenses the palmar fascia, flexes the wrist, and may assist with elbow flexion	Elbow extension, forearm supination, wrist extension
Flexor digitorum superficialis	Common flexor tendon of medial epicondyle of humerus, UCL of elbow, and deep antebrachial fascia	Flexes the PIP joints of the second through fifth digits; assists with MP and wrist flexion	Elbow extension; forearm supination; wrist extension; and MP, PIP, and DIP extension of the fingers

DIP, Distal interphalangeal; *MP,* metacarpophalangeal; *PIP,* proximal interphalangeal; *UCL,* ulnar collateral ligament.

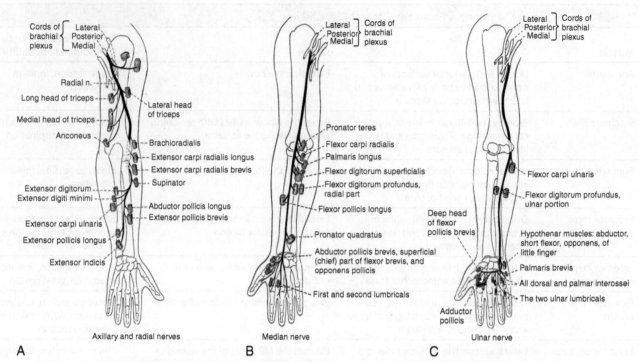

FIG. 3.8 (A) Axillary and radial nerves. (B) Median nerve. (C) Ulnar nerve. (From Jenkins DB. *Hollinshead's Functional Anatomy of the Limbs and Back.* 6th ed. Philadelphia, PA: WB Saunders; 1991.)

brachial plexus regions. The selection of muscles to be evaluated should include wrist and finger extensors as well as those muscles that are responsible primarily for elbow extension, elbow flexion with the forearm in neutral position, supination, and thumb extension. In addition to wrist drop, common postural changes for radial nerve injuries at rest may be increased forearm pronation and thumb adduction.

When identifying the muscles that are innervated by the median nerve, the same approach could be used. Fig. 3.8B provides a visual representation of the muscles innervated by the median nerve. You may notice that several **extrinsic muscles**, those muscles that originate outside of the hand, are innervated by the median nerve. In some cases, the musculotendinous system can cross the elbow, the wrist, the fingers, and the thumb. In addition, there are several **intrinsic muscles**, those muscles that originate in the hand, which are innervated by the median nerve and provide movements to the thumb, the index, and the middle fingers. In a median nerve injury at the wrist, the motor loss to the abductor pollicis brevis, opponens pollicis, and a portion of the flexor pollicis brevis presents with loss of bulk to the thenar eminence. The loss of muscle tone from the median nerve innervated muscles increases the dominance of the ulnar nerve innervated muscles. The thumb is drawn into CMC adduction at rest, a posture called the **ape hand position**. The orientation of the thumb CMC joint changes to a flat posture, the flexor pollicis longus is without balance at the MP joint. With this loss of intrinsic abductor tension, the IP joint of the thumb is then persuaded into flexion. Weakened tip and chuck pinch may be present. Fig. 3.9 illustrates the mapping of postural imbalances created from the absence of the median nerve at the wrist. Important landmarks are changes in the orientation of the nail, the prominent head of the index MP joint, and the flat space between the index and thumb.

The muscles innervated by the ulnar nerve are identified in Fig. 3.8C. Motor function is supplied to a wrist flexor, finger

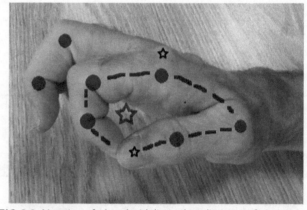

FIG. 3.9 Mapping of a hand with limited median nerve function. (Photo Lori DeMott.)

flexors to the ring and small fingers, and to many intrinsic muscles of the fingers and thumb. Compression of the ulnar nerve at the elbow can result in reduced grip from weakened FDP of the ring and small fingers and lateral pinch from weakened adductor pollicis. Recognizing patterns of muscle imbalance based on the nerve distribution provides a picture of function very different from that picture obtained from a generalized manual muscle test and/or standardized testing such as the use of dynamometers and pinch gauge.

The default position of the hand and wrist at rest is described as the normal resting hand position. In this posture the wrist is positioned in approximately 30 degrees of extension, the MP and IP joints of the fingers are in approximately 45 degrees of flexion, and the fingers abduct and converge toward the radius. At rest, the posture of the thumb joints is CMC abduction, MP flexion, and IP extension. The balanced relationship between the wrist, fingers, and thumb demonstrates the principle of

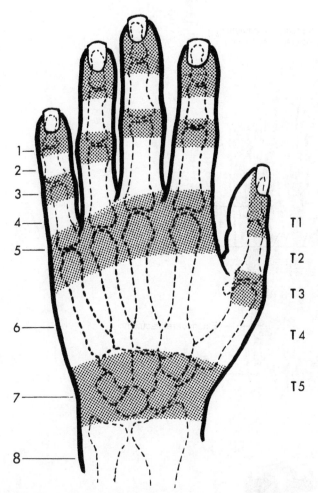

FIG. 3.10 Extensor tendon zones as defined by the Committee on Tendon Injuries for the International Federation of the Societies for Surgery of the Hand. (From Fess EE, Gettle K, Phillips C, et al. *Hand and Upper Extremity Splinting: Principles and Methods.* 3rd ed 3. St Louis, MO: Mosby; 2005.)

tenodesis. That is, the **length-tension** of the musculotendinous structures and the ability of the extrinsic tendons to freely glide within their sheaths to create movements at distal joints as a result of passive wrist repositioning. In the absence of active muscular contraction, flexion of the fingers and thumb occurs with wrist extension and extension of the fingers and thumb occurs with wrist flexion. A wrist-produced tenodesis can be beneficial in providing gross grasp, prehension, and release for individuals who lack C7 innervation, amplitude, and tensile strength from tendon transfers.[15] However, subtle limitations in tenodesis can result from joint and soft-tissue problems, such as musculotendinous shortening, poor wrist patterns, and extrinsic tendon adhesions.[15] In the event where normal joint range of motion and length-tension of the musculoskeletal structures are present, the focus of the functional anatomy screen should be on the quality of **tendon gliding** through sheaths with the expectation of fluid distal joint flexion and extension. Different scenarios occur when adhesions are present at different locations in the arm and hand.

As mentioned before, the EDC crosses the elbow, the forearm, the wrist, and the fingers. In addition to considering the length of a musculotendinous unit, the location of the extensor tendons is useful to appreciate the role of other structures that can impact tenodesis and tendon gliding.[15] Fig. 3.10 identifies the eight locations, or zones, of the extensor tendons. Another important contribution to the function of extensor tendon gliding is the presence of six compartments created by the deep layers of the dorsal fascia. Fig. 3.11 shows the tendons that are located in each of the numbered dorsal compartments of the wrist. Testing the independent movement of each extensor tendon by compartment provides a clearer picture of the effectiveness of tendon excursion through the dorsal pulley system and can supplement the findings of a more generic range of motion or manual muscle test. A functional anatomy screen at zone VI for the extensor tendons may show changes at rest for the MP joints of the fingers with increased extension. With movement, passive and active limitations of wrist flexion and exaggerated finger extension can be observed.

Similarly, an appreciation of the extensor tendons to the fingers in zones II–IV provides a different perspective of how location impacts tendon gliding. In Fig. 3.12, the extensor mechanism of a finger PIP joint is presented in a dorsal and lateral view with digital MP flexion and extension. One can see the balance that must occur between the intrinsic and extrinsic muscle groups so that full extension of a digit can occur. To assess the contribution of the extrinsic musculature with PIP extension, the wrist and the MP joints can be stabilized in extension. In this position, the power of the intrinsic muscles is minimized. When the PIP joint is held in extension and the DIP joint is actively flexed, the lateral bands are passively stretched, which ultimately facilitates balanced extension between the PIP and the DIP joints. Knowledge of the extensor tendon anatomy, location by zone, and presence of surrounding structures is an important consideration in your assessment of the hand.

At rest, a functional anatomy screen for the extensor tendons in zones II–IV can present with imbalances in PIP and DIP extension. An injury to the palmar plate at the PIP joint results in loosening of the volar supporting structures resulting in unchecked pull of the extensor tendon, increased dorsal orientation of the lateral bands, and hyperextension of the PIP joint. This imbalance results in a change of the PIP joint axis, loss of mechanical advantage, and flexion bias of the distal phalanx. At rest, the digit is observed in PIP joint extension and DIP joint flexion. The normal resting balance of flexion cascade in the MP, PIP, and DIP joints is also lost, as seen in the advanced swan neck deformity.

The finger flexors have similarities and contrasting differences from the extensor tendons. Fig. 3.13 illustrates the five flexor tendon zones to the fingers and three flexor tendon zones to the thumb. Zone IV contains the structures within the carpal tunnel, and Fig. 3.14 provides a cross-sectional view of their anatomy. When examining excursion of the flexor tendons in this zone, the carpal tunnel contents can be assessed from superficial to deep. The FDS to the middle and ring fingers would be the most superficial structure, followed by the FDS to the index and small fingers, and finally the FDP to all of the fingers. Two other structures are contained within the carpal tunnel, the flexor pollicis longus and the median nerve, as well as the synovium, which encases and lubricates the flexor tendons. It can be useful to isolate the excursion of flexor tendons by zones. For example, injuries in zone IV that are more superficial, such as burns, may have more effect on the FDS compared to injuries that are deeper, such as distal radius fractures. A functional anatomy screen for the flexor tendons in zone IV can show exaggerated tenodesis or increased finger flexion with increased wrist extension.

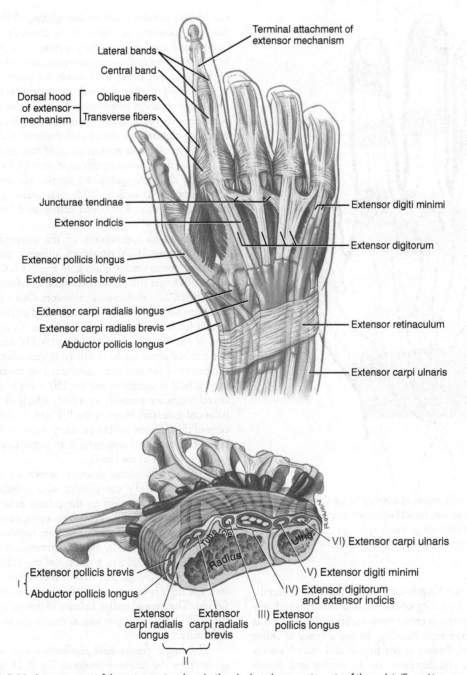

FIG. 3.11 Arrangement of the extensor tendons in the six dorsal compartments of the wrist. (From Neuman D. *Kinesiology of the Musculoskeletal System: Foundations for Rehabilitation.* 2nd ed. St Louis, MO: Mosby; 2010.)

Further considerations become evident in flexor tendon zones I–II. At this level the relationship between the FDP and the FDS changes. Prior to entering zone II, the FDP is deep to the FDS. In zone II, the FDP passes through the bifurcation of the FDS, which can be visualized in Fig. 3.15. It becomes very important to isolate each tendon when assessing its excursion. When testing the FDS, the effects of the FDP must be eliminated by the examiner holding the DIPs of the nontested fingers in extension and allowing each individual finger to actively flex at only the PIP joint. When testing the FDP, the PIP joint can be supported in extension to allow only DIP flexion. In this way, isolated range of motion exercises can facilitate the independent function of these two important flexor tendons to the hand. A functional anatomy screen for the flexor tendons in zones I–II can reveal imbalances, such as insufficient flexion of the DIP joint with full fisting of the hand.

Shoulder and Upper Limb

The glenohumeral joint depends on the rotator cuff muscles for support, rather than on the bones or ligaments. Fig. 3.16 shows the relationship of the rotator cuff muscles, which include the subscapularis, the supraspinatus, the infraspinatus, and the teres minor. The glenohumeral joint is a ball-and-socket synovial joint that

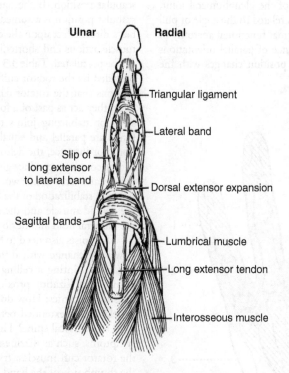

Ulnar — Radial

- Triangular ligament
- Lateral band
- Slip of long extensor to lateral band
- Dorsal extensor expansion
- Sagittal bands
- Lumbrical muscle
- Long extensor tendon
- Interosseous muscle

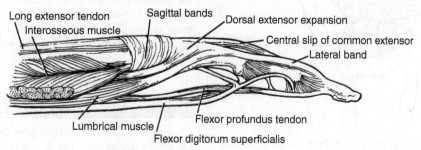

Long extensor tendon
Interosseous muscle
Sagittal bands
Dorsal extensor expansion
Central slip of common extensor
Lateral band
Lumbrical muscle
Flexor profundus tendon
Flexor digitorum superficialis

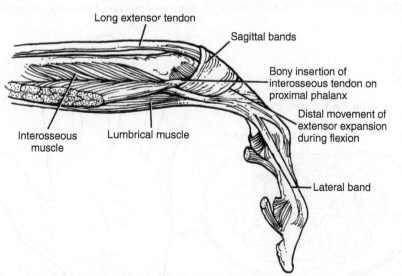

Long extensor tendon
Sagittal bands
Bony insertion of interosseous tendon on proximal phalanx
Distal movement of extensor expansion during flexion
Interosseous muscle
Lumbrical muscle
Lateral band

FIG. 3.12 Extensor mechanism of the finger in dorsal and lateral views. The bottom image shows distal movement of the extensor expansion with metacarpophalangeal joint flexion. (From Fess EE, Gettle K, Phillips C, et al. *Hand and Upper Extremity Splinting: Principles and Methods.* 3rd ed. St Louis, MO: Mosby; 2005.)

moves in multiple axes. The motion of the glenohumeral joint, provided by the rotator cuff muscles, is related to the angle of pull for each muscle. A quick screen of normal functional anatomy in a standing resting posture is the presence of parallel orientations for the hand and scapula. The hand position changes with the

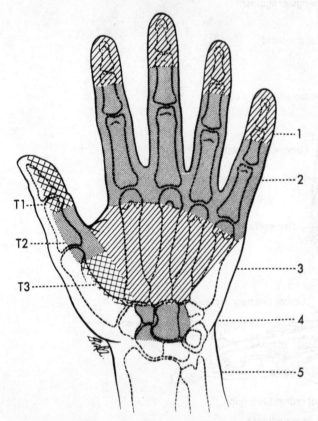

FIG. 3.13 Flexor tendon zones of the hand. (From Kleinert HE, Schepel S, Gill T. Flexor tendon injuries. *Surg Clin North Am.*1981;61(2):267-286.)

scapular position. If the hand position is pronated, an abducted scapular position is assumed. Consequently, the abducted scapula has a direct effect upon the origin and insertion of the rotator cuff muscle actions and shortening or lengthening of these structures can be postulated. Table 3.3 identifies the locations of and motions provided by the rotator cuff muscles.[2] In addition to the primary motions that the rotator cuff muscles have on the glenohumeral joint, they act as part of a force couple. **Force couples** are responsible for stabilizing joints through muscle co-contractions. The forces are parallel and equal in magnitude but opposite in direction. For instance, the deltoid and supraspinatus muscles work as a force couple to produce glenohumeral abduction or flexion. The deltoid and teres minor work as a force couple to produce depression and stabilization of the humeral head. Another force couple is the deltoid muscle and the rotator cuff muscles for depression of the humeral head and flexion of the humerus.[11]

Therapists also need to keep in mind the impact of forces and how they change with different positions and/or postures. For instance, painting a ceiling requires scapulothoracic and glenohumeral stabilization proximally to hold the limb in flexion. The question becomes: How do the forces change when the position is held for an extended period of time with the addition of the head and cervical spine? This could result in a variety of possible symptoms, such as dizziness, core lumbar pain, impingement of the rotator cuff muscles, triceps weakness, or sensory changes in the thumb side of the hand. Therefore when treating clients with rotator cuff injuries, therapists need to consider the entire kinematic chain, all the forces applied to the upper quadrant, and the context of movement, not just the isolated motion of shoulder flexion.[16]

Head and Neck

Observations of static postures provide valuable information of the body's resting tone, the default zero resting balance. A quick screen of functional anatomy can be done by observing structures

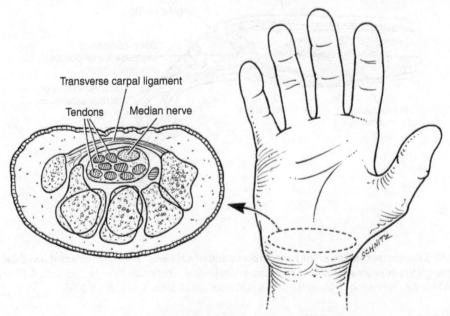

FIG. 3.14 Cross-sectional view of the carpal tunnel anatomy. (From Fess EE, Gettle K, Phillips C, et al. *Hand and Upper Extremity Splinting: Principles and Methods.* 3rd ed. St Louis, MO: Mosby; 2005.)

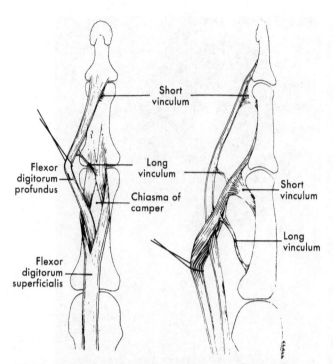

FIG. 3.15 The flexor digitorum profundus lies deep to the flexor digitorum superficialis (FDS) until the level of the MP joint where the FDS bifurcates. (From Schneider LH. *Flexor Tendon Injuries.* Boston, MA: Little Brown; 1985.)

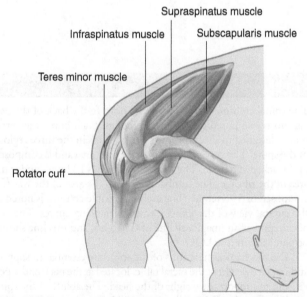

FIG. 3.16 The rotator cuff muscles. (From Cummings NH, Stanley-Green S, Higgs P. *Perspectives in Athletic Training.* St Louis, MO: Mosby; 2009.)

TABLE 3.3	Location and Motion of Rotator Cuff Muscles	
Muscle	**Location**	**Motion**
Supraspinatus	*Proximal attachment:* Supraspinous fossa of scapula *Distal attachment:* Superior facet of greater tubercle of humerus	Abduction and rotation
Subscapularis	*Proximal attachment:* Subscapular fossa *Distal attachment:* Lesser tubercle of humerus	Medial rotation and adduction
Infraspinatus	*Proximal attachment:* Infraspinous fossa of scapula *Distal attachment:* Middle facet of greater tubercle of humerus	Lateral rotation
Teres minor	*Proximal attachment:* Superior part of lateral border of scapula *Distal attachment:* Inferior facet of greater tubercle of humerus	Lateral rotation

from the sagittal and coronal planes. Anatomical knowledge of normal muscle location and length are correlated to the observed postural structures, the combined alignment of all joints, and is the critical analysis needed for functional motor assessment. In a standing position, from the anterior view, horizontal symmetry of the eyes, ears, and shoulders from right to left is noted. From the posterior view, the position of the head and shoulders should not deviate laterally from the imaginary plumb line (line of gravity [LOG]). Normal posture is observed when the LOG passes through the external auditory meatus, the bodies of the cervical spine, the acromion, and anterior to the thoracic spine. Fig. 3.17 identifies the mapping specific to normal and forward head positions. Disparities exist between the two head positions. Compared to the normal head position, imbalances in the pathological posture are identified by three visible landmarks; the position of the chin, ear, and scapula. Abnormal posture impacts the neuromuscular system and has a kinematic effect on the upper limb.

In summary, the observations of static posture and observations of active movements of the upper limb are needed due to the additional tension created on the neurovascular bundle in the upper quadrant of the body.[17] Common adverse symptoms of the sensory, motor, or vascular systems are localized burning, cramping, or cooler skin temperature identified throughout the limb at rest or more commonly caused by movement. When provocative movements are repeated over time, the temporary symptoms caused by the compression of the neurovascular bundle can become frequent or constant and somewhat unrelenting. Fig. 3.18 shows common claviculocostal sites where increased neurovascular pressure occurs with upper body movement. The symptoms that occur at these sites are often referred to as **thoracic outlet syndrome**. anatomy.[11,19]

Cervical alignment is necessary for sound neurological and vascular function in the shoulder, arm, and hand. The normal relationships of bone, ligaments, disks, vasculature, and nerves provide the cervical spine with valuable mobility that other segments of the spinal column do not possess. The cervical spine supports the head and allows rotation from side to side, flexion and extension, lateral flexion to each side, and all the motions in between. While the locations of the structures are designed to provide increased mobility at the cervical level, they are also vulnerable to injuries because of these anatomical relationships.

Alignment of vertebrae, muscle, and soft tissues provides normal blood flow within the vertebral artery and the vertebral and deep cervical veins, ensuring adequate blood flow and drainage for the cervical structures related to upper limb function. Also, alignment of these structures facilitates normal conduction and excursion of nervous tissue in nerves C1 to C8. Fig. 3.19

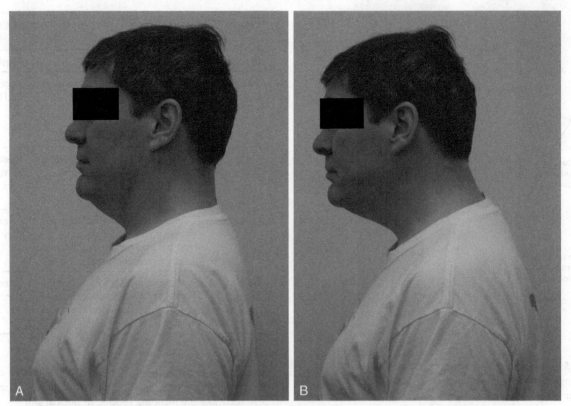

FIG. 3.17 Mapping of normal (A) and forward (B) head positions. (From Sahrmann SA. *Movement System Impairment Syndromes of the Extremities, Cervical and Thoracic Spines: Considerations for Acute and Long-Term Management.* St Louis, MO: Elsevier Mosby; 2011.)

illustrates the anterior rami of nerves C5 to T1, which form the brachial plexus and innervate the entire upper limb.

Symptoms of cervical misalignment may appear distal to the primary injury site and present as sensory, motor, or autonomic dysfunction. For example, forward head posture can be the cause of head, neck, shoulder, or mid and lower back pain as well as distal paresthesias. When the head moves forward, the axis of reference shifts, the cervical spine is pushed into compensatory extension, and the neck extensors shorten. Another postural fault is observed with the rounded shoulder posture found in many clients while sitting at their computers or while texting on a cell phone screen. The forward head impacts the cervical and thoracic spine that directly presents with a compensatory scapular position. An elevated, abducted, and upwardly rotated scapula influences the axis of the glenohumeral joint by changing the balance of the rotator cuff muscles. The orientation of the glenoid fossa is altered, leaving the humerus in more forward and internally rotated position. In time, a cascading chain of events occurs as the pectoralis minor, serratus anterior, and upper trapezius muscles shorten as seen in Fig. 3.20. The extrinsic muscle origins of the thoracic vertebrae, ribs, and scapula also contribute to an elevated and upward scapular position. This adaptive shortening of soft tissue has been associated with nerve compression as the nerve plexus exits the scalenes to the thoracic outlet and influences the limb, contributing to sensory disturbances distally. Table 3.4 describes other disorders that result from misalignment of the cervical spine and can result in conditions that impair upper limb function.

Trunk and Lower Limb

The spinal column extends from the head to the back of the pelvis and is composed of 24 separate bones. Each bone, the vertebra, is designed to meet specific specifications in the three regions of the spine. The cervical section is the neck area and is composed of 7-stacked vertebrae. The thoracic spine has 12 bones and is the area of the ribcage. The lumbar region, in the area of the waist, is composed of 5 vertebrae. The arching flexible column is noted in the sagittal view of the spine, forming balancing curves. The axis of the spine is an imaginary line of C1 to L5, and this line should be parallel with the LOG.

The mechanical functions of the spine are essential to support and transfer weight at the sacral table, located at the back of the pelvis, and to support the weight of the head. The ability of the spine to adjust from inefficient alignment will influence overall function as the freedom of movement is reduced. During compensatory misalignment, the altered postural deficit changes and a reduction in the available movement of the kinematic chain develops. The relational force from the ground can be absorbed in the vertebral bodies and disks of the spine during sitting, standing, walking, running, and jumping. When the spine is not aligned, muscles and ligaments must take part in the absorption of the reaction forces, which can lead to undue muscular strain and pain.

The erector spinae is a large complex muscle that arises from the sacrum and runs up the spine, fanning out as it attaches up the spine, to form a series of smaller muscles. These are interlaced

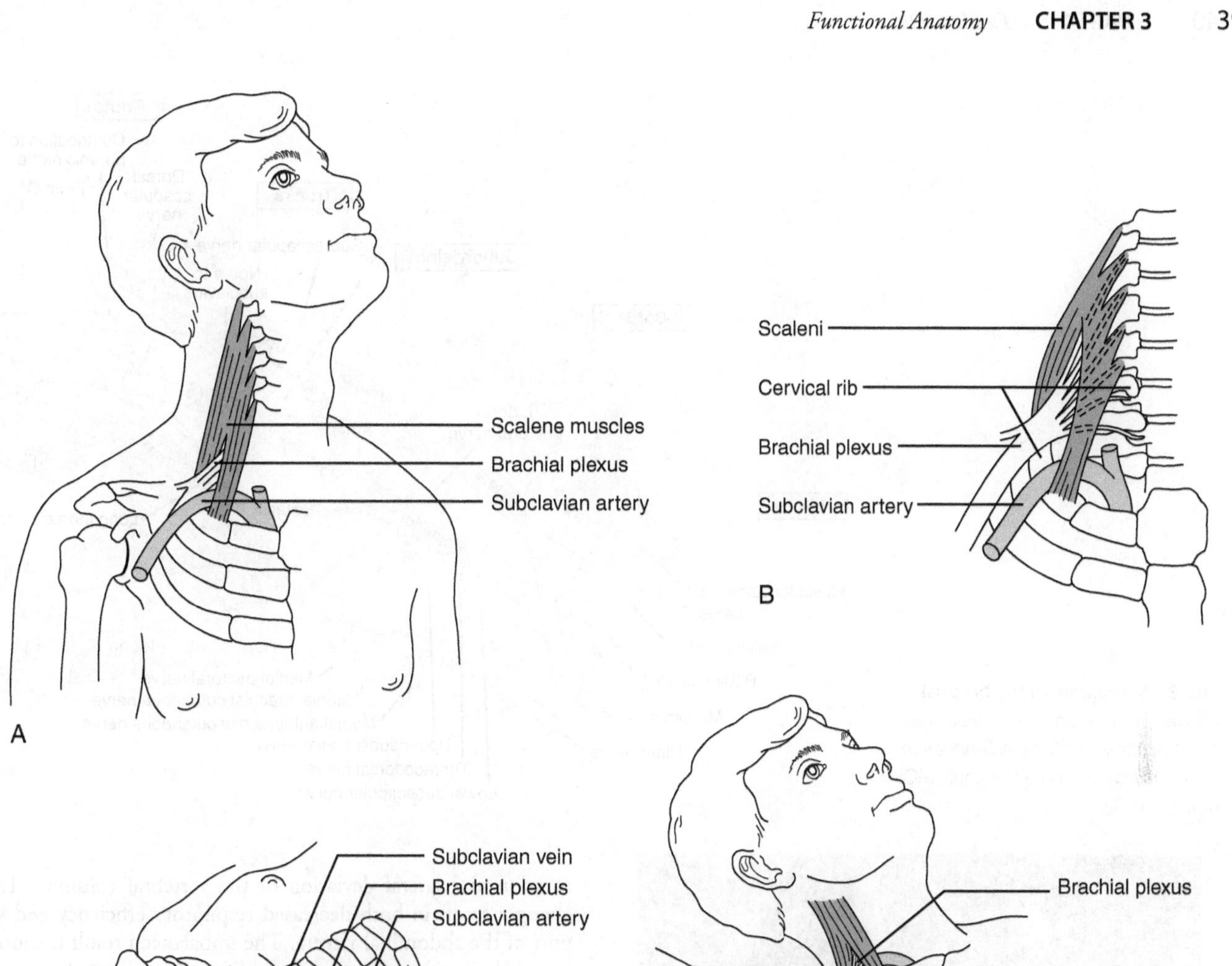

FIG. 3.18 Common claviculocostal sites where increased neurovascular pressure occurs. (A) Scalenus anterior syndrome. (B) Cervical rib syndrome. (C) Costoclavicular syndrome. (D) Hyperabduction syndrome. (From Cummings NH, Stanley-Green S, Higgs P. *Perspectives in Athletic Training*. St Louis, MO: Mosby; 2009.)

with the neck muscles that run down from the head. The erector spinae are joined by the smaller deeper muscles between vertebrae and are responsible for both back extension and flexion.

The transverse abdominis, internal obliques, and external obliques are three layers of muscle that protect internal organs. These muscles are responsible for most trunk control and movement. The rectus abdominus, which runs vertically from the pubis symphysis to the sternum, flexes the trunk and resists extension against gravity. The obliques provide both lateral flexion and rotation, which occur simultaneously. Full rotation of the spine requires coordination of the internal and external obliques on opposite sides of the body.

The quadratus lumborum and the iliopsoas are posterior abdominal wall muscles. The quadratus, with their fibers mostly vertical, acts to laterally flex or extend the spine. The psoas major

and iliacus make up the iliopsoas, and these two muscles combine to form a tendon that attaches to the inferior trochanter of the femur. The iliopsoas bends the hips and pulls the pelvis forward. When lying on the back, the iliopsoas will pull the trunk up to sitting once the shoulders are off the ground. The iliopsoas primarily flexes the hip, but also serves to maintain the lordotic curve of the lumbar spine, is used in sitting balance, and laterally flexes the spine[3,14] Further postural changes ensue within the pelvic and abdominal cores and are associated with the musculoskeletal changes of the low flat-back posture (posterior tilt), elongated and weakened hip flexors, and shortened hip extensors and anterior abdominals.

The cross-sectional weakness of the external obliques on one side and of the internal oblique on the other allows separation of the costal margin from the opposite iliac crest, resulting in

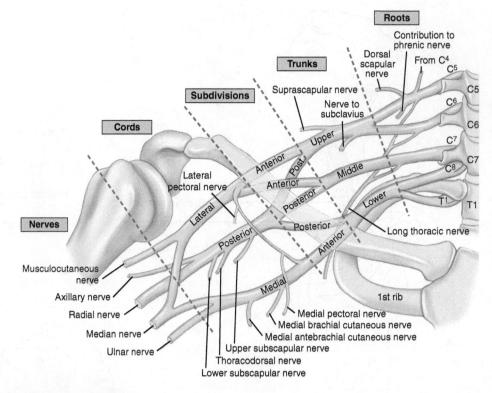

FIG. 3.19 Diagram of the brachial plexus. (From Neuman D. *Kinesiology of the Musculoskeletal System: Foundations for Rehabilitation.* 2nd ed. St Louis, MO: Mosby; 2010.)

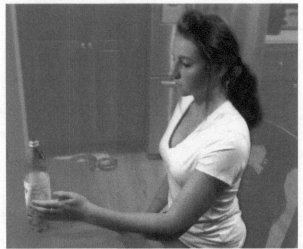

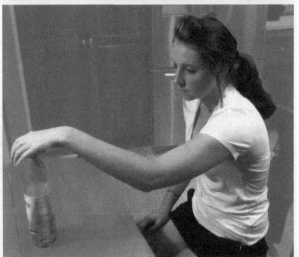

FIG. 3.20 Reaching capacity expected for a client with and without balanced muscle control of the scapulothoracic joint. (Photo Lori DeMott.)

rotation and lateral deviation of the vertebral column.[3] These changes result in both decreased respiratory efficiency and support of the abdominal viscera. The imbalanced result is shortening of the anterior fibers of the obliques muscles and causes the thorax to be depressed anteriorly, contributing to flexion of the trunk. In standing, this is seen as a predisposition toward kyphosis and depressed chest, then can lead to kinematic changes to the motoric reach patterns. These same findings of core imbalance occur in the sway back posture with anterior deviation of the pelvis and postural deviations of the thorax.

The hip joint serves as a central pivot point for the body as a whole. The femoral joint is a large ball and socket that allows simultaneous triplanar movements. These three planes are the imaginary lines passing through the body (in an anatomical position) that represent the dynamic planes of motion through which the human body is capable of moving. The functional demand of the hip musculature requires strong and specific activation to support the body over one limb.[21]

Assessment of Posture

Both occupational therapists and physical therapists should be assessing posture as it relates to upper extremity function. The Occupational Therapy Practice Framework (OTPF), in accordance with the World Health Organization (WHO), identifies client/person factors that affect performance skills as the interrelationship of body functions and structures.[20] In many pathological conditions of illness or injury, the intrinsic nature of the neuromusculoskeletal system (functions and structures) is essentially visible during resting and dynamic body postures. Therefore the assessment of key postural markers of skeletal landmarks, joint angles, and muscle trajectories throughout the upper limb provides an understanding of relative skeletal alignment. The posture analysis is the basis for comparing the normal default of

TABLE 3.4	Common Cervical Injuries and Disorders and Resulting Impairment	
Anatomical Structure	**Injury or Disorder**	**Symptoms**
Vertebrae	Subluxation, instability, fracture; abnormal bone development; arthritis; displacement; degenerative changes; stenosis; bony spurs	Disruption of sensory, motor, or vascular function throughout the UE
Muscle	Weakness; tightness; imbalance; hypertonicity or hypotonicity; spasm; overstretching; sprain or strain	Compression of nervous tissue characteristically results in numbness, pain, paralysis, and loss of function; vascular compression characteristically results in moderate pain and swelling[3]
Soft tissue	Disk protrusion, lax ligament; ligament avulsion; degeneration or thickening of dura; adhesions	Disruption of sensory and motor function throughout the UE
Vasculature	Compression; constriction; mechanical irritation; congestion; reflex response; hemorrhage; stretching	Sympathetic symptoms associated with circulation can manifest in UE; decreased blood flow to UE tissues; temperature changes; pain; edema; decreased healing time
Nerve root and nerves	Decreased movement and elasticity; compression; strain, irritation, axonotmesis, severance	Pain at point of entrapment or along distal distribution in UE; decrease in or loss of sensation, motor control, or strength in UE; decreased UE deep tendon reflexes; decreased UE muscle tone; trophic changes in UE; sensation of deep pain; pain that radiates over shoulders and arms

UE, Upper extremity.

TABLE 3.5	Neurovascular Symptoms Associated With Upper Body Movement		
Body Part	**Motion**	**Result**	**Symptoms**
Shoulder	Depression	*Peripheral nerve:* Stretching of upper and middle trunks of brachial plexus over scalene muscle; pulling of lower trunks into angle formed by first rib and scalene tendon	Numbness and pain, particularly over ulnar distribution; pain worse at night because of positioning; intensity fluctuates throughout the day; arm fatigue, weakness, finger cramps, tingling, numbness, cold hand, areas of hyperesthesia, atrophy, tremor, and/or discoloration of hand
		Blood vessel: No compression of subclavian artery	
	Retraction	*Peripheral nerve:* No compression	
		Blood vessel: Compression of subclavian vein by tendon of subclavian muscle, not by clavicle	
	Abduction and retraction	*Peripheral nerve:* Clavicular compression on brachial plexus	
		Blood vessel: Clavicular compression of subclavian artery against scalene muscle	
Scapula	Retraction	*Peripheral nerve:* Compression of brachial plexus at point where it passes between clavicle and first rib	
		Blood vessel: Compression of subclavian artery at point where it passes between clavicle and first rib	

body conformation to that of abnormal alignment, the essence of functional anatomy. Using a comparative analysis of the predicted to observed postures allows for the identification of specific anatomical mechanical imbalances. Critical analysis of the way muscles essentially load a joint due to length and strength (e.g., short, long, weak, strong) is critical to choosing the most appropriate intervention.

As therapy professionals, we rely on our knowledge and synthesis of the functional anatomy as a determinant in grading the success of our client's ability to move and perform daily tasks. Many times, a client's base of support influences their upper limb kinematics. In standing, the base of support is controlled by the foot position (space and control), and in

sitting the core initiates pelvic tilt and contributes to forward head position and ultimately the kinematic hand position during reach.

Fundamentally and simplistically, the observation and assessment of the body's alignment is a measure of how the neuromusculoskeletal system is performing. The concept of balance and movement can provide a greater understanding of human anatomy and the contributions of soft-tissue impairment. The key point is that postural assessment gives the therapist the ability to evaluate overall muscle balance and responses of the body to internal and environmental stresses. The therapist then determines if the observed fault correlates to the client's adverse symptoms and/or functional limitations.

It is important that clients think more about what they want to do and less about how they want to do it. Frequently, inefficient functional movements lead to adaptive straining of joints with subsequent overloading or shortening of the surrounding ligaments and muscles. The correlation between movement efficiency and dysfunction are seen in individuals with degenerative joint pathology and neuropathy. When clients present with functional limitations and pain, understand that this is the body's response to problems within the kinematic chain. As the first line of defense, movement is altered unconsciously to reduce pain. When one joint has a reduced arc of motion, the action of adjacent joints is to reduce stress, strain, and pain through adaptation. An adaptation response may then create abnormal neuromusculoskeletal forces. Whether a client's complaints are global and diffuse or pinpoint and local, we should not be fooled into assigning the source of pathology to a specific body structure. We must always consider the kinematic chain and the interrelatedness of all involved structures. Altered body kinematics and imbalances in the neuromusculoskeletal alignment can cause mechanical pathology. The result is often the client's chief complaint: that is, it "hurts."

◎ Clinical Pearl

It is important to understand that the upper extremity is a *component* of a complex system; the client's complaints of pain or weakness may not be the source of the pathology.

Hand therapists must understand functional anatomy and fine-tune clinical observation skills. Observing "functional" balance as clients move through both resting and dynamic postures will assist us in determining the cause of pain and movement inefficiencies. Our clients' functional anatomy, consisting of postures and movement patterns, will contribute to our understanding of movement restrictions that affect their satisfaction in performing everyday activities. Proficient evaluation skills are imperative to effective collaboration with clients and the provision of client-centered practice that emphasizes meaningful episodes of care.[9] Above all, accurate assessments direct the choice of interventions that produce the best outcomes for our clients.

During the initial client interview, the therapist can simultaneously assess body posture and the quality of balance in the neuromusculoskeletal structures. Observation can be performed with the client in static resting positions while sitting, standing, and lying down, as well as during spontaneous dynamic movements when the client first shakes our hand, takes off their coat, walks, sits down, or completes paperwork. Observation during these activities provides the first quick functional anatomy screen. The client's posture and any adaptive kinematic responses observed centrally at the core as well as in the distal limb may provide useful information to explain the client's physical complaints.

Resting and dynamic postural assessments assist in developing a plan of care that provides a clear relationship between the desired improvements of the neuromuscularskeletal balances and functional tasks. A systematic approach using a functional anatomy screening of the core and distal joints of the body combines the knowledge of kinematic chains, tissue imbalances, and compensatory movements in the recovery of the upper limb from disease and trauma.[21]

◎ Clinical Pearl

Understanding alignment and musculoskeletal balance will direct treatment interventions to improve body structure/position for the goal of promoting the client's satisfaction in activity and participation. Functional anatomical positions of a client in context can be identified to minimize primary and secondary complications and ultimately provide efficiency of desired movement during meaningful activity.

- In the presence of a noted imbalance, when do we support, strengthen, or stretch the joint of concern? What are the soft tissue structures that are to be influenced by our interventions?
- What may occur if we strengthen into the direction of the imbalance?
- Can a therapist use strengthening to overcome a joint contracture?
- In what situations can proximal alignment/orientation improve or limit distal control?
- How can pain-free and increased functional range improve a client's functional outcome measures?

CASE STUDIES

CASE STUDY 3. 1 ■ Thumb CMC Joint Instability Posture

Condition: Thumb CMC joint osteoarthritis, etiology is either bone impingement or ligament laxity as the instigator to progressive degeneration. The thumb CMC joint, which has a relative incongruent bone interface, relies heavily on ligamentous, intrinsic, and extrinsic muscle stabilizers for the extensive mobility required for functional movements. The loss of the stable base of control of the thumb CMC joint is the core concept of progressing imbalance and functional deformity.

Scenario: When opening jars or bottles, or turning a key, a 55-year-old female, right-handed dominant, would complain of tenderness and pain at the base of her right thumb. More recently, she's concerned with dropping objects and fatigue with handwriting and reports that she feels weaker for most grasp and pinch activities. She is a schoolteacher and enjoys vegetable gardening and playing cards. Most recently, she went to her orthopedic doctor and was told her she has osteoarthritis at the CMC joint of her thumb.

Standard Posture	The ideal alignment of the thumb in a resting posture is observed with the thumb CMC joint in balanced abduction, extension, and MP joint flexion and IP joint neutral extension	In the lateral view, the line of stability is envisioned through the radius, metacarpal head bisecting the midline of the nail. In the anterior to palmar view, the CMC joint rests in relative extension, MP joint flexion, and IP joint extension.
		During active contraction for functional tip pinch and grasp, the CMC joint moves into flexion and abduction. The MP joint flexed position contribution CMC joint alignment.
Skeletal Imbalance	Resting and dynamic positions present with various degrees of CMC joint adduction, supination, and MP joint extension. The pathomechanics of instability can be observed in both resting and active positions. Postures observed are seen in the thumb's physical appearance of the pronounced bony base of the first MP (rounded hump) appearance to the advanced collapse of thumb adduction and MP joint extension.	The thumb carpometacarpal CMC joint, a biconcave-convex saddle joint, consists of the articulation between the first metacarpal of the thumb and the trapezium carpal bone. In early stages, a common articular wear pattern observed in radiographic analysis is in the dorsoradial quadrant of the trapezium being significantly more degenerated.[1] In advanced stages, the CMC joint exhibits more severe joint narrowing, with osteophytes and debris greater than 2 mm in size.[2] In advanced stages of CMC imbalance, the MP joint is stressed and may present with arthritic changes, due to the unfortunate position of a broken kinematic chain.
Muscle Imbalance	Ligament: anterior oblique ligament (AOL) dorsoradial subluxation of CMC joint – AOL becomes attenuated Adductor pollicis: shortens – reduces web space Abductor pollicis brevis; weakness Opponens pollicis: weakness subsequent loss to pulp pinch patterns First dorsal interossei (FDI): weakness contributes to instability, functions as a distraction stabilizer to counteract the dorso-radial forces of lateral pinch and grip.[3] Extensor pollicis longus: inefficiency due to kinematic chain alteration Flexor pollicis longus: unopposed hyperflexes the thumb IP joint during pinch	What emerges from the research is that CMC-OA is likely to be promoted by joint impingement resulting from thumb pronation.[1] The CMC joint lacks bony confinement, there are various ligaments that play a role in stabilizing, the most important ligament for stability, is the anterior oblique (also known as 'beak') ligament. Adaptive shortening: The CMC joint collapse imbalance is described in this chapter, as when the joint surface permits a dorsal gliding shift leaving the standard axis point. The abductor pollicis longus may pull strongly, and the whole metacarpal and the whole thumb moves proximally. Without the intrinsic stability (ligamentous and articular), the thumb adductor shortens and pulls without the antagonist abductor pollicis brevis.
Compensation	Thumb CMC MP IP, zigzag deformity anterior to posterior, proximal to distal	The moment arm of tendons and skin become totally altered. High contact stresses through pinch initiate and/or exacerbate imbalance of the CMC, MP, and IP joints. Thumb CMC joint instability dorsal subluxation primary change to axis of motion.
Occupations	Work, leisure, ADLs and social participation	Tasks specific: writing using pen, holding cards, using tools in garden, dressing wearing closes with zippers and small buttons
Assessments: Impairment based Performance based Self-report outcome	Radiograph Grind test Goniometry (Kapandji Index) Manual muscle test (APB, OP, FDI) Sensory testing Pain assessment Functional posture PRO measure	Classification of OA of the CMC joint (X ray) Grind test + result indicative of OA[4,5] Active range of motion CMC (thumb joint active ROM measurements appear to have higher measurement error than other joints when measuring patients with first CMC joint OA)[6] Visual analogue scale Disability of arm, shoulder, hand

| Therapy interventions | *Occupation based* | Adaptions to restrictions of grasp and pinch, education of joint protection and use of adaptive equipment during ADL/iADL tasks (card holder, button assist)
Practices offload activity (ergonomic tools and adaptive grasp pattern) in handwriting, opening jars, and pulling weeds.[7] |
| | *Therapeutic procedures*
Orthosis intervention
a. Corrective rest position
b. Functional stability
Dynamic Stability
Program | a. Thumb MCP joint flexion unloads volar surface of trapezium (30 degrees of MCP joint flexion causes 60% dorsal shift of contact along trapezium).[8]
b. Provide stability for functional use[9]
Encourage joint motion and tissue elasticity (cartilage nutrition and joint lubrication) to restore web space with stretch to the adductor pollicis. Maintain functional strength using isometric exercises pinch and grasp. Promote joint stability with neuro reeducation that conditions muscles to absorb damaging impact loads in balance.[10,11] |

ADL, Activities of daily living; *APB*, abductor pollicis brevis; *CMC*, carpometacarpal; *FDI*, first dorsal interosseous; *iADL*, independent activities of daily living; *IP*, interphalangeal; *MP*, metacarpophalangeal; *OA*, osteoarthritis; *OP*, opponens pollicis; *PRO*, patient reported outcome; *ROM*, range of motion.

Sources

1. Koveler M, Lundon K, McKee N, Agur A: The human first carpometacarpal joint: osteoarthritic degeneration and 3-dimensional modeling, *J Hand Ther* 17(4):393–400, 2004.
2. Gillis J, Calder K, Williams J: Review of thumb carpometacarpal arthritis classification, treatment and outcomes, *Can J Plast Surg* 19(4):134–138, 2011.
3. McGee C, O'Brien V, Van Nortwick S, Adams J, Van Heest A: First dorsal interosseous muscle contraction results in radiographic reduction of healthy thumb carpometacarpal joint, *J Hand Ther* 28(4):375–380, 2015. quiz 381 https://doi.org/10.1016/j.jht.2015.06.002.
4. Kennedy CD, Manske MC, Huang JI: Classifications in brief: the Eaton-Littler classification of thumb carpometacarpal joint arthrosis, *Clin Orthop Relat Res* 474(12):2729–2733, 2016.
5. Model Z, Liu AY, Kan L, Wolfe SW, Burket JC, Lee SK: Evaluation of physical examination tests for thumb basal joint osteoarthritis, *Hand* 11:108–112, 2016.
6. Jha B, Ross M, Reeves SW, Couzens GB, Peters SE: Measuring thumb range of motion in first carpometacarpal joint arthritis: the inter-rater reliability of the Kapandji Index versus goniometry, *Hand Therapy* 21(2):45–53, 2016. https://doi.org/10.1177/1758998315616399.
7. O'Brien VH, McGaha JL: Current practice patterns in conservative thumb CMC joint care: survey results, *J Hand Ther* 27(1):14–22, 2014. https://doi.org/10.1016/j.jht.2013.09.001.
8. Armbruster EJ, Tan V: Carpometacarpal joint disease: addressing the metacarpophalangeal joint deformity, *Hand Clin* 24(3):295–299, 2008. https://doi.org/10.1016/j.hcl.2008.03.013.
9. Moulton MJ, Parentis MA, Kelly MJ, Jacobs C, Naidu SH, Pellegrini Jr VD: Influence of metacarpophalangeal joint position on basal joint-loading in the thumb, *J Bone Joint Surg Am* 83(5):709–716, 2001.
10. O'Brien VH, Giveans MR: Effects of a dynamic stability approach in conservative intervention of the carpometacarpal joint of the thumb: a retrospective study, *J Hand Ther* 26(1):44–51, 2013. https://doi.org/10.1016/j.jht.2012.10.005.
11. Valdes K, Marik T: A systematic review of conservative interventions for osteoarthritis of the hand, *J Hand Ther* 23(4):334–351, 2010.

CASE STUDY 3.2 ■ Forward Head Rounded Shoulders (FHRS) Posture

Condition: Upper back and neck pain and headache
Scenario: A graduate student had a final exam and studied for three days in a row. While studying, she sat in her front room on a couch or on her bed reading and writing. She changed positions when she was uncomfortable, yet she describes mostly looking down at her laptop in a long leg sitting position. While taking the exam, she complained of a headache and upper back and neck pain.

Standard posture	Ideal alignment of head and neck in which the head is balanced and maintained with minimal effort	In side view, the perpendicular line of reference (in sit or stand) coincides with the lobe of the ear to the anterior aspect of the humeral head.
		In the posterior view, the line of reference is the line from the midline of the head to the cervical spinous process. The head is not tilted upward or downward and is not rotated or sideways off the midline.
Skeletal Imbalance	Forward head, cervical extension Ossous anatomy: The base of the skull forms joints with the atlas (C1, first cervical vertebral body) and the axis (C2, Second cervical vertebral body) at the occipital-C1 articulation and the C1-C2 articulation.	Atlantooccipital (AO) joint (combined flexion and extension 10–15 degrees of normal motion) Atlantoaxial (AA) joints (rotation) (50 degrees of normal rotation) C3-C7 zygapophysial (facet joints) (40 degrees of flexion, 25 degrees of extension) Lateral view of forward head demonstrated an increase cervical angle and reduced lordosis.[1]
Muscle Imbalance	Flexor neck muscles: longus capitis, longus colli, and rectus capitis anterior	Elongated and weak
	Extensor neck muscles: Rectus capitis obliques, posterior minor, and major	Adaptive shortening: Forward head posture and reduced cervical lordosis were seen more in younger patients with spontaneous neck pain (cite)
		In movement, these muscles are aided by the sternocleidomastoid, anterior scalene, suprahyoids, and infrahyoids.

Compensation	Abducted scapula, thoracic spine kyphosis	The upper trapezius, when shortened, results in an elevation of the shoulder girdle, which contributes to the cervical spine extension and leads to the rounded shoulder kyphosis of the thoracic spine.
Occupations	Education Social participation Work Sleep	Study results demonstrate that mentally challenging computer work increases perceived anxiety, cardiac demand, and forward head posture in asymptomatic office workers. The pain in more proximal areas of the posterior neck may be related to extreme forward head postures while working at the computer.[1]
Assessments	Wall test Functional posture Assessment Goniometry MMT in supine Sensory testing Pain assessment	Posture assessment[2] Shoulder (AROM) was measured using a universal goniometer. Goniometric measurement of shoulder ROM has demonstrated fair to good reliability.[3]
Therapy Interventions	Occupation based (Alignment in occupations) Therapeutic procedure	Education in sleep preparation and position computer ergonomics, education in body mechanics during occupations (e.g., anterior pelvic tilt, chin tuck, and neck lengthening), stand to sit shifting 20-min intervals
	Stretch and strengthen for balance	Restore neuromuscular balance for the adaptive shortening of the FHRS: stretch shortened muscles and strengthen weak muscle groups

AROM, Active range of motion; *MMT,* manual muscle test, *ROM,* range of motion.

Sources

1. Sun A, Yeo HG, Kim TU, Hyun JK, Kim JY: Radiologic assessment of forward head posture and its relation to myofascial pain syndrome, *Ann Rehabil Med* 38(6):821–826, 2014.
2. Kendall F, McCreary E, Provance P, Rodgers M, Romani W: *Testing and Function with Posture and Pain,* Lippincoll Williams & Wilkins, 2005.
3. Hayes K, Walton JR, Szomor ZL, Murrell GA: Reliability of five methods for assessing shoulder range of motion, *Aust J Physiother* 47(4):289–294, 2001.

References

1. Donatelli RA, WM: *Orthopedic physical therapy,* ed 4, 2010. St Louis, MO, Elsevier Health Sciences.
2. Thigpen CA, Padua DA, Michener LA, et al.: Head and shoulder posture affect scapular mechanics and muscle activity in overhead tasks, *J Electromyogr Kinesiol* 20:701–709, 2010.
3. Kendall FP, McCreary EK, Provance PG: *Muscles: testing and function with posture and pain,* Baltimore, MD, 2005, Lippincott Williams & Wilkins.
4. Brand PW, Hollister A: *Clinical mechanics of the hand,* St. Louis, MO, 1993, Mosby Year Book.
5. Walsh MT: Interventions in the disturbances in the motor and sensory environment, *J Hand Ther* 25:202–218, 2012, quiz 219.
6. Topp KS, Boyd BS: Peripheral nerve: from the microscopic functional unit of the axon to the biomechanically loaded macroscopic structure, *J Hand Ther* 25:142–151, 2012, quiz 152.
7. O'Driscoll SW, Horii E, Ness R, et al.: The relationship between wrist position, grasp size, and grip strength, *J Hand Surg Am* 17:169–177, 1992.
8. Hung CH, Lin CY: Using concept mapping to evaluate knowledge structure in problem-based learning, *BMC Med Educ* 15(1):212, 2015, https://doi.org/10.1186/s12909-015-0496-x.
9. Federolf PA: A novel approach to study human posture control: "principal movements" obtained from a principal component analysis of kinematic marker data, *J Biomech* 49(3):364–370, 2016, https://doi.org/10.1016/j.jbiomech.2015.12.030.
10. McHenry MJ: There is no trade-off between speed and force in a dynamic lever system, *Biol Lett* 7(3):384–386, 2011, https://doi.org/10.1098/rsbl.2010.1029.
11. Singla D, Veqar Z: Association between forward head, rounded shoulders, and increased thoracic kyphosis: a review of the literature, *J Chiropr Med* 16(3):220–229, 2017. https://doi.org/10.1016/j.jcm.2017.03.004.
12. Sun A, Yeo HG, Kim TU, Hyun JK, Kim JY: Radiologic assessment of forward head posture and its relation to myofascial pain syndrome, *Ann Rehabil Med* 38(6):821–826, 2014.
13. Neumann DA: Kinesiology of the hip: a focus on muscular actions, *J Orthop Sports Phys Ther* 40:82–94, 2010. https://doi.org/ 10.2519/jospt.2010.3025.
14. Fess EE, Gettle KS, Philips CA, Janson JR: *Hand and upper extremity splinting: principles and methods,* St. Louis, MO, Mosby Inc, 2004.
15. Hurov J: Anatomy and mechanics of the shoulder: review of current concepts, *J Hand Ther* 22(4):328–343, 2009.
16. Pratt N: Anatomy of nerve entrapment sites in the upper quarter, *J Hand Ther* 18(2):216, 2005.
17. Rybski M: *Kinesiology for occupational yherapy,* Thorofare, NJ, 2012, SLACK.
18. Novak CB, Mackinnon SE: Repetitive use and static postures: a source of nerve compression and pain, *J Hand Ther* 10:151–159, 1997.
19. Novak CB: Physical therapy management of thoracic outlet syndrome in the musician, *J Hand Ther* 5:73–79, 1992.
20. Occupational Therapy Practice Framework: Domain and process (3rd Edition), *Am J Occup Ther* 68(Suppl 1):S1–S48, 2017, https://doi.org/10.5014/ajot.2014.682006.
21. American Occupational Therapy Association, Inc: *Musculoskeletal disorders. AOTA Critically Appraised Topics and Papers Series,* 2016. Retrieved from https://www.aota.org/~/media/Corporate/Files/Secure/Practice/CCL/MSD/CAT_MSD_Exercise.pdf.

4 Evaluation of the Hand and Upper Extremity

Linda J. Klein

The client's initial evaluation sets the stage for successful rehabilitation. Evaluation establishes rapport, determines areas of functional deficit, and serves as the foundation for treatment and recovery. Only with an accurate assessment can the therapist determine the best course of treatment for the client's condition. A number of assessment processes and clinical assessment skills are needed to perform a thorough evaluation (Fig. 4.1). The main areas of assessment for the injured hand include pain, wound and scar status, vascular status, range of motion (ROM), swelling, sensation, strength, current and previous use of orthoses, and functional limitations including self-rated impairment assessment. A screening of proximal motion, strength, and posture are important to have a full understanding of deficits in the distal upper extremity. Periodic reevaluations are necessary to show progress, identify new or remaining problems, and redirect goals.

Using an evaluation summary form is helpful (see Appendix 4.1). The form will guide you through each step of the assessment, ensuring that you do not forget any areas. Defer specific areas of the evaluation when it is not appropriate to perform them at a certain time in the tissue-healing process or if the client simply cannot tolerate these procedures. Sometimes an additional form is needed for a complete assessment. For example, the evaluation summary form should have an area listed as sensation even though a separate form is used for sensory tests (for example, the Semmes-Weinstein monofilament test or two-point discrimination test). On the evaluation summary form, give a brief description that indicates where the client perceives altered sensation, including numbness, tingling, burning, or hypersensitivity. Then use the Semmes-Weinstein monofilament, two-point discrimination, or other sensation forms for more specific and objective information.

The evaluation summary form promotes clinical reasoning and assists the therapist's organization of thoughts and communication with a thorough and logical progression of categories.

Interview

Obtaining a History

Before assessing the function of the client's hand, obtaining a history of the injury or symptoms that bring the client to therapy is essential. Understanding the onset of symptoms (for example trauma versus gradual) is essential. Next, ask about any prior medical intervention. Has there been surgery? An injection? X-ray, magnetic resonance imaging, or computed tomography scan? Nerve study? Cast immobilization? Use of orthoses? Medication? Manual tests by the physician? Or has there been no intervention by the physician except to send the client to therapy for the therapist's expertise in evaluation and treatment?

Understanding previous care that the client has experienced helps in a number of ways. It gives the client confidence that you understand what has been done, and it builds trust because in many cases you can explain what the physician was attempting to determine with various tests. A client who trusts you is more likely to participate fully in the evaluation and rehabilitation process. In addition to the history of the injury or condition, you must understand the individual's pertinent medical history because many medical conditions, such as diabetes or peripheral vascular disease, affect the healing process. Assessing comorbidities is now required as part of the evaluation documentation.

Observation

During the initial process of meeting new clients and discussing their history and symptoms, use your observation skills. Observe the client's nonverbal communication,

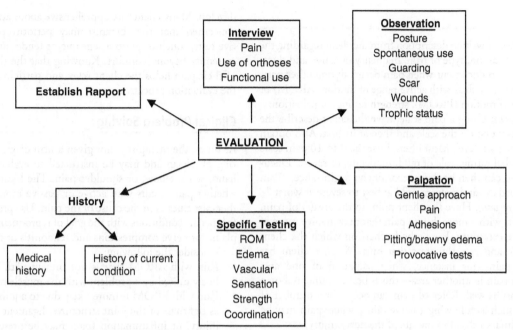

FIG. 4.1 Summary of the evaluation process. *ROM,* Range of motion.

including facial expressions and body language, as well as how the client holds and uses the injured extremity and trunk. The client often guards the injured extremity at the time of initial evaluation, possibly as a subconscious protection from pain. I also have seen situations in which the client guards the extremity or exaggerates limitations, such as strength or motion, during the evaluation to be sure that the therapist recognizes and appreciates the extent of deficit. In these cases, it is sometimes possible to observe them functioning at a higher level during a spontaneous situation than during the formal assessment. For example, a client with an elbow injury who lacks 40 degrees of elbow extension during formal assessment can sometimes be seen extending the elbow significantly further while removing or putting on their coat. Another example is the client who guards the hand by holding it close to the body during the assessment but uses the hand more freely with gestures during informal discussion.

Observe differences in posture and use of the upper extremity in spontaneous situations compared with formal assessment. This gives clues regarding the client's comfort with the extremity. Use different approaches to elicit the best response from clients who are not comfortable moving freely. In my experience, most clients with abnormal posturing (guarding) are unaware of their upper extremity positioning and are eager to change. In contrast, facilitating positive engagement by clients who may be consciously controlling their responses in therapy is more challenging. I have had some success reminding these clients that continued therapy is contingent on their progress. I have found that having a nonjudgmental attitude, pointing out inconsistencies between formal testing and observation, is the most effective approach in this situation. Reinforce that your goal is to work with the client toward recovery, as this will maximize the client's positive involvement in the rehabilitation process.

In discussing each section of the evaluation, I will describe the tools and process of the evaluation. I will also point out inconsistencies and difficulties to be aware of, and discuss when portions of the evaluation should be deferred.

BOX 4.1   Pain Scales

- *Numeric analog scales*: A line with equal markings from 0 to 5, 0 to 10, or 0 to 20 is used to indicate the perceived level of pain at the initial evaluation compared with periodic re-evaluations.
- *Visual analog scale*: Provide the client with a 10-cm line drawn vertically on paper with one end labeled "no pain" and the other end labeled "pain as bad as it could be." The client marks the location and level of pain, and the examiner later divides the line into 20 equal portions to determine the distance from zero to the client's pain mark.
- *Verbal rating scale*: Client describes their pain with four to five descriptive words (for example, mild, moderate, or severe).
- *Graphic representation*: The client marks his or her pain location and type on a body chart.
- *Pain questionnaire*: Written pain questionnaires are available that obtain more information about the client's pain, such as the McGill or McGill short-form Pain Questionnaire, described in detail in the references.[1,2] Although more time consuming, the knowledge of the content of specific questionnaires may be helpful to develop your skills in discussing pain during an evaluation.

Assessment of Pain

Equipment

No equipment is necessary, but you may choose to use a pain scale during initial evaluation to summarize the client's overall perception of pain. Numerous pain scales are available (Box 4.1).[1,2]

Methods

Obtain a verbal or written description from the client regarding the level of pain, location, type of pain, frequency or cause, and duration of pain. Also document when pain occurs during other parts of the evaluation, such as with active range of motion (AROM) or passive range of motion (PROM), strength testing, or palpation:

- *Level of pain*: Using a pain scale, have the client describe the pain at its worst on the scale and then at its best. Also obtain an average pain level. Most often, I use the 0-to-10 pain scale or the verbal rating scale of mild, moderate, or severe. Documentation can then be done accordingly; for instance, "Pain is described as varying from mild at best to severe at worst."
- *Location of pain*: Have the client point to the area(s) of pain. For clients with a more diffuse pain that may involve more of the upper extremity, I use a body chart on which the client can circle and rate the areas that hurt. When a client has referred pain—for instance, when palpation of one area results in pain in another area—this is best documented on a body chart as well. Referred pain can occur for a number of reasons, such as following a nerve injury where pain may be felt proximal or distal to the site of the nerve injury.
- *Type of pain*: Ask the client to describe the pain as throbbing, aching, sharp, stabbing, shooting, burning, or hypersensitive to light touch.
- *Frequency or cause of pain*: Determine whether the pain is constant or intermittent. Have the client describe when the pain occurs and what seems to cause the pain. This information is helpful in determining a diagnosis if the physician has not provided a firm diagnosis.
- *Duration of pain*: Determine how long the pain has been present.

> ### ◎ Clinical Pearl
>
> Pain in an area for longer than 6 months is often classified as chronic pain, as opposed to acute pain experienced following a recent injury.

- *Chronic pain*: Chronic pain is often associated with depression, anxiety, and other psychological involvement and may be best helped by a team approach with specialists in the area of chronic pain management.
- *Pain levels*: Note pain levels that occur during the evaluation, such as pain during AROM, PROM, or strength testing. For instance, my evaluation might state, "Strength: Grip strength right hand 100#, left hand 50# with moderate pain identified in left volar wrist with grip." I may have a goal to reflect this in my initial evaluation note, such as "Increase left hand grip strength to 75# without pain." Tendonitis is more frequently associated with painful AROM than painful PROM. Thus detailed information about pain during evaluation becomes part of the clinical reasoning and treatment process.

Discussion

I usually begin my assessment of a new client's injury by discussing the client's pain and reassuring the client that the evaluation is not intended to worsen the pain. As soon as the client has the opportunity to tell me about his or her pain, I see a level of relief develop. Many clients are apprehensive about attending therapy, concerned that the therapist may perform painful provocative tests, touch or grasp a sensitive or tender area, or move the extremity beyond comfort. Knowing that the therapist is aware of their pain helps the client relax and participate in the rest of the evaluation process.

Clinical Problem Solving

At times, the therapist is not given a firm diagnosis by the referring physician and may be instructed to evaluate and treat for hand, wrist, elbow, or shoulder pain. The location of pain and whether pain occurs with active or passive motion can give the therapist clues as to the cause of the pain. Use provocative testing for specific conditions with the goal of reproducing the pain complaint for nerve compressions and tendonitis or tendinopathy.

Consider the following:

- Pain with AROM that is not present with PROM is most likely caused by a problem with the muscle or tendon.
- Pain with PROM is more likely due to a joint problem, such as tightness of the joint structures, ligament injury, cartilage injury, or inflammation (pain may be present equally with AROM in these situations).
- When a joint is limited in motion because of pain, and pain is present with distraction of the joint but not compression of the joint, pain is most likely due to a ligament or joint capsule being stretched with distraction and relieved with compression.
- If pain is present with compression of the joint but is relieved with distraction, pain is more likely due to a problem at the joint surface, such as thinning or loss of cartilage, inflammation within the joint, or other abnormality such as a bone spur.

Precaution. *Aggressive clinical problem-solving methods can be used safely only when the physician has allowed AROM and PROM as part of treatment. These methods are not appropriate in the acute phase following a tendon, nerve, or ligament repair or tendon transfer.*

Wound Assessment

Open wounds can be intimidating. Breaking the assessment down to wound size, depth, color, drainage, and odor is helpful. When wounds are closed, it is appropriate to skip this section and go on to scar assessment.

Consider the following:

- *Size:* Measure length and width of the wound with a ruler. Consider tracing the wound for future comparison using transparent calibrated grids. Do not touch the wound with the ruler or other measuring device unless the item is sterile.
- *Depth:* Wound depth may be measured with a sterile cotton swab if the client and therapist are comfortable with this procedure.
- *Color:* Open wounds can be categorized as red, yellow, or black.[3,4] Many wounds have a combination of these colors, and wounds progress through stages of these colors.
- *Red wound:* Wound characterized by moist and healthy **granulation tissue.** Color ranges from pink to red. Granulation tissue is new connective tissue with tiny blood vessels that forms in a healthy wound bed. It is a prerequisite for wound healing.

- *Yellow wound:* Wound characterized by soft and sticky **slough.** Color ranges from cream to yellow. Slough is a type of necrotic (dead) tissue. It is a moist composite of fibrin, bacteria, dead cells, and wound exudate that adheres to the wound bed. Slough in the wound increases risk for infection and must be removed.
- *Black wound:* Wound characterized by semifirm to hard **eschar.** Color ranges from grey to black. Eschar is a type of necrotic tissue that is dryer than slough, adheres to the wound bed, and has a spongy or leather-like appearance. Eschar in the wound increases risk for infection, physically splints the wound open, and must be removed before a wound will heal.

◎ Clinical Pearl

Wounds almost always have more than one color present at one time. Treat the worst stage first; that is, progress from treatment of black to yellow, and then treat yellow to red.

- *Drainage (also known as **exudate**):* Attempt to quantify the amount of drainage (mild, moderate, heavy) and color of drainage. Thin watery drainage that is clear to very light pink in color is normal in small amounts. Cloudy thin drainage that is yellow to tan in color may indicate infection. Thick drainage that is green, brown, tan, or yellow is never normal and indicates infection.
- *Odor:* Note any odor emanating from the wound. Unpleasant odors often indicate infection. Likewise, a very sweet-smelling wound can be a sign of infection.
- *Temperature:* Compare periwound (tissue surrounding the wound) temperature with temperature of an unaffected area. Surface thermometers or temperature tapes can be used for this. Warmer periwound temperature could indicate infection.

◎ Clinical Pearl

If there is any question of infection, have the wound examined by a physician.

Scar Assessment

The characteristics to assess for scar status include color, size, whether it is flattened or raised, and the presence of **adhesion** (attachment) to underlying or surrounding tissue.

Consider the following:
- *Color:* Scars usually begin as deep red and gradually become lighter as time progresses.
- *Size:* Use a ruler to measure the length and width of the scar.
- *Flat/raised:* Use observation and palpation to assess how far the scar is raised above the skin level, and describe it using terms like mild or moderate. Sometimes the superficial scar may be flat but there may be a lump under the skin. This happens most commonly on the dorsum of the hand or wrist with a lump under the surface scar that is a thickening composed of a combination of scar and fluid. This lump of scar and fluid can be described by size and height (for example, "Dorsal incisional scar is 3cm in length along the third meta-

carpal, with a thickened area under the skin of 3 mm in height and 2–3 mm in width surrounding the scar.")
- *Adhesions:* Assessment of adhesions of surface scars to underlying tissue is done by observation and palpation. Some adhesions can be seen during active motion. When the adhesion is on the dorsal hand or wrist, or the volar wrist/forearm, the scar is often seen to dip deeper, or dimple, when active motion is attempted, because of adhesions from the superficial scar to underlying fascia and tendons. Also assess adhesions of skin to underlying tissue by palpation. Attempt to slide or lift the scar tissue and compare it to the surrounding uninjured tissue. Describe the level of adhesion as mild, moderate, or severely adherent.

Precaution. *Respect the level of healing of a new scar and the tissue to which it may adhere. Avoid aggressively attempting to move scar tissue within the first week following suture removal or when a portion of the wound is still open. Doing so may damage fragile healing tissue or could reopen the wound. Avoid strong scar manipulation over a tendon during assessment or treatment in the early phase of tendon healing.*

Vascular Status Assessment

A basic vascular evaluation of the hand can be done by observation (color or **trophic** changes, pain level), palpation (pulse, capillary refill assessment, modified Allen's test), and temperature assessment. Blood flow to the hand can be affected by proximal injury or diagnoses, such as thoracic outlet syndrome, injury to the hand itself, or conditions like Raynaud's phenomenon.

Observation

Observation includes assessment of color and trophic changes in the hand. Increased levels of white (**pallor**), blue (**cyanosis**), or red (**erythema**) coloration of the skin are the most common changes noted.

◎ Clinical Pearl

Arterial interruption usually produces a white or grayish discoloration of the affected area (pallor), whereas venous blockage produces a congested, purple-blue color.[5] Dusky blue may indicate chronic venous insufficiency. Redness may indicate loss of outflow of blood from the hand, but it may also be an indication of a normal inflammatory phase of wound healing or the presence of infection.

Trophic changes are changes in the texture of the skin and nail. Changes in the trophic status can occur from sympathetic nerve or vascular issues. Note the presence of increased dryness or moisture of the skin in the involved hand during the initial evaluation. Also note the presence of open wounds or necrotic tissue. Reevaluate these items frequently for improvement.

Pain is present in two-thirds of clients with upper extremity vascular disease.[6] Pain may be described as aching, cramping, tightness, or cold intolerance. Pain may be associated with activity that exposes the upper extremity to vibration, cold, or repetition.

Precaution. *Close monitoring of color and temperature change is important, and communication with the referring physician is* *recommended if abnormalities are worsening or not improving. Causes of vascular abnormalities are numerous, and in-depth evaluation and testing by the physician may be indicated.*

Palpation Tests of Vascular Status

Capillary Refill Test

To perform the capillary refill test, place pressure on the distal portion of the volar finger or over the fingernail of the digit until tissue turns white.[5,6] Capillary refill time is the number of seconds it takes for the color to return to normal after the pressure is released. Normal capillary refill time is less than 2 seconds, and the time can be compared with the same digit on the opposite hand or with uninjured digits.

Peripheral Pulse Palpation

Place light pressure over the radial artery or ulnar artery just proximal to the wrist crease to gain information about the strength of the pulse or blood flow to the hand.[6,7] If the pulse is weaker in one wrist than the other, there may be a potential problem with blood flow proximal to the wrist.

Modified Allen's Test

The modified Allen's test assesses the status of the blood supply within the hand through the ulnar and radial arteries of the wrist.[5-8] To perform the test, place firm pressure over the radial and ulnar arteries just proximal to the wrist crease. Instruct the client to make a tight fist and then open the fingers repeatedly until the palm turns white. Then instruct the client to relax the fingers to a partially opened position. Release the pressure from one side of the wrist, allowing blood flow through one of the arteries. Record the time it takes for the color to return to normal in the hand. Repeat the process, releasing pressure from the artery on the opposite side of the wrist. Record the time it takes for the color to return to normal in the hand. A normal response is 5 seconds or less and can be compared to the opposite extremity to confirm a normal response time for that individual.

Surface Temperature Assessment

Surface thermometers can be used to compare forearm temperature to fingertip temperature. If the forearm is at least 4°C (39°F) warmer than the fingertip surface, it may indicate vascular compromise. Assess Raynaud's phenomenon with a temperature assessment that measures the temperature of the involved fingertip(s) after being in a warm room (24°C [75°F]) for 30 minutes and then after being immersed in ice water for 20 seconds. Record the time it takes to return to the baseline temperature. The normal time for return to body temperature is within 10 minutes, but clients with Raynaud's phenomenon will take much longer.

Range of Motion Assessment

Assessment of ROM in this chapter is limited to the forearm, wrist, fingers, and thumb. A variety of ways to assess ROM are

available; thus using recognized reference sources for technique is recommended when learning to perform ROM testing.[9-11] All ROM of the forearm, wrist, and hand is performed with the client in the seated position. Clinical problem solving that interprets the cause of the limited ROM (joint stiffness, **intrinsic tightness** that limits simultaneous metacarpophalangeal [MP] extension and interphalangeal [IP] flexion, and **extrinsic tendon tightness** that limits composite wrist and digit motion in the same direction) is important for determining the most appropriate treatment plan.

Methods

Passive Range of Motion

PROM is the ability of a joint to be moved through its normal arc of motion while relaxed, with motion being performed by an outside source such as the therapist's hand, the client's opposite hand, or gravity. Limitations in PROM indicate a problem within the joint (for example, stiffness caused by capsular or ligamentous tightness, decreased joint space, or bone spur). PROM may also be limited by tightness of the muscle/tendon group opposing the passive motion (for example, a tight or adherent extensor muscle/tendon will prevent full passive or active flexion).

Precaution. *Traumatic injuries to the bone or joint in the acute phase of healing, or as determined by the physician, are limited to AROM with no PROM allowed. Forceful PROM by an outside source could reinjure the healing bone or ligament. Following a tendon repair in the early phase of tendon healing, PROM in the direction that would stretch the tendon is not allowed.*

Active Range of Motion

AROM is motion of a joint caused by musculotendinous contraction, most often from a voluntary muscle contraction. Limitations in AROM can result from a number of causes. Some of these causes include weakness of the muscle, loss of tendon continuity, adhesions of the tendon preventing its motion, inflammation or constriction of the tendon, decreased tendon mechanical efficiency because of loss of pulley (bowstringing), and disrupted nerve supply to the muscle.

Precaution. *AROM using a repaired tendon (that is, contracting a repaired muscle/tendon) is not allowed following many tendon repairs or tendon transfers in the acute phase of tendon healing. This restriction lasts for approximately the first 4 weeks after the repair unless the type of repair performed by the surgeon allows use of an immediate active-motion protocol. Please refer to Chapters 26, 27, and 28.*

You must recognize that AROM or PROM may also be limited by pain. If the client describes pain during ROM testing, note this on the evaluation form.

When there is no medical limitation regarding use of AROM and PROM, it is important to do the following:
- Measure both passive and active motion for information that helps determine the cause of limitation.
- Compare ROM to the other hand to learn what is normal for that individual.
- Measure ROM at a consistent time or sequence in the treatment session (for example, always before or always after exercise) for a more accurate reading of improvement.

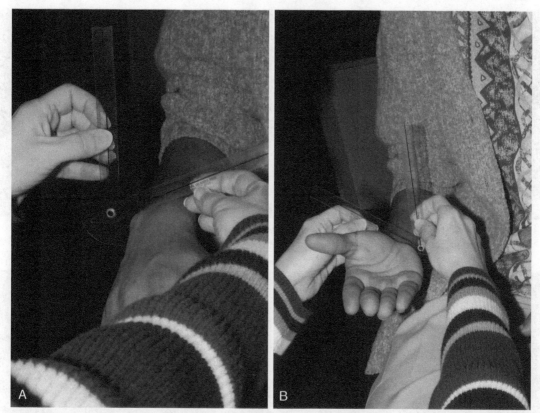

FIG. 4.2 (A) Pronation as measured with a standard 6-inch goniometer, demonstrating axis of motion on the dorsal distal ulna. (B) Supination as measured with a standard 6-inch goniometer, demonstrating axis of motion on the volar distal ulna.

- When measuring ROM of the fingers, be consistent in positioning the hand and proximal joints. For instance, it is more difficult to perform finger flexion when the wrist is flexed compared with when the wrist is extended. When the extensors are adherent, each individual digital joint measured alone or independently will flex further than when all three finger joints are flexed at the same time.

Total Active Motion

Total active motion (TAM) is used to describe the full arc of active motion of the digit(s). TAM is measured as the total flexion of all three finger joints, subtracting any loss of full extension at all finger joints:

$$(MP + PIP + DIP \text{ flexion}) - (MP + PIP + DIP \text{ extension loss}) = TAM$$

where *MP* is metacarpophalangeal, *PIP* is proximal interphalangeal, and *DIP* is distal interphalangeal.

> ◎ *Clinical Pearl*
>
> Use TAM when reporting ROM in situations where tendon adhesions limit motion and composite motion is more limited than individual joint motion.

Total Passive Motion

Total passive motion (TPM) is the same process as TAM but is measured passively. This can be helpful to document the presence of adhesions.

> ◎ *Clinical Pearl*
>
> When flexor tendon gliding is limited by adhesions, TPM will be better than TAM.

Standard plastic goniometers work well for measurement. Large goniometers (12¼ inches) are recommended for the larger elbow and shoulder joints. Standard goniometers (6–7 inches) are used for measuring the forearm and wrist (Figs. 4.2 and 4.3). They can be cut down in length to measure finger ROM (Fig. 4.4). Metal finger goniometers are available at a higher cost and do not have the benefit of transparency when lateral placement is needed. Electronic and computer system goniometers are available at a much higher cost. For the wrist, I prefer the 6-inch goniometer with rounded ends because it allows dorsal placement on the wrist for flexion and extension (Fig. 4.5).

Hyperextension of the fingers is recorded with a plus sign (+), loss of full extension with a minus sign (–). When standard placement of the goniometer is not used because of scar, swelling, or wound, document the modified placement of the goniometer for future reference to allow for accurate comparative measurements.

Forearm Range of Motion

Consider the following for forearm ROM:
- Motions of the forearm are pronation and supination.
- Starting position is with the arm adducted at the side, elbow flexed to 90 degrees, forearm and wrist neutral.

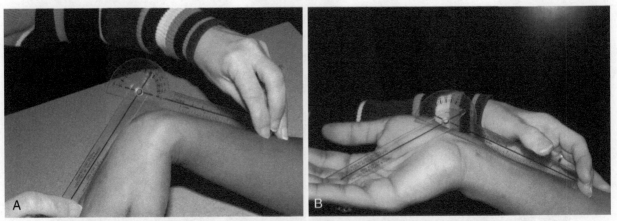

FIG. 4.3 (A) Wrist flexion measured dorsally over the central wrist with a standard 6-inch goniometer. (B) Wrist extension measured along the volar surface over the central wrist with a standard 6-inch goniometer.

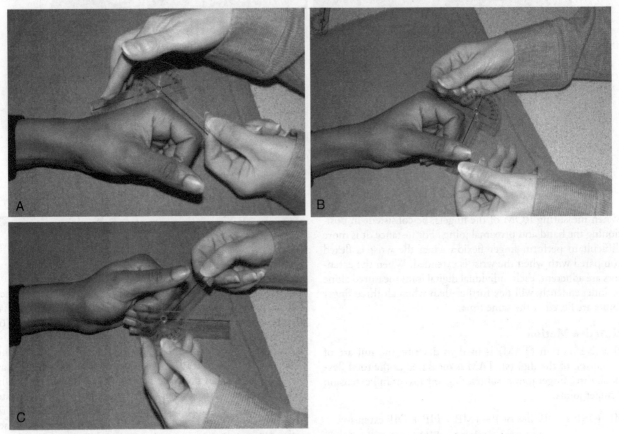

FIG. 4.4 Finger flexion measured dorsally with a standard 6-inch goniometer that has been cut down in length. (A) Demonstrates metacarpophalangeal flexion; (B) demonstrates proximal interphalangeal flexion; and (C) demonstrates distal interphalangeal (DIP) flexion. Note the placement of the goniometer arms to allow DIP flexion to be measured in a composite flexion position.

- Axis of motion is the ulnar edge of the forearm, dorsally for pronation, and along the volar surface for supination.
- Placement of the goniometer is with both arms of the goniometer across the distal forearm, dorsally with axis placed at the lateral edge of the dorsal ulna for pronation, and along the volar surface of the distal forearm, with axis placed at the lateral edge of the volar ulna for supination.
- To measure pronation, one arm of the goniometer stays in place in the starting position (straight up), while the other

arm of the goniometer stays in contact with the dorsal distal forearm as it moves into pronation. The stationary arm of the goniometer, which stays in the starting position, is now straight up and should be aligned with the humerus if the client has maintained the correct starting position of the trunk and arm. The moving arm of the goniometer is to stay flat on the dorsum of the distal forearm, flush with the center of the distal forearm, between the ulna and radius (see Fig. 4.2A).

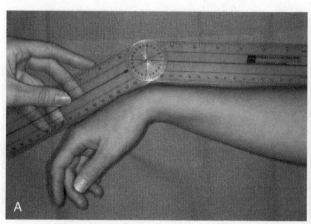
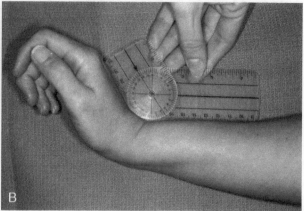

FIG. 4.5 (A) Alternate goniometer for wrist flexion, measured dorsally over the central wrist. (B) Alternate goniometer with rounded ends used for wrist extension measured dorsally over the central wrist.

- To measure supination, one arm of the goniometer stays in place in the starting position (straight up), while the other arm stays in contact with the volar distal forearm as it moves into supination. The stationary arm of the goniometer, which stays in the starting position, is now straight up and should be aligned with the humerus if the client has maintained the correct starting position of the trunk and arm. The moving arm of the goniometer is flush on the center of the volar forearm on the flattest portion of the midvolar forearm (see Fig. 4.2B).
- While some sources identify the starting position of the goniometer as straight down, this will give an inaccurate result if the humerus is not perfectly straight up and down. If the humerus is not straight up and down due to body composition or compensation by leaning, I prefer to align the stationary arm of the goniometer with the humerus. This will provide an accurate measurement of forearm motion in relation to the humerus. It is important to perform the test in the same manner on retest.
- Frequent errors are made when measuring pronation and supination by allowing the goniometer to overturn and measure more along the distal radius or underturn and measure more along the distal ulna, rather than correctly on the middle section of the distal forearm. Other common errors are to allow the client to lean or move the arm away from the starting position of humeral adduction against the side of the body. Feedback from an experienced therapist is helpful when learning to measure forearm motion.

Wrist Range of Motion

Consider the following for wrist ROM:
- Motions of the wrist are flexion, extension, radial deviation, and ulnar deviation.
- Starting position is with wrist neutral.
- Axis of motion is the center of the wrist.
- Placement of the goniometer according to American Society of Hand Therapists recommendations are along the volar surface for extension, dorsally for flexion, and dorsally for radial deviation and ulnar deviation. Lateral placement is appropriate when scar or swelling make dorsal or volar placements inaccurate.
- To measure flexion, place one arm of the goniometer along the dorsum of the forearm and the other arm along the third metacarpal on the dorsum of the hand (see Fig. 4.3A).

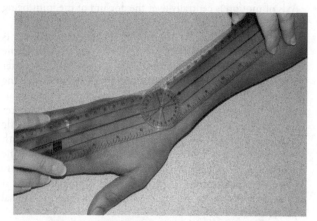

FIG. 4.6 Wrist ulnar deviation measured dorsally.

- To measure extension, place one arm of the goniometer along the volar forearm and the other arm along the third metacarpal on the palmar side of the hand (see Fig. 4.3B).
- To measure radial and ulnar deviation, with hand flat on a table surface, place the goniometer flat on its side, one arm of the goniometer on the dorsum of the forearm, axis at the center of the wrist, and the other arm of the goniometer along the third metacarpal (Fig. 4.6).

Volar placement of the goniometer on the palm to measure wrist extension may be difficult because the goniometer does not lay flat on the many curves in the palm. A goniometer with rounded ends (see Fig. 4.5), which is available in many therapy supply catalogs, allows dorsal placement of the goniometer to measure flexion and extension of the wrist.

Digital Range of Motion

The MP, proximal interphalangeal (PIP) joints, distal interphalangeal (DIP) joints of the fingers, and MP and IP joints of the thumb are measured with the same procedure and are described together next:
- Motions of the finger and thumb MP and IP joints are flexion and extension. The MP joints of the fingers also perform abduction and adduction, and although this can be assessed with goniometric measurements,[11] a tracing of the hand with the fingers fully abducted is also an effective way to show change over time.
- Starting position for measuring flexion and extension of the digit is extension. Neutral wrist is recommended for consistency in procedure.

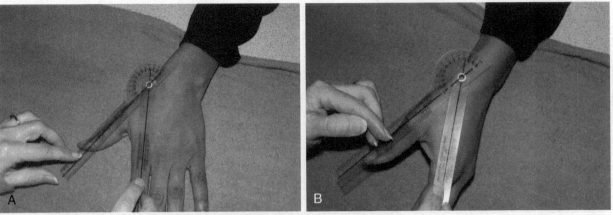

FIG. 4.7 (A) Thumb carpometacarpal (CMC) radial abduction measured dorsally with a standard 6-inch goniometer. (B) Thumb CMC palmar abduction measured radially with a standard 6-inch goniometer.

- Axis of motion is centrally over the dorsum of the joint being measured.
- Placement of the goniometer for all finger measurements is on the dorsal surface. The MP joint is measured with one arm of the goniometer along the metacarpal, and the other arm of the goniometer along the proximal phalanx, with the axis at the dorsal MP (see Fig. 4.4A). Placement of the goniometer for the PIP joint is with one arm of the goniometer on the proximal phalanx and the other arm on the middle phalanx (see Fig. 4.4B). Placement for the DIP joints is with one arm of the goniometer on the middle phalanx and the other arm on the distal phalanx (see Fig. 4.4C). Alternate placement of the goniometer is laterally along the finger if there is a lump or other abnormality preventing dorsal placement.
- To measure motion, note the maximal extension at each joint, and when moving into flexion, move the distal arm of the goniometer to maintain its position on the dorsum of the finger section noted before. Note the degree of flexion attained. If loss of full extension is present, record it with a minus sign (–); for example, –25 to 50 degrees MP motion means there was a loss of 25 degrees of extension and the joint was able to flex to 50 degrees of flexion. For hyperextension, use a plus sign (+): +25 to 50 degrees MP motion means there is 25 degrees of hyperextension at the MP joint and the joint was able to flex to 50 degrees of flexion.

Hyperextension is difficult to measure with the standard 6-inch goniometer or 6-inch goniometer cut down in length, and lateral placement is necessary for this measurement. The goniometer style with rounded ends described in the discussion section of wrist ROM (see Fig. 4.5) can be used to measure hyperextension of the digit joints with dorsal placement.

> ◎ **Clinical Pearl**
>
> Measurement of each digit with the hand placed in full composite flexion and then full extension (TAM) is important during the initial evaluation.

Each joint may be near normal if measured in isolation, but significant limitation in ROM may be evident when total active flexion and extension are measured, due to tendon gliding or scar tissue limitations. The TAM of the digit measured in composite flexion and extension indicates the functional limitations of

motion. Functional limitations of motion also can be demonstrated by measuring the distance, during a composite fist, from the fingertip pulp to the distal palmar crease of the hand.

Thumb Carpometacarpal Joint

Consider the following:
- Motions include palmar abduction, radial abduction, adduction, and opposition.
- Axis of motion is the intersection of lines extending down the first and second metacarpals on the dorsal radial aspect of the hand.
- Starting position is with the forearm pronated with hand flat on table for radial abduction or with the ulnar side of the hand on the table, forearm neutral for palmar abduction or opposition. The thumb is adducted when it is flat along the side of the index finger.
- Placement of the goniometer is with one arm placed along the second metacarpal and the other arm placed along the first metacarpal, dorsally for radial abduction and radially for palmar abduction. The axis of the goniometer will be located at the first carpometacarpal (CMC) joint, where the first metacarpal articulates with the trapezium and trapezoid.
- To measure radial abduction, the goniometer arm placed over the second metacarpal is stationary, and the goniometer arm placed over the first metacarpal moves, staying in alignment over the first metacarpal as the thumb moves into radial abduction (Fig. 4.7A).
- To measure palmar abduction, the goniometer arm placed on the radial side of the second metacarpal is stationary, and the goniometer arm placed on the dorsal first metacarpal moves, staying in alignment over the first metacarpal as the thumb moves into palmar abduction (Fig. 4.7B).
- Opposition can be assessed in a number of ways. One source suggests measuring opposition as the distance between the thumb tip and the base of the small finger.[10] Still another suggests having the patient touch the tip of the small finger with the thumb and assessing whether the nail of the thumb is perpendicular to the nail of the small finger and parallel to the plane of the metacarpals.[11] Because there are a number of different ways to assess opposition, it is important to define the method used in the documentation and be consistent when retesting.

Thumb CMC joint ROM testing is difficult to perform consistently because placement of both arms of the goniometer is done using visual judgment of the therapist. Placing the goniometer arms correctly over the first and second metacarpal with the axis at the CMC joint can be difficult, and practice with an experienced therapist is recommended.

Clinical Problem Solving

When ROM of the digits is limited, it is important to determine whether the limited ROM is due to joint stiffness, extrinsic tendon tightness or adhesions, or intrinsic tightness. Perform this type of assessment as soon as active and passive motion is allowed because it dictates the most appropriate type of treatment by determining the limiting structure(s).

Follow these steps:

Step 1: Measure and record composite flexion and composite extension of the digits with the wrist in neutral to slight extension.

Step 2: Compare composite flexion and extension of the fingers with the wrist fully extended and fully flexed (to determine whether extrinsic tendon tightness or adhesions are present).

Step 3: Screen ROM of each finger joint separately with the proximal joints supported in neutral (to determine whether limited motion is isolated to the joint, regardless of the position of the proximal joints).

Step 4: Perform passive motion of the digits. Comparison of passive motion to active motion provides information regarding tendon adhesions that may be limiting active motion.

The following is a description of the causes of finger joint motion limitations in each of the screened positions:

- If AROM of a joint is the same as PROM, and the motion is the same regardless of the position of proximal joints, the limitation is due to joint stiffness.
- If passive flexion is better than active flexion, the limited active flexion is due to weak or paralyzed flexor muscles, or flexor tendon adhesion or rupture.
- If passive extension is better than active extension, the limited active extension is due to weak or paralyzed extensor muscles, extensor tendon adhesion, extensor tendon subluxation, or extensor tendon rupture.
- If active and passive flexion is equal, and flexion is better with the proximal joint(s) in extension than with the proximal joint(s) in flexion, the limited flexion is due to extrinsic extensor tendon tightness or adhesions.
- If active and passive extension is equal and extension is better with the proximal joint(s) in flexion than extension, the limited extension is due to extrinsic flexor tendon tightness or adhesions.
- If the IP joints of the finger can be flexed passively further with the MP joint flexed than when the MP joint is extended, the limitation is due to intrinsic tightness.

Treatment plans can be made accordingly. For example, when limited flexion is due to tight or adherent extensor tendons, treatment should address the extensor tendon length and ability to glide, not the motion at individual joints. This type of situation occurs frequently following an open reduction and internal fixation of a metacarpal fracture with scar tissue adhesions to underlying extensor tendons. My treatment choice would include applying heat over the hand that is placed in a composite flexion position with a wrap that supports the flexed fingers in a comfortable stretch. Following the heat treatment with the tissue in its lengthened position, manual techniques would include massage to the dorsal scar that is adherent to the extensor tendons and ROM exercises emphasizing composite flexion of the fingers distal to the site of adhesion. I would not choose to do joint mobilization or individual joint stretches, or heat to an individual joint. However, if the assessment shows individual joint stiffness, my treatment choice would include joint mobilization (when passive motion is allowed), modalities to the limiting joint structures, as well as AROM and PROM of the individual joint and composite motion to encourage functional use of the injured hand.

Swelling

Swelling of the hand occurs after every surgery or injury to some extent and is the normal response of the body to injury, bringing cells that are important for healing to the injured area. Normal reduction of swelling begins within 2 weeks of the injury or surgery but may take a number of months to complete. Excessive edema or edema that is not decreasing gradually but instead remains in an area longer than 2 weeks can become problematic because it becomes more like gel, interfering with joint and tendon motion and functional use of the hand.

Precaution. *Awareness of edema and assessment of the amount and characteristics of edema present are critical.*

As discussed in Chapter 8, numerous types of swelling occur in the extremity. Inflammatory edema that occurs after injury, surgery, or other insult is initially fluid but over time may become spongy and eventually fibrotic and thus more resistant to methods aimed at reducing the swelling.

Amount of Swelling

The amount of swelling in the hand and wrist is assessed most often using circumferential and volumetric measurements. The characteristics of edema typically are evaluated by observation and palpation.

Volumetric Displacement

Equipment

Volumeter kits available in supply catalogs include a volumeter tank, a collection beaker, and a graduated cylinder for measuring the displaced water. Hand volumeters and arm volumeters are available.

Method

Always use the same level surface for each test. The client's hand must be free of jewelry or other objects. If jewelry cannot be removed, document that fact.

Follow these steps[12]:

Step 1: Fill the volumeter with room-temperature water to the point of overflow, to allow an accurate starting point. Allow excess water to flow out into the collection beaker, and then empty the beaker.

Step 2: Position the hand so that the palm faces the client and the thumb faces the spout of the volumeter. Keep the hand as vertical as possible; avoid contact with sides of volumeter

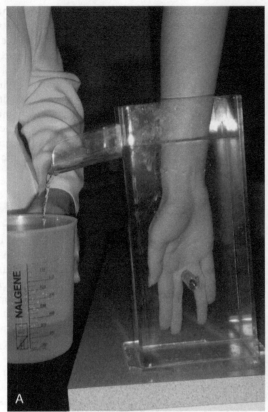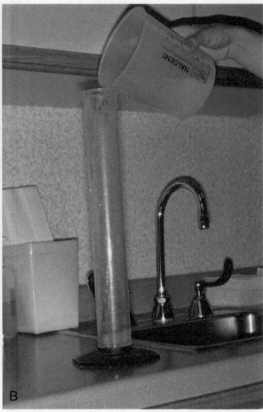

FIG. 4.8 (A) Edema measurement using the volumeter. The water that is displaced by immersion of the hand and distal forearm into the volumeter overflows into a collection beaker. (B) Volumeter measurement is completed when the water from the collection beaker is poured into a graduated cylinder for accurate reading.

(surfaces that are too high prevent the client from placing the arm straight down into the volumeter).

Step 3: Lower the hand slowly into the volumeter until the dowel in the volumeter is firmly seated between the middle and ring fingers. Collect the displaced water in the collection beaker. Hold the hand still in the volumeter until water stops dripping into the beaker (Fig. 4.8A).

Step 4: Pour the displaced water from the collection beaker into the graduated cylinder for final measurement (Fig. 4.8B).

Step 5: Repeat the previous steps if you would like to average results for increased accuracy.

Step 6: Compare the volume to that of the other hand to determine a relative normal for the individual and to determine whether a systemic increase in volume is occurring. The difference between the two extremities is the most valuable information because there is a normal daily variance in volume, even in uninjured extremities. This test has been determined to be accurate to 5 mL, or 1% of the volume of the hand. Therefore a 10-mL difference is considered a significant change from one measurement to the next.[13]

Precaution. *Volumetric measurement should not be performed with open wounds, with an unstable vascular status, casts, external fixators, percutaneous pins, or other nonremovable supports or attachments to the extremity.*

Discussion

To increase reliability of volumetric testing, it has been helpful in my experience to use a waterproof marker to mark the spot on the forearm at the edge of the water when it is lowered into the water on the first trial. When swelling is reduced, it is possible for the hand and forearm to be lowered further into the volumeter because the web space between the fingers that is used as a stopping point against the dowel may deepen as swelling reduces. Thus, there are times when I see a significant decrease in edema of the hand; however, because the forearm is lowering deeper into the volumeter, there is little if any change in the volumetric reading. Ensuring that the hand and forearm are lowered to the same depth on each repeat test minimizes this variable.

Circumferential Measurement

Equipment

Tape measure or tape measure/loop for finger circumference is available from therapy supply sources. When measuring circumference, identify the area being measured in relation to anatomic landmarks, and use the same amount of tension on the tape measure for each test.

Method

Follow these steps:

Step 1: Apply tape measure around area to be measured.

Step 2: Tighten lightly (Fig. 4.9).

Step 3: Record the circumference. Be sure to note exactly where tape was placed, for example 4 cm proximal to radial styloid, around radial styloid and distal ulna, proximal phalanx, or PIP joint. Note positioning, such as elbow flexed or extended, wrist neutral, or fingers relaxed or extended.

Discussion

Consistency of repeat measurements with a tape measure is difficult because the tightness with which the tape measure is applied can vary with each application. Having the same therapist perform repeat measurements can help improve reliability in testing.

Characteristics of Edema

Observation

The skin becomes shiny and tauter with loss of wrinkles or joint creases when there is an increase in swelling. A description of the appearance of the skin should be documented. The evaluation form may have a checklist to choose from a variety of options, such as shiny, dry, and partial or full loss of joint creases. The color of the skin is also helpful to document and can be described as having increased redness (erythema), bluish tinge (cyanosis), or pallor (loss of normal color).

Palpation

Pressure with the examiner's finger into the swollen area may allow an indent into the swelling and may provide feedback as to the firmness of the swelling. If the examiner's finger is able to push into a soft edema fairly quickly, it is characterized as **pitting**

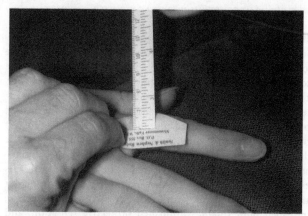

FIG. 4.9 Edema measured using circumferential finger tape available in therapy supply catalogs.

edema. Pitting edema is made up of large amounts of free fluid in the tissue that can be displaced by pressure, leaving a pit that slowly fills back up when the pressure is removed[14] (Fig. 4.10).

As the edema becomes spongier and gel-like, the pit will refill more slowly than fluid edema. As time goes on, if the edema becomes very firm, it will decrease the ability of the fluid to move out of the way with pressure and no longer will be pitting. This type of firmer edema is called **brawny edema**. Brawny edema is usually caused by the interstitial fluid becoming clogged, preventing it from moving easily.[12] The terms *mild, moderate,* and *severe* can be used to quantify the extent of the pitting or brawny characteristic; however, this is a subjective observation made by the examiner.

Sensation

Static Two-Point Discrimination

The static two-point discrimination test measures **innervation density** (the number of nerve endings present in the area tested). Flexor zones I and II are tested (the area between the distal palmar crease and the fingertips). Two-point discrimination determines the ability to discern the difference between one and two points and relates to clients' ability to determine not only *if* they can feel something but also *what* they are feeling.

Equipment

The devices used for this test are the Disk-Criminator or the Boley gauge, which are available in therapy supply catalogs.

Method

Follow these steps[15,16]:

Step 1: Instruct the client to respond to each touch, with vision occluded, by saying "one point" or "two points."

Step 2: Support the client's hand to avoid movement of fingers when touched by the point(s). Putty commonly is used as a support for the fingers.

Step 3: Occlude the client's vision. Begin at 5 mm. Touch the client's fingertip with one or two points, randomly applied (Fig. 4.11).

Step 4: The force of the touch pressure is just to the point of blanching, in a longitudinal direction to avoid crossing digital nerve innervation in the finger, perpendicular to the skin.

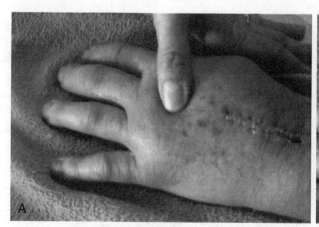
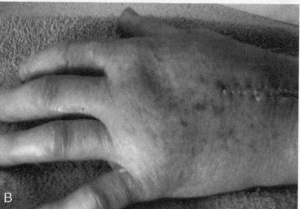

FIG. 4.10 (A) and (B) Pitting edema is seen when pressure from the examiner's finger leaves an indent, or "pit," when removed.

Step 5: Increase or decrease the distance between the two points. If the client is unable to discriminate two points correctly at 5 mm, increase the distance between the points. If the client is able to discriminate two points correctly at 5 mm, decrease the distance, and continue until you have determined the smallest distance the client can discriminate as two points.

Step 6: Begin distally and work proximally from fingertips to distal palmar crease.

Discussion

Seven out of 10 correct responses in one area are required to establish a reliable "correct response" score. Box 4.2 describes two-point discrimination scoring.

Moving Two-Point Discrimination

According to Dellon,[17] moving two-point discrimination always returns earlier than static two-point discrimination after nerve laceration, and it approaches normal 2–6 months before static two-point discrimination. This test is used to determine progress in return of sensation following nerve injury.

Equipment

The device used for this test is the Disk-Criminator, or Boley gauge.

Method

Follow these steps[17]:
Step 1: Describe the test to the client.
Step 2: Fully support the client's hand.

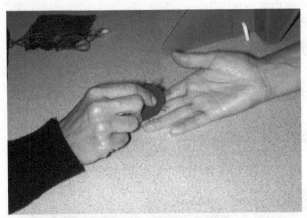

FIG. 4.11 Two-point discrimination test is performed with the points placed longitudinally onto the skin of the fingertips with pressure just to the point of blanching.

BOX 4.2   Static Two-Point Discrimination Scoring[15,16]

1–5 mm = Normal
6–10 mm = Fair
11–15 mm = Poor
One point perceived = Protective sensation only
No points perceived = Anesthetic

Step 3: Occlude the client's vision.

Step 4: Instruct the client to respond with either "one" or "two" to the stimulus provided.

Step 5: Application is from proximal to distal on the volar distal phalanx of the fingertip. The points are longitudinal to the axis of the finger and are placed perpendicular to the skin. Move the points along the fingertip only, from proximal to distal. Speed has not been addressed.

Step 6: Begin with a distance of 5–8 mm and increase or decrease as needed.

Step 7: Lift the points off the tip of the finger. Do not allow the points to come off the tip of the finger separately because this gives the client information that it was two points.

Discussion

Seven out of 10 correct responses are needed for an accurate response. Two millimeters is considered normal moving two-point discrimination. A common error is to press too hard during the testing process, and inconsistency in amount of pressure placed on the device and skin is the main problem with reliability of this test.

Touch/Pressure Threshold Test (Semmes-Weinstein Monofilament Test)

This test determines light touch thresholds. The test is effective in identifying impairments in nerve compression injuries.

Equipment

The Semmes-Weinstein Pressure Aesthesiometer Kit is available in catalogs with 5 or 20 monofilaments. The monofilaments are color-coded, with green monofilaments indicating light touch within normal limits, blue monofilaments indicating diminished light touch, purple monofilaments indicating diminished protective sensation, and red monofilaments indicating loss of protective sensation. If only the largest monofilament is felt, it indicates deep pressure sensation only; and if the largest monofilament is not felt, it indicates that light touch sensation is "untestable" (Table 4.1).[15] The five-monofilament screening kit contains the largest monofilament in the categories of normal, diminished light touch, diminished protective sensation, and the smallest and largest monofilament in the loss of protective sensation category.

TABLE 4.1	Semmes-Weinstein Monofilament Categories/Scoring[15]	
Color Code	**Definition**	**Monofilament Size Range**
Green	Normal light touch threshold	1.65 to 2.83
Blue	Diminished light touch	3.22 to 3.61
Purple	Diminished protective sensation	3.84 to 4.31
Red	Loss of protective sensation	4.56 to 6.65
Untestable	Unable to feel largest monofilament	—

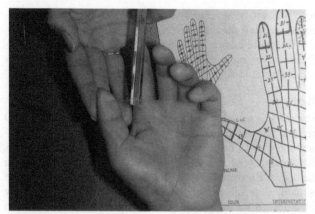

FIG. 4.12 Semmes-Weinstein monofilament test measures touch force threshold.

Method

Follow these steps[15]:

Step 1: Describe the test to the client.

Step 2: Support the client's hand on a rolled towel to prevent the fingers from moving with the touch.

Step 3: Occlude the client's vision with a screen or folder.

Step 4: Instruct the client to respond with "touch" each time a touch is felt.

Step 5: Begin with the largest monofilament in the normal category (2.83). Proceed to larger monofilaments if there is no response.

Step 6: For the smaller monofilaments, sizes 1.65 to 4.08 (green and blue categories), the filament needs to be applied for three trials. One correct response to the three trials is considered a correct response. All larger monofilaments are applied only one time for each trial.

Step 7: Begin testing distally and move proximally.

Step 8: Apply the monofilament perpendicular to the skin until the monofilament bends. Apply it slowly (1–1.5 seconds) to the skin, hold for 1 to 1.5 seconds, and then lift slowly (1–1.5 seconds) (Fig. 4.12).

Step 9: Record on a hand map the monofilament size that the client correctly perceives.

Localization of Light Touch

The localization of light touch test is used to determine functional ability to locate touch on the hand.[15] The ability to localize light touch returns after light touch threshold and impairment can cause significant problems following a nerve repair.

Equipment

The equipment needed is the Semmes-Weinstein monofilament (the smallest monofilament to be determined intact on threshold testing described previously). If monofilaments are not available, a cotton ball or pencil eraser has been used. It is important to use the same item for retests.

Method

Follow these steps:

Step 1: Describe the test to the client. The client is to open his or her eyes and point to the location the touch was felt after the stimulus is given.

Step 2: Provide a light touch stimulus to an area. Place a dot on the hand map where the stimulus was placed.

Step 3: Following the client's response, if touch is felt in another place than given, draw an arrow pointing to the location the client felt touch from the location given. If the client did feel touch where given, draw the dot alone.

Additional Tests

Additional tests for assessing sensation are the following[15]:

- *Ninhydrin test*: Used to evaluate sudomotor or sympathetic nervous system function. It does not require a voluntary response from the client and therefore can be used for children or individuals with cognitive impairments. Ninhydrin spray is a clear agent that turns purple when it reacts with a small concentration of sweat. The individual's hand is cleansed and air dried for at least 5 minutes. The fingertips are then placed on bond paper for 15 seconds and traced. The paper is sprayed with the ninhydrin spray reagent and dried according to directions. The prints are then sprayed with the ninhydrin fixer reagent, and areas where sweat is present will appear as dots. The test identifies areas of distribution of sweat secretion after recent complete peripheral nerve lesions. No sweat will be present in a particular nerve's innervation area after a complete nerve laceration.

- *O'Riain wrinkle test*: Used to evaluate sympathetic nervous system function or recovery following a complete nerve lesion. Denervated palmar skin does not wrinkle when soaked in 42°C (108°F) water for 20 to 30 minutes, as normal skin will.

- *Vibration*: Used to determine frequency response of mechanoreceptor end organs. Tuning forks of 30 and 256 cps are most frequently used. It has been noted that there is currently no equipment that controls for force and technique.[15]

- *Moberg's pick-up test*: Used to determine tactile gnosis, or functional discrimination. Using specific small objects, the client picks the objects up with each hand and is timed with vision and without vision. The time to place the objects in the box with and without vision is recorded, and the quality of movement and use or disuse of specific digits is observed.

Discussion

Although it is helpful to be aware of the battery of sensory evaluations described, a standard screening of sensation is limited to one or two assessments. I recommend use of the Semmes-Weinstein monofilaments for nerve compressions (such as carpal tunnel or cubital tunnel syndrome), and monofilaments, two-point discrimination testing, and functional test (such as Moberg pickup test) following a nerve injury or laceration. Following a nerve laceration, touch threshold (Semmes-Weinstein monofilaments) will show an improvement before the ability to discriminate touch (two-point discrimination).

Coordination

Coordination is the ability to manipulate items in the environment. This ranges from gross coordination to fine coordination tasks. A large number of standardized coordination tests are available with methodology available for each test. Standardized coordination tests include O'Connor Dexterity Test, Nine-Hole

Peg Test, Jebsen-Taylor Hand Function Test, Minnesota Rate of Manipulation Test, Crawford Small Parts Dexterity Test, and the Purdue Pegboard Test.[18] A simple test for a quick screening of coordination is the Nine-Hole Peg Test.[18,19] This test is standardized yet allows use of a commercially available or low-cost homemade board and pegs. The Jebsen-Taylor Hand Function Test assesses functional tasks, such as writing, as well as the ability to manipulate large and small items.[18,20] The methodology is available with each test and will not be specified in this chapter because of the number of tests available. Use of a standardized test is helpful for clients whose injuries affect their coordination due to weakness, pain or nerve injury.

Strength Testing

Grip and Pinch Strength Testing

Grip and pinch strength testing is the standard method used for decades to determine functional grasp and pinch strength. The tests are used initially and in periodic retests to demonstrate improvement in hand strength. Contraindications are noted in the following discussion.

Contraindications

Do not perform these tests when resistance has not yet been approved by the referring physician. Grip and pinch strength testing are maximally resistive tests. Testing is contraindicated before full healing following a fracture, ligament repair, tendon laceration, or tendon transfer of the forearm, wrist, or hand, or as determined by the referring physician.

Precaution. *An acute joint, ligament, or tendon injury or sprain of a digital joint or wrist are contraindications for maximal grip or pinch strength testing until resistive exercises are appropriate.*

For any traumatic injury, I defer testing of grip or pinch strength until resistive exercises or strengthening have been approved by the referring physician. For a gradual-onset condition or injury (such as tendinopathy or carpal tunnel syndrome), I will test strength at the time of initial evaluation, even though my initial treatment plan may not include strengthening until the level of pain decreases. At the time of initial evaluation for this type of condition, I modify the instructions and tell the client to stop grasping when mild pain occurs to prevent an increase in pain following use of the test, and I document when pain does occur with the test. Determination of initial grip and pinch strength for tendinopathy or nerve compressions is important to determine future progress.

Clinical Pearl

Before performing strength testing, always ask yourself whether there are any healing tissues that can be damaged by this test.

Grip Strength Test

Equipment

To assess grip strength, the Jamar dynamometer is recommended by the American Society for Surgery of the Hand and the American Society of Hand Therapists.[18,21] The test has been determined to be accurate and reliable. Annual calibration is recommended and should be done more often in high-use settings. Do not ignore calibration. Pinch meters are commercially available; however, no one specific type is endorsed by the aforementioned associations.

Method

The client is seated with shoulder adducted, elbow flexed to 90 degrees, forearm neutral, and wrist in 15 to 30 degrees of extension and 0 to 15 degrees of ulnar deviation. The therapist places the dynamometer in the client's hand while gently supporting the base of the dynamometer, and instructs the client to squeeze as hard as possible. Grip force should be applied smoothly for at least 3 seconds, with at least 15 seconds of rest between repetitions.[18,21]

Consider the following:
- *Standard grip test*: Three trials on the second handle-width setting. Use the average as the test result.
- *Five-level grip test*: One trial on each of the five handle-width settings. This test is used to determine a bell curve when graphed. The strongest grip is almost always on the second or third handle-width setting. The weakest grips normally occur at the most narrow and widest settings, with scores on the middle three handle settings falling between the strongest and weakest scores, assimilating a bell curve. When the five handle setting scores show a flat line when graphed (readings at all handle settings are almost the same) or when there is an up/down-up/down type of curve, it is possible your client did not provide maximal effort during testing.
- *Rapid-exchange grip test*: The examiner rapidly moves the dynamometer, alternating from the client's right to left hands, for 10 trials to each hand. This test had been thought to prevent voluntary control of grip strength by the client, making it more difficult for a client to self-limit the grip response or provide less than maximal effort.[22] More recently, Shechtman and colleagues[21,23-25] have articulated well-founded concerns about the methods with which clinicians interpret sincerity of effort during grip testing. Their work provides some thought-provoking findings on the topic.

Discussion

Normative data exists for grip and pinch strength testing.[26] In addition, comparison to the client's opposite, uninjured extremity provides individualized normative information.

Pinch Strength Test

Equipment

The device used is the pinch gauge (styles vary).

Method

With the client seated, elbow flexed to 90 degrees with arm adducted at side, and forearm neutral, proceed as follows[18]:
- *Lateral pinch (key pinch)*: Place the pinch meter between the radial side of index finger and thumb and instruct the client to pinch as hard as possible.
- *Three-point pinch (three jaw chuck pinch)*: Place the pinch meter between the pulp of the thumb and pulp of the index and middle fingers. Instruct the client to pinch as hard as possible.

- *Two-point pinch (tip-to-tip pinch)*: Place the pinch meter between the tip of the thumb and tip of the index finger and instruct the client to pinch as hard as possible.

Discussion

Repeat each test three times and calculate an average. Calibrate equipment at least annually.

Manual Muscle Testing

It is essential to test manual muscle strength and document for improvement when there is weakness related to a nerve injury or compression. Identifying the strength of various muscles along a specific nerve distribution helps determine the level of nerve injury and improvement over time. Measurement of manual muscle strength also is helpful in order to document improvement when weakness is present because of disuse, such as after prolonged immobilization.

Equipment

Manual muscle testing is a form of strength testing that measures the client's ability to move the body part being tested against gravity and, if able to move fully against gravity, to maintain the position against the examiner's resistance. Thus the only equipment needed is a reference book and a form on which to record the results.

Method

Manual muscle testing is performed according to methods documented in numerous sources. Strength is graded according to normal, good, fair, poor, and trace strength definitions—with fair strength defined as the ability to move the body part through its full available range against gravity, although not able to tolerate any additional resistance. Also acceptable is a number grading system where 5 corresponds to normal, 4 to good, 3 to fair, 2 to poor and 1 to trace strength. Description of the method of applying resistance to each muscle of the hand, wrist, and forearm is beyond the scope of this chapter. An excellent reference for specific testing procedures for each muscle is found in *Muscles: Testing and Function* by Kendall et al.[27] I recommend use of a form designed for manual muscle testing with the muscles listed in relation to their nerve innervation, as described in this reference.

Discussion

Manual muscle testing is contraindicated in the same situations as for grip and pinch strength testing, or when pain prevents full effort by the client. Because manual muscle testing is a maximally resistive test, any injury with healing tissues (bone, ligament, and tendon) that could be reinjured should not be tested until determined to be safe by the referring physician or the appropriate time after surgery allows resistance.

Precaution. *Finger or thumb tendon repairs are not sufficiently strong to test until 14 weeks after surgery.*

Use of Orthoses

Many clients have obtained their own orthoses or have been given a prefabricated orthotic by their physicians. Determine the use of any orthoses and the amount of time and activities during which they are worn. This information is helpful in determining the client's functional limitations and allows you to offer insight into the appropriate use of orthoses for the client's condition.

Functional Ability

Functional ability is an area that should be assessed as part of every evaluation. This portion of the evaluation is important for determining functional goals with the client and for documenting those goals for the insurance company. Determining difficulty in daily activities helps you set goals in conjunction with your clients' needs and gives clients confidence that you are working together toward common and meaningful goals. Following documentation of the status of pain, wounds/scars, ROM, sensation, and strength, the functional ability statement becomes a reflection of the way that the previously noted deficits affect the client's daily life.

Equipment

Use of a client self-report outcome measure is recommended. Please see Chapter 5 for specific information about appropriate measures. A checklist to help clients think of areas in which they are successful or in which they have difficulty is also helpful. Categories such as self-care skills, meal preparation, home management (outdoor and indoor), and vocational tasks can be included (Appendix 4.1).

Method

Functional use of the affected extremity is assessed through discussion with the client, simulation of activities, and/or completion of a self-report outcome measure. A client with an injured hypersensitive finger may have difficulty with fine motor coordination. In this case, specific tasks such as writing, buttoning clothes, and tying shoes may be limited. At the opposite end of the spectrum, an extremity may be almost completely nonfunctional because of the presence of a cast, limitations due to injury, or restrictions following recent surgery. In these cases, it is impossible to list all the functional tasks that are limited, and it may be more appropriate to report the limitations as, "Unable to use the right upper extremity for any functional tasks other than support of a light object using the forearm."

In some situations, time limitations may preclude an in-depth assessment of all areas of the upper extremity in one session. A screening of some sections may be done with a full assessment deferred to the next session. For instance, I may screen the area of sensation by asking about the client's sensation and may defer monofilament or two-point discrimination testing to the next visit.

Summary

Awareness of the areas to include in a thorough evaluation is enhanced by use of an evaluation summary form (see Appendix 4.1), which facilitates the logical progression through the steps of the evaluation.

Precaution. *Awareness of situations in which it is unsafe to perform certain assessments is essential.*

Much evaluation is done by observation. Effectiveness as a therapist is enhanced when the therapist takes the time to communicate well with a new client during the evaluation. This occurs not only by describing the process of the assessments but also by listening as the client attempts to communicate verbally and nonverbally. The information gained during the assessment process is the foundation on which the treatment plan rests. Likewise, the connection between the therapist and each new client is the foundation on which the client's confidence in the therapeutic process rests. Both are equally important.

References

1. Fedorczyk JM: Pain management: principles of therapist's intervention. In Skirven TM, Osterman AL, Fedorczyk JM, editors: *Rehabilitation of the hand and upper extremity*, ed 6, Philadelphia, PA, 2011, Elsevier Mosby, pp 1461–1470.
2. Walton D: Pain. In *Clinical assessment recommendations*, ed 3, American Society of Hand Therapists, 2015, pp 47–70.
3. Cuzzell JZ: The new red yellow black color code, *Am J Nurs* 88(10):1342–1346, 1988.
4. von der Heyde RL, Evans RB: Wound classification and management. In Skirven TM, Osterman AL, Fedorczyk JM, editors: *Rehabilitation of the hand and upper extremity*, ed 6, Philadelphia, PA, 2011, Elsevier Mosby, pp 219–232.
5. Seiler III JG: *Physical examination of the hand. Essentials of hand surgery. American society for surgery of the hand*, Philadelphia, PA, 2002, Lippincott Williams & Wilkins, pp 23–48.
6. Taras JS, Lemel MS, Nathan R: Vascular disorders of the upper extremity. In Mackin EJ, Callahan AD, Skirven TM, editors: *Rehabilitation of the hand and upper extremity*, ed 5, St. Louis, MO, 2002, Mosby, pp 879–898.
7. Drudi L, MacKenzie K. Differential diagnosis of upper extremity ischemia. In: Dieter R, Dieter Jr. R, Dieter III R, Nanjundappa A, eds. *Critical limb ischemia*. Cham, 2017, Springer International Publishing Switzerland, pp 79-93.
8. Hay D, Taras JS, Yao J: Vascular disorders of the upper extremity. In Skirven TM, Osterman AL, Fedorczyk JM, editors: *Rehabilitation of the hand and upper extremity*, ed 6, Philadelphia, PA, 2011, Elsevier Mosby, pp 825–844.
9. Gibson G: Goniometry. In *Clinical assessment recommendations*, American Society of Hand Therapists, 2015, pp 71–80.
10. Seftchick JL, Detullio LM, Fedorczyk JM, et al.: Clinical examination of the hand. In Skirven TM, Osterman AL, Fedorczyk JM, editors: *Rehabilitation of the hand and upper extremity*, ed 6, Philadelphia, PA, 2011, Elsevier Mosby, pp 55–71.
11. Berryman Reese N, Bandy WD: *Joint range of motion and muscle length testing*, ed 3, St Louis, MO, 2017, Elsevier.
12. Villeco JP: Edema: therapist's management. In Skirven TM, Osterman AL, Fedorczyk JM, editors: *Rehabilitation of the hand and upper extremity*, ed 6, Philadelphia, PA, 2011, Elsevier Mosby, pp 845–857.
13. Waylett-Rendall J, Seibly D: A study of the accuracy of a commercially available volumeter, *J Hand Ther* 4(1):10–13, 1991.
14. Colditz JC: Therapist's management of the stiff hand. In Skirven TM, Osterman AL, Fedorczyk JM, editors: *Rehabilitation of the hand and upper extremity*, ed 6, Philadelphia, PA, 2011, Elsevier Mosby.
15. Bell Krotoski JA: Sensibility testing: history, instrumentation, and clinical procedures. In Skirven TM, Osterman AL, Fedorczyk JM, editors: *Rehabilitation of the hand and upper extremity*, ed 6, Philadelphia, PA, 2011, Elsevier Mosby, pp 894–921.
16. Dellon AL, Mackinnon SE, Crosby PM: Reliability of two-point discrimination measurements, *J Hand Surg Am* 12(5 Pt 1):693–696, 1987.
17. Dellon AL: The moving two-point discrimination test: clinical evaluation of the quickly adapting fiber/receptor system, *J Hand Surg* 3:474–481, 1978.
18. Fess EE: Functional tests. In Skirven TM, Osterman AL, Fedorczyk JM, editors: *Rehabilitation of the hand and upper extremity*, ed 6, Philadelphia, PA, 2011, Elsevier Mosby.
19. Mathiowetz V, Volland G, Kashman N, et al.: Adult norms for the nine-hole peg test of finger dexterity, *Am J Occup Ther* 39(6):386–391, 1985.
20. Jebsen RH, Taylor N, Trieschmann RB, et al.: An objective and standardized test of hand function, *Arch Phys Med Rehabil* 50(6):311–319, 1969.
21. Schectman O, Sindhu BS: Grip assessment. In *Clinical assessment recommendations*, American Society of Hand Therapists, 2015, pp 1–8.
22. Hildreth DH, Breidenbach WC, Lister GD, et al.: Detection of submaximal effort by use of the rapid exchange grip, *J Hand Surg Am* 14(4):742–745, 1989.
23. Shechtman O: Using the coefficient of variation to detect sincerity of effort of grip strength: a literature review, *J Hand Ther* 13:25–32, 2000.
24. Taylor C, Shechtman O: The use of rapid exchange grip test in detecting sincerity of effort, part I: administration of the test, *J Hand Ther* 13(3):195–202, 2000.
25. Shechtman O, Taylor C: The use of rapid exchange grip test in detecting sincerity of effort, part II: validity of the test, *J Hand Ther* 13(3):202–210, 2000.
26. Mathiowetz V, Kashman N, Volland G, et al.: Grip and pinch strength: normative data for adults, *Arch Phys Med Rehabil* 66(2):69–74, 1985.
27. Kendall FP, McCreary EK, Provance PG, et al.: *Muscles testing and function with posture and pain*, ed 5, Baltimore, MD, 2005, Lippincott Williams & Wilkins.

Evaluation Summary Form

History of Injury/Condition _____

_____

Pertinent Medical History: _____

Pain Level   0 – 1 – 2 – 3 – 4 – 5 – 6 – 7 – 8 – 9 – 10   At best____Worst____
                    (mild)   (intolerable)
Description (Circle all that apply):
   Sore   Aching   Throbbing   Burning   Sharp   Stabbing   Radiating
Location: _____
Frequency: Intermittent (Occasional   Frequent) / Constant
         At rest   With use   With exercise   Other_____

Scar   Location:_____
    Raised/Flattened   Color:_____
Adhesions (circle one):   Adherent   Partially adherent   Non-adherent

Wound (circle one):   Closed   Eschar   Sutured   Open
Wound color: Red   Yellow   Black   Combination   Size:_____
Location: _____
Drainage Amount and Color: _____

Vascular Status   Color (circle one):   Normal/Pink/Red/Blue/White/Mottled
Trophic: Normal   Dry/Moist   Shiny/Dull   Location: _____
Peripheral Pulse Strength/Quality: Right _____ Left _____
Capillary Refill Time: _____ Location: _____
Allen'sTest: _____
Surface Temperature: Location/Degrees _____
Fingertip Pulp Changes: Narrowing/Thickened/Other: _____

Fixation Devices   Pins (Internal/Protrude through skin) _____
Screw(s) _____ Plate _____
External Fixation _____ Other _____

Use of Orthotics (Describe Orthotic and Times of Use) _____

<u>**Swelling**</u>

<u>Visual Inspection</u> (circle one)
Not significant
Mild
Moderate
Moderate +
Severe

<u>Volumetric Measurements</u>
Injured hand: _____ mL
Noninjured hand: _____ mL
Difference: _____ mL

<u>Pitting/Brawny</u> Location: _____

<u>**Circumferential Measurements (cm)**</u>

	Right	Left
Forearm (Location_____)		
Hand (MCP)		
Wrist		
Digit (Circle)	Thumb IF MF RF SF	Thumb IF MF RF SF
Proximal Phalanx		
PIP joint		
Middle Phalanx		
DIP joint		

<u>**Range of Motion**</u>

		Right	Left			Right	Left
Shoulder	Flexion			**Index Finger**	MP		
	Extension				PIP		
	Ext Rot				DIP		
	Int Rot			**Middle Finger**	MP		
Elbow	Flexion				PIP		
	Extension				DIP		
Forearm	Supination			**Ring Finger**	MP		
	Pronation				PIP		
Wrist	Extension				DIP		
	Flexion			**Small Finger**	MP		
	Radial Dev				PIP		
	Ulnar Dev				DIP		
Thumb MP				**Thumb CMC**	Radial Abd		
Thumb IP					Palmar Abd		

Sensation

Circle One: Intact   Hypersensitive   Tingling   Numb   Frequency: Intermittent/Constant

Occurrences: With use / At rest / Prolonged position / Repetitive use / At night

Semmes-Weinstein monofilament / Two-point discrimination / Other (see separate forms)

STRENGTH	Right	Left
Grip		
Lateral pinch		
2 point pinch		
3 point pinch		

Five-level or rapid exchange grip if indicated—see separate form

Manual muscle test if indicated—see separate form

Coordination

Observation: _____

Test Results (see separate form)

Functional Use   Patient has difficulty with the following (circle all that apply):

Self-Care	*Home Management*
Dressing	Washing dishes
Fasteners	Mealpreparation
Eating	Laundry
Bathing	Openingcontainers
Hygiene	Cleaning—light
Hair care	Cleaning—heavy (floors, tub)
Other	Lawn/outdoor maintenance
Driving/starting vehicle	Grocery shopping
Opening doors	Computer use
Writing	

Vocational (Describe)   *Avocational* (Describe)

Computer use,   Hobbies, gardening

assembly, heavy lifting

Other_____   Other_____

5 Assessment of Functional Outcomes

Bridget Hill
Andrea Bialocerkowski

Selecting an appropriate outcome measure is extremely challenging but central to evidence-based practice. An appropriate outcome measure is essential to monitor client progress, aid in clinical decision making, and evaluate the effectiveness of treatment, but how do we decide when a measure is appropriate or right for our measurement purposes? The renowned physicist William Thomson, better known as Lord Kelvin, once said, '*When you can measure what you are speaking about, and express it in numbers, you know something about it; but when you cannot measure it, when you cannot express it in numbers, your knowledge is of a meagre and unsatisfactory kind.*'[1] It is relatively simple to use a measuring device such as a dynamometer to assign a number to grip strength, or a goniometer to measure joint range of motion in degrees. These types of devices produce scores that can be objectively evaluated,[2] but can we assign a score to less tangible constructs such as day-to-day use of the arm or a client's participation in society? And if this is possible, how do we ensure that the outcome measure is appropriate to quantify these complex constructs?

Choosing an outcome measure to assess day-to-day use of the arm is complicated for a variety of reasons. First, there are many different types of outcome measures, each having different measurement properties and demands on the client and the clinician. Second, the arm works in different ways throughout the day. We use the arm to stabilize, reach, grasp, and manipulate objects when performing basic life tasks.[3] In addition, each arm or hand is used in a variety of different ways for any given activity.[4] Activities may be bimanual or unimanual. To perform bimanual activities, the two arms frequently adopt different roles: (a) the arms and hands may work symmetrically, as when carrying a tray or pushing an object with both hands; (b) the arms and hands may work asymmetrically but cooperatively, as when pouring water from a jug to a glass; or (c) the arms and hands may perform very separate diverse activities, as when holding a bag while opening a door.[5] Further, the dominant hand is used more often while the nondominant arm and hand usually performs an orientation or stabilizing role when the two arms work collaboratively.[5]

For these reasons, the impact of an injury may vary dependent on whether it involves the dominant or nondominant arm. Evidence suggests that those with severe injury or long-term disability may change their hand dominance over time or live primarily with the use of only one arm.[6,7] As a result, people with severe long-term injuries can become so proficient at using compensatory techniques that they rate themselves as being the same or less disabled as somebody with far less severe functional loss.[8] For example, Baltzer et al. demonstrated that unilateral arm amputees reported similar levels of disability to people with Dupuytren's contracture, thumb osteoarthritis, or finger amputation when assessed by the Disability of the Arm, Shoulder and Hand (DASH).[9] By the very nature of these disparate conditions, greater disability would be expected in the amputee group. However, while the DASH is a patient-reported outcome measure that evaluates function and disability, it does not differentiate between the use of the affected or unaffected arm. It is therefore more likely assessing compensation for people with severe long-term injury.[8]

At times it can be useful to know how people manage day to day by whatever strategies they normally use. However, results that assess change over time from outcome measures that do not attribute responses to the affected arm cannot be attributed to an intervention directed specifically at the injury.[7,10] Moreover, it is biologically plausible that a person can make significant functional improvements by learning to write or becoming adept at washing their hair with the preinjury nondominant hand while avoiding using the injured arm entirely.

All these factors mean that assessment of the arm requires a range of tools that target different aspects of arm use. The clinician must have a clear understanding of what it is they wish to assess, some knowledge of psychometric properties of outcome measures, and a wide range of outcome measures to choose from in order to select the appropriate one for their needs. This chapter provides information to address this fundamental knowledge required by hand therapists.

International Classification of Functioning Disability and Health

To clearly define the variable being assessed, outcome measures must be based on a conceptual framework that underpins the relationship between the items contained in an outcome measure and the concepts measured.[11] One framework regularly used to underpin the development of new outcome measures and to classify existing ones is the International Classification of Functioning Disability and Health (ICF).[12] Based on a biopsychosocial model, the ICF identifies three levels of human functioning:

1. Level of the body and body parts (i.e., body functions and body structures including body systems and anatomical parts of the body). Impairments are problems with body functions or body structures
2. Level of the whole person (i.e., activity or the execution of a task or action by an individual). Activity limitations are difficulties a person may have in executing activities
3. Level of the whole person in a social context (i.e., participation). Participation restrictions are problems an individual may experience in real-life situations

Historically, health care professionals, including hand therapists, have used measures of body function, in particular strength, sensation, and range of motion, to monitor client outcomes and to evaluate the effectiveness of interventions (i.e., level 1 functioning). There is, however, growing evidence that impairment variables are not accurate in predicting how an individual may use their arm and hand to perform day-to-day activities.[13-17] Therefore it is important to measure outcomes in terms of activities and participation.

Two qualifiers are used to classify information about activities and participation [12]:

- The "performance" qualifier describes what a person does in their day-to-day environment, including the social context or lived experience. Performance qualifiers reflect how the person manages in their own environment using multiple strategies including compensatory techniques or assistive devices, and reflects the barriers that influence day-to-day life. They are reported directly by the person, usually via patient-reported outcome measures or goal-setting tools.
- The "capacity" qualifier describes the ability of a person to execute a task or action in a standardized environment, at one time point. This usually occurs outside their lived experience, in a clinical setting, and without the use of compensation or assistive devices. This means that the capacity qualifier identifies the highest level of function possible without environmental adaptation. Outcome measures that quantify capacity usually involve the performance of specific tasks that are observed and rated by a clinician (e.g., the Jebsen Test of Hand Function[18] or the Box and Block[19]).

The gap between capacity and performance provides an indication of environmental barriers that may limit a person's function.[12]

Performance outcomes are increasingly being recognized as pivotal to understanding the impact of an injury on an individual and have a direct influence on the clinical decision-making process.[20,21] Unlike timed or observer-rated measures completed in an artificial setting that may or may not be translated to the day-to-day lived experience, patient-reported outcomes reflect change in a patient-centered model of health care delivery.

The ICF consist of over 1400 different items.[12] To make it more applicable for daily use by clinicians, core sets of items have been developed as a guide to the variables that should be measured for various diagnoses. To describe functioning in people with hand conditions, there are two core sets—the Comprehensive (CCS-HC)[22,23] and Brief Core Set (BCS-HC).[24] Both contain ICF categories from all ICF components. New outcome measures have been developed based on the CCS-HC, such as the Brachial Assessment Tool (BrAT),[25] or existing ones can be linked to the core sets, for example the DASH.[26,27] Linking items in outcome measures to the appropriate core set facilitates direct comparison with other outcome measures,[26,28] as well as analyses of whether the items cover the full scope of day-to-day activities and roles.

Patient-Reported Outcome Measures

As noted above, patient-reported outcomes are increasingly being accepted as key to a client-centered approach. Large clinical trials now use patient-reported outcome measures as the primary outcome to determine treatment effectiveness.[11,20,29,30] Some funding bodies have mandated their use.[31]

Tools designed to assess a patient-reported outcome are called patient-reported outcome measures.[11] Many have been designed to cover a wide range of variables that directly impact the individual. Patient-reported outcome measures may be specific to one diagnosis and contain items that relate only to that condition. In contrast, joint- or region-specific measures can be used for a range of diagnoses confined to one joint or region of the body, such as the arm. Finally, generic measures such as those that address health-related quality of life are appropriate to use for people with a wide array of diagnoses including neurological, orthopedic, or cardiorespiratory conditions.[32] Outcome measures may be unidimensional, assessing only one construct, or multidimensional, with a number of modules designed to assess many aspects of health in one measure.

Choosing an Outcome Measure

Choosing a measure from the vast array of possibilities can seem daunting. For example, Roe and Østensjø[33] linked 17 shoulder-specific questionnaires to the ICF. However, a systematic approach should be used, and there are a wide variety of resources available to assist clinicians. There are four steps to selecting an appropriate outcome measure[32,34]:

1. Determine the clinical or research requirements. Define what it is you wish to measure. Determine the type of outcome measure you wish to use (i.e., region specific versus disease specific versus joint specific).
2. Source a measure that is based on a sound framework and underlying construct that aligns with your requirements.

3. Look for evidence of the measure's reproducibility, validity, and responsiveness to change for your diagnostic group.
4. Investigate the burden of assessment on all stakeholders (i.e., is the measure expensive to use, does it take a long time to complete or score, etc.?).[34]

Region-Specific Patient-Reported Outcome Measures

Region-specific patient-reported outcome measures are designed for use with a wide range of diagnoses, injury severity, and interventions.[32] A number have been designed specifically for the upper limb. Information regarding these outcome measures has been summarized and tabulated in Table 5.1; however, it should

be noted that research on the psychometric properties of these measures is continuously evolving and is not detailed in this chapter.

The Disabilities of the Arm Shoulder and Hand (DASH).[9]

The DASH is the most widely used and studied upper limb outcome measure.[35,36] It was developed in the early 1990s to quantify physical function and symptoms in people with a cross section of upper extremity disorders. It conceptualizes the upper limb as a single working unit.[37] The 30 items in the DASH have been linked to 63 ICF categories from all levels of functioning, except body structure and environment.[27,38] It assesses six domains: daily activities, symptoms, social function, pain, sleep,

TABLE 5.1	Summary of Outcome Measure Properties						
Measure	Number of Items	Item Generation / Reduction	Type of Response	Dimensions	Translated	Scoring	Recall Period
DASH	30 plus 8 items specific to work and sport / music	Items from 13 existing scales, expert opinion and pretesting with 20 patients	5-point scale	Multidimensional	Multiple languages	Higher score = greater disability	1 week
Quick DASH	11 plus 8 items specific to work and sport/music	Reduction of original DASH items	5-point scale	Multidimensional	Multiple languages	Higher score = greater disability	1 week
M²DASH	18 items	Reduction of original DASH items	5-point scale	Multidimensional	Unknown	Higher score = greater disability	1 week
UEFI	20 items	Items from existing measures, 40 patient self-reported scales and expert opinion	5-point scale	Activity limitations Participation restrictions	No	Higher score = better function	Today
ULFI	25 items plus 5 patient specific activities & a VAS of patient status	Items from 71 existing PROM Reduced by specificity to the UL or HRQOL, peer and patient	3-point categorical response	Multidimensional	Multiple languages	Higher score = greater disability	Last few days
CTQ	11 items symptom specific scale 8 item functional status scale	Panel of experts including surgeons rheumatologists and patients	5-point scale	2 separate modules not added	Multiple languages	Higher score = greater disability	24- hour period in the last 2 weeks
WORC	21 items in 5 modules	Items from existing outcome measures, 30 people with RCD and experts	VAS 100 mm long	Multidimensional	Multiple languages	Higher score = greater disability	1 week
ABILHAND	27 items	Items from existing questionnaires, authors expertise & 18 people with RA	3-point response Interview based	Activity limitations	Multiple languages	Higher score = greater manual ability	Last 3 months
ASES	15 items in 2 modules	Research committee of the ASES and member input	VAS & 4-point scale	Multidimensional	Multiple languages	Higher score = less pain and disability	Not indicated

Continued

TABLE 5.1	Summary of Outcome Measure Properties—cont'd						
Measure	Number of Items	Item Generation / Reduction	Type of Response	Dimen- sions	Translated	Scoring	Recall Period
CMS	4 modules, pain, ADL, ROM and power	No indication	VAS, categorical responses, goniometer & power	Multidimen- sional	Multiple languages	Higher score = better shoulder function	Not indi- cated
PRWE PRWHE	15 items in 2 modules	Survey of experts and patients	Scale 0–10	Multidimen- sional	Multiple languages	Higher score = greater pain or disability	Past week
MHQ	37 items in 6 modules for L and R hand			Multidimen- sional	Multiple languages	Higher score = better hand function & greater pain.	Past week ADL & pain; 4 weeks work
SPADI	13 items in 2 modules	4 experts	Scale 0–10	Multidimen- sional	Multiple languages	Higher score = greater pain or disability	Last week
GAS	NA	NA	5-point	Individual- ized		Higher score = greater achieve- ment	Present
COPM	Up to 5 indi- vidual goals	NA	Scale 1–10	Individual- ized	Multiple languages	Higher score = better perfor- mance and satisfaction	Typical day
PSFS	3 individual goals	NA	VAS (0–10)	Individual- ized	Multiple languages	Higher score = less activity limitation	Today

ASES, The American Shoulder and Elbow Surgeons standardized assessment form; *CMS*, constant Murley score; *COPM*, Canadian occupational performance measure; *CTQ*, carpal tunnel questionnaire; *DASH*, disabilities of the arm, shoulder and hand; *GAS*, goal attainment scaling; *MHQ*, Michigan hand questionnaire; *M²DASH*, Manchester-modified disabilities of the arm, shoulder and hand; *NA*, not applicable; *PRWE*, patient-rated wrist evaluation; *PRWHE*, patient-rated wrist hand evaluation; *PSFS*, perfor-mance specific functional scale; *QuickDASH*, quick disabilities of the arm, shoulder and hand; *SPADI*, shoulder pain and disability index; *UEFI*, upper extremity functional index; *ULFI*, upper limb functional index; *WORC*, Western Ontario Rotator Cuff Index; *VAS*, visual analogue scale; *PROM*, patient-reported outcome measure; *UL*, upper limb; *HRQOL*, health-related quality of life; *RCD*, rotator cuff disease; *RA*, rheumatoid arthritis; *ADL*, activities of daily living; *ROM*, range of motion; *L*, left; *R*, right.

and confidence.[26,27,38] Two additional four-item options are available to assess work and sport/music. Despite the widespread use of the DASH, there are a number of issues:

- Relationship of the DASH to lower limb injury. Dowrick and colleagues demonstrated that the DASH measures disability in individuals with lower limb as well as arm injuries.[39] They hypothesize this may occur as a number of tasks require some lower limb ability. For example, pushing open a door requires walking to the door.
- Measurement of compensation. Responses are not attributed to the affected limb, and people are requested to respond based on their ability, irrespective of how they perform the task. As a result, responses are more likely to represent com-pensation rather than actual use of the affected limb.
- Multidimensionality. While designed to measure a single factor termed "symptoms and physical function," the DASH is multidimensional. Further, a number of authors have reported multidimensionality in the activity items. Using Rasch analysis, Franchignoni et al identified two sets of activ-ities they termed "shoulder range of motion" and "manual functioning,"[40,41] while Lehman et al identified two sets of activity items that they termed "gross motor involving the whole arm" and "fine motor using factor analysis."[42] Scores

resulting from multidimensional measures should be inter-preted with caution, as it is unclear which factors have led to the observed change.[43,44]

- Recent factor and Rasch analyses of the DASH have shown that responders have problems differentiating between "mild," "moderate," and "severe" levels of difficulty. This impacts the validity of the measure.[41,45] Further, a number of authors have reported that some items appear to be misfits in that they are not related to the underlying construct. These include item 21 "sexual activity" (also the most frequent item not responded to) and item 26 "tingling."[40,42]
- As a region-specific questionnaire, specificity and responsive-ness of the DASH are lower than that for outcome measures that are joint or diagnosis specific.[46]

QuickDASH

The DASH is considered relatively long, as it contains 30 items. Moreover, some studies have suggested item redundancy, as some items tend to measure the same concept.[47] An 11-item abbrevi-ated version, the QuickDASH, was developed in 2005.[47] While the QuickDASH offers advantages over the DASH, evidence on the comparability of the two outcome measures is conflicting.

Angst and coworkers believed that these outcome measures were not comparable, as they measure different constructs.[48] In this study, despite producing the same scores as the DASH, the QuickDASH was found to have underestimated symptoms (i.e., reporting lower severity) and overestimated function (i.e., reporting less disability) in people with specific joint disorders. MacDermid and colleagues, meanwhile, suggested that the QuickDASH may be a valid surrogate for the DASH in people undergoing total shoulder arthroplasty and rotator cuff repair.[17] The results of a systematic review on the QuickDASH suggested that there is evidence of appropriate reliability and validity and moderate evidence to support its structural validity.[49] However, there is strong evidence that does not support its responsiveness to change. This calls into question the ability of the QuickDASH to accurately measure change over time. As the QuickDASH is derived from the DASH items, it also has many of the same issues.

Manchester-Modified DASH (M²DASH)[50]

Dowrick and colleagues demonstrated that the DASH is affected by disability of the lower limbs.[39] To counter this, Khan and coworkers developed the 18-item M²DASH.[50,51] The M²DASH offers an advantage over both the DASH and QuickDASH, as it has removed items that may involve lower limb use, including "push open heavy door," "carry objects," and "recreational activities" that are not sedentary. However, it retains some of the same issues as the DASH. As the M²DASH is not attributed to the affected limb, it potentially measures compensation rather than actual use of the affected limb. It is also multidimensional so scores must be viewed with caution.

Upper Extremity Functional Index (UEFI)[52]

Designed to assess upper extremity function in individuals with hand and upper extremity disorders, the UEFI is a 20-item patient-reported outcome measure developed in the late 1990s.[52] All items are attributed to the affected limb, indicating that the UEFI is less likely to assess compensatory techniques. However, it still contains an item "open a door," which may be influenced by lower limb ability. Hamilton and Chesworth published a 15-item interval version of the UEFI, as the original 20-item version was not supported by the Rasch model.[53] Five items were deleted: "Sleeping," "Usual hobbies," "Dressing," "Throwing a ball," and "Tying and lacing shoelaces."[54]

Upper Limb Functional Index (ULFI)[55,56]

The ULFI is an upper limb functional patient-reported outcome measure published in 2010. Designed to assess upper limb status and impairment, it has 25 items that address activity limitations and impairments.[55,56] Responses are attributed to the affected arm. The ULFI has been translated into a number of languages. It is multidimensional—containing items that assess impairments including pain, sleep, mood, activity limitations, and participation restrictions. Thus the total score should be viewed with caution.

Condition-Specific Outcome Measures

The measures discussed in the previous section are all classified as region-specific measures designed to be used on clients with a variety of diagnoses. Condition-specific outcome measures, however, are designed to be more focused on one particular diagnosis or health condition. Condition-specific measures are usually found to be more responsive to change for populations with that condition.

Carpal Tunnel Injury

The Carpal Tunnel Questionnaire (CTQ) is the most frequently used outcome measure for carpal tunnel syndrome.[57] First published in 1993 by Levine et al., the CTQ is comprised of two modules: an 11-item Symptom Specific Scale (SSS) and an 8-item Functional Status Scale (FSS). The two module scores are not summed and either can be used in its own right. The CTQ contains items that assess unimanual and bimanual tasks as well as one dominant activity—writing. While it is multidimensional, each scale is scored and interpreted separately. When compared to region-specific measures, the CTQ has been reported to be more responsive to change for people with carpal tunnel syndrome.[58]

Rotator Cuff Disease

Many patient-reported outcome measures have been used to evaluate outcomes in people with rotator cuff disease.[59] The most frequently reported outcome measure in the literature is the Western Ontario Rotator Cuff (WORC).[60] Designed as a multidimensional measure of five domains (physical symptoms, sports and recreation, work, lifestyle, and emotions) the WORC is comprised of 21 items, each scored on a visual analog scale (VAS). A number of limitations of the WORC have been documented, including a lack of evidence on the specificity of the items in each domain. Additionally, the VAS scoring system has been reported as complex, which has increased the response and scoring burden. However, the WORC appears to be the most responsive of the patient-reported outcome measures for rotator cuff disease.[61]

Joint-Specific Outcome Measures

Joint-specific outcome measures contain items that are designed to assess activities related to one joint.

ABILHAND[62]

The ABILHAND was designed as a measure of bimanual ability for adults with rheumatoid arthritis undergoing wrist fusion. This outcome measure is specific to the wrist joint. The ABILHAND is administered during an interview with the clinician and is not considered a self-report outcome measure. As a measure of only bimanual activities, the ABILHAND does not have issues with face validity and is unlikely to be influenced by compensation. However, scoring can only be completed online, and the ABILHAND must be completed in conjunction with the clinician, increasing user burden.

The American Shoulder and Elbow Surgeons Standardized Assessment Form (ASES)[63]

The ASES was developed by the American Shoulder and Elbow Surgeons' research committee to assess functional limitation and pain at the shoulder. It is comprised of two sections: (1) a physician assessment of impairment, and (2) a self-report section that addresses pain and activities of daily living. Pain is assessed on a VAS (0 "no pain" to 10 "worst pain"). Eight items assess activity limitation and two address participation restrictions (work and sport/leisure). As a multidimensional measure, scores should be viewed with caution. A standardized assessment of elbow function designed in a similar fashion is also available.[64]

Constant-Murley Score (CMS)[65,66]

The CMS is recommended by the European Society for Shoulder and Elbow Surgery (ESSES) to assess shoulder function. It is divided into four modules: pain, activities of daily living, active range of motion, and strength. Pain is assessed on a VAS (0 "no pain" to 10 "maximum pain you can experience"). Four items assess activities of daily living—occupation, leisure/recreation, sleep, and painless arm use. Pain-free active range of motion is measured using a goniometer, and strength is measured at 90 degrees of shoulder abduction using a dynamometer or a calibrated spring balance.[66] As a measure that includes objective assessment of impairment and self-report of activities, the CMS offers advantages over other outcome measures. However, as a multidimensional scale, scores should be viewed with caution. Further, the CMS lacks standardization of the testing procedures, which is evidenced by the wide variation in testing protocols used in published studies.[67]

Michigan Hand Outcome Questionnaire (MHQ)[68]

The MHQ is a hand-specific outcome measure designed for people with conditions or injury to the hand or wrist. The MHQ has six modules that measure hand function, activities of daily living (ADLs), pain, work performance, aesthetics, and satisfaction with hand function. The 57 items can be completed as a self-report outcome measure, or a clinician may administer them to the client. The MHQ offers a number of advantages including responses attributed to the left or right wrist/hand, and a section on aesthetics, which is important for some clients. Scoring, however, is complicated and can increase clinician burden. Some studies have also indicated item redundancy.[68] To counter this, a brief 12-item version has been developed.[69]

The Patient-Rated Wrist Evaluation (PRWE)[70] and Patient-Rated Wrist Hand Evaluation (PRWHE)[71]

The PRWE was developed to assess pain and functional disability in people with wrist disorders. It comprises 15-items divided into two modules: pain and function. The pain module has five items, each scored from 0 "no pain" to 10 "worst ever pain." The function module contains 10 items: 6 assess activity limitations and 4 assess usual activities, including personal care, household work, work, and recreation. Each of these items are scored from 0 "no difficulty" to 10 "unable to do."

The PRWHE was based on the PRWE to assess people with hand conditions. The same items and scoring system were used; however, the term "wrist" was replaced by "wrist/hand." Both the PRWE and PRWHE have been subjected to Rasch analysis,[43,72] where it was found that both measures lack a true two-module structure. In addition, analysis identified that people have difficulty distinguishing between response options.

The Shoulder Pain and Disability Index (SPADI)[73]

The SPADI was developed to assess shoulder pain and disability. The 13-item outcome measure assesses 2 modules: pain (5 items) and disability (8 items). Factor analysis of the SPADI has confirmed two factors based on the pain and disability modules.[74,75] The SPADI uses a numerical rating scale from 0 "no pain/no difficulty" to 10 "worst pain imaginable/so difficult it requires help."[76] The SPADI score is a product of a multidimensional measure and should therefore be viewed with caution.

Patient-Derived Outcome Measures

All the outcome measures discussed in this chapter thus far use a set of items that must be answered by each person, even if the responder feels they have little or no relevance to them. Patient-derived outcome measures circumnavigate this through goal setting or problem identification to reflect the impact of disease or injury on them as individuals. Although normally said to be relatively simple to use clinically, goal setting requires a degree of skill on the part of the clinician. One criticism of these types of measures is that comparison of results between people can be difficult as the activities nominated invariably differ. However, group results can be calculated.

Canadian Occupational Performance Measure (COPM)[77]

The COPM is designed to capture a person's self-perception of performance in everyday living over time in three areas: self-care, productivity, and leisure. Using semistructured interviews, clients identify activity goals that they wish to achieve in each of the three areas. The five most important goals are then identified. Each goal is rated for performance and satisfaction. The COPM can be time consuming and difficult to administer as goals can be hard to establish. The COPM is copyrighted and must be purchased prior to use.

Goal Attainment Scaling (GAS and GAS-light)[78]

GAS is a mathematical technique for quantifying the attainment of goals by applying a score to the achievement of a goal. When setting the goals using the SMART principle (Specific, Measurable, Attainable, Realistic and Timely), it is important to establish the criteria for successful achievement of each goal that is agreed to by all stakeholders. Each expected outcome must be objective and measurable. Each goal is then rated and weighted for importance and difficulty. The GAS can be scored by computer using an electronic calculation sheet in Microsoft Excel. The GAS is client centered; however, it does require some experience on the part of the clinician to establish clear, well-structured goals with all stakeholders and is time consuming to complete. Further, clinicians are often reluctant to give clients negative scores when goals are not achieved. The "GAS-light" model was consequently developed to encourage the inclusion of goal attainment as part of the clinical decision making.

Patient Specific Functional Scale (PSFS)[79]

The PSFS can be used to quantify activity limitation and functional outcomes for individuals with any orthopedic condition. The PSFS asks people to nominate up to three important activities that they currently experience difficulty performing because of their condition. They then rate each activity on a numerical rating scale from 0 "unable to perform activity" to 10 "able to perform activity at the same level as before injury or problem." At follow-up, difficulty associated with each activity is rated again on the same scale. The PSFS has been found to have appropriate levels of reliability, validity, and responsiveness to change at an individual level but cannot be used to compare at a group level.[80]

How to Find an Outcome Measure

Outcome measures can be identified in a variety of ways. Systematic reviews have been published on the psychometric properties of patient-reported outcome measures for hand injuries,[28,81] shoulder instability,[82] shoulder function,[33,36] upper limb trauma,[83,84] nerve injury,[85,86] amputation,[87,88] and arthritis.[89,90] Websites have been developed that are dedicated to providing information on a wide range of outcome measures, including the following:

- Rehabilitation Measures Database: https://www.sralab.org/rehabilitation-measures
- Patient Reported Outcome Measurement group: http://phi.uhce.ox.ac.uk
- American Academy of Orthopedic Surgeons: https://www.aaos.org/Quality/Performance_Measures/Patient_Reported_Outcome_Measures/?ssopc=1
- Physiopeadia: https://www.physio-pedia.com

Some of the more established outcome measures may have a dedicated website that provides information about the measure and its scoring, for example:

- DASH: http://www.dash.iwh.on.ca
- COPM http://www.thecopm.ca
- ABILHAND: http://www.rehab-scales.org/abilhand.html
- MHQ: http://mhq.lab.medicine.umich.edu

User manuals can also be sourced via the Internet, for example the GAS: https://www.kcl.ac.uk/nursing/departments/cicelysaunders/attachments/Tools-GAS-Practical-Guide.pdf.

Finally, word of mouth from experts in the field can provide additional information, particularly on new or emerging outcome measures.

Measurement Properties

Finding an outcome measure is the first part of the puzzle. Next, it is important to demonstrate that the outcome measure chosen has proven psychometric properties for the condition of interest. The outcome measure should be reproducible, valid, responsive to change, and should not excessively burden the client or the clinician. Historically, there has been some confusion on measurement properties of outcome measures and how they are defined.[91] For the purposes of this chapter, the terminology developed by researchers at the Consensus-Based Standards for the Selection of Health Measurement Instruments (COSMIN) initiative will be used.[92-95]

Reproducibility

First, measures need to be reproducible. Reproducibility is comprised of two different but essential components, reliability and agreement.

Reliability is defined as "the proportion of the total variance in the measurements that is due to true differences between people."[96] In practice, this means that the measure will produce the same results on different occasions in a sample that has not changed in status, and is able to detect differences in people over time that are the result of true change not measurement error.[97] The most appropriate type of reliability for patient-reported outcome measures is test–retest reliability, where one sample of individuals completes the same test on two separate occasions, and their results are compared. Frequently calculated statistics that are used to convey the magnitude of reliability include the Intraclass Correlation Coefficient (ICC) or a weighted Kappa ≥0.70.[98] Values close to 1 indicate greater reliability in scores.

Agreement is the degree to which scores are identical. Agreement statistics—for example, the standard error of measurement (SEM) and minimal detectable change (MDC) or limits of agreement, are expressed in the same units as the outcome measure, are related to absolute error, and aid in the understanding and interpretation of results of the outcome measure over time.[99] It is beyond the scope of this chapter to explain how agreement statistics are derived. However, there are a number of very useful texts in this area including those by Streiner and Norman,[100] Portney and Watkins,[2] and De Vet.[91]

To ensure items are measuring similar things (i.e., the same underlying variable), it is important that items correlate moderately with each other and with the total score.[100] Internal consistency reliability is a measure of the scale's homogeneity.[2,91] However, items that correlate too highly may be repeatedly measuring the same thing, contribute little to the overall result, and could potentially be redundant.[101] Look for a Cronbach alpha between 0.07 and 0.95, as evidence of an appropriate level of internal consistency.[98]

Validity

While a measure may have appropriate reliability (i.e., it is relatively free from error and able to discriminate between people), it may not be valid.[2,100,102] For example, the box and block test is a reliable tool of unilateral gross manual dexterity. However, no inferences can be drawn from it as to how the person uses their arm/hand to perform day-to-day tasks.[19] Validity is defined as: "The extent to which an instrument measures what it is intended to measure."[96] When an outcome measure quantifies what is intended, meaningful inferences can be drawn from the results obtained. Validity contains three separate but important measurement properties[92]:

1. Content validity: "The degree to which the content of a patient-reported outcome instrument is an adequate reflection of the construct to be measured." Content validity is key to any patient-reported outcome measure, and lack of content validity will affect all other measurement properties.[95] Content validity also contains face validity defined as "the degree to which the items of a measure look as though they are an adequate reflection of the construct to be measured." While face validity cannot be statistically evaluated, it is very important.
2. Construct validity: "The degree to which the scores of a patient-reported outcome instrument are consistent with hypotheses based on the assumption that the patient-reported outcome instrument validly measures the construct to be measured." As previously discussed, defining a construct that is not tangible can be difficult. One way to test the assumed

underlying construct is to determine the association between two outcome measures. Measures believed to assess the same construct have "convergent validity," while those believed to measure different constructs have "divergent validity."[91]

3. Criterion validity: The degree to which the scores of a patient-reported outcome instrument are an adequate reflection of a gold standard. The COSMIN checklist recognizes that gold-standard patient-reported outcome measures do not exist,[103] except when comparing a shortened version of an existing measure with the original measure, such as the QuickDASH with the DASH.

Responsiveness

Outcome measures need to be able to detect change over time (i.e., they should be responsive if they will be used to document client progress).[2,91] Moreover, the score needs to change in proportion to the person's actual change, remain stable if their status has not changed, and be meaningful to all stakeholders.[2] The COSMIN panel defines responsiveness as: "The ability of an instrument to detect change over time in the construct to be measured."[91] As with reliability, there is no consensus as to which statistical test best assesses responsiveness.[91] The COSMIN checklist recommends that the results are in accordance with hypotheses, or the receiver operating curve area under the curve is ≥0.70.[94]

Clinical Utility/Feasibility

Based on the discussion above, you have now identified a group of outcome measures that could be feasible to use in your clinical setting. These outcome measures evaluate the underlying variable you wish to measure, have appropriate psychometric properties for your diagnostic group, and the items look appropriate to all stakeholders. To make a final choice on which one to use, there are a number of other considerations that can assist the decision-making process (Table 5.2).

1. The time it takes to administer and score an outcome measure is important in the clinic setting. Most patient-reported outcome measures are relatively simple to administer and score. However, some, like the ABILHAND, are scored online or require specific scoring software such as the MHQ. These outcome measures require more time to access and use a computer, which may make them less practical for daily clinical use.

2. Method of administration. While it has been demonstrated that there is usually equivalence between paper/pencil and electronic versions of outcome measures,[104] it is recommended that evidence to support this notion be provided by the developers of the measures.[105]

3. Dealing with missing responses is important, and information on handling this issue should be freely available, easily understood, and enacted.

4. Response options for items may be an odd or even number. An even number of responses forces responders to make a choice, while an odd number allows a neutral response. De-Vellis suggested that neither format is superior to the other.[106] However, some people may not like being forced to make a decision. In contrast, if a neutral response is chosen, it may be unclear what the responder intended.

5. Some outcome measures can be expensive to use, require a license, or are difficult to obtain. For example, the COPM can only be obtained online and requires the purchase of a manual as well as copies of the paper-based outcome measure.

6. Proxy responses. The relationship between client and proxy responses remains unclear. While proxy results can lead to higher response rates, the trend to more negative responses from proxies needs to be acknowledged.[107]

7. Translation. The majority of outcome measures have been designed in the English language, both British and American English. Translating outcome measures is complicated and requires a clearly defined forward and backward translation using native speakers.[108] Language differences are extremely subtle but incredibly important. Consequently, there are British English versions of the DASH[109] and Short Form-36, both originally developed in American English.[110]

8. Individual literacy and the readability of any outcome measure is important. A number of tools exist that can assist in determining readability, including Gunning Fog and the Flesch-Kincaid Scale. The recommended minimum literacy level to understand outcome measures is grade 6 or 12 years of age.[111] The Gunning Fog can be calculated online and the Flesch-Kincaid is available through Microsoft Word.

To quantify some of these factors, Connell and Tyson developed a simple method to determine if a tool is feasible to use in practice.[34] A score ≥8/10 is considered to be a feasible tool.

Summary

Choosing an outcome measure is not easy. However, a systematic approach can assist in the decision-making process. The following list outlines the key points covered in this chapter:
- A clear definition of the variable being measured that matches what you wish to assess.
- A clear definition of the conceptual framework that underpinned the item generation for the outcome measure chosen.
- A clear definition of the population for whom the outcome measure is intended.
- A clear outline of the statistical analyses that underpined the outcome measure development, including a priori hypotheses where appropriate.
- A clear report of the psychometric properties of the outcome measure including an evaluation and appropriate levels of reproducibility (including reliability and agreement statistics), content and construct validity, and responsiveness to aid in interpretation of scoring.
- Instructions that match the intended use, for example to assess change attributed to the affected limb or how a person performs activities regardless of how they complete the task.
- A variety of unimanual and bimanual activities that cover the spectrum of arm use.
- A clearly defined recall period that matches the intended purpose of the outcome measure.
- Consistent response options that match the purpose of the assessment.
- Clear instructions on how to complete the outcome measure, including recall period and limb attribution.

TABLE 5.2 Feasibility and Content Validity

Measure	Time to Complete	Cost	Specialist Training	Tool Portable	Attribute Affected	Uni/ Bimanual Activities	Dominant Limb Activities	Normative Values
DASH	5–7 mins	Free	No	Yes	No	Uni and Bimanual	Yes	Yes
Quick DASH	<5 mins	Free	No	Yes	No	Uni and Bimanual	Yes	Yes
M2DASH	<5 mins	Free	No	Yes	No	Uni and Bimanual	Yes	No
UEFI	5 mins	Free	No	Yes	Yes	Uni and Bimanual	No	No
ULFI	<3 mins	Free	No	Yes	Yes	Uni and Bimanual	Yes	No
CTQ	<10 mins	Free	No	Yes	Yes	Uni and Bimanual	Yes	Yes
WORC	Not documented	Free	No	Yes	Yes	Uni and Bimanual	Yes	No
ABILHAND	<10 mins	Free	Yes	Briefcase	NA	Bimanual	No	Yes
ASES	<5 mins	Free	No	Yes	L & R	Uni and Bimanual	Yes	Yes
CMS	Unknown	Equipment	Yes	No	L & R	Uni and Bimanual	No	Yes
MHQ	15 mins	Requires a license	No	Yes	L & R	Uni and Bimanual	No	Yes
PRWE, PRWHE	<5 mins	Free	No	Yes	Yes	Uni and Bimanual	Yes	Yes
SPADI	<5 mins	Free	No	Yes	Yes	Uni and Bimanual	No	No
Gas	Individual	Free	Yes	Yes	NA	NA	NA	NA
Gas light	Individual	Free	Yes	Yes	NA	NA	NA	NA
COPM	30–45 mins	Free copies & manual	Yes	Yes	NA	NA	NA	NA
PSFS	Individual	Free	No	Yes	NA	NA	NA	NA

DASH, Disabilities of the Arm, Shoulder and Hand; QuickDASH, Quick Disabilities of the Arm, Shoulder and Hand; M2DASH, Manchester-modified Disabilities of the Arm, Shoulder and Hand; UEFI, Upper extremity Functional Index; ULFI, Upper Limb Functional Index; CTQ, Carpal Tunnel Questionnaire; WORC, Western Ontario Rotator Cuff Index; ASES, The American Shoulder and Elbow Surgeons standardized assessment form; CMS, Constant Murley Score; MHQ, Michigan hand Questionnaire; PRWE, Patient-rated Wrist Evaluation; PRWHE, Patient-rated Wrist Hand Evaluation; MHQ, Michigan hand Questionnaire; SPADI, Shoulder Pain and Disability Index; GAS, Goal attainment Scaling; COPM, Canadian Occupational Performance Measure; PSFS, Performance Specific Functional Scale; L, Left; R, Right; NA Not applicable

- Clear instructions on how the outcome measure is scored, how long scoring takes, and how to manage missing responses.
- Clear instructions on how the measure should be delivered (e.g., paper based, electronic, or interview).
- Minimal responder and assessor burden (feasibility score of >8[34]).

- Good face validity; items need to look right to all stakeholders.

Measurement is anything but simple. Taking time to review all the available outcome measures and matching the right one to the clinical or research need is not an easy process, but it is central to ensuring effective evidence-based practice.

References

1. Thomson W: Lecture on electrical units of measurement, *Popular Lectures* 1:73, 1883.
2. Portney L, Watkins G: *Foundations of clinical research applications to practice*, ed 3, Upper Saddle River, NJ, Pearson Prentice Hall, 2009.
3. Barreca S, Gowland C, Stratford P, Huijbregts M, Griffiths J, Torresin W, et al.: Development of the chedoke arm and hand activity inventory: theoretical constructs, item generation, and selection, *Top Stroke Rehabil* 11(4):31–42, 2004.

4. Kilbreath SL, Heard RC: Frequency of hand use in healthy older persons, *Aust J Physiother* 51(2):119–122, 2005.

5. Kimmerle M, Mainwaring L, Borenstein M: The functional repertoire of the hand and its application to assessment, *Am J Occup Ther* 57(5):489–498, 2003.

6. Mancuso CA, Lee SK, Dy CJ, Landers ZA, Model Z, Wolfe SW: Expectations and limitations due to brachial plexus injury: a qualitative study, *Hand* 10(4):741–749, 2015.

7. Mancuso CA, Lee SK, Dy CJ, Landers ZA, Model Z, Wolfe F: Compensation by the injured arm after brachial plexus injury, *Hand* 4(11):410–416, 2016.

8. Baltzer H, Novak CB, McCabe SJ: A scoping review of disabilities of the arm, shoulder, and hand scores for hand and wrist conditions, *J Hand Surg* 39(12):2472–2480, 2014.

9. Hudak PL, Amadio PC, Bombardier C: Development of an upper extremity outcome measure: the DASH (disabilities of the arm, shoulder, and hand), *Am J Ind Med* 29(6):602–608, 1996.

10. Hill B, Bialocerkowski A, Williams G: Do patient reported outcome measures capture actual upper limb recovery? *Int J Rehabil Res* 21(12):558–559, 2014.

11. FDA: *Guidance for industry, patient-reported outcome measures: use in medical product development to support labelling claims*, Rockville, MD, 2009, Department of Health and Human Services, Food and Administration, Centre for Drug Evaluation and Research.

12. WHO: International Classification of Functioning, *Disability and Health,* Geneva, 2001.

13. Wahi Michener SK, Olson AL, Humphrey BA, Reed JE, Stepp DR, Sutton AM, et al.: Relationship among grip strength, functional outcomes, and work performance following hand trauma, *Work* 16(3):209–217, 2001.

14. Bialocerkowski AE, Grimmer KA, Bain GI: Validity of the patient-focused wrist outcome instrument: do impairments represent functional ability? *Hand Clin* 19(3):449–455, 2003.

15. Farzad M, Asgari A, Dashab F, Layeghi F, Karimlou M, Hosseini SA, et al.: Does disability correlate with impairment after hand injury? *Clin Orthop Relat Res* 473(11):3470–3476, 2015.

16. Nota SPFT, Bot AGJ, Ring D, Kloen P: Disability and depression after orthopaedic trauma, *Injury* 46(2):207–212, 2015.

17. Macdermid JC, Khadilkar L, Birmingham TB, Athwal GS: Validity of the QuickDASH in patients with shoulder-related disorders undergoing surgery, *J Orthop Sports Phys Ther* 45(1):25–36, 2015.

18. Jebsen RH, Taylor N, Trieschmann RB, Trotter MJ, Howard LA: An objective and standardized test of hand function, *Arch Phys Med Rehabil* 50(6):311–319, 1969.

19. Mathiowetz V, Volland G, Kashman N, Weber K: Adult norms for the box and block test of manual dexterity, *Am J Occup Ther* 39(6):386–391, 1985.

20. Rolfson O, Eresian Chenok K, Bohm E, Lübbeke A, Denissen G, Dunn J, et al.: Patient-reported outcome measures in arthroplasty registries: Report of the patient-reported outcome measures working group of the international society of arthroplasty registries: part I. Overview and rationale for patient-reported outcome measures, *Acta Orthop* 87:3–8, 2016, https://doi.org/10.1080/17453674.2016.1181816.

21. Black N: Patient reported outcome measures could help transform healthcare, *BMJ* 346(7896), 2013, https://doi.org/10.1136/bmj.f167.

22. Rudolf KD, Kus S, Chung KC, Johnston M, Leblanc M, Cieza A: Development of the international classification of functioning, disability and health core sets for hand conditions results of the world health organization international consensus process, *Disabil Rehabil* 34(8):681–693, 2012, https://doi.org/10.3109/09638288.2011.613514.

23. Kus S, Dereskewitz C, Wickert M, Schwab M, Eisenschenk A, Steen M, et al.: Validation of the comprehensive international classification of functioning, *Disability and Health (ICF) Core Set for Hand Conditions Hand Therapy* 16:58–66, 2011.

24. Kus S, Oberhauser C, Cieza A: Validation of the brief international classification of functioning, disability, and health (ICF) core set for hand conditions, *J Hand Ther* 25(3):274–287, 2012.

25. Hill B, Pallant J, Williams G, Olver J, Ferris S, Bialocerkowski A: Evaluation of internal construct validity and unidimensionality of the brachial assessment tool, a patient-reported outcome measure for brachial plexus injury, *Arch Phys Med Rehabil* 97(12):2146–2156, 2016, https://doi.org/10.1016/j.apmr.2016.06.021.

26. Forget NJ, Higgins J: Comparison of generic patient-reported outcome measures used with upper extremity musculoskeletal disorders: linking process using the international classification of functioning, disability, and health (ICF), *J Rehabili Med* 46(4):327–334, 2014, https://doi.org/10.2340/16501977-1784.

27. Drummond AS, Sampaio RF, Mancini MC, Kirkwood RN, Stamm TA: Linking the disabilities of arm, shoulder, and hand to the international classification of functioning, disability, and health, *J Hand Ther* 20(4):336–344, 2007.

28. van de Ven-Stevens LAW, Graff MJL, Selles RW, Schreuders TAR, van der Linde H, Spauwen PH, et al.: Instruments for assessment of impairments and activity limitations in patients with hand conditions: a European delphi study, *J Rehabil Med* 47(10):948–956, 2015, https://doi.org/10.2340/16501977-2015.

29. MacDermid JC: Patient-reported outcomes: state-of-the-art hand surgery and future applications, *Hand Clin* 30(3):293–304, 2014, https://doi.org/10.1016/j.hcl.2014.04.003.

30. Dang A, Mendon S: The role of patient reported outcomes (PROs) in healthcare policy making, *Sys Rev Pharm* 6(1):1–4, 2015.

31. Dawson J, Doll H, Fitzpatrick R, Jenkinson C, Carr AJ: Routine use of patient reported outcome measures in healthcare settings, *BMJ* 340(7744):464–467, 2010.

32. Bryant D, Fernandes N: Measuring patient outcomes: a primer, *Injury* 42(3):232–235, 2011.

33. Roe Y, Østensjø S: Conceptualization and assessment of disability in shoulder-specific measures with reference to the International Classification of Functioning, Disability and Health, *J Rehabil Med* 48(4):325–332, 2016.

34. Connell LA, Tyson SF: Clinical reality of measuring upper-limb ability in neurologic conditions: a systematic review, *Arch Phys Med Rehabil* 93(2):221–228, 2012.

35. Smith MV, Calfee RP, Baumgarten KM, Brophy RH, Wright RW: Upper extremity-specificmeasures of disability and outcomes in orthopaedic surgery, *J Bone Joint Surg—Series A* 94(3):277–285, 2012.

36. Roy JS, Macdermid JC, Woodhouse LJ: Measuring shoulder function: A systematic review of four questionnaires, *Arthritis Care Res* 61(5):623–632, 2009.

37. Kennedy C, Beaton D, Solway S, McConnell S, Bombardier C: *The DASH and QuickDASH outcome measure user's manual*, ed 3, Toronto, ON, 2011, Institute for Work and Health.

38. Dixon D, Johnston M, McQueen M, Court-Brown C: The disabilities of the arm, shoulder and hand questionnaire (DASH) can measure the impairment, activity limitations and participation restriction constructs from the International Classification of Functioning, Disability and Health (ICF), *BMC Musculoskelet Disord* 9, 2008, https://doi.org/10.1186/1471-2474-9-114.

39. Dowrick AS, Gabbe BJ, Williamson OD: Does the presence of an upper extremity injury affect outcomes after major trauma? *J Trauma* 58(6):1175–1178, 2005.

40. Franchignoni F, Giordano A, Ferriero G: On dimensionality of the DASH, *Mult Scler* 17(7):891–892, 2011, https://doi.org/10.1177/1352458511406909.

41. Franchignoni F, Giordano A, Sartorio F, Vercelli S, Pascariello B, Ferriero G: Suggestions for refinement of the disabilities of the arm, shoulder and hand outcome measure (DASH): a factor analysis and rasch validation study, *Arch Phys Med Rehabil* 91(9):1370–1377, 2010.

42. Lehman LA, Woodbury M, Velozo CA: Examination of the factor structure of the disabilities of the arm, shoulder, and hand questionnaire, *Am J Occup Ther* 65(2):169–178, 2011.

43. Packham T, Macdermid JC: Measurement properties of the patient-rated wrist and hand evaluation: Rasch analysis of responses from a traumatic hand injury population, *J Hand Ther* 26(3):216–224, 2013.

44. Strauss ME, Smith GT: Construct validity: Advances in theory and methodology, *Ann Rev Clin Psychol* 5:1–25, 2009, https://doi.org/10.1146/annurev.clinpsy.032408.153639.

45. Cano SJ, Barrett LE, Zajicek JP, Hobart JC: Beyond the reach of traditional analyses: using rasch to evaluate the DASH in people with multiple sclerosis, *Mult Scler* 17(2):214–222, 2011.

46. Angst F, Goldhahn J, Drerup S, Aeschlimann A, Schwyzer H-K, Simmen BR: Responsiveness of six outcome assessment instruments in total shoulder arthroplasty, *Arthritis Rheum* 59(3):391–398, 2008.

47. Beaton DE, Wright JG, Katz JN, Amadio P, Bombardier C, Cole D, et al.: Development of the QuickDASH: comparison of three item-reduction approaches, *J Bone Joint Surg—Series A* 87(5):1038–1046, 2005.

48. Angst F, Goldhahn J, Drerup S, Flury M, Schwyzer HK, Simmen BR: How sharp is the short QuickDASH? A refined content and validity analysis of the short form of the disabilities of the shoulder, arm and hand questionnaire in the strata of symptoms and function and specific joint conditions, *Qual Life Res* 18(8):1043–1051, 2009, https://doi.org/10.1007/s11136-009-9529-4.

49. Kennedy CA, Beaton DE, Smith P, Van Eerd D, Tang K, Inrig T, et al.: Measurement properties of the QuickDASH (disabilities of the arm, shoulder and hand) outcome measure and cross-cultural adaptations of the QuickDASH: a systematic review, *Qual Life Res* 22(9):2509–2547, 2013.

50. Khan WS, Jain R, Dillon B, Clarke L, Fehily M, Ravenscroft M: The M2 DASH—Manchester-modified disabilities of arm shoulder and hand score, *Hand* 3(3):240–244, 2008.

51. Khan WS, Dillon B, Agarwal M, Fehily M, Ravenscroft M: The validity, reliability, responsiveness, and bias of the Manchester-modified disability of the arm, shoulder, and hand score in hand injuries, *Hand* 4(4):362–367, 2009.

52. Stratford PW, Binkley JM, Stratford DM: Development and initial validation of upper extremity functional index, *Physiother Can* 53(4):259, 2001.

53. Hamilton CB, Chesworth BM: A Rasch-validated version of the upper extremity functional index for interval-level measurement of upper extremity function, *Phys Ther* 93(11):1507–1519, 2013.

54. Chesworth BM, Hamilton CB, Walton DM, Benoit M, Blake TA, Bredy H, et al.: Reliability and validity of two versions of the upper extremity functional index, *Physiother Can* 66(3):243–253, 2014.

55. Gabel CP, Michener LA, Burkett B, Neller A: The upper limb functional index: development and determination of reliability, validity, and responsiveness, *J Hand Ther* 19(3):328–349, 2006.

56. Gabel CP, Michener LA, Melloh M, Burkett B: Modification of the upper limb functional index to a three-point response improves clinimetric properties, *J Hand Ther* 23(1):41–52, 2010.

57. Levine DW, Simmons BP, Koris MJ, Daltroy LH, Hohl GG, Fossel AH, et al.: A self-administered questionnaire for the assessment of severity of symptoms and functional status in carpal tunnel syndrome, *J Bone Joint Surg—series A* 75(11):1585–1592, 1993.

58. Jerosch-Herold C, Leite JCdC, Song F: A systematic review of outcomes assessed in randomized controlled trials of surgical interventions for carpal tunnel syndrome using the international classification of functioning, disability and health (ICF) as a reference tool, *BMC Musculoskelet Disord* 7:96, 2006.

59. Huang H, Grant J, Miller B, M Mirza F, Gagnier J: A systematic review of the psychometric properties of patient-reported outcome instruments for use in patients with rotator cuff disease, *Am J Sport Med* 43(10):2572–2582, 2015.

60. Kirkley A, Alvarez C, Griffin S: The development and evaluation of a disease-specific quality-of-life questionnaire for disorders of the rotator cuff: the western Ontario rotator cuff index, *Clin J sport Med* 13(2):84–92, 2003.

61. St-Pierre C, Desmeules F, Dionne CE, Frémont P, MacDermid JC, Roy J-S: Psychometric properties of self-reported questionnaires for the evaluation of symptoms and functional limitations in individuals with rotator cuff disorders: a systematic review, *Disabil Rehabil* 38(2):103–122, 2016, https://doi.org/10.3109/09638288.2015.1027004.

62. Penta M, Thonnard JL, Tesio L: Abilhand:a Rasch-built measure of manual ability, *Arch Phys Med Rehabil* 79(9):1038–1042, 1998.

63. Richards RR, An K-N, Bigliani LU, Friedman RJ, Gartsman GM, Gristina AG, et al.: A standardized method for the assessment of shoulder function, *J Shoulder Elbow Surg* 3(6):347–352, 1994, https://doi.org/10.1016/S1058-2746(09)80019-0.

64. King GJ, Richards RR, Zuckerman JD, Blasier R, Dillman C, Friedman RJ, et al.: A standardized method for assessment of elbow function. Research Committee, American Shoulder and Elbow Surgeons, *J Shoulder Elbow Surg* 8(4):351–354, 1999.

65. Constant CR, Murley AHG: A clinical method of functional assessment of the shoulder, *Clin Orthop Relat Res* 214:160–164, 1987.

66. Constant CR, Gerber C, Emery RJH, Søjbjerg JO, Gohlke F, Boileau P: A review of the constant score: modifications and guidelines for its use, *J Shoulder Elbow Surg* 17(2):355–361, 2008.

67. Roy JS, MacDermid JC, Woodhouse LJ: A systematic review of the psychometric properties of the constant-Murley score, *J Shoulder Elbow Surg* 19(1):157–164, 2010.

68. Chung KC, Pillsbury MS, Walters MR, Hayward RA: Reliability and validity testing of the Michigan hand outcomes questionnaire, *J Hand Surg* 23(4):575–587, 1998.

69. Waljee JF, Kim HM, Burns PB, Chung KC: Development of a brief, 12-item version of the Michigan hand questionnaire, *Plast Reconstr Surg* 128(1):208–220, 2011.

70. MacDermid JC, Turgeon T, Richards RS, Beadle M, Roth JH: Patient rating of wrist pain and disability: a reliable and valid measurement tool, *J Orthop Trauma* 12(8):577–586, 1998.

71. MacDermid JC, Tottenham V: Responsiveness of the disability of the arm, shoulder, and hand (DASH) and patient-rated wrist/hand evaluation (PRWHE) in evaluating change after hand therapy, *J Hand Ther* 17(1):18–23, 2004.

72. Esakki S, MacDermid JC, Vincent JI, Packham TL, Walton D, Grewal R: Rasch analysis of the patient-rated wrist evaluation questionnaire, *Arch Physiother* 8:5, 2018, https://doi.org/10.1186/s40945-018-0046-z.

73. Roach K, Budiman-Mak E, Songsiridej N, Lertratanakul Y: Development of a shoulder pain and disability index, *Arthritis Care Res* 4(4):143–149, 1991.

74. Tveitå EK, Sandvik L, Ekeberg OM, Juel NG, Bautz-Holter E: Factor structure of the shoulder pain and disability index in patients with adhesive capsulitis, *BMC Musculoskelet Disord* 9:103, 2008, https://doi.org/10.1186/1471-2474-9-103.

75. Hill CL, Lester S, Taylor AW, Shanahan ME, Gill TK: Factor structure and validity of the shoulder pain and disability index in a population-based study of people with shoulder symptoms, *BMC Musculoskelet Disord* 12:8, 2011, https://doi.org/10.1186/1471-2474-12-8.

76. Williams Jr JW, Holleman Jr DR, Simel DL: Measuring shoulder function with the shoulder pain and disability index, *J Rheumatol* 22(4):727–732, 1995.

77. Law M, Baptiste S, McColl M, Opzoomer A, Polatajko H, Pollock N: The Canadian occupational performance measure: an outcome measure for occupational therapy, *Can J Occup Ther* 57(2):82–87, 1990.

78. Turner-Stokes L: Goal attainment scaling (GAS) in rehabilitation: a practical guide, *Clin Rehabil* 23(4):362–730, 2009, https://doi.org/10.1177/0269215508101742.

79. Stratford PW, Gill C, Westaway M, Binkley JM: Assessing disability and change on individual patients: a report of a patient-specific measure, *Physiother Can* 47:238–263, 1995.

80. Horn K, Jennings S, Richardson G, van Vliet D, Hefford C, Haxby Abbott J: The patient-specific functional scale: psychometrics, clinimetrics, and application as a clinical outcome measure, *J Orthop Sports Phys Ther* 42(1):30–42, 2012, https://doi.org/10.2519/jospt.2012.3727.

81. van de Ven-Stevens LA, Munneke M, Terwee CB, Spauwen PH, van der Linde H: Clinimetric properties of instruments to assess activities in patients with hand injury: a systematic review of the literature, *Arch Phys Med Rehabil* 90(1):151–169, 2009, https://doi.org/10.1016/j.apmr.2008.06.024.

82. Rouleau DM, Faber K, MacDermid JC: Systematic review of patient-administered shoulder functional scores on instability, *J Shoulder Elbow Surg* 19:1121–1128, 2010.

83. Jayakumar P, Williams M, Ring D, Lamb S, Gwilym S: A systematic review of outcome measures assessing disability following upper extremity trauma, *J Am Acad Orthop Surg Glob Res Rev* 4:e021, 2017, https://doi.org/10.5435/JAAOSGlobal-D-17-00021.

84. Dowrick AS, Gabbe BJ, Williamson OD, Cameron PA: Outcome instruments for the assessment of the upper extremity following trauma: a review, *Injury* 36:468–476, 2005.

85. Hill B, Williams G, Bialocerkowski A: Clinimetric evaluation of questionnaires used to assess activity after traumatic brachial plexus injury in adults: a systematic review, *Arch Phys Med Rehabil* 92:2082–2089, 2011.

86. Novak CB, Anastakis DJ, Beaton DE, Katz J: Patient-reported outcome after peripheral nerve injury, *J Hand Surg-Am* 34(2):281–287, 2009, https://doi.org/10.1016/j.jhsa.2008.11.017.

87. Resnik L, Borgia M, Silver B, Cancio J: Systematic review of measures of impairment and activity limitation for persons with upper limb trauma and amputation, *Arch Phys Med Rehabil* 98:1863–1892, e14, 2017.

88. Wright V: Prosthetic outcome measures for use with upper limb amputees: a systematic review of the peer-reviewed literature, 1970 to 2009, *J Prosthet Orthot* 21(Suppl 9):P3–P63, 2009, https://doi.org/10.1097/JPO.0b013e3181ae9637.

89. Hendrikx J, de Jonge MJ, Fransen J, Kievit W, van Riel PL: Systematic review of patient-reported outcome measures (PROMs) for assessing disease activity in rheumatoid arthritis, *RMD Open* 2(2):e000202, 2016, https://doi.org/10.1136/rmdopen-2015-000202.

90. Dziedzic KS, Thomas E, Hay EM: A systematic search and critical review of measures of disability for use in a population survey of hand osteoarthritis (OA), *Osteoarthr Cartil* 13:1–12, 2005.

91. De Vet HCW, Terwee CB, Mokkink LB, Knol DL: *Measurement in medicine: a practical guide*, Cambridge, UK, 2011, Cambridge University Press.

92. Mokkink LB, Terwee CB, Patrick DL, Alonso J, Stratford PW, Knol DL, et al.: The COSMIN study reached international consensus on taxonomy, terminology, and definitions of measurement properties for health-related patient-reported outcomes, *J Clin Epidemiol* 63:737–745, 2010.

93. Mokkink LB, Terwee CB, Patrick DL, Alonso J, Stratford PW, Knol DL, et al.: The COSMIN checklist for assessing the methodological quality of studies on measurement properties of health status measurement instruments: an international delphi study, *Qual Life Res* 19:539–549, 2010.

94. Prinsen CAC, Mokkink LB: COSMIN guideline for systematic reviews of patient-reported outcome measures, *Qual Life Res* 27(5):1147–1157, 2018, https://doi.org/10.1007/s11136-018-1798-3.

95. Terwee CB, Prinsen CAC, Chiarotto A, Westerman MJ, Patrick DL, Alonso J, et al.: COSMIN methodology for evaluating the content validity of patient-reported outcome measures: a delphi study, *Qual Life Res* 27:1159–1170, 2018, https://doi.org/10.1007/s11136-018-1829-0.

96. Mokkink LB, Prinsen CAC, Bouter LM, de Vet HCW, Terwee CB: The consensus-based standards for the selection of health measurement instruments (COSMIN) and how to select an outcome measurement instrument, *Braz J Phys Ther* 20:105–113, 2016.

97. Bialocerkowski AE, Bragge P: Measurement error and reliability testing: Application to rehabilitation, *Int J Ther Rehabil* 15(10):422–427, 2008.

98. Terwee CB, Bot SDM, de Boer MR, van der Windt DAWM, Knol DL, Dekker J, et al.: Quality criteria were proposed for measurement properties of health status questionnaires, *J Clin Epidemiol* 60:34–42, 2007.

99. Kottner J, Audige L, Brorson S, Donner A, Gajewski BJ, Hrobjartsson A, et al.: Guidelines for reporting reliability and agreement studies (GRRAS) were proposed, *J Clin Epidemiol* 64:96–106, 2011.

100. Streiner DN, Cairney GR, Health J: *Measurement scales a practical guide to their development and use*, ed 4, New York, NY, 2015, Oxford University Press.

101. Boyle GJ: Does item homogeneity indicate internal consistency or item redundancy in psychometric scales? *Pers Individ Dif* 12:291–294, 1991.

102. Hernaez R: Reliability and agreement studies: a guide for clinical investigators, *Gut* 64(7):1018–1027, 2015.

103. Mokkink LB, Terwee CB, Knol DL, Stratford PW, Alonso J, Patrick DL, et al.: The COSMIN checklist for evaluating the methodological quality of studies on measurement properties: a clarification of its content, *BMC Med Res Methodol* 10, 2010, https://doi.org/10.1186/1471-2288-10-22.

104. Gwaltney CJ, Shields AL, Shiffman S: Equivalence of electronic and paper-and-pencil administration of patient-reported outcome measures: a meta-analytic review, *Value in Health* 11(2):322–333, 2008. https://doi:10.1111/j.1524-4733.2007.00231.x.

105. Coons SJ, Gwaltney CJ, Hays RD, Lundy JJ, Sloan JA, Revicki DA, et al.: Recommendations on evidence needed to support measurement equivalence between electronic and paper-based patient-reported outcome (PRO) measures: ISPOR ePRO good research practices task force report, *Value Health* 12(4):419–429, 2009. https://doi:10.1111/j.1524-4733.2008.00470.x.

106. DeVellis RF: *Scale development: theroy and applications*, ed 3, Thousand Oakes, CA, 2003, Sage.

107. Graham C: Incidence and impact of proxy response in measuring patient experience: secondary analysis of a large postal survey using propensity score matching, *Int J Qual Health Care* 28:246–252, 2016.

108. Wild D, Grove A, Martin M, Eremenco S, McElroy S, Verjee-Lorenz A, et al.: Principles of good practice for the translation and cultural adaptation process for patient-reported outcomes (PRO) measures: report of the ISPOR Task Force for Translation and Cultural Adaptation, *Value Health* 8:94–104, 2005.

109. Hammond A, Prior Y, Tyson S: Linguistic validation, validity and reliability of the British English versions of the disabilities of the arm, shoulder and hand (DASH) questionnaire and QuickDASH in people with rheumatoid arthritis, *BMC Musculoskeletal Disord* 19(1):118, 2018, https://doi.org/10.1186/s12891-018-2032-8.

110. Jenkinson C, Stewart-Brown S, Petersen S, Paice C: Assessment of the SF-36 version 2 in the United Kingdom, *J Epidemiol Community Health* 53:46–50, 1999.

111. Perez JL, Mosher ZA, Watson SL, Sheppard ED, Brabston EW, McGwin G, et al.: Readability of orthopaedic patient-reported outcome measures: is there a fundamental failure to communicate? *Clin Orthop Relat Res* 475(8):1936–1947, 2017.

6 Hand Coordination

Cynthia Cooper
Colleen West

Background

The hand is a perceptual entity that has been described as an information-seeking organ. Its use provides individuals with the ability to interpret and analyze tactile properties, such as shape, size, and texture. Hand use also enables us to manipulate objects in order to identify and handle them effectively. Using coordinated hand function, we manually explore and recognize the relationship of objects to our bodies and to gravity.[1]

Functional hand skills require tactile-proprioceptive and visual information, but if the somatosensory functions are good, then visual feedback is not mandatory. Hand skills include reach, grasp, carry, voluntary release, in-hand manipulation, and bilateral hand use. The latter two hand skills are considered to be the most complex. The radial digits are considered to be the skill side (manipulative side) of the hand, while the ulnar digits are considered to be the stability side of the hand.

Definitions[2]

Reach is defined as moving and extending the arm for placing or grasping an object. **Grasp** is attaining an object with the hand. **Carry** is transporting an object in the hand to another place. **Voluntary release** is intentionally letting go of an object in the hand at a specific place and time. **In-hand manipulation** means adjusting an object in the hand after grasping it. **Bilateral hand use** means using two hands together in order to accomplish an activity. Developmentally, bilateral hand use follows unilateral hand use. Examples of bilateral hand use could be steering a bicycle or throwing a large ball. **Bimanual hand use** means each hand does something different during the activity. Examples of bimanual hand use are tying shoelaces or cutting with scissors.

Hand movements are classified as nonprehensile and prehensile. **Nonprehensile movements** use the fingers or the entire hand to lift or push an object. **Prehensile movements** incorporate grasping an object and can be subdivided into two purposes: precision grasp and power grasp. **Precision grasp** uses opposition of the thumb to the fingertips. Power grasp uses the whole hand with thumb flexion or abduction according to the control level required for the task.

Another classification system differentiates grasp by the inclusion or exclusion of thumb opposition. Hook grasp, power grasp, and lateral pinch do not incorporate thumb opposition. **Hook grasp** is useful for sustaining grip during activities such as holding the handle of a briefcase or carrying a bucket of water. **Power grasp** is useful for controlling objects, such as tools. Using a hairbrush employs power grasp with oblique positioning of the object in the hand and more flexion of the ulnar digits than of the radial digits. **Lateral pinch** is useful when one needs power to manipulate or hold a small object. Lateral pinch is utilized when one turns a key in a lock.

Tip pinch and palmar grasp differ from hook grasp, power grasp, and lateral pinch because they do incorporate thumb opposition. **Tip pinch** is demonstrated by touching the tip of the thumb to the tip of the index finger while all joints of the thumb and index finger are partially flexed, forming a circle. Patients with anterior interosseous nerve injury are unable to perform tip pinch because they lack the function of the thumb's flexor pollicis longus and the index finger's flexor digitorum profundus.

Palmar grasp is further categorized into standard, cylindrical, disk, and spherical grasps. With **cylindrical grasp**, flattening of the transverse arch facilitates holding the fingers against an object. In **disk grasp**, there is metacarpophalangeal (MP) hyperextension and finger abduction that is adjusted according to the object's size. When we open a jar, the hand stabilizing the jar utilizes a cylindrical grasp, while the hand opening the lid uses a disk grasp. **Spherical grasp** occurs with wrist extension, digital abduction, and some MP and interphalangeal (IP) flexion, as in holding a tennis ball. This prehension pattern requires control and balance of the intrinsic and extrinsic muscles.

Pinches are classified according to the number of digits involved. **Two-point pinch,** also called **pad-to-pad pinch** or **pincer grasp,** occurs when the thumb opposes the index finger pad only. **Three-point pinch**, also called **three-jaw chuck** grasp, occurs when the thumb opposes the index and middle finger pads simultaneously. This pinch provides better prehension stability than does two-point pinch.

Manipulation Patterns

There are five types of in-hand manipulation patterns. In order to perform these patterns, individuals must be able to control the palmar arches of their hand. The pattern types are finger-to-palm translation, palm-to-finger translation, shift, simple rotation, and complex rotation. Varying definitions of finger-to-palm translation are offered in the literature. Exner[2] defines **finger-to-palm translation** as the grasping of an object with the thumb and finger pads and then moving the object into the palm. This is exemplified by the activity of picking up a button with the thumb and fingers and then moving the button into the palm. **Palm-to-finger translation** occurs in the opposite direction and is more difficult to perform. It is performed when a person has coins in their palm, and they move one coin from the palm to the finger pads in preparation for inserting the coin into a slot. **Shift** is demonstrated when an object that is being held on the radial aspect of the hand is moved linearly on the finger surface in order to reposition it on the finger pads. Repositioning a pen after grasping it is an example of shift. **Simple rotation** occurs when an object is turned or rolled less than or equal to 90 degrees in the finger pads. Opening a small bottle cap is an example of simple rotation. **Complex rotation** is similar to simple rotation, but the object is rotated 180 to 360 degrees. Turning a pencil in order to use the eraser end is an example of complex rotation. **In-hand manipulation with stabilization** is defined as the performance of any in-hand manipulation pattern while stabilizing other objects in the same hand.

Clinical Pearl

Having excellent range of motion (ROM) or good somatosensory function does not guarantee good coordination. For hand therapy clients, coordination activities that look easy may in fact be quite challenging, particularly for their nondominant extremity.

Clinical Pearl

Fine motor skills result from combinations of various factors including excellent control of finger motions, but it is the impact of the central nervous system that truly provides the foundation for specialized hand use.[3]

Grading Coordination Activities

Clinical Pearl

Developmentally, prehension precedes manipulation.

Coordination activities may be graded from gross motor control to fine motor control; from handling of rubbery or textured objects to handling of smooth, slippery, or wet objects; from activities near the body to activities farther away from the body; from use of proximal support to no proximal support; from gravity-assisted to gravity-eliminated to anti-gravity positions; and from nonresistive to resistive.

Examples

See Figs 6.1 through 6.20 for examples of coordination exercises.

Conclusion

Through complex sensorimotor capabilities of hand use, motion is transformed into function. Adding coordination activities to hand therapy treatment provides a way to transform objective clinical improvements such as increased range of motion (ROM) into meaningful gains of hand function and use.[4]

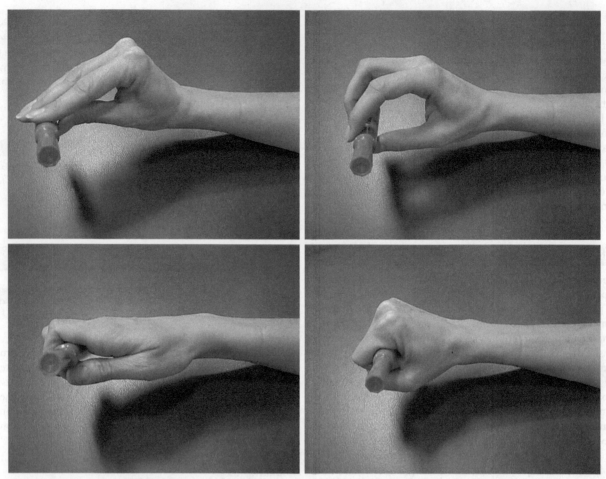

FIG. 6.1 Finger-to-palm translation. (Copyright Cynthia Cooper and John Evarts.)

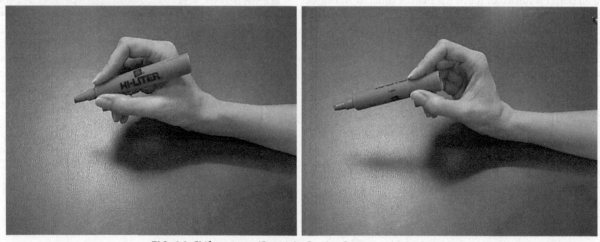

FIG. 6.2 Shift or scoot. (Copyright Cynthia Cooper and John Evarts.)

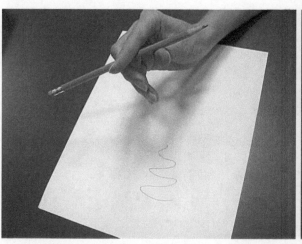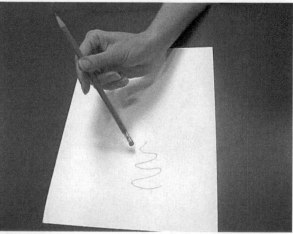

FIG. 6.3 Complex rotation. The fingers change position from one side of the pencil to the other side in order to flip/rotate the pencil. (Copyright Cynthia Cooper and John Evarts.)

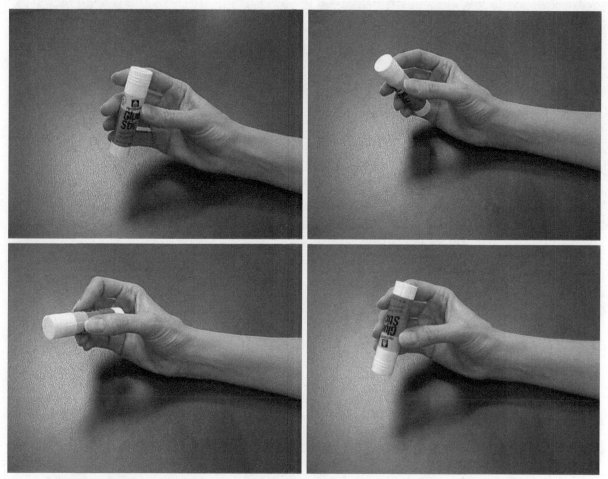

FIG. 6.4 Complex rotation in steps. The thumb stays on the same side of the object and the fingers manipulate the object to spin/rotate it. (Copyright Cynthia Cooper and John Evarts.)

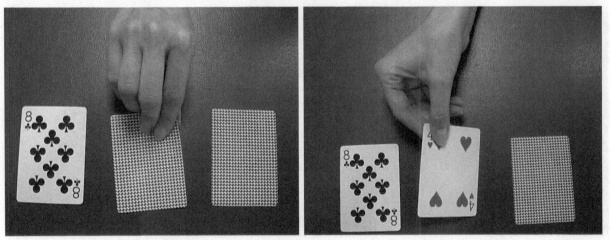

FIG. 6.5 Card flip. (Copyright Cynthia Cooper and John Evarts.)

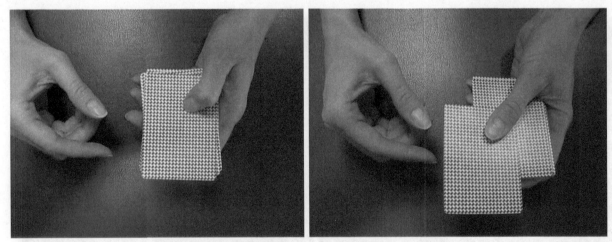

FIG. 6.6 Dealing cards. (Copyright Cynthia Cooper and John Evarts.)

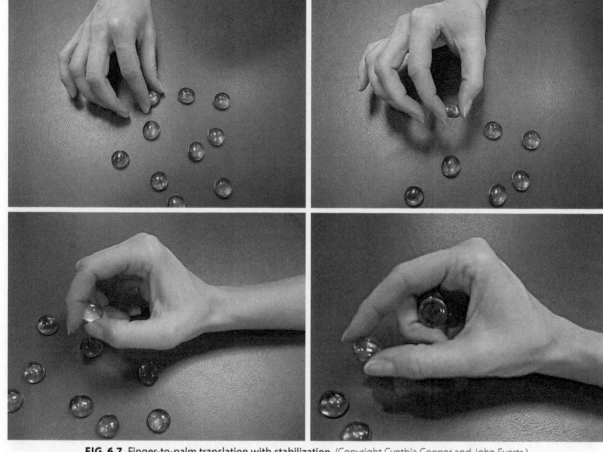

FIG. 6.7 Finger-to-palm translation with stabilization. (Copyright Cynthia Cooper and John Evarts.)

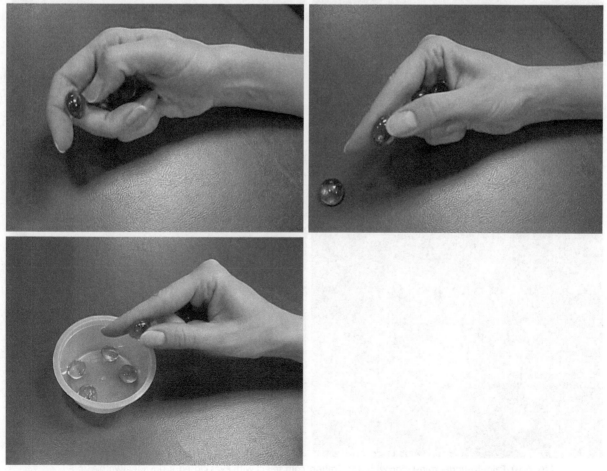

FIG. 6.8 Palm-to-finger translation with stabilization. (Copyright Cynthia Cooper and John Evarts.)

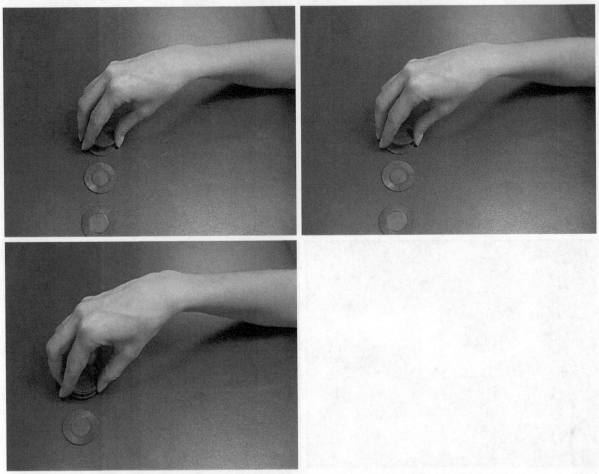

FIG. 6.9 Stacking checkers and graded release. (Copyright Cynthia Cooper and John Evarts.)

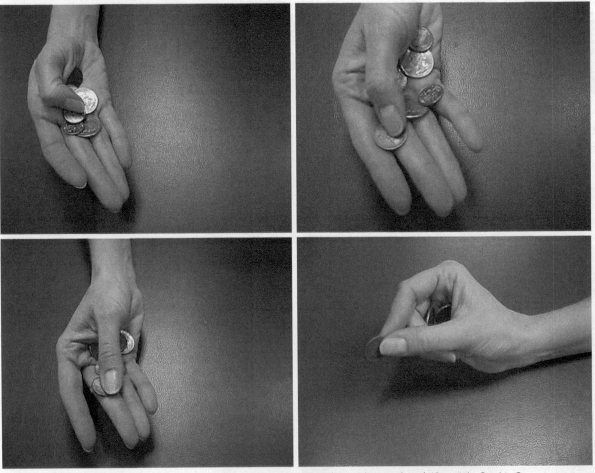

FIG. 6.10 Palm-to-finger translation with stabilization, coin select with eyes closed. (Copyright Cynthia Cooper and John Evarts.)

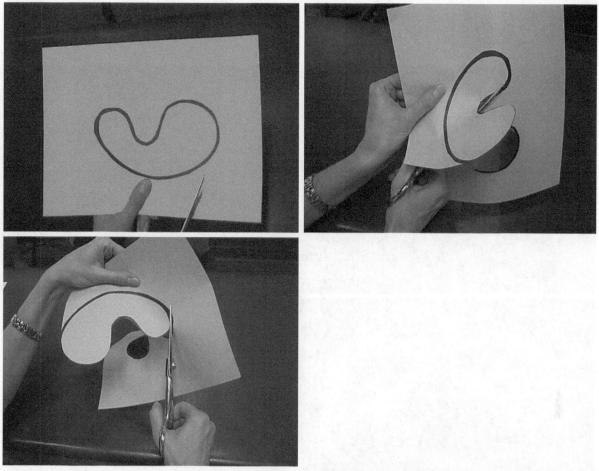

FIG. 6.11 Bimanual task: scissors. (Copyright Cynthia Cooper and John Evarts.)

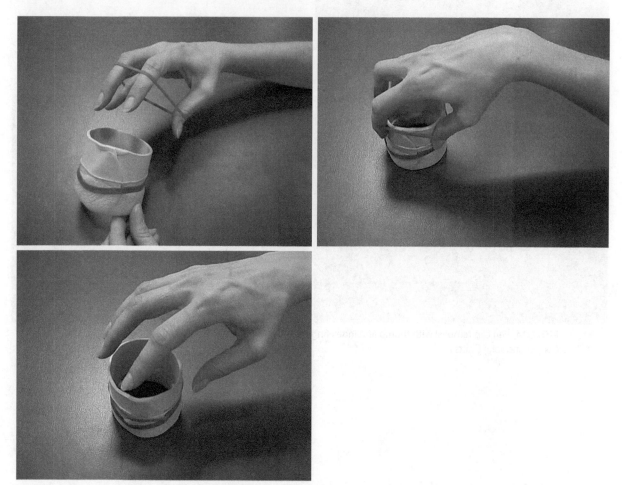

FIG. 6.12 Rubber band graded release. (Copyright Cynthia Cooper and John Evarts.)

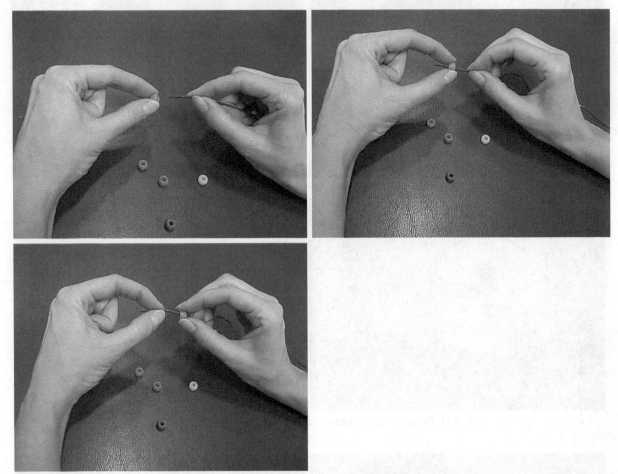

FIG. 6.13 Stringing. (Copyright Cynthia Cooper and John Evarts.)

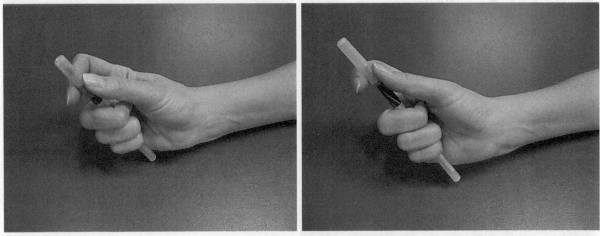

FIG. 6.14 Pen cap removal with thumb and index fingers while holding pen in the hand. (Copyright Cynthia Cooper and John Evarts.)

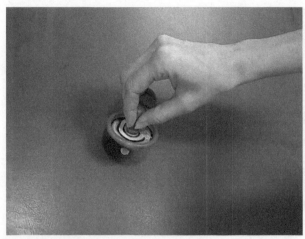

FIG. 6.15 Pincer grasp to spin a top. (Copyright Cynthia Cooper and John Evarts.)

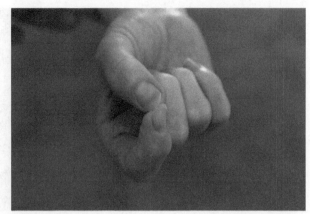

FIG. 6.16 Flicking fingernails. (Copyright Cynthia Cooper and John Evarts.)

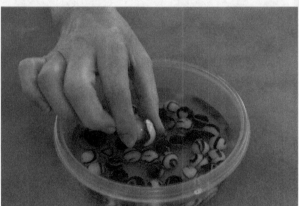 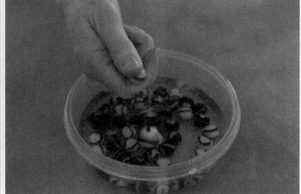

FIG. 6.17 Finger-to-palm translation of slippery marbles in water. (Copyright Cynthia Cooper and John Evarts.)

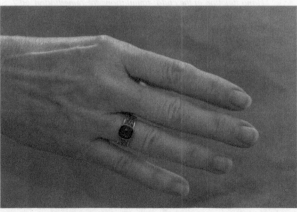 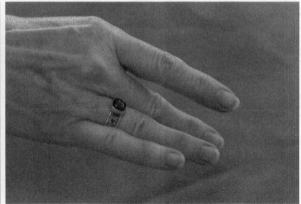

FIG. 6.18 Rolling a ring around on the finger using the two adjacent fingers. (Copyright Cynthia Cooper and John Evarts.)

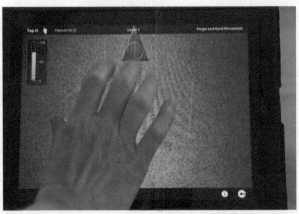

FIG. 6.19 Dexteria application for iPad. (Copyright Cynthia Cooper and John Evarts.)

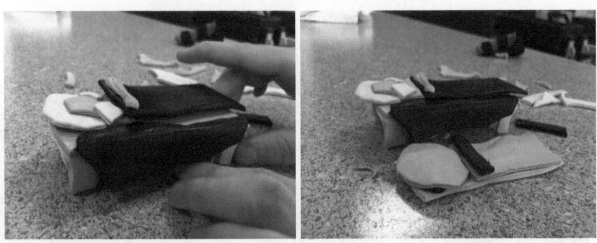

FIG. 6.20 Young girl with juvenile rheumatoid arthritis making a trundle bed out of thermoplastic scraps. (Copyright Cynthia Cooper and John Evarts.)

References

1. Cermak SA: Perceptual functions of the hand. In Henderson A, Pehoski C, editors: *Hand function in the child: foundations for remediation*, ed 2, St. Louis, MO, 2008, Mosby, pp 63–88.
2. Exner CE. Evaluation and interventions to develop hand skills. In: Case-Smith J, O'Brien JC, eds. *Occupational therapy for children*. ed 6. Maryland Heights, MO, 2010, Mosby; pp 275–324.
3. Rao AK: Cognition and motor skill. In Henderson A, Pehoski C, editors: *Hand function in the child: foundations for remediation*, ed 2, St. Louis, MO, 2006, Mosby, pp 101–113.
4. Cooper C, West CG: *Coordination Activities for Hand Therapy Patients*, Boston, 2008, (Unpublished work, poster presented at the American Society of Hand Therapists Annual Meeting). Retrieved from: http://evarts.net/ASHT-2008/ASHT_2008_Cooper_poster.pdf. [Accessed 16 April 2013].

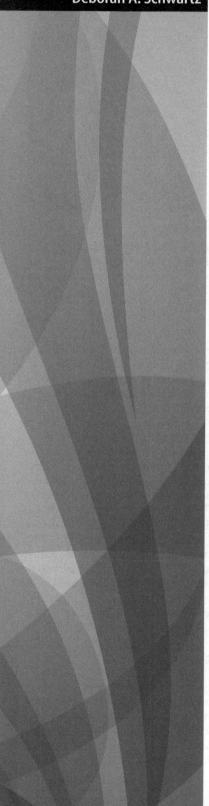

7

Orthoses: Essential Concepts

Deborah A. Schwartz

Introduction

This chapter provides an introduction to orthotic fabrication principles and techniques for upper extremity rehabilitation. Orthoses are custom-made or prefabricated devices used to optimize body functions and structures and help promote an individual's participation in activities and roles.[1] In most treatment settings, including hospitals, skilled nursing facilities, outpatient rehabilitation centers, hand therapy clinics, and school settings, there is an opportunity for therapists to assess clients' needs for orthotic intervention. A recent systematic review by Roll and Hardison provides evidence to support orthotic intervention for clients with arthritis, general hand pain, carpal tunnel, and other musculoskeletal conditions.[2] Goals of orthotic use include, but are not limited to, pain relief, functional positioning, and postoperative immobilization. Orthotic fabrication is an important therapeutic intervention that requires advanced knowledge and practice. This chapter will focus on custom-made orthoses for the upper extremity.

Getting Started in Orthotic Fabrication

Orthotic fabrication is a skill that develops through practice and repetition. It takes time to become skilled. You must have a sound understanding of anatomy, kinesiology, biomechanical principles, and psychosocial concepts to fabricate orthoses for your clients. You should understand tissue healing and have an appreciation for both simple and complex diagnoses and conditions that affect the upper extremity.[1] You must also understand the characteristics of a wide variety of low temperature thermoplastics (LTTPs) available for orthotic fabrication. In addition, you need to develop clinical reasoning skills to determine how an orthosis will benefit each individual client and their specific condition/diagnosis. Be patient with yourself as you develop the necessary skills to include this important intervention in your treatment regimen. You will become more and more adept with every orthosis you design and mold, and you will develop improved skill through multiple practice sessions and applications. Take every opportunity to observe others, attend orthotic fabrication courses, watch instructional videos, and practice orthotic fabrication on your friends, family members, and even on yourself! You will be amazed at how quickly you can master the skills of designing, cutting, and molding orthoses if you devote the necessary time to learn the basics.

Who Needs Orthoses?

Therapists may fabricate orthoses for clients needing conservative management of hand conditions or for protection immediately after trauma or postsurgical interventions. Therapists working with clients in skilled nursing facilities, inpatient departments, and pediatric settings may fabricate orthoses for clients requiring functional aids or assistance with positioning of fingers and extremities. These types of orthoses are usually constructed from LTTPs and typically require frequent adjustments and modifications in order to keep up with clients' changing medical requirements.

Types of Orthoses

Orthoses can be divided into two categories: **orthoses for immobilization** and **orthoses for mobilization.** Orthoses for immobilization exert a static force on a specific body part. An example of this would be an immobilized wrist joint in a wrist cock-up orthosis (Fig. 7.1B). There are no moveable parts in the orthosis, and the wrist joint itself is at rest in the orthosis. On the other hand, orthoses for mobilization are constructed with moveable

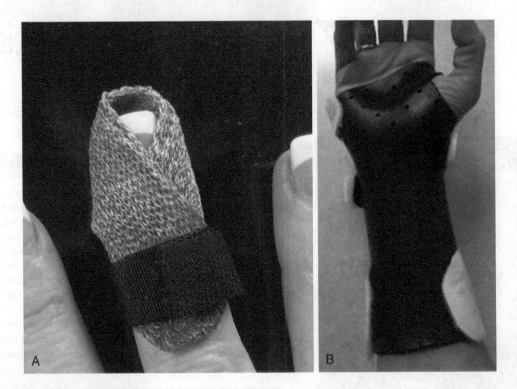

FIG. 7.1 (A) Mallet orthosis. **(B)** Volar wrist cock up orthosis.

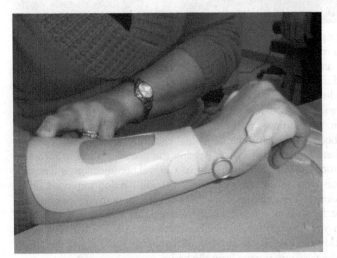

FIG. 7.2 Dynamic wrist orthosis with coils.

components and can be adjusted depending on the specific construction type and purpose of the orthosis.[1] Orthoses for mobilization can be further categorized into dynamic, static progressive, and serial static orthoses. **Dynamic** orthoses incorporate elastic components, coils, or springs that allow movement of the client's joint(s) while wearing the orthosis (Fig. 7.2). These orthoses might be indicated in postoperative treatment protocols, to assist with weak muscles, or to increase passive joint range of motion. **Static progressive** orthoses include inelastic components that typically pull on stiff joints or other tight tissues to allow progressive changes in joint position. This can be an effective intervention when someone has a very stiff joint after trauma or surgery (Fig. 7.3A and B).[1] A **serial static** orthosis is worn by a client over a specific time period and is then remolded to accommodate positive changes in joint motion or positioning (Fig. 7.4). The goals are quite different for orthoses for immobilization versus orthoses for mobilization. You should always consider the goal of

your orthosis before you begin to design and fabricate it on your client. The goal should be the first thing you consider.

Goals of orthoses for immobilization and mobilization are highlighted in Box 7.1 and Box 7.2.

Naming of Orthoses

In the past, therapists have attempted various classification and naming systems to give a sense of organization to the construction and fabrication of different orthoses, formerly known as splints.[1] This was done in an effort to establish a more standardized naming system for communication between therapists who fabricate orthoses and the physicians who prescribe them. Despite attempts at standardizing the nomenclature, many traditional names of orthoses have endured. Some therapists and physicians will still use traditional nomenclature when ordering or discussing the appropriate orthosis for a client. It is important to understand that traditional orthoses' names generally indicate specific body part(s) to include and specific positioning to be achieved during fabrication of the orthosis. For example, a resting hand orthosis typically includes the forearm, wrist, fingers, and thumb in specific postures (Fig. 7.5). The wrist is positioned in slight extension, the fingers are resting in slight flexion, and the thumb is positioned in wide abduction. A long opponens orthosis will include the wrist and the thumb, while the short opponens orthosis leaves the wrist free. Take the time to familiarize yourself with the common names of orthoses and the joints and positioning they comprise, as outlined in Table 7.1.

Reimbursement for Orthoses

Although therapists don't typically think of what we do in terms of cost and pricing, it is critical to understand that billing and reimbursement for orthoses are important considerations in our use of this intervention. L codes were introduced by the Centers for Medicare and Medicaid Services (CMS) to describe the various orthoses fabricated by therapists. L codes are found in

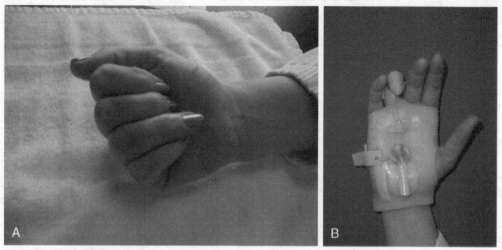

FIG. 7.3 **(A)** Stiff finger after injury. **(B)** Static progressive orthosis for stiff finger.

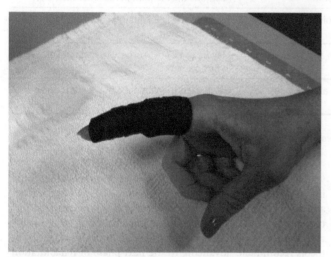

FIG. 7.4 Serial static orthosis for proximal interphalangeal joint flexion contracture.

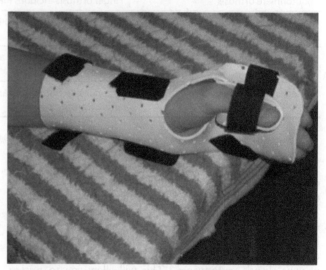

FIG. 7.5 Resting hand orthosis.

BOX 7.1   Goals of Orthoses for Immobilization

- Symptom relief
- Protection and positioning
- Maximize function
- Improve and/or preserve joint alignment
- Contracture management
- Block and/or transfer muscle force

BOX 7.2   Goals of Orthoses for Mobilization

- Remodel long-standing dense mature scar tissue
- Elongate soft-tissue contractures
- Increase passive joint range of motion
- Substitute for weak or absent muscle
- Provide resistance for exercise
- Maintain intraarticular fracture reduction

---

the Healthcare Common Procedure Coding System (HCPCS) Level II manual. The CMS website at https://www.cms.gov/dme posfeesched/ offers information on billing for orthoses.[1] Orthoses provided by a therapist require a prescription and/or certificate of medical necessity signed by the referring physician in order to receive reimbursement from insurance companies.

Critical Thinking/Clinical Reasoning

As the treating therapist, you should always use your critical thinking and clinical reasoning skills when evaluating clients for an orthosis. *Do not fabricate an orthosis just because a physician's prescription requests it!* Begin by evaluating your client and looking at all of the variables that make this individual unique. Client variables include, but are not limited to, diagnosis, wound status, physical and mental status, age, motivation, intelligence, culture, activities of daily living (ADLs), instrumental activities of daily living (IADLs), work activities, leisure activities, family/caregiver support, and distance from the clinic. Consider client roles and their ability to perform these roles in a variety of contexts. How will an orthosis impact the client's performance? Will it help them engage in activities that currently cause pain? Will it

TABLE 7.1   Names of Common Upper Extremity Orthoses

Orthosis Name	Include These Joints	Positioning
Resting hand orthosis	Forearm, wrist, fingers and thumb	Resting posture: Wrist in extension, thumb in abduction, MCP joints in flexion and PIP and DIP joints in slight flexion
Short opponens/short thumb spica orthosis	Thumb CMC/ MP joints	Positions the thumb in functional abduction and opposition
Long opponens/long thumb spica orthosis	Wrist and thumb CMC/ MP joints	Positions the wrist in functional extension and the thumb in functional abduction and opposition
Dorsal block orthosis	Dorsal surface of forearm, wrist and fingers (and thumb)	Wrist in neutral or some flexion*, MCP joints in maximum flexion, PIP and DIP joints in 0 degrees extension
Wrist cock-up orthosis	Forearm and wrist joint up to distal palmar crease	Positions the wrist in functional position of 20–30 degrees extension
Boutonniere orthosis	Finger orthosis includes PIP joint	Positions the PIP joint in maximal extension
Mallet orthosis	Finger orthosis includes DIP joint	Positions the DIP joint in neutral or slight hyperextension
Posterior elbow orthosis	Posterior side from upper arm and includes entire forearm	May be used post-surgery to maintain elbow in flexion
Anterior elbow orthosis	Anterior side from upper arm and includes entire forearm	Often used to maintain elbow extension and/or limit elbow flexion

*Check with referring physician.

CMC, Carpometacarpal; *DIP*, distal interphalangeal; *MCP*, metacarpophalangeal; *PIP*, proximal interphalangeal.

eventually lead to improved performance and independent functioning? Should the orthosis be part of the overall treatment plan and for what duration of wear?[3] Most importantly, how will you evaluate the benefits and success of your orthotic intervention? It is important to include a functional evaluation and a client self-directed functional scale as part of the overall initial assessment of your client's performance.[4] This will allow you to reassess performance after your client has worn the orthosis. Your client can then reevaluate their own performance to see if they think the orthosis has improved their functional abilities. The Patient Rated Wrist Hand Evaluation (PRWHE) and the Disabilities of the Arm Shoulder and Hand (DASH) are two tools often used for this assessment.

Indications for the use of Orthoses

Therapists fabricate orthoses to prevent pain in inflamed joints (as for clients with arthritis) or to position a body part to reduce paresthesia (as for clients with nerve compression syndromes). Therapists fabricate orthoses to protect joints after fractures or surgeries.[1] Therapists also fabricate orthoses to maintain length of tissues (as for clients with high tone) or position joints for improved function (as for clients with hypermobile joints). There are many ways in which orthoses can benefit our clients. In order for therapists to receive reimbursement for orthotic fabrication, insurance companies require that a physician prescribe an orthosis. The therapist's documentation must also support a need for the orthosis and the specific benefit a client gains from its use. You must provide supporting information in your documentation such as the client's age, gender, occupational status, and current diagnosis. You must also document the medical history of

your client, including any previous injuries or surgeries that could influence the outcome of the present condition. Include the dates and names of any recent medical or surgical procedures. Dates of pertinent procedures provide critical information in terms of current tissue healing and expected progress. Many treatment protocols recommend advancing to the next phase of rehabilitation based on expected tissue healing.

> **◉ Clinical Pearl**
>
> Take care to record pertinent injury and surgical dates accurately. Keep a calendar at your treatment table to count how much time has elapsed from the injury/surgery date to the present. This time frame will help guide your treatment because it will indicate how much tissue healing has likely occurred to date. Remember, however, that time frames and protocols are only guidelines. They do not take the place of good clinical reasoning and judgement.

The physician's prescription will often indicate the type of orthosis the physician wants fabricated, and will give direction for positioning key joints. However, this is not always the case! You may receive a prescription that reads, "Wrist pain: Evaluate, splint, and treat." You can always call the physician's office to verify the specific orthosis requested, and you *should* call the physician if you have questions or doubts as to which orthosis might be the best option. Experienced clinicians often use their clinical reasoning skills and knowledge of procedures and diagnoses to select the most appropriate orthotic design. Novice therapists might want to discuss the selection of the most appropriate orthosis with more experienced colleagues.

What to Ask the Physician

Most referring physicians will welcome the opportunity to discuss a client's case and continued care with the treating therapist. Try to find a convenient time to approach the physician. Have your questions and concerns ready. Ask about the client's diagnosis or surgical procedure if you are unfamiliar with these, or if you have additional concerns about the client's status. Ask about the specifics of the prescribed orthosis, which joints to include, and whether alterations to the standard orthosis need to be considered. Ask about the recommended duration of wear and any changes to the standard protocol the physician normally uses. Ask if the physician has any concerns about advancing the client through the treatment protocol. If you have special insights or information about the client and their reactions to treatment, it is helpful to discuss these with the physician as early as possible.

Precautions and Contraindications to Orthotic Interventions

If you have any concerns regarding the health status of your client or concerns regarding the status of their involved extremity, bring this up with the physician immediately. If the wound appears more red or swollen than you would expect, or if the skin appears to be necrotic, or if the sutures are not intact, it is imperative that you contact the physician's office prior to fabricating the prescribed orthosis. Do not fabricate the orthosis until you have discussed the situation with the physician! An orthotic intervention can usually wait, but treatment for an infection or worsening medical condition cannot.

If the client presents with an unclear diagnosis or the physician's prescription does not match what you would expect in the client's situation, take time to make the appropriate phone call. If you are unsure, ask the physician specific questions regarding the details of the proposed orthosis. Before you begin orthotic fabrication, know exactly which joints to include in the orthosis, which joints are allowed to move, what is the expected orthotic wearing schedule, and what is the expected outcome of the orthotic intervention.

Clinical Examples of Orthoses for Immobilization

Orthoses for immobilization may provide a safe and comfortable support or may improve positioning for function. It is critical to understand the specifics of each diagnosis and the underlying anatomy to appreciate the exact positioning of the extremity in the orthosis and how it may benefit your client. Here are some examples of orthoses for specific conditions.

Arthritis

For clients with rheumatoid arthritis (RA) or osteoarthritis (OA), orthoses offer resting and positioning relief from inflamed joints and tissues.[5] A commonly prescribed orthosis is the short opponens orthosis for immobilization of the carpometacarpal (CMC) and metacarpophalangeal (MP) joints of the thumb (Fig 7.6). There is moderate evidence to support this orthosis' effectiveness for reducing pain and improving function. Clients

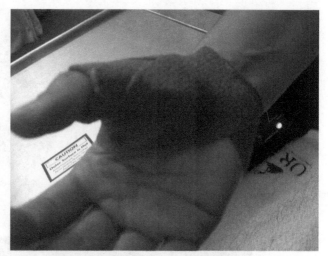

FIG. 7.6 Short opponens orthosis for thumb arthritis.

with arthritis might also display deformities of the fingers, such as swan neck deformity, boutonniere deformity, or ulnar drift[6] (Fig. 7.7A–D). Orthoses can be extremely helpful in positioning the fingers for function if the deformity is still passively correctable.

Carpal Tunnel Syndrome

Clients with carpal tunnel syndrome have compression or irritation of the median nerve in the wrist and often complain of numbness and tingling in the median nerve distribution of the hand. Irritation of the median nerve can occur with repeated wrist and finger movements. Prolonged wrist flexion places pressure on the median nerve at the wrist. There is some evidence that a wrist cock-up orthosis with the wrist positioned in neutral may help alleviate symptoms, especially if worn while sleeping[7,8] (see Fig. 7.1B).

Mallet Finger

A mallet finger deformity occurs when the terminal portion of the extensor tendon over the distal interphalangeal (DIP) joint becomes disrupted. Disruption of the extensor tendon in this location results in the DIP joint dropping into flexion. The client loses the ability to actively straighten the tip of the finger. Orthotic intervention consists of immobilizing the DIP joint in neutral or slight hyperextension for a period of 6 to 8 weeks to allow healing to occur[9] (see Fig. 7.1A). *No flexion of the DIP joint is allowed during this 6- to 8-week period.* Many therapists provide their clients with two orthoses to allow for bathing while wearing one and then switching to the other orthosis to allow for drying.

◎ *Clinical Pearl*

To prevent accidental flexion of the DIP joint while switching from one mallet finger splint to another, teach your client to place their hand on a table (palm down) while sliding mallet finger splints off and on.

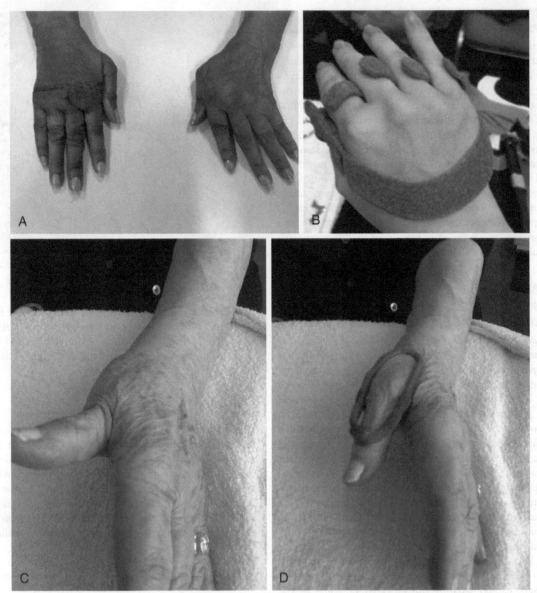

FIG. 7.7 **(A)** Ulnar drift. **(B)** Antiulnar drift orthosis. **(C)** Thumb MCP joint subluxation. **(D)** Anti–swan neck orthosis for thumb MCP joint.

Stroke

The use of orthoses in the treatment of clients with neurological involvement will sometimes be part of an overall management strategy. Wrist and hand orthoses may help decrease pain and improve or maintain range of motion. The use of orthoses may have a role in prevention or treatment of contractures.[10] The effectiveness of orthotic intervention is improved by providing an individualized approach to each client in determining the most appropriate wearing schedule and orthotic design.[11]

Clinical Examples of Orthoses for Mobilization

Dynamic Orthosis for Radial Nerve Palsy

Radial nerve palsy occurs with injury to the radial nerve in the arm. Clients lose the ability to actively extend the wrist and meta-carpophalangeal (MCP) joints of the hand. Daytime wear of a

dynamic orthosis improves a client's functional hand use.[12] A properly designed orthosis assists with wrist and finger extension and lets the client use their hand in many activities of daily living while awaiting nerve recovery. A radial nerve palsy orthosis is similar to the orthosis used following MCP joint replacement surgery (Fig. 7.8).

Static Progressive Orthosis for Limited Finger, Wrist, Forearm, or Elbow Motion

Custom-made static progressive orthoses can be added to the treatment protocol of clients with decreased active motion or stiffness following injury or surgery. Many studies have shown that static progressive orthoses are effective for increasing passive motion of the elbow, forearm, wrist, and digits[13] (Fig. 7.9, see also Fig. 7.3B). Active exercises and functional activities should follow a wearing session of this type of orthotic.

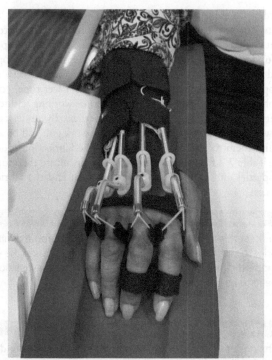

FIG. 7.8 Dynamic extension orthosis used for post-operative MCP joint arthoplasties.

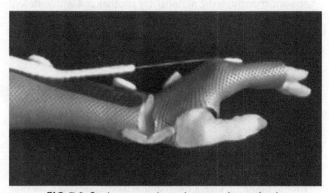

FIG. 7.9 Static progressive wrist extension orthosis.

Serial Static Orthosis for Proximal Interphalangeal Flexion Contracture

Stiffness of the finger joints is a common problem following surgical procedures and traumatic events. The proximal interphalangeal (PIP) joint is particularly prone to stiffness and often develops a flexion contracture, or the inability to fully extend even with manual force. PIP joint flexion contractures are typically treated with serial static orthoses. The PIP joint is placed at its maximal end-range extension, and the orthosis is then molded around the joint to maintain this position. The client wears the orthosis full time for several days and then returns to the therapy clinic for removal of the orthosis, repositioning of the PIP joint at its new end-range extension position, and remolding of the orthosis. This is repeated until the joint is able to fully extend or stops showing improvement[14] (see Fig. 7.4).

During the course of your studies to become a physical or occupational therapist, you learned the basics of upper extremity anatomy and kinesiology. You studied physiology, physics, and psychology. Fabricating and using orthotics effectively requires full integration of knowledge from all of these fields, as well as keeping up with information that becomes available with new research.[15] This section reviews a few key points related to the knowledge base that you must acquire to appropriately fabricate and utilize orthotics in your therapy practice.

Anatomy, Kinesiology, and Physiology

You need a good working knowledge of this trifecta. This means you must be familiar with all bony structures/arches, muscle innervations, and nerve/blood vessel pathways of the upper extremity. Know what areas are prone to nerve compression, blood vessel compression, and bony prominence irritation by ill-fitting orthoses and straps. Use the joints and digital creases as important landmarks in orthotic fabrication. Orthoses should fully support the intended joint but not impede motion of adjacent joints. Make sure to trim orthotic edges just proximal to creases to allow full flexion, especially at the distal palmar crease (DPC). This line needs to be angled ulnarly, reflecting the shorter length of the ulnar metacarpals.

You should understand common conditions that affect the upper extremity, as well as medical, surgical, and therapy protocols used to treat these conditions. Familiarize yourself with the effects of medications that might be prescribed. Medications can affect the integrity of skin and wound healing, which in turn could affect your use of orthotics in those cases.

The Importance of Understanding Tissue Healing

Be aware of the time frames for both soft-tissue and bone healing. Orthotic intervention directly correlates with the phases of tissue healing. In general, during the acute **inflammatory phase,** tissues should be positioned for support and rest using orthoses that immobilize. During the **proliferative phase**, the tensile strength of the injured tissues increases. Active motion may be initiated in this phase and the focus of orthotic intervention is continued protection of soft-tissue structures and their associated repairs while allowing for intervals of active exercises. During this phase, orthoses might be used to restrict joint motion in specific directions while allowing motion in other directions. And, periodically, the orthosis might be modified for improved positioning during this phase. During the **maturation phase,** you will begin to encourage your clients to move more, increase their participation in functional activities, and add movement against resistance. Orthotic interventions during this phase might address limitations in joint motion. Remember to monitor the client's extremity. You may elect to revise or maintain the orthotic intervention based on what you observe during the healing process. Do not make changes based solely on the calendar, but on your assessment of the client's needs.

Orthoses for mobilization are typically introduced during the maturation phase of healing to encourage and promote movement, tissue remodeling, and collagen realignment. These types of orthoses are particularly helpful when joints are stiff or soft tissues are shortened from lack of motion.

The Importance of Understanding the Impact of Low-Load Prolonged Stress and Total end Range Time

When adding orthoses for mobilization to a client's treatment, there are two important concepts to consider: **low-load prolonged stress** and **total end range time (TERT)**.[1]

Low-load prolonged stress refers to providing low amounts of stress over prolonged periods of time to help with tissue remodeling along lines that encourage motion. Application of large amounts of tension may cause an inflammatory reaction to reoccur and delay healing, and too little tension might result in minimal to no tissue remodeling. The key to success is knowing how much tension to apply and when to do so. Orthoses designed to correct digital joint contractures apply between 100 to 300 grams of traction, although very few therapists measure this force.[16] However, therapists can learn to be very good at reading signs of too much force applied to stiff joints: edema, pain, skin blanching, vascular problems, reddened skin, and tingling. Be watchful and make appropriate adjustments to orthoses when necessary.

TERT refers to the total amount of time a client wears the mobilization orthosis to increase passive range of motion in a stiff joint.[13] A typical protocol for wear of a static progressive orthosis might be for 30 minutes, 3 times per day, and this TERT equals 90 minutes.[13] If you have instructed your client to wear their orthosis for 20 minutes, 5 times per day, then the TERT equals 100 minutes. Always look at the TERT as reported by your client when evaluating the effectiveness of the orthosis and encourage your client to increase the TERT before making changes to the level of force applied.

Physics and Mechanical Principles

Orthoses act as levers on the extremity and should firmly support the intended body part. Typically, orthoses are constructed so that they encompass two-thirds the length of the forearm and half the circumference of the forearm to evenly distribute the weight of the limb. Orthoses offer three points of contact with the extremity. The middle force is applied at the joint axis, and the two opposing forces are placed as far away as possible from this point in order to stabilize the intended joint while also distributing force. Longer lever arms are more effective at providing stability and support.

Padding bony prominences prior to orthosis fabrication ensures that the structures are protected from pressure. Orthotic contact with bony prominences can also be removed after fabrication by heating up the specific spot on the orthosis and bumping out or enlarging the area of contact.

Properties of Thermoplastics

Therapists typically utilize LTTPs for orthotic fabrication. These are thermoplastics that are activated in hot water (145–165°F [63–74°C]) or by dry heat, and become soft and moldable in a relatively short time. They can be easily cut and then molded on the extremities, and they will maintain that shape as they cool and

harden. There is a wide variety of LTTPs on the market. Therapists can chose LTTPs with specific properties/characteristics that enable different types of orthotic fabrication. It is important to understand the terminology used to describe these properties and to appreciate the differences between them. Every LTTP property has advantages and disadvantages. Over time, you will probably develop your own preferences for working with certain thermoplastics and thermoplastic properties.. By understanding how these properties and characteristics work you will be able to utilize them to your advantage during the fabrication process.[17] See Table 7.2 for information on low temperature thermoplastic properties and how these benefit the client and the fabrication process.

Clinical Pearl

Preheat thicker thermoplastics (1/8″, 1/12″) for about a minute prior to cutting out the pattern. A little heating makes the thermoplastic much easier to cut. Thinner thermoplastics do not need to be preheated prior to cutting.

Clinical Pearl

Thinner or perforated thermoplastics heat up and cool down quicker than thicker or solid thermoplastics. This means that thinner and perforated thermoplastics have a relatively shorter working time. If you are having difficulty molding with one specific thermoplastic material, try another one with different properties. You will eventually find a thermoplastic that works for you. All thermoplastics come in a variety of thicknesses and perforation patterns, as well as in solid (no perforations).

Clinical Pearl

Coated thermoplastics and noncoated thermoplastics each have advantages and disadvantages. It is easier to attach outriggers to noncoated thermoplastic materials. Coated thermoplastics will pop apart when cooled, and this is sometimes desirable when trying to make an orthosis with an adjustable thumb opening. Check the manufacturer's directions for how to remove the coating, when desired.

Clinical Pearl

When working with thermoplastics possessing excellent memory, remember to let the orthosis fully cool and harden before removing it from the extremity, or it might lose its shape.

Work Space, Equipment, and Materials

Orthotic fabrication should be performed in a designated work space in your clinic. You will need a countertop or work table, a storage area, and access to water and electrical outlets. Basic equipment for orthotic fabrication includes a splint pan or other device for heating water, a heat gun, sharp scissors, a utility knife or box cutter, wire cutters, a hole punch, an awl or marker, and a goniometer. Along with sheets or boxes of thermoplastics, you

TABLE 7.2 Properties of Low-Temperature Thermoplastics

Property/Characteristic	What it Means	Intended Use
Rigidity	The strength of the material	High rigidity is necessary for large splints, specific diagnoses such as spasticity, and splints projecting large forces
Memory	Ability of the material to return to its original size and shape after being stretched	This is an important concept when frequent remolding of the splint will be necessary, as in serial splinting to increase extension or flexion over time. Memory makes the material more cost efficient.
Conformability	The way the material conforms to the shape of the hand	Materials with high drapability work best with gentle handling as they conform easily to the arches or bony prominences. Materials with low drapability require firm handling and are recommended for larger splints where this moldability is less important.
Resistance to stretch	The amount of resistance the material gives to being stretched when heated	High resistance means you must work slowly and steadily to stretch the material. Low resistance to stretch means you need to work more quickly and carefully control the material as it stretches.
Coating	A coating may be applied to certain materials to make them easier to work with and less likely to adhere together where no adherence is desired	Coated materials do not bond easily to attachments without having the coating removed. Noncoated materials have very good bonding to themselves and other attachments.

will need "loop" or neoprene material for strapping and adhesive backed "hook" for adhering the straps to the orthoses.

Foam and adhesive-backed padding materials are available for placement inside the orthosis and are often applied for comfort over bony prominences. Make sure to bump out or stretch the thermoplastic surface to create space for padding. Adding padding without creating space for it will increase pressure on a bony prominence, which is exactly what you want to avoid. Neoprene sheeting material is an excellent addition to many orthoses when used for strapping or as part of the orthosis. Neoprene can be adhered directly to thermoplastic surfaces by heating the material with the heat gun and making it sticky.

Safety

Orthotic fabrication involves working with heat and sharp tools. Both require extreme caution and supervision around clients. This is especially important when children or cognitively impaired people are nearby. Consider your own clients as well as those of your coworkers. Tools such as utility knives and scissors should not be left unattended on the table or countertop. Heat guns should be pointed away from people and objects when on, and should never be left running unattended on high settings. Make sure to close splint pan lids when you walk away. *Always check the temperature of heated material prior to placing it on your client!* It is easy to accidentally burn yourself or your client if you are not vigilant about safety in the clinic.

Therapists treating hand conditions should take care to protect their own bodies when fabricating orthoses for clients. Use good tools and sharpen your scissors often. Remember to preheat thicker materials prior to cutting so that you do not damage your own hands. When fabricating an orthosis on a client, avoid leaning excessively over the table or awkwardly over the client. These positions put a lot of strain on a therapist's back and neck. Always try to obtain easy access to the client's extremity. Position the

client at the corner of a table, as this might be the easiest way to get close. Use gravity to assist you in orthotic fabrication by letting the material rest on top of the extremity as opposed to holding it up and in place. Sometimes the client will need to be placed supine to achieve this. Be creative when positioning your clients. A different position may be more comfortable for the client and easier for you as well. Utilize all the principles of good body mechanics and ergonomics that you learned as part of your basic training to become an occupational or physical therapist.

Orthotic Fabrication Steps

Therapists follow several key steps in order to successfully fabricate orthoses. These are outlined in **Box** 7.3. More experienced therapists might skip pattern making, but novice therapists should stick to this routine in order to be as accurate as possible.

⊙ *Clinical Pearl*

Dip open scissors in hot water from the splint pan (or run the scissor blades over hot air from a heat gun) prior to cutting through adhesive-backed "hook" to prevent scissor blades from becoming caked with sticky glue. The heated metal will prevent glue from sticking.

What to Tell Your Client

Clients must understand the benefits of wearing their orthosis and know the expected time frame for achieving results. Determine your client's specific orthotic-wearing schedule based on the diagnosis, treatment protocol, and client's individual needs. It is critical to explain the purpose of the orthosis to your client and to make sure they are aware of the wearing schedule. Document the client's agreement with the treatment plan and have them repeat

BOX 7.3   Orthotic Fabrication Steps

1. Draw an orthotic pattern around your client's hand on a paper towel.
2. Carefully cut out the pattern and check the fit by placing the paper pattern on the client's hand.
3. Make adjustments to the paper pattern as needed.
4. Select the appropriate thermoplastic material. Trace the pattern on the thermoplastic sheeting, briefly heat up the thermoplastic to soften it just enough for easy cutting, then carefully cut out the orthosis inside the traced pattern markings.
5. Place the cut out orthosis back in the splint pan to fully activate the material.
6. Position your client's hand/wrist in the desired position.
7. Remove the activated orthosis from the hot water and gently dry with a towel.
8. Check the temperature before placing the orthosis on your client. Mold into the desired position. Let fully harden and cool before removing.
9. Mark excess areas and trim. Round all sharp edges. Flair the proximal edge by dipping in hot water and pushing it outward slightly with your thumb.
10. Add straps and check the fit on your client. Make sure your client can take it off and put it on correctly.

back to you the wearing schedule and benefits of the orthosis. Put this schedule in writing, and have the client keep a home record of orthotic use. The goals of the orthosis will only be met if the orthosis is worn according to plan.

Precautions

Explain to the client that the orthosis might lose its shape if left near a heat source. Explain that all orthotic adjustments should be performed by a therapist in the clinic (*never by the client or a family member at home*) so that the shape is not adversely altered in any way. Verify with the physician whether the client should shower with the orthosis on or off. Supply extra "hook" and

"loop" straps as needed. Offer clients stockinette sleeves to wear underneath the orthosis. Alternately, suggest that the client use a colorful sock with the toe area cut off and a hole cut for the thumb.

Encouraging Adherence to Prescribed Orthotic Use

Clients may be more willing to adhere to the orthotic component of the treatment plan if they understand the benefit and purpose of orthoses and have some choice in their design. When possible, allow clients to choose the color of orthotic materials, and add stickers or colorful duct tape as decorations. Adding bling in the form of inexpensive plastic jewels, puppet eyes, or stickers will often enhance the orthotic experience for clients. This is especially true for children and adolescents, but also for some adults! Ensure that the orthosis is comfortable. Take the time to smooth edges and trim straps. Let the client know how important the orthosis is by striving for a cosmetically appealing and well-fitting finished product.

◎ *Clinical Pearl*

Remember to round all corners of the orthosis and all corners of the straps to give a finished look to the orthosis and to prevent sharp and pointed edges from scratching your client.

Summary

The successful fabrication of orthotics for clients is extremely rewarding, but it requires careful thought, application of knowledge, and lots of practice! Take the time to challenge yourself and experiment with different materials and different patterns while you explore this process. An orthosis is one of the few visual representations of your skills as a therapist. It accompanies your client home and in to the community, and will be the topic of conversation among his/her family and friends. Commit yourself to mastering this important skill so that your orthotics are both therapeutically effective and aesthetically pleasing.

References

1. Jacobs ML, Coverdale J: Concepts of orthotic fundamentals. In Jacobs MA, Austin NM, editors: *Orthotic intervention for the hand and upper extremity: splinting principles and process*, Philadelphia, PA, 2014, Lippincott Williams & Wilkins, pp 2–25.
2. Roll SC, Hardison ME: Effectiveness of occupational therapy interventions for adults with musculoskeletal conditions of the forearm, wrist, and hand: a systematic review, *Am J Occup Ther* 71(1), 2017. 7101180010p1-7101180010p12.
3. American Occupational Therapy Association: Occupational therapy practice framework: domain and process, 3rd edition, *Am J Occup Ther* 68:S1–S48, 2014. org/10.5014/ajot.2014.682006.
4. Von der Heyde R, Droege K: Assessment of functional outcomes. In Cooper C, editor: *Fundamentals of hand therapy: clinical reasoning and treatment guidelines for common diagnoses of the upper extremity*, St. Louis, MO, 2013, Elsevier Health Sciences.
5. Valdes K, Naughton N, Algar L: Linking ICF components to outcome measures for orthotic intervention for CMC OA: a systematic review, *J Hand Ther* 29(4):396–404, 2016.
6. Beasley J: Osteoarthritis and rheumatoid arthritis: conservative therapeutic management, *J Hand Ther* 25(2):163–172, 2012.
7. Page MJ, Massy-Westropp N, O'Connor D, Pitt V: Splinting for carpal tunnel syndrome, *Cochrane Database of Syst Rev* 7:CD010003, 2012, https://doi.org/10.1002/14651858.CD010003.
8. Hall B, Lee HC, Fitzgerald H, et al.: Investigating the effectiveness of full-time wrist splinting and education in the treatment of carpal tunnel syndrome: a randomized controlled trial, *Am J Occup Ther* 67(4):448–459, 2013.
9. Cook S, Daniels N, Woodbridge S: How do hand therapists conservatively manage acute, closed mallet finger? A survey of members of the British Association of Hand Therapists, *Hand Ther* 22(1):13–25, 2017.
10. Chazen LA, Franzsen D: Expert opinion on splinting adult patients with neurological injuries, *S Afr J Physiother* 46(2):4–9, 2016.
11. Kilbride C: *Splinting for the prevention and correction of contractures in adults with neurological dysfunction: practice guideline for occupational therapists and physiotherapists*, London, UK, 2015, College of Occupational Therapists, Association of Chartered Physiotherapists in Neurology.

12. McKee P, Nguyen C: Customized dynamic splinting: orthoses that promote optimal function and recovery after radial nerve injury: a case report, *J Hand Ther* 20(1):73–88, 2007.

13. Schwartz DA: The current evidence for static progressive orthoses for the upper extremity, *ASHT Times* 22:4, 2016.

14. Uğurlu Ü, Özdoğan H: Effects of serial casting in the treatment of flexion contractures of proximal interphalangeal joints in patients with rheumatoid arthritis and juvenile idiopathic arthritis: a retrospective study, *J Hand Ther* 29(1):41–50, 2016.

15. Austin NM: Anatomic principles. In Jacobs MA, Austin NM, editors: *Orthotic intervention for the hand and upper extremity: splinting principles and process*, Philadelphia, PA, 2014, Lippincott Williams & Wilkins, pp 26–46.

16. Austin GP, Jacobs ML: Mechanical principles. In Jacobs MA, Austin NM, editors: *Orthotic intervention for the hand and upper extremity: splinting principles and process*, Philadelphia, PA, 2014, Lippincott Williams & Wilkins, pp 66–83.

17. Austin NM: Equipment and materials. In Jacobs MA, Austin NM, editors: *Orthotic intervention for the hand and upper extremity: splinting principles and process*, Philadelphia, PA, 2014, Lippincott Williams & Wilkins, pp 84–106.

8 Fundamentals of Edema Management

Aida E. Olvera-Dyckes

Edema (oedema) is a common condition after upper extremity injury or surgery. Dorsal hand edema causes the skin to tighten, forcing the metacarpophalangeal (MP) joints into hyperextension and the interphalangeal (IP) joints into flexion. As a consequence, the collateral ligaments of all the joints tighten and the volar plates of the proximal interphalangeal (PIP) joints shorten. The arches of the hand are lost and the thumb becomes adducted and extended.

> ◎ *Clinical Pearl*
>
> Without early intervention from a therapist, the anatomical response to hand edema can result in fixed contractures with fibrotic changes of tissues and shortening of musculotendinous units.

Edema versus Swelling

Many people use the terms *swelling* and *edema* interchangeably, but they are not technically synonymous. Swelling is an enlargement of tissue that can occur for many reasons, for example a tumor, excess fluid, infection (pus), or inflammation. Edema refers specifically to an excessive amount of fluid in the interstitial space (space between the cells). So, edema manifests as swelling. Hand edema is not seen by the naked eye until interstitial fluid volume has increased over 30% beyond normal.[1]

> ◎ *Clinical Pearl*
>
> Localized swelling due to hemorrhage or infection is not edema.

Edema is often described relative to its mechanism of injury, location, and pathogenesis. There are several classifications of edema, including acute, mild, brawny, pitting, and lymphedema. This chapter focuses on peripheral edema, which is the edema that occurs in the extremities.

Biological Mechanism of Edema Formation

There is normally a balance of fluid moving into and out of the vessels on a cellular level. This balance is based on **Starling's equilibrium,** which refers to the movement of fluid across capillary walls and which is affected by hydrostatic pressure and oncotic pressure in the capillaries and in the interstitium. The movement of fluid is usually balanced so that there is a steady state in the sizes of the intravascular and interstitial compartments. Edema occurs when the balance is disrupted.[2] If either the capillary hydrostatic pressure increases and/or the oncotic pressure is reduced, more movement of fluid from the intravascular to the interstitial spaces will take place.

Edema Related to Wound Healing

One of the most important tasks of managing wounds and edema is identifying **inflammation**. Inflammation may be a sign of infection and presents as a localized area of soft-tissue redness and swelling. The area is often warm to the touch and painful. When an infection is suspected, the therapist should alert the physician immediately. In the presence of infection, therapeutic intervention should be paused until the therapist has clearance from the physician to continue treating. Physical agent modalities, manual edema mobilization, and many other treatments are contraindicated when there is infection.

Types of Edema

Pitting edema is present when the pressure of a finger makes an indentation that persists after the finger pressure is removed. The indentation is not permanent; the depression slowly refills with fluid from the surrounding tissues. Pitting edema may be related to problems with the kidneys, heart valves, and low protein levels.[3] It can also be caused by trauma, localized problems with the veins, pregnancy, and certain medications. This type of edema is often simply due to an accumulation of water and is easily treated with movement, cold modalities, elevation, and light compression.

Nonpitting edema (also known as **brawny edema)** is firm to the touch because the tissue is fibrotic. When chronic, the skin in the involved area can become thickened and brown in color. Nonpitting edema is composed of fluid that is more protein-rich and static—making this type of edema more difficult to treat.

Lymphedema is a condition that occurs when lymph fluid has difficulty draining properly due to damage or a blockage in the lymphatic system. This type of edema can be either pitting or nonpitting. The lymphatic network can be altered by infection, radiation therapy, surgery, parasitic infection, and trauma. With lymphedema, protein-rich fluid accumulates in the interstitial spaces of the skin and subcutaneous tissue. This condition is incurable but it can be managed with appropriate treatment. Manifestations of chronic lymphedema are abnormal skin changes and an increased risk of infection. Complications are more common in clients who are unable to obtain proper medical care.

Measuring Edema

Edema can be measured using volumetry, figure-of-eight measurement, or circumferential measurement.[1]

Volumetry: This is a method of determining the volume of a hand or arm by immersing the limb in a container full of water and then measuring the amount of water that is displaced.

Figure-of-Eight: This method of measuring edema utilizes a flexible tape measure. The therapist wraps the tape measure around the hand in a figure-of-eight pattern at specific anatomical landmarks.

Circumferential Measurement: This method uses a flexible tape measure. The therapist wraps the tape measure once around the hand/limb in a circular pattern at specific anatomical landmarks.

Volumetric measurement is considered the gold standard for measuring edema. Both the figure-of-eight and circumferential techniques are useful when it is not appropriate to immerse the limb in water (for example, if there is a wound). By placing a thin gauze covering over the wound, the therapist is able to obtain a measurement while protecting the wound. However, one of the problems with these two methods is that therapists use varying amounts of force when pulling the tape measure around the hand/limb. To address this problem, some therapists use a force gauge to standardize the force applied to the tape measure.

> **◎ Clinical Pearl**
>
> Edema can fluctuate due to factors such as activity level, time of day, and fluid retention. To most objectively measure changes in edema, try to have the same therapist measure the client at the same anatomical position, using the same measuring tool, at the same time of day.

Edema Management

Edema can be treated using a variety of techniques including elevation, active range of motion (AROM), manual edema mobilization, compression, taping, and modalities.

Elevation: Elevation of the limb is commonly recommended for individuals with upper extremity edema. Elevation helps because gravity assists with fluid drainage. The most effective position for upper extremity elevation is as follows: elbow higher than the shoulder, wrist higher than the elbow, and hand higher than the wrist. Additionally, the elbow should be more extended than flexed. This position for elevation should be used as long as it is not medically contraindicated. This sequential positioning pattern creates a pathway for fluid drainage.

AROM: Active movement promotes fluid drainage and discourages the formation of adhesions. The type and frequency of AROM exercises should be customized to each client's injury/surgery and medical contraindications.

Manual Edema Mobilization (MEM): This technique treats edema based on the anatomy and physiology of the lymphatic system. The lymphatic system is the only pathway for interstitial proteins to return to circulation and it is a key player in fluid homeostasis.[4] Interstitial fluid persists due to protein molecules that attract water. At 6 to 12 days postinjury or surgery, these molecules are too large to be reabsorbed through the arteriovenous system. Therefore they must be returned through the lymphatic system. MEM includes light proximal-to-distal then distal-to-proximal mobilization of the skin done in specific patterns and segments, massaging over lymph node(s) proximal to the edema, and promoting flow in the anatomic direction of the lymphatic pathways. This facilitates the removal of excess fluid and interstitial protein molecules that continue to attract water if they are not recirculated.[5]

MEM can be very effective for clients with persistent edema following upper extremity trauma or surgery who have intact but overwhelmed lymphatic systems. It is not designed to be used with clients who have damaged lymphatic systems or for clients with primary lymphedema (a form of lymphedema not caused by another medical condition). Contraindications for MEM include infection, blood clots, congestive heart failure, renal failure, and cancer.[6,7]

> **◎ Clinical Pearl**
>
> When using hands-on techniques to reduce edema, use very light pressure (just enough pressure to gently move the skin). Deep or heavy massage pressure collapses the lymphatic network and is counterproductive or even injurious.

Compression: External compression provides counterpressure and compensates for the lack of elasticity in edematous tissues and thereby improves circulation. Compression helps reinforce tissue hydrostatic pressure and facilitates venous and lymphatic flow. Using compression in the acute phase of healing is thought to limit the amount of space available for excess fluid to accumulate during the fibroblastic phase of healing. Compression is thought to decrease the fibroblastic synthesis of collagen by decreasing blood flood. This in turn causes local hypoxia, slowing down the development of scar tissue and fibrosis. In the later stages of healing, compression assists with edema management by reducing net filtration. Compression wrapping of brawny edema softens fibrotic connective tissue and scar tissue.

Contraindications to the use of compression include severe arterial insufficiency, deep vein thrombosis, heart failure, uncontrolled hypertension, severe peripheral neuropathy, and active tuberculosis.

Be aware that compression that is too tight actually damages the lymphatic system. A well-fitted compression garment promotes light skin traction during active movement, and this stimulates lymphatic flow. If creases are still visible in the skin 20 to 30 minutes after removing an edema glove or elastic tubular stockinette, then the compression is too tight and a looser-fitting garment should be used.

Types of Compression

Edema Gloves: Edema gloves provide gentle compression. These gloves are typically fabricated from nylon and spandex. The glove should provide 15 to 25 mm Hg pressure in order to stimulate the superficial lymphatic system, promoting edema reduction. Custom and off-the-shelf gloves in various sizes are available. Gloves should be designed to extend only to the middle phalanges to allow sensory input and integration of the hand into activities of daily living. It is very important that gloves not be too tight, especially at the distal edges, as this can cause worsening of distal edema.

Elastic Tubular Stockinette: Elastic tubular stockinette provides gentle compression. It is made of a cotton/rayon blend with rubber latex yarn. Caution should be used with clients who have latex allergies. The elastic tubular stockinette can be cut to size.

Edema gloves and elastic tubular stockinette are reusable. Clients can wash the garments with warm soapy water and then air-dry them. These garments are often used for general edema, burns, strains, sprains, and soft-tissue injuries. Elastic tubular stockinette can be worn in combination with an edema glove. It is common practice to give the client two pairs of edema gloves and two sets of elastic tubular bandages, one to wash and one to wear. It is important to closely monitor the skin for marks indicating that the garments are too tight. A safe guideline is that therapists should be able to get their finger inside a tubular sleeve. If you can't, it is too tight.[6,8]

String Wrapping: String wrapping is an outdated edema management technique that is still sometimes used and therefore deserves to be mentioned. It was originally thought to be a way of using distal to proximal compression to move edema out of the hand. However, we now know that the terminal portion of the lymphatic system is very delicate. *Too much pressure, such as the pressure used with string wrapping, damages the lymphatic tissues. For this reason, string wrapping should **not** be used.*

Short-Stretch Bandaging: Short-stretch bandages stretch 20% of their original length. In this way they differ from ACE elastic bandages, which stretch 140% to 300% of their original length. Short-stretch bandaging is a compression technique used to manage lymphedema. It is also used in manual edema mobilization. The techniques of use exceed the scope of this chapter, but readers are encouraged to pursue outside information about the use of short-stretch bandaging in the treatment of edema.

Kinesiology tape: Kinesiology tape can be applied to increase lymphatic and vascular flow, thereby reducing edema and diminishing pain. The tape is thinner and more elastic than conventional tape and can be stretched 120% to 140% of its original length. Kinesiology taping is designed to raise the epidermis, reducing the pressure on the mechanoreceptors below the dermis. This is proposed to reduce pain. Kinesiology tape is reported to have a beneficial effect on lymphatic and venous circulation by raising the epidermis, thereby decreasing the pressure in the dermis and promoting lymphatic drainage through its mechanical action during movement. The theory is that when applied on stretch, kinesiology tape can lift the skin away from the muscle, creating space between the layers of fascia. Blood vessels, lymphatic vessels, and certain nerves are found in the fascia. By lifting the skin away from the muscle, kinesiology tape changes the pressure differential underneath the skin, allowing for improved perfusion of the area with ground substance, which includes the water and proteins responsible for the lubrication and nutrition of the connective tissue cells. Contraindications include allergic reactions to adhesive tape, open wounds, presence of a deep vein thrombosis, infection, peripheral neuropathy, and active cancer.[9]

Contrast Baths: It has been suggested that contrast baths produce a "pumping effect" contributing to edema reduction. The rationale provided is that contrast baths may help reduce pain and stiffness by activating vasodilation and vasoconstriction via muscle contraction.[10] However, a randomized controlled study of contrast baths on patients with carpal tunnel syndrome did not find any significant effect on hand volume with use of contrast baths.[11] A systematic review of the effectiveness of contrast baths concluded that although its use may increase the temperature of skin and blood flow superficially, there was conflicting evidence on its effect on edema.[12] Contraindications for use of contrast baths include open wounds, poorly controlled epilepsy, hypertension, and diabetes.

Intermittent Pneumatic Compression (IPC): IPC is often a modality of choice for treating lymphedema. It can also be effective for reducing posttraumatic edema, especially in the inflammatory phase of healing.[13] The pump consists of a sleeve with multiple pressure compartments that encompass the entire limb. Once placed on the extremity, the chambers of the pump are sequentially inflated, working distal to proximal. This sequential compression moves the edematous fluid into the lymphatic system, which in turn pushes the venous blood proximally. The pumping motion encourages normal circulatory action by stimulating extracellular drainage and fluid clearance. Contraindications include congestive heart failure, deep vein thrombosis, inflammatory phlebitis, a history of pulmonary embolism, active infection, lymphangiosarcoma, and nonhealed fracture.

Electric Stimulation: Muscle contractions are imperative for lymphatic flow. When a client is unable to perform effective active muscle contractions to assist in the drainage of the lymphatic and venous systems, electric stimulation can be helpful. Muscle contractions stimulate venous and lymphatic circulation. Current intensity must be high enough to elicit a muscle contraction. The client should be encouraged to actively contract their muscles simultaneously with the electrical stimulation. Treatment time is usually 20 minutes, with a cycle of 5 seconds on and 5 seconds off. High-voltage pulsed current and medium-frequency alternating current are commonly used. Contraindications are pregnancy, cancer, cardiac pacemaker or other implanted electrical stimulators, active tuberculosis, thrombophlebitis, thrombosis over the carotid sinus, and active hemorrhage.[14]

Cryotherapy: Cold therapy is often beneficial for the reduction of acute edema, especially in the inflammatory phase of healing. Cold therapy includes ice packs, gel wraps, and cold-water baths. Physiological exposure to cold activates vascular permeability, promotes vasoconstriction, and reduces local blood flow. This in turn decreases prostaglandin synthesis and histamines, thus reducing swelling and pain. Contraindications include but are not limited to deep vein thrombosis, thrombophlebitis, impaired sensation, nerve regeneration, impaired circulation, and chronic wounds.[1]

Summary

This chapter has presented a selection of techniques commonly used to treat edema. Elevation and appropriate active movement are very powerful methods to prevent and reduce edema. Edema-reducing modalities are an adjunct to treatment and must be selected cautiously using sound clinical reasoning. Edema control is key to successful clinical outcomes and should be among the highest of priorities in the hand therapist's plan of care.

References

1. Villeco JP: Edema: Therapist's management. In Skirven TM, Osterman AL, Fedorczyk JM, Amadio PC, editors: *Rehabilitation of the hand and upper extremity*, ed 6, Philadelphia, PA, 2011, Elsevier Mosby, pp 845–857.
2. Fauci AS et al: *Harrison's principles of internal medicine*, ed 18, New York, NY, 2012, McGraw Hill.
3. Colditz JC: Therapist's management of the stiff hand. In Skirven TM, Osterman AL, Fedorczyk JM, Amadio PC, editors: *Rehabilitation of the hand and upper extremity*, ed 6, Philadelphia, PA, 2011, Elsevier Mosby, pp 894–921.
4. Levick JR, Michel CC: Microvascular fluid exchange and the revised starling principle, *Cardiovasc Res* 87:198–210, 2010.
5. Artzberger SM: Hand manual edema mobilization: overview of a new concept in hand edema reduction, *SAJHT* 1:1–6, 2003.
6. Artzberger S: Edema reduction techniques: a biologic rationale for selection. In Cooper C, editor: *Fundamentals of hand therapy: clinical reasoning and treatment guidelines for common diagnoses of the upper extremity*, ed 2, St. Louis, MO, 2014, Mosby, pp 35–50.
7. Artzberger SM, Priganc VW: Manual edema mobilization: an edema reduction technique for the orthopedic patient. In Skirven TM, Osterman AL, Fedorczyk JM, Amadio PC, editors: *Rehabilitation of the hand and upper extremity*, ed 6, Philadelphia, PA, 2011, Elsevier Mosby, pp 868–881.
8. Villeco JP: Edema: a silent but important factor, *J Hand Ther* 25(2):153–162, 2012.
9. Bassett KT, Lingman SA, Ellis RF: The use and treatment efficacy of kinaesthetic taping for musculoskeletal conditions: a systematic review, *N Z J Physiother* 38(2):56–62, 2010.
10. Stanton DEB, Bear-Lehman J, Graziano M, Ryan C: Contrast baths: what do we know about their use? *J Hand Ther* 343–346, 2003.
11. Janssen RG, Schwartz DA, Velleman PF: A randomized controlled study of cointrast baths on patients with carpal tunnel syndrome, *J Hand Ther* 22:200–208, 2009.
12. Stanton DEB, Lazaro R, MacDermid JC: A systematic review of the effectiveness of contrast baths, *J Hand Ther* 22:57–70, 2009.
13. Zaleska M, Olszewski WL, Jain P, et al.: Pressures and timing of intermittent pneumatic compression devices for efficient tissue fluid and lymph flow in limbs with lymphedema, *Lymphat Res Biol* 11(4):227–232, 2013.
14. Shapiro S, Ocelnik M: Electrical currents for tissue healing. In Cameron MH, editor: *Physical agents in rehabilitation: from research to practice*, ed 4, St. Louis, MO, 2013, Elsevier Saunders, pp 267–272.

9 Physical Agent Modalities in the Hand Clinic

Kendyl Brock Hunter

Introduction

Physical agent modalities (PAMs) are defined as those modalities that produce a biophysiological response using light, water, temperature, sound, electricity, or a mechanical device.[1] PAMs are used to help reduce inflammation, promote healing, provide pain relief, alter collagen extensibility, modify muscle tone, and enhance muscle function.[2] We almost always see modalities listed in a hand therapy client's plan of care.

It can be difficult for some hand therapists to decide which, if any, modalities will enhance treatment and provide more promising clinical outcomes. Although scientific studies cannot conclusively support the efficacy of some modalities, many hand therapists are convinced by anecdotal evidence that PAMs are helpful in treating a variety of issues. As such, the use of PAMs is integral to the practice of hand therapy, and modalities are a part of most hand therapists' clinical "tool box." This chapter provides an overview of the modalities commonly used in hand therapy as well as general guidelines and practical tips for their clinical application.

General Precautions When Using Physical Agent Modalities

Before using any modality, it is important to get a thorough medical history from your client to ensure you do not inadvertently harm them. As a general rule, modalities should be closely monitored (and sometimes avoided) if there is compromised sensation, circulation, cognition, or ability to communicate. Additionally, certain rehabilitation protocols – for example, tendon repair protocols – prohibit the use of some modalities during parts of the healing process. *The use of modalities with clients who have active deep vein thrombosis, thrombophlebitis, and hemorrhagic conditions is contraindicated and requires physician clearance before proceeding.[3] Likewise, electrical stimulation and ultrasound are contradicted in the presence of electronic implants, pregnancy (over the low back, abdomen, and pelvic area), and cancer (over the area of malignancy).[2]*

Thermal Modalities

Classification of Thermal Modalities

Thermal modalities can be categorized by how they transfer heat. The three primary mechanisms of heat transfer include conduction, convection, and conversion. Each method of heat transfer involves different properties that affect energy absorption and depth of tissue treatment. Heat is typically absorbed by human tissue to depths of 1 to 5 cm. Thermal modalities causing absorption up to a depth of 3 cm are generally classified as **superficial heating agents**, while modalities causing a deeper level of absorption, 2 to 5 cm, are classified as **deep heating agents**.[4]

Conduction is the transfer of heat by direct molecular collisions. Hot packs and paraffin both transfer heat by conduction. These are stationary heat sources that make contact with the body and transfer heat energy to tissues. These modalities are superficial heating agents and can be used to heat tissue up to 2 cm in depth.[3]

Convection is the transfer of heat by forced movement or agitation. Fluidotherapy transfers heat by convection as heated particles of cellulose are air-blown around a body part like a dry whirlpool. Fluidotherapy is also a superficial agent, but it results in higher levels of heat absorption by internal structures due to a constant temperature during treatment.

BOX 9.1   Effects of Heat

Mild heat: 98–101°F (37–38°C) reduces mild inflammation and increases metabolism

Moderate heat: 101–103°F (38–39°C) decreases pain and muscle spasm

Vigorous heat: 103–113°F (39–45°C) increases tissue compliance to stretch[7]

Conversion is mechanical energy converted to heat. Ultrasound converts electrical energy to acoustic energy in the form of sound waves. These sound waves are transferred to tissue where molecules in the tissue start to move and, under the right conditions, heat up. Continuous wave ultrasound can heat tissue up to 5 cm in depth and is therefore considered a deep heating agent.[4]

Choosing Your Heating Agent

Thermal modalities are commonly used in therapy clinics as well as in the home. Typically, we find that clients love heat. Heat "feels good," but what does it really do? Clinically, it decreases tissue tightness and joint stiffness, provides pain relief, decreases muscle spasm, promotes relaxation, increases blood flow, and facilitates tissue healing (Box 9.1). Therapeutic heating levels range from 98 to 113°F (37–45°C) and penetrate to depths of 1 to 2 cm with hot packs, paraffin, and Fluidotherapy, and 2 to 5 cm with ultrasound.[3]

Heat should be avoided the first 24 to 48 hours after an injury or surgery during the initial inflammatory phase of healing. Thereafter heat modalities can be appropriate, but therapists should be cautious when applying heat to areas with vascular instability or to areas with impaired sensation. Convection heat modalities, such as Fluidotherapy, provide systemic heating that will affect the entire body. Individuals with conditions that may be affected by systemic heating should be monitored closely or avoid these modalities altogether.[4] Hot packs and paraffin provide localized heat and are a good choice to use on specific body parts when systemic heating could be an issue for a client.

Depending on the therapeutic goal, a variety of heat modalities may be used. Fluidotherapy allows for active movement and is a great choice when you want your client to perform exercises while the heat modality is in use. Fluidotherapy also provides a sensory component and can be helpful with desensitization. However, Fluidotherapy can be more complicated to use with clients who have open wounds (requires a sealed dressing), and it can be drying to the client's skin. Hot packs and paraffin are both moist heating agents and are great choices when your client has dry skin that needs a little added moisture. Moist heat is often more soothing than dry heat. However, the client is basically static during treatment with hot packs and paraffin unless the therapist provides an external stretch. Each heating agent has a place and a purpose. It is important to design your treatment plan in accordance with the client's needs.

Fluidotherapy

This modality was originally developed using ground corn husks as a medium to transfer heat energy. The medium, now granulated cellulose particles, is circulated by warm air to simulate a water whirlpool. Thus, Fluidotherapy is often referred to as a **dry whirlpool**.

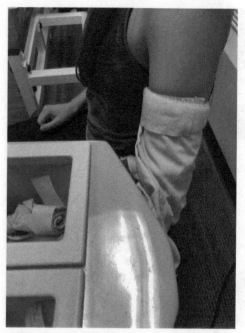

FIG. 9.1 Fluidotherapy.

In addition to allowing clients to actively move during the heating process, Fluidotherapy also provides a sensory component for those clients requiring sensory reeducation. Another advantage of Fluidotherapy is that clients can tolerate temperatures as high as 120°F (49°C), whereas the traditional water whirlpool is generally only tolerated to 105°F (41°C). As with any thermal modality, monitor clients with vascular or nerve compromise carefully.

Fluidotherapy is a nonrestrictive modality that allows clients to move their hand or arm while heated cellulose particles are circulating around the body part (Fig. 9.1). The convection form of heat transfer provides for more heat absorption than other superficial heat modalities. Be cautious when using Fluidotherapy with clients who are prone to swelling or have conditions where high heat should be avoided.[6] Typical treatment temperatures range from 102 to 118°F (39–48°C). A good starting point is 115°F (46°C). Clients can usually tolerate this temperature, and it can be adjusted up or down according to client preference or treatment goals.

Tell your client, "This is a dry whirlpool, it simulates water, but the media is sand-like cellulose particles. The heat will make it easier and more comfortable to move while exercising in the machine. If you have sensory issues, it will help normalize nerve function. There is a fan inside that blows the cellulose particles around, but the fan blades are enclosed in a box so they won't hurt you. I have also placed a sponge (or other items) inside for you to find and manipulate."

◎ Clinical Pearl

Always inform your client when you have added foreign objects to the Fluidotherapy machine, as it is alarming for clients to blindly encounter unexpected objects in the cellulose medium. Some clients have reported thinking there was a mouse or snake inside the machine! Also, adding a dryer sheet to the cellulose particles can help with static electricity during drier weather (and it makes the hand therapy clinic smell wonderful!).

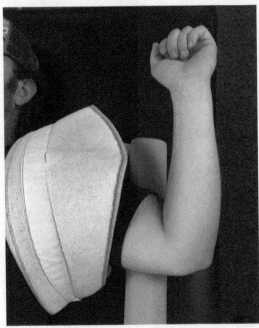

FIG. 9.2 Heat and Stretch: Hot pack coupled with external rotation and gravity assist. Note that the client is lying on the hot pack, and the posterior aspect of the pack may require more padding.

Hot Packs

Hot packs are quite versatile and have been shown to help with reducing pain and improving motion and function when applied prior to exercise.[7] They are a good warm-up for clients in the clinic in preparation for exercise and therapeutic activity, and are readily available for clients to use on their own at home. Though beneficial, most insurances do not allow therapists to bill for the application of hot packs, so many therapists have their clients arrive before the scheduled treatment time to warm up with this modality.

To ensure your client receives adequate heating without burning, it is important to place a folded towel or two between the body part to be treated and the hot pack. Hot packs are heated in a hot water bath that is approximately 160°F (71°C). The amount of insulation (padding) you should use over the hot pack is dependent on the condition of your client and the current temperature of the hot pack. In a busy clinic, hot packs are hotter in the early morning than they are toward noon. This is because the packs never sit in the hot water bath long enough to return to their maximum temperature between uses. Similarly, this concept applies directly after lunch when hot packs have had a chance to fully heat up for at least 30 minutes during a break in treatment activity. The packs will be hotter directly after lunch than they will be later in the afternoon.

If the client is lying on a hot pack (Fig. 9.2) or pressure is applied to an area over a hot pack, additional padding may be necessary. Be aware that air acts as an insulator, so consider the condition of your clinic's towels when deciding how much toweling to use around hot packs. Fluffy new towels hold more air and provide very good heat insulation when wrapped around hot packs. It may take a little longer for your client to feel the heat and the heat will not be as intense, but the hot pack will stay warm longer than if thinner towels are used. Towels that are worn-thin offer less insulation, provide faster and more intense heating, and allow the hot pack to cool down faster.

Tell the client, "This is a moist hot pack. It is gel-filled and heated in a very warm water bath. It is insulated with a cover, and toweling is added for hygiene and comfort. You should begin to feel the heat in a few minutes. The heat should be comfortable and soothing. Please inform me immediately if the hot pack feels too hot. Every client tolerates heat differently. I don't want it to burn you, and it can if you don't let me know it's getting uncomfortable." *Be aware that after a hand injury, clients' sensory heat regulators can be "off." Check your clients' skin frequently throughout the heating process to assure it isn't getting too red.*

Clients can make their own hot packs for use at home from a variety of common items such as field corn, cherry pits, and rice. Essential oils can be added for a pleasant olfactory experience. Have clients fill a sock, small pillowcase, or kitchen towel and sew it closed. Instruct clients to heat the hot pack in the microwave for 30-second intervals until a comfortable temperature is reached.

> ### Clinical Pearl
>
> Heating dry rice in a microwave will create a moist heat effect. This is true for both rice-based hot packs and loose rice in a bowl. Heated rice bowls allow clients to exercise in the rice while receiving heat. The rice also provides a sensory component for clients requiring sensory reeducation.

Paraffin

A paraffin bath is a mixture of paraffin wax and mineral oil. It is a practical modality that is relatively easy to use both in the clinic and at home. Paraffin is a moist heating agent that provides an even distribution of heat and assists in the lubrication of dry tissue. One of the benefits of paraffin is its low cost and versatility. It is a great modality for clients with painful arthritis, healed burns, and stiff joints. Paraffin temperatures typically range between 113 and 130°F (45–54°C). Treatment times range from 15 to 20 minutes.[8]

Clients must wash their hands before using the clinic's paraffin bath because the bath is shared by clients. Removing rings, bracelets, and watches also helps keep the paraffin clean. Paraffin should never be used on a hand with open wounds. Ask the client to dip their hand until it is fully submerged in the paraffin bath, and then to repeat this four to eight times. Once achieved, wrap the hand with a protective barrier such as plastic wrap, aluminum foil, plastic grocery bags, or plastic bread bags. This will help hold the heat in. To prolong the heat for an even longer period, place an oven mitt or towel over the barrier wrap. Once the wax has cooled (about 20 minutes), have the client remove the wax and use it as a therapy tool while it is still pliable. Manipulating the paraffin wax is a good activity for improving fine motor coordination and strength.

Tell the client, "Paraffin is a mixture of wax and oil and is used to heat your tissues. It helps decrease joint stiffness, prepares your hand for activity, and provides pain relief. The wax will feel quite warm during your first dip, but after that it should be comfortable. It takes about 20 minutes for the wax to cool, and then we will remove it. You should not feel a burning sensation, but if you do, let me know and I will remove the wax immediately." *Always throw used paraffin in the trash. Do not reuse paraffin in the clinic because this is unhygienic.*

⊙ *Clinical Pearl*

Taping the hand before dipping it in paraffin (Fig. 9.3) helps stretch tight structures. If you use this technique, always check to make sure the paraffin has not pooled at the tips of the fingers because that can cause a burn.

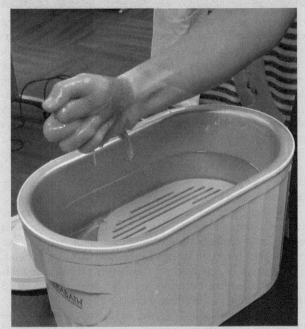

FIG. 9.3 Hand taped and then dipped in paraffin to provide a combination of heat and stretch.

⊙ *Clinical Pearl*

Commercial paraffin baths are readily available, inexpensive, and are a great home modality. Commercial paraffin wax is available in many beauty supply stores, drug stores, and online. There are many online recipes for do-it-yourself paraffin baths, but recommending these to your clients could be a liability, as paraffin is highly flammable. Play it safe and recommend only the commercial units.

Continuous-Wave Ultrasound

Ultrasound works by converting electrical energy into sound energy that, when introduced into tissue, elicits a type of molecular activity that produces biophysical changes.[9] Ultrasound can be used to assist with pain management, tissue and bone healing, edema reduction, and circulation.[5] The effects of this modality, either thermal or mechanical, depend on whether ultrasound is delivered in continuous wave or pulsed mode. Pulsed ultrasound is used when we desire the mechanical benefits but not heat. Continuous-wave ultrasound is used when we are trying to heat deeper structures. See Box 9.2 for the thermal and mechanical effects of therapeutic ultrasound. Continuous-wave (thermal mode) ultrasound is considered a deep heating agent, as it can penetrate tissues to depths of 5 cm (depending on the frequency selected).

Ultrasound energy is absorbed best by collagen-rich structures such as ligaments, tendons, fascia, joint capsules, and scar tissue. It is commonly used for conditions involving these structures. Ultrasound does not work well on muscle tissue because muscles are so

BOX 9.2   Effects of Ultrasound

Thermal Effects[4]:
- decreased muscle spasm and guarding
- decreased pain perception
- increased tissue extensibility in collagen-rich structures
- increased blood flow and nerve conduction velocity
- mild inflammatory reactions

Mechanical Effects[5]:
- decreased inflammation
- stimulation of tissue regeneration
- soft-tissue and bone repair
- alterations in cell membrane permeability and cellular activity

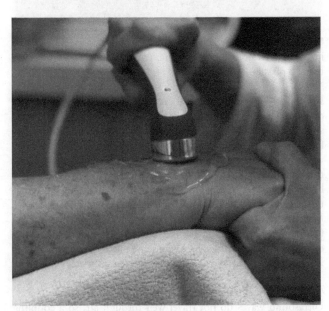

FIG. 9.4 Combining manual stretching with thermal ultrasound.

vascular. Heat dissipates quickly in muscle tissue and is unable to reach the high temperature levels needed for therapeutic results.[9]

When we use ultrasound, we need to consider that the treatment area must be very specific—no larger than two to three times the **effective radiating area (ERA).** The ERA is roughly two times the size of the soundhead. If the goal of applying thermal ultrasound is to assist with elongating tissue, then manual therapy should be performed throughout the treatment and immediately after (Fig. 9.4). Research suggests that there is a limited amount of time in which heated tissue is at an optimal temperature for stretch and elongation. This is referred to as the **stretching window**, and it is a very short time period (3–7 minutes).[10] As one would expect, superficial structures lose heat faster than deeper ones.

Setting Up the Ultrasound Machine

When setting the ultrasound machine parameters, the therapist selects a continuous sound wave (100% duty cycle). Continuous ultrasound means that the sound wave energy is entering the body without interruption. The ultrasound machine must be set to continuous mode in order to produce thermal effects.

The therapist then selects a wave frequency of either 1 MHz or 3 MHz depending on the target tissues depth. For deeper

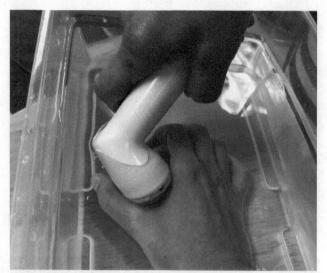

FIG. 9.5 When treating an uneven surface or bony area, water immersion ultrasound is the treatment of choice. Note that the container is plastic—NOT metal.

structures, 1 MHz (1,000,000 cycles per second) is a slower frequency and will penetrate tissue to depths of 5 cm. For more superficial structures, 3 MHz (3,000,000 cycles per second) is a faster frequency and will only target tissue to three cm in depth.

Because soundwaves lose energy and focus as they travel through tissues, treatment at the 1 MHz frequency can require higher intensities to reach the desired therapeutic temperature at the target tissue. The 3 MHz frequency is three times faster than 1 MHz and provides a very focused amount of energy to more superficial tissue. Therefore the intensity setting used with a 3 MHz frequency can be lower to achieve the same therapeutic temperature. Intensity is documented as watts per square centimeter (W/cm^2).

Application Techniques

Ultrasound waves do not travel well through air, so a coupling agent is necessary to facilitate transfer of energy from the soundhead to the target tissue. The most common coupling agents are commercial aqueous solutions, water, or pharmaceutical compounding agents. Removing body lotions and clipping body hair in the treatment area will also aid in the transfer of energy and improve the effectiveness of ultrasound treatment.

It is important to ensure that the soundhead is flush with the area being treated and that the entire soundhead is in contact with the skin. This requires using an appropriately sized soundhead. The hand often requires smaller soundheads than other body parts. *The therapist should keep the soundhead moving in small circles at a steady rate, roughly 4 cm per second, to reduce the risk of disrupting blood flow and causing tissue damage.*

When treating an uneven surface or bony area, water immersion is the method of choice (Fig. 9.5). To perform this technique, both the soundhead and the treatment area are immersed in a container of water. *It is important to use a plastic or glass container, and not one made of metal.* Metal has the potential to reflect energy and increase the heat intensity during this type of ultrasound treatment. During water immersion, the soundhead should be moved parallel to the treatment area at approximately 1 cm from the surface of the skin. If air bubbles accumulate on the soundhead during treatment, they should be quickly wiped off to ensure better penetration of the sound energy.

Tell the client, "Ultrasound is a form of sound energy that is absorbed by tissues and causes cell activity. It helps relax tight tissues, reduces pain, softens scars, and promotes wound healing."

Cryotherapy

Cryotherapy refers to the application of ice or other cooling agents to the body for the purpose of therapeutic cooling. Therapeutic cooling temperatures range from 32 to 65°F (0–18°C). The use of this modality dates back to 2500 BC. The Greek word "cryotherapy" is comprised of two words: "cryo" meaning cold, and "therapy" meaning to cure or heal. Lowering the temperature of body tissue to therapeutic levels helps reduce pain and edema.[5] Because so many hand injuries and conditions are accompanied by pain and swelling, cold therapy is often used to help treat a variety of diagnoses. However, *never use cold therapy on someone with compromised circulation such as in the setting of Raynaud syndrome or peripheral vascular disease.* Cold therapy causes vasoconstriction and will aggravate these problems.

Cold therapy comes in a variety of forms, including ice massage, cold packs, and ice baths. Topical agents such as Biofreeze (a menthol-based analgesic) will enhance the cooling sensation and can be applied before or during cryotherapy treatment. Depending on the type of cold modality used, energy transfers at a different rate. Therefore treatment times can range from 5 to 45 minutes depending on the desired cooling effect.

When a cold modality is applied to the skin, there is a typical sequence of events that occurs. First, the skin becomes red **(hyperemia)**. This is followed by a burning sensation, then a deep ache, and finally the relief of numbness **(analgesia)**.[13] Once the client reports that the treatment area is numb, the therapist should remove the cooling agent to avoid tissue damage or frostbite. Although ice is an antiinflammatory and a pain reliever, it also decreases blood flow and slows nerve conduction.[14] Clients with compromised nerve function will often report a noxious painful sensation outside the predictable cooling response and may not tolerate cold modalities. Any abnormal response should be noted in your clinical assessment.

Tell the client, "Cold therapy usually works really well for pain relief, but you have to endure some discomfort to get the benefit. You can expect to feel cold first, followed by burning, then deep aching, and THEN numbness. If you can tolerate the cold until you are numb, this treatment will probably give you very good temporary relief from pain."

♡ *Tips from the Field*

- An ice massage will cool tissue much quicker than a cold pack.
- To enhance the cooling effect of ice wrapped in a towel, wet the towel.
- A sealed plastic bag partially filled with ice and water conforms better to the hand than ice cubes or crushed ice alone, and it improves the skin and intramuscular cooling effect.[12]
- Coupling a cooling agent with compression results in deeper depths of cooling.
- Adipose tissue (fat) increases the amount of time it takes to cool underlying muscle, as well as the length of time it takes for the muscle to return to its baseline temperature after treatment.[3] For example, it takes 10 minutes to produce a 13°F decrease in temperature in muscle underlying 1 cm of adipose tissue. Con-

versely, 60 minutes is required to achieve the same temperature change in the presence of 3 to 4 cm of adipose tissue.[4]

> ### ◎ *Clinical Pearl*
>
> Ice packs can be made with plastic resealable bags of varying sizes using a ratio of one part rubbing alcohol to three parts water. The rubbing alcohol prevents the water from fully freezing, and the result is a slushy cold pack that conforms well to the contours of the hand.

Electrical Stimulation

Electrical stimulation (also called e-stim) is frequently used when treating the upper extremity. Typically, the goal is to reduce pain and edema, increase circulation, assist in wound healing, or facilitate muscle function.[17] The term **electrical stimulation** is an umbrella term that covers different types of stimulation used to accomplish various therapeutic tasks. These applications are differentiated by the type of electrical current each uses.

Common applications of e-stim used in the hand therapy clinic include neuromuscular electrical stimulation (NMES), functional electrical stimulation (FES), Russian current, high-voltage pulsed current (HVPC), and transcutaneous electrical nerve stimulation (TENS). NMES, FES, and Russian stimulation are used to help promote tendon excursion, muscle reeducation, and strengthening. HVPC helps with wound healing, scar remodeling, and pain management. TENS is used for pain management.

> ### ◎ *Clinical Pearl*
>
> Some theorize that the better hydrated one is, the better one's body responds to electrical therapies.

How It Works

In order to understand how e-stim works, we need to understand how nerve fibers respond to electrical current. First, let's look at **waveform**. A waveform depicts the characteristics of electrical current.[17] Waveforms can be monophasic, biphasic, or polyphasic. A monophasic waveform depicts current flowing in one direction. A biphasic waveform depicts current flowing in two opposing directions. A polyphasic waveform is a bidirectional wave with three or more phases in bursts. Different applications of e-stim use different waveforms.

Now, let's look at the amount of current used in e-stim treatment. In the simplest terms, nerve fiber response is dependent on the amount of stimulation we apply. Larger amounts of electrical stimulation will elicit a greater response than smaller amounts of stimulation. In this context, the two key factors that affect the amount of applied current is the **pulse frequency** and **pulse/phase duration**.

A pulse is essentially a flow of electrical current that occurs and then stops. The shorter the pulse the less the stimulus and therefore less recruitment of tissue.[17] The pulse frequency is the frequency in which these pulses of electricity are generated—sometimes called "rate" and expressed in pulses per second (pps). Duration is the amount of time the electrical current is available and is expressed in microseconds (μsec) (Fig. 9.6).

It might be helpful to think about the amount of current used in e-stim by using a chocolate cake analogy. Using this analogy,

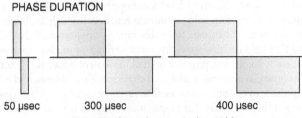

PHASE DURATION

50 μsec   300 μsec   400 μsec

FIG. 9.6 Phase duration/pulse width.

the duration is the size of the cake piece and the frequency is the number of bites taken. The bigger the cake piece and the greater the frequency of bites, the more calories we ingest. The same thing applies to e-stim parameters. The longer we allow electrical current to flow and the more frequently we allow bursts of electrical current, the more fibers we will stimulate.

Not only do nerve fibers respond differently to various waveforms and amounts of current, but different types of nerves depolarize at different rates. Sensory nerves are the most sensitive and are stimulated first. This is followed by motor nerve stimulation, and finally pain fiber stimulation. The sensitivity and speed of stimulation also depends on the diameter of the nerve and the depth of the nerve in relationship to the electrode. Fortunately, for currently practicing hand therapists, many commercial e-stim units have been engineered and programmed to target specific nerve types. This makes it easier for us to elicit the clinical response that we desire during treatment.

> ### ◎ *Clinical Pearl*
>
> Where we place electrodes influences how deep the current will flow. Electrodes placed closer to each other recruit more superficial fibers, while electrodes placed farther apart recruit deeper fibers.[15]

Using Electrical Stimulation for Muscle Reeducation, Strengthening, and Tendon Excursion

In order to produce either a voluntary or electrically induced muscle contraction, the motor nerve serving a particular muscle must be fully or partially intact. It is important to understand that while electrical stimulation is a useful tool for improving muscle function, stimulating a motor nerve does not create a normal physiological muscle contraction. Therefore we must be cautious when applying this modality.

E-stim will recruit all motor units at once, and large type II fast-twitch fibers are stimulated first. This is different from what occurs during a voluntary muscle contraction. During a voluntary muscle contraction, motor unit recruitment is staggered: type I fibers are stimulated first and are followed by type II fibers. Type II muscle fibers fatigue very quickly, so in order to have a well-balanced contraction when using this modality (and to help delay the onset of muscle fatigue), it is important for the client to attempt to contract their muscles during the active phase of electrical stimulation.[3]

Neuromuscular Electrical Stimulation and Functional Electrical Stimulation

NMES and FES are commonly used in hand therapy to help strengthen and reeducate muscles and to promote tendon excursion. They are clinical tools used to help regain normal muscle function and movement. Clients with both orthopedic and neurological conditions who need to enhance muscle function through facilitation or inhibition will benefit from this type of application.[17] NMES and FES help decrease spasticity, increase range of motion, increase muscle strength, and promote normal movement patterns.[17] There are numerous protocols available to target specific problems, and it is important to customize treatment to meet the specific needs of your client. However, a detailed presentation of this is beyond the scope of this chapter. Readers are encouraged to seek out further education on using e-stim for a variety of applications.

NMES and FES work in a similar fashion, so the terms are often used interchangeably. However, using the terms interchangeably is technically inaccurate. FES is actually a subcategory of NMES. FES is the use of e-stim to substitute for an orthotic device while performing a functional activity. The primary goal is improved function, not specific improvements in motion and strength. The difference between NMES and FES is subtle and relates to the goal of the treatment.

The client should be actively engaged in treatment in order to get the best results from FES and NMES. Engagement is easily achieved during FES treatment because the client is performing a functional task while the e-stim is aiding with functional movement. However, the engagement aspect can get lost when using e-stim in the form of straightforward NMES to improve muscle strength, tendon excursion, or to decrease spasticity. Therefore it is important to educate clients about why they are receiving e-stim and to encourage them to focus on the ultimate outcome of improved function. If the goal is to reduce spasticity, have the client focus on relaxing during the inactive phase of the treatment. If you are working on enhancing tendon excursion and strength, ensure that the client is trying to contract their muscles during the active phase of the treatment.

Symmetrical biphasic current, asymmetrical biphasic current, and Russian current are the three most common waveforms used for this type of electrical stimulation. All are useful for muscle recruitment. Muscle size and anatomical placement of the muscle will determine which current is best suited for your needs. The symmetrical biphasic waveform is used most often and produces equal current flow from each electrode. If the goal is gross muscle recruitment, for example all the wrist extensors, this would be a good choice. By changing the duration, frequency, and intensity, the therapist can alter the amount of nerve fiber recruitment and quality of the resulting muscle contraction. Figs. 9.7A–F demonstrate different motor units recruited simply by changing the waveform and duration. The electrode placement stays constant.

The asymmetrical biphasic waveform is the current of choice when we want to recruit small muscles. It has more versatility than symmetrical biphasic or Russian current. Since this current is asymmetrical, the current flow is not equal; one electrode will provide for more recruitment than the other. This is beneficial when trying to isolate and stimulate specific muscles. The advantage to the asymmetrical waveform is that by changing the lead wires the muscle recruitment changes as well. Usually, the black lead wire has a stronger output of electrical current and the red lead has less-strong output. Therefore place the black lead wire where you want to produce a stronger muscle contraction.

Russian Current

Russian stimulation sounds strong, and it is. The Russians originally developed this form of e-stim to enhance their athletes' performance. Whether it actually does so or not is still up for debate. However, Russian current is a widely recognized modality and is often used to augment strengthening efforts. Russian current is defined by its unique 2,500 Hz carrier sine wave with burst modulation, which is quite strong. Many hand therapists are reluctant to use Russian current due to its strength, and theorize that the distal muscles of the forearm are too small to tolerate such a strong current if the goal is to achieve an isolated recruitment of muscles. However, Russian current can be beneficial for recruiting type II fibers and weak or atrophied muscles. Changing the duty cycle will modify the strength of the current.

Using Electrical Stimulation for Wound Healing and Scar Remodeling

High-Voltage Pulsed Current

HVPC is a monophasic twin peak current commonly known as **high volt**. It has been shown to help with both acute and chronic edema, pain, wound healing, and muscle reeducation for small-sized muscles.[18,19] Because it is a monophasic current, electrode placement is important. As a general rule, the red lead is the treatment electrode and the black lead the dispersive electrode.[18] However, always check the operator's manual to ensure this applies to the machine you are using.

A variety of electrode options are available when using high volt: standard reusable carbon, water bath, electromesh glove (Fig. 9.8), and custom aluminum foil (Fig. 9.9). If possible, the dispersive electrode should be twice the size of the active electrode to provide the most comfort during treatment. The polarity is programmed in the machine. Clinicians can get confused thinking that by switching the wires the polarity is changed. This is not the case with HVPC. Changing the lead wires changes the treatment electrode. Depending on your treatment objectives, the current will be set as either positive or negative. The negative polarity has been shown to be beneficial for addressing acute inflammation, infected wounds, debridement of nonviable tissue in wounds, and muscle reeducation.[18,19] The positive polarity is reportedly more comfortable and is used for pain management, treating chronic edema, and for scar tissue management.

Using Electrical Stimulation for Pain Management

Transcutaneous Electrical Nerve Stimulation

TENS is an electrical modality used by therapists for pain management. The majority of clients seen in the hand clinic report some type of pain, and this must be managed in order for the client to fully participate in the hand therapy program. Although TENS is the term coined for using electrical current to manage pain, there is nothing magical about the current. All e-stim units can be used to control pain. What sets TENS current apart is the pulse duration and intensity. TENS has several applications—each based on a different pain control theory—that are used to modulate different types of pain (Fig. 9.10). These are discussed below.

⊙ *Clinical Pearl*

Studies have concluded that caffeine may reduce the effectiveness of TENS for pain management. However, the exact amount of caffeine one must consume to cause this effect has not been determined.[16]

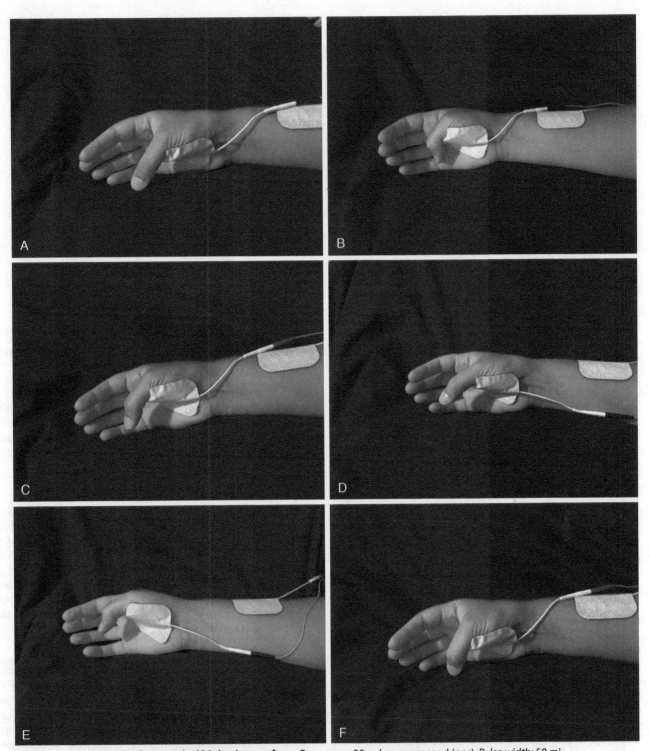

FIG. 9.7 **(A) Symmetrical biphasic waveform.** Frequency: 35 pulses per second (pps). Pulse width: 50 microseconds (μsec). Action achieved: thumb palmar abduction with metacarpophalangeal (MCP) flexion and slight interphalangeal (IP) flexion. **(B) Asymmetrical biphasic waveform.** Frequency: 35 pps. Pulse width: 50 μsec. Lead placement: Black distal, red proximal. Action achieved: strong thumb MCP and IP flexion without abduction. **(C) Asymmetrical biphasic waveform.** Frequency: 35 pps. Pulse width: 50 μsec. Lead placement: red distal, black proximal. Action achieved: slight thumb palmar abduction, MCP flexion, and increased IP flexion (gross opposition). **(D) Symmetrical biphasic waveform.** Frequency: 35 pps. Pulse width: 300 μsec. Action achieved: thumb abduction with MCP flexion and IP flexion. **(E) Asymmetrical biphasic waveform.** Frequency: 35 pps. Pulse width: 300 μsec. Lead placement: black distal, red proximal. Action achieved: slight thumb abduction with MP flexion and strong IP flexion. **(F) Asymmetrical biphasic waveform.** Frequency: 35 pps. Pulse width: 300 μsec. Lead placement: red distal, black proximal. Action achieved: gross opposition with slight distal pronation.

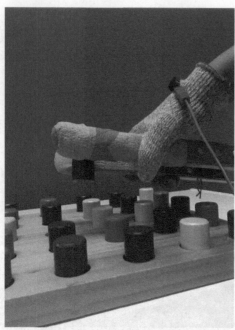

FIG. 9.8 Electromesh glove used during high-voltage pulsed current treatment to minimize pain and swelling during active hand use.

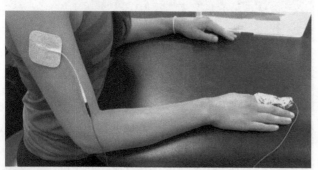

FIG. 9.9 Custom aluminum foil electrode made of wet gauze or paper towels covered with aluminum foil. Used for circumferential stimulation during high-voltage pulsed current.

Gate Control Theory and Conventional High-Rate TENS

Using TENS in this manner is beneficial for treating clients postoperatively or with other types of acute pain. The parameters should be set for a short pulse duration (50–150 μsec) and a high frequency (80+ pps) to provide maximal sensory stimuli without eliciting a muscle contraction. The sensory stimulation helps prevent pain signals from reaching the brain. Treatment time is typically continuous for 20 to 60 minutes. Acute painful conditions such as sprains, fractures, soft-tissue trauma, and tendon and ligament repairs are appropriate for this type of electrical stimulation.

Central Biasing Theory (Acupuncture/Trigger Point Theory)

Using TENS in this way is meant to hyperstimulate a trigger point with the goal of reducing the painful nodule.[16] Trigger points are commonly found in clients with frozen shoulders and various tendinopathies. A trigger point is defined as a focused hyperirritable area within a taut band of muscle that, when digitally stimulated, causes significant pain. The parameters for

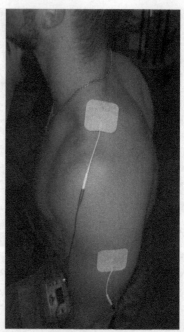

FIG. 9.10 Transcutaneous electrical nerve stimulation for management of a supraspinatus trigger point with referred pain.

a TENS trigger point application is a short pulse duration (10 μsec) with a high frequency (80 pps) with an on-time of 30 to 60 seconds. The stimulation should be quite intense—almost noxious—but should not elicit a contraction. Treatment time is 20 to 60 minutes.

Opiate Pain Control Theory

Chronic pain is difficult to manage and can be debilitating. Another TENS application to help individuals manage their pain utilizes the opiate pain control theory, where e-stim is used to produce the body's natural endorphins to help minimize an individual's pain.[20] Parameters for this application would be a longer pulse duration (200+ μsec) with a low frequency (1–5 pps) and an on-time of 20 to 45 seconds. Intensity is set to maximum tolerance and a slight muscle contraction is acceptable with this application. Treatment time is 20 to 60 minutes.

◎ *Clinical Pearl*

Clients come up with all sorts of ideas after using e-stim units in the clinic. It is not uncommon for the occasional client to report trying to rig up their own home unit using an alkaline or lithium battery. *Strongly discourage this, as it can be dangerous!* Safe and inexpensive e-stim units are available for purchase online without a physician's prescription.

CASE STUDY

Sarah, a 53-year-old phlebotomist in a medical office, is referred to hand therapy with a diagnosis of bilateral thumb carpometacarpal joint osteoarthritis and generalized hand pain. She denies any other medical conditions. Range of motion is limited at the distal interphalangeal joints of the index fingers, middle fingers, and thumbs due to pain and swelling, and Herberden nodules are present on the index and middle fingers. Pinch is weak in both hands. Sarah is having difficulty performing her job duties due to the pain in her hands. She says that stiffness is at its worst in the morning, and her pain increases as the day progresses. This problem is limiting her ability to manipulate small objects in the home and at work.

Things to consider when determining your treatment plan:

1. Are there any medical conditions that would prevent using physical agent modalities with this client?

No, there is nothing reported in her medical history that would prevent application of a modality.

2. Would the client benefit from one or more physical agent modalities to address her dysfunction?

Yes. Osteoarthritis can be effectively managed with a variety of physical agent modalities. It is important to determine the client's primary concerns and then develop a treatment plan based on the client's input. Sarah is very bothered by morning stiffness, so heat modalities would be a good way to start her day. Heat would help decrease tightness and improve her hand flexibility for morning tasks. This can be achieved with warm water, paraffin, or hot packs. All are easily obtained and can be used in the home. Ice massage or a cold pack may be beneficial at the end of the day, since Sarah reports pain and swelling as the day progresses.

In the hand therapy clinic, ultrasound, HVPC, or Fluidotherapy could also be used to address swelling, pain, and stiffness. It is also important to educate your client about joint protection, address any orthoses needs, and provide a comprehensive home exercise program.

3. What is the expected outcome?

Within a week or two the client should be reporting less pain, less swelling, and better joint flexibility. It is important to stress to the client that osteoarthritis is a condition that must be managed on a daily basis, and that developing a self-management strategy is the key to success.

References

1. Cameron MH: Introduction to physical agents and how they are used. In Cameron MH, editor: *Physical agents in rehabilitation: from research to practice*, ed 3, St. Louis, MO, 2009, Saunders Elsevier Inc.
2. Bellew JW: Therapeutic modalities past, present, and future: their role in the patient care management model. In Bellew JW, Michlovitz SL, Nolan Jr TP, editors: *Modalities for therapeutic intervention*, ed 6, Philadelphia, PA, 2016, F.A. Davis Company.
3. Starkey C: *Therapeutic modalities*, ed 4, Philadelphia, PA, 2013, F.A. Davis Company.
4. Kenny GP, Yardley J, Brown C, Sigal RJ, Jay O: Heat Stress in older individuals and patients with common chronic disease, *Can Med Asso J* 182(10):1053–1060, 2010.
5. Hartzell TL, Rubinstein R, Herman M: Therapeutic modalities—an updated review for the hand surgeon, *J Hand Surg* 37(A):597–621, 2012.
6. Rennie S, Michlovitz SL: Therapeutic heat. In Bellew JW, Michlovitz SL, Nolan Jr TP, editors: *Modalities for therapeutic intervention*, ed 6, Philadelphia, PA, 2016, F.A. Davis Company.
7. Patwardhan TY, Mhatre BS, Mehta A: Efficacy of superficial heat therapy as an adjunct to therapeutic exercise program in rehabilitation of patients with conservatively managed distal end radius fractures, *Indian J Physiother Occup Ther* 9(2):102–107, 2015.
8. Dilek B, Gozum M, Sahin E, Bayder M, Ergor G: Efficacy of paraffin bath therapy in hand osteoarthritis: a single-blinded randomized controlled trial, *Arch Phys Med Rehabil* 94:642–649, 2013.
9. Cameron MH: Ultrasound. In Cameron MH, editor: *Physical agents in rehabilitation: from research to practice*, ed 3, St. Louis, MO, 2009, Saunders Elsevier Inc.
10. Draper D, Castel C, Castel D: Rate of temperature increase in human muscle during 1 MHz and 3 MHz continuous ultrasound, *J Ortho Sports Phys Ther* 22:142–150, 1995.
11. Lake D: Therapeutic ultrasound. In Bellew JW, Michlovitz SL, Nolan Jr TP, editors: *Modalities for therapeutic intervention*, ed 6, Philadelphia, PA, 2016, F.A. Davis Company.
12. Dykstra J, Hill HM, Miller MG: Comparisons of cubed ice, crushed ice, and wetted ice on intramuscular and surface temperature changes, *J Athl Train* 44(2):136–141, 2009.
13. Fruth SJ, Michlovtiz SL: Cold therapy modalities. In Bellew JW, Michlovitz SL, Nolan Jr TP, editors: *Modalities for therapeutic intervention*, ed 6, Philadelphia, PA, 2016, F.A. Davis Company.
14. Algafly A, George K: The effects of cryotherapy on nerve conduction velocity, pain threshold, and pain tolerance, *Br J Sports Med* 41:365–369, 2007.
15. Bellow JW: Clinical electrical stimulation. In Bellew JW, Michlovitz SL, Nolan Jr TP, editors: *Modalities for therapeutic intervention*, ed 6, Philadelphia, PA, 2016, F.A. Davis Company.
16. Liebano RE: Mechanisms of pain and use of therapeutic modalities. In Bellew JW, Michlovitz SL, Nolan Jr TP, editors: *Modalities for therapeutic intervention*, ed 6, Philadelphia, PA, 2016, F.A. Davis Company.
17. Doucet BM, Lam A, Griffin L: Neuromuscular electrical stimulation for skeletal muscle function, *Yale J Bio Med* 85:201–215, 2012.
18. Bellew JW: Clinical electrical stimulation: application and techniques. In Bellew JW, Michlovitz SL, Nolan Jr TP, editors: *Modalities for therapeutic intervention*, ed 6, Philadelphia, PA, 2016, F.A. Davis Company.
19. Shapiro S: Electrical currents. In Cameron MH, editor: *Physical agents in rehabilitation: from research to practice*, ed 3, St. Louis, MO, 2009, Saunders Elsevier Inc.
20. Cameron MH: Pain. In Cameron MH, editor: *Physical agents in rehabilitation: from research to practice*, ed 3, St. Louis, MO, 2009, Saunders Elsevier Inc.

10 Tissue-Specific Exercises for the Upper Extremity

Peggy Stein
Lori Falkel

Clinical decisions in hand therapy are made with foundational knowledge of anatomy, physiology, kinesiology, and pathology. Additionally, hand therapists must strive to understand how the client's experience of injury affects them in a psychosocioeconomic context. In this regard, rehabilitation of hand injuries is complex and multifaceted. However, the seemingly mundane task of choosing an exercise program for a client should be simple and straightforward, right? As it turns out, a client's participation in activity and therapeutic exercise requires careful guidance to restore mobility and power to the hand.

Mobility and power are two of the main concepts of the Core Set for Hand Conditions[1] developed by the International Classification of Functioning, Disability and Health (ICF) research branch of the World Health Organization. These core set concepts correlate to the musculoskeletal function and structures within the ICF classification system.[2] Our understanding of the complexities of hand function, comorbidities, and client-related factors helps develop safe, client-specific exercise instruction.

Tissue-specific exercise progression is the science of prescribing an accurate dosage of exercise. Tissue-specific exercise allows us to use our knowledge of exercise physiology to address specific pathological tissue conditions. With proper knowledge, exercise can be a therapist's area of expertise. When designing an exercise program to promote the recovery of the target tissue, the therapist needs to consider multiple variables. These variables include the appropriate resistance; the repetitions and sets that will promote the desired response; the speed, frequency, breaks, and duration of exercise; the appropriate positioning of the client; and the precise range of motion. Proper exercise equipment, to provide support, can be critical for restoration of physiological motion. The types of muscle work (for example, concentric, eccentric, and isometric) are also important considerations.

The Ola Grimsby Institute developed Scientific Therapeutic Exercise Progressions (STEP), which is a concept of dosing exercises according to specific pathological conditions and tissue tolerance of individuals. STEP is based on principles of medical exercise therapy and addresses musculoskeletal dysfunctions with respect to their histological, biomechanical, and neurophysiological significance. Readers interested in learning more about this specific approach are encouraged to seek more information from the Ola Grimsby Institute, which offers courses on a range of subjects related to exercise and therapy.

This chapter will highlight related concepts foundational to critical thinking and problem solving during treatment/intervention planning.

Joint Dysfunction

Joint dysfunction occurs because of a compromise in connective tissue integrity. This may result from capsular, ligamentous, or cartilaginous issues. If the joint dysfunction is capsular, joint swelling will be present. A ligamentous injury has point tenderness. In cartilage, symptoms of joint dysfunction present as an inability to withstand compressive forces. The result of these changes is altered mobility. Joint dysfunction can be labeled as **hypomobility, hypermobility,** or **instability.** A joint is hypomobile when movement takes place about a physiological axis but is less than normal. A hypermobile joint has greater than normal motion around a physiological axis. Joint instability is motion around a nonphysiological axis.[3] All synovial joints can be categorized by a joint mobility grading system[3] (Table 10.1).

Musculoskeletal Dysfunctions

The two main causes of musculoskeletal dysfunctions are acute trauma and cumulative trauma. *Acute trauma* is associated with an excessive contraction (muscle strain) or an

TABLE 10.1 Joint Mobility Grading Scale

Grade	Joint Mobility	Treatment
0	Ankylosed	Surgery/no mobilization treatment
1	Considerable limitation	Articulation/avoid exercise and manipulation
2	Slight limitation	Joint mobilization/self-mobilization
3	Normal	No treatment needed
4	Slight increase	Postural correction/ADLs and ANLs/check for hypomobility/taping/self-stabilization
5	Considerable increase	Postural correction/bracing/taping/self-stabilization/ADLs and ANLs/check for hypomobility/dry needling/sclerosing injections
6	Pathologically unstable	Surgery/no mobilization treatment

ADLs, Activities of daily living; *ANLs,* activities of nightly living.

BOX 10.1 Traits That Have Been Shown to Increase Risk for Fractures

Slender build
Fair skin
Family history of osteoporosis or osteoporotic fracture
Small muscle mass
Sedentary lifestyle
Small peak adult bone mass (approximately age 35)
Low calcium intake
Cigarette smoking
Excessive consumption of protein, sodium, and alcohol
One or more osteoporotic fracture(s)
A situation that increases the likelihood of falling (that is, wet floor, throw rugs, or small pets)

BOX 10.2 Common Age-Related Changes Affecting Bone Loss

Gradual increase in parathyroid hormone secretion as a result of chronic calcium deficiency
Decreased intestinal absorption of elemental calcium
Lower circulating calcitonin
Decreased sunlight exposure and dietary vitamin D intake
Decreased ovarian function causing altered estrogen balance

externally applied force. Chronic overload, or *cumulative trauma*, is associated with prolonged static work, stress, and often reduced aerobic activity. Other chapters in this textbook provide an overview of specific musculoskeletal dysfunctions, including fractures (Chapters 21 and 23), peripheral nerve injuries (Chapter 20), and tendon injuries (Chapters 26, 27, and 28).

Clinical Pearl

A large percentage of clients who have cumulative trauma injuries are deconditioned because of a sedentary job or lifestyle.

Comorbidities Associated With Increased Prevalence of Musculoskeletal Dysfunction

Comprehensive treatment that addresses the whole client, rather than just an extremity, is the aim of client-centered care. Many clients have comorbidities to consider when developing a treatment plan. Some of the more common diseases that are associated with lowered tolerance of the musculoskeletal system are osteoporosis, arthritis, diabetes, hypothyroidism/hyperthyroidism, gastric ulcer, chronic/recurrent infections, colitis, and cardiovascular and respiratory diseases.

Osteoporosis

An estimated 30 million Americans have osteoporosis. This disease is responsible for 1.5 million individuals sustaining bone fractures per year (200,000 wrist fractures, 300,000 hip fractures, and 300,000 non–wrist extremity fractures). Osteoporosis costs more than $18 billion per year in health care expenses and lost productivity. Bone mass attains a peak in males and females at approximately 30 to 35 years of age, with total bone mass beginning to decline 5 to 10 years later. Boxes 10.1 and 10.2 list traits and age-related changes associated with osteoporosis.[4,5]

Males are less affected by osteoporosis than females, and several factors can affect bone resorption levels. A lack of weight bearing and activity in antigravity muscles changes the resorption rate, as does excessive thyroid and parathyroid hormones. Corticosteroids also have an impact. Determinants of bone mass and loss are genetic, mechanical, or hormonal. Genetics can cause large-boned individuals to gain a relative immunity to osteoporotic fractures. The mechanics of bone density can aid in the prevention of fractures, but can also be a possible cause. Increased loading leads to increased bone mass, and decreased loading leads to decreased bone mass.

Exercise for Prevention/Treatment of Osteoporosis

Exercise can help prevent or slow down bone loss, improve posture, and increase overall fitness. For clients who are at risk for osteoporosis, having a bone density test before starting an exercise program is recommended. Box 10.3 lists factors to consider when selecting exercise for individuals with osteoporosis.[6]

Although walking is the best of all the options listed in Box 10.3, those clients who are unable to tolerate walking because of comorbidities or advanced osteoporosis have other options. These options generate muscle tension, which provides needed stress to bone. To prevent injury, individuals with advanced osteoporosis should avoid the exercises listed in Box 10.4.

Client Education for Osteoporosis

Education of the client on what impact osteoporosis will have on his or her life and what the client can do to prevent fractures or falls is important. Teach clients about proper body mechanics by demonstrating proper posture. When teaching lifting and

---

BOX 10.3   Some Considerations for Exercise Selection

- Weight-bearing activities and strength training are ideal for bone stimulation.
- Increased strength improves balance and decreases the risk of falls.
- Walking is ideal because it is weight bearing, dynamic, and repetitive.
- Swimming or cycling use less weight-bearing forces and are less effective than walking.
- Nonimpact loading may cause damage to weakened bone.

BOX 10.4   Contraindicated Exercises for Advanced Osteoporosis

Vigorous aerobic workout
Exercises that require twisting or bending
Abdominal machines
Biceps-curl machines
Rowing machines
Tennis
Golf
Bowling

---

carrying techniques, show the client how to hold loads close to the body. Explain that strengthening exercises improve balance and decrease the risk of falling. Address fall prevention. Wearing of proper shoes, removal of throw rugs, sufficient lighting, and use of handrails decrease the risk of a fall or fracture.

Precaution. *Avoid forceful, unguarded motions, such as opening a stuck window or bending forward to lift a heavy object. Instead, teach clients how to squat when lifting.*

Arthritis

Arthritis presents concerns for exercise participation due to characteristic joint disfunction and pain. Erosive osteoarthritis is more prevalent, often due to trauma or misuse of the hands; the base of the thumb and distal joints of the fingers are often affected.[7] Rheumatoid arthritis (RA) is a systemic autoimmune disorder prevalent in less than 1% of the population, with joint involvement of the wrist, thumb, and metacarpophalangeal (MP) joints.[7,8] Addressing exercise early in the disease process helps manage symptoms.[8] With RA, the joints are particularly fragile and may develop subluxation, synovitis, swan neck, boutonniere, or mallet deformities. Exercises that maintain joint mobility and soft-tissue excursion through active motion, such as intrinsic stretches and tendon glides, are indicated.[8] Chapter 29 in this textbook provides more detail about arthritis management.

Metabolic Conditions

Diabetes causes the production and use of insulin in the body to be impaired. This results in an abundance of sugar in the bloodstream. With diabetes, the pancreas secretes little or no insulin (type I diabetes) or the body becomes resistant to the action of insulin (type II diabetes). If the disease is not treated, the level of sugar in the bloodstream builds up and leads to diabetic complications, such as peripheral neuropathy and changes in vision.

The thyroid gland affects all aspects of metabolism. The thyroid releases hormones that regulate heart rate, the strength of bones, how quickly calories are burned, and sensitivity to heat/cold. If the thyroid gland is underactive or overactive (hypothyroidism/hyperthyroidism), medical treatment is necessary to avoid complications.[4]

Exercise Considerations in the Presence of Comorbidities

Always use caution and discretion when prescribing the intensity of exercise. A thorough evaluation provides the necessary information regarding cardiovascular compromise or other risk factors such as pulmonary disease, diabetes mellitus, hypertension, obesity, peripheral vascular disease, arthritis, and renal disease.[9]

Precaution. *An exercise program may not be recommended for uncontrolled diabetes. A rigorous strengthening or aerobic exercise program, in this case, may cause a hyperglycemic effect because cellular absorption of glucose is restricted. Insulin-dependent diabetic clients may need to decrease insulin or increase carbohydrate intake when exercising. They should monitor their glucose more frequently when starting an exercise program. For this client population, the exercise should be dosed at a lower level of intensity and duration initially and should progress at a much slower rate.*[4]

Histology of Collagen, Bone, and Cartilage

Collagen

Collagen is the fundamental component of the connective tissues of the body, including fascia, fibrous cartilage, tendons, ligaments, bones, joint capsules, blood vessels, adipose tissue, and dermis. Collagen is the most abundant protein in the human body. It accounts for approximately 30% of all protein. Before 1970, researchers believed that all collagen was identical. Now, 19 types of collagen are known that are differentiated by their protein composition. Type I and type II together compose approximately 90% of human connective tissue. Type III collagen is produced first, in the initial reparative phase of healing, before type I collagen. Type III collagen also is found in arteries, the liver, and the spleen.[6]

Type I collagen constitutes about 90% of total body collagen. Type I collagen is found in bone, tendon, fascia, fibrous cartilage, derma, and sclera. This collagen is synthesized by **fibroblasts, osteoblasts,** and **chondroblasts.** Its primary function is to resist tension.

Type II collagen is found in hyaline and elastic cartilage and intervertebral disks. Type II collagen is synthesized by chondroblasts. Its primary function is to resist intermittent pressure.

Fibroblasts produce type I collagen fibers that are found in tendons, ligaments, and joint capsules. **Procollagen**, the precursor of collagen, is produced in the endoplasmic reticulum and is made up of polypeptide chains of lysine, glycine, and proline. **Tropocollagen** is the basic molecular unit of collagen fibrils and is found in the interstitial spaces; this collagen is the building block of collagen. The bonds of procollagen and tropocollagen are weak and easily deformed or ruptured. One must understand that collagen bonds are remodeled from mobilization or exercise.

Fibroblasts also produce **glycosaminoglycans**. These are **proteoglycans**, the fundamental components of connective tissue, which make up the **extracellular matrix** of tendons, ligaments, and articular cartilage. **Imbibition** is the primary nutritional source for avascular tissues, such as tendons, ligaments, cartilage, and vertebral disks. When tension/pressure increase, fluid is forced out of tissue and the volume of the tissue decreases. This causes an increase in the concentration of proteoglycan substances and an increase in osmotic pressure, which in turn produces imbibition. Glycosaminoglycans provide the fibers with nutrition via imbibition and lubrication. They allow space for elastic deformity of the tissue.[6] The half-life of glycosaminoglycans is 1.7 to 7 days. Immobilization for more than 1.7 to 7 days causes a 50% decrease in glycosaminoglycans. Therefore lubrication is decreased, and the elastic range of collagen is decreased. A decrease in glycosaminoglycans causes a decrease in nutrition, which damages the tissue.

Bone

Bone is the protective and supportive framework that has rigid and static, elastic and dynamic properties. The properties and geometry of bone can be altered in response to internal and external stress, and in response to mineral demands. Bone has plastic qualities; it absorbs and stores compressional forces and transmits tensile forces. Bone also has elastic qualities. Long bone can deform up to 5%. The ability of bone to deform decreases with age.

Bone is composed of approximately 5% water and approximately 70% minerals (calcium hydroxyapatite, phosphate, magnesium, sodium, potassium, and fluoride carbonate); approximately 20% organic compounds, mostly type I collagen; and approximately 5% non-collagenous proteins. Osteoblasts are the functional building blocks of the **osteoid matrix**; they are located only at the surface of bone tissue. **Osteocytes** are mature osteoblasts. **Osteoclasts** are responsible for bone dissolution and absorption. Bone homeostasis balances synthesis, dissolution, and absorption with the forces that are applied on the skeleton.[10]

Cartilage

Cartilage is a semirigid connective tissue that is less dense and more elastic than bone. The functional unit of cartilage is the chondrocyte. Chondroblasts are immature **chondrocytes**, and they produce the **ground substance** or extracellular matrix of cartilage. This extracellular matrix consists of glycosaminoglycans and type II collagen. Water composes 65% to 80% of articular cartilage. Like fibroblasts, chondroblasts synthesize collagen and glycosaminoglycans when stimulated by mechanical tension. Mature cartilage is avascular and lacks nerve supply. Cartilage gets nutrition through imbibition. The mechanical forces of motion stimulate imbibition and removal of waste products.

The three types of cartilage are the following:

1. *Hyaline cartilage*: The most common and found on articular surfaces of peripheral joints, sternal ends of the ribs, nasal septum, larynx, and tracheal rings
2. *Elastic cartilage*: Found in the epiglottis, laryngeal cartilage, walls of eustachian tubes, external ear, and auditory canal
3. *Fibrocartilage*: Found in intervertebral disks, some articular cartilage, the pubic symphysis, dense connective tissue in joint capsules, ligaments, and the union of tendons to bone.

The two primary functions of articular cartilage are to promote motion between two opposing bones with minimal friction and wear and to distribute the load applied to the joint surfaces over as great an area as possible.[11]

Optimal Stimulus for Regeneration of Collagen, Bone, and Cartilage

Collagen

The optimal stimulus for fibroblastic function in the regeneration of collagen is modified tension along the line of stress. This modified tension is not to exceed the level of tension that the newly formed polar bonds of tropocollagen can withstand. The tropocollagen is an immature precursor to the stronger, more resilient collagen. Once a certain level of tension is exceeded, tissue breakdown will occur instead of proliferation.

Precaution. *If tension exceeds this critical level, the signs and symptoms will be pain, inflammatory reaction, muscle guarding, decreased range of motion or loss of flexibility, and secondary scarring.*[6]

Bone

The optimal stimulus for osteoblastic production in the regeneration of bone is modified compression in the line of stress. Wolff's law states that bone will change its internal architecture according to the forces placed upon it.

Precaution. *Abnormal shear force may cause a pseudarthrosis.*

Pseudarthrosis or "false joint" occurs at the site of nonunion. Shearing force stimulates undifferentiated mesenchymal cells to produce cartilage, and a false joint may be created at the fracture site.[10] **Osteophytes** are bony outgrowths that develop as the body attempts to provide stability or to repair itself.

Cartilage

The optimal stimulus in the regeneration of cartilage is intermittent compression/decompression with glide. Joint movement (shear) is necessary to distribute synovial fluid over the cartilaginous surface and provide oxygen and other necessary nutrients. Intermittent compression forces the extracellular fluid within the joint to be compressed into the cartilage matrix. With joint immobilization, an alteration in joint mechanics and a decrease in the normal contact areas of cartilage occur. This eventually leads to joint dysfunction, hypomobility or hypermobility, and muscle guarding.

Precaution. *The body responds to the stresses placed upon it. With abnormal stresses, there will be dysfunctional remodeling. This manifests as joint degeneration, osteophytes, bone spurs, or pseudarthrosis.*[10]

Effects of Immobilization Versus Early Mobilization

> **Clinical Pearl**
>
> Early mobilization within a pain-free range of motion promotes faster healing of connective tissue, stronger collagen bonds, reduced scar tissue adhesions, and improved collagen fiber orientation.

BOX 10.5   Home Exercise Program

The home exercise program should do the following:
1. Provide modified tension in the line of stress. Initially, this will be accomplished by performing light muscle contractions to move the joint through the full available pain-free range of motion.
2. Avoid reinjury. *Any exercise or activity that causes pain is an indication of tissue trauma.*
3. Provide the proper dosage. Give specific instructions about the number of repetitions, sets, breaks, positioning, and speed of exercises.
4. Indicate the frequency of exercise. This depends on healing time frames, intensity, volume, comorbidities, and the tolerance to stress of the tissue. Be clear in the instructions to the client about the frequency of exercise. Initially this may be three or more times per day, but with increased exercise stress, there will be a decrease in frequency.
5. Supply adequate nutritional support. Explain the importance of eating a balanced diet and drinking a sufficient amount of water to stay hydrated. A well-balanced diet combined with exercise promotes healthy tissue.

After 9 weeks of immobilization, there is 14% loss of total collagen, and by 12 weeks, there is a 28% loss. The half-life of collagen is 300 to 500 days. For this reason, under normal physiological conditions, it takes between 1 and 2 years for full healing to occur. Immobilization of cartilage causes a decrease in thickness and number of collagen bundles, a decrease in proteoglycan content, an increase in water content, a decrease in load-bearing capacity, softening of the articular surface, decrease in tensile strength of cartilage, and a decrease in oxygen content. To decrease these adverse effects of immobilization, one should institute an exercise model of high repetitions with low to no resistance. This model increases the oxygen content within the tissues by improving blood flow and imbibition. For maximal benefit, mobilization exercises should be performed several times a day.[6] A home exercise program helps accomplish these goals. Box 10.5 lists the qualities of a good home exercise program.

Neurophysiology

Muscle Spindles

Muscle spindles are proprioceptors that consist of intrafusal muscle fibers enclosed in a sheath (spindle). They run parallel to the extrafusal muscle fibers and act as receptors that provide information on muscle length and the rate of change in muscle length. The spindles are stretched when the muscle lengthens. This stretch causes the sensory neuron in the spindle to transmit an impulse to the spinal cord, where it synapses with alpha motor neurons. This causes activation of motor neurons that innervate the muscle. The muscle spindles determine the amount of contraction necessary to overcome a given resistance. When the resistance increases, the muscle is stretched further, and this causes spindle fibers to activate a greater muscle contraction.[12]

Golgi Tendon Organs

Golgi tendon organs (GTOs) are proprioceptors that are located in the tendon adjacent to the myotendinous junction. They are arranged in series with the extrafusal muscle fibers. They are sensitive to stretch but are activated most efficiently when the muscle shortens. The GTO transmits information regarding muscle tension as opposed to length. Neural input from the GTO causes an inhibition of muscle activation. This provides a protective mechanism to avoid development of excessive tension.[12]

Joint Mechanoreceptors

Four types of **mechanoreceptors** are found in the synovial joint capsules. Mechanoreceptors have a significant effect on muscle tone and pain sensation locally and distally along segmental innervations. The number of mechanoreceptors decreases with age. By age 70 the total number of receptors has decreased by about 50%, depending on factors such as genetics and activity level.[13]

Type I mechanoreceptors are found in the superficial layers of the joint capsule between the collagen fibers. A large percentage of the type I mechanoreceptors is found in the joints of the neck, hip, and shoulder. They have a great effect on the coordination of the tonic muscle fibers. They are slow-adapting and inhibit pain. They fire during movement and for about 1 minute after movement stops. They provide postural and kinesthetic awareness (awareness of the position of the body or body part in space). They are active in the beginning and end-range of collagen tension.

Type II mechanoreceptors are found in deep layers of joint capsules. A high concentration of the type II mechanoreceptors is found in the joints of the lumbar spine, hand, foot, and temporomandibular joint. They are fast adapting and pain inhibiting. They fire during movement and continue to fire until about 0.5 seconds after movement stops. They do not respond to stretch but are activated in beginning and midrange of collagen tension. They have more effect on the phasic muscle fibers and **kinesthesia**.

Type III mechanoreceptors are located in the deep and superficial layers of the joint capsules and ligaments. They are slow adapting and inhibit muscle tone in response to stretch at the extreme end-range of tension. They provide kinesthetic information, but their role is less understood than the type I and II mechanoreceptors.

Type IV mechanoreceptors are located in joint capsules, blood vessels, articular fat pads, anterior dura mater, ligaments of the spine, and connective tissue. They are not found in muscle. They fire when excessive levels of tension are reached in the collagen, and they warn of tissue trauma. They function as pain-provoking, nonadapting, high-threshold receptors. They fire continuously until the injurious stimulus is removed. They are provoked by excessive stretch, inflammation, high temperature (38–42°C or 100.4–107.6°F), or respiratory and cardiovascular distress.[13]

Pain has been defined by the International Association for the Study of Pain as an unpleasant emotional disorder evoked by sufficient activity in the nociceptive system and associated with real or potential tissue damage.[14] The irritation causing the pain may be due to immobilization, physical trauma, infection, or emotional tension.

Precaution. *Pain is a protective mechanism. Pain is not a warning that something is about to go wrong; it has already gone wrong! Pain is the way the body alerts the brain that an irritation to the tissue has occurred. For this reason, one must remember to exercise within a pain-free range of motion. In this case, feeling bad is a good thing because it is how your body communicates. Listen to the body.*

Traumatology

The response of the body to trauma is predictable and consistent, regardless of the tissue involved or the mechanism of injury. Trauma sets off a highly organized response involving chemical, metabolic, permeability, and vascular changes at a cellular level in preparation for tissue repair.

Phases and Time Frames of Healing

The initial response to a traumatic event is irritation, lasting for 5 to 6 hours. Vasomotor constriction occurs in the first few seconds. An immediate release of chemical vasodilators occurs. These dilators are also transmitters for the nociceptive (pain) system. The vasodilation increases the hydrostatic pressure because of increased capillary permeability. Clinicians rarely can influence this phase because of its immediate occurrence.

The next stage of healing is the acute stage, which lasts for 1 to 3 days depending on the vascularity of the tissue. During this time frame, a migration of the larger cell bodies through the wall of the vessel occurs. Subsequently, blood flow increases to the area, increasing hydrostatic pressure and increasing bleeding. The large proteins leak out of the capillary, causing a shift in osmotic pressure with resultant pulling of fluid out of the capillary. Venous stasis occurs distal to the traumatized area, and edema results.

The third stage of healing is the subacute stage. The subacute stage begins with the settled stage, where muscle spasming occurs over the next 3 to 5 days. Bleeding is no longer present. Oxygen and macrophages are present. Walling off of the capillary occurs, which makes waste removal difficult. This leads to secondary healing or scarring. Externally applied heat in the settled stage promotes stasis and inflammatory exudates. The preferred method of heating tissue is internally. Initiating movement with low-resistance exercise produces friction and naturally generates heat. This promotes increased blood flow.

The final stage is the chronic stage. Tissue becomes strongly chemical bonded (**covalent bonds**) and matures at 9 to 12 months. At this stage the tissue becomes nonelastic and cannot be deformed. Mature scar tissue may cause pain. Clinically, concentrate on increasing the tolerance of the tissue to tension about the scar by use of controlled stress through properly dosed exercises.

Tissue-specific exercise in the subacute stage provides the optimal stimulus for the removal of **metabolites**, which are products of metabolism, from the tissue. Muscle contraction is necessary to transport metabolites from the cell and provide oxygen/nutrition to the area. Increased vascularization accomplishes this goal. This is achieved through many repetitions of properly dosed exercise with minimal resistance while avoiding excessive tissue tension. In other words, the muscle contractions with proper exercise facilitate formation of capillaries, blood flow, and removal of metabolites.

Stages of Repair

The stages of repair can be categorized into three phases: inflammation, repair, and remodeling. During the inflammatory phase, the white blood cells/macrophages destroy cellular debris, synthesize fibronectin, and produce protein and fiber. During the repair stage, collagen is produced, and during the remodeling stage, the fibroblasts orient longitudinally within 28 days and repair is complete between 128 and 135 days. **Myofibroblasts** (involved in tissue reconstruction) are active from 5 to 21 days after trauma to up to 9 months. During the initial remodeling, a random configuration of collagen fibrils occurs. This arrangement provides minimal strength. During the maturation phase, the mechanical strength increases with remodeling and organization of fibers with modified tension in the line of stress.[6]

Muscle Physiology

◎ *Clinical Pearl*

Strength is related to fiber diameter, not fiber type.

Type I muscle fibers are smaller in diameter than type II muscle fibers. Muscle recruitment progresses from smaller to larger diameter. **Tonic muscles** fire first because they are the primary dynamic joint stabilizers. Their nutrition mainly comes from the delivery of oxygen. They are predominantly type I or slow-twitch muscles and are responsible for sustaining proper joint **arthrokinematics** over time.[15]

Tonic Versus Phasic Muscles

Tonic muscles initiate the easy work; they are better adapted for endurance exercise than **phasic muscles** because they have more capillaries, mitochondria, and metabolic enzymes (Table 10.2). With long-distance running, the tonic muscles are primarily responsible for work because they are adapted for aerobic activity. The phasic muscles are recruited to participate if the load is too great or if it is increasing. They are better suited for short-duration activities that are of higher intensity. They also begin to participate if the light work has lasted for 2 to 3 hours, as seen with marathon runners who sprint when approaching the finish line. Phasic muscles are anaerobic and contract at a higher speed and with greater force of contraction; they fatigue more quickly than tonic muscles do.

The tonic muscle fibers atrophy almost immediately when immobilized after injury because they depend primarily on oxygen for metabolism. Therefore exercise to improve vascularization provides the oxygen necessary to nourish the tonic system.

Habitually overloading a system will cause it to respond and adapt. The rate of protein synthesis in a muscle is related directly to the rate of amino acid transportation into the cell. Amino acids transported into the muscle are influenced by the intensity and the duration of the muscle tension. Conversely, muscle atrophies as a result of disuse, immobilization, guarding associated with pain, or starvation.[15,16]

TABLE 10.2   Comparison of Tonic and Phasic Muscle Fibers

Tonic	Phasic
Red: High myoglobin concentration	White: Lower myoglobin concentration
Slow twitch: 10–20 impulses per second	Fast twitch: 30–50 impulses per second
Type I	Type II
Arthrokinematic	Osteokinematic
Bipenate	Fusiform
Antigravity	—

Types of Muscle Work and Training Effects

Isometric muscle contraction is the production of muscle tension without a change in muscle length or joint angle. The tension in the **cross-bridges** (the portion of myosin filament that pulls the actin filaments toward the center of the sarcomere during muscle contraction) is equal to the resistive force, thereby maintaining constant muscle length.

Concentric muscle contraction is muscle shortening as the muscle produces tension while the insertion moves toward the origin. Movement occurs in the same direction as the tension and joint motion because the contractile force is greater than the resistive force. Based on the **sliding filament theory**, the cross-bridges on the myosin filament attach to the active site on the actin filament. When all the muscle cross-bridges shorten in a single cycle, the muscle shortens by approximately 1%. Muscles have the capacity to shorten up to 60% of their resting length; therefore the contraction cycle must be repeated multiple times.[17]

Eccentric muscle contraction is muscle lengthening as the muscle produces tension and the insertion moves away from the origin. The net muscle movement is in the opposite direction of the force of the muscle because the contractile force is less than the resistive force. Eccentric contractions require less energy than concentric contractions and are thought to be responsible for some aspect of postexercise muscle soreness. The cross-bridges of myosin stay attached to the active sites while the resistance is lowered. It may be the actual "tearing" away of the cross-bridges while resisting the lowering of a heavy resistance that results in the delayed-onset muscle soreness.[17,18]

Exercise

Functional Qualities of Exercise

Coordination refers to quality of motion. With atrophy of the tonic system, coordination is the first functional quality to be lost because the tonic muscles are the primary dynamic stabilizers of the joints. Therefore coordination must be the first functional quality to be restored. With an increase in speed or an increase in resistance comes a need for increased coordination. Normalization of a reflex disturbance, which is abnormal action of the cell, tissue, organ, or organism caused by overstimulation or understimulation, requires 5000 to 6000 repetitions. The repetitions

are necessary to regain optimal coordination of movements about a physiologic axis.[16]

Endurance is the capacity to maintain an intensity of exercise for a prolonged period. Endurance requires continuous restoration of energy sources. Tonic muscles primarily require oxygen from the vascular system for their nutrition. Phasic muscles require glucose and body fat for their nutrition. Because the tonic system is the first to atrophy, due to of muscle guarding and decreased motor recruitment, endurance is the quality that will increase nutrition through vascularization. Endurance exercise also promotes removal of waste products and prevents continued firing of the type IV mechanoreceptors caused by an abnormal chemical environment. Exercise dosage for endurance and vascularization requires many repetitions (3 sets of 24) with low resistance.[16]

Speed is the time it takes to cover a fixed distance. Speed equals distance divided by time. With an increase in speed of movement is an increase in inertia, and overcoming this inertia requires a higher level of coordination. Speed of movement ultimately must be functional. During the initial phases of healing, coordination is not sufficient to exercise safely at a fast/functional speed.[19]

Volume refers to the total amount of weight lifted in a workout. The weight per repetition determines the appropriate volume per set. Heavy weights cannot be lifted for many repetitions in a set. Volume can be determined by multiplying the number of repetitions by the number of sets times the weight lifted per repetition. For instance, 3 sets of 25 repetitions with 5 pounds would be calculated as $3 \times 25 \times 5$ lbs = 375 lbs of volume. If other sets also are performed with different amounts of weight, the volumes per set are calculated and then all are added together to obtain the total workout volume.[20]

Strength is the maximal force that a muscle or group of muscles can generate against a resistance at a given speed. Strength can be tested as a measure of 1 RM (resistance maximal). Strength training is performed at a percentage of 1 RM. For strength training, the number of repetitions decreases as the resistance increases. Increased resistance produces an increase in tissue tension and a decrease in blood flow to the capillaries during the muscle contraction, as well as an increase in blood flow when the exercise is over. Therefore only a few repetitions are performed. For pure strength gains, 85% of 1 RM (3 sets of 6) are performed. However, when there is muscle atrophy after immobilization, strength gains are realized at 30% to 40% of 1 RM.[19-22]

Power is the ability to overcome resistance over a specific distance in a fixed time frame. Work equals force multiplied by distance. Power equals work divided by time. Power lifting is generally not a functional requirement for clients. However, increased power is necessary to perform a task at a faster rate. Power is therefore a critical component of exercise for clients.[23]

Dosing

Exercise initially is dosed based on the physiology of the type I muscle fibers and their depletion of nutrients in a state of guarding.

> **◉ Clinical Pearl**
>
> Clinically, the first goal of dosing exercise is to deliver oxygen to the muscles, elicit no pain, and perform many repetitions.

Initially, focus on sustaining slow, coordinated movement around a physiological axis. Ultimately, progress toward a fast/functional speed while maintaining coordination and providing optimal stimulus for regeneration of the specific tissue(s) in lesion.[16] Resistance should be objective and measurable, physiological, and adjusted to the tissues participating (see explanations of these concepts later in this chapter). Training with free weights or a pulley system is easier to quantify and provides a more specific resistance throughout the entire range of motion than elastic bands.

Starting Positions

Determining a starting position depends on tolerance of the specific tissues to stress. Gravity assists, resists, or is eliminated, depending on what the tissue can tolerate while working in a pain-free synergy about a physiological axis.

Precaution. *If there is pain while exercising against the force of gravity, position the limb in a posture that eliminates the effects of gravity.*[16]

If necessary, to complete a pain-free arc of motion, the limb can be positioned so that the motion to be performed is assisted by gravity. This way, the antagonists, muscles that work in opposition to the prime movers, generate motion instead of the painful agonists, or prime movers.

Range of Motion

Initially, localize motion to a specific joint in a specific direction with controlled range of motion maintained throughout the arc. Monitor the tension on noncontractile tissues. Watch for controlled, normal physiological motion, and educate the client to avoid compensatory motion while exercising. Adjust the resistance to allow for acceleration toward maximal length-tension range and deceleration away from it. Quality of motion, while avoiding pain-provoking end-ranges, dictates quantity.[19]

Work Capacity/Effects of Aging

An individual's sustainable work capacity is approximately 30% of that person's available energy. The remaining 70% of the stored energy in the body is needed for protein synthesis and maintenance of tissue (Fig. 10.1). The amount of energy available for maintenance, repair, and regeneration of tissue decreases with age. With age, it takes less activity to dip into the 70% of energy reserve that is so necessary for tissue synthesis and repair (Fig. 10.2).

Precaution. *With an older client population, take care not to over exercise, or the risk for breakdown of collagen tissue and problems, such as tendinopathy will increase.*[16]

Calculating Dosage

In 1948, DeLorme defined the term **resistance maximal** (RM). This is the resistance that a group of muscles can overcome once. RM, a measure of strength, combines with Holten's concentric curve to develop correct dosing of exercise for a client as outlined in the following section. In the 1950s the Norwegian, Oddvar Holten, developed a curve that estimated guidelines for dosing repetitions/resistance for concentric work (Fig. 10.3).[16,24]

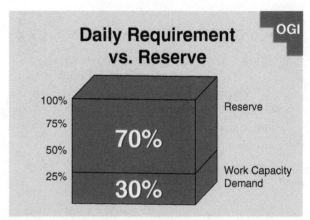

FIG. 10.1 Total daily energy requirements. *(Used with permission from the Ola Grimsby Institute.)*

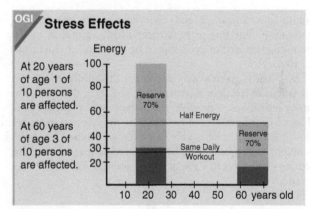

FIG. 10.2 Effects of age on energy requirements. *(Used with permission from the Ola Grimsby Institute.)*

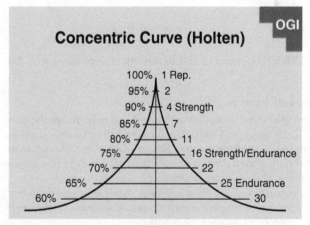

FIG. 10.3 Holten diagram. Rep., Repetitions. *(Used with permission from the Ola Grimsby Institute.)*

Calculating Resistance by Percentage of 1 RM

Repetitions of Exercise

Because 1 RM is the maximum resistance that can be overcome once, this resistance has a high risk of causing further injury to the already compromised tissue. When dosing an exercise program initially, the first functional qualities desired are to

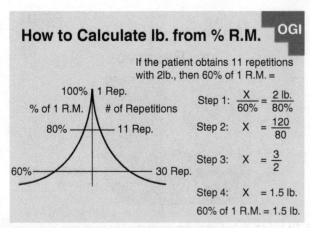

FIG. 10.4 Example for calculating exercise dose. *(Used with permission from the Ola Grimsby Institute.)*

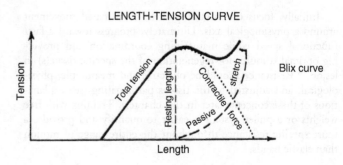

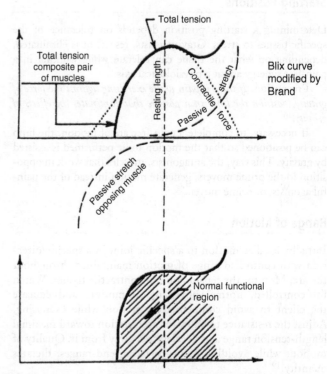

FIG. 10.5 Length-tension curve. *(From Brand PW, Hollister A. Clinical Mechanics of the Hand. St Louis, 1999, Mosby. In: Trumble. Principles of Hand Surgery and Therapy. Philadelphia, 2000, W.B. Saunders.)*

promote vascularization and endurance while maintaining coordination. For this to be accomplished, according to the Holten diagram, the exercise should be dosed at 30 repetitions (Fig. 10.4).[16,24]

The client is given a weight that the therapist predicts will cause fatigue in less than 30 repetitions. The client then performs as many repetitions as possible before the onset of fatigue, pain, or loss of coordination. As an example, the client is provided with a 3-lb weight and is able to perform 16 repetitions with this weight before becoming fatigued or experiencing pain (16 repetitions correlates to 75% of 1 RM according to the Holten diagram).

Therefore

$$\frac{x}{60} = \frac{3}{75}$$

$$x = \frac{180}{75}$$

$$x = 2.4 \ lb$$

This client should be able to perform 30 repetitions with 2.4 lbs.

Speed of Exercise

Speed of exercise is another component that may change the dosage. Increased speed causes an increase in inertia and requires more coordination to execute. Oxygen debt is also important to avoid during exercising to provide the type I muscle fibers with nutrition while they are in a state of guarding.

Precaution. *If the client's respiratory rate is increasing during the exercise, then the speed of exercise must be decreased or there must be a longer break between sets or both.*

To increase the total number of repetitions while maintaining an accurate dose, increase the number of sets. It has been determined that to go from one set to three sets without changing the resistance, the number of repetitions must be decreased by 15% to 20%. By doing this, 1 set of 30 repetitions now becomes 3 sets of 24 to 25 repetitions. The amount of time between sets is determined by how long it takes the client to return to **a steady state respiratory rate** (equilibrium of the respiratory system). This is necessary to avoid oxygen debt.

When using pulleys to exercise the upper extremity, if the weight of the limb alone exceeds 60% of 1 RM, then a counterweight may be used to de-weight the arm. Other ways to decrease the weight of the limb for proper dosage are to position it in a gravity-eliminated position or even a gravity-assisted position.[16,24]

Length-Tension Relationship and Implications to Exercise

Blyx,[25] a Swedish physiologist, defined **muscle fiber length equilibrium** as the length the muscle will maintain when it is unaffected by outside forces. Muscle force production varies depending on the angle of the muscle in the arc of motion. The length/tension curve identifies the length at which a muscle generates the most contractile tension (Fig. 10.5). This length is influenced by histological, biomechanical, and neurophysiological factors. Histologically, the overlap of actin and myosin filaments is most extensive toward the midrange of motion. Biomechanically, the angle of the tendon insertion into the bone dictates where the greatest tensile strength will occur. The greatest amount of force is achieved when the moment arm for a muscular force is perpendicular to the lever arm. Neurophysiologically, the joint mechanoreceptors influence muscle facilitation around the joint. Type I and type II mechanoreceptors fire at the beginning of range. Type II alone fires at midrange, and type I fires at the end-range of capsular tension.[13]

The clinical importance of the length/tension concept can be discussed in terms of concentric and eccentric aspects.

Concentric Aspects

When working concentrically with pulleys, set the rope perpendicular to the lever arm at 20% into the lengthened range of the muscle that is going to do the work. If using free weights, position the limb where it is perpendicular to the force of gravity, when the lever arm is at 20% into the lengthened range of motion.

Eccentric Aspects

When working eccentrically, have the maximal resistance set perpendicular to the lever arm at 20% to 30% into the shortened range of the muscle that is going to do the eccentric work. The length/tension concept reveals that muscle produces the least amount of power at the beginning and end-ranges. When activated, the muscle contraction accelerates toward the midrange and decelerates away from it. The variability of speed is an important component of all activities of daily living. Because activity is task specific, the variables of speed and resistance throughout the range of a contraction are important for fiber recruitment and physiological coordination.[26,27]

Formulation and Progression of an Exercise Program

When formulating an exercise program for treatment of hypomobility or hypermobility, start by identifying the specific problems that exist. Examples of these problems are the following:

- The complaint of pain
- Muscle guarding of the tonics (rotator cuff)
- Decreased endurance, and limited range of motion (external rotation [ER] > abduction [ABD] > internal rotation [IR])
- Articular compression
- Decreased synovium/decreased articular cartilage nutrition
- Decreased mechanoreceptor input in the capsule
- Compensatory motion

Once an examination has been completed, establish functional or measurable goals that address the identified problems. The following suggestions are several possible goals for the client:

- Decrease pain with arm elevation (1 to 10 scale)
- Increase endurance with exercise (time and repetitions) and with functional work/avocation activities (time)
- Increase range of motion (specific planes of motion and to accomplish functional activities)
- Educate/improve posture to promote proximal stability and improved arthrokinematics of the glenohumeral joint (at work, with activities, time frames)

Identify treatment approaches to resolve the goals:

- *Decrease pain and guarding*: Distraction of the joint to fire type I mechanoreceptors

---

BOX 10.6 Considerations for Exercise Program

Equipment: Consider using pulleys, benches, bolsters, and wedges for positioning; straps, free weights, and de-weighting devices.

Ropes: Consider the range of motion, and set the rope perpendicular to the lever arm and parallel to the muscle fiber.

Pulley: Should be single, double, concentric, or eccentric.

Starting positions: Consider recommending supine, prone, side lying, sitting, standing, non–weight bearing, weight bearing, arm supported, or unsupported.

Movement range: Consider recommending full range of motion; inner, outer, or midrange of motion.

Weight: Consider the functional quality that is desired and what percentage of 1 RM is needed to accomplish that. (In this case, the functional qualities most likely would be endurance and vascularization.) Also take into account the body/limb position, gravity, and quality of motion when determining weight.

Dosage: The number of repetitions and sets is determined by the desired functional qualities. These include coordination, vascularization, endurance, strength, and power.[7,23]

Speed: This will vary, but early in the rehabilitation, when working on vascularization and endurance, it is important to follow respiratory rate at steady state to avoid oxygen debt. Speed should increase as coordination and function increase.

Rest: Breaks between sets are determined by respiratory rate. As the client starts to increase strength (x resistance + x repetitions), the rest breaks will increase. As resistance increases, the frequency of exercise decreases as well (three times per week).

Education: Instructions to the client must be specific. Demonstration of the exercise first or even guiding the client's limb through the arc of motion that is desired is often helpful. Use verbal, visual, and tactile cues as necessary.

RM, Resistance maximal.

- *Increase joint mobility*: Compression/decompression with gliding for cartilage, modified tension in the line of stress for joint capsule
- *Hydrate/lubricate cartilage*: Compression/decompression with glide
- *Increase proprioception*: Modified tension in the line of stress

Consider client and equipment needs before starting exercises. Box 10.6 outlines different aspects of an exercise program. Consider precautions and contraindications when implementing an exercise program.

Precaution. *Comorbidities (such as cardiac or pulmonary disease, specific physician protocol, and other medical/surgical considerations) must dictate exercise decisions.*

Progressions of Hypomobilities

Progressions of hypomobile joints has four stages (Table 10.3).

TABLE 10.3	Progression of Hypomobilities Stages I to IV	
Stage	**Procedures**	**Goals**
Stage 1	Many repetitions	Increase endurance
	Low speed	Increase circulation
	Minimal resistance	Increase exercise ability
	Outer range of motion	Avoid overexertion
Stage II	Increase repetitions	Increase endurance
	Increase speed	Increase fast coordination
	Do not increase resistance	
Stage III	Stabilizing exercise in the gained range of motion	Increase strength in the gained range of motion
	Concentric and eccentric	
Stage IV	Coordinate tonic and phasic function throughout physiologic range of motion	Functional stability

TABLE 10.4	Progression of Hypermobilities Stages I to IV	
Stages	**Procedures**	**Goals**
Stage I	Many repetitions	Increase endurance
	Low speed	Increase circulation
	Minimal resistance	Increase exercise ability
	Beginning or midrange of motion	Avoid overexertion
Stage II	Increase repetitions	Increase strength
	Include isometric contractions in inner range of motion	Increase sensitivity to stretch
Stage III	Submaximal (80% RM) resistance concentrically and eccentrically	Increase dynamic stability in the gained range of motion
	Include isometric contractions in the full range of motion (except the outer range)	
Stage IV	Coordinate tonic and phasic function throughout physiologic range of motion	Functional stability

RM, Resistance maximal.

Stage I

Stage I begins with many repetitions to address coordination. Following the Holten diagram, 60% of 1 RM promotes vascularization. This is dosed at 3 sets of 25 repetitions. Fifty percent of one RM helps decrease joint edema. Beginning with 40% of 1 RM may be necessary when the amount of muscle fiber atrophy present is significant. Start at a slow speed with minimal resistance to maintain coordinated movement and help decrease inflammation. Work into the outer, pain-free range of motion to promote stimulation of fibroblasts and production of glycosaminoglycans. This stage of exercises stimulates joint mechanoreceptors and GTOs to inhibit pain and guarding. Begin with the joint in a resting position and provide support of bolsters or other equipment as needed to promote quality of motion around a physiological axis. Start with concentric contractions initially to increase vascularity.[26]

Stage II

Have the client progress to stage II when the functional quality of coordination and vascularization is achieved. Signs for progressing to this stage are a decrease in complaint of pain, increased range of motion, increased speed of exercise, decreased muscle guarding, and less fatigue experienced by the client.

The goal of stage II is to increase endurance and speed. This is accomplished by increasing the number of sets and the number of exercises. With increased coordination, increase the speed of exercise. Do not increase resistance. At this point, remove the supportive bolsters so that the client can begin stabilizing proximally while improving the mobility of the hypomobile joint. Histological changes that take place in stage II are improved nutrition to the joint cartilage through decreased viscosity of synovial fluid associated with the increase in speed.[26]

Stage III

Have the client progress to stage III when pain has resolved, full range of motion is regained, and when speed and coordination have increased. For the newly gained range of motion, there must be dynamic stability. This means that the musculotendinous units are strong enough to maintain controlled, physiological mobility. Concentric and eccentric contractions in the newly gained range of motion promote functional stability. In stage III the resistance is increased to 60% to 80%, and the repetitions are decreased to 10 to 15 repetitions to promote strength/endurance. Begin triplanar motions by exercising in proprioceptive neuromuscular facilitation (PNF) patterns. Add isometric contractions in the newly gained end-range of motion to promote strength.

Stage IV

Have the client progress to stage IV when the client is able to increase the speed of exercise and still maintain coordination. Absence of delayed-onset muscle soreness is also an indication that it is time to progress to the next level. Stage IV emphasizes functional exercises and retraining for activities of daily living, essential job functions, and sport-specific activities. Exercises are performed through a full range of motion at up to 80% to 90% of 1 RM at a functional speed in order to achieve the functional quality of power.[19]

Progressions of Hypermobilities

Exercise progressions for hypermobile joints have four stages (Table 10.4).

Stage I

Stage I for joint hypermobility is identical to stage I for hypomobility with one major exception. With a hypomobility the exercises are dosed to promote increased mobility, whereas with a hypermobility the goal is to increase stability. Therefore exercises for hypermobility are performed in the beginning and midrange of motion so that coordination can be maintained while developing stability.

Stage II

In stage II, increase repetitions, number of sets, and number of exercises. Add closed kinetic chain and slow plyometric exercises to increase sensitivity to stretch. Continue to perform exercise in a single plane of motion, and increase speed as coordination permits.

Stage III

In stage III, increase resistance to 80% of 1 RM and decrease the number of repetitions to promote strength. Perform concentric and eccentric contractions for increased stability in the physiological range of motion. Add a set of 1 isometric contraction at 75% to 85% of **1 IM (isometric maximum)**. This contraction should be held for 15 seconds. Fast **plyometrics** (when an eccentric contraction is immediately followed by a concentric contraction) for recruitment of the muscle spindle helps increase sensitivity to stretch and aids in stability. Triplanar motion can start in stage III for promotion of functional stability.

Stage IV

Hypermobility progression in stage IV is equivalent to that for hypomobility. The exercises become more functional, and you should focus more on retraining for a job, activities of daily living, or sport. Increase the resistance to improve the qualities of power and speed.[19]

Monitoring of Vital Signs

Monitoring of vital signs is a reliable, valid, and meaningful way of measuring clients' response to exercise. It takes practice to become accurate with monitoring vital signs and to understand the significance of these values. Taking a resting heart rate, blood pressure, respiratory rate, and oxygen saturation (SpO2) only measures the body systems at rest. To get baseline measurements, take vital signs before, during, and after exercise or activity. Doing this provides critical information about how the body is responding to the exercise loads placed upon it, as well as how well it recovers from the stress of exercise.

Precaution. *Proper dosing of exercise can improve the efficiency of the cardiovascular system, whereas overdosing may cause irreversible damage.*

Heart rate/pulse may be altered by many medications and diseases. When this is the case, as in clients who are taking beta blockers or with congestive heart failure, monitoring of the heart rate in response to exercise may provide inaccurate or misleading information. In such cases, one must use other forms of measuring the response of the body to exercise.[4,9]

Rate of Perceived Exertion

Gunner Borg established the Borg scale (rate of perceived exertion, or RPE) in 1962. The RPE is a subjective measurement of how hard clients think they are exercising. The RPE has been

TABLE 10.5	Borg Rate of Perceived Exertion Scales
Borg Scale	**Newer Scale**
6	0 Nothing at all
7 Very, very light	0.5 Very, very weak
8	1 Very weak
9 Very light	2 Weak
10	3 Moderate
11 Fairly light	4 Somewhat strong
12	5 Strong
13 Somewhat hard	6
14	7 Very strong
15 Hard	8
16	9
17 Very hard	10 Maximal
18	
19 Very, very hard	
20	

proved to be a valid and reliable way of measuring exertion during exercise and functional activities. The original scale was based on numeric values that ranged from 6 to 20, with 6 being a perception of minimal effort, as in relaxing in a chair, and with 20 describing maximal effort, as in running up a steep hill. Target RPE is between 11 and 13 (fairly light to somewhat hard). This is a pace that could be maintained for at least a 15-minute workout. Breathing would be labored; one could carry on a conversation but likely would prefer not to do so. In more recent years, a modified RPE scale has become popular. This newer version is based on a 0 to 10 value system. Zero is equivalent to work at rest, and 10 is maximal exertion. Some find this modified scale easier to use. Table 10.5 gives the Borg RPE scales.[9]

Training Modes

Cardiovascular warmup not only gets the heart and lungs prepared for exercise, but it also is the healthy, natural way of preparing tissue for more vigorous, tissue-specific exercise. The warmup may consist of 5 to 15 minutes of walking on the treadmill or riding on a stationary bike or upper body ergometer. This type of warmup increases blood flow, heart rate, deep muscle/tissue temperature, and respiratory rate with a decrease in joint synovial fluid. This means of increasing circulation may be the wise choice as opposed to the passive hot pack application for tissue warming.

Core/proximal stabilization exercises are essential components of all phases of exercise and activities of daily living. For normal physiological movement to take place, there must be distal mobility on proximal stability.

Precaution. *Increased mobility at the expense of proximal stability equates to compensatory or nonphysiological movement.*

Therefore proper posture and core stabilization exercises are an appropriate component of the hand therapist's repertoire.

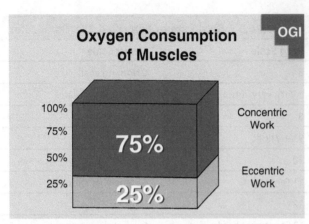

FIG. 10.6 Oxygen consumption of muscles.

Concentric exercise requires three times as much energy as does eccentric exercise. Most of the energy of the body is stored in muscle mass. Seventy percent of the stored energy is used to maintain all vital organ function. Thirty percent of the stored energy is used to carry out functional daily activities. If a person regularly exceeds the 30% of energy reserved for activities of daily living and dips into the 70% reserved for vital organs, pathological conditions of the collagen will result. This may be manifested as a tendonitis, for example. To promote healing, when dosing initially for concentric exercise, it is best to require many repetitions with light resistance. Doing so will increase oxygen to the injured tissue by increasing its blood flow (Fig. 10.6).[15]

Isometric exercise occurs when a muscle contracts without joint motion. A strengthening effect for the muscle occurs at the angle the joint assumes during the contraction and at 20 degrees on either side of that angle. For example, if the biceps are isometrically contracted with the elbow at 90 degrees, a strengthening effect will result from 70 to 110 degrees. This is a safe way to begin strengthening after an injury if the isometric exercises are performed in a pain-free range. Isometric exercises can be performed at varying angles and can be dosed at different intensities. The amount of force that can be maintained by an isometric contraction for 1 second is 1 IM. In rehabilitation, therapists dose isometric contractions at a percentage of 1 IM. Percentage of isometric resistance is dosed in relation to holding time. For example, 60% of 1 IM can be held from 50 to 60 seconds; 80% of 1 IM for 20 to 30 seconds; 90% of 1 IM can be maintained for 10 seconds.[15]

Open and closed kinetic chain exercises play an important role in rehabilitation of the upper extremity. Most functional activities of the upper extremity are **open chain.** Movement occurs from muscle origin to insertion, and the terminal joint is free. With **closed chain** exercises, movement occurs from muscle insertion to origin, and the terminal joint is constrained in a fixed position.[28]

Client Education

To increase compliance with exercise programs, it is essential to educate clients on why they are doing each component of the exercise program and what is being accomplished.

○ Clinical Pearl

Explain that the exercises that are dosed at high repetitions are to improve vascularization and endurance.

Movement is life, and conversely lack of movement will lead to tissue destruction. Many repetitions in a pain-free range of motion help increase blood flow, which in turn brings more oxygen to the injured tissue. The body gets nutrition through the oxygen in the blood.

Precaution. *Avoid pain because pain indicates that the tissue is being irritated. With tissue irritation there will be more pain, which leads to muscle guarding, inflammation, and a decrease of blood flow/nutrition to the area.*

Emphasize quality of motion. The body responds to the stress placed upon it. Maintaining proper posture and body mechanics during exercises and throughout the day and night will result in optimal health. Encourage clients to keep a journal of their activities and home exercise program. This is often helpful for accountability and guidance for upgrades. Include exercises for the opposite upper extremity[29] and uninvolved joints for comprehensive treatment. Finally, do transition the client with quality community resources to continue the progression gained with hand therapy and to maintain health status.[30,31]

CASE STUDIES

CASE STUDY 10.1 ■ EXERCISE PROGRESSION

History

TP is a 36-year-old left-hand dominant female secretary who spends 8 hours a day working on the computer and talking on the telephone. Also, she is attending night school and studying nursing. Because of limited free time, she reports that she has not been participating in any regular exercise program. She admits that she has gained quite a bit of weight over the last year. TP often studies in bed at night, propped up by pillows, until she falls asleep. She presents to therapy reporting that her right lateral elbow has been painful for approximately 3 months. She does not recall sustaining any injury. She notes that the pain in her elbow becomes more intense over the course of the workday. Upon questioning, she does recall that she often awakens during the night with numbness and tingling into the "whole hand."

Clinical Evaluation Findings

TP reports frustration because she has had 1 month of therapy for her elbow, and she feels that it has not improved but rather has gotten worse. She states that her therapy has consisted of hot packs, ultrasound, and stretching exercises. She also was provided with a wrist orthosis and tennis elbow strap.

Her evaluation was remarkable for rounded shoulder with a forward head (RSFH) posture, sixth cervical vertebra–facilitated segment (causing increased tone along the C6 distribution), pain to palpation at the origin of the extensor carpi radialis brevis, pain at end-range elbow extension, decreased grip on the right (because of pain), and pain with resisted wrist extension. After explaining the findings and outlining the treatment plan, the therapist established goals for therapy with TP, and she agreed to comply.

An ergonomic evaluation of the workstation was performed. Recommendations for computer monitor, keyboard height, and chair adjustments were made. New mouse placement and style were reviewed. A phone headset was ordered.

TP was instructed in some postural exercises, including pectoralis stretches, chin tucks, neck stretches, and gentle brachial plexus/

peripheral nerve glides. The postural strengthening exercises included wall letters and scapular retraction and depression exercises. TP agreed to perform these exercises during breaks at work and at home.

TP agreed to start walking daily, beginning with 15 minutes a day at a comfortable pace while maintaining good posture. Duration of the walks is to increase by 2 minutes a week over the next 2 months, as she is able. Speed of gait is also to increase as TP becomes more comfortable and acclimated to her walking program.

The first therapy treatment was spent evaluating TP, and educating her on the different components of her present complaints. Explanations were provided on how posture, work, and exercise habits contributed to the elbow pain and how she could address this responsibly. She was provided with the foregoing home exercise program and was dosed for her clinical elbow exercise program.

The first stage of exercise was dosed with the physiology of the tonic muscle fiber of the elbow in mind. Three months of muscle guarding resulted in some tonic muscle atrophy, degeneration of collagen, and alteration in joint mechanics leading to a decrease in normal contact areas of cartilage. The optimal stimulus for regeneration of collagen is modified tension in the line of stress, and the optimal stimulus for regeneration of cartilage is compression/decompression with glide. Following the stage I protocol for hypomobility, it was determined that TP could tolerate 21 repetitions of concentric wrist extension against gravity before pain set in.

On the second visit, treatment commenced. All exercises were dosed at 3 sets of 25 repetitions to promote vascularization and endurance while maintaining coordinated movement around a physiological axis throughout a full pain-free arc of motion. TP warmed up on the upper body ergometer for 12 minutes at 120 rpm (revolutions per minute), forward and backward to avoid fatigue.
1. Concentric wrist flexion, with forearm supported on a table.
2. Concentric wrist extension, with forearm supported on a table.
3. Pronation, with forearm supported on a table.
4. Supination, with forearm supported on a table.
5. Elbow flexion/extension, with forearm supported on a table.

After finishing the foregoing 375 repetitions, the home exercise program was reviewed to ensure that the exercises were being performed correctly. Treatment concluded with an ice massage. TP reported fatigue but no pain.

TP returned to therapy 2 days later reporting that she had been compliant with her home exercises, walking program, and working on proper posture throughout the day/night. Her complaint of pain had decreased approximately 25%, and the "numbness and tingling" in the hand had resolved. TP went through the foregoing exercise program again and then was scheduled for one visit per week in therapy to make upgrades in the program as necessary. She also agreed to add the dosed exercises to her current home exercise program.

One week later, she returned to the clinic and reported compliance and denied any problems with her exercises. She stated that the exercises were taking much less time now than they were originally. TP described minimal complaint of elbow pain during the workday and no more symptoms at night. The exercises were upgraded because she now could tolerate 30 repetitions.
1. Wrist extension against gravity.
2. Wrist flexion against gravity.
3. Pronation with 1 lb.
4. Supination with 1 lb.
5. Elbow flexion—recumbent seated position flexion with 2 lbs.
6. Elbow extension in prone with 2 lbs.

TP agreed to continue with her home exercise program, adding the new upgrades with the 3 sets of 25 each.

Result of Care
On the following week, TP called to cancel her future therapy appointments. She reported no elbow pain in the previous 4 days and that because of time constraints she felt that she could continue with her independent exercise program and make upgrades appropriately.

CASE STUDY 10.2 ■

History
RJ is a 42-year-old right-hand dominant male carpenter who sustained an injury to his left shoulder 3 weeks before presenting for therapy. He reports that when unloading his truck at the job site early one morning, he lost his footing and started to fall backward off the truck. At the time, he was holding his toolbox in his right hand. As he was falling, he reached out with the left hand and grabbed on to a long 4×4 that was sticking out of the bed of the truck. He reports that "it happened so fast," but he is sure that he did not actually fall onto the shoulder or bump it on anything. Over the next 2 hours, he found it difficult to do his job because of left lateral and posterior shoulder pain. He decided to go to the nearby urgent care facility when the pain did not resolve over the course of the day. X-ray films were taken, and no fracture was noted. Over the next 2 weeks, RJ tried to persevere at work and apply ice to the shoulder whenever he could. He returned to the physician because his shoulder "just wasn't getting any better."

Clinical Evaluation Findings
Magnetic resonance imaging confirmed a near full-thickness tear of the supraspinatus and partial tear of the infraspinatus. Therapy evaluation ruled out any cervical spine involvement. Manual muscle testing of the left shoulder revealed 3/5 grade strength of the supraspinatus and 4/5 grade strength of the infraspinatus. There was a positive sulcus test at zero degrees, positive Hawkins-Kennedy sign, and positive external rotation lag sign with the supraspinatus at greater than 10 degrees and with the infraspinatus at less than 10 degrees. The evaluation confirmed the magnetic resonance imaging findings, and it was determined that RJ had a right shoulder impingement with an underlying hypermobility because of the rotator cuff tear.

Goals of Therapy
The goals of therapy were as follows:
1. Decrease pain.
2. Resolve muscle guarding.
3. Restore functional range of motion around a physiological axis.
4. Increase endurance/strength of the rotator cuff.

Initial Treatment
Exercises were selected for stage I hypermobilities:
1. Start with a warmup exercise, such as the upper body ergometer for 10 minutes at 120 rpm.
2. Dose with many repetitions initially to increase endurance and circulation to the type I muscle fibers of the rotator cuff (3 sets of 25).
3. Begin with slow speed to promote coordinated movement about a physiological axis.

4. Choose starting positions that are in the inner range of motion to maintain stability from inner to midrange of motion.
5. Support the limb with equipment, as necessary, to aid with preserving proper joint arthrokinematics.

The following exercises were selected for RJ's shoulder rehabilitation:

1. Scapular retraction
2. Internal rotation
3. External rotation
4. Abduction
5. Lateral pull downs
6. Triceps
7. Biceps

RJ's first treatment was spent evaluating and testing to determine the appropriate resistance to achieve the functional qualities of vascularization and endurance while maintaining coordination and quality of motion without eliciting pain. The outer range of motion initially was avoided because of instability. On return visits, he performed 3 sets of 25 repetitions for all of the foregoing exercises. He took rest breaks between sets. For each exercise the pulley rope was set perpendicular to the lever arm at 20% into the lengthened range of motion and parallel to the muscle fiber. Concentric contractions were performed initially, and between each repetition, the weight stack was let down to remove tension.

CONTINUING CARE

RJ was scheduled for therapy 3 times per week for 4 weeks. On his third treatment, he was noted to be moving through his exercise program more quickly, maintaining coordination, and reporting no pain with exercise and decreased pain overall. He then was dosed for four more exercises.

1. Horizontal adduction
2. Horizontal abduction
3. Extension
4. Flexion

On the fifth visit, RJ began stage II for hypermobility. Slow plyometrics were added with a 1-lb ball tossed against a wall, catching it with the left hand. Closed chain exercises were initiated by performing wall pushups. He started to perform (2 sets of 25) concentric contractions and one set of isometric contractions in the inner to midrange of motion. The isometric contractions were dosed at 60% to 70% of 1 IM, which is a 40- to 60-second hold.

By the eighth visit, RJ was able to progress to stage III. Exercises were upgraded to include concentric contractions at 80% of 1 RM for 2 sets of 10 repetitions and one set of isometric contractions in the mid to outer (stable) range at 85% of 1 IM for a 10- to 15-second hold. Fast plyometrics were performed to recruit the muscle spindle. He started to incorporate diagonal (proprioceptive neuromuscular facilitation) patterns into his exercise routine as well.

RESULT OF CARE

In the fourth week, Robert's rehabilitation introduced some retraining of some of his essential job functions. At that time, he was released back to full duty and was discharged from therapy. He decided to join a local gym and continue with his established exercise routine.

References

1. ICF Research Branch: *Icf core set for hand conditions*, 2017. Available: https://www.icf-research-branch.org/icf-core-sets-projects2/other-health-conditions/development-of-icf-core-sets-for-hand-condition.
2. World Health Organization: *Classifications*, 2017. Available: http://www.who.int/classifications/icf/en/.
3. Grimsby O, Rivard J, Kring R: Models of pathology in orthopaedic manual therapy. In Grimsby O, Rivard J, editors: *Science, theory and clinical application in orthopaedic manual physical therapy: applied science and theory*, vol. 1. Taylorsville, UT, 2008, The Academy of Graduate Physical Therapy, Inc., pp 161–224.
4. Goodman CC, Snyder TE: *Screening for endocrine and metabolic disease. Differential diagnosis for physical therapists: screening for referral*, St Louis, MO, 2007, Saunders Elsevier.
5. Carmona RH, Beato C, Lawrence A: *Bone health and osteoporosis: a report of the surgeon general*, Rockville, MD, 2004, Department of Health and Human Services.
6. Grimsby O, Rivard J, Kring R: Exercise for collagen repair. In Grimsby O, Rivard J, editors: *Science, theory and clinical application in orthopaedic manual physical therapy: applied science and theory*, vol. 1. Taylorsville, UT, 2008, The Academy of Graduate Physical Therapy, Inc., pp 33–65.
7. Beasley J: Osteoarthritis and rheumatoid arthritis: conservative therapeutic management, *J Hand Ther* 25:163–172, 2012.
8. Porter B, Brittain A: Splinting and hand exercises for three common hand deformities in rheumatoid arthritis: a clinical perspective, *Curr Opin Rheumatol* 24(2):215–221, 2012, https://doi.org/10.1097/BOR.0b013e3283503361.
9. ACSM: *American College of Sports Medicine: guidelines for exercise testing and prescription*, ed 8, Philadelphia, 2009, Lippincott Williams & Wilkins.
10. Grimsby O, Rivard J: Exercise for bone repair. In Grimsby O, Rivard J, editors: *Science, theory and clinical application in orthopaedic manual physical therapy: applied science and theory*, vol. 1. Taylorsville, UT, 2008, The Academy of Graduate Physical Therapy, Inc., pp 19–31.
11. Grimsby O, Rivard J: Properties of cartilage. In Grimsby O, Rivard J, editors: *Science, theory and clinical application in orthopaedic manual physical therapy: applied science and theory*, vol. 1. Taylorsville, UT, 2008, The Academy of Graduate Physical Therapy, Inc., pp 67–82.
12. Hunter GR, Harris RT: Structure and function of the muscular, neuromuscular, cardiovascular and respiratory systems. In Baechle TR, Earle RW, editors: *Essentials of strength training and conditioning*, ed 3, Omaha, NE, 2008, Human Kinetics, pp 3–12.
13. Grimsby O, Rivard J: Clinical neurophysiology. In Grimsby O, Rivard J, editors: *Science, theory and clinical application in orthopaedic manual physical therapy: applied science and theory*, vol. 1. Taylorsville, UT, 2008, The Academy of Graduate Physical Therapy, Inc., pp 137–158.
14. *Classification of chronic pain*, Seattle, WA, 1994, IASP Press.
15. Grimsby O, Rivard J, Kring R: Muscle physiology. In Grimsby O, Rivard J, editors: *Science, theory and clinical application in orthopaedic manual physical therapy: applied science and theory*, vol. 1. Taylorsville, UT, 2008, The Academy of Graduate Physical Therapy, Inc., pp 107–135.
16. Grimsby O, Rivard J, Kring R: Exercise prescription. In Grimsby O, Rivard J, editors: *Science, theory and clinical application in orthopaedic manual physical therapy: applied science and theory*, vol. 1. Taylorsville, UT, 2008, The Academy of Graduate Physical Therapy, Inc., pp 347–392.
17. Cipriani DJ, Falkel JE: Physiological principles of resistance training and functional integration for the injured and disabled. In Lee AC, Quillen WS, Magee DJ, et al.: *Scientific foundations and principles of practice in musculoskeletal rehabilitation*, St Louis, MO, 2007, Saunders Elsevier.
18. Cheung K, Hume P, Maxwell L: Delayed onset muscle soreness: treatment strategies and performance factors, *Sports Med* 33:145–164, 2003.
19. Grimsby O, Rivard J, Kring R: Functional qualities and exercise dosage. In Grimsby O, Rivard J, editors: *Science, theory and clinical application in orthopaedic manual physical therapy: applied science and theory*, vol. 1. Taylorsville, UT, 2008, The Academy of Graduate Physical Therapy, Inc., pp 325–344.

20. Peterson MD, Rhea MR, Alvar BA: Maximizing strength development in athletes: a meta-analysis to determine the dose-response relationship, *J Strength Cond Res* 18:377–382, 2004.
21. Baechle TR, Earle RW, Wathen D: Resistance training. In Baechle TR, Earle RW, editors: *Essentials of strength training and conditioning*, ed 3, Omaha, NE, 2008, Human Kinetics, pp 405–407.
22. Wolfe BL, LeMura LM, Cole PJ: Quantitative analysis of single vs multiple set programs in resistance training, *J Strength Cond Res* 18:35–47, 2004.
23. Harman E: The biomechanics of resistance exercise. In Baechle TR, Earle RW, editors: *Essentials of strength training and conditioning*, ed 3, Omaha, NE, 2008, Human Kinetics, pp 73–78.
24. *Medical exercise therapy*, Oslo, 1996, Norwegian MET Institute.
25. Blyx M: Blyx curve, *Scand Arch Physiol* 93–94, 1892.
26. Grimsby O, Rivard J, Kring R: Exercise progression. In Grimsby O, Rivard J, editors: *Science, theory and clinical application in orthopaedic manual physical therapy: applied science and theory*, vol. 1. Taylorsville, UT, 2008, The Academy of Graduate Physical Therapy, Inc., pp 431–472.
27. Ratamess NA, et al.: Progression models in resistance training for healthy adults, *Med Sci Sports Exerc* 687–708, 2009.
28. Brumitt J: Scapular-stabilization exercises: early-intervention prescription, *Athletic Therapy Today* 11(5):15–18, 2006.
29. Magnus C, et al.: Cross-education for improving strength and mobility after distal radius fractures: a randomized controlled trial, *Archives of Physical Medicine and Rehabilitation* 94(7):1247–1255, 2013.
30. Rimmer J: Getting beyond the plateau: bridging the gap between rehabilitation and community-based exercise, *PM R* 4:857–861, 2012.
31. Rimmer J, Lai B: Framing new pathways in transformative exercise for individuals with existing and newly acquired disability, *Disabil Rehabil* 39(2):173–180, 2017.

11

Saba Kamal

Clinical Reasoning and Problem Solving in Upper Extremity Rehabilitation

Clinical reasoning and critical thinking occur when a clinician thinks creatively, uses reflection, and engages in analytical thinking in order to implement interventions that promote successful outcomes.[1] Hand therapists should make treatment decisions based on an understanding of pathology, surgical procedures, the healing mechanism of human tissues, and the psychosocial impact of injury and dysfunction on individuals. As such, every chapter in this book includes information about these factors to assist the newer hand therapist in appropriate and individualized treatment planning. This chapter briefly outlines the basic concepts underlying clinical reasoning; and readers are encouraged to give special attention to these factors when studying the chapters on common diagnoses of the upper extremity.

Wound Healing

Soft tissues heal in a predictable manner in healthy individuals. Healing is characterized by three phases: (1) the inflammatory phase; (2) the proliferative phase; and (3) the maturation phase—collectively known as the **healing cascade**. This cascade of events works to clean up the wounded area, fill in the soft-tissue defect, and strengthen the covering of the defect. Understanding the wound healing process can assist hand therapists in evaluating clients and planning a course of treatment independent of cookie-cutter protocols, thus prescribing an individualized and customized program to fit each person's injury and specific needs. The phases of healing are complex and overlapping, but in the most basic of terms look like this:

The inflammatory phase begins at the moment of injury or surgery and usually lasts a couple weeks. The purpose of this phase is to clean up the wound. If wounds are complicated by necrosis and/or infection, the inflammatory phase is prolonged and wound healing is delayed. Wounds will stay in the inflammatory phase until the wound bed is clean of debris and infection.

◎ Clinical Pearl

Hand therapy goals related to wound healing are to minimize swelling and scar tissue formation, to control cellular injury, and to establish a clean wound bed for repair.

The proliferative phase begins within 3 to 4 days of the initial injury/surgery and may continue for up to 6 weeks. The purpose of this phase is to fill in the soft-tissue defect and cover the wound bed. The proliferative phase is characterized by angiogenesis, granulation, wound contraction, and epithelialization. Collagen synthesis is the hallmark of this phase; and the proliferative phase is associated with deposition of scar tissue. However, this tissue is not strong because the collagen fibers are random in their orientation. This is the phase when joint stiffness and tissue adherence begin to occur. Joint end feel will be soft, and the cross linkages of scar will be weak.

> **◎ Clinical Pearl**
>
> Appropriate controlled stress along physiological axes at this stage allows collagen fibers to align themselves more functionally. Prioritize edema control, gentle range of motion (ROM), joint mobilization, and scar management to promote good alignment of the collagen fibers and to help prevent scar tissue adhesions.

The maturation phase is the final stage of wound healing. The purpose of this phase is to strengthen the wound's covering (with a combination of collagen and epithelium, known as scar). It occurs from as early as day 21 and may continue for years. This is when type III collagen is replaced by type I collagen.

> **◎ Clinical Pearl**
>
> Wound strength may increase for up to 2 years after injury, and during this time scar tissue is active. Active scar tissue is malleable. Therapists can capitalize on this with scar management techniques and use of orthoses designed to elongate and flatten the scar.

There are a multitude of factors that can affect the rate and quality of tissue healing. Circulation, debris in the wound bed, infection, chemical stress, temperature of the wound bed, amount of moisture in the wound, nutrition, age, and medications all contribute to an individual's unique cascade of healing. For example, medications such as anticoagulants, antiplatelet aggregation medications, nonaspirin nonsteroidal antiinflammatory medicines (NSAIDs), and steroids may interfere with platelet activation, angiogenesis, and collagen production. Steroids, which are immunosuppressive, inhibit macrophage levels, reduce immunocompetent lymphocytes, decrease antibody production, and diminish antigen processing. Protein malnutrition and insufficient calorie intake are also detrimental to wound healing. Irradiation and chemotherapy can cause delayed healing and increase the risk of tissue breakdown.[2]

The hand therapist must be on constant alert for all factors affecting tissue healing. After injury or surgery, therapists use their understanding of physiology and pathology to identify signs of infection. A good example of this is the scenario of an infected flexor tendon sheath. We use Kanavel's four cardinal signs of flexor tenosynovitis to identify this condition: (1) uniform digital swelling; (2) flexed digital posture; (3) pain with passive digital extension; and (4) pain with palpation along the flexor tendon sheath.

Peripheral Nerve Repair

Hand therapists are learning more about the interplay between the central nervous system (CNS) and the peripheral nervous system (PNS) due to recent increases in research in this area. In particular, we know that this interplay between the CNS and the PNS can affect wrist stability and function, as well as people's perception of pain. These are very important concepts to grasp and to integrate into treatment planning following every injury or surgery to the upper extremity.

> **◎ Clinical Pearl**
>
> People who are younger in age and whose nerve injuries are more distal on the extremity have better outcomes.[3]

> **◎ Clinical Pearl**
>
> In prioritizing the treatment plan when multiple structures are involved, remember that protection of bony injury supersedes nerve, ligament, and tendon repairs.

Edema and Internal Scar Tissue Formation

According to Dr. Paul Brand, edema is scar in evolution, and if it is left untreated, it will result in adaptive shortening, adhesions, and joint contractures.[4-7] Edema routinely occurs during acute inflammatory reactions from infections, traumatic injury, or surgery. Edema can also be present from decreased mobility or immobilization, systemic diseases, and local infections.

Hand therapists must make early and aggressive edema control a priority when treating any injury or surgery to the upper extremity. Because prolonged swelling may lead to stagnation of fluid and result in formation of scar tissue and adhesions (thus affecting function), early management of edema is critical to improving outcomes in rehabilitation of the upper quadrant.

Stiffness

The typical stiff hand posture is characterized by the metacarpal joints in extension due to pooling of edema in the dorsum of the hand with resulting stress applied to the extrinsic extensor mechanism.[4,8,9] The proximal interphalangeal (PIP) and distal interphalangeal (DIP) joints are in a flexed posture with the edema stress creating a tenodesis effect on the extrinsic flexors from the fabric bias stress on connective tissue.[10]

The stiff hand posture can be extremely problematic due to shortening and adherence of the collateral ligaments of the metacarpophalangeal (MP), PIP, and DIP joints.[11] This may lead to insufficient glides of contractile tissues (tendon, muscle) and stress deprivation of noncontractile tissues (joint capsule, ligamentous structures).[7,12,13] Restrictions such as these may result in joint contractures, tendon adhesions, and long-lasting functional limitations. Preventing stiffness from occurring is always preferable to treating established stiffness.

Stiffness, once established, must be approached with the eye of a detective to decipher the hidden problems. Hand therapists use knowledge of anatomy, physiology, kinesiology, and physics to determine the etiology and pathology of stiffness, as well as to determine appropriate interventions to reverse it. For example, one concept we utilize with orthotic intervention for stiffness is TERT (total end range time). TERT refers to the idea that gentle sustained stress over longer periods of time lengthens tissues more effectively than forceful mobilization for shorter periods.

Cosmetic Scar

The look and feel of external scarring is important because it affects how clients feel about their injury, their recovery, and occasionally their self-image. In addition to cosmesis, scar management is important for functional recovery. Hand therapists work with their clients to prevent adhesion of the skin to the underlying structures and to maximize joint range of motion in the presence of scar. An understanding of the different types of scar tissue is helpful for developing a treatment plan.

Hypertrophic scars are visible and elevated scars that do not spread into surrounding tissues and that often regress spontaneously.[14] These scars are characterized by proliferation of the dermal tissue with excessive deposition of fibroblast-derived extracellular matrix proteins, especially collagen, over long periods and by persistent inflammation and fibrosis.[15]

Keloids are firm, mildly tender scars with a shiny surface and occasional telangiectasia (dilated small blood vessels). The epithelium is thinned and there may be focal areas of ulceration.[16] The color is pink to purple and may be accompanied by hyperpigmentation.[16] Keloids form at the area of injury but grow beyond the original area of injury or the original margin of scar. In this way they differ from hypertrophic scars, which do not exceed the boundaries of the original trauma.

> ◎ **Clinical Pearl**
>
> Aggressive hand therapy that encourages high levels of force and repetition can keep tissue in a sustained inflammatory state and can even cause an inflammatory state in mature tissue, thus creating excessive scar tissue.[17,18]

Experienced hand therapists approach upper extremity rehabilitation more gently than one might expect. Even clients are sometimes surprised that (proper) hand therapy does not induce a lot of pain. Tissues respond best to slow and gentle forces. We want to keep inflammation to a minimum in order to avoid excessive scar tissue formation, both internally (adhesions) and externally (cosmesis). It is helpful to teach clients that sharp pain is an indicator of tissue damage and should be avoided; however, some discomfort during stretching is required to improve flexibility, motion, and function.

Range of Motion

ROM limitations can occur for a variety of reasons. Again, hand therapists use knowledge of physiology, anatomy,

kinesiology, and physics to identify the source of the limitation and then develop a reason-based intervention plan to address it. Sometimes limitations are due to certain muscle groups, intrinsic versus extrinsic hand muscles, for example. When assessing this, we know that the position of the proximal joints directly impacts the length–tension relationship of the extrinsic muscles thereby affecting distal joint positions.[13]

ROM limitations can also be due to limited neural gliding. The neural system is composed of a mechanical component and a physiological component. The mechanical component is the ability of the nerve to move in relation to the surrounding tissues, and the physiological component provides the blood flow to the nerves.

Edema, scar tissue, and pain all affect how individuals move as well as how *far* they move. Furthermore, any limitation to a body structure may present with pain, inflammation, and sensory involvement further preventing or limiting movement of the joint or body part.[19-22] Hand therapists help clients break this cycle of motion-limiting events.

> ◎ **Clinical Pearl**
>
> Active range of motion (AROM) evaluates contractile tissue function. Passive range of motion (PROM) evaluates noncontractile tissue.[6,7]

In summary, this chapter has highlighted the basic concepts underlying clinical reasoning. The goal of this textbook is to help new hand therapists understand these concepts and how they relate to specific diagnoses and conditions. An understanding of these concepts will enable the reader to be selective and effective in the treatment of individuals with upper extremity problems. Readers are encouraged to give special attention to these factors when studying the chapters in this textbook.

References

1. Bittencourt GKGD, Crossetti MGO: Theoretical model of critical thinking in diagnostic processes in nursing, *Nurs* 11(Suppl 1):563–567, 2012.
2. Arem AJ, Madden JW: Effects of stress on healing wounds: I. Intermittent noncyclical tension, *J Surg Res* 20(2):93–102, 1976.
3. Griffin MF, et al.: Peripheral nerve injury: principles for repair and regeneration, *Open Orthop J* 8(Suppl 1: M10):199–203, 2014.
4. Brand PW, Hollister AM: *Clinical mechanics of the hand*, ed 2, St Louis, 1993, Mosby Yearbook.
5. Brand PW, editor: *Clinical mechanics of the hand*, St. Louis, 1985, Mosby.
6. Brand PW: Mechanical factors in joint stiffness and tissue growth, *J Hand Ther* 8(2):91–96, 1995.
7. Brand PW, Hollister AM: *Clinical mechanics of the hand*, ed 3, St Louis, 1999, Mosby.
8. Kaltenborn FM: *Manual mobilization of the joints*, ed 7, Minneapolis, 2011, Orthopedic Physical Therapy Products.
9. Kapandji AI: *The physiology of the joints*, ed 6, Philadelphia, 2007, Churchill Livingstone Elsevier.
10. McKee P, Hannah S, Priganc VW: Orthotic considerations for dense connective tissue and articular cartilage—the need for optimal movement and stress, *J Hand Ther* 25(2):233–243, 2012.
11. Hertling D, Kessler R: *Management of common musculoskeletal disorders: physical therapy principles and methods*, Lippincott Williams & Wilkins, 1996.
12. Brand PW: Hand rehabilitation: management by objectives. In Hunter JM, Schneider LC, Mackin E, editors: *Rehabilitation of the hand*, ed 2, St Louis, 1984, Mosby.

13. Riordan DC: A walk through the anatomy of the hand and forearm, *J Hand Ther* 8(2):68–78, 1995.
14. English RS, Shenefelt PD: Keloids and hypertrophic scars, *Dermatol Surg* 25(8):631–638, 1999.
15. Atiyeh BS: Nonsurgical management of hypertrophic scars: evidence-based therapies, standard practices, and emerging methods, *Aesthetic Plast Surg* 31(5):468–492, 2007.
16. Al-Attar A, Mess S, Thomassen JM, Kauffman CL, Davison SP: Keloid pathogenesis and treatment, *Plast Reconstr Surg* 117(1):286–300, 2006.
17. Wang J, et al.: Toll-like receptors expressed by dermal fibroblasts contribute to hypertrophic scarring, *J Cell Physiol* 226(5):1265–1273, 2011.
18. Hirshowitz B, et al.: Silicone occlusive sheeting (SOS) in the management of hypertrophic scarring, including the possible mode of action of silicone, by static electricity, *Eur J Plast Surg* 16(1):5–9, 1993.
19. Shacklock M: Neurodynamics, *Physiotherapy* 81(1):9–16, 1995.
20. Shacklock MO: *Clinical neurodynamics: a new system of neuromusculoskeletal treatment*, Oxford, UK, 2005, Butterworth Heinemann.
21. Butler DS: *The sensitive nervous system*, Adelaide, Australia, 2000, Noigroup Publication.
22. Ellis RF, Hing WA: Neural mobilization: a systematic review of randomized controlled trials with an analysis of therapeutic efficacy, *JMMT* 16(1):8–22, 2013.

12 Fundamentals of Client–Therapist Rapport

Goldie Eder
Renee B. Lonner

This chapter introduces the psychological and emotional factors that affect a client's motivation to participate in hand therapy and suggests ways to maximize treatment outcomes based on this understanding. Most medical professionals, over time, come to appreciate that the same type of injury will impact clients differently, depending on each client's unique context. Understanding the client's context, including their psychological makeup, what shapes their beliefs about themselves and their condition, and what their beliefs are about their ability to recover, can help hand therapists set more realistic treatment goals with the client. Additionally, this type of insight can help therapists build the kind of rapport with their clients that leads to a more positive and constructive working relationship and that feels more productive to the therapist, resulting in better treatment outcomes.

Understanding the Psychological Impact of Illness and Injury

While there are a number of particular factors affecting each individual with whom hand therapists work, there are some generalizations that are worth considering about the psychological impact of illness or injury on an individual. Usually, clients who present for hand therapy feel a sense of vulnerability. Having an injury to the hand, which causes temporary or permanent, and for some, extensive, impairment of daily functioning, causes most clients to feel a sense of helplessness and loss. However, individuals have different **psychological defenses** or "protections" that they employ. Some common emotional reactions are anger, fear, helplessness, shame, victimization, blaming oneself or blaming others, avoidance and withdrawal, and/or a sense of defeat and hopelessness. On the other hand, other clients have the general trait of **resilience**, expect to recover, and show an "I'm going to beat this!" kind of attitude.

When the hand therapist meets the client, she/he will have read the medical record or obtained information directly from the referring physician that includes background information on the condition or injury. For example, the therapist may know that the condition occurred because of a repetitive work injury, sporting accident, or surgery. This kind of information is useful, of course, but it is essential to ask the client about *their* understanding of what has happened to their hand and how it has impacted them, both in terms of their physical functioning and how they are feeling on an emotional level about the condition or injury.

> ### ⊙ *Clinical Pearl*
> Establishing rapport begins the first time you meet your client. Greet clients with a smile, establish and use their preferred name, and give them your undivided attention.

It is important not to make assumptions about how the client is reacting to their injury and what the injury means to them; rather, "curiosity" about the client's perceptions is a more productive approach. In the world of mental health counseling, this approach is simply called "starting where the client is." As hand therapists, we can observe and listen carefully to the client tell their story; and based on their narrative, we can then start to make some hypotheses as to what they are undergoing, how they view their problems, and what capacity for change they seem to have.

An important step in understanding the psychological impact of the medical condition, and eventually establishing rapport, is "testing" these hypotheses by a process called **active listening**. This approach means that we stop the client at points in the story to ask them to clarify their meaning about a specific issue; for example, "When you told me that your hand was injured as a result of a rear-end collision, it sounded like you felt at fault for the accident – could you explain that part to me?"

Active listening conveys to the client that we are working to see the issues from their point of view. Thus, we are attempting to form a **therapeutic alliance** with the client so that they are able to participate actively with us in their care and treatment. While a hand therapist is not a client's psychotherapist, there is a clear psychological dimension to this relationship. If the client feels that the therapist is "on their team" and understands what they are going through, they will be more likely to develop trust in the therapist. That foundation can lead to better cooperation with the treatment plan and an improved clinical outcome. Empathy and trust are essential for the client to place themselves in the hand therapist's care so that the healing work can begin.

◎ Clinical Pearl

Active listening is a way to communicate to the client that you are interested in a *connection* with them, not a relationship based on control. This kind of listening and engagement can bridge the gap between therapist and client.

Building a Therapeutic Alliance

The word "empathy" comes from the Latin roots "em," meaning "into" and "pathos," meaning "pain." So as healers, we "go into" the client's pain with them in the relational stance we assume. This stance or attitude puts us "side by side" with our client in terms of showing them we are sensitive to their feelings. Leston Havens, MD, a mentor to many psychotherapists at Cambridge Health Alliance in Massachusetts, modeled this stance by sitting next to the client, rather than facing him/her, when he would demonstrate how to interview. He talked about wanting to create the feeling for the client that it was the therapist and the client looking out at the world together, from the same vantage point, and discovering together how to approach a difficult situation and cope more successfully with it.[1,2]

This idea can be usefully applied to establishing rapport with clients who have a physical condition or injury as well. Even though in hand therapy the therapist is often facing the client across a treatment table, one can, by nonverbal expressions and verbalizations, create the impression that the therapist empathizes with the client's experience and is "by their side" in working to treat the condition. This empathic stance is the foundation from which to build client trust and hope and makes it much more likely that the client will follow specific treatment recommendations (including those they need to follow at home!).

◎ Clinical Pearl

Empathy, identifying oneself mentally with (and so fully comprehending) another person, is more difficult and much more meaningful to communicate than sympathy.

A more recently developed approach in health care that addresses the issue of gaining client engagement is **motivational interviewing (MI)**. This approach was initially developed for a client population seen as largely "involuntary" and noncompliant with treatment recommendations—alcohol and drug abusers—but is now successfully used with clients presenting with a broad range of issues. Motivational interviewing is a unique clinical style that is designed to assist the client in identifying their own motivation and self-interest in following a treatment plan.

According to Rollnick, Miller, and Butler, in their book about this therapeutic approach,[3] "MI is not a technique for tricking people into doing what they do not want to do. Rather, it is a skillful clinical style for eliciting from patients their own motivations for making behavior changes in the interest of their health. It involves guiding more than directing, dancing more than wrestling, listening at least as much as telling. The overall 'spirit' has been described as collaborative, evocative, and honoring of patient autonomy" (p. 6).

For therapists, the four principles of this "guiding" style in MI are:

1. to resist our desire to set things right;
2. to understand and explore the client's own motivations;
3. to listen with empathy;
4. to empower the client, encouraging hope and optimism.

According to Rollnick et al. (p. 4), "These four principles can be remembered with the acronym RULE: Resist, Understand, Listen and Empower."[3]

The authors[2] describe that a good guide will get to know the client and ask where the person wants to go, and then inform the person about options and see what makes sense to them. Effective guides must listen to and respect what the person wants to do while offering help and encouragement.

Clients who present as pessimistic or even hopeless about their capacity to improve present a challenge for even the most experienced therapist. They seem resistant or even noncompliant, and the therapist can come to feel that a power struggle, and not treatment, is the primary "content" of the appointments. However, it is important to remember that this defensive stance usually comes from fear—the client's fear that they will not be able to recover or improve, that they are trapped and helpless. When a hand therapist encounters this dynamic with a client, it is useful for the therapist to imagine a time when they felt scared and powerless, as if they would not be able to overcome a situation. That memory can help the therapist imagine, remember, and empathize with the client's emotional experience.

MI is one method for reducing the distance between the "expert" therapist and their client, thus hopefully, reducing resistance and paving the way to engagement. It is important to remember that even if the hand therapist is relatively new and lacking confidence that experience brings, the client is likely to view the therapist as the one with the knowledge and power in the situation.

◎ Clinical Pearl

Client resistance to treatment recommendations should be seen as an opportunity for dialogue, rather than as simply a frustrating problem. It is a signal for the therapist to pause and ask the client for help in understanding the feelings that are behind the resistance. Slowing down at this point can actually speed things up.

Both John Rolland[4] and Arthur Kleinman,[5] psychiatrists who work with individuals and families experiencing serious medical conditions, discuss how a person's (or family's) beliefs about medical conditions in general, and specific injuries or conditions in particular, can determine what explanation or meaning they create about their situation. These psychiatrists point out that it is important for patients and their families to create meaning when someone suffers a physical impairment, because this type of loss can destroy our common (and defensive) belief that the body is invulnerable. Creating meaning in these situations helps people develop a sense of mastery over their circumstances. This sense of competence is essential to the client's ability to utilize the therapist's technical skills. It is sometimes a major challenge to move a client toward believing that their effort can result in increased functionality and decreased pain in their disabled hand, either by strengthening it or by learning how to adapt and "move smarter." Medical professionals tend to think of the issue from a biological/physiological/anatomical perspective, but most clients think about their condition from a functional or experiential viewpoint. In addition, conditions and injuries to the hand that require therapy accrue meaning on societal and cultural levels.

It is the individual/human and societal factors that form what psychotherapists call the **psychosocial context** of a medical condition. Clients, of course, are more than their hand—they are people with thoughts and feelings about their conditions. These factors form each individual's psychosocial context and may influence the client's participation in treatment as much as the nature of the injury or the deterioration caused by a degenerative disease. This "backdrop" is the reason why taking time to find out about the client's situation before the occurrence of the impairment can benefit the therapeutic alliance. Hand therapists are experts in conducting a functional assessment of the client's hand, but if the client is not "on board" with the process, chances are they will not participate effectively in the treatment program.

How to Introduce Hand Therapy – What to Say to the Client

While it is not necessary to follow a script to introduce yourself and the concept of hand therapy, it may be helpful to have some specific concepts in mind when meeting with a new client:

"Hello, Ms./Mr. Smith. I am Jane, your occupational/physical therapist. Today we are going to start working together on treating your hand injury/condition. First, I will be assessing the nature and extent of your impairment and then will be employing/teaching you a number of techniques to help you strengthen your hand/reduce pain/adapt your movements in ways that help. Our sessions will each last ___ minutes. I may use some modalities (e.g., electric stimulation, ultrasound, or the like) and we will do some exercises that you can practice here and later do at home. Your asking questions, providing me with information, and our collaborating in your care will be key to your improvement. It will be helpful for me to know how and when your injury/condition occurred and what you are physically experiencing. I will do my best to explain the specific suggestions I am making for you, and it is very important that you tell me if I am not clear or you do not understand. Please ask as many questions as you would like. Treatment always works best when there is a dialogue between client and therapist."

In this early process, the therapist is setting up an environment where the client feels invited to participate in a project that both they and the therapist will find rewarding. This does not mean being spuriously cheerful and minimizing the work ahead,

but rather indicating to the client that the therapist is interested in them as a person, that the therapist really understands their current suffering, and that the therapist believes that the skills and tools offered will help them in their recovery.

Being a "Hope Merchant"

How a therapist handles hope in the relationship between her/himself and a client is a matter worthy of some reflection. Just as clients are now routinely assessed on a pain scale, there is an argument to be made that similarly, a new client should be routinely assessed for their level of hope. This way, the subject is out in the open between the hand therapist and the client.

For some people, the only acceptable or positive outcome is the full restoration of physical functioning that existed prior to the impairment. Anything short of this will precipitate intolerable feelings of loss and anger. Other people will be more adaptable and flexible in their expectations and feel satisfied if they regain some increased mobility or ability. The client's personality style and/or external factors, such as feeling a practical need to resume work quickly, can drive these kinds of perceptions.

Jerome Groopman, a hematologist-oncologist, describes in his book, *The Anatomy of Hope: How People Prevail in the Face of Illness*,[6] his journey as a physician treating people with life-threatening illnesses. Dr. Groopman talks about the ethical dilemmas he experienced in his relationships with his patients, in which he felt a responsibility to be straightforward and honest about their prognosis. He then experienced a serious and disabling back injury himself and learned about the importance of hope first-hand.

For years following the injury, until he began a supervised rehabilitation program at a local hospital, he was severely limited in his activities. He recounts how, during his rehabilitation program, he began to try to balance the pain from the exercises with visions of activities that brought his life meaning, such as walking to a pond with his young daughter and experiencing her joy at encountering frogs. He decided that he would engage in this positive visualization process, and eventually he recovered significant function in his back. He attributes his recovery to developing a store of hope that allowed him to push himself beyond his comfort zone, performing his exercises even when there was pain.

A hand therapist can be a pivotal "hope merchant" in that they not only model a "can do" attitude, but they also have concrete techniques that can help clients improve range of motion, improve strength, reduce pain, and improve function.

◎ *Clinical Pearl*

A sense of hope is an essential element of hand rehabilitation, and the therapist may need to be the primary carrier, even briefly, if the client feels hopeless.

CASE STUDY

Jane is a 30-year-old single woman with a genetic disorder, Ehlers-Danlos syndrome (EDS), which can cause hypermobility in wrist and other joints, as well as shoulder dislocations. Jane's father, a physician, first diagnosed his daughter during her adolescence; she had several surgeries during this period, including a wrist surgery with insertion of a plate. After 6 years the plate became dislodged, causing her pain and discomfort. Consultation with her hand surgeon resulted in a recommendation to have the plate removed, which she did. Jane accepted a referral and recommendation for hand therapy after initial recovery from her surgery. Initially, she presented as informed, relieved to have the surgery over, and optimistic about achieving her goal of "recovering my strength in my right hand and returning to my life," adding "I know I will always have to be careful with my body because of the EDS, but it's not nearly as disabling as a traumatic brain injury or mental illness can be."

The hand therapist was then, understandably, surprised when Jane only minimally performed her home exercises program, thus delaying recovery of motion and strength in the wrist. At the fifth visit, the therapist felt that Jane's attitude had changed since starting therapy. She seemed distracted and preoccupied, impatient to finish the therapy session, and informed the therapist that, in fact, she almost did not come to the appointment that day. The therapist remembered that on the client's medication list she had seen Lamictal, a medication used as an antiseizure medication or a mood stabilizer. She had not discussed the medication with the client, as she felt it would be intrusive and would make the client feel uncomfortable. Also, the hand therapist remembered Jane's comment in the first session about traumatic brain injury or mental illness being much harder to deal with, and she formed a hypothesis in her mind that perhaps Jane was more stressed or depressed than she had originally appeared. The therapist also wondered about the client's use of pain medication and how that was possibly interacting in an adverse way with Jane's psychotropic medication. The therapist consciously thought about the need to be curious about this apparent change of attitude, without prematurely judging or assuming what had happened with the client.

The therapist paused before starting the planned therapy activity, commented that she felt rushed, and brought herself and Jane cups of water. She calmly noted that it was not her usual practice to interrupt the session for a water break, smiled at Jane, and said she thought both she and Jane could use one. Jane looked surprised, but thanked the therapist for the water and looked at the table and then began to look at the scar on her arm. The therapist asked Jane what she thought about how her arm looked, and Jane noted that she felt like it was red and angry, like she felt some days. The therapist asked if that reaction had to do with her feelings about having a genetic disease that could possibly affect her long term, or if she was feeling discouraged about something else or even depressed. Jane looked away, then took a swallow of water and told the therapist that she and her partner had just decided to split up and she was going to have to move, as they lived in his home. She said she also felt anxious about having to return to her job where she worked with clients with cognitive limitations and impulsive behavior and she was concerned that someone might impulsively bang into her and reinjure her arm or hand. Additionally, she worried that she could not take additional time off from work, beyond the month of medical leave she had requested for the surgery, because she needed the income to secure a new place to live. She did not know how she was going to move once she found a place because she could not really lift things yet, but she was uncomfortable staying with her boyfriend because she felt sad about losing the relationship.

The therapist became concerned that she had opened a "Pandora's box" of issues for Jane and imagined her supervisor overhearing the conversation with disapproval or at least impatience

that she return to the work of hand therapy. When Jane paused, the therapist said that she was honored that Jane felt enough trust to tell her honestly what she was contending with in her life. She said that she had remembered that Jane had commented in their first session that hand therapy would be easier than dealing with traumatic brain injury or mental illness, and that perhaps Jane was discouraged that something she had anticipated handling more easily (her physical recovery after surgery) was now proving harder in the face of the unexpected personal stressors. She said she wondered if Jane felt overwhelmed from having to deal with the unpredictability of the EDS as well as mood issues, and that perhaps now the loss of her relationship made her feel hopeless. The therapist felt a great deal of empathy for Jane, but also felt concern that if Jane did not do her home exercises and recover the use of her arm, this client would be in an even more vulnerable position. She proposed that they return to the hand therapy activity, and that Jane continue to talk about what she was going through while doing this.

As they returned to the hand therapy activity, the therapist asked Jane if she had a "talk therapist" and whether she thought her medications were working well. She continued and said, with a smile, that she admired that Jane worked in a field where she was helping others and she (the therapist) knew what it was like to have days when it felt harder than usual to give of oneself. Jane said she really appreciated the hand therapist being open with her because then it was easier for her to admit that she was minimizing her problems and needed to return to seeing her talk therapist, whom she had not seen since her surgery. Jane said that she did not take her prescription pain medication after the surgery and that most days she tried controlling the pain with ibuprofen. She admitted there were days where the pain was almost intolerable—but she was afraid to add any opioid medication because of her history of substance abuse before her bipolar disorder was diagnosed in college. Jane worried that Vicodin could be a gateway to her returning to substance abuse. Toward the end of the session, the therapist talked about a plan for the coming week. She and Jane agreed that Jane would practice the exercises for just 10 minutes before she left for work and 20 minutes when she returned home in the evening. The hand therapist asked if it would be useful for Jane to contact her psychotherapist during the coming week and make an appointment, and Jane responded affirmatively. Also, the hand therapist suggested that Jane do something for herself that would feel like a return to her pre-surgery routine. The therapist then asked Jane if she had a vision of some pleasurable, peaceful place where she had felt a sense of well-being and beauty. Jane recalled a swing under a big tree at her grandmother's house where she went each summer as a child, where she could relax and dream in peace. The therapist suggested that when Jane did her exercises, she picture herself on the swing in the summer air under the shade of the big tree, feeling stronger and more relaxed with each whoosh up and back.

Jane's adherence to her home exercise program significantly improved after this discussion. Jane completed her course of hand therapy with the outcome of excellent hand function. The hand therapist also had a very positive outcome in that she realized she could adjust her expectations and the strategy she used to motivate a client based on what emerged in the course of treatment. Her increased appreciation of the value of compassion, empathy, and rapport made her feel competent in helping this client move toward full recovery.

References

1. Havens L: Sullivan and the heart. In *a safe place: laying the groundwork of psychotherapy*, Cambridge, MA, 1989, Harvard University Press.
2. Havens L: Empathic language. In *making contact: uses of language in psychotherapy*, Cambridge, MA, 1989, Harvard University Press.
3. Rollnick S, Miller WR, Butler CC: Motivational interviewing: principles and evidence. In *motivational interviewing in health care: helping patients change behavior*, New York, NY, 2008, Guilford Press.
4. Rolland JS: Family health and illness belief systems. In *families, illness, and disability: an integrative treatment model*, New York, NY, 1994, Basic Books.
5. Kleinman A: *The illness narratives: suffering, healing, and the human condition*, New York, NY, 1988, Basic Books.
6. Groopman J: Exiting a labyrinth of pain. In *the anatomy of hope: how people prevail in the face of illness*, New York, NY, 2004, Random House.

13 Facilitating Adherence to the Plan of Care

Lisa O'Brien
Luke Steven Robinson

Introduction

In this chapter, we explain the difference between the terms **adherence** and **compliance** and highlight the risks and costs associated with treatment nonadherence. We summarize the evidence for adherence-enhancing strategies tested with individuals with hand and upper limb conditions, and we provide a model that helps therapists understand why some clients struggle to stick to their plan of care. Finally, we discuss practical evidence-based approaches to enhance client adherence.

Adherence Versus Compliance

Understanding the Difference Between the Terms Adherence and Compliance

Confusingly, the terms **adherence** and **compliance** are often used interchangeably in the medical and therapeutic literature. A detailed description of the differences between these terms is discussed in Meichenbaum and Turk's classic textbook[1] and can be summarized as:

Compliance is the "extent to which patients obey and follow instructions, prescriptions and proscriptions outlined by their treating health practitioner," whereas

Adherence implies an "active, voluntary and collaborative involvement by the patient in a mutually acceptable course of behavior to produce a preventative or therapeutic result."

The World Health Organization's adherence project defines adherence as "the extent to which a person's behavior—taking medication, following a diet and/or executing lifestyle changes—corresponds with agreed recommendations from a health provider."[2] The word **agreed** is the keystone of this statement, as adherence requires the client to agree with the recommendations, and then stick to the agreed regimen to achieve optimum clinical benefit. The term **adherence** is intended to be nonjudgmental and does not imply blame on the part of the client, prescriber, or treatment.

It is also important to understand their different connotations and inferences, mainly in the role the client adopts. **Compliance** places the client in a passive role of treatment recipient who takes instruction from the doctor or treating health practitioner. The power balance in the practitioner–client relationship is heavily slanted toward the practitioner in this instance. In contrast, the client's role in **adherence** is that of an informed consenter, in that they understand and decide to follow the chosen intervention or advice in order to achieve the best possible clinical benefit.[3] The power relationship shifts toward the client in this instance,[4] but the balance of power is still with the health practitioner.

Why the Term *Adherence* Is a Better Fit With Hand Therapy

The terms we use to describe client behavior are important. In a hand clinic, you may hear some clients described as "noncompliant" if they miss crucial appointments, don't complete their exercises as recommended, or arrive either without their orthosis or with some unauthorized or unsafe modifications to it. The underlying assumption behind the term **noncompliant** is that any negative consequences are likely to be the client's own fault. This reflects an outdated medical and health care ideology, in which health care practitioners assume the role of experts and clients are expected to simply obey the experts' recommendations. A review of the medical, nursing, and therapy literature of the 20th century concluded that the term **compliance** used in this context was synonymous with physician control.[5] The control ideology, however, does not sit comfortably with physical and occupational therapy training and our professions' commitment to client-centered practice. While it is important that clients wear their orthosis, complete graded exercise programs, avoid unsafe use of the limb during the healing phase, and attend appointments, hand therapists need to consider how the individual will manage their necessary occupations (self-care, work, and leisure) during the recovery phase. We also need to establish an agreement with our clients so that they understand *how* they can complete necessary activities while still avoiding potential risks. We will therefore use the preferred term **adherence** rather than compliance throughout this chapter.

Why Is Adherence to the Hand Therapy Plan of Care Important?

People with acute hand and upper limb injuries who adhere to their plan of care have better functional outcomes.[6,7] They also have a lowered risk of requiring potentially costly secondary surgery for preventable deformities, contractures, and reinjury of tissues.[8] It is reported that the percentage of people who adhere to their agreed hand therapy plan for the required time is between 32% and 60.5%.[7,9-12] However, the true rate is likely to be lower in practice, as it can be a very difficult construct to measure accurately. It may also be context dependent; a person may manage well when surrounded by cues and reminders (for example, during their inpatient hospital stay) but may forget to adhere to their therapy program when they return home, where it may become a lower priority.

When Is Someone Deemed Nonadherent?

Some researchers treat adherence as a dichotomous variable (i.e., a specific client is rated as either adherent or nonadherent).[13,14] Others describe varying levels of nonadherence[10,12,15] that may span from: (a) never adhered to any aspect of treatment; (b) adhered with some but not other aspects; (c) initially adhered but relapsed over time; to (d) inappropriate or overadherence. Newer definitions of nonadherence adopt a "threshold" approach,[16] defining a set point of exercises sessions completed, appointments attended, or hours of orthosis time below which the desired therapeutic or preventative effect is unlikely to be achieved.

A Multidimensional Concept of Adherence

Nonadherence with health interventions is recognized as a significant problem worldwide, and the literature exploring the determinants of adherence is extensive, prompting the World Health Organization to undertake a major critical review of the evidence in 2003.[2] As a result of this, the Multidimensional Adherence Model was created (see Fig. 13.1), which groups the key predictors of adherence into five dimensions and factors: (1) social/economic, (2) health care system, (3) condition related, (4) therapy related, and (5) patient-related factors. This model states that the ability to follow treatment is impacted by more than one barrier, and interventions to improve adherence need to address *all* relevant factors.

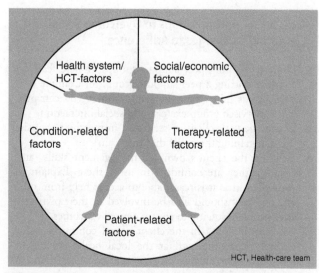

FIG.13.1 The five dimensions of adherence. HCT, ***. *(Reprinted with permission from World Health Organization. Sabaté, E. Adherence to Long-Term Therapies: Evidence for Action. Geneva, Switzerland: World Health Organization; 2003, p 27).*

These dimensions will now be defined and applied to hand therapy contexts.

Social/Economic Factors

Social/economic factors include race (and cultural beliefs), poverty, illiteracy, unemployment, lack of social supports, distance from treatment facility/outlet, family dysfunction, the cost of travel/treatment, and age. While no consistent relationship between social and economic factors and adherence has been identified in hand surgery and therapy literature, it is likely that factors such as access to services in the local community, lack of family support, and cost of treatment (and associated travel to clinics) could have an impact for some clients. Examples of interventions that have been shown to work for people with chronic hand conditions such as rheumatoid arthritis are peer support groups.[17] These group programs are thought to work by promoting sharing of experiences regarding management of the condition/disease, and engendering the client's sense of responsibility and self-efficacy. They can also reduce the burden on health care providers, improve client self-management skills, and integrate overall care provision. Box 13.1 outlines interventions to overcome social and economic challenges to adherence.

Health System/Health Care Team Factors

This dimension includes the client–provider relationship, continuity of care, training of health care providers, and length of follow-up. One qualitative study of the client experience of traction therapy for complex finger joint fractures[18] found that those who trusted their treatment providers (most importantly the hand therapist, but also the surgeon) and were provided with clear and consistent education were more likely to follow the orthosis and exercise program. A systematic review of the literature on the effect of client–practitioner interaction on adherence in people with arthritis[19] found evidence that affective tone (including the client's perception of the practitioner's attitude, and whether

---

BOX 13.1   Interventions to Overcome Social and Economic Challenges to Adherence

- Using/developing peer support groups. Where feasible, consider starting a peer support group, for example brachial plexus injury or wrist groups where you can provide supervised group exercise and social interaction.
- Encourage your client to seek help from others or assist them in gaining the belief that they can.[40]
- Building the client's own self-management skills, and ensuring they are confident in using these. Explain to your client that it is reasonable to accept help from others, but they should also be involved in their own creative problem solving to ensure desired outcomes.[40]
- Capacity building in the client's local community (for example, coaching staff at the local health service in monitoring the client's progress and engaging them in suitable activities).

BOX 13.2   Interventions to Overcome Health Care Team/System Challenges to Adherence

- Ensuring continuity of care—the entire health care team should give the same messages, delivered in the same way.
- Encouraging the client's own sense of self-efficacy.
- Eliciting the client's perceptions, expectations, wants, and needs in the early stages of the therapeutic relationship so that these can be addressed and incorporated into the treatment plan.
- Specific skill development/staff training in adherence management to enable health care team members to better design and implement interventions that have been shown to improve treatment adherence.
- Development of clinical tools for assessing and addressing the potential for nonadherence in each client.

BOX 13.3   Interventions to Overcome Condition-Related Challenges to Adherence

- Ensuring that therapists are able to identify the signs and symptoms of comorbidities that may affect adherence, such as depression, anxiety disorders, substance abuse or cognitive impairment, and be prepared to refer the client for assessment and support if necessary.
- Ensuring that support or treatment for comorbidities is in place. This may involve contact with the treating doctor, referral to counselling services, or mobilizing the client's own support systems (i.e., friends and family, peer support groups).
- Providing clear "plain language" verbal and written education about the therapy program. All written materials should have consumer involvement in their preparation, and should be written in active voice using short sentences and common words rather than technical jargon. Therapists should provide information regarding the expected prognosis and rate of progress for the specific condition, and a clear rationale for treatment at each stage.

---

adequate time was spent with them) and the client's belief in the benefit of a particular treatment had a significant positive impact. A systematic review conducted by this chapter's authors in 2017[20] found that behavioral approaches that encourage self-efficacy are likely to be useful in achieving treatment adherence in populations with chronic upper limb conditions. Box 13.2 outlines interventions to overcome health care team and health system challenges to adherence.

Condition-Related Factors

These factors include symptom severity, level of disability, prognosis, and the availability of effective treatment. They also extend to comorbidities such as depression and substance abuse, as these play an important role in modifying the individual's ability to adhere to treatment. Few studies of acute hand injuries have examined the impact of comorbidities and adherence, and results have been conflicting. For example, one study found no relationship between adherence and drug and alcohol abuse, psychiatric illness, and previous brain injury on adherence with orthoses in an acutely brain-injured population[21]; however, the literature on adults with acute burns has found a strong association between preinjury alcohol intake, drug dependency, and psychiatric illness and treatment adherence.[22,23] Box 13.3 outlines interventions to overcome condition-related challenges to adherence.

Therapy-Related Factors

Therapy-related factors include how long the person needs to continue with therapy, how complex or multistep their regimen is, interference with daily living tasks, potential pain, discomfort, or other adverse effects, and how long before the client will notice any benefits. It also encompasses the availability of support services to assist with any of the above factors. In a group of patients undergoing dynamic skeletal traction for complex finger fractures, the perceived complexity of treatment, interference with daily occupations (e.g., working, dressing, and sleep), and availability of support (especially pain relief) exerted the most significant influence on adherence.[18] For orthosis wear, immediate benefit, such as pain relief, can also improve adherence,[15] as can orthosis comfort[24,25] and visual appearance (and visibility to others),[26-28] including the ability to wear it comfortably with the client's usual clothing.

Meaningful occupation-based interventions can also improve treatment adherence[29,30] and there is emerging evidence that they achieve superior results on measures of range of motion, pain, strength, and functional ability when compared to traditional therapeutic exercise programs.[31-33] Box 13.4 outlines interventions to overcome therapy-related challenges to adherence.

Patient/Client-Related Factors

Client factors encompass their own knowledge, motivations, beliefs, and expectations, as well as their physical, sensory, and psychological resources. Hand therapists may assume that: (a) clients should be motivated to follow their care plan, and (b) they should be able to do so if provided with the correct

BOX 13.4   Interventions to Overcome Therapy-Related Challenges to Adherence

- Ensuring orthoses are comfortable and aesthetically acceptable to the client. Therapists are encouraged to ask themselves "Would I be happy to wear this orthosis myself 24/7?" Therapists should ensure an open dialogue with their clients so that they can report any issues with discomfort at any time.
- Taking photos or videos of the correctly worn orthosis and home exercise programs to assist with recall after leaving the clinic setting.
- Incorporating meaningful activity into therapy programs wherever possible. For example, a client with an interest in video games or gardening may use these activities with appropriate guidance and instruction to facilitate increases in strength and/or range of motion.
- Preparing clients for the fact that exercise may be painful or uncomfortable in the early stages after an acute injury, but this does not signify further damage.
- Liaising with the medical staff to ensure preemptive analgesia in the early stages post injury.
- Giving examples of how other clients have successfully adapted activities of daily living without compromising splint adherence.

BOX 13.5   Interventions to Overcome Patient/Client-Related Challenges to Adherence

- Ensuring that interventions go beyond the provision of advice and prescriptions. It is well established that education alone is a weak intervention. The client may benefit from a follow-up phone call a few days after the appointment, or the use of a smartphone or tablet application such as www.rehabminder.com/, which guides them through their home program.
- Promoting optimism, providing enthusiasm, providing a "reality check," and reinforcing the client's power to influence their own outcome.
- Activating the client's own resources, such as family members, caregivers, friends, and co-workers, to reinforce therapy goals.
- Specific skill development for therapists in behaviorally based interventions that can be incorporated into daily practice.

information about their plan and the risks of not doing so. These assumptions, however, need to be questioned. Let's use the example of advising a client not to smoke during the postoperative recovery phase. While most clients will understand that smoking impairs tissue healing due to its constrictive effects on small blood vessels, this will not necessarily translate into adherence. Some may not be sufficiently motivated to change their behavior, or may simply perceive that they are incapable of making the change. The second assumption that information alone will result in adherence is also potentially dangerous, as many clients may feel overwhelmed, in pain, or distracted at the time they receive information. Most people can only retain five to nine new pieces of information, and they may have reached overload by the time they attend your clinic. One study found that only 42.5% of patients (none of whom had cognitive impairments) remembered being told that they could not remove their orthosis following surgery to repair flexor tendons.[34] While some authors have suggested applying adhesive labels to orthoses (similar to the instructions on a medicine bottle) detailing wear and exercise routines[35] or cognitive screening for elders who appear to have memory problems,[36] care must be taken to avoid patronizing or alienating your client. We recommend only using these strategies in cases where cognitive disability is strongly suspected or (in the case of the label) if the orthosis application is the responsibility of caregivers.

Clients' beliefs about their own power to influence the outcome condition, as well as their expectations regarding suitable treatment, have been shown to be important influencers of adherence.[18,37] As therapists, we should promote optimism and reinforce the client's abilities and resources, including family members, caregivers, and friends who could assist with therapy goals. Therapists should also avoid using language that might discourage the client's own sense of control and hope, such as "this

is one of the worst cases I've treated" or "you will get a very poor outcome unless you work very hard on your therapy and attend all your appointments." Box 13.5 outlines interventions to overcome client-related challenges to adherence.

Interventions to Improve Adherence With Hand Therapy Plan of Care

While there are few studies into the effectiveness of adherence-enhancing interventions for hand therapy clients, this is an important and growing area. At present, there is insufficient evidence for interventions (other than the behavioral approaches mentioned earlier in this chapter) aimed at improving adherence in acute upper limb injuries and conditions. The evidence from similar patient populations tells us that supervised or individualized exercise therapy and self-management techniques can enhance exercise adherence for adults with chronic musculoskeletal pain, as can specific adherence-enhancing strategies such as positive reinforcement, goal setting, and self-monitoring plans or logbooks.[38] There is also evidence that providing both verbal and well-designed written health information to clients and/or significant others on discharge from the acute hospital setting may improve treatment adherence.[39]

Summary

If we are truly acting as client-centered practitioners, we must move toward replacing the term **compliance** with that of **adherence**. We also need to stop blaming clients when they do not follow their programs, as that is unhelpful at best and, most likely, incorrect or only part of a much more complex story. Although nonadherence is a behavior observed in an individual client, it is important to recognize that the causes are not just client related.

"[Nonadherence] occurs in the context of treatment-related demands that the patient must attempt to cope with. These demands are characterized by the requirement to learn new behaviors, alter daily routines, tolerate discomforts and inconveniences, and persist in doing so while trying to function effectively in their various life-roles."[2]

There are many opportunities to influence adherence by adapting our own approach (and that of our team) and our interventions, including (but not limited to) the use of specific counselling approaches, building the client's own self-management skills, ensuring continuity of care, incorporating meaningful activity, and more client-centered design of orthoses.

References

1. Meichenbaum D, Turk D: *Facilitating treatment adherence*, New York, 1987, Plenum Press.
2. World Health Organization: *Adherence to long-term therapies: evidence for action*, Geneva, Switzerland, 2003, World Health Organization.
3. Dunbar-Jacob J: Models for changing patient behavior, *Am J Nurs* 107:20–25, 2007.
4. Joffe H: Adherence to health messages: a social psychological perspective, *Int Dent J* 50:295–303, 2000.
5. Trostle J: Medical compliance as an ideology, *Soc Sci Med* 27:1299–1308, 1988.
6. Lyngcoln A, Taylor N, Pizzari T, Baskus K: The relationship between adherence to hand therapy and short-term outcome after distal radius fracture, *J Hand Ther* 18:2–8, 2005.
7. O'Brien LJ, Bailey MJ: Single blind, prospective, randomized controlled trial comparing dorsal aluminum and custom thermoplastic splints to stack splint for acute mallet finger, *Arch. Phys. Med. Rehabil* 92:191–198, 2011.
8. O'Brien L: Adherence to therapeutic splint wear in adults with acute upper limb injuries: a systematic review, *Hand Therapy* 15:3–12, 2010.
9. Cole T, Underhill A, Kennedy S: Adherence behavior in an acute pediatric hand trauma population: a pilot study of parental report of adherence levels and influencing factors, *J Hand Ther* 29:299–306, 2016.
10. Groth G, Wilder D, Young V: The impact of compliance on the rehabilitation of patients with mallet finger injuries, *J Hand Ther* 7:21–24, 1994.
11. Sandford F, Barlow N, Lewis J: A study to examine patient adherence to wearing 24-hour forearm thermoplastic splints after tendon repairs, *J Hand Ther* 21:44–53, 2008.
12. Walker WC, Metzler M, Cifu DX, Swartz Z: Neutral wrist splinting in carpal tunnel syndrome: a comparison of night-only versus full-time wear instructions, *Arch Phys Med Rehabil* 81:424–429, 2000.
13. Feinberg J: Effect of the arthritis health professional on compliance with use of resting hand splints by patients with rheumatoid arthritis, *Arthritis Care Res. (Hoboken)* 5:17–23, 1992.
14. Hall RJ: Treatment of metacarpal and phalangeal fractures in noncompliant patients, *Clin Orthop Relat Res* 31–36, 1987,Jan.
15. Paternostro-Sluga T, Keilani M, Posch M, Fialka-Moser V: Factors that influence the duration of splint wear in peripheral nerve lesions, *Am J Phys Med Rehabil* 82:86–95, 2003.
16. Jansons PS, Haines TP, O'Brien L: Interventions to achieve ongoing exercise adherence for adults with chronic health conditions who have completed a supervised exercise program: systematic review and meta-analysis, *Clin Rehabil* 31:465–477, 2017.
17. Taal E, Rasker J, Wiegman O: Group education for rheumatoid arthritis patients, *Semin Arthritis Rheum* 26:805–816, 1997.
18. O'Brien L, Presnell S: Patient experience of distraction splinting for complex intra-articular finger fractures, *J Hand Ther* 23:249–259, 2010.
19. Feinberg J: The effect of patient-practitioner interaction on compliance: a review of the literature and application in rheumatoid arthritis, *Patient Educ Couns* 11:171–187, 1988.
20. Cole T, Robinson L, Romero L, O'Brien L: Effectiveness of interventions to improve therapy adherence in people with upper limb conditions: a systematic review, *J Hand Ther*, 2017.
21. O'Brien L, Bailey M: Determinants of compliance with hand splinting in an acute brain injured population, *Brain Inj* 22:411–418, 2008.
22. Anwar M, Majumder S, Austin O, Phipps A: Smoking, substance abuse, psychiatric history, and burns: trends in adult patients, *J Burn Care Rehabil* 26:493–501, 2005.
23. Juzl E, Leveridge A: The hand: burns. In Prosser R, Connolly W, editors: *Rehabilitation of the hand and upper limb*, Eastbourne, 2003, Butterworth Heinemann, pp 66–74.
24. Agnew P, Maas F: Compliance in wearing wrist working splints in rheumatoid arthritis, *Occupational Ther J Research* 15:165–180, 1995.
25. Callinan N, Mathiowetz V: Soft versus hard resting hand splints in rheumatoid arthritis: pain relief, preference, and compliance, *Am J Occup Ther* 50:347–353, 1996.
26. Manigandan C, Bedford E, Ninan S, Gupta AK, Padankatti SM, Paul K: Adjustable aesthetic aeroplane splint for axillary burn contractures, *Burns* 31:502–504, 2005.
27. Spoorenberg A, Boers M, Linden S: Wrist splints in rheumatoid arthritis: a question of belief? *Clin Rheumatol* 13:559–563, 1994.
28. Basford JR, Johnson SJ: Form may be as important as function in orthotic acceptance: a case report, *Arch Phys Med Rehabil* 83:433–435, 2002.
29. Colaianni D, Provident I: The benefits of and challenges to the use of occupation in hand therapy, *Occup Ther Health Care* 24:130–145, 2010.
30. King Tn: Hand strengthening with a computer for purposeful activity, *Am J Occup Ther* 47:635–637, 1993.
31. Guzelkucuk U, Duman I, Taskaynatan M, Dincer K: Comparison of therapeutic activities with therapeutic exercises in the rehabilitation of young adult patients with hand injuries, *J Hand Surg Am* 32:1429–1435, 2007.
32. Daud AZC, Yau MK, Barnett F, Judd J, Jones RE, Nawawi RFM: Integration of occupation based intervention in hand injury rehabilitation: a randomized controlled trial, *J Hand Ther* 29:30–40, 2016.
33. Hardison ME, Roll SC: Factors associated with success in an occupational rehabilitation program for work-related musculoskeletal disorders, *Am J Occup Ther* 71, 2017. 7101190040p7101190041–7101190040p7101190048.
34. Kortman B: Patient recall and understanding of instructions concerning splints following a zone 2 flexor tendon repair, *Aust Occup Ther J* 39:5–11, 1992.
35. Hough M, Gregson M, Southern S: The splint prescription, *Br J Plast Surg* 55:537, 2002.
36. Cooper C: Maximizing therapist effectiveness with geriatric hand patients, *J Hand Ther* 6:205–208, 1993.
37. Brus H, van de Laar M, Taal E, Rasker J, Wiegman O: Compliance in rheumatoid arthritis and the role of formal patient education, *Seminars in Arthritis and Rheumatology* 26:702–710, 1997.
38. Aitken D, Buchbinder R, Jones G, Winzenberg T: Interventions to improve adherence to exercise for chronic musculoskeletal pain in adults, *Aust Fam Physician* 44:39, 2015.
39. Johnson A, Sandford J, Tyndall J: Written and verbal information versus verbal information only for patients being discharged from acute hospital settings to home, *The Cochrane Library*, 2003.
40. Hannah SD: Psychosocial issues after a traumatic hand injury: facilitating adjustment, *J Hand Ther* 24:95–103, 2011.

14

Narratives in Hand Therapy*

Cynthia Cooper

Statement of the Problem: The Illness Experience

Hand therapists and clients do not always use the same end points to define the client's recovery as a success. Clinicians may include in their definitions of success measures of reductions in disease and impairment, whereas clients tend to measure their success in terms of recovery of function.[1] Given the strong correlation between disability and mood, stress, and beliefs, and the usually more limited correlation with disease or impairment,[2] a client's physical problem, such as a hand injury, cannot be separated from the personal experiences that give the problem its meaning. The meaning a problem or injury embodies for a client is idiosyncratic, circumstantial, and personal. The illness experience can help explain how a person's diagnosis affects their life.[3,4,5] Narrative medicine helps therapists treat the illness experience, not just the disease. This involves listening empathetically, trying to imagine how the situation feels to the client, and also how it changes the client's life and story.[6]

Narrative Example of the Illness Experience

Martha's Story

An 80-year-old retired woman fell while walking and fractured her left dominant distal radius. She elected cast treatment and healed with some malalignment. She presented for hand therapy 3 months later with a stiff, edematous, dysesthetic hand and wrist. She relied on her right hand for self-care. She told the hand therapist that she loved to take walks but had not resumed this activity.

Therapist Reflection

Through conversation, Martha revealed that her morning walk was not just for exercise. She explained that it could take her more than 2 hours to walk around the block because she paused and visited her friends and neighbors along the way. Walking was her social outlet, and her illness experience had disrupted it.

Solution

With further discussion, her hand therapist helped her explore ways to reestablish sufficient confidence to resume taking walks. She gradually incorporated arm exercises into her walking.

Narrative Message

The client was very pleased to be able to resume walking. Recovering her social connection helped her reconnect with her preinjury experiences and gave her a renewed sense of hopefulness about restoring her involvement in other activities as well.

Introduction to Narrative Medicine

Dr. Rita Charon's appreciation that a substantial portion of medicine involves the exchange of stories motivated her to earn a PhD studying narrative in English literature while she was active in her primary care practice. Finding that her improved

*This chapter is a modified reprint of Cynthia Cooper's article for the Journal of Hand Therapy, Volume 24, Issue 2, pages 132-139, April 2011.

understanding of narrative helped her better connect with her patients, she developed this aspect of her practice and coined the term **narrative medicine**. Absorbing and interpreting the patient's story and being able to retell that story and give it form and meaning helped her and her patients realize the complexity of the illness experience, creating new possibilities for healing.[7] The narrative approach asks health providers to absorb, interpret, recognize, and be moved by patients' stories.

Operationally, narrative medicine looks like casual conversation between the provider and client. The provider uses communication techniques that elicit personal and meaningful information from the client. Both the client and the provider are engaged in the exchange, with the provider listening actively, reflecting, maintaining eye contact, avoiding interruptions, and asking open-ended questions.[8] Clients feel listened to by being given opportunities to convey personal and emotional aspects of their illness.

When we listen to clients' stories, we collaborate with them and can empower them to create new life stories. In other words, providers who facilitate the unfolding of clients' stories[6] help them become authors of their lives, which restores or enhances a sense of control.[9] To do this requires engagement with the client. In other words, just listening is not enough; the therapist must also be engaged in the interaction.[10]

Another aspect of the practice of narrative medicine is the process of reflection. Charon[10] describes the "reflective space" that leads to a fresh or clearer version of the meaning of one's story. When therapists state the clients' narrative back to the client, they show that they are listening and reflecting.

The **narrative fallacy** occurs when we create a story that confirms our flawed interpretation of a circumstance.[11] When clients' stories are reinforcing their illness, pain, or disability, therapists can help develop a more accurate, adaptive, and enabling story. For example, a client who is having trouble performing range of motion soon after tenolysis surgery for fear of hindering healing may do better when encouraged to adopt the more accurate and adaptive narrative of performing range of motion to remodel soft tissue and prevent adhesions.

Emotional Labor

Practicing narrative medicine is not easy. It requires emotional labor. Emotional labor occurs when clinicians regulate the emotions they display to convey a desired professional image.[12] Narrative medicine helps physicians (and therapists) become more supportive as colleagues, enhancing self-reflection that fosters greater sensitivity to the complexity of people's lives. In this way, narrative medicine promotes a sense of physician (and therapist) society, where individual client stories matter.[10]

Regulating one's emotional display while looking sincere can be challenging at times, such as when a client's ideas about the injury are very dissimilar to the clinician's. Understanding the importance and strength of one's intuition can help depersonalize these disagreements and keep the relationship from becoming adversarial. It is not that the client lacks respect for your views as the expert; it is just that—right or wrong—they value and respect their own intuition and gut feelings more than your expert advice.

Narrative Example of Emotional Labor

Jack's Story

An active 60-year-old male executive sustained a radial collateral ligament injury to his right dominant small finger proximal interphalangeal joint while bicycling, which was one of his favorite activities.

Therapist Reflection

Jack loved to ride his bicycle. When discussing his progress and the typical timeline for recovery, he was shocked to learn that it could take longer than 2 weeks for him to recover from his injury. He could not accept this and demanded that he recover normal range of motion and resolution of all symptoms in 2 weeks' time.

Solution

The therapist helped him explore other activities to do temporarily while recovering, which helped him occupy his time more effectively, and the hand team provided enthusiasm and encouragement for his progress.

Narrative Message

This client was used to being in charge in all aspects of his life, and he was going stir-crazy not being able to perform his usual high-demand athletic activities.

Procedural Reasoning Versus Interactive Reasoning

Narrative medicine emphasizes interactive over procedural reasoning. **Procedural reasoning** is where an expert uses structured actions (procedural knowledge) to accomplish goals. Procedural reasoning is used to decide what treatment to use at what frequency or intensity.[13,14] There is a certain comfort in having procedures and rules for care, but when providers use only procedural reasoning, evaluation and treatment may resemble a cookbook approach. By comparison, when providers collaborate with clients to understand their unique needs, it is called **interactive reasoning**.[13,15] Interactive reasoning looks like a social interaction but is actually a purposeful process that helps the therapist understand the client while also building rapport.[13] Interactive reasoning uses the client interaction to bring to light and amplify information that is relevant to recovery.[4] This is facilitated when the therapist elicits the client's story and appreciates the client's emotional tone and nonverbal communication.[6] By eliciting and restating the client's narrative, both the client and therapist come to a better understanding of how the client makes sense of their illness experience.[14,16] This insight can create new opportunities for addressing the illness.

Narrative Example of Interactive Reasoning

Ms. Jones' Story

A young woman was experiencing nonspecific pain related to typing at work. She was taught postural exercises by a hand therapist as part of a program to help her be more comfortable at work. She returned to the therapist reporting that she had not performed her postural exercises as instructed, although she could demonstrate that she understood them.

Therapist Reflection

After confirming her desire for relief of symptoms, Ms. Jones noted that she was feeling self-conscious because she had been gaining weight, and she was concerned that practicing better posture would make her look heavier and "less attractive." The consequent discussion of weight management options was meaningful to the client. Once she started participating in a program for weight reduction, she might be willing to practice better posture as well.

Solution

Ms. Jones' narrative helped the therapist understand the lack of follow-through. Elucidation of the client's experience of the illness and suggested treatments improved the therapist's connection with the client and led to useful support and guidance with participation in a weight reduction program.

Narrative Message

What looked like noncompliance was not straightforward refusal to follow suggestions. This client was not able to practice better posture at work if it made her feel like she looked heavier.

Mechanistic Paradigm Versus Phenomenological Paradigm

A study of clinical reasoning among occupational therapists identified two paradigms of treatment: the **mechanistic paradigm** and the **phenomenological paradigm**. The mechanistic or Newtonian paradigm assumes that humans work much like machines. This has also been referred to as the **biomedical model**. It is provider or expert centered and has an authoritarian nature with the provider telling the client what to do. Objective measures and quantitative language typify this paradigm. The therapist focuses on measurable improvement in impairments rather than on the client's quality of life and function/disability. In the mechanistic approach, the therapist is in control of the treatment process and the measures of success, and the client is expected to comply with the therapist's instructions and derive satisfaction from improvements in the measures.

The phenomenological paradigm places emphasis on how things appear to be as being as important, or more important, than how things actually are. This paradigm centers on the client's experience of their illness and promotes shared decision making. Subjective measures and qualitative language represent this paradigm.[17] This is also referred to as the **biopsychosocial** in contrast to the biomedical model of medicine.

In this model, the therapist sees the whole person, not just the injured part or the pathophysiology (disease). There is collaboration between client and therapist, and the clients' interests, abilities, and motivation are considered when working together to make decisions about treatment.[18] The therapist understands the impact of the illness on the client's life and addresses this while also performing the tissue-specific interventions of mechanistic care. The effort involved in this more holistic approach is well worth it—the clients' compliance is reported to be greater when they are encouraged to tell their stories.[19]

Narrative Example of Phenomenological Paradigm

Emily's Story

A female music professor found it difficult to play her instrument because of pain in her left wrist. Her pain increased after operative treatment of an ulnar styloid nonunion and triangular fibrocartilage complex defect.

Therapist Reflection

Emily told the hand therapist that music was her passion and "her life."

Solution

Working within this narrative, the therapist addressed the uniquely personal and symbolic (that is, phenomenological) aspects of her illness by suggesting that she bring her flute to hand therapy and by incorporating the functional demands of playing the flute in her hand therapy program.

Narrative Message

Emily found it very distressing that she could not even assemble, let alone play, her flute because of the pain in her wrist. She later told the therapist that bringing her flute to therapy was very important for her because it was like bringing her best friend to therapy for support.

The Medical History Is Only Part of the Story

Clients' lives and experiences are complex and multifaceted. Time constraints may force therapists to focus on the medical history, but this should not preclude our efforts to learn more about the client. The use of a narrative approach broadens awareness of our clients' illness experience. Hand therapists and other medical providers may feel required to focus on pathology. Clinical conversations tend to emphasize impairments and symptoms. Mattingly[6] refers to this as chart talk. An alternative is to place emphasis on the client's story. The use of storytelling in narrative medicine leads to greater appreciation of the complexity of the illness experiences and promotes more client-centered care.

Narrative Example of Learning More of the Story

Mrs. Smith's Story

A middle-aged woman with hearing impairment and cochlear implants was sent to hand therapy with a diagnosis of left-hand numbness. Nerve conduction studies were normal. Her symptoms were vague, variable, and not characteristic of a specific disease. When Mrs. Smith was encouraged to tell her story, she revealed that she had recently been to the emergency department with uncontrolled right hand and upper extremity spasms and had been told that her symptoms were "psychological." She expressed concern to her physicians that she wondered if she might have multiple sclerosis. She has been told by her doctors that because of her cochlear implants, she is not a candidate for a computed tomographic scan.

Therapist Reflection

During her visits to the hand therapist, Mrs. Smith explained that she works two jobs, her son's friend recently committed suicide, and her daughter was missing the year in school because of illness. She also explained that her hearing diminished as a young girl at a time when her parents were divorcing and she was being taken care of by her older sister who "yelled all the time." The patient describes spontaneously losing her hearing, but after a few years she experienced some return of hearing. After seeing many experts, she was diagnosed with hearing impairment of psychological origin.

Solution

When therapists feel that clients' stories are difficult to relate to and hard to imagine, they should draw on their resources of professional behaviors and think of these differences as an opportunity to react sensitively and to be moved by the life challenges and adversities that are revealed in clients' stories. Doing so can clarify the differences between impairment and disability, disease and illness, increasing empathy and decreasing frustration. It can also help the therapist place realistic limits on their role without taking hope from the client.

Narrative Message

The narrative approach requires therapists to try to understand what it must be like to be in the client's situation.[20,21] It is easiest to experience empathy with clients who are similar to ourselves.[12]

Stories Are Not Trivial

What looks like idle chitchat in the clinic may in fact be essential for uncovering and incorporating narrative in hand therapy. A brief remark or detail from a client may seem to be trivial from the mechanistic viewpoint but may be quite significant from the phenomenological viewpoint. Said more plainly, a detail that seems trivial from a physical point of view may actually be very important to that client from a psychological point of view.[4]

Narrative Example of a Seemingly Small Detail

Rebecca's Story

A 64-year-old female sustained an embarrassing fall in public with resulting right dominant shoulder pain and rotator cuff tendinopathy. Her pain worsened during her initial therapy sessions. She changed providers and was diagnosed with complex regional pain syndrome. She received multiple stellate ganglion blocks, along with other medications and attended hand therapy after her blocks. She developed severe stiffness of her wrist and digits. Her hands were edematous and dysesthetic. In the client's words, "I thought I would be cured after the first injection, even though I had been told otherwise, so it was disappointing when I was not dramatically better all of a sudden." She further commented, "It is exhausting to hurt all the time. And my pain affects my entire family. I have learned to appreciate those who have to live with constant pain."

Therapist Reflection

Before the fall, Rebecca had been very independent. She was widowed and had raised five children on her own. She told the therapist, "I was used to taking charge of things. It is very difficult to have to rely on others to help with driving, dressing, and personal care. This cannot be me."

Solution

The therapist provided extra time for conversation and discussion with Rebecca. She made good functional improvement over time and valued the opportunity to tell her story.

Narrative Message

Having to rely on others was extremely difficult for Rebecca, who was proud of her independence and self-sufficiency. Talking helped her recognize this and led to her being able to receive help from friends temporarily. In her words, "I am the type of person who has to talk about things. Physicians typically do not have time to do that. It has made a big difference for me to be able to listen, learn, and talk in hand therapy."

Hand Therapy Can Help Even if It Cannot Cure

Hand therapists need to know their limitations, but even with limitations, the listening skill can stimulate powers of self-healing for the client. Narrative medicine helps therapists have an impact on clients' well-being beyond the upper extremity. An underacknowledged but substantial part of hand therapy involves the mind and the spirit of the client. Therapists who present a positive and respectful regard establish more of the rapport needed to elicit clients' stories.[22] Some clients' stories are so sad or complex that the hand therapist may feel overwhelmed. It will help to remember that therapists are not expected to solve all the clients' problems. It is amazing how effective it can be just to listen. Even in the most challenging of clinical cases, details will surface in clients' stories that open new avenues for problem solving, leading to productive hand therapy interventions and experiences.

Narrative Example of Helping Without Curing

Mrs. Miller's Story

An elderly client was referred to hand therapy with bilateral wrist tendinitis and trapeziometacarpal arthrosis. She had a medical history including lung cancer, diabetes, balance disorders, and chronic pain. The hand therapist provided several interventions with minimal relief of pain.

Therapist Reflection

Mrs. Miller had weathered multiple illnesses in the past. She had surely developed strategies that helped her through these prior challenges.

Solution

Attention was focused on the Mrs. Miller's illness experience. The therapist encouraged her to describe the strengths she drew on in difficult times.

Narrative Message

This client's stories led to an exploration of strategies for temporary pain relief. The client acknowledged that hand therapy had not been able to cure her pain, but it had helped her manage and live with her pain.

Clients as Actors in Their Real Worlds

A hand injury may disrupt an entire life. Therapists who appreciate this can help clients mend the disruption. By seeking information from the client and then modifying therapy goals accordingly, a truly individualized treatment program is achieved.[4] Narrative medicine helps therapists create experiences for clients that give them identities other than that of an ill person, instead becoming actors in their real worlds.[6]

Narrative Example of Idiosyncratic and Personal Intervention

Jean's Story

A middle-aged woman fractured her distal radius in a fall while hiking. She did not go to a doctor until more than a week after the injury. The fracture was displaced and was treated with external fixation and percutaneous pin fixation. She told the hand therapist that she was bipolar and had attention-deficit disorder and other psychiatric diagnoses. During some of her therapy sessions, she was medicated and lethargic. It was frequently difficult for her to maintain her attention and focus at the hand therapy sessions.

Therapist Reflection

Jean required a unique and very nontraditional approach to hand therapy. She told the hand therapist that she loved to dance and that she would like to perform "theatrical dances" in hand therapy to express herself.

Solution

Jean performed dances in which she used her entire body, and she received the stretch and stimulation to the upper extremities that she needed.

Narrative Message

Traditional hand therapy did not fit this client's narrative. Hand therapy by way of dancing allowed her to choreograph and accomplish her hand therapy in her own world and way.

Listening

Listening to a client's story is one aspect of their healing.[23] When clients describe their stories, it is therapeutic because finding words helps contain the disorder and its associated worries, while also providing a sense of control over the chaos of illness or injury.[7] There are some situations where simply listening helps clients with their pain more successfully than the actual physical treatment.

Narrative Example of Listening

Patty's Story

A 30-year-old right dominant female dishwasher was referred to hand therapy with a diagnosis of right arm pain. She reported that an aggressive coworker who "had hurt other employees before" had maliciously shoved a crate of dishes forcefully into her, hitting her right forearm. X-rays and magnetic resonance imaging were normal.

Therapist Reflection

Patty presented with an intense expression of pain, wincing and moaning even when her arm was at rest. She told the therapist that she had been transferred by her employer from another state and had not been told that she would have a significant pay cut with the transfer. For this reason, she had to work 60 hours per week to make ends meet. She described a crowded and underresourced living situation with family members and her children.

Solution

After having an opportunity to talk about herself, she stated that her pain was improved and that by listening, the hand therapist had helped her more than anyone else had.

Narrative Message

This client had no one to confide in. Simply having an opportunity to express problems and frustrations and be listened to can help quiet an illness.

Enter the Client's Subjective World

Narratives do not always have to reveal deeper psychological issues but may also assist the therapist in interventions, such as complicated ergonomic analysis. The art of hand therapy occurs when we allow clients to guide us to and through their problems.[24] To do this, our clients must have time to talk.[25] Yerxa[21] encourages us to enter the subjective world of our clients and to welcome the complexity of human nature.

Narrative Example of Entering the Client's Subjective World

Mrs. Clark's Story

A 35-year-old woman who was wheelchair bound because of complications from surgery for a heart problem resulting in incomplete quadriplegia as a teenager presented with nonspecific right dominant wrist and hand pain. She is a certified recreational therapist and an administrator at a center for independent living, where she also teaches independent living skills. There was no objective impairment but 9/10 pain in response to palpation of the A-1 pulley of the right long finger. There was crepitus with composite digital flexion but no locking in composite flexion. She had no edema and no sensory complaint. She did demonstrate pain at the metacarpophalangeal (MP) joint of the right long finger, which was worse with passive MP hyperextension and hyperflexion, positions she used with transferring from wheelchair to bed and when crawling on the floor, which she did regularly at home. In addition, she had inconsistent vague pain at the ulnar right wrist that was worst when keying at the computer—a task that was necessary for work.

Therapist Reflection

When asked what she thought had caused or contributed to her right upper extremity pain, Mrs. Clark identified two factors: propelling her manual wheelchair and transferring from her wheelchair to her bed. When asked if she could perform transfers with more neutral MP joint positioning, she felt strongly that this would not be possible for various reasons. Splinting options were offered as part of a comprehensive treatment program, but she had particular needs and requests that were, frankly, contrary to the textbook solutions.

Solution

Ergonomic recommendations were made to accommodate the extremes of motion that Mrs. Clark used with propelling her wheelchair and transferring to her bed. In addition, nontraditional splints were made to help with soft-tissue protection.

Narrative Message

Through narrative, clients may show us how to help them achieve their goals, sometimes in unconventional ways.

Conclusion

The practice of narrative medicine allows clients' stories to unfold so that their hand therapy care can be made personal and meaningful to them. This article applies the concepts of narrative

medicine to hand therapy. The illness experience is explained, along with background on the development of narrative medicine. Obstacles to practicing narrative medicine, such as emotional labor, are addressed. Procedural reasoning is compared with interactive reasoning, and mechanistic versus phenomenological paradigms are discussed. Case examples based on the author's clinical experience are provided to illustrate a narrative approach and methods of interaction that elicit self-healing powers among our hand therapy clients.

> ### Clinical Pearl
>
> The recommendations below are based on the author's personal experience and on the literature[26]:
> - Try to listen initially in the visit without interruption.
> - Do not condescend or criticize clients when they express their views or beliefs.
> - Ask clients and escorts open-ended questions about their view of the problem. For example, "Tell me more," "Is there anything else?" "This must be very difficult."
> - Be yourself with the client, and trust your feelings.

References

1. Kleinman A: Clinical relevance of anthropological and cross-cultural research: concepts and strategies, *Am J Psychiatry* 135:427–431, 1978.
2. Vranceanu A-M, Cooper C, Ring D: Integrating patient values into evidence-based practice: effective communication for shared decision-making, *Hand Clin* 25:83–96, 2009.
3. Mattingly C, Fleming MH: *Clinical reasoning*, Philadelphia, 1994, F.A. Davis.
4. Mattingly C: What is clinical reasoning? *Am J Occup Ther* 45:979–986, 1991.
5. Jackson J: Living a meaningful existence in old age. In Zemke R, Clark F, editors: *Occupational science: the evolving discipline*, Philadelphia, 1996, F.A. Davis, pp 339–361.
6. Mattingly C: The narrative nature of clinical reasoning, *Am J Occup Ther* 45:998–1005, 1991.
7. Charon R: Narrative medicine: a model for empathy, reflection, profession, and trust, *JAMA* 286:1897–1902, 2001.
8. Boyle D, Dwinnell B, Platt F: Invite, listen, and summarize: a patient-centered communication technique, *Acad Med* 80:29–32, 2005.
9. Frank G: Life histories in occupational therapy clinical practice, *Am J Occup Ther* 50:251–264, 1995.
10. Charon R: *Narrative medicine: honoring the stories of illness*, New York, 2006, Oxford University Press.
11. Taleb NN: Nassim Nicholas Taleb, Wikipedia (website), http://en.wikipedia.org/wiki/Nassim_Taleb. [Accessed 21 March 2009].
12. Larson EB, Yao X: Clinical empathy as emotional labor in the patient-physician relationship, *JAMA* 293:1100–1106, 2005.
13. Higgs J, Jones M: *Clinical reasoning in the health professions*, ed 2, Burlington, VT, 2000, Butterworth/Heinemann.
14. Schell BAB, Schell JW: *Clinical and professional reasoning in occupational therapy*, Baltimore, MD, 2008, Lippincott Williams & Wilkins.
15. Fleming MH: The therapist with the three-track mind, *Am J Occup Ther* 45:1007–1014, 1991.
16. Mallinson T, Kielhofner G, Mattingly C: Metaphor and meaning in a clinical interview, *Am J Occup Ther* 50:338–346, 1995.
17. Gillette NP, Mattingly C: Clinical reasoning in occupational therapy, *Am J Occup Ther* 41:399–400, 1987.
18. Brody H: The biopsychosocial model, patient-centered care, and culturally sensitive practice, *J Fam Pract* 45:585–587, 1999.
19. Barrier PA, James T-C, Jensen NM: Two words to improve physician-patient communication: what else? *Mayo Clin Proc* 78:211–214, 2003.
20. Yerxa EJ: Seeking a relevant, ethical, and realistic way of knowing for occupational therapy, *Am J Occup Ther* 45:199–204, 1991.
21. Yerxa EJ: Confessions of an occupational therapist who became a detective, *Br J Occup Ther* 63:192–199, 2000.
22. Pipe TB: Fundamentals of client-therapist rapport. In Cooper C, editor: *Fundamentals of hand therapy: clinical reasoning and treatment guidelines for common diagnoses of the upper extremity*, ed 1, St Louis, 2006, Mosby, pp 126–140.
23. Charon R: Narrative Medicine Creates Alliance with Patients, Medscape Med Students (website), http://www.medscape.com/viewarticle/520704. [Accessed 20 May 2010].
24. Morris MB, Morris B: Personalized Medicine and Patient-Centric Learning: a Core Requirement for Informed Decision Making, Medscape Per Med (website), http://www.medscape.com/viewarticle/576151. [Accessed 20 May 2010].
25. Marvel MK: Soliciting the patient's agenda: have we improved? *JAMA* 281:283–287, 1999.
26. Branch WT, Malik TK: Using "windows of opportunities" in brief interviews to understand patients' concerns, *J Am Med Assoc* 269:1667–1668, 1993.

15 Utilization of Therapy Assistants in Hand Therapy

Luella Grangaard

Today's health care environment has many demands that impact delivery of services. These include ever-increasing referrals (due, in part, to aging Baby Boomers), the rising cost of health care service delivery, the limited availability of specialized services, and the rising cost of educating health care providers. Simply put, there are just not enough resources to meet current demand. The use of service extenders—such as physician assistants, occupational therapy assistants, and physical therapist assistants—has increased to meet these needs. Hand therapists around the world need to be aware of legislation, regulations, and reimbursement guidelines that direct how services are to be delivered and how to appropriately utilize assistants.

For example, in the United States, many third-party payers reimburse services provided by physician assistants at a lower rate than that of the physician. Specifically, Medicare (the United States federal program that provides health care to people age 65 or older and certain younger disabled individuals) reimburses services provided by physician assistants at 85% of the physician fee schedule. This type of tiered reimbursement model for physical and occupational therapy services is currently being proposed by legislation affecting Medicare. Additionally, Tricare (the United States Department of Defense's health care program for military families) currently does not reimburse for services provided by occupational/physical therapy assistants, even if the services are supervised by a therapist. The future of these policies is uncertain, but could certainly affect how other third-party payers decide to reimburse for services provided by assistants. Regulatory and reimbursement climate changes such as these have the potential to affect how therapy assistants are used in the future, at least in some countries.

That being said, a knowledgeable and well-trained assistant can significantly augment the care provided in a hand therapy program. This chapter will discuss utilization of therapy assistants and suggests ways to develop a team to effectively deliver quality hand therapy services. For clarity, this chapter uses the term **assistant** to mean an occupational therapy assistant (OTA) or a physical therapist assistant (PTA). It is understood that all are professional therapy practitioners and that semantics vary. This chapter is heavily slanted to address issues in the United States. However, this author hopes that readers will find common points of interest and concerns applicable to practice anywhere in the world.

Legislation, Regulations, and Guidelines Affecting Delivery of Care

In the United States, therapy assistants need a license to practice in many states. The professions of occupational therapy and physical therapy each have separate and unique practice acts in each state. Some practice acts and corresponding regulations outline details of the supervisory relationship between the therapist and the assistant. These statutes and regulations may also dictate acceptable ratios of assistants to therapists, the frequency and type of clinical supervision required for assistants, how assistants and therapists should each document client care, and how the therapy team should document collaboration between service providers. Both therapists and assistants have a professional and legal responsibility to understand the laws that govern therapy practice in their state.

When the hand therapy team at an organization is comprised of both physical and occupational therapy practitioners, complying with laws governing practice can get confusing. This is especially true for laws governing clinical supervision of assistants by therapists. In this type of situation, hand therapists must remember that "hand therapy" is not a separate profession. Hand therapy is a subspecialty of both occupational and physical therapy, and each professional is governed by their own license. While all hand therapy staff can be administratively managed by either an occupational or a physical therapist, when it comes to providing direct client care, each professional must act within their legal scope of practice. Thus, OTAs must be clinically supervised by an occupational therapist and follow an occupational therapy plan of care. PTAs must be clinically supervised by a physical therapist and follow a physical therapy plan of care. Furthermore, *how* that clinical supervision looks depends entirely on each profession's practice act in that particular state. Laws and regulations for each profession are different, and the role delineation between an occupational therapist and an OTA may look quite different from the role delineation between a physical therapist and a PTA, even within the same hand therapy department. It is very important to remember that an occupational therapist cannot sign clinical notes written by a PTA, and a physical therapist cannot sign clinical notes written by an OTA. These types of issues need to be taken into consideration when deciding on staffing and supervision. Professional associations and licensing boards have position papers, guidelines, statutes, and regulations that address appropriate supervision practices to assist with management of staff.

Developing a Respectful and Effective Team Relationship

We know that the therapist performs the evaluation, establishes goals with input from the client, and formulates the treatment plan. The assistant is responsible for implementing the plan as directed by the therapist. However, the therapist and the assistant can and should collaborate on client care. Some clinics have written clinical guidelines or protocols to help guide the treatment plan based on diagnosis. The term *collaboration* has many definitions, but in this setting it means cooperation between two or more parties who are working together toward a common goal. In this case, the parties are the therapist, the assistant, and the client. The common goal is rehabilitation of the client's hand. Considerations when developing a therapist/assistant treatment team differ based on the amount of experience the therapist and the assistant each has in hand therapy, as well as the skill level and expertise of each practitioner.

◉ Clinical Pearl

The therapist has the final say about all treatment decisions, as it is the therapist who is ultimately responsible for client care. However, collaboration with the assistant plays a big part in the decision-making process. It is extremely helpful to have a second set of eyes and additional insight into the client's performance.

It is the responsibility of both the therapist and the assistant to ensure that appropriate quality and frequency of supervision occurs in order to provide safe and effective therapy services. This means that each practitioner needs to be aware of their own skill level and limitations. The following are general principles of supervision[1]:

1. To ensure safe and effective hand therapy, it is the responsibility of the therapist and assistant to recognize when supervision is needed and to seek supervision that supports the current and advancing levels of competence.
2. The specific frequency, methods, and content of supervision are dependent on the:
   a. Complexity of client needs
   b. Number and diversity of clients
   c. Skills of the therapist and assistant

d. Type of practice setting
e. Requirements of the practice setting
f. Other regulatory requirements

As indicated above, a variety of factors will dictate supervision requirements. These factors can also highlight areas of additional training that team members may require. In addition, basic teamwork skills are necessary for clinical and professional success when therapists and assistants work together. These skills include the ability to communicate effectively, to graciously provide and receive constructive feedback, to openly acknowledge team member skill levels, and to eagerly collaborate. Individual character traits of integrity, kindness, reliability, respectfulness, and honesty are also important to the therapy team.

◉ Clinical Pearl

A team is strongest with good communication and respect among team members.

Clients are sensitive to the subtleties of communications and relationships among coworkers, whether these are therapist to therapist or therapist to assistant. A therapy clinic is a professional environment, and all team members should show respect for each other and appreciation for each other's work, no matter the professional title. Clients recognize and appreciate a friendly, collegial, caring, and professional environment. Clients will also quickly identify tension and lack of respect between colleagues in the work environment. The therapeutic relationship between the client and hand therapy team, including the client's satisfaction and perception of quality of care, is easily affected by team member interactions. Clients often share their hand therapy experiences with physicians and friends, so a negative experience can hinder referrals, while a positive experience will likely result in increased referrals. At the time of the initial evaluation, the therapist should explain that the client may work with other therapists and assistants throughout the course of treatment, but that everyone works together as a team. Explain that, "Even though you may work with other practitioners here at the hand clinic, there will be no difference in the quality of care."

◉ Clinical Pearl

When issues arise during treatment with clients, both the therapist and the assistant need to find a discreet way to communicate with each other. It is generally not a good idea to discuss differences of opinion in front of the client. Care should appear seamless and cohesive.

Promoting Clinical and Professional Growth of Assistants

Every member of the hand therapy team, including assistants, should be encouraged to grow both clinically and professionally. Continuing education, whether it be through peer presentations, journal clubs, or formal workshops, will help team members develop strong individual clinical competencies. In addition, it is important for all practitioners to belong to their professional association(s) and/or specialty professional group (for example, the American Society of Hand Therapists). These professional organizations provide excellent resources for issues surrounding clinical treatment, evidence-based practice, billing, and documentation. In addition, membership in these organizations provides opportunities for networking with other practitioners, accessing special-interest groups, and participating in study groups. Some therapists and assistants actively seek a mentor within their professional organization who will provide support and guide development of skills.

It is the professional responsibility of both the therapist and the assistant to maintain a high level of clinical skill. All practitioners should be utilizing evidence-based techniques and methods. Critical thinking should be based in physiology and anatomy. To assure that these skills are in place, shared responsibility for continuing education of the hand therapy team is critical. Both therapists and assistants can organize and lead journal clubs, as well as attend and share information from continuing education courses. Senior members of the hand therapy team, whether therapists or assistants, can act as mentors by providing team direction with suggestions for clinical topics of focus. All team members should be open to change and continued learning, as best practices do evolve over time.

Summary

Hand therapy is a specialized service provided by both therapists and assistants who may be occupational or physical therapy practitioners. All providers must be aware of the regulations guiding delivery of service. It is the professional responsibility of the provider, whether therapist or assistant, to be aware of their own skills and limitations. The hand is very complicated. Advanced training, continuing education, evidence-based treatments, and good clinical reasoning are all required for good client outcomes. A therapy team that communicates effectively, is respectful of team members, and is clinically skilled can have great client outcomes.

CASE STUDY

Scenario 1: Both the therapist and the assistant are inexperienced in hand therapy. Both practitioners should obtain continuing education, study, join professional associations for guidance, and reach out to other hand therapy practitioners in the community for mentoring. It is also helpful to collaboratively develop a structured and defined clinical reasoning tool to assure clear communication. Develop a relationship with referring physicians and physician assistants. Regarding the client's status, if you have a question, ask. Good communication will develop trust and lead to a good working relationship with your referral source.

Scenario 2: An inexperienced therapist is working with an experienced assistant. This is a complicated situation because the inexperienced therapist is ultimately responsible for the client's care and for clinical supervision of the assistant. The assistant cannot evaluate the client and cannot develop the treatment plan, nor can they supervise the therapist. However, the therapist and assistant can collaborate on the evaluation and treatment plan. Use the assistant as a resource. This is a situation where good communication is extremely important. Collaborate with each other and respect each other's skill level in order to develop a trusting supervisory relationship.

Scenario 3: An experienced therapist working with an inexperienced assistant. The therapist can help train the assistant utilizing any protocols, guidelines, and competencies that are facility specific and/or physician specific. It is important to supervise closely, to communicate, and to model appropriate behaviors. Develop a structured system for clinical review and for discussing clinical reasoning. This will help ensure that all areas of the client's care are covered and that issues are communicated appropriately. Both members of the team need to be on the same page.

References

1. American Occupational Therapy Association: Guidelines for supervision, roles, and responsibilities during the delivery of occupational therapy services, *Am J Occup Ther* 68(Suppl 3), S16–S22, 2014 https://doi:10.5014/ajot.2014.686S03.

16 Some Thoughts on Professionalism

Luella Grangaard

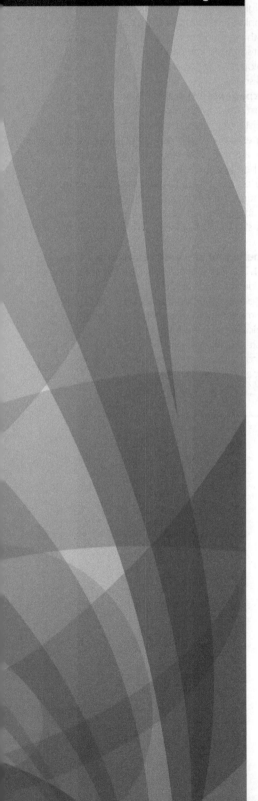

What is Professionalism?

Professionalism is the responsibility of every health care provider. Often professionalism is outlined in a code of ethics or code of conduct published by a regulatory body or professional organization as a guide for the right way to do things. Professionalism is the incorporation and operationalization of these codes into daily behaviors. Professionalism has many components that include, but are not limited to, expertise, respect, responsibility, honesty, and conduct.

Expertise is demonstrated by the skilled performance of those activities for which one is trained, and the achievement of competency on a continual basis to assure high standards are maintained. This is often validated through an accreditation of some type. It is important to regularly engage in continuing education in order to update skills and maintain expertise in hand therapy.

Respect is the portrayal of admiration for, or recognition of the value of, the client and the health care team. This includes how the care provider communicates with the client and other members of the care team. Acting in this manner often results in reciprocated respect for the individual care provider and the profession as a whole.

Responsibility is demonstrated by independently making appropriate decisions, being accountable, and ensuring that tasks and duties are addressed appropriately.

Honesty assures that all actions are fair, law abiding, and of good character.

Conduct is reflected in daily actions and interactions with clients and colleagues that are appropriate and proper. This includes professional appearance, tone of voice, facial expressions, and body language.

How Is Professionalism Demonstrated?

- Putting the client's needs first
- Listening to and collaborating with the client
- Being trustworthy
- Taking pride in your work
- Taking initiative by identifying and implementing changes that improve efficiency and clinical care
- Arriving to work on time and seeing your clients on time
- Knowing the limits of your expertise and being honest about this, including admitting when you don't know something and asking for help when you need it
- Communicating with the referring physician
- Being open to constructive feedback
- Being supportive of the team
- Assuring that you are providing skilled, evidence-based care
- Maintaining competency by participating in continuing education and reviewing current professional literature
- Being aware of and adhering to your organization's policy about receiving gifts from clients
- Being aware of and adhering to laws about socializing or doing business with clients

♡ Tips from the Field

- Greet clients and colleagues with a smile, even if you are not feeling particularly happy. Doing this might actually make you feel better.
- Be hopeful with clients and pleasant with colleagues. Your clients and colleagues will notice and appreciate your attitude.

- Present a harmonious team-front to clients, even if there are differences to be ironed out in private. Be professional with your colleagues in both mannerism and speech.
- Do not discuss politics or religion with clients.
- Do not engage in any outside business activity with clients.
- Do not date clients, their family members, or their caregivers.
- Be open to constructive feedback from the care team.
- Do not feel obliged to socialize with colleagues outside of work. Prioritize a good working relationship that focuses on clients' needs and harmony in the workplace.
- If the workload is skewed, try to help each other when possible.

Summary

As hand therapists, everything we do is for the client. Lack of professionalism can affect client care. Approaching clients with expertise that is current and evidence based will help produce the best possible outcomes. Respect assures that our behaviors send the message that we care. This, in turn, adds value to what we do and positively represents all professionals who provide hand therapy services. Being responsible communicates to the client and our team that we will be accountable and can act independently to make the best decisions for our clients. Honesty in action and communication creates a relationship based on trust, and this trust strengthens the client–therapist relationship. Conduct is how we behave with our clients and our colleagues. When therapy providers are professional, there are a number of benefits beyond improved client–therapist relationships and great therapeutic outcomes. Professionalism communicates quality and promotes the value of hand therapy to the public and to other health care providers. This, in turn, improves the visibility of this specialty area of practice, increases demand for services, and draws more therapists to hand therapy practice. As the number of skilled hand therapists increases, client access to specialized care will become more widespread. The bottom line is that both the public and the practice area of hand therapy benefit from professionalism.

CASE STUDIES

Since the majority of hand therapy professionals do practice in a professional manner, analyzing case examples of nonprofessional behavior is often the easiest way to examine the concept of professionalism. Review the following scenarios and consider the questions that follow.

CASE STUDY 16.1 ■

Bonnie is a hand therapist who thinks she has excellent orthotic fabrication skills. When a co-worker's client returns to the clinic after not showing for appointments the past 3 weeks, Bonnie assesses the client's orthosis and notices that it no longer fits well due to clinical changes in the client's forearm and hand over the 3-week absence. Bonnie states to the client, "This orthosis was made poorly and does not fit well. In fact, it is causing damage to your tissues. I'll fix it for you and talk to the other therapist about the poor quality of her orthotic work."

Question: How could she have worded this more professionally?

CASE STUDY 16.2 ■

George is a therapist who believes that hand therapy should be painful. He imposes painful forces on delicate finger joints during passive range of motion (PROM) and tells clients that this will help them. His clients frequently have flare responses with pain, edema, and stiffness. He yells at his clients to "Relax!" while he performs painful PROM of their digits.

Questions: Is this an issue of professionalism or is it a lack of clinical understanding? What type of communication skills would be more effective in helping a client relax?

17 Wound Care

Christine M. Wietlisbach

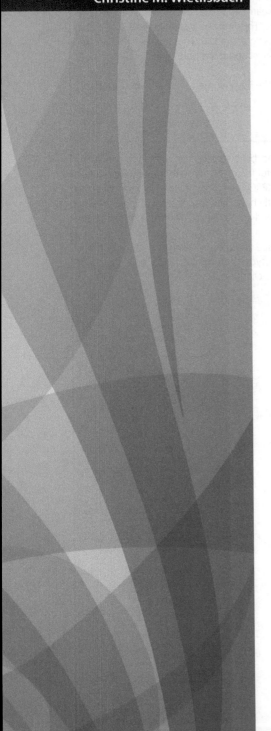

Introduction

Therapists specializing in upper extremity rehabilitation see and treat a wide variety of wounds, including abrasions, lacerations, skin tears, blisters, punctures or penetrations, human-animal-insect bites, degloving, surgical incisions, open surgical wounds, burns, and skin grafts. The significance of this aspect of hand therapy cannot be understated. Understanding how to properly care for an upper extremity wound gives you the ability to reduce pain and swelling, speed wound closure, and minimize scar tissue formation. When these factors are controlled, your client is much more likely to participate in all other aspects of the hand therapy program that lead to a successful outcome.

Both the American Occupational Therapy Association (AOTA) and the American Physical Therapy Association (APTA) definitively state that wound care is within the scope of practice of occupational therapists and physical therapists, respectively.[1-2] Many occupational therapy and physical therapy legislative practice acts also include wound care within our scope of practice, but laws vary with regard to what specific wound care procedures can be performed by therapists in certain jurisdictions. As such, you should always consult your licensing board on the legal parameters of providing this service.

This chapter introduces the basics of effective wound care. You will learn how wounds heal, the many factors that can influence wound healing, how to cleanse and debride wounds, and how to choose dressings that maintain an optimal environment for wound healing. Additionally, you will learn how to measure, describe, and document wounds along the healing continuum. This chapter does not cover the specifics of treating burns or skin grafts. These are special-circumstance wounds, and while many principles of basic wound care will also apply to burns and skin grafts, the appropriate handling of these wounds is more complicated and beyond the scope of this chapter.

Diagnosis

For the purposes of this chapter, we will consider a wound as any sort of open traumatic or surgical damage to the skin. The skin consists of two layers: the **epidermis** and the **dermis** (Fig. 17.1).

The epidermis is the outermost surface of the skin. It is avascular and made up primarily of **keratinocytes**—cells that produce the protein keratin. Although it is only about 0.5 mm thick, the epidermis is a rather dense and tough covering that helps shield the body from infection, trauma, and rapid dehydration.

The dermis lies directly below the epidermis, is about 3 mm thick, highly vascular, and made up mostly of **fibroblasts.** Fibroblasts are cells that produce collagen and elastin, which give skin strength and flexibility. Other cells found in the dermis include **macrophages** that destroy debris and bacteria within the skin, and **mast cells** that secrete substances that initiate inflammation to help fight infection. The dermis helps regulate body temperature, protects the body from infection when foreign substances break through the epidermis, and provides sensory information via receptors located there.

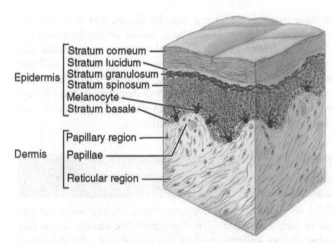

FIG. 17.1 The skin consists of two layers: the epidermis and the dermis. *From* Today's Medical Assistant, *2009.*

Timelines and Healing

Normal Wound Healing

When the skin is wounded, it normally undergoes a predictable sequence of events consisting of three overlapping phases: inflammation, proliferation, and maturation (also called remodeling). Collectively, these three phases are known as the **wound healing process**. This process is a very complicated vascular and cellular response to tissue injury. What follows here is a very basic description of these events. Understanding the wound healing process can assist you in evaluating and planning a course of treatment for upper extremity wounds.

Inflammation is the initial response to tissue injury. During the **inflammatory phase of wound healing**, the body is working to control blood loss and to clean the wounded area. Blood loss is controlled, in part, when the blood vessels in the injured area immediately constrict. This is known as **vasoconstriction.** At the same time, a protein-based fluid leaks out of the vessels and swelling begins at the injury site. Additionally, the body begins sending specialized clean-up cells to the area that work to break down and destroy damaged tissue, foreign matter, and bacteria. Within about 30 minutes, mast cells release histamine, which causes blood vessels to open, or **vasodilate.** This vasodilation pushes more fluid into the tissue spaces and causes increased pain, swelling, and discoloration (red, blue, or purple) in and around the wound.

The inflammatory phase begins the moment of injury and continues until the injured area is free of debris and bacteria. It is a normal and necessary phase of tissue healing. The reported wound healing timeline varies in the literature, but the acute inflammatory phase usually lasts 2 days to 2 weeks. During this time, physicians and therapists should strive to control only *excessive* inflammation and edema because these issues result in severe pain and potentially decreased circulation, which can cause further tissue damage. However, it is important to remember that some amount of inflammation and swelling is normal and necessary to prepare the wound for the proliferative phase of healing.

The **proliferative phase of wound healing** begins once the injured area is clean and free from damaged tissue, foreign matter, and bacteria. At this point, the body starts repairing (filling-in) the open space created by the wound. Proliferation consists of granulation, angiogenesis, wound contraction, and epithelialization. Granulation occurs when the body forms a matrix of connective tissue, including collagen, in the wound bed. This tissue is known as **granulation tissue** and builds on itself to fill the "hole" of the wound. **Angiogenesis** is the growth of new blood vessels. Very small capillary networks are formed in the granulation tissue of the wound and give healthy wounds their distinctive pink-red color. **Wound contraction** occurs when specialized cells in the wound bed act to pull the edges of the wound together. Finally, epithelial cells migrate across the top of the granulation tissue and completely cover the wound. This is known as **epithelialization.** The proliferative phase may take up to a few weeks to complete. It is completed more rapidly in a moist and protected environment, which becomes important for you to remember when choosing appropriate wound dressings. This will be discussed later in the chapter.

Newly epithelialized wounds are still quite fragile and must go through the **maturation phase of wound healing** (also called the remodeling phase). During this final phase, water and amino acids are squeezed out of the granulation tissue matrix as collagen fibers continue to be produced. This new tissue, dense with collagen, is called **scar tissue**. Scar tissue is not as elastic or as cosmetically appealing as skin, but it serves as an adequate wound cover.

> **◉ Clinical Pearl**
>
> Although scar tissue becomes stronger over time, at full maturity it is only about 80% as strong as skin. The maturation phase of wound healing can take up to 2 years to complete. Throughout the maturation phase, collagen fibers change and reorient as a result of stress in and around the wounded area. During this time, therapists can influence final scar quality through the tension of exercise and orthoses, as well as with scar mobilization techniques.

Factors Affecting Wound Healing

Although most wounds progress through the three phases of healing without incident, there are certain factors that can influence both the rate and quality of healing. These factors include:

- Circulation
- Debris in the wound bed
- Infection
- Chemical stress
- Temperature of the wound bed
- Amount of moisture in and around the wound
- Medications and other medical conditions
- Nutrition
- Age

Neither the therapist nor the client has control over all factors affecting wound healing. However, to the extent that it is possible, all factors that can be modified to improve wound healing should be addressed. Familiarizing yourself with these variables will help you and your clients create an optimal environment for wound healing. Understanding these variables will also help explain why some wounds take longer to heal.

Adequate circulation is essential to wound healing. Wounds will not heal unless an adequate supply of oxygenated blood reaches the wound bed. Many things can reduce blood flow to the hands, such as peripheral vascular disease, diabetes, smoking,[3] excessive edema, and mechanical stress from orthoses or dressings. It is the therapist's responsibility to assure that all wound dressings and orthoses fit correctly. Dressings that are wrapped too tightly or orthoses that cause pressure areas can affect circulation in the hand.

In addition to having adequate circulation, a wound must be clean before it can heal. A wound is considered "clean" when it is free from infection and debris. **Wound debris** is anything embedded in the wound bed that should not be there: sutures, gauze fibers, dog hair, dead tissue, and so on. When a wound is infected or contains debris, the body's natural reaction is to clean it up by initiating an inflammatory response, sending specialized clean-up cells to the area that work to destroy foreign matter and bacteria. The wound will remain stuck in the inflammatory phase of healing until it is clean. As a hand therapist, you play an important role in monitoring wounds for infection and in removing debris from the wound bed to facilitate more rapid healing.

Chemical stress occurs when a toxic substance makes contact with granulation tissue forming in the wound bed. Cells that make up granulation tissue are very fragile and must be treated with care. When chemical stress occurs, the new cells die, and this slows the rate of wound healing. Many products that have traditionally been used to clean wounds, such as hydrogen peroxide and povidone-iodine, are **cytotoxic** and can kill tissue cells.[4] You must use care in choosing wound-cleansing products and educate your clients to do the same. Sterile water and saline solution are ideal cleansing agents for clean wounds, as they are not cytotoxic.

The temperature of the wound bed also influences healing. Wounds heal best when the wound surface temperature is kept relatively constant and close to the normal core body temperature range of 36 to 38°C (96.8–100.4°F).[5] The temperature of the wound bed drops, on average, 2 degrees Celsius (3.6°F) when dressings are removed and the wound is cleansed with room-temperature saline. It can take up to 3 hours for the temperature of a wound to return to predressing-change temperature once a new dressing is applied.[6] Strategies that reduce the frequency of dressing changes help keep the wound warm and the temperature more constant, and this assists with healing.

Another factor that assists with wound healing is moisture balance. A wound that is either too wet or too dry will not heal as quickly as a properly balanced moist wound. A moist wound provides the optimal environment for cell growth and migration of epithelial cells over the wound bed. Wounds with a high level of **exudate** (drainage) can become too wet, and this often leads to breakdown of the wound bed and surrounding skin. Wounds with little or no exudate can become too dry, and this slows the action of regenerative cells in the wound.[7]

◎ *Clinical Pearl*

Selecting the right dressings to balance wound moisture is the key to promoting efficient wound healing.

Finally, there are a few factors specific to the uniqueness of each client that will affect wound healing. Wounds in younger clients tend to heal more quickly than wounds in older clients. This is generally due to the presence of medical conditions, medications, and inadequate nutritional intake more likely to be found in older clients. However, when these factors are present in younger clients, the effect on wound healing is the same. Chronic

diseases, such as peripheral vascular disease and diabetes, will slow wound healing. Clients with cancer or acquired immune deficiency syndrome (AIDS), or those with autoimmune disorders who require immunosuppressive drug therapy, will also demonstrate slower wound healing.[8] Additionally, clients with chronically poor nutritional intake will demonstrate less efficient wound healing because malnutrition affects cell production, collagen synthesis, and wound contraction.[9]

Nonoperative Treatment: Basic Wound Management

With so many variables affecting wound healing, what can you do to help heal your clients' wounds? We already know that some factors affecting healing are out of both the therapist's and the client's control. However, there are a few factors that we can manipulate to facilitate more efficient wound healing. It is helpful to think of basic wound management in terms of the three hallmarks of therapy-assisted wound care: (1) wound debridement, (2) proper wound cleansing, and (3) maintenance of proper moisture balance in and around the wound.

Wound Debridement

Debridement is the removal of necrotic tissue from a wound so that healthy tissue is exposed in the wound bed. Remember, a wound will not heal as long as it contains debris. It will be stuck in the inflammatory phase of wound healing until it is clean. Dead tissue is a type of wound debris, and it can take two forms: slough or eschar. **Slough** is a moist composite of fibrin, bacteria, dead cells, and exudate. It is whitish or yellowish in color and usually somewhat adhered to the wound in the form of stringy tissue. **Eschar** is dead tissue that is usually hard and dry but will occasionally be moist in appearance. It is black in color and firmly attached to the wound.

Both slough and eschar are breeding grounds for bacteria and increase the risk of wound infection. Removal of this devitalized tissue will both speed healing and reduce the risk for wound infection, so it is generally one of the first actions that should be considered as part of the wound care plan. However, not all wounds should be debrided. Any wound in an area where blood flow is impaired should be debrided cautiously, if at all. **Precaution.** *You should always discuss with the physician any plans to debride a wound in an area with compromised circulation.*

There are four traditional methods of wound debridement: autolytic, enzymatic, sharp, and mechanical. Autolytic debridement should be the method of choice in the hand therapy clinic. Occasionally, you may need to resort to enzymatic or sharp debridement. Mechanical debridement is no longer used by most therapists and physicians, and it should be avoided.

Autolytic debridement occurs when the body breaks down necrotic tissue on its own. We can encourage this by choosing wound dressings that keep the wound moist and trap the body's natural enzymes that break down dead tissue. Film and hydrogel dressings are excellent for promoting autolytic debridement. A discussion of these and other dressings will be covered later in this chapter. Autolytic debridement is comfortable and usually effective, but it can take longer to accomplish than the other methods of debridement. Therapists should take care to maintain a proper moisture balance when using this method. A wound that is too wet can result in macerated wound edges, which is a weakening of healthy tissue around the wound caused by too much fluid absorption. Everyone has seen macerated skin; it is white, wrinkly, and fluid-logged. **Macerated** periwound skin can easily break down and cause a wound to enlarge.

Enzymatic debridement uses topical enzymes to break down slough and eschar. Therapists should check their practice laws for legal guidance on the application of topical medications. Some jurisdictions do not allow therapists to do this. The most widely used enzymatic treatment is collagenase ointment, which is sold under the brand name Santyl and is available with a physician's prescription. Collagenase ointment is applied to necrotic tissue once or twice daily and is covered with a dressing. Very dry eschar should be cross-hatched first to help the enzymes penetrate the tissue. Enzymatic debridement is **selective debridement**, in that it breaks down necrotic tissue without harming healthy granulation tissue in the wound bed. This method is very effective, but may cause some discomfort and irritation in clients who are sensitive to the enzyme.

Sharp debridement is the use of any sharp instrument, such as scissors or a scalpel, to selectively remove necrotic tissue. Again, therapists should refer to their practice laws for legal guidance on this. Some jurisdictions allow occupational and/or physical therapists to perform sharp debridement, other jurisdictions do not. Sharp debridement is the fastest and most effective method of debridement, but it should only be done by a skilled clinician. Once you cut something out, it is permanent. It can sometimes be difficult for an inexperienced therapist to distinguish between adipose tissue, slough, and tendon. If in doubt, never cut! This method of debridement can also be uncomfortable for the client and may require topical or local anesthetic. Because of these factors, many therapists defer sharp debridement to the physician.

Mechanical debridement is the removal of dead tissue using methods such as whirlpool agitation, high-pressure fluid irrigation, or wet-to-dry dressings. Wet-to-dry dressings are made by wetting gauze and inserting it into the wound. The gauze is allowed to dry inside the wound for a few days, then it is ripped out quickly so that tissue within the wound is pulled out along with the gauze. This method will, of course, remove some necrotic tissue every time it is performed. The problem is that any new granulation tissue forming in the wound bed is also pulled out with the gauze. Removing healthy tissue along with dead tissue is called **nonselective debridement**, and it is disruptive to wound healing. Mechanical debridement methods, especially wet-to-dry dressings, slow wound healing and are unnecessarily painful for clients. Therefore they are not recommended. There are much more comfortable and effective methods to debride wounds in the hand clinic.

Sometimes you will utilize a combination of debridement methods. For example, the physician may surgically remove most of the necrotic tissue, and you will then remove the rest with autolytic or enzymatic debridement. No matter what form of debridement you employ, the goal is always the same. You want to remove all devitalized tissue so that only a healthy, well-vascularized, pink-red wound bed remains.

There is one more thing to mention about preparing the wound for healing by removing unwanted tissue. A healthy wound bed is pink-red. However, there is a certain type of tissue that forms in the wound bed that is red colored but undesirable. This tissue develops when there is an overgrowth of granulation tissue, possibly due to infection or excessive moisture in the wound.[10] It is called **hypergranulation tissue**.

Hypergranulation tissue looks like shiny, deep-red balls of tissue that grow taller than the wound margins. Some therapists think it looks like little red raspberries. The tissue is soft and will often bleed easily when touched. This tissue must be treated in order for the wound to heal normally. An effective way to treat this tissue is to apply silver nitrate to the hypergranular areas.[10,11] Use silver nitrate sticks and roll the treatment end of the stick over the abnormal tissue. As you treat the tissue, it will turn gray in color. After treating with silver nitrate, you can bandage the wound as you normally would. Repeat the procedure at each dressing change until the hypergranulation tissue is controlled.

Wound Cleansing

Wounds should be cleansed every time the dressing is changed. The purpose of cleansing the wound is to remove loose debris and surface contaminants from the wound bed. Gauze fibers, loose sutures, liquefied necrotic tissue, and bacteria are all commonly found in wounds and must be washed out. Ideally, this should be done without causing trauma to any new tissue forming in the wound bed. The therapist must decide two things: (1) what solution to use to cleanse the wound, and (2) how to apply the solution.

The best solutions for cleansing wounds in the hand clinic include normal saline, sterile water, and drinkable tap water.[12] Avoid using solutions such as hydrogen peroxide, Dakin's solution, povidone iodine/Betadine, soap, or bleach on clean wounds. These solutions contain chemicals that are toxic to granulation tissue, and use of these solutions will slow wound healing. Using a product like hydrogen peroxide is only appropriate for cleaning cuts and scrapes immediately after an injury. Hydrogen peroxide is fine for cleaning a superficial *dirty wound* once or twice. However, once that wound is free of injury-related debris like dirt, asphalt, and grass, it should be cleansed with saline, sterile water, or drinkable tap water so as not to impede the healing process.

> **Clinical Pearl**
>
> A good rule of thumb is to never cleanse a *clean* wound with anything you would not be willing to put in your eye.

The method you use to apply the cleansing solution is also important. You want to use enough pressure to remove surface debris and contaminants without causing trauma to any new tissue forming in the wound bed. To date, research has failed to identify the ideal method of wound cleansing.[13] However, most practitioners have discarded the practice of whirlpool wound cleansing and replaced that method with syringe irrigation. Syringe irrigation is more convenient and carries less risk of cross-contamination between clients than whirlpool cleansing does. Much of the available literature indicates that wounds seen by the hand therapist should be irrigated with pressures at or below 8 psi.[13,14] A 35-mL medical syringe with a 25-gauge needle will produce 4 psi, and a 35-mL/19-gauge combination will produce 8 psi.[15] This equipment is readily available in most health care settings. You can cleanse all wounds in the clinic with either of these syringe/needle combinations filled with saline, sterile water, or drinkable tap water.

Maintenance of Moisture Balance: Choosing the Right Dressing

Moisture in the wound bed is critical to efficient wound healing. A moist wound will heal much faster than a wound that is either too wet or too dry. Maintaining an appropriate moisture balance depends on one thing: your choice of wound dressing. Every wound is different and will require different dressings or dressing combinations to keep it moist. If a wound has a lot of exudate, you will want to choose a dressing that can absorb the drainage. On the other hand, if a wound is too dry, you will want to choose a dressing that will add moisture to the wound bed.

Choosing the right dressing is somewhat of an art form that requires practice. The more wounds you see, the better you will get at selecting the right dressing. However, understanding the different categories of available dressings, and the characteristics of each, will help guide you.

Dressings are sometimes described as nonocclusive, semiocclusive, or totally occlusive. This nomenclature has to do with the relative ability of a dressing to block water, water vapor, and bacteria from passing through the dressing. A completely **nonocclusive dressing** will allow the free passage of water, vapor, and bacteria. A completely **occlusive dressing** will not allow any passage of water, vapor, or bacteria. A **semiocclusive dressing** falls in the middle of this continuum—generally allowing the passage of water vapor but not water or bacteria. In truth, there is no completely occlusive or completely nonocclusive dressing, but dressings are described with the term that most accurately describes their ability to keep water, vapor, and bacteria from passing through.

When occlusive dressings first arrived on the scene, many physicians feared that their use would cause infection. This myth is still prevalent in some settings. However, research has shown that occlusive dressings do *not* increase the risk for infection.[17] The goal is to find a dressing that will keep bacteria out, retain some moisture, but still absorb any excess fluid if needed.

Standard dressing choices generally fall into the following categories: transparent films, impregnated low-adherence dressings, hydrogels, hydrocolloids, gauze, foams, and alginates. There are other types of specialty dressings available, but the typical hand therapist will make their selection from these standard dressing choices. Every medical supply company has these types of dressings available, but they will be identified by different brand names. When looking for a specific type of dressing, ask your supplier for the brand names of the available dressings in that category. The dressing categories described below are listed in order from least absorptive to most absorptive.[18-21]

Transparent Films

These versatile dressings are exactly what they sound like: thin, see-through films (Fig. 17.2). Films come in a variety of shapes and sizes and easily conform to the contours of the hand. They adhere right to the skin and can be used either as a **primary**

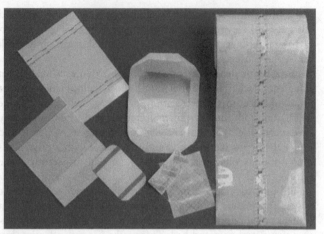

FIG. 17.2 Transparent film dressings. (*From Acute and Chronic Wounds, 2007.*)

dressing (making contact with the wound) or as a **secondary dressing** (holding a primary dressing in place). Transparent films are semiocclusive in that they are permeable to water vapor but impervious to liquids and bacteria.[19] Therefore they are waterproof in the shower and good at keeping bacteria out of the wound. One advantage of using a transparent film as a primary dressing is that it allows us to see the wound without removing the film. Additionally, films are nonabsorptive, and because these dressings hold most moisture in, they are excellent for promoting autolytic debridement of slough or moist eschar. Transparent films must be changed if too much fluid builds up under the film and starts to leak out the edges. However, dry or very-low-draining wounds can tolerate a film dressing in place for up to 7 days.

Brand names of transparent films include OpSite (Smith & Nephew), Tegaderm Transparent Film (3M), and Suresite (Medline).

Impregnated Low-Adherence Dressings

These nonocclusive to semiocclusive dressings are designed to make contact with the wound and reduce sticking and tearing of wound tissue during dressing changes. Low-adherence dressings are almost always used at the time of surgery in preparation for the first postoperative dressing change. These dressings are generally made of gauze or mesh impregnated with paraffin or a petroleum-based ointment, and they require a secondary dressing to keep them in place. A few low-adherence dressings contain antibacterial agents, and there is some evidence that application of these particular types of nonstick dressings in the operating room reduces the risk of surgical-site infections, including methicillin-resistant *Staphylococcus aureus* (MRSA) infections.[22] Impregnated low-adherence dressings are indicated for use in the hand clinic when the wound is very superficial, not draining much, and expected to heal without incident in a matter of several days. They are easy to use and conform well to the contours of the hand.

Brand names include Adaptic (Johnson & Johnson) and Xeroform (Kendall).

Hydrogels

Hydrogels are nonocclusive to semiocclusive dressings made mostly of water and are available in sheet, impregnated gauze, or gel form (Fig. 17.3). They are designed to hydrate wounds,

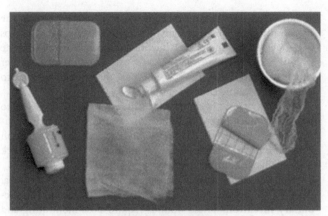

FIG. 17.3 Hydrogels.

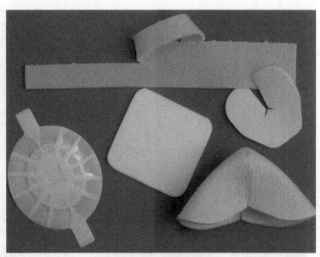

FIG. 17.4 Foam dressings.

but some newer hydrogels have additives that allow them to also absorb a little exudate while keeping wounds moist.[20] Hydrogels are very soothing and can therefore offer some pain relief. They are excellent for promoting autolytic debridement, especially of small amounts of eschar. Hydrogels, in all forms, can easily be kept in place on the hand with a secondary dressing. Hydrogels usually need to be replaced every 24 to 72 hours, but this will depend on how much exudate, if any, is being produced by the wound.

Brand names include Intrasite Gel and SoloSite Wound Gel (Smith & Nephew) and Tegaderm Hydrogel Wound Filler (3M).

Hydrocolloids

Hydrocolloid dressings are occlusive to semiocclusive and are made of ingredients like cellulose, gelatin, and pectin. Hydrocolloids create a gel-like substance over the wound bed as it absorbs exudate.[21] Some wound experts claim that this gel is resistant to bacterial growth while holding on to natural growth factors in the wound exudate that assist with efficient wound repair.[20] Hydrocolloids absorb moderate amounts of exudate while hydrating the wound bed, so they can assist in autolytic debridement. These dressings come in a variety of shapes, sizes, and thicknesses. Depending on the specific hydrocolloid, it may or may not conform well to the contours of the hand. However, hydrocolloid adhesive is stronger than in most dressings, so it can usually stand alone without a secondary dressing. The strong adhesive around the edge of the dressing helps keep fluids and bacteria from entering. Additionally, hydrocolloids feel cool and comforting to the client, so they are well received. One thing to be aware of is that hydrocolloids take on an unpleasant odor when they absorb exudate. During dressing changes, this odor is very noticeable and is sometimes mistakenly interpreted as a sign of infection.[20] When using hydrocolloids, be sure to cleanse the wound thoroughly before assessing for infection.

Brand names include DuoDERM (ConvaTec), Tegaderm Hydrocolloid (3M), and RepliCare (Smith & Nephew).

Gauze

Woven gauze is the most widely available and probably the most commonly used dressing material in the hand clinic. Every hand therapist has worked with gauze. It comes in a variety of sizes and forms, from pads to rolls. It is easy to obtain, moderately absorptive, and easy to work with. Gauze can be used to clean around wounds, to pack wounds, and to cover wounds. It can

be inexpensive to use if not many dressing changes are needed. Gauze is an important material in every hand therapist's clinic.

The problem with using gauze as a primary dressing is that it cannot easily create a moist wound environment on its own because it is relatively nonocclusive. Some therapists try to wet gauze with saline to keep wounds moist, but it is difficult to gauge how much moisture is needed to create that optimal healing environment. Often, we add too much water and end up with macerated wound edges. Other times, we add too little water and the dressing becomes dry and adhered to the wound—causing trauma to the wound bed during the next dressing change. Gauze also tends to shed its fibers. If we do not thoroughly irrigate wounds between dressing changes, fibers left behind can irritate the wound and slow healing.

When it comes to upper extremity wound care, gauze works best for loosely packing larger wound cavities and as a secondary dressing for keeping other types of dressings in place. When packing wounds, you should try to have any gauze in direct contact with the wound bed be the low-adherence impregnated type of gauze. Standard dry gauze is fine for packing the remainder of the wound cavity. When gauze is used to pack a wound, sterile gauze should be used. If gauze is used as a secondary dressing over a wound, clean gauze can be used. Sterile gauze has been processed to kill all living germs and microorganisms, and it is usually packaged in units of one dressing per package. Clean gauze is not sterile, but it is free from environmental contaminants such as dirt and other foreign material. Multiple rolls of clean gauze are usually contained within one package.

Brand names include Kerlix (Kendall) and Kling (Johnson & Johnson).

Foams

Foam dressings are made of mostly polyurethane and are used to absorb moderate amounts of exudate[21] (Fig. 17.4). Some foams can adhere directly to the wound area, while other foams require a secondary dressing to hold them in place. The thicker foams can even provide a little protective cushioning over the wound. Additionally, most are semiocclusive in that the outer cover of foam dressings is usually waterproof and will act as a bacterial barrier.[20] However, one of the difficulties with using foam dressings is that, despite the wide variety of shapes and sizes available, they never seem to conform well to the contours of the hand.

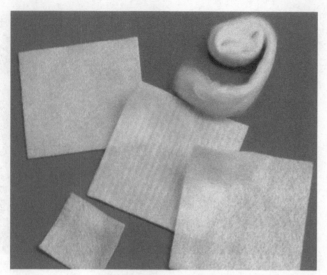

FIG. 17.5 Alginate dressings.

Brand names include Allevyn (Smith & Nephew), PolyMem (Ferris), and Mepilex (Molnlycke).

Alginates

Alginate dressings are nonocclusive to semiocclusive, highly absorbent, and made to manage moderate to large amounts of exudate (Fig. 17.5). These dressings are made primarily of seaweed derivatives, and the fibers are spun into ropes or sheets. As the alginate absorbs fluid, it is converted to a gel that provides moisture to the wound bed. Alginates always require a secondary dressing to keep them in place. Alginates conform well to the contours of the hand. In rope form, they are also great for filling small, draining wound cavities.

During dressing changes, you must be sure to irrigate the wound thoroughly to remove all of the alginate before applying a new dressing. If you find that not all the alginate has gelled, you are either changing the dressing too soon or the wound is not draining enough to warrant an alginate dressing. It is important to reserve alginates only for moderately to severely draining wounds. Using an alginate on a wound with minimal exudate will dry out the wound bed.

Brand names include AlgiSite M (Smith & Nephew), Sorbsan (Bertek), and SeaSorb (Coloplast).

Operative Treatment

Almost every wound we see in the hand clinic has first been addressed by a physician. When a client presents to a physician with a wound, the physician must decide how to best clean and prepare the wound so that it can heal. In the case of trauma-related hand wounds, the wound is often part of an environment that includes tendon and nerve injuries. Traumatic and infected wounds often need to be addressed in surgery before the client is followed by a therapist in the hand clinic. Some clients will require more than one surgical procedure to address wound issues throughout the course of hand therapy.

A common procedure performed by hand surgeons is surgical irrigation and debridement. During this procedure, the client is placed in a sterile environment within the surgical suite and administered an anesthetic. Intravenous antibiotics are usually administered during the procedure to help treat or reduce the risk of infection. The surgeon will then use a scalpel and forceps to remove any wound debris, including nonviable tissue, and the wound is thoroughly irrigated with saline. Assuming no other structures need repair, the surgeon must then decide whether to close up the wound or leave it open.

When a wound is closed with sutures or staples, it is said to heal by **primary intention.** Since the wound edges are approximated (brought together), these wounds heal by fibrous adhesion with little to no granulation tissue formation. Healing is quick and usually without incident.

When a surgeon leaves the wound open and allows it to heal through the granulation process, this is called healing by **secondary intention.** These wounds require close monitoring and skilled wound care to assure they heal without complications. Deep open wounds are traditionally loosely packed to assure they heal from the inside out. The common understanding is that if a wound is allowed to close over too early, the inside cavity is susceptible to abscess and infection. There is some evidence that wound packing may be unnecessary,[23] but more research is required to validate this assertion.

Some clinicians rely on the use of negative pressure therapy, like a vacuum-assisted closure (VAC) device, to assist with healing large open wounds. Wounds do tend to granulate better with the use of negative pressure therapy,[24] but the disadvantage for using these devices with hand wounds is that the cumbersome tubing and machine must stay attached to the hand at all times. Because this interferes so drastically with hand function, many hand therapists use VAC for only the most difficult wounds or for wounds on people who are substantially immobilized in the hospital—as in the case of severe trauma victims.

Occasionally, a surgeon will leave a wound open after the irrigation and debridement procedure with the plan to return the client to surgery for wound closure in a few days. This is known as **delayed primary wound closure**, and the wound is said to heal through **tertiary intention.** This is most commonly done for very dirty or infected wounds. The surgeon will want to wait a few days before closing the wound to make sure all infection is under control and healing is underway.

? Questions to Discuss With the Physician

Close collaboration between the referring physician and the hand therapist is strongly encouraged during hand rehabilitation, and this is especially true when wound care is part of the treatment plan. With regard to the client's wound, you will want to have the following types of discussions:

• If you start to notice any signs of infection, ask the physician to evaluate. If an infection is present, it is important to start medical treatment as soon as possible. Common wound infections include those caused by MRSA, Streptococcus pyogenes (strep), and *Pseudomonas aeruginosa.* Wound infections generally require systemic antibiotics.

• Also, know that sometimes a wound will not heal and no one suspects infection because the wound is not red, inflamed, odorous, or draining pus. Although typical signs of infection are usually present, occasionally the only sign of infection is the nonhealing wound. If wound healing stops progressing for a couple of weeks, contact the physician and discuss the possibility of infection. The physician may want to culture the wound to see if it is indeed infected.

- If there is an infection, ask if it is okay to move the joints surrounding the infected area. Some physicians will want to limit movement until an infection is controlled, for fear of spreading the infection. It depends on the physician, the type of the infection, and the severity of the infection.
- If debridement is necessary, discuss the type of debridement you plan to perform.
- Autolytic debridement should be your first choice, but the physician will need to know that this type of debridement may take some time to complete. If the physician wants faster debridement, then you will need to discuss either enzymatic or sharp debridement. Enzymatic debridement requires a prescription enzyme. Sharp debridement may require a topical anesthetic. If you are at all uncomfortable or feel you do not have the skill to perform sharp debridement, you must speak up. Sharp debridement may need to be performed by the physician.
- If the wound is covered with eschar, but the underlying tissue has decreased circulation, discuss the pros and cons of debridement with the physician. In the case of poor blood flow to the wound area, immediate debridement is not always a good idea. Other medical interventions, like revascularization surgery, may need to be considered first.
- It is also worth noting that debridement of uninfected dry fingertip necrosis caused by vascular insufficiency, such as in clients with Raynaud disease, systemic lupus erythematosus, and scleroderma, is rarely performed. In these unfortunate cases, the usual course of treatment is to allow the fingertip to autoamputate.
- If a physician asks for a less-than-ideal wound treatment, offer a wound care plan that meets the current standard of care. There is usually more than one way to accomplish wound care goals.
- Therapists still get orders for wet-to-dry dressings and for whirlpool treatments. In these instances, you have a responsibility as a licensed clinician to discuss better alternatives for wound debridement and cleansing with the physician. Once a physician is aware of more effective and safer options, they will almost always agree with your plan of care.
- If a wound just is not healing and infection has been ruled out, discuss the client's lab work with the physician.

The following lab values are indicators of malnutrition or poorly controlled blood sugar and may indicate that nutritional status is interfering with wound healing[11]:

Serum albumin levels below 3.5 g/dL
Serum prealbumin levels below 16 mg/dL
Serum transferrin levels below 170 mg/dL
Total lymphocyte count (TLC) below 1800/mm^3
Blood glucose levels greater than 110 mg/dL

While malnutrition is a rare factor in clients coming to an outpatient hand clinic, you may see malnutrition interfering with wound healing in hospitalized patients or residents of long-term care facilities. When nutrition might be a factor in poor wound healing, a dietitian should be part of the care team.

( ) What to Say to Clients

You will want to give your clients as much information as possible so that they become partners in the wound-healing effort. Many clients have misconceptions about wound healing, but once educated, most will do everything possible to help their wounds heal.

The following topics should be discussed with every client who has a wound.

Schedule for Dressing Changes

As the therapist, you will decide how frequently to change the dressing(s). If you see clients in an outpatient setting, you will decide if the dressing changes will be done at home or in the clinic. Many things factor into your decision: how much the wound is draining, which dressings you plan to use, the client's anxiety about the wound, the client's ability to follow directions, support systems available to the client, and reimbursement issues. The more wounds you treat, the better you will get at making this decision.

Once you decide how often the dressing(s) should be changed, clearly communicate this to your client. Make it very clear that the dressing(s) should not be changed more frequently unless they become soiled or saturated. In the event that the dressing(s) must be changed early, have a plan and communicate this to your client. If your client is an outpatient, decide if the client should come into the clinic for a dressing change or if they should go ahead and change the dressing(s) at home. You can say, "I am going to see you back here in the clinic in a couple of days. I want you to keep the dressing(s) clean and dry. If the drainage from your wound starts to seep through the dressing(s), or if you accidentally get your dressing(s) wet or very dirty, I want you to call me as soon as possible so that we can have you come in for a dressing change."

Cleansing

One of the biggest misconceptions therapists encounter has to do with wound cleansing. If your client will be doing dressing changes at home, make it very clear that only saline, sterile water, or drinkable tap water should be used to cleanse the wound. Many clients are surprised to learn that hydrogen peroxide or soap should not be used to cleanse open wounds. Educate your clients that using these substances will slow the healing process by killing healthy cells that build granulation tissue. Because we do not give out needles and syringes for home wound cleansing, clients performing home dressing changes usually cleanse their wounds with drinkable tap water running slowly from the faucet or a squeeze-bottle contact lens saline solution. Tell your clients, "I want you to rinse your wound well every time you change your dressing. Put your hand under warm (not hot) slow-running tap water, or rinse the wound by squeezing contact lens saline solution from a bottle. Rinse the wound for 30 seconds. Do not use anything else to clean your wound. Some things, like hydrogen peroxide and soap, actually slow down healing by killing 'good' cells that are helping close the wound."

Moist Wound Healing

The second biggest misconception that therapists encounter concerns moist wound healing. Most of us were taught as children to expose our wounds to the air and sun in order to dry them. Our parents and grandparents told us that this would help our wounds heal faster. We now know that this could not be farther from the truth. You must educate your clients on the efficacy of moist wound healing. All you usually need to say is, "Research has shown that moist wounds heal faster than dry wounds, and moist wound healing occurs when wounds stay covered. Keep your dressing on and try not to change it any more often than we have discussed."

> ○ **Clinical Pearl**
>
> If you need help convincing your client to keep their wound covered, let them know that a moist wound heals with less scarring, and therefore will look better when fully healed.[25] Many clients care a lot about cosmesis, and will adhere to a plan of care that is more likely to result in a better-looking scar.

Hygiene

Clients need to know that it is important for their dressings to stay clean and dry between dressing changes (unless you are using a waterproof dressing, like a transparent film). Most dressings are not waterproof and must be covered by a plastic bag during bathing. A wet dressing is a breeding ground for bacteria and can cause maceration of the skin around the wound. Clients who are sports enthusiasts should also be cautioned about exercising. Body sweat can saturate a dressing from the inside out. *Whatever the cause, a dressing that is wet to the touch must be changed.* Tell your client, "You must keep your dressing dry to help avoid infection and skin breakdown. Cover it with plastic in the shower, and try to avoid house-cleaning tasks that involve water. Also, avoid activities that will cause you to sweat a lot. Sweating can make your dressing wet from the inside out. Just remember—if your dressing is wet to the touch, it must be changed."

Additionally, although dressings are designed to keep debris and bacteria out of the wound, clients must use common sense in their daily activities. Not many upper extremity dressings can withstand the stress of activities like cleaning the garage, working in the yard, or changing the oil in the car. If a dressing gets too dirty or too worn from activity, there is an increased risk for wound infection. *A dirty or damaged dressing must be changed.* Say, "You must protect your dressing from damage to reduce the risk for infection. Avoid heavy hand use for things like cleaning, working in the yard, or working with heavy equipment. If your dressing gets dirty or worn, it must be changed."

> ○ **Clinical Pearl**
>
> Teach your clients this trick for keeping dressings dry in the shower: Wrap the hand/dressing in a small towel before covering everything with a plastic bag. Seal the plastic bag around the arm with hypoallergenic tape. If any water leaks inside the bag, it will be absorbed by the towel, not the dressing!

Cigarette Smoke

If your client smokes cigarettes, you should educate them that nicotine decreases the delivery of oxygen to tissues and can increase the risk for wound-healing complications.[26] Smoking just one cigarette can reduce blood flow to the hand.[3] You should encourage your clients to temporarily stop smoking until their wound is healed. However, for many clients, this is not a realistic expectation. If you get the sense that your client will not stop smoking during the wound-healing process, you should tell your client that if they cannot stop smoking entirely, there may be some benefit in cutting back on the number of cigarettes smoked per day. Most clients are willing to at least cut back on smoking until their wound is healed. You can say, "I am not going to give you a lecture about smoking, but you should know that your wound will heal better if you stop—or at least cut back—on your smoking until your wound is healed. Smoking just one cigarette decreases oxygen to the hand, and your wound needs all the oxygen it can get to heal."

Diet

Although we are not dieticians, we can encourage our clients with wounds to eat well and drink plenty of fluids. Tell your clients, "Try to eat a balanced diet and drink plenty of water right now. Nutrition plays an important role in wound healing. Your wound especially needs protein to heal."

Signs and Symptoms of Infection

All clients should be educated about the signs and symptoms of infection. If a client does have any indication that an infection may be present, encourage them to call the physician immediately. You should use plain and simple language with your clients. Say, "These are the signs and symptoms of infection that I want you to watch for: feeling generally unwell, running a fever, increased pain in the wound area, redness around the wound, red streaks leading away from the wound, warmth in the wound area, a bad odor coming from the wound, or any discharge that is white, thick, and yellow or greenish/blue." Tell your clients not to be shy about reporting a possible infection because it is important to catch infections early. Say, "If you suspect you have an infection, call your doctor or me right away—even if you are not sure. I would rather you be safe than sorry. Wound infections can be serious and we must catch and treat them early."

> **Evaluation Tips**

Wound evaluation is important for treatment planning, for documenting the progression of wound healing, and for communicating with other caregivers. You must know what you are looking at and how to record it. Additionally, your assessment methods and terminology must remain consistent in order to accurately track progress. Never rely on your memory to gauge the progress of a wound. Wound evaluation is the basis for every intervention you choose, so the wound must be evaluated at every dressing change.

A good evaluation of an upper extremity wound will include the following:
- The location and size of the wound
- The condition of the periwound skin and wound margins
- Wound characteristics (for example, granulation tissue, hypergranulation tissue, debris, or dead tissue)
- The amount of wound exudate
- Any signs or symptoms of infection

Location and Size of Wound

When describing the location of a wound, do so in terms of anatomical position. For example, "The wound is on the anterior medial aspect of the distal forearm, 2 cm proximal to the pisiform." The more precise you can be, the better.

The size of the wound is usually recorded in millimeters or centimeters. Size is described in terms of length, width, and depth. There are a couple of ways to measure length and width. Some therapists will sit across from their client and view the wound in terms of a clock face. The length of the wound would be the measurement from 12 o'clock to 6 o'clock; the width of the wound would be the measurement from 9 o'clock to 3 o'clock. Another way to measure length and width is to measure the longest proximal to distal points of the wound, and then the widest medial to lateral points of the wound. Whichever way you choose to measure wound length and width, always do it the same way. This will assure consistency of comparative wound size over time.

Wound depth is measured by inserting a moistened sterile cotton-tipped applicator (that is, a sterile cotton swab) into the deepest part of the wound. Next, slide your gloved fingers down the length of the applicator until your fingers are at the level of the surrounding intact skin. Keep holding the applicator in this spot while lifting the applicator out of the wound. Measure the distance between the tips of your fingers to the tip of the cotton applicator. This is your wound depth.

Occasionally, in the forearm or upper arm, you will notice that a wound is very deep in a particular direction. If you gently try to push a moistened sterile cotton-tipped applicator into this area, you will note a narrow and deep hole—like a small tunnel that runs away from the main part of the wound. This is a condition called **tunneling.** Tunnels create open areas called "dead space" and increase the risk of abscess formation, so you want to keep the tunnel very clean. Record the depth of the tunnel as the distance that the sterile applicator can be gently inserted into the hole. Record the location of the tunnel using the clock face method. For example, "There is a 3 cm tunnel at 7 o'clock."

Condition of Periwound Skin and Wound Margins

When you look at the edges of the wound, you want to note its color and condition. Healthy wound margins look pink and flat. This tells you that epithelial tissue is being generated at the wound margins and that the wound is healing normally. If the wound margins appear grey or slightly turned under, that is a sign that the wound is not healing in a timely or efficient manner.

Wound margins should be firmly attached to the tissue underneath. If you notice that there is space under the wound edge, this is known as **undermining.** Undermining is another sign that the wound is not healing efficiently. There is a breakdown of tissue under the wound margins, and the result is a relatively smaller wound opening with a larger wound underneath. It is difficult to see undermining, so if you do not clearly see that the wound edges are attached to the wound, try to gently slip a moistened sterile cotton-tipped applicator horizontally under the wound edge. If you have undermining, record the depth of the undermining as the distance that the sterile applicator can be pushed under the wound edge. Record the location of the undermining using the clock face method. For example, "There is 1 cm of undermining between 4 and 7 o'clock."

The skin around the wound, or **periwound skin,** should be skin-colored or maybe a little pink. Redness, inflammation, or hardening of the periwound skin could indicate infection. Small lesions of the periwound skin could indicate damage from adhesive dressings. If the periwound skin is soft and white, this indicates that the skin has absorbed too much fluid. We call this **macerated skin,** and it is the result of wound exudate not being adequately absorbed by the wound dressing. Macerated skin is fragile and easily damaged. If the epidermis around the wound starts to break down, we call this **denuded skin.**

Wound Characteristics

One of the simplest ways to describe the wound itself is to use the "red-yellow-black" system. To use this method, simply estimate what percentage of the wound is covered by each color. For example, "The wound is 50% red, 25% yellow, and 25% black." In this system, red represents a healthy wound bed, yellow represents slough, and black represents eschar. This is a common method of describing wounds, and many health care professionals who treat wounds understand this terminology.

Digital photos are extremely helpful in documenting what the wound and periwound skin looks like. When using a digital camera to record wound-healing progression, be as consistent as possible with your picture-taking technique. For example, always taking the picture after cleansing and/or debriding the wound. Use the same camera and camera settings for all photos, and try to take the picture from the same distance and angle every time. Always include a client identifier, date, and scale reference (like a centimeter tape measure) in every picture. Finally, try to approximate the same lighting conditions for each picture if possible.

> ### ⊙ Clinical Pearl
>
> Do not use a flash when using a digital camera to record the image of a wound. You will be able to see more detail when the flash is turned off.

Wound Exudate

Wound exudate should be described in terms of type and amount. Terms used to describe the type of exudate are based on the color and consistency of the discharge. Color can range from clear to red to tan to green. Consistency can range from thin and watery to very thick and creamy. The following terms to describe exudate are commonly used and well understood by health care professionals:

- Serous—clear and watery. This is normal.
- Serosanguinous—thin and pink. This is normal.
- Sanguinous—thin and bright red. This may or may not be normal, depending on the amount and type of tissue in the wound bed.
- Purulent—thick or thin, tan to yellow. This is a sign of possible infection.
- Foul purulent—thick, yellow to green, bad odor. This is a sign of infection.

Remember if you are using a hydrocolloid dressing, you will notice a thick, foul-smelling gel during dressing changes. This is normal and needs to be cleansed away before you can assess for foul purulent discharge.

The amount of wound exudate can range from none to large amounts. Describing the amount of drainage is subjective, but the following terms are typical:

- None—dry wound
- Scant amount—wound is moist but not draining
- Minimal amount or moderate amount—easily managed with your standard dressing choices
- Large amount—requires alginate dressing to control drainage
- Copious amount—so much drainage that it is difficult to manage with any dressing; this is rare

Infection

The cardinal signs and symptoms of infection include increased pain, foul odor, purulent drainage (pus), **erythema** (redness), **calor** (warmth), **induration** (hardening) around the wound, **lymphangitic streaking** (red streaks), **malaise** (feeling unwell), and **febricity** (fever). When documenting signs and symptoms of infection, it is acceptable and common to use lay terms so that what you are seeing is very clear to all members of the team. Only the physician can formally diagnose an infection. However, you are the care provider who sees the wound most often. It is your responsibility to assess for signs and symptoms of infection every time you see your client. If you have any indication that a wound is infected during your assessment, this should be immediately reported to the referring physician.

◎ Clinical Pearl

Not all infections smell bad. A wound that smells sweet and has a distinctive neon-green discharge is very likely infected with *Pseudomonas aeruginosa*.

Diagnosis-Specific Information That Affects Clinical Reasoning

In summary of what we have already learned in this chapter, clinical reasoning in wound care is guided by the following principles:

1. Moist wound healing is the standard of care. Choose the right dressing(s) to create a moist wound environment.
2. A wound will not heal until it is free of anything that should not be there: dead tissue, dressing debris, hypergranulation tissue, and so on. Strive to create a wound bed that is a healthy pink-red in color.
3. The regenerating wound bed is fragile. Do not stress a healing wound with cytotoxic chemicals, high-pressure irrigation, or dressings that stick to the wound bed.
4. Infection must be identified and addressed early. Assess for infection at every dressing change and report any signs to the physician immediately.
5. Above all, do no harm. Never cut anything from an open wound that has not been positively identified.

♡ Tips from the Field

If you are able to assimilate everything presented in this chapter, you will have the basic skills necessary to care for your clients' upper extremity wounds. However, here are a few more pieces of advice:

1. Keep in mind that even if wound care is legally within your scope of practice, you still must be competent to provide the service. Most licensing laws include language stating that therapists must be competent to perform any service within their scope of practice. No one wants to find themselves in front of a licensing board or jury box supporting a claim of competence to provide wound care services, but this does happen. Most of us get very little information about wound care in school. Therefore you will want to gain additional knowledge and skill in this area through postprofessional continuing education courses and/or mentorship. Keep all documentation of your training in wound care in a safe place.

2. Keep the lines of communication open with your referring physicians. Ask for help if you need it and educate when you must. Never allow yourself to be pressured into providing a wound care procedure that you know is not the standard of care.
3. It is absolutely critical to keep exposed tendons moist. Hydrogel in gel form works great for this. If a tendon is allowed to dry, it will be damaged beyond repair. Monitor these clients closely.

➢ Precautions and Concerns

When you perform wound care procedures, you will want to keep yourself and your clients safe from cross-contamination by using **standard precautions.** *Standard precautions are basic infection prevention guidelines and include the following: (1) hand hygiene, (2) use of personal protective equipment, (3) proper cleaning and use of medical equipment, (4) and proper environmental cleaning.*[27]

You should perform proper hand hygiene before and after donning gloves for a wound care procedure. Using alcohol-based hand rub is the preferred method of hand decontamination except when your hands are visibly soiled, in which case soap and water should be used. During the wound care procedure, you should wear whatever personal protective equipment is needed to protect you from contact with your clients' body fluids. This will always include clean or sterile gloves, and may include disposable gowns, face masks/shields, and goggles. Any medical equipment that will come in contact with the wound itself (for example, scalpels, forceps) should be single use or properly sterilized between clients. Equipment that will not come in contact with the wound (such as bandage scissors) should be disinfected between clients. Finally, all tabletops and client chair armrests should be disinfected between clients.

There has been a long-standing debate in the literature regarding the use of sterile gloves versus nonsterile (clean) gloves for clinical wound care outside of the surgical suite. A majority of the evidence suggests that there is no difference in infection rates or wound healing based on the use of either sterile or clean gloves.[28] However, proponents of using sterile gloves will point out that the evidence is not clearly convincing, and recommend erring on the side of caution by using sterile gloves for all dressing changes.[29] More research is needed in this area. Many hand therapists use clean gloves for all but their most high-risk clients. Sterile gloves should always be used if a client is immune compromised, has a resistant infection, or has a history of multiple infections.

One thing that you can do to reduce the chance of contaminating a wound is to apply dressings using a "no-touch" technique. It works like this:

- Don a pair of clean gloves, and remove your client's "dirty" dressing.
- Remove your gloves, decontaminate your hands with an alcohol-based hand rub, and then apply a fresh pair of gloves.
- Do not touch anything except the new dressing materials and a decontaminated pair of bandage scissors.

This technique works best with an assistant present to open the dressing packaging. After your assistant opens the packaging, you can reach in and grab the sterile dressing that will make contact with your client's wound. Only a sterile dressing should make contact with the wound bed. You don't

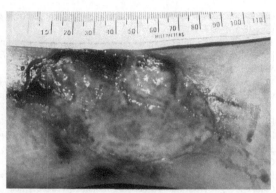

FIG. 17.6 Upper extremity wound resulting from trauma.

want to open the package yourself because the outside of the package may be contaminated, but the inside of the package will be sterile. After the wound bed is covered with the sterile dressing, any secondary dressing that is required can be clean/nonsterile. However, continue with the no-touch technique until all the dressings have been applied.

> **◎ Clinical Pearl**
>
> If you do not have anyone to assist you with dressing changes, you can still do a no-touch technique by gloving-up and carefully opening all packaging to expose the new dressings inside. Do not touch the new dressing material at this point. Place the open packages on a clean surface. Then, remove your gloves, decontaminate your hands, and apply fresh gloves. Now, the packages will be open so that you can reach over and grab the new dressings as needed.

CASE STUDY

Wound Assessment ■

Fig. 17.6 represents a typical upper extremity wound resulting from trauma. Wounds like this can be seen on the forearms of clients who have been in high-speed motorcycle accidents. Upon presentation, you note the wound to be tricolored (although you cannot see it in

this black-and-white picture!). It contains approximately 80% slough (yellow), 15% eschar (black), and 5% granulation tissue (pink-red). The wound appears to be very superficial, although you will not know for sure that there is no tunneling or cavities under the eschar until the black tissue has been removed. When documenting the size of this wound, measure the longest proximal to distal point of the wound and call that the wound "length." Then, measure the widest medial to lateral point of the wound and call that the wound "width." The periwound skin looks healthy—a pinkish tan color. There is little discharge, and the wound does not have a foul odor. Based on these observations, you would not suspect a wound infection at this point.

Treatment Planning

In order for this wound to heal, you must remove the eschar and slough from the wound bed. Your goal is to remove all dead tissue until only healthy pink-red granulation tissue is present. The safest and easiest way to try to remove the eschar and slough is through autolytic debridement. You can encourage the body to break down its own dead tissue by choosing a dressing that keeps the wound moist. At first, there will be some trial and error as you look for the most effective dressing. Because this wound is superficial and has little discharge, you might first try applying a transparent film over the wound. Irrigate the wound well with sterile saline, pat it dry with a sterile piece of gauze, and then use a "no-touch" technique to apply the transparent film. Your client should keep this dressing in place until they return in 3 to 5 days. Transparent films are waterproof in the shower, so your client may shower with the dressing in place. When your client returns to the clinic, remove the transparent film and note how much of the dead tissue has liquefied under the dressing. Irrigate the wound with saline and decide on the most appropriate dressing to try next. If there has been little change in the amount of eschar and slough, you need to add moisture and might consider a little hydrogel under the transparent film. If there was a lot of liquification of dead tissue under the film and the periwound skin is turning white, the wound is now too wet. You may need to change the film dressing more frequently. At each dressing change, continue to choose dressings based on the amount of moisture in and around the wound. Once the eschar and slough are gone, continue to use dressings that keep the wound moist until it is completely healed. Monitor for any sign of infection or nonhealing at each dressing change, and report these situations to the referring physician.

References

1. American Occupational Therapy Association: The role of occupational therapy in wound management, *Am J Occup Ther* 72(Suppl 2):7212410057, 2018. Downloaded from http://ajot.aota.org. [Accessed 16 December 2018].
2. News Now Staff, American Physical Therapy Association: New APTA resource on active wound care management available online, PT in Motion for members of the American Physical Therapy Association (website). http://www.apta.org/PTinMotion/NewsNow/2011/7/14/WoundManagementFAQs/. [Accessed 2 July 2012].
3. Mosely LH, Finseth F: Cigarette smoking: impairment of digital blood flow and wound healing in the hand, *Hand* 9(2):97–101, 1977.
4. Wilson JR, Mills JG, Prather ID, et al.: A toxicity index of skin and wound cleansers used in vitro fibroblasts and keratinocytes, *Adv Skin Wound Care* 18:373–378, 2005.
5. Alvarez OM, Rogers RS, Booker JG, et al.: Effect of noncontact normothermic wound therapy on the healing of neuropathic (diabetic) foot ulcers: an interim analysis of 20 patients, *J Foot Ankle Surg* 42:30–35, 2003.
6. McGuiness W, Vella E, Harrison D: Influence of dressing changes on wound temperature, *J Wound Care* 13:383–385, 2004.
7. Okan D, Woo K, Ayello EA, et al.: The role of moisture balance in wound healing, *Adv Skin Wound Care* 20:39–53, 2007.
8. Hess CT: Checklist for factors affecting wound healing, *Adv Skin Wound Care* 24:192, 2011.
9. Langemo D, Anderson J, Hanson D, et al.: Nutritional considerations in wound care, *Adv Skin Wound Care* 19:297–303, 2006.
10. Hampton S: Understanding overgranulation in tissue viability practice, *Br J Community Nurse* 12:S24–S30, 2007.
11. Myers BA: *Wound management: principles and practice*, New Jersey, 2004, Prentice Hall.
12. Fernandez R, Griffiths R: Water for wound cleansing, *Cochrane Database Syst Rev* 15:CD003861, 2012.
13. Chatterjee JS: A critical review of irrigation techniques in acute wounds, *Int Wound J* 2:258–265, 2005.
14. Hess CT: *Wound care*, ed 5, Philadelphia, 2005, Lippincott, Williams & Wilkins.

15. Stevenson TR, Thacker JG, Rodeheaver GT, et al.: Cleansing the traumatic wound by high pressure syringe irrigation, *JACEP* 5(1):17–21, 1976.

16. US Department of Health and Human Services: Quick Reference Guide for Clinicians: Pressure Ulcer Treatment Clinical Practice Guideline, HHS.Gov Archive (Online Archive from 1994 December 21): http://archive.hhs.gov/news/press/1994pres/941221a.txt. Accessed May 6, 2013.

17. Panuncialman J, Falanga V: The science of wound bed preparation, *Surg Clin N Am* 89:611–626, 2009.

18. Fulton JA, Blasiole KN, Cottingham T, et al.: Wound dressing absorption: a comparative study, *Adv Skin Wound Care* 25:315–320, 2012.

19. Worley CA: So, what do I put on this wound? Making sense of the wound dressing puzzle: part III, *Medsurg Nursing* 15:251–252, 2006.

20. Worley CA: So, what do I put on this wound? Making sense of the wound dressing puzzle: part II, *Medsurg Nursing* 15:182–183, 2006.

21. Worley CA: So, what do I put on this wound? Making sense of the wound dressing puzzle: part I, *Medsurg Nursing* 15:106–107, 2006.

22. Mueller SW, Krebsbach LE: Impact of an anti-microbial-impregnated gauze dressing on surgical site infections including methicillin-resistant Staphylococcus aureus infections, *Am J Infect Control* 36:651–655, 2008.

23. Kessler DO, Krantz BS, Mojica M: Randomized trial comparing wound packing to no wound packing following incision and drainage of superficial skin abscesses in the pediatric emergency department, *Pediatr Emerg Care* 28:514–517, 2012.

24. Taylor CJ, Chester DL, Jeffery SL: Functional splinting of upper limb injuries with gauze-based topical negative pressure wound therapy, *J Hand Surgery* 36:1848–1851, 2011.

25. Wigger-Alberti W, Kuhlmann M, Ekanayake S, et al.: Using a novel wound model to investigate the healing properties of products for superficial wounds, *J Wound Care* 18(3):123–128, 2009. 131.

26. Bartsch RH, Weiss G, Kastenbauer T, et al.: Crucial aspects of smoking in wound healing after breast reduction surgery, *J Plast Reconstr Aesthet Surg* 60:1045–1049, 2007.

27. Centers for Disease Control and Prevention: Guide to Infection Prevention for Outpatient Settings: Minimum Expectations for Safe Care, CDC.gov Healthcare-Associated Infections (Website Article Written May 2011): http://www.cdc.gov/HAI/settings/outpatient/outpatient-care-guidelines.html. Accessed August 13, 2012.

28. Flores A: Sterile versus non-sterile glove use and aseptic technique, *Nurs Stand* 23(6):35–39, 2008.

29. St Clair K, Larrabee JH: Clean versus sterile gloves: which to use for postoperative dressing changes? *Outcomes Manag* 6(1):17–21, 2002.

18 Common Shoulder Diagnoses

Mark Butler

Introduction

Positioning the hand in space to allow for interaction with the environment is the primary function of the shoulder. Accordingly, dysfunction of the shoulder complex often results in profound impairment of the entire upper extremity (UE).[1] The shoulder will compensate for decreased mobility of the wrist and elbow, which can lead to shoulder dysfunction as the individual tries to perform normal activities of daily living (ADLs). *When treating a client with elbow or wrist dysfunction, the therapist needs to monitor the health of the shoulder.* Therefore a thorough understanding of the shoulder is imperative for therapists treating clients with UE dysfunction.

◎ Clinical Pearl

The shoulder has the greatest range of motion (ROM) of any joint in the body. This ROM is the result of the aggregate movement of a series of articulations that comprise the shoulder complex. These articulations work in concert to provide a unique balance between mobility and stability, with the emphasis on mobility. A shift in this balance often results in (or can be caused by) the pathological processes we will review in this chapter.

Anatomy

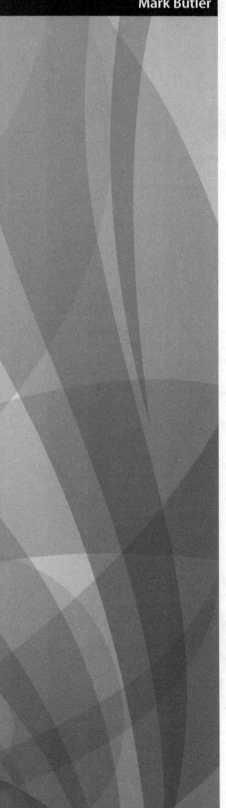

The shoulder complex consists of:
- three bones: the humerus, the clavicle, and the scapula
- three joints: the glenohumeral (GH), acromioclavicular (AC), and sternoclavicular (SC)
- one "pseudo joint": the scapulothoracic (ST) articulation

Glenohumeral Joint

The GH joint is a multiaxial, synovial, ball-and-socket joint that moves around three axes of motion: internal/external rotation around a vertical axis, abduction/adduction around a sagittal axis, and flexion/extension around a frontal axis (Fig. 18.1). The humeral head forms roughly half a sphere, with the glenoid fossa forming the socket component of the joint. The glenoid fossa covers only one-third to one-fourth of the humeral head (Fig. 18.2). The glenoid labrum, a ring of fibrocartilage, surrounds and deepens the glenoid socket by about 50% and increases joint stability by increasing humeral head contact 75% vertically and 56 % transversely.[2]

The **open packed position** (joint position in which the capsule and ligaments are most lax and separation of joint surfaces are greatest) of the GH joint is 55 degrees of abduction and 30 degrees of horizontal adduction. The **close packed position** (joint position in which the capsule and ligaments are under the most tension with maximal contact between joint surfaces) of the joint is full abduction and lateral rotation. At rest, the humerus sits centered in the glenoid cavity; with contraction of the rotator cuff (RC) muscles, the humeral head translates anteriorly, posteriorly, superiorly, inferiorly, or any combination of these movements. These translations are very small, but full motion of the GH joint is impossible without them, as the combined actions of the RC muscles contribute to the overall stability of the GH joint during ROM.[3] It is the motion of the GH joint that contributes the most to shoulder movement.

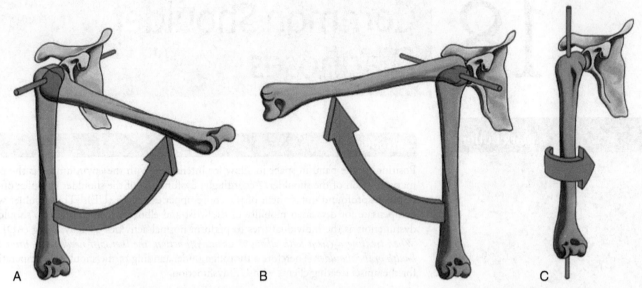

A   B   C

FIG. 18.1 The three degrees of freedom of the glenohumeral joint. (A) Flexion/extension. (B) abduction/adduction. (C) internal/external rotation. *(From Standring S. Gray's Anatomy. (e-book) 40th ed. St Louis, MO: Churchill Livingstone; 2012.)*

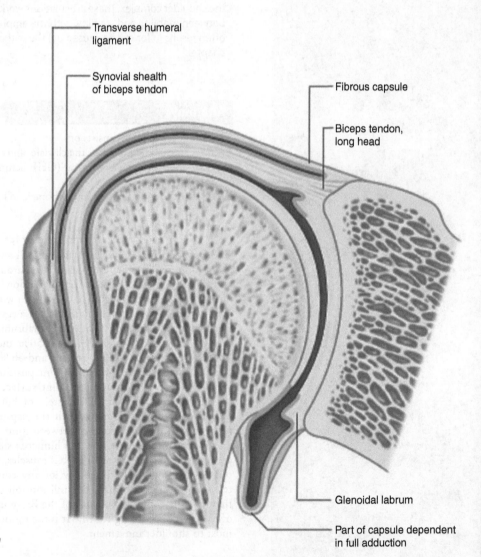

Transverse humeral ligament

Synovial shealth of biceps tendon

Fibrous capsule

Biceps tendon, long head

Glenoidal labrum

Part of capsule dependent in full adduction

FIG. 18.2 Coronal section of the left shoulder joint through the long head of the biceps tendon. *(From Putz R, Pabst R. Sobotta—Atlas of Human Anatomy Single Volume Edition: Head, Neck, Upper Limb, Thorax, Abdomen, Pelvis, Lower Limb. 14th ed. St Louis, MO: Elsevier; 2008.)*

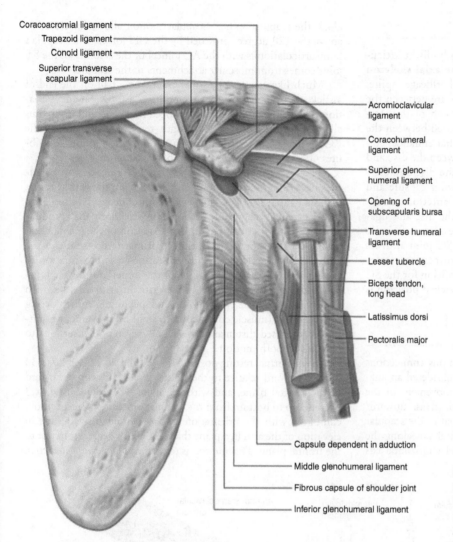

Coracoacromial ligament
Trapezoid ligament
Conoid ligament
Superior transverse scapular ligament

Acromioclavicular ligament
Coracohumeral ligament
Superior gleno-humeral ligament
Opening of subscapularis bursa
Transverse humeral ligament
Lesser tubercle
Biceps tendon, long head
Latissimus dorsi
Pectoralis major

Capsule dependent in adduction
Middle glenohumeral ligament
Fibrous capsule of shoulder joint
Inferior glenohumeral ligament

FIG. 18.3 Anterior aspect of the left shoulder showing the joint capsule and acromioclavicular ligaments. *(From Standring S. Gray's Anatomy. (e-book) 40th ed. St Louis, MO: Churchill Livingstone; 2012, p. 802.)*

Acromioclavicular Joint

The AC joint is a **plane synovial joint** (joint with a synovium lined capsule and relatively flat surfaces) that augments the ROM of the GH joint as this is the joint around which the scapula moves. The bones that comprise the AC joint are the acromion process of the scapula and the distal end of the clavicle. The AC joint moves around three axes resulting in three **degrees of freedom** (direction or type of motion at a joint): pure spin around a longitudinal axis for abduction/adduction of the shoulder, a vertical axis for protraction/retraction of the shoulder, and a horizontal axis for shoulder elevation/depression.

The AC and coracoclavicular (CC) ligaments support the AC joint (Fig. 18.3). The AC ligaments contribute the least to joint stability; they function mainly to support the joint capsule and check anterior/posterior translation of the clavicle on the acromion. The AC ligaments are damaged in grade I shoulder separations. The CC ligaments have no attachment to the acromion and consist of the conoid and trapezoid ligaments. They transmit scapular motion to the clavicle and check superior clavicular displacement.[4] As all fibers of the upper trapezius insert on the clavicle,[5] the CC ligaments play an integral role in the transmission of force from the upper trapezius to the scapula.[6] Complete rupture of these ligaments represents a grade III separation, resulting in a step deformity at the AC joint (Fig. 18.4).

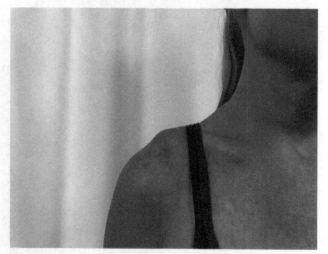

FIG. 18.4 Chronic grade III acromioclavicular separation showing step deformity indicating disruption of the coracoclavicular ligaments.

The open packed position for the AC joint is with the arm by the side. The close packed position is at 90 degrees of shoulder abduction.

Sternoclavicular Joint

The sellar (saddle) shaped SC joint is the only direct articulation between the shoulder complex and the **axial skeleton** (skeletal components consisting of the skull, ribcage, spine, and pelvis). The articulations of the SC joint are between the medial end of the clavicle, the clavicular notch of the sternum, and the cartilage of the first rib. Interposed between the clavicle and the sternum is an articular disc that enhances stability of the joint (Fig. 18.5). Movement between the disc and clavicle is greater than movement between the disc and sternum. The joint is further stabilized by the joint capsule and ligaments that primarily check superior and anterior translation.[7] The SC joint is stabilized so well by the disc and ligaments that trauma to the clavicle usually results in fracture instead of dislocation.[8] The motion of the SC joint mirrors that of the AC joint: elevation/depression, protraction/retraction, and rotation (spin). The open packed position for the SC joint is with the arm by the side. The close packed position is full UE elevation.

Scapulothoracic Articulation

As the scapula has no direct bony or ligamentous connections to the thorax, the ST articulation cannot be considered an anatomical joint. Scapular movement results in movement of the shoulder girdle. These movements are described as: upward/downward rotation around an axis perpendicular to the scapular body, internal/external rotation around a vertical axis along the medial border, and anterior/posterior tilt around a horizontal axis

along the scapular spine.[9] Scapular motion allows for elevation above the 120 degrees provided by the GH joint.[2] The scapula's bony articulation is with the AC joint, but the stability of the ST joint comes from muscular attachments to the scapula.

Much like a street performer balancing a ball on the end of a stick, the scapula must change position during shoulder elevation to keep the humeral head balanced in the glenoid fossa, thus allowing for the most efficient length–tension relationship of the RC. With shoulder elevation, scapulothoracic motion contributes 40 to 50 degrees to humerothoracic elevation.[10]

This movement of the scapula is the result of **force couples** between groups of muscles that run from the thorax to the scapula (Table 18.1). A force couple is defined as two resultant forces of equal magnitude in opposite directions that produce rotation of a structure. The upward rotation of the scapula that occurs during shoulder elevation is primarily the result of the **concentric** (muscle contraction resulting in approximation of the origin and insertion) actions of the upper and lower trapezius and the lower portion of the serratus anterior muscles, with the levator scapulae, rhomboids and pectoralis minor acting **eccentrically** (muscle contraction to stabilize movement resulting in increased distance between the origin and insertion) to produce smooth motion.

In the normal resting position the scapula sits angled 20 to 30 degrees forward relative to the frontal plane, 20 degrees forward in the sagittal plane, and with the medial boarder angled at 3 degrees top to bottom from the spinous processes. This position, combined with the orientation of the glenoid fossa, results in elevation of the arm in a plane that is 30 to 45 degrees anterior to the frontal plane. This motion is termed *scapular plane abduction*

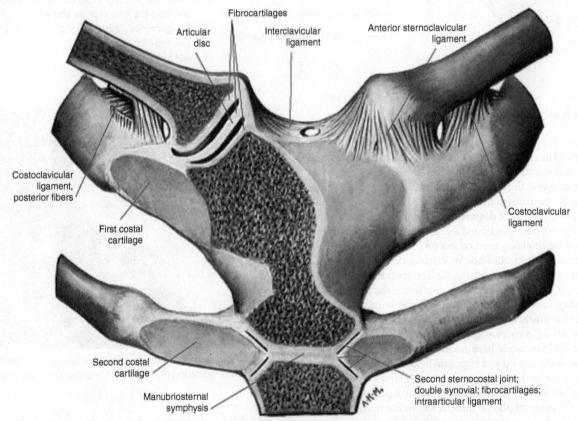

Fibrocartilages

Articular   Interclavicular   Anterior sternoclavicular
disc   ligament   ligament

Costoclavicular
ligament,
posterior fibers

First costal
cartilage

Costoclavicular
ligament

Second costal
cartilage

Second sternocostal joint;
double synovial; fibrocartilages;
intraarticular ligament

Manubriosternal
symphysis

FIG. 18.5 Sternoclavicular joints: Right joint in coronal section. *(From Standring S. Gray's Anatomy. (e-book) 40th ed. St Louis, MO: Churchill Livingstone; 2012, p. 802.)*

or **scaption**.[11] The scapula extends from the level of the T2 spinous process to the T7 or T9 spinous process based on size. Since the ST articulation is not an anatomical joint, there is no close or open packed position.

Movement	Concentric Force Couple	Eccentric Stabilizers
Upward rotation (GH elevation)	Upper trapezius Lower trapezius Serratus anterior	Levator scapulae Rhomboids Pectoralis minor
Retraction	Trapezius Rhomboids	Serratus anterior Pectoralis major Pectoralis minor
Protraction	Serratus anterior Pectoralis major Pectoralis minor	Trapezius Rhomboids
Elevation	Upper trapezius Levator scapulae	Serratus anterior Lower trapezius
Depression	Serratus anterior Lower trapezius	Upper trapezius Levator scapulae
Downward rotation	Levator scapulae Rhomboids Latissimus dorsi Pectoralis minor	Upper trapezius Lower trapezius Serratus anterior

TABLE 18.1   Scapular Force Couples

GH, Glenohumeral.

Proximal (Cervical) Screening

Because of the proximity of the cervical spine to the shoulder, the cervical spine must be screened for contribution to the client's symptoms. It is essential to the screening process to have a basic understanding of cervical anatomy and of the structures that refer symptoms to the shoulder and UE.

Anatomy

The cervical structures that refer symptoms to the shoulder and entire UE that are cleared via cervical screening are the following:
- Cervical nerve roots
- Cervical discs
- Cervical facets
- Cervical intrinsic soft tissue (muscles, ligaments, joint capsules)
- Cervical extrinsic musculature

Cervical Nerve Roots

The C4 to C7 nerve roots supply structures that overlie or comprise the shoulder complex (Fig. 18.6). The C5 and C6 nerve roots innervate most of the GH joint structures with the C4 nerve root innervating the AC joint.

Because of their location and path of travel, the cervical nerve roots are susceptible to injury. A **disc herniation** (damage to the annular wall of the disc resulting in disc deformity as the nucleus displaces into the lesion) can entrap the nerve root against the

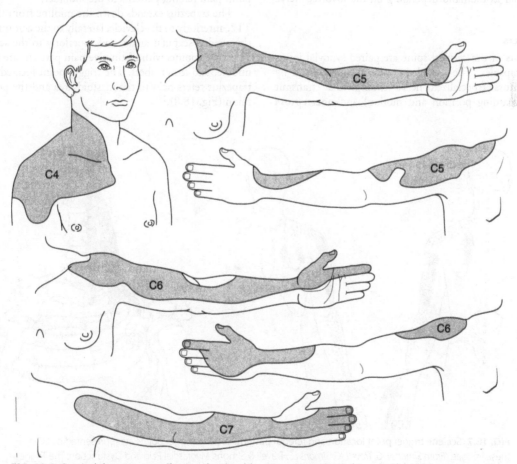

FIG. 18.6 Cervical dermatomes affecting the shoulder. *(From Magee DJ. Orthopedic Physical Assessment. 5th ed 5. Philadelphia, PA: Saunders; 2008, p.183.)*

vertebral lamina and encroach upon the dorsal root ganglion. Hypertrophy of the facet joints, spurring of the vertebral end plates, and spurring of the **uncinate processes** (wing-like projections from the superior portion of the cervical vertebrae that articulate with the inferior portion of the vertebrae above) will narrow the **intervertebral foramen (IVF)** (bony canal that contains the spinal nerve), resulting in compression of the cervical nerve roots. Degenerative loss of cervical disc height further enhances this process.

Cervical Discs

The cervical spine contains five discs, with the most superior disc located between C2 and C3, and the most inferior disc located between C7 and T1. The disc consists of three parts: the **annulus fibrosis** (multilayered ligamentous exterior of the disc), the **vertebral end plate** (cartilaginous interface between the vertebral disc and the vertebral body), and the **nucleus pulposus** (pulpy semiliquid center of the disc). The cervical discs are morphologically quite different from lumbar discs, as they essentially lack a posterior annular wall.[12] The posterior longitudinal ligament mainly supplies that role. Also, the cervical disc develops horizontal annular clefts or tears in the lateral portion by age 15 that progressively extend across the back of the disc.[12] It is likely due to these differences that the cervical discs degenerate more quickly than the lumbar discs.[13]

The onset of neck and arm pain with cervical disc herniation is usually insidious and often starts in the neck and medial scapular border before radiating to the shoulder and arm. Symptoms can spread as far as the hand depending on the involved nerve root.

Cervical Facets

The **facet joints** of the cervical spine are paired synovial joints with fibrous capsules. The capsules are heavily innervated by **mechanoreceptors** (specialized nerve endings that transmit information regarding position and motion) and **nociceptors**

(specialized nerve endings that transmit noxious stimuli), which likely modulate protective muscle reflexes that are important in preventing joint instability and degeneration.[14]

Studies of normal individuals with neck pain demonstrate pain referral patterns from the cervical facets to the cervical and shoulder regions.[15,16] These studies demonstrate a consistent pain referral pattern to the top and lateral parts of the shoulder, extending to the inferior border of the scapula from the C6-C7 facet joints.

Cervical Intrinsic Soft Tissue

The intrinsic soft-tissue structures of the cervical/thoracic region include the muscles that do not originate or insert on the clavicle or scapula. Of these muscles, the scalenes demonstrate **trigger point** (palpable taut muscle bands that refer pain when compressed) pain referral patterns to the shoulder (Fig. 18.7). There are substantial anatomical variations in the attachments of the scalene muscles. In general, the proximal portions attach to the transverse processes of the cervical vertebrae. The distal attachments of the anterior and medial scalenes are the first rib; the distal attachment of the posterior scalene is the second rib. The trigger points refer pain to the anterior lateral aspect of the shoulder and medial scapular border.[17]

Cervical Extrinsic Muscle

The extrinsic muscles are those that have attachments to the shoulder structures (scapula and clavicle) and cervical spine. Of these, the trapezius and levator scapulae demonstrate trigger point pain referral patterns to the shoulder.

The trapezius extends down the midline from the occiput to T12, anteriorly to the clavicle, laterally to the acromion and superior medial scapular angle, and superiorly to the scapular spine. Six trigger points with distinctive pain patterns are in the upper, middle, and lower fibers. The trigger point located in the lower trapezius refers pain to the mastoid area and the posterior acromion (Fig. 18.8).[17]

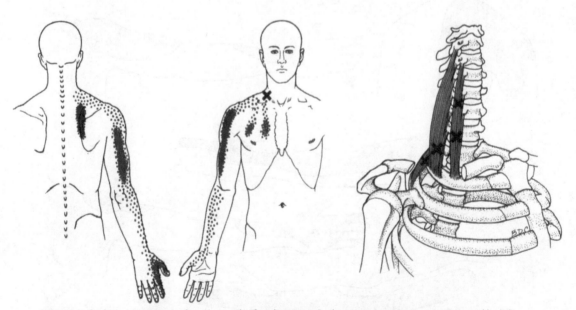

FIG. 18.7 Scalene trigger point location and referral pattern. Scalene trigger points are represented by "X" in these images. *(From Simons DG, Travell JG, Simons LS.* Travell & Simons' Myofascial Pain and Dysfunction: The Trigger Point Manual. *Vol. 1, 2nd ed. Baltimore, MD: Lippincott Williams & Wilkins; 1998, p. 506.)*

The levator scapulae attaches proximally to the transverse processes of the first four cervical vertebrae and distally to the superior medial scapular angle. The trigger point refers pain to the angle of the neck and often projects to the posterior aspect of the shoulder (Fig. 18.9).[17]

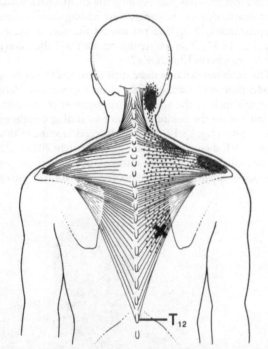

FIG. 18.8 Lower trapezius trigger point location (represented by "X") and referral pattern. *(From Simons DG, Travell JG, Simons LS. Travell & Simons' Myofascial Pain and Dysfunction: The Trigger Point Manual. Vol. 1, 2nd ed. Baltimore, MD: Lippincott Williams & Wilkins; 1998.)*

Diagnosis and Pathology

The primary goal of the cervical screening examination is to efficiently screen for cervical pathology that may be contributing to or causing shoulder symptoms. If screening indicates cervical pathology, the examiner must perform further testing of the cervical spine. There are numerous examination procedures described in the literature that are beyond the scope of this chapter. *The following screening procedures are not a substitute for a complete examination of the cervical spine.*

Cervical Screening Examination

Range of Motion Testing—Intrinsic Versus Extrinsic Restrictions

Having your client perform active movements of the cervical spine is an excellent beginning point for the screening examination. By changing the relative position of the shoulder and cervical spine during testing, you can begin to differentiate between intrinsic and extrinsic restrictions to cervical motion.

Your client performs the basic motions of the cervical spine (flexion/extension, rotation, lateral flexion) from a corrected neutral seated posture with the arms unsupported. Next, they perform the same motions in a crossed arm position (Fig. 18.10). You can see this on the YouTube video link at https://youtu.be/Kj29biHyCz4.

While sitting upright, your client grasps as close to their AC joints as possible then relaxes their arms and shoulders, letting their arms rest against their chest wall. This position effectively elevates the scapulae, and by having the client grasp their shoulders, the scapular elevators can relax. An improvement in ROM in this position implicates the extrinsic cervical structures as

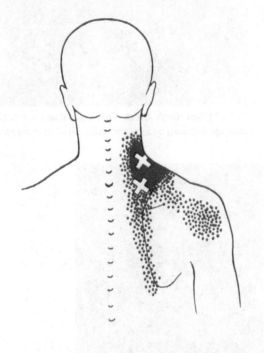
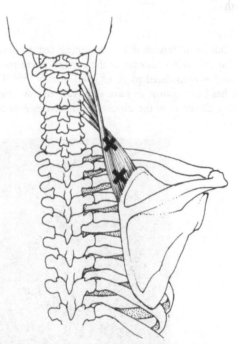

FIG. 18.9 Levator scapulae trigger point location (represented by "X" in these images) and referral pattern. *(From Simons DG, Travell JG, Simons LS. Travell & Simons' Myofascial Pain and Dysfunction: The Trigger Point Manual. Vol. 1, 2nd ed. Baltimore, MD: Lippincott Williams & Wilkins; 1998.)*

contributing to motion loss. No change in motion implicates the intrinsic structures. However, the extrinsic structures may still be limiting motion. The test is designed to rule out intrinsic restrictions if a difference exists between the two test positions.

Repeated Motion Testing—The Search for a Directional Preference

Repeated motion testing is the basis of the McKenzie model of examination. By having your client perform the cervical motions of protrusion, retraction, retraction plus extension, flexion, lateral flexion, and rotation in groups of 5 to 10 repetitions, the therapist looks for a **directional preference**.

A directional preference exists if any of these movements centralize and/or decrease your client's symptoms and/or improve any ROM restrictions. It is important to note that with centralization, your client's proximal pain levels may intensify.

> ◉ **Clinical Pearl**
>
> Worsening and or peripheralization of the client's distal symptoms indicate cervical pathology.[18]

Test Clusters to Detect Cervical Radiculopathy

Since the cervical nerve root is the most likely structure of the cervical spine responsible for **cervicobrachial pain** (shoulder and arm pain originating from the cervical region),[19] screening for cervical nerve root pathology is critical in ruling out the cervical spine as a source of shoulder pain. An optimum group of four test items was identified by Wainner et al.[20] that, if present, produced a **post-test probability** (the probability of the condition being present compared to pretesting) of 90%. These items were the Spurling's test, cervical distraction test, cervical rotation less than 60 degrees toward the involved side, and the upper limb neurodynamic test (ULNT) (described in the section on Thoracic Outlet Syndrome/Brachial Plexopathy).

Spurling's Test

Spurling's test has been described as a screening test to detect cervical radiculopathy (CR) (disease of the cervical nerve roots) in numerous studies considered to be of good quality.[20-23] The Spurling's test has been shown to have moderate to low **sensitivity** (few if any clients with the disease will have negative test

results; a negative test rules out the condition) and moderate to high **specificity** (all persons who do not have the disease will have negative test results; a positive test rules in the condition).

Although variations of this test are common, Spurling[24] originally described the test performed with the client seated and the examiner passively side bending the client's neck toward the symptomatic side to end-range, next adding axial compression of approximately 7 kg directed toward the base of the cervical spine (Fig. 18.11). You can see this on the YouTube video link at https://youtu.be/nFKbnDDKg28.

The examiner executes these steps sequentially, stopping with reproduction or worsening of the client's symptoms. Variations of the test include the additional movements of extension and rotation toward the painful side prior to adding compression of cervical spine (Fig. 18.12).[23] With the cervical spine in this position, the IVF diameter closes by approximately 70%,[25] decreasing the available space for an inflamed nerve root; the presence of a space-occupying lesion (such a disc herniation or osteophytic

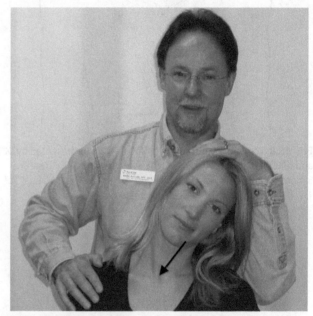

FIG. 18.11 Spurling's A test. Consists of lateral cervical flexion to end-range followed by axial compression of approximately 7 kg.

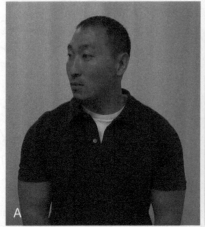
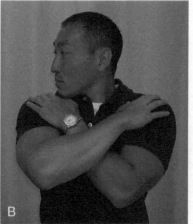

FIG. 18.10 Cervical rotation testing. (A) Arms at rest. (B) Cross-arm position.

spur) will intensify the test result. Axial loading at the end-range of extension, lateral flexion, and rotation also stresses the facet joints, provoking symptoms if pathology is present.

Cervical Distraction Test

The examiner performs this test seated at the head of the plinth with the client supine. The examiner grasps the client's chin and occiput, flexes their neck to a position of comfort, and applies an axial distraction force of approximately 14 kg through the occiput (Fig. 18.13). You can see this on the YouTube video link at https://youtu.be/ASPy_8nTsG4.

A positive test results in reduction or elimination of the client's symptoms. With distraction of the cervical spine in this manner, the IVF diameter increases by approximately 120%, effectively relieving pressure on the inflamed nerve root and resulting in symptom reduction.[25]

Cervical Rotation Range of Motion

The examiner performs this test utilizing a standard goniometer. The examiner stands behind the client seated in a chair with back support to stabilize the thoracic spine. The examiner positions the axis of the goniometer over the vertex of the client's head, the stationary arm of the goniometer perpendicular to the client's shoulders, and the movable arm in line with the client's nose (Fig. 18.14). Rotation ROM of 60 degrees or less toward the involved side results in a positive test.

Thoracic Outlet Syndrome/Brachial Plexopathy

The term *thoracic outlet syndrome* (TOS) encompasses an assortment of clinical entities involving the shoulder region. The thoracic outlet provides the pathway for the neural and vascular structures to and from the upper limb; therefore pathology

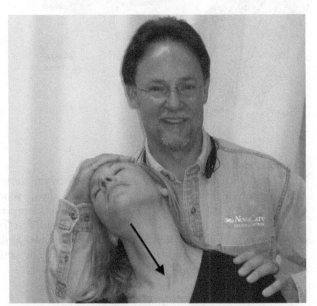

FIG. 18.12 Spurling's B test. Consists of lateral cervical flexion to end-range—cervical extension to end-range with the addition of axial compression here of approximately 7 kg, or adding ipsilateral rotation followed by axial compression.

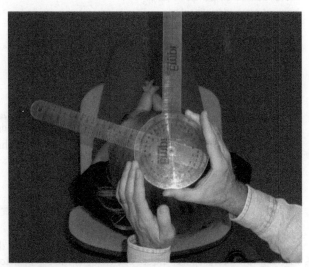

FIG. 18.14 Cervical rotation range-of-motion measurement technique.

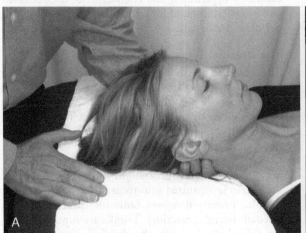 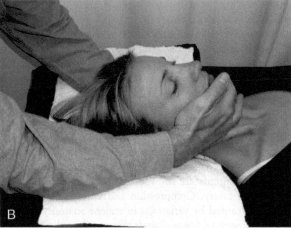

FIG. 18.13 Cervical distraction test. (A) Therapist hand position on client's occiput. (B) Final hand position with the addition of 14 kg axial traction pull.

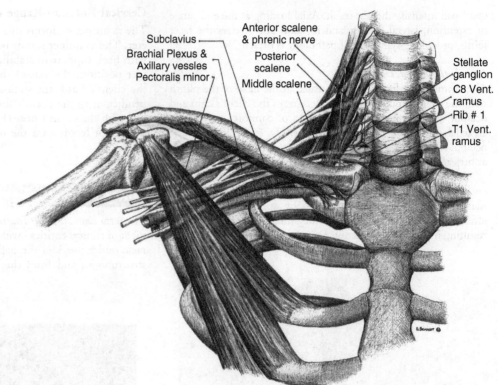

FIG. 18.15 The thoracic outlet. *(From Edgelow PI. Neurovascular consequences of cumulative trauma disorders affecting the thoracic outlet: a patient-centered treatment approach. In: Donatelli RA, ed. Physical Therapy of the Shoulder. 4th ed. St Louis, MO: Churchill Livingstone; 2004. Courtesy of Peter Edgelow.)*

Labels in figure: Subclavius; Brachial Plexus & Axillary vessels; Pectoralis minor; Anterior scalene & phrenic nerve; Posterior scalene; Middle scalene; Stellate ganglion; C8 Vent. ramus; Rib # 1; T1 Vent. ramus

of this area has profound and often disabling results. As vascular presentations of TOS are relatively uncommon (3%–5%), the great majority of TOS clients, in fact, have brachial plexopathies.[26]

Anatomy

The Thoracic Outlet

The thoracic outlet (TO) can be divided into four regions: the sternocostovertebral space, the scalene triangle, the costoclavicular space, and the pectoralis minor (coracopectoral) space. Each region has distinct boundaries, contents, and potential pathologies that result in neurovascular compression and/or entrapment (Fig. 18.15).

Sternocostovertebral Space

The sternocostovertebral space is bordered anteriorly by the sternum, posteriorly by the spinal column, and laterally by the first rib. The contents are the roots of the plexus—the subclavian artery and vein, jugular vein, and neck lymphatics. Compression of the contents is usually caused by tumors of the lung (Pancoast), thymus, parathyroids, and lymph nodes.

Scalene Triangle

The scalene triangle is bordered anteriorly by the anterior scalene, posteriorly by the middle scalene, and inferiorly by the first rib. The contents are the roots and trunks of the plexus and subclavian artery. Compression and entrapment of these structures are caused by variations in scalene anatomy and the presence of congenital fibrous bands that may interdigitate with the plexus.[27]

Costoclavicular Space

The costoclavicular space is bordered superiorly by the clavicle and inferiorly by the first rib. The contents are the divisions of the plexus and the subclavian artery and vein. Compression of these structures between the clavicle and first rib occurs because of postural deficits, resulting in shoulder girdle depression, clavicular and first rib fractures, and the presence of a cervical rib.

Pectoralis Minor (Coracopectoral) Space

The coracopectoral space is bordered superiorly by the coracoid process, anteriorly by the pectoralis minor, and posteriorly by the chest wall. The contents are the cords of the plexus and the subclavian artery and vein. Compression of these structures is caused by hypertrophy and contracture of the pectoralis minor and hyperabduction of the arm as they are pulled up against the pectoralis minor tendon.

The Brachial Plexus

The brachial plexus is netlike in design, which allows for individual neurons from the spinal nerves to eventually reach their respective peripheral nerve. It also serves as a force distributor to dissipate traction forces from the peripheral nerve, helping prevent traction injuries of the lower cervical nerve roots.

Although anatomical variations exist, the brachial plexus is consistent in its organization. Moving proximal to distal, the plexus is organized into roots (C5 to T1); trunks (upper, middle, lower); divisions (anterior, posterior); and cords (medial, lateral, posterior). Trunks are supraclavicular; cords are infraclavicular with the divisions occurring under the clavicle.

Diagnosis and Pathology

Nearly a dozen surgical and medical specialties see TOS clients. Unfortunately, these various specialties have disparate views regarding diagnosis and treatment of the condition. The most up-to-date thoughts on TOS are that it is comprised of five discrete subgroups: (1) arterial vascular, (2) venous vascular, (3) true neurologic, (4) traumatic neurovascular, and (5) disputed.[26] Groups 1 to 4 are rare and beyond the scope of this chapter. The disputed subgroup is fairly common and primarily involves the brachial plexus. As a result, a wide range of clinical presentations are common and confusing to clinicians.[26,28]

Vascular Component

The diagnosis of TOS versus brachial plexopathy is somewhat controversial. TOS, being a syndrome, by definition is a collection of symptoms related to pathology of an anatomical space (the thoracic outlet). Brachial plexopathy is pathology of a specific anatomical structure (the brachial plexus). The vascular component of TOS ought to be diagnosed via vascular studies because there is often a sympathetic nervous system component to the brachial plexopathy that presents clinically with vascular symptoms.

Unfortunately, the clinical tests for vascular compromise that are advocated in the literature (such as the Adson's and Wright's tests, which rely on obliteration of the radial pulse while in the test position) have a high incidence (as high as 87%) of positive results in normal individuals.[28-33] Therefore drawing conclusions based on the results of these clinical tests should be questioned.

Neural Component—Brachial Plexopathy

Due to the paucity of diagnostic tests that detect mild to moderate brachial plexopathies, the best way to identify a brachial plexopathy is through careful and thorough evaluation. This should include a detailed history as to the onset of symptoms and mechanism of injury. Onset of symptoms is often traumatic in nature, with trauma involving forced lateral cervical flexion with

the shoulder held in a fixed position (as in a seat belt injury), or forced depression of the shoulder combined with forced lateral cervical flexion (as in a sports injury, such as "burner" syndrome), or even dislocation of the shoulder. Symptoms may be delayed for months as adhesions form between the neural tissue and surrounding nerve bed. This leads to restricted **neural mobility** (the ability of the neural structures to adjust to changes in the nerve bed length through a combination of gliding and elongation), ultimately resulting in loss of UE motion and function.

Onset can be insidious in nature, with genetic and morphological predisposition combined with poor postural and movement habits leading to the development of the condition. During the growth phase into adolescence, the scapulae gradually descend along the posterior thorax, with the descent being greater in women. A strain with resulting weakness of the scapular suspensory muscles that lengthen during this process is associated with the development of brachial plexopathy. This helps explain the rarity of insidious-onset brachial plexopathy before puberty and the increased incidence of the disease in women.[34]

Clients with brachial plexopathy will often complain of unilateral headaches in the occipital region with facial pain from the angle of the jaw to the zygomatic region to the ear. They may complain of shoulder and chest wall pain from the trapezius ridge down the medial border of the scapula, in the supra/infraclavicular fossa, and from the sternum to the axilla to the epigastric region. These clients are often seen in the emergency room for a suspected cardiac event but misdiagnosed with costal chondritis or gastritis.[35]

Clinical Pearl

Arm and hand involvement often include complaints of pain, paresthesias, and weakness. A strong clue that the plexus is involved is that these symptoms do not follow dermatomal or peripheral nerve distributions. Other strong indications that the plexus is involved are intolerance to overhead activities, reports of dropping objects, cramping of the hand intrinsics while writing, waking with a "dead arm," and intolerance of straps across the top of the shoulder.

Timelines and Healing

Full recovery from a brachial plexus injury is rare. However, clients can often achieve enough of a reduction in symptoms to allow for a return to restricted activity. The level of restriction is related to the severity of the original injury, **neural sensitization** (activation of the small diameter pain fibers within the nerve itself),[36] and the amount of **intraneural** (contained within the nerve) and/or **perineural** (between the nerve and the nerve bed) scarring. This is a lifelong injury, and clients must be instructed in management of the condition. The condition is characterized by periods of high and low neural irritability based on an individual's activity level and degree of pathology. Because these clients have experienced an injury to the nervous system, many progress to a condition known as **central sensitization** (loss of brain-orchestrated pain inhibitory mechanisms and hyperactivation of ascending pain pathways).[37] Specifically, the problem is not just due to a peripheral nerve injury, but symptoms are driven from changes within the brain—not a bottom up, but a top-down issue. This way of looking at clients with chronic nerve pain has led to treatments that take advantage of the brain's **neuroplasticity** (the ability of the brain to adapt and change neuronal connections based on a variety of stimuli) and are beyond the scope of this chapter.

Nonoperative Treatment

The theme that provides the underpinning of treatment for brachial plexus injuries is that the nerves need three conditions to optimize healing: (1) space, (2) motion, and (3) slack. The most important step to begin healing is teaching your client how not to irritate the injured plexus. Through neural mobility assessment, clients can be taught where the safe boundaries of motion are. If your client can follow these movement guidelines and plexus irritation drops to a stable level, they can attempt to regain plexus mobility through gliding and stretching exercises. As plexus mobility improves, the safe boundaries of motion increase, resulting in improved function.

Clients must be taught how to breathe using the diaphragm, minimizing the use of the scalenes, and they must be instructed in safe sleeping positions to avoid stretching or compressing the plexus. *Most importantly, your client must be taught to maintain a posture that minimizes stress on the brachial plexus while maximizing the apertures of the thoracic outlet.*

These clients will rarely tolerate conventional weight training at the gym, but guided exercises to strengthen the scapular stabilizers and elevators are essential. With direct supervision, clients can use resistance bands and/or weights to strengthen the upper, middle, and lower trapezius, as well as the levator scapulae, rhomboids, and serratus anterior. Doing the exercises in sets of three repetitions allows the therapist and client to assess for increased plexus irritation signs between sets, thereby avoiding overstressing the thoracic outlet contents.

Clients can regain scapular proprioception through visual feedback exercises. The client stands facing the mirror while performing scapular motions, targeting points of the clock. With 12 o'clock being superior, 9 o'clock anterior, and 3 o'clock posterior; your client symmetrically elevates the shoulders to the 12 o'clock, 1 o'clock, and 2 o'clock positions. You can see this on the YouTube video link at https://youtu.be/LUuD90aJ3tQ.

These are performed in straight lines of motion as smoothly as possible. After each cycle, your client assesses their level of irritation and adjusts the exercise accordingly.

Your client performs gliding and stretching exercises in front of the mirror as well. They begin the glide exercise with the arms against their side and elbows flexed to 90 degrees with their palms facing up. Next, they elevate the shoulders while slowly extending the elbows. To bias the medial and lateral cords of the plexus via the median nerve, the client maintains supination while extending the wrists (Fig. 18.16). You can see this on the YouTube video link at https://youtu.be/YPkFiBR8POg.

To bias the posterior cord of the plexus via the radial nerve, your client pronates their forearms and flexes their wrists (Fig. 18.17).

Your client begins the stretch exercise with the palm of their hand brought to eye level in front of their face, and the elbow held close to the body. While maintaining the hand at eye level, your client moves their shoulder into abduction and external rotation with the wrist held in supination. Again, keeping the hand at eye level, your client slowly extends their elbow just until a stretch is felt or a slight increase in symptoms occurs. At this point, they back off slightly on the elbow extension and alternately flex and extend their wrist three times (Fig. 18.18). You can see this on the YouTube video link at https://youtu.be/Mgh9OMxeAyk.

The client attempts to straighten their elbow further with each cycle of the exercise. The nerve gliding variation of this exercise consists of cervical lateral flexion toward the ipsilateral arm with wrist extension. You can see this on the YouTube video link at https://youtu.be/YPkFiBR8POg.

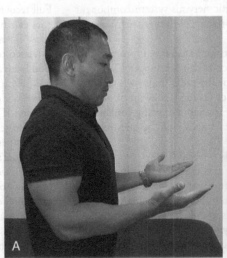
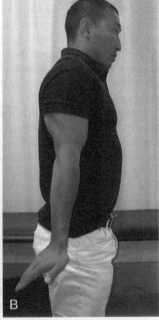

FIG. 18.16 Nerve glide biasing the medial and lateral cords via the median nerve. (A) Starting and ending position. (B) Midpoint of the glide.

The glide and stretch exercises are performed in sets of three.

The client performs all exercises from a neutral posture position. They achieve this by lifting their sternum through increasing their lumbar lordosis and elevating their ribcage. This effectively corrects the forward head–rounded shoulder posture, relieving stress from the thoracic outlet contents.

Clients who demonstrate tight scalenes and tight pectoralis minor muscles must be taught stretching exercises. Since these muscles lie against the brachial plexus, the therapist must watch for an increase in the client's symptoms during stretching. The rule of threes works here as well—sets of three stretches held for three seconds. As your client demonstrates good tolerance to the stretch, the stretch can be held for longer periods and/or the number of sets can be increased.

Many of the scalene stretches described in the literature and in exercise kits often stretch the brachial plexus and should therefore be avoided. They usually instruct the client to depress their shoulder while stretching, frequently causing further irritation to the injured plexus. *The scalenes, which have no attachment to the shoulder and are intrinsic to the cervical and thoracic regions, should be stretched with the shoulder held elevated, thereby relieving tension from the brachial plexus during stretching. Anchoring*

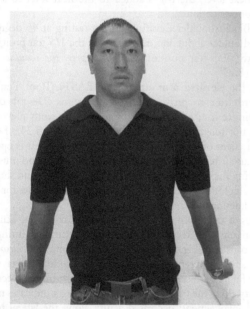

FIG. 18.17 Midpoint of the nerve glide biasing the posterior cord via the radial nerve.

the first rib at its sternal attachment further enhances the scalene stretch (Fig. 18.19). You can see this on the YouTube video link at https://youtu.be/RY-_UygbkK8.

The doorway stretch is ideal for stretching the pectoralis minor (Fig. 18.20). An important component of this stretch is the addition of the shoulder shrug before stepping into the doorway. This initiating maneuver serves two purposes: first, lifting the shoulders increases the origin-to-insertion length of the pectoralis minor, enhancing the stretch; second, lifting the shoulders increases the aperture of the costoclavicular space by elevating the clavicle away from the first rib, minimizing the potential for neurovascular compression once the stretch is commenced. *Having the client perform nerve glides (as previously described) between each stretch helps minimize neural irritation that may occur because of tissue stretching.*

Operative Treatment

The primary goal of TOS surgery is decompression of neurovascular contents or **neurolysis** (the removal of scar tissue from the nerve) of the entrapped brachial plexus. Clients who fare the best are those with confirmed vascular or neurological compromise in the thoracic outlet via diagnostic testing.[38] Unfortunately, surgical outcomes have been disappointing; therefore surgery is reserved as a last resort.[28,39] The most common procedures are transaxillary first rib resection and **supraclavicular scalenectomy** (surgical removal of the anterior scalene) with neurolysis.

> ◎ **Clinical Pearl**
>
> Maintaining postoperative neural mobility is imperative because the formation of perineural scarring will entrap the plexus, leading to a poor surgical outcome. Neural mobilization exercises should begin as soon as the client is stable (usually within the first 3 postoperative days).

> ? **Questions to Ask the Doctor**
>
> **Postoperative Clients**
> - How soon can ROM exercises begin?
> - Are there any restrictions to movement of the neck or shoulder?

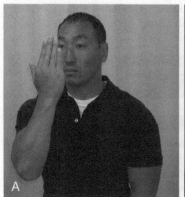
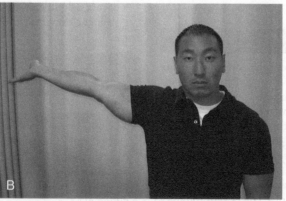

FIG. 18.18 The oscillating brachial plexus nerve stretch. (A) Starting position and ending position. (B) Maximal stretch position.

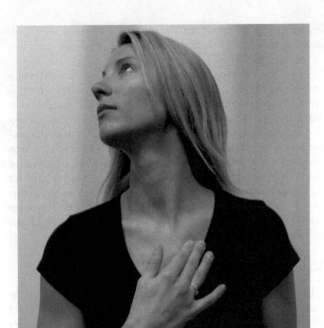

FIG. 18.19 Scalene stretch of the left scalenes. Note stabilization of the first rib to enhance the stretch and protect the brachial plexus.

( ) *What to Say to Clients*

About the Condition

"Here is a drawing of your thoracic outlet. You can see the nerves and blood vessels that supply the arm travel through here. The areas of possible damage are here in your neck (the scalenes), between the collar bone and first rib, and under the muscles of your chest wall (pectoralis minor)."

About the Home Exercise Program

"In order for you to move your arm comfortably, your nerves must be able to slide through the thoracic outlet smoothly. You may have developed restrictions that prevent this from happening. Maintaining good posture is critical because you place excessive strain on the nerves with poor posture habits. Your exercises are designed to reinforce proper posture and help the nerves slide through the thoracic outlet, much like sliding a string through a straw."

"Your postural exercises should be performed hourly to help reinforce good postural habits. Set your cell phone to 'beep' on the hour to remind you to exercise. Your gliding and stretching exercises should be performed a minimum of three times a day. Tie these exercises to meal times so you will remember to do them."

Evaluation Tips

- Assess your client's ability to achieve the corrected posture position.
- Check for asymmetry of scapular/shoulder position.
- Look for swelling over the supraclavicular fossa.
- Monitor your client's UE for evidence of **autonomic instability** (sympathetic nervous system irritation) during testing, such as reticular mottling, color changes, and temperature changes.
- Palpate along the course of the brachial plexus and peripheral nerves for tenderness and evidence of a **Tinel's sign** (production of tingling or paresthesia with percussion over the nerve).

- Neural mobility testing of the brachial plexus can be graded as follows[40] (Fig. 18.21). (You can see this on the YouTube video link at https://youtu.be/H8tCH1PqP-Y.)
  - 0/5: Shoulder in internal rotation, elbow flexed to 90 degrees with arm across stomach, wrist and fingers in neutral (Fig. 18.21A)
  - 1/5: Shoulder in neutral, elbow flexed to 90 degrees, wrist and fingers in neutral (Fig. 18.21B)
  - 2/5: Shoulder in approximately 110 degrees of abduction, neutral rotation, elbow flexed to 90 degrees, wrist and fingers in neutral (Fig. 18.21C)
  - 3/5: As above with the shoulder in approximately 90 degrees of external rotation, forearm in supination, and fingers in neutral (Fig. 18.21D)
  - 4/5: As above with the elbow extended to 0 degrees (Fig. 18.21E)
  - 5/5: As above with the wrist and fingers extended to end-range (Fig. 18.21F)
  - Use +/− for positions between each grade. If movement into the test position is less than halfway to the next grade position, the (+) is added to the level achieved. If the position achieved is more than halfway but falls short of the next level, the (−) is added to the next level to aide in documentation.
- Block shoulder elevation during testing at 45 degrees of shoulder abduction moving from the 1/5 test position to the 2/5 test position; *do not depress the shoulder* (Fig. 18.22)
- Use the **elevated arm stress test (EAST)** (Roos Test) and record time to provocation of symptoms. Described as a 3-minute test;[41] in my experience, clients with plexopathy will not tolerate more than 1 minute (Fig. 18.23). Having your client open/close their hands during the test is optional because it tests for fatigue of the forearm and hand muscles.
- During the myotomal screen, focus on scapular and shoulder muscles for upper trunk lesions, and hand intrinsics for lower trunk lesions.
- Using a safety pin flagged with tape to check for acuity to sharp sensation keeps the level of pressure applied during testing constant (Fig. 18.24). Clients with brachial plexopathy will show differential sensation of the middle finger versus ring finger with carpal or cubital tunnel syndrome. Decreased acuity along the medial half of the ring finger indicates medial cord involvement; decreased acuity along the lateral half of the ring finger indicates lateral cord involvement.[35] Differences found with testing of the ring finger concurrent to positive findings of the long finger could indicate the presence of a **double or multiple crush syndrome** (areas of more than one compressive lesion along the injured nerve).

Diagnosis-Specific Information That Affects Clinical Reasoning

◎ *Clinical Pearl*

Clients who cannot tolerate the corrected posture position, have a positive EAST result in less than 30 seconds, and/or neural mobility of the plexus lower than 3/5 have a poorer prognosis because they will easily irritate their condition during ADLs.

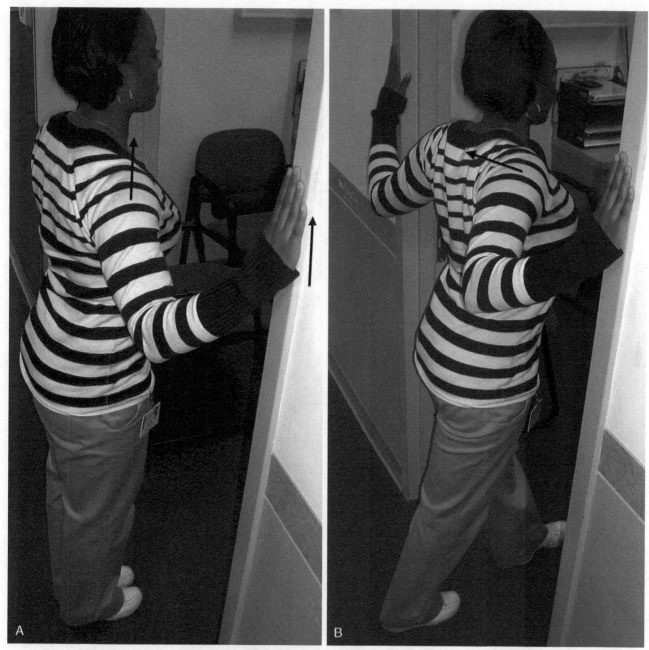

FIG. 18.20 The doorway stretch. (A) The client stands with their toes in line with the doorway opening. They shrug their shoulders and raise their hands along the doorframe to shoulder height, or just below the point of symptom provocation, whichever happens first (as shown by the arrows). (B) While holding this posture, the client takes a half step into the doorway. This creates shoulder motion in the direction of the arrow, producing a stretch to the soft tissue of the chest wall.

Achieving these basic parameters should be the initial goals of treatment. Base the speed and intensity of the rehabilitation program on your client's level of symptom irritability/stability. Inform clients with chronic restrictions that they may experience increased symptoms for up to 48 hours after treatment. *If the client's level of posttreatment irritation persists for greater than 48 hours, the intensity of the treatment needs to be decreased.*

♡ **Tips from the Field**

Constantly stress proper posture when clients are in the clinic. Instruct clients to notice the poor posture of people they encounter during the day and to use these observations as a reminder to correct their own posture. *The inability of a client to achieve stable symptoms at correct posture is one of the best predictors of treatment failure.*

Clients often complain that their home exercises increase their symptoms. Have clients demonstrate their home program on a regular basis and correct any modifications they have made. Adjust the amount of movement during the home exercises to keep symptoms stable.

The application of heat prior to exercise may help calm symptoms. Riding the stationary bike for 10 to 15 minutes while using proper posture with the involved arm supported (if needed) is an excellent warm-up exercise.

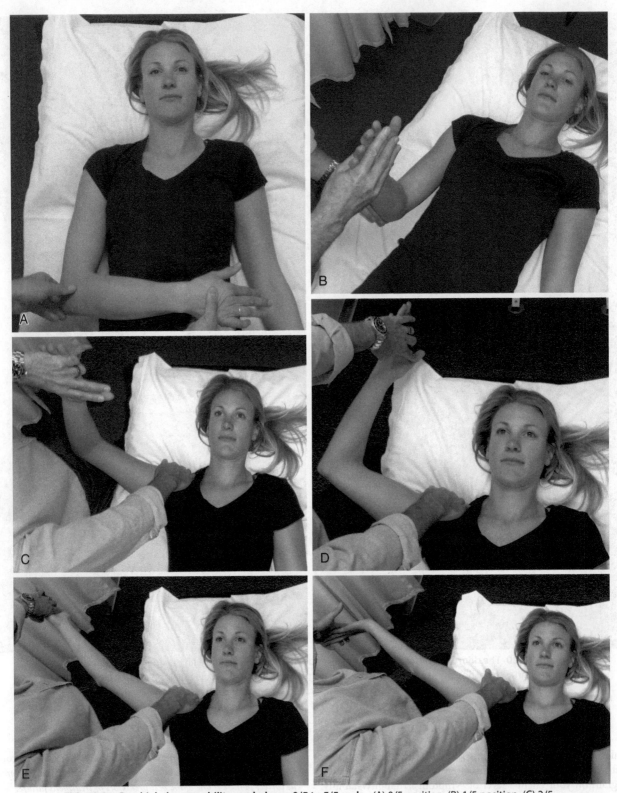

FIG. 18.21 Brachial plexus mobility graded on a 0/5 to 5/5 scale. (A) 0/5 position. (B) 1/5 position. (C) 2/5 position. (D) 3/5 position. (E) 4/5 position. (F) 5/5 position.

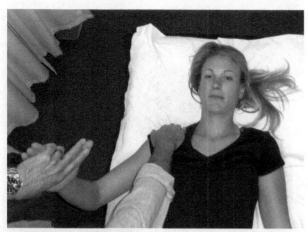

FIG. 18.22 Blocking shoulder elevation at 45 degrees of abduction prevents shoulder hiking, which will reduce neural tension and affect the testing outcome, reducing test-retest reliability.

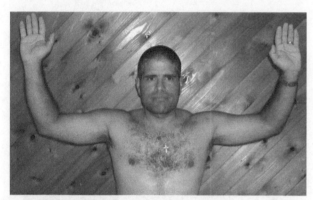

FIG. 18.23 Test position for the elevated arm stress test, or Roos test.

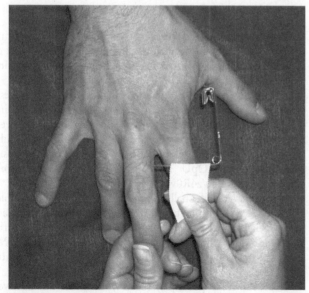

FIG. 18.24 Example of a tape-flagged safety pin used to maintain constant pressure to check for sensation difference between the medial and lateral aspect of the long finger.

> **Precautions and Concerns**

- *Avoid overstretching the brachial plexus during treatment.*
- *Be careful with overhead exercise, such as wall pulleys.*
- *When clients use the upper body ergometer (UBE), monitor their posture and be alert for provocation of symptoms.*
- *Progress strengthening exercises cautiously.*
- *Watch exercise positions to avoid overstressing the brachial plexus.*

Proximal Humerus Fracture

Anatomy

Proximal humerus fractures are the most common fracture of the humerus and may involve the articular surface, greater tuberosity, lesser tuberosity, or the surgical neck. These four regions are described as the four major fracture fragments that occur and are the basis of the classification systems for proximal humerus fractures.[42,43]

Diagnosis and Pathology

The majority of proximal humerus fractures occur as a direct result of a fall on the involved shoulder in the elderly population, or a direct blow to the humeral region, and are stable one-part fractures involving the surgical neck of the humerus.[42,44]

One-part fractures, as classified by the Neer system, are described as no fracture fragments being displaced more than 1 cm and no more than 45 degrees of angulation. Two-part fractures exceed these position limits and can involve the humeral head and surgical neck or the humeral head and greater tuberosity. Three- and four-part fractures involve the humeral head, greater tuberosity, and lesser tuberosity.[42,43]

Timelines and Healing

One-part fractures are initially treated by sling immobilization for 1 to 3 weeks. Clients can start passive movements when the humeral shaft and head move as a unit, which can be as early as a couple of days.[42] Two- to four-part fractures, being more complex, usually require 4 to 6 weeks of immobilization, except in clients with hemiarthroplasties, who begin passive range of motion (PROM) exercises on postoperative day one.

Nonoperative Treatment

Your client begins treatment while still in the immobilizer by performing gripping exercises and active range of motion (AROM) of the elbow and wrist to prevent edema and joint stiffness. Once clinically stable, your client starts PROM exercises in the clinic, and pendulum and tabletop PROM exercises at home. They should continue to wear the sling immobilizer in public and while sleeping for support and protection the first 6 weeks post injury or surgical repair.

The therapist can start more aggressive stretching and the client begins AROM exercises around 4 to 6 weeks. The focus here should be on proper glenohumeral and scapulothoracic movement to prevent the substitution patterns of early scapular elevation and trunk leaning to achieve UE elevation. *Substitution patterns discourage proper recruitment of the rotator shoulder muscles, so they need to be avoided at all costs.*

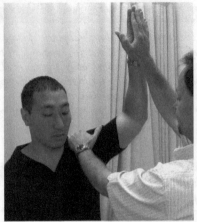

FIG. 18.25 Range-of-motion exercise with the client mirroring the therapist while the therapist stabilizes the shoulder to prevent early scapular elevation.

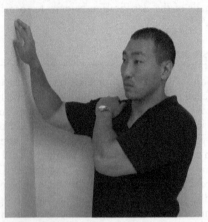

FIG. 18.26 Wall walking exercise with the client self-stabilizing to prevent early scapular elevation.

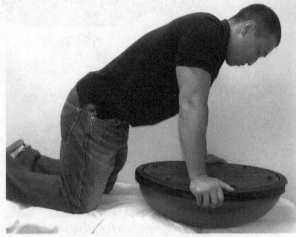

FIG. 18.27 Example of closed chain exercise for the shoulder in quadruped on a rocker surface.

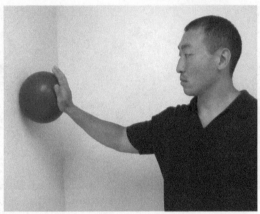

FIG. 18.28 Example of closed chain exercise for the shoulder rolling a weighted ball against the wall.

The therapist plays a significant role here by having the client perform hand-to-hand active assisted range of motion (AAROM) progressing to AROM mirroring exercises in a seated position while the therapist prevents early scapular elevation (Fig. 18.25). You can see this on the YouTube video link at https://youtu.be/qfd29vRf0HQ.

Once your client understands the movement concept, they can perform the same exercise through self-scapular stabilization and wall walking (Fig. 18.26). You can see this on the YouTube video link at https://youtu.be/hg9M1EKAAps.

These motions are performed in the scapular plane initially to provide the rotator cuff muscles the best length–tension relationship to encourage coordinated activity.

At 8 to 12 weeks postinjury/repair, your client can begin resisted strength training. The focus is on the rotator cuff muscles and scapular stabilizer/force couple muscles. *Therapist-provided manual resistance in diagonal planes of motion is essential at this stage of the program to encourage functional movements and to discourage substitution movements.*

A mixture of open and closed chain exercises must be included at this stage because the shoulder functions in both situations. **Open chain exercises** are defined as working against resistance where the extremity is free to move in space resulting in movement of the distal segment. **Closed chain exercises** are defined as working against resistance with the extremity working against a stationary or mobile but motion-constrained object or surface. Closed chain exercises impart a degree of stability during the exercise motion.

Closed chain exercises include wall pushups, seated press-ups, weight shifting in quadruped, prone press-ups resting on elbows, and advanced exercises including box walk-overs in a press-up position. You can see this on the YouTube video links at https://youtu.be/hg9M1EKAAps and https://youtu.be/RYeu-exHOpU and https://youtu.be/jCItG9Ub3AI and https://youtu.be/z4R0vcfJJgo

Variations include ball rolling against the wall or tabletop and use of a tilt board for weight bearing in quadruped (Figs. 18.27 and 18.28). You can see this on the YouTube video links at https://youtu.be/vhB7FmOHSMs and https://youtu.be/aa5fmARTzA4 and https://youtu.be/C_STdGMVYyQ.

If at 12 weeks postinjury/repair your client has achieved functional ROM and normal movement patterns, they can begin **plyometric** (exercises that link strength and speed of movement to produce an explosive-reactive type of muscle response). You can see this on the YouTube video link at https://youtu.be/g-0pi8Ov3LY.

They can also begin sport-specific activities to prepare them for return to full function. It is therefore important to understand your client's goals of rehabilitation and their **premorbid** (prior to injury) activity level.

Operative Treatment

Proximal humerus fractures graded as two- to three-part will usually require surgical intervention of open reduction internal fixation (ORIF) to reduce the displaced fracture fragments. **Hemiarthroplasty** (prosthetic replacement of one joint surface) is usually indicated to replace the avascular, compromised humeral head in four-part fractures.

? Questions to Ask the Doctor

Regarding Postoperative Clients

- What structures were repaired? Ask for a copy of the operative report.
- How soon can active motion start?
- When can my client begin lifting weights?

Regarding Nonoperative Clients

- When can my client begin to take off the sling?
- How much longer does my client need to wear the sling to sleep?
- How soon can my client begin moving their shoulder?
- When can my client begin lifting weights?

( ) What to Say to Clients

About the Injury

If the fracture is classified as one-part: "Your fracture is considered stable, so you are allowed to begin moving your arm while the healing process continues. In fact, the motion will help the healing process. All motions must be passive – meaning motion provided by the therapist, by gravity, or on a supported surface such as a tabletop. You must not attempt to raise your arm by itself for the next couple of weeks because this could affect the healing fracture."

If the fracture has been surgically repaired or if it is a two-part fracture and is now considered stable: "Your doctor has determined that the fracture is healed enough to begin motion exercises. Movement will make a big difference in how quickly you recover, and it is critical to your recovery."

About Exercise

"You need to move your arm as often and as much as possible. The motion helps lubricate the joint and keeps it healthy."

If your client is doing tabletop exercises: "By using your fingers to pull your arm forward, you will avoid stressing your shoulder during this exercise. Keep your shoulder relaxed while moving; at the end of tolerable motion, rest your hand flat on the table surface while you sit back upright, dragging your arm back to the starting position."

If your client is doing pendulum exercises: "Do your exercises next to a table or counter. Using the table for support with your uninjured arm, bend at the waist as far as you can and let your injured arm swing forward as if it were a piece of rope. Now rock your body side-to-side and in circles. Get your arm swinging just as you would do with your hand to swing a rope side-to-side or in a circle."

For all ROM exercises: "It is not how hard you push your stretches, but how often you stretch and how much cumulative time you spend at the end of the motion that counts. Try for a minimum of 15 minutes of total end-range time by doing 50 stretches a day, each held for 20 seconds."

Evaluation Tips

Take PROM measurements with your client seated. Make sure motions are slow and gentle because your client will be very apprehensive about moving their arm. Often, when you attempt to return your client's arm to neutral after full elevation, they will experience sharp pain as the deltoid and humeral head elevators reflexively contract. By having your client actively lower their arm against your resistance, this reflex is inhibited and the motion will be considerably more comfortable.

Measure functional internal rotation (IR) by seeing which bony landmark on the pelvis or spinous process your client can touch with their thumb (for example, anterior superior iliac spine [ASIS], iliac crest, posterior superior iliac spine [PSIS], L5, and so on).

Diagnosis-Specific Information That Affects Clinical Reasoning

The type of fracture directly affects how aggressively you can rehabilitate your client. Obtaining this information from the doctor is crucial. This information is also available from radiology and operative reports.

◎ Clinical Pearl

Alignment of the humeral head to the shaft will affect how much ROM the client will ultimately recover. For example, if the shaft is in 45-degree extension relative to the humeral head, the client's expected flexion ROM will be 135 degrees (180 degrees – 45 degrees = 135 degrees). The same holds true for rotational deformities.[44]

♡ Tips From the Field

Clients starting therapy a few weeks after a one-part proximal humerus fracture will usually be apprehensive about moving their arm due to fears about fracture instability. There are two ways to calm their fears. First, tell them that as you rotate their arm, the humeral head will not move if the fracture is unstable. Have them place their hand over their injured humeral head while you gently rotate the arm from internal rotation to external rotation; they should feel the humeral head move. The second and rather novel technique involves using a stethoscope. Explain to your client that sound will not travel across an open fracture. Have your client listen through the stethoscope placed on the humeral head of their healthy shoulder while you tap on their lateral epicondyle. Do the same to their injured shoulder where the intensity of sound should be the same. This will often decrease a client's apprehension about moving their shoulder.

Scapular position and posture have a direct effect on shoulder ROM. These clients must be given postural exercises as previously described for brachial plexus clients.

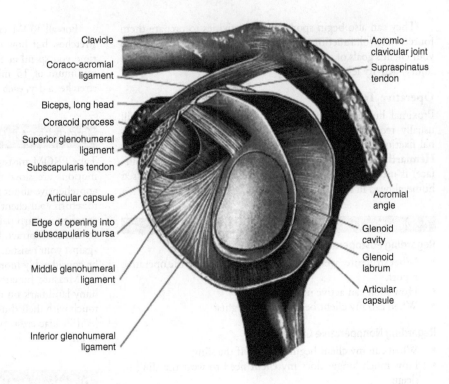

Clavicle

Coraco-acromial
ligament

Biceps, long head

Coracoid process

Superior glenohumeral
ligament

Subscapularis tendon

Articular capsule

Edge of opening into
subscapularis bursa

Middle glenohumeral
ligament

Inferior glenohumeral
ligament

Acromio-
clavicular joint

Supraspinatus
tendon

Acromial
angle

Glenoid
cavity

Glenoid
labrum

Articular
capsule

FIG. 18.29 Interior view of the left shoulder joint, looking into the glenoid fossa and joint capsule. *(From Putz R, Pabst R. Sobotta—Atlas of Human Anatomy Single Volume Edition: Head, Neck, Upper Limb, Thorax, Abdomen, Pelvis, Lower Limb. 14th ed. St Louis, MO: Elsevier; 2008.)*

> ## ❯ Precautions and Concerns

- *RC injuries are often overlooked at the time of injury. Watch for evidence of rotator cuff tear (RCT) during rehabilitation.*
- *These clients are at a high risk of developing **adhesive capsulitis** (frozen shoulder [FS]). Movement must be the basis of any therapy program.*
- *Many of these clients will have a concurrent axillary nerve or brachial plexus injury. Screen for this during the initial examination by checking sensation over the deltoid (axillary distribution) and by asking if the client is experiencing paresthesias in the hand or arm (possible brachial plexus involvement).*

Frozen Shoulder/Adhesive Capsulitis

Anatomy

The fibrous capsule that envelopes the GH joint is lined with synovial tissue. It is attached medially to the glenoid margin and encompasses the glenoid labrum and long head of the biceps. Laterally it attaches to the anatomical neck of the humeral head near the articular surface. The inferior portion attaches laterally about 1 cm distal to the articular surface on the humeral shaft. The capsule is slack enough that the GH joint surfaces can be distracted up to 3 cm.[2]

The capsule has three distinct thickened areas known as the glenohumeral ligaments (superior, middle, and inferior) that help stabilize the GH joint. These ligaments become taut at various portions of GH motion, as their fibers run in both radial and circular directions. During abduction and rotation, the capsule becomes shortened, producing both a compressive and centering force of the humerus on the glenoid.[45] During abduction and rotation, the inferior GH ligament forms a sling providing anterior, posterior, and inferior stability to the joint. With the arm at rest, this portion of the capsule forms the dependent axillary pouch, which is often obliterated with FS (Figs. 18.29 and 18.2).

The coracohumeral ligament extends from the base of the coracoid process as two bands that blend with the capsule running to the greater and lesser tuberosities. Parts of the ligament form the tunnel for the biceps tendon and reinforce the **rotator interval** (the region between the superior edge of the subscapularis and anterior edge of the supraspinatus tendons).

The tendons of the subscapularis, supraspinatus, infraspinatus, and teres minor fuse with the lateral part of the joint capsule forming the RC. With contraction of the RC muscles, the lax capsule is pulled away from the movement path of the humeral head preventing capsular impingement.[2]

Diagnosis and Pathology

The terms *adhesive capsulitis* and *frozen shoulder* are used interchangeably in the literature. The condition is characterized by a progressive loss of GH range of motion usually in the capsular pattern of external rotation being most limited, followed by abduction and internal rotation. Magnetic resonance imaging (MRI) studies demonstrate capsular thickening with loss of the axillary recess.[46,47] The disease appears to be periarticular, with little to no capsular adhesions found during arthroscopic examination.

The condition is found in 2% to 5% of the US population,[48] most commonly in the fourth through sixth decades of life.[49] However, one author[50] who has studied this disease extensively feels it is overdiagnosed. Bunker provides a compelling argument that the prevalence of FS is about 0.75%. It is more common among women, with one study reporting women comprising 70% of all FS clients.[49] FS is usually classified as primary or secondary adhesive capsulitis with the course of the disease following three phases: the freezing phase, the frozen phase, and the thawing phase.[48,49,51,52]

Primary Adhesive Capsulitis

Primary FS is idiopathic in nature. There is considerable debate over the pathogenesis of FS, with possible causes being inflammatory, immunological, endocrine alterations, or biochemical. Research has shown a possible genetic predisposition for developing FS.[53] This form of the disease is overrepresented in clients with diabetes, with rates three to six times that of the non-diabetic population.[51]

Histological findings in clients with primary FS reveal active fibroblastic proliferation of the coracohumeral ligament and rotator interval with an absence of inflammation or synovial involvement, much like that of **Dupuytren's disease** (disease process resulting in thickening and contracture of the palmer fascia).[47] In examining the hands of 58 clients with FS, Smith et al. found that 30 patients had a pit, nodule, or band of Dupuytren's contracture.[54] Bunker noted the same finding in 58% of clients with frozen shoulder.[50]

Secondary Adhesive Capsulitis

Secondary FS is characterized by a precipitating event (such as surgery or trauma to the shoulder) or specific shoulder pathology (such as bursitis, impingement syndrome, or tendonitis). Although the same pattern of motion loss occurs, these clients may not go through all the stages of freezing, frozen, and thawing.[52]

The Freezing Phase

This phase is characterized by shoulder pain interrupting sleep, pain with ADLs (such as brushing one's hair or tucking in one's shirt), and often pain at rest. It is difficult to distinguish FS pathology from that of rotator cuff tendonitis, shoulder bursitis, or impingement syndrome.

Examination of your client during this phase reveals ROM to be close to full, with pain occurring often before the end of motion. Palpation reveals nonspecific tenderness at the anterior, lateral, and posterior aspects of the shoulder. Strength is often normal or slightly decreased, with pain on resisted testing.

Clients tend to limit the use of the affected extremity because all movements are painful, leading to further loss of motion. Over the next 2 to 9 months, the pain subsides and the client is left with the typical FS—pain occurring at the end of motion.

The Frozen Phase

This phase may last up to 1 year. It is characterized by distinct pathological movement patterns as your client attempts to substitute scapulothoracic motion to compensate for the lack of GH mobility. In this phase, pain occurs with stretching of the joint capsule at the end of motion.

The Thawing Phase

This phase is characterized by a gradual return of motion and lasts up to 26 months. The ability of clients to regain full motion after the thawing phase is unclear in the literature. In an earlier study, Shaffer et al.[55] reported that 30% of primary FS clients exhibited some degree of motion loss compared to the uninvolved shoulder at an average follow-up of 7 years. Vastamaki et al.[56] was more optimistic, reporting 94% of clients with primary FS achieved

motion and function equal to their uninvolved side without treatment.[56]

Timelines and Healing

As noted earlier, there are average time lines for each phase of the disease. The majority of individuals complete the thawing phase within 18 months to 3 years from onset.[56]

Nonoperative Treatment

There is no evidence to suggest that modalities (such as ultrasound or interferential electric stimulation) affect the outcome of the disease. In fact, the use of passive modalities may prolong recovery.[49] Treatment should be directed at the process occurring during each phase of the disease. *Overstretching the capsule during the freezing phase may enhance the inflammatory process stimulating further capsular fibrosis.* When the joint has progressed to the frozen and thawing phases, the stretching exercises can be more aggressive. *However, pushing to the point that reinitiates the inflammatory process should be avoided.*[52]

The role of the occupational therapist (OT) in assisting clients with bilateral FS in ADL modifications or adaptive equipment for grooming, bathing, and dressing cannot be overestimated. Clients with unilateral FS may benefit from workstation modification to help them remain productive during the protracted course of the disease.

The use of intraarticular corticosteroid in the freezing phase may be helpful in stabilizing the synovial tissue, allowing for better tolerance to stretching exercises.[57]

Operative Treatment

For FS cases that fail to progress after protracted conservative treatment, manipulation under anesthesia and arthroscopic release of the GH capsule ligaments are two of the most common surgical interventions. Of the two, arthroscopic release of the anterior glenohumeral ligament and coracohumeral ligament currently has the most promising outcome.[58]

? Questions to Ask the Doctor

Postoperative Clients
• What was the intraoperative ROM?

() What to Say to Clients

About the Injury

"Here is a diagram of your shoulder, and this is the joint capsule. Normally the capsule is loose and develops a redundant pouch at the bottom when your arm is at your side. Having this extra capsule space allows you to raise your arm above your head. Think of your shoulder capsule as an accordion with its folds glued together. That accordion is unusable, since it cannot expand; your shoulder is restricted in motion and function as well."

About Exercises/Activities of Daily Living

"Moving your shoulder regularly to the end of comfortable motion helps prevent motion loss. Avoid positions and activities that cause your shoulder to hurt for more than a few minutes afterward. Sleeping on your back is the best position. If you must sleep on your side, keep your arms to your sides (if possible) to prevent shoulder irritation. Using a body pillow may help you find a comfortable sleeping position."

"You have to watch your posture. Having your shoulders rounded will place more stress on the supportive tissue and will slow the healing process."

Evaluation Tips

- Take careful baseline and follow-up ROM measurements with your client supine to stabilize the trunk and scapula. This will allow for careful tracking of the progress of the condition.
- Loss of rotation must be present for a diagnosis of FS. Specifically, loss of ER must be observed. The loss of IR without the loss of ER constitutes glenohumeral internal rotation deficit (GIRD), which is not clinically the same as FS.[59]
- If all passive and resisted motions are painful throughout the ROM, your client is still in the freezing stage.
- If resisted motion is pain free and pain occurs only at end ROM, your client is in the frozen or thawing phase.

Diagnosis-Specific Information That Affects Clinical Reasoning

The intensity of the therapy program is directly proportional to the phase of the condition. The primary treatment goal of the freezing phase is to prevent motion loss. The primary treatment goal of the frozen and thawing phase is to restore functional ROM.

♡ Tips from the Field

Proper posture and normal **scapular kinematics** (scapular movement in sequence and proportion to humeral movement) must be stressed at all times during exercise. Clients with FS quickly develop the pathological motion of early scapular elevation to raise their arm. This movement pattern can lead to secondary cervical problems, further complicating the recovery process.

➤ Precautions and Concerns

- *Do not push ROM during the freezing phase to the point of pain that lasts more than a few minutes. This will only enhance the inflammatory and fibrosing process.*
- *These clients must avoid self-imposed immobilization.*

Glenohumeral Instability

Anatomy

GH instability could be considered the antithesis of adhesive capsulitis. Laxity of the GH joint is a quality that allows full ROM; however, *laxity is not synonymous with instability.* When laxity leads to pain with loss of power and shoulder function, then GH instability exists.

The concepts and structures that contribute to GH stability can be categorized as static and dynamic. The static stabilizers

TABLE 18.2   TUBS Versus AMBRII

TUBS or "Torn Loose"	AMBRII or "Born Loose"
Traumatic etiology	**A**traumatic or microtrauma with no specific episode
Unidirectional instability	**M**ultidirectional instability may be present
Bankart lesion is the pathology	**B**ilateral: asymptomatic shoulder is also loose
Surgery is required	**R**ehabilitation is the treatment of choice
	Inferior capsular shift
	Interval between the supraspinatus and subscapularis closed surgically if conservative measures fail

have a larger role when the shoulder is at rest, while the dynamic stabilizers playing a larger role when the shoulder is in motion.

The static restraints include **negative intracapsular pressure** (air pressure inside the joint capsule being lower than pressure outside the capsule), the suction effect of the glenoid labrum acting on the humeral head like a "plunger," and cohesion-adhesion between the wet smooth surfaces of the humeral head and glenoid fossa. The orientation of the humeral head and glenoid fossa contribute to the static stability of the GH joint as well. With proper postural positioning of the scapula, the dynamic stabilizers need minimal effort to maintain GH congruency.[2]

The dynamic restraints include the RC, which provides a compressive and positioning force, and, to a certain degree, the long head of the biceps tendon. Although the GH ligaments are passive structures, they are under relatively little tension with the shoulder at rest. These ligaments serve as a restrictive leash to check force and limit ROM at various positions of the GH joint during movement. Of these ligaments, the inferior GH ligament is the most crucial to dynamic GH stability. As mentioned in the section covering adhesive capsulitis, during abduction and rotation, the inferior GH ligament forms a sling providing anterior, posterior, and inferior stability to the joint, affording stability when the GH joint is potentially at its most vulnerable position for dislocation.

Diagnosis and Pathology

Two major categories are useful in understanding shoulder instability. They are known by the acronyms of AMBRII and TUBS.[59] The major points of each are summarized in Table 18.2. The pathology and treatment of AMBRII and TUBS shoulders are quite different.

AMBRII shoulders have no history of dislocation or subluxation. The client's major complaint is pain with activity, usually in overhand throwing motions. This pain is often a result of **impingement** (compression of soft tissue between bony structures), which is related to the client's inability to adequately stabilize the ST and/or GH joint due to RC pathology, capsular laxity, and altered **proprioception** (awareness of joint position).[60] Budoff et al. described this condition as primary instability leading to secondary impingement.[61]

Primary instability is often a combination of global capsular laxity and pathological imbalances of the RC and shoulder muscles. Weak and/or proprioceptively compromised RC muscles cannot effectively oppose the upward pull of the deltoid muscle during UE elevation. The result is superior migration of

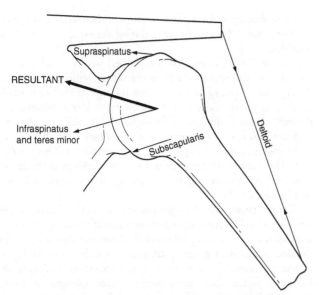

FIG. 18.30 Force couple between the rotator cuff and deltoid resulting in inferior glide of the humeral head during elevation of the arm. *(From Donatelli RA, ed.* Physical Therapy of the Shoulder. *4th ed. St Louis, MO: Churchill Livingstone; 2004. Courtesy of Peter Edgelow.)*

the humeral head and impingement of the greater tuberosity and RC against the underside of the acromion and coracoacromial (CA) ligament (Fig. 18.30).

TUBS shoulders have a history of dislocation, usually in the anterior direction. The mechanism of injury is a fall or blow to the arm while in the position of abduction and ER. Recurrent subluxation or dislocation results when the client places their arm in the position of injury, leading to apprehension and dysfunction. These clients often have a resulting **Bankart lesion**, which consists of damage to the anterior GH capsule glenoid labrum and possibly the glenoid. They also may have a **Hill-Sachs lesion**, which consists of an osseous defect of the posterolateral portion of the humeral head, caused by traumatic anterior dislocation. Both conditions usually require surgery to restore stability to the GH joint.

Between these categories of shoulder instability are a group of shoulder pathologies related to asymmetrical capsular tightness.[62] This occurs from the excessive distraction force on the GH joint during the deceleration phase of throwing leading to thickening and contracture of the posterior-inferior portion of the capsule.[63] The sequelae of this asymmetrical capsular tightening is a loss of GH internal rotation, resulting in a cascade of events that may lead to impingement syndrome as well as pathology of the biceps tendon, labrum, and RC.[59,64]

The long head of the biceps tendon helps stabilize the GH joint during the overhand throwing motion.[2] The unstable and asymmetrically tight shoulder places extra stress on the biceps tendon leading to bicipital tendon irritation and **superior labrum anterior to posterior (SLAP) lesions**.[64] The SLAP lesion is hypothesized to be a result of increased torsional force from the biceps tendon that "peels back" the biceps and posterior labrum from the glenoid rim.[65] The SLAP lesion then enhances the dynamic and static instability of the already unstable shoulder. All the conditions described above can contribute to the development of impingement syndrome and RC disease, described in next section.

Timelines and Healing

For the client with a nonsurgical unstable shoulder, 4 to 8 weeks of rehabilitation is common. The length of rehabilitation depends on the client's ability to gain control of the instability. Once stable, they are released to a sustained home exercise program that they will continue indefinitely. Surgically corrected unstable shoulders require more time for rehabilitation. After a period of immobilization lasting 2 to 4 weeks, 3 to 6 months of rehabilitation is common. These clients will also require a sustained home exercise program. Most postoperative clients report that it takes 6 months to 1 year before their shoulder feels "normal."

Nonoperative Treatment

Treatment focuses on strengthening the RC and scapular stabilizers. Strengthening starts with shoulder isometrics in the safe position of the arm at the side. The motions include resisted shoulder flexion/extension, internal/external rotation, abduction/adduction, and elbow flexion and extension. While performing isometrics, it is important that clients "set" their scapula against their ribcage in a corrected posture position to engage the scapular stabilizers.

Once the client demonstrates fair to good control of the instability, the next step is progression to isotonic exercises in a subimpingement range using light resistance and high repetitions. For clients with anterior instability, the focus is on strengthening the internal rotators, adductors, and biceps. For clients with global instability, the focus is on the RC, scapular stabilizers, deltoid, biceps, and triceps.

It is essential at this stage to incorporate open and closed chain exercises as previously described for proximal humeral fractures. The intensity of the closed chain exercises can be increased by using weighted medicine balls against the wall, by moving the body into a more horizontal position, or even working off the exercise ball while in a prone UE weight-bearing position.

Therapist-applied manual resistance can be used throughout each phase of the rehabilitation process. Starting with isometrics and AAROM and then progressing to concentrics and eccentrics, the therapist controls the speed of movement and amount of force. The major benefit of manual resistance is the immediate feedback the therapist receives from the client during a therapy session.

For clients with posteroinferior capsule restrictions, stretching exercises to restore IR are critical. Use of towel-behind-back stretches and the sleeper stretch work well (Fig. 18.31).

Operative Treatment

Surgical correction of the multidirectionally unstable shoulder should be considered only after a minimum of 3 months of conservative therapy has failed.[66] Two surgical procedures most often recommended in the literature are the **open inferior capsular shift** (surgical detachment and superior advancement of the inferior GH ligament)[67] and **arthroscopic capsular plication** (suturing folds into the GH capsule).[68] Each of these procedures has advantages and disadvantages.

There is greater surgical morbidity with the open inferior capsular shift, but the repair has good and predictable outcomes and allows for repair of the glenoid fossa if needed. Surgeons usually recommend the open inferior capsular shift procedure for

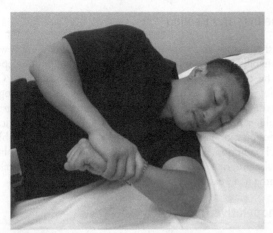

FIG. 18.31 Example of the sleeper stretch. Gentle pressure applied in the direction of internal rotation while the body weight stabilizes the scapula.

moderate-to-severe multidirectional instability (MDI) with concurrent injury to the glenoid fossa. They recommend arthroscopic capsular plication for mild-to-moderate MDI without involvement of the glenoid fossa. In cases of mild-to-moderate MDI, the open and arthroscopic techniques yield comparable results, with less morbidity occurring with the arthroscopic procedure.[67]

For clients with traumatic anterior dislocation, the need for surgical repair of the Bankart lesion varies based on the client's age and the physical demands on the shoulder. Rates of recurrent dislocation were highest in clients younger than 30, with rates ranging from 79% to 100%. Conservative therapy had little effect on reducing rates of recurrence. Therefore clients younger than 30 and those over 30 who perform UE labor-intensive jobs should consider surgical repair.[69]

? Questions to Ask the Doctor

Nonoperative Clients
- What is the nature and direction of the instability?
- Are there any secondary pathologies that need to be addressed (rotator cuff tear, SLAP lesion, and so on)?
- Is this client a surgical candidate?

Operative Clients
- What type of repair was performed? Ask to see an operative report.
- What are the ROM restrictions?
- How soon can the client begin strengthening exercises?
- Do you have a specific postoperative protocol for rehabilitation?

( ) What to Say to Clients

About the Injury

"Your shoulder is a ball-and-socket joint with the ball much larger than the socket. This design allows for a lot of motion, but your shoulder must rely on the muscles and ligaments to keep the joint stable."

For the AMBRII client: "Because the ligaments that support your joint are so loose, your rotator cuff muscles need to work much harder to keep the joint stable. When they fatigue, the ball

is able to slide up and pinch the tendons of the rotator cuff against the bony roof of your shoulder during throwing and overhead activities."

For the TUBS client: "When you fell with your arm out to the side, the ball was forced from the socket, which likely caused damage to the rim of the socket and the supportive ligaments in the front of the shoulder. As a result, your shoulder is unstable, and the ball can easily slip out of the socket if you raise your arm out to the side as if you were going to throw a ball. As your shoulder heals, you must avoid this position, or the problem will keep occurring. There is a chance that even if you avoid this position during your recovery, the damage is great enough that your shoulder will remain unstable."

For the client with the tight posterior capsule: "Because of the way your shoulder has adapted to the stress of throwing, you have developed tightness in a portion of the ligaments that support the shoulder joint. As a result, your joint has a decreased ability to internally rotate. This restriction causes abnormal motion of the ball in the socket when your shoulder is under the stress of throwing, resulting in pain and loss of function."

About Exercises

For the AMBRII client: "Your exercises are designed to compensate for your unstable shoulder by increasing the strength, coordination, and endurance of your rotator cuff and scapular stabilizing muscles. This exercise program is a lifelong commitment because if the weakness returns, your shoulder problems will return as well."

For the TUBS client: "Your exercises strengthen the muscles around your shoulder to support the damaged part of the joint. You must follow the motion restrictions carefully during exercise to avoid disrupting the repair process."

For the client with the tight posterior capsule: "You need to regain the internal rotation motion of your shoulder to restore normal function. The stretches work best if performed frequently. Three sets a day is not enough. You should try for a minimum total of 15 minutes of stretch time each day. Remember, it is not how hard you push the stretch, but how much time you spend at the end of the motion that counts."

Evaluation Tips

- Screening for general connective tissue laxity utilizing the Beighton scale (Table 18.3) assists in identifying the degree of hypermobility your client exhibits. Clients scoring greater than 4/9 are considered hypermobile (Fig. 18.32).[70,71]
- For the unstable shoulder, the goals are to find the direction(s) of instability and to reproduce the client's symptoms. Client feedback during examination is critical.
- The client must be as relaxed as possible during examination because muscle guarding will hide the degree of instability.
- Various tests are described in the literature to test for shoulder instability. Basic tests to check for the direction of instability are as follows:
  - **Anterior and posterior drawer tests:** The client is supine for both tests. For the anterior test, the therapist stands facing the client and fixes the client's hand in the therapist's opposite axilla (Fig. 18.33). By holding the client's arm to be tested in this manner, the client can relax their arm. The therapist grasps the humeral head with the hand opposite the client (the same side holding

TABLE 18.3 Beighton Score for Assessing Hypermobility

Beighton Scale Item	Highest Possible Score*	Criteria for a Positive Sign
Passive hyperextension of fifth finger	2	>90 degrees
Passive thumb opposition to forearm	2	Thumb touches forearm
Elbow hyperextension	2	>10 degrees
Knee hyperextension	2	>10 degrees
Standing trunk flexion with knees fully extended	1	Both palms flat on floor

*Each item is scored bilaterally, except for standing trunk flexion. A score greater than 4/9 is considered positive for hypermobility

the client's hand in the axilla) while stabilizing the scapula and clavicle with the other. Next, the therapist applies an anterior subluxing force to the humeral head while assessing the amount of humeral head movement. You can see this on the YouTube video link at https://youtu.be/a0pyuk9EbiY.

- For the posterior test, the therapist stands level with the affected shoulder and grasps the client's proximal forearm while flexing the client's elbow to 120 degrees. The therapist then positions the client's shoulder in 80 to 120 degrees of abduction and 20 to 30 degrees of forward flexion (Fig. 18.34A). The therapist stabilizes the client's scapula with the opposite hand while resting their thumb over the humeral head (Fig. 18.34B). To perform the test motion, the therapist horizontally adducts the client's arm while simultaneously applying a posterior oblique pressure to the humeral head tangential to the glenoid fossa. If instability exists, the therapist will be able to sense the humeral head's movement as it subluxes posteriorly. The therapist then compares the amount and quality of movement to the opposite side for both tests.[72] You can see this on the YouTube video link at https://youtu.be/B36nIXLe2Eo.
- Sulcus sign test: With the client seated and their arm supported in 20 to 50 degrees of abduction, the therapist pulls inferiorly on the client's arm. A depression of more than a finger width resulting between the acromion and humeral head indicates a positive test. This test indicates MDI (Fig. 18.35).[73] You can see this on the YouTube video link at https://youtu.be/0JF5XmITTfY.
- Apprehension test: With the client supine, the therapist moves the client's shoulder into 90-degree abduction and end-range ER. If with the application of over pressure the client experiences apprehension but not pain, the test is considered positive for anterior instability.[74]
- Relocation test: With the client positioned as at the end of the apprehension test, the therapist applies posteriorly directed pressure from the anterior aspect of the humeral head. The test is positive if the client's apprehension disappears. This test helps confirm anterior instability.[74]

Diagnosis-Specific Information That Affects Clinical Reasoning

The direction of the instability dictates the course of treatment as described earlier. Consequently, you must have a clear understanding of your client's instability pattern. *Applying an incorrect exercise and stretching program may enhance your client's pathology.*

Many of these clients have impingement and/or SLAP lesions as well. If a SLAP lesion is present, your client may need to avoid rotary exercises with the arm above shoulder height. In these cases, overhead throwing exercises are contraindicated.

♡ *Tips From the Field*

- **Proprioception exercises** (activities to enhance position and movement sense/control of the scapula and shoulder complex) need to be stressed with these clients.
- Manually resisted exercises in diagonal patterns at various speeds using concentric and eccentric force are a valuable component of the rehabilitation program.
- Have your client perform UE exercises to strengthen the rotator cuff while concurrently working on balance while in quadruped, sitting, kneeling, and standing.
- Stress proper posture as described earlier.

➤ *Precautions and Concerns*

- *Do not perform end-range or grade IV joint mobilization or stretches on clients with MDI.*
- *Clients with anterior instability need their posterior capsule mobilized. Avoid stretching the anterior capsule.*
- *Pay close attention to ROM restrictions for postoperative clients.*

Rotator Cuff Disease

Anatomy

After neck and back pain, shoulder pain is the third most common musculoskeletal disorder. Up to 70% of shoulder disorders are related to RC disease.[75] The structures of the shoulder that are involved in RC disease include the muscles of the RC, the long head of the biceps tendon, the subdeltoid-subacromial bursa, and CA arch.

The supraspinatus, infraspinatus, and teres minor make up the greater tuberosity attachments of the RC. The subscapularis attaches to the lesser tuberosity. All the RC muscles work together to stabilize the head of the humerus in the glenoid fossa during shoulder motion while their tendons form a cuff that surrounds the humeral head.

Along with their primary role of stabilizing the GH joint, each muscle of the RC imparts specific motion to the humeral head. The supraspinatus is an abductor, the infraspinatus is an external rotator, the teres minor is an external rotator and weak adductor of the humerus, and the subscapularis is an internal rotator and the strongest of the RC muscles (Figs. 18.36 and 18.37).

The stabilizing role of the long head of the biceps tendon was reviewed previously in the section on glenohumeral instability. As the arm elevates overhead, the head of the humerus glides along the biceps tendon as it sits in the bicipital groove between the greater

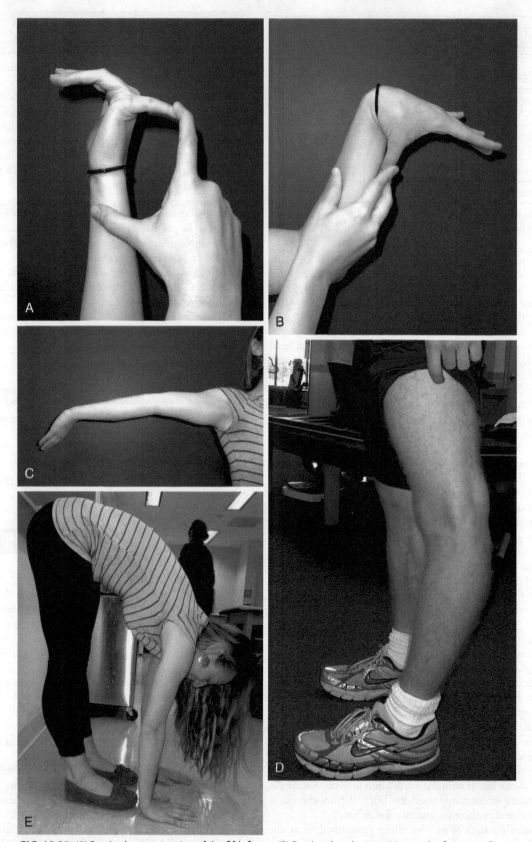

FIG. 18.32 (A) Passive hyperextension of the fifth finger. (B) Passive thumb opposition to the forearm. (C) Elbow hyperextension. (D) Knee hyperextension. (E) Standing trunk flexion with the knees extended.

and lesser tuberosities. The long head of the biceps plays a role in shoulder flexion, as well as forearm flexion and supination.

The subdeltoid-subacromial bursa is a smooth serosal (a smooth membrane that secretes lubricating fluid that reduces friction) sac that sits between RC tendons and the CA arch. Above, it is adherent to the underside of the deltoid, CA ligament, and the acromion. Beneath, it is adherent to the RC and greater tuberosity. This structure provides a cushioning and low friction interface between the convex humeral head and RC as they rotate below the concave CA arch during arm elevation.

The CA arch consists of the anteroinferior aspect of the acromion process, the inferior surface of the AC joint, and the CA ligament. This structure forms a roof over the rotator cuff and humeral head.[11] It not only serves as an attachment site for the deltoid and subdeltoid-subacromial bursa, but it also provides superior stability and protection to the GH joint.

Diagnosis and Pathology

There are two major hypotheses about the etiology of RC disease. One is based on extrinsic causes, and the other is based on

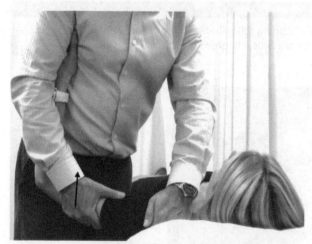

FIG. 18.33 Starting position for the anterior drawer test. The arrow indicates the direction of force applied by the therapist while performing the test.

intrinsic causes. Current evidence demonstrates that both contribute to the disease process and are affected by age, postural habits, movement quality, and activity level.

Extrinsically caused lesions result from the repeated impingement of the RC tendon against different structures of the GH joint. Neer[76] describes impingement between the long head of the biceps and supraspinatus tendons and the CA arch during UE elevation, resulting in lesions on the bursal side of the RC. His three-stage classification of impingement syndrome is still used today (Table 18.4). Bigliani et al.[77] described three types of acromion morphology (Fig. 18.38) with cadaver studies demonstrating a 70% incidence of RC tears in subjects with a Type III acromial shape and a 3% incidence in subjects with a Type I acromial shape. Walch et al.[78] described a type of impingement between the supraspinatus and infraspinatus tendons in the late cocking phase of throwing on the glenoid rim, resulting in lesions on the articular side of the RC.

Intrinsically caused lesions result from age-related degeneration of the RC tendon. These lesions are related to the vascularization of the RC and are on the articular side of the tendon.[11,60,61] Lindblom was the first to describe an area of hypovascularity of the supraspinatus tendon where it attaches to the greater tuberosity.[79] Codman referred to the same area as the "critical zone," as it appeared to be at greater risk of developing a tear.[80]

As most RC tears are partial-thickness tears,[81] the condition is often progressive in nature and can lead to a full-thickness lesion. As tendon fibers fail, they retract because the RC is under constant tension. This process leads to at least four adverse effects[82]:
- Increased load on intact neighboring fibers—leading to their potential failure
- Loss of muscle fibers attached to bone—leading to decreased strength and function of the RC
- Intact tendon blood supply placed at risk by distorted anatomy from fiber failure—leading to progressive ischemia and tendon degeneration
- Loss of tendon repair potential as the tendon is exposed to joint fluid containing lytic enzymes, which inhibit hematoma formation that would facilitate healing

Usually beginning in the supraspinatus tendon, the tear may progress to involve the infraspinatus tendon. Once this occurs, the RC's ability to stabilize the humeral head in the glenoid fossa is severely compromised leading to superior migration under the

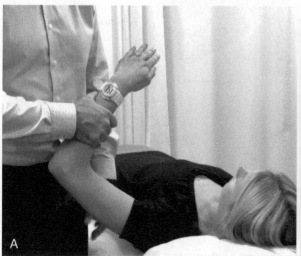
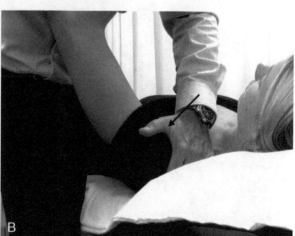

FIG. 18.34 (A) Starting position for the posterior drawer test. (B) Hand position for performing the test. The arrow indicates the direction of force applied by the therapist while performing the test.

unopposed pull of the deltoid. Humeral head superior migration loads the long head of the biceps tendon leading to tendinopathy and potential failure. Traction spurs develop at the CA ligament attachment on the acromion through repeated loading from the upward displacement of the humeral head, leading to further RC damage. This damage allows the RC tendon to slide down below the axis of joint rotation. Much like a boutonnière deformity of the finger, the buttonholed RC becomes a humeral head elevator

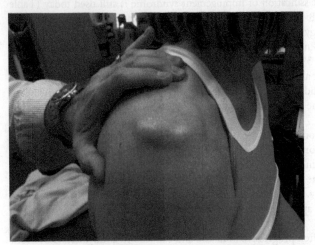

FIG. 18.35 Example of a positive Sulcus sign test.

instead of a depressor. The RC is then ineffective as a humeral head stabilizer, and the individual is unable to elevate their arm above a horizontal position.

Timelines and Healing

Recovery from RC pathology is extremely variable due to multiple presentations of the disease. If the case is uncomplicated, such as a tendonitis, the condition can stabilize in 2 to 6 weeks. If secondary pathologies are present (such as frozen shoulder, impingement, instability, and RC tear), recovery time lengthens considerably. Complex cases may take up to 1 year to resolve with or without surgical intervention.

Nonoperative Treatment

Initial treatment focuses on rest and antiinflammatory modalities to stabilize the disease process. Early ROM exercises (such as, pendulum and wand-assisted elevation in the scapular plane to avoid impingement) help moderate pain through the analgesic effect of mechanoreceptor stimulation.

> ◎ **Clinical Pearl**
>
> Maintaining full pain-free internal rotation and external rotation are critical to preventing frozen shoulder.

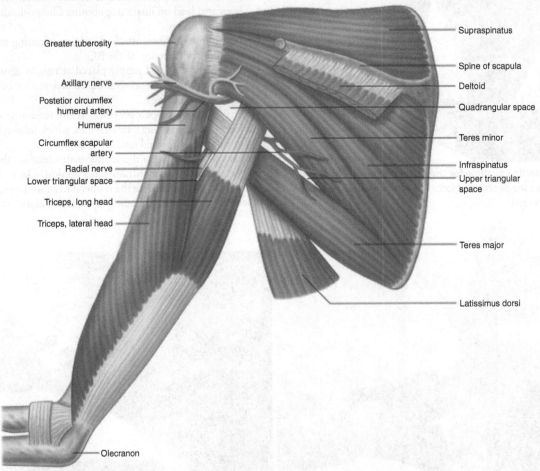

Greater tuberosity
Axillary nerve
Postetior circumflex humeral artery
Humerus
Circumflex scapular artery
Radial nerve
Lower triangular space
Triceps, long head
Triceps, lateral head
Olecranon

Supraspinatus
Spine of scapula
Deltoid
Quadrangular space
Teres minor
Infraspinatus
Upper triangular space
Teres major
Latissimus dorsi

FIG. 18.36 Dorsal muscles of the shoulder, including the supraspinatus, infraspinatus, and teres minor of the rotator cuff. *(From Standring S. Gray's Anatomy. (e-book) 40th ed. St Louis, MO: Churchill Livingstone; 2012, p. 839.)*

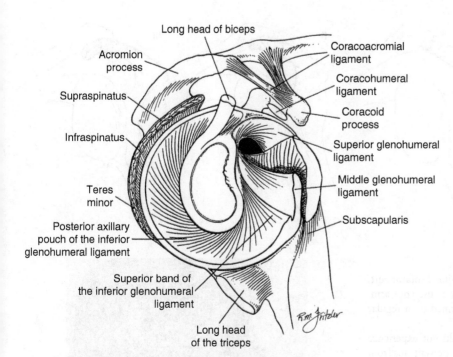

FIG. 18.37 Internal view of the right shoulder joint. The tendons of the rotator cuff and long head of the biceps are indicated. *(From Dutton M. Dutton's Orthopaedic Examination, Evaluation, and Intervention. 3rd ed. Philadelphia, PA: McGraw Hill Medical; 2012, p. 409.)*

TABLE 18.4   Neer's Three-Stage Classification of Impingement Syndrome

Stage	Age Range	Pathology
I	<25 years	Reversible edema and hemorrhage from excessive overhead use
II	25-40 years	Irreversible fibrotic changes to the rotator cuff following repeated episodes of mechanical inflammation
III	>40 years	Bone spurs and tears (complete and incomplete) of the rotator cuff and long head of the biceps tendon

Strengthening of the healthy portion of the RC and scapular stabilizer muscles, usually in the motions of shoulder IR, adduction, and extension, is safe and encourages the stabilizing function of the RC. The use of isometrics and resistance band exercises are effective during this portion of the program. As pain levels decrease and RC function improves, the next step is to strengthen the UE elevators and external rotators. Throughout this process, you must stress muscle balance and proper scapular kinematics. Incorporating open/closed chain and manual exercises, like those described for proximal humerus fracture and for glenohumeral instability, complete the exercise program.

You should focus on strengthening the scapular force couples once your client demonstrates good control of the RC muscles. The addition of sport- and activity-specific exercise is usually the final phase of the rehabilitation program.

Operative Treatment

Indications for RC surgery are the presence of a full or partial tear that has not responded to a course of conservative care and that interferes with the client's ADLs. RC surgery is rapidly evolving as more physicians perform complex repairs through the arthroscope.

Arthroscopic debridement for freshening the frayed, partially torn RC tendon stimulates healing. For full-thickness tears, the surgeon debrides the tear edges and then closes the defect to provide a foundation to regain RC strength and shoulder function. Acromioplasty is often performed at the time of RC repair to decompress the subacromial space and to prevent impingement of the repaired structures.

Most postoperative therapy programs include a 2- to 4-week period of immobilization while the tissues stabilize. The client then starts therapy to regain ROM. For the next 2 to 3 weeks, ROM progresses from passive to active motion exercise. At approximately 8 to 10 weeks postoperative, the client begins strengthening exercises and follows the program for the nonoperative client listed earlier.

❓ Questions to Ask the Doctor

Nonoperative Clients

- Are there any concurrent pathologies (instability, impingement, and so on)?
- Is surgery a possibility?

Operative Clients

- What structures were repaired? Try to obtain an operative report
- Do you have a specific rehabilitation protocol?
- Are there any ROM restrictions or precautions?
- How soon can strengthening begin?

( ) What to Say to Clients

About the Injury

"Your shoulder relies on the rotator cuff muscles to stabilize the head of the humerus in the socket and to prevent the humeral head from being pinched against the roof of your shoulder when you raise your arm. Your rotator cuff is damaged, so this protective function has been interrupted, placing your shoulder at risk. If the problem progresses, you may lose the ability to raise your arm."

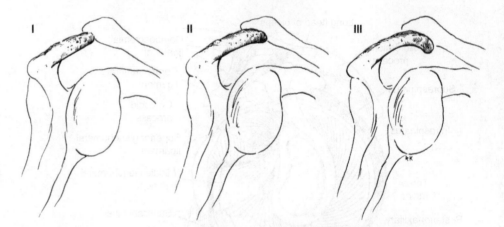

FIG. 18.38 Acromion morphology types I, II, and III. *(From Jobe CM. Gross anatomy of the shoulder. In: Rockwood CA, Matsen FA III. eds.* The Shoulder. *Philadelphia, PA: WB Saunders; 1990.)*

About Exercise

"By strengthening the healthy portions of your injured rotator cuff, there is a good chance you can regain the ability to use your arm. The exercises are specific and need to be performed on a regular basis."

"While performing the exercises, you should not experience sharp sudden pain when raising your arm up. To prevent this from occurring, you must lead the motion with the thumb side of your hand while keeping the point of your elbow facing the ground throughout the motion. Before raising your arm, you must correct your posture (as described in the section on thoracic outlet syndrome/brachial plexopathy). By following these movement precautions, you will minimize the chance of pinching the rotator cuff under the bony roof of your shoulder."

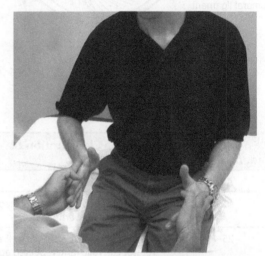

FIG. 18.39 Quick screening position test for full-thickness rotator cuff (RC) tears involving the supraspinatus and infraspinatus. A positive test is pictured. The right shoulder moves into abduction and internal rotation on resisted external rotation, as the deficient RC cannot stabilize against the action of the deltoid.

Evaluation Tips

There is a multitude of tests to detect RC disease. The following tests are included because they are easy to perform and because research indicates they have reasonable sensitivity and specificity.

- A quick screening test to detect a large RC tear involving the supraspinatus and infraspinatus is to resist ER with the client's shoulder in neutral and their elbow flexed to 90 degrees. In the presence of a large RC tear, the unopposed deltoid will abduct their arm while their hand dips into IR (Fig. 18.39).[85]
- Client positioning to palpate the RC insertions are as follows[84]:
  - Supraspinatus: With the dorsum of your client's hand resting on their posterior iliac crest, palpate just inferior to the anterior aspect of the acromion (Fig. 18.40).
  - Infraspinatus: With your client's shoulder in ER and their elbow brought to their navel, palpate just inferior to the posterior aspect of the acromion (Fig. 18.41).
  - The long head of the biceps tendon: With your client's arm held in IR and the forearm resting on a pillow in the client's lap, the tendon should lie in the **deltopectoral interval** (the sulcus formed by the medial border of the deltoid and the lateral edge of the pectoral muscle belly) (Fig. 18.42).
  - Subscapularis: With your client positioned as above, bring their shoulder to neutral rotation. Palpate the lesser tuberosity and tendon in the deltopectoral interval (Fig. 18.43).

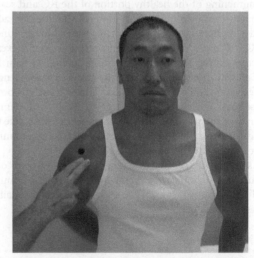

FIG. 18.40 Palpation position for the supraspinatus insertion. The black dot indicates the anterior aspect of the acromion process.

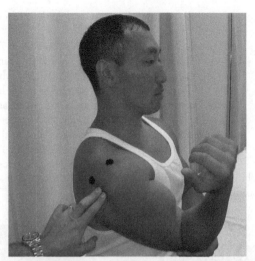

FIG. 18.41 Palpation position for the infraspinatus insertion. The black dots indicate the posterior and anterior aspects of the acromion process.

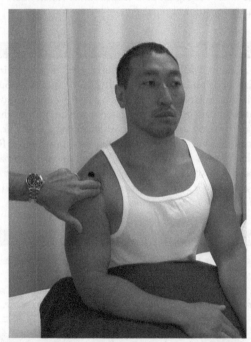

FIG. 18.42 Palpation position for the biceps tendon in the deltopectoral interval. The black dot indicates the anterior aspect of the acromion process.

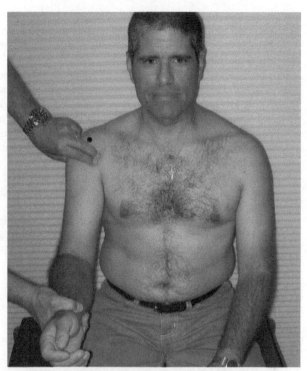

FIG. 18.43 Palpation position for the subscapularis insertion in the deltopectoral interval. The black dot indicates the anterior aspect of the acromion process.

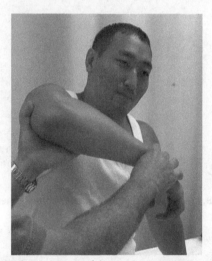

FIG. 18.44 End test position of the Hawkins-Kennedy impingement test.

- Shoulder impingement is a sign of RC disease. The Hawkins-Kennedy and Neer impingement tests are useful in detecting this pathology.[85]
  - Hawkins-Kennedy test[85,86]: With the client's shoulder flexed to 90 degrees, bring their shoulder into full IR. This drives the greater tuberosity under the CA arch and will elicit pain if impingement is present (Fig. 18.44). You can see this on the YouTube video link at https://youtu.be/CkxDKNX_CU0.
  - Neer impingement test[85,86]: Passively flex the client's shoulder to end-range of motion. Positioning their shoulder in IR at the start of the test enhances the impingement of the RC on the underside of the anterior third of the acromion and CA ligament (Fig. 18.45). You can see this on the YouTube video link at https://youtu.be/M218dpojAJM.
- Isometric testing of the specific muscles of the RC and the long head of the biceps aids in detecting tendinopathy. These tests include the Jobe or "empty or full can" tests, the Patte test, the Gerber lift-off test, and the Speed's test.
  - The Jobe or "empty or full can" tests: The client's arms are brought to horizontal in the scapular plane with their shoulder in IR for "empty can" (see this on the YouTube video link at https://youtu.be/peEvU1mXlUY) or 45 degrees externally rotated with the thumb point up for the "full can" test (see this on the YouTube video link at

https://youtu.be/1puSk4gOrSc). Next, apply downward pressure while your client provides isometric resistance. Weakness or the inability to hold this position implicates the supraspinatus (Fig. 18.46).[87]

- The Patte test: The client's arm is positioned in 90 degrees of abduction with neutral rotation in the scapular plane. Apply pressure at their wrist to resist shoulder ER while stabilizing the client's arm at the elbow. Weakness and/or pain implicates the infraspinatus (Fig. 18.47).[88] You can see this on the YouTube video link at https://youtu.be/ZrmlzoRFkYg.
- The Gerber lift-off test: Position the client's arm so the dorsum of their hand rests against their posterior iliac crest. Have the client actively raise their hand 2 to 5 inches from their back while you apply resistance (Fig. 18.48). You can see this on the YouTube video link at https://youtu.be/xMupIO-nSSs.

A client's inability to apply pressure or hold their hand in this position implicates the subscapularis.[88,89]

- The Speed's test: Position the client's shoulder in 70 to 90 degrees of flexion with their elbow in extension, and their forearm in supination. Resist shoulder flexion while palpating the long head of the biceps tendon in the bicipital groove. A painful response implicates the long head of the biceps (Fig. 18.49).[83] The test can also be performed without tendon palpation. You can see this on the YouTube video link at https://youtu.be/i3695fGzLb4.
- There is no resistance test specific to isolating the teres minor.
- While performing these tests, watch for patterns that support specific locations of RC lesions.

Diagnosis Specific Information That Affects Clinical Reasoning

The existence of a RC tear does not always lead to surgery. Many clients function well with MRI-confirmed RC deficits. Clients who are unable to regain pain-free shoulder function are the best candidates for surgical repair.[87]

Tips from the Field

Good palpation skills aide substantially in differentiating subacromial-subdeltoid bursitis from RC tendonitis. The bursa lies beneath the therapist's finger when palpating the supraspinatus and infraspinatus insertions as described earlier. Since the bursa is a relatively fixed structure, its position changes little during arm movement. Conversely, the palpation locations for the RC tendons change with arm movement. A pain response with palpation implicates both structures. *When your client returns their arm to the resting position, the pain will remain constant if the bursa is the source and will decrease if the RC tendons are the source.*

Precautions and Concerns

- *Watch for a tight posterior capsule with these clients and treat accordingly.*
- *In clients showing impingement signs, care must be taken to avoid impinging the shoulder during overhead exercise.*

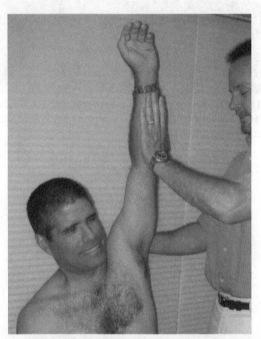
FIG. 18.45 End test position of the Neer impingement test.

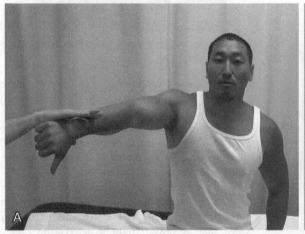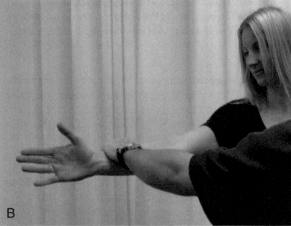
FIG. 18.46 (A) Test position for isometric testing of the supraspinatus or the "empty can" test. (B) "Full can" test position.

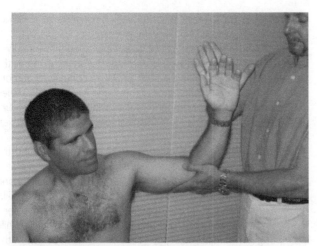

FIG. 18.47 Test position for the Patte test for isometric strength of the infraspinatus and teres minor.

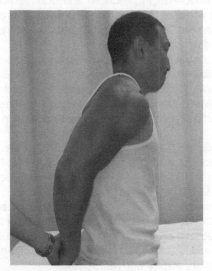

FIG. 18.48 Test position for the Gerber lift-off test for isometric strength of the subscapularis.

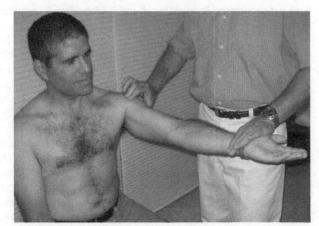

FIG. 18.49 Speeds test for pathology of the long head of the biceps tendon and superior glenoid labrum.

- *Monitor for excessive scapular elevation during UE elevation. Abnormal movement patterns must be avoided.*
- *Discourage clients from sleeping on their involved side, as this often increases the chance for impingement.*

CASE STUDIES: COMMON SHOULDER DIAGNOSES

CASE STUDY 18.1 ▪

John is a 48-year-old right dominant stockbroker, nonsmoker, who presented with a diagnosis of mild brachial plexus stretch injury. He reported symptoms of headache in the C2 distribution, anterior chest wall pain on the left, pain in the left anteriolateral neck extending to the angle of his jaw and to the anterior aspect of his shoulder. He noted occasional swelling with flushing of the left side of his face, extending to his ear. This symptom became more prevalent when his left upper quarter pain was high. He was experiencing slight numbness of digits one to three and arm pain on the inside of the proximal humerus of the left UE while sitting at his desk and with overhead activities. He reported difficulty combing his hair because of arm pain.

Symptoms began 2 months ago when he decided to return to surfing after a 15-year hiatus. He stopped surfing about 1 month ago because his face, chest wall, and arm symptoms would increase dramatically during and for days after time spent on his board.

He had a thorough cardiac workup and was cleared. X-rays and MRI of the cervical spine were unremarkable. He is in excellent physical shape, with an unremarkable past medical history.

On exam, he demonstrated a drooped left shoulder with a forward-head-rounded-shoulders posture. Cervical ROM was limited 25% only for rotation and lateral flexion to the right. Crossed-arm cervical ROM test showed no improvement in motion. Shoulder ROM was limited in flexion to horizontal by arm pain, with IR and ER being full. RC strength was at 5/5 bilaterally and pain free on testing. There was muscle spasm in the suboccipital region, across the trapezius ridge, and along the medial scapular boarder.

Palpation at the left supraclavicular fossa was tender with spread of pain into the side of the face to the ear. Palpation at the left infraclavicular fossa and neurovascular bundle was painful with an increase of left UE symptoms. Tinel's sign was positive in the same areas.

There was decreased sensitivity to pin prick of the thumb, index, and radial side of the long finger on the left. Roos (EAST) test was positive immediately. Neural mobility of the brachial plexus was at 2–/5 on the left with increase of left upper quarter symptoms and 5/5 on the right.

Impressions

Based on clinical presentation, John demonstrated evidence of an upper trunk lateral cord brachial plexopathy with decreased plexus mobility restricting UE elevation. Cervical motion loss implicated scalene tightness.

Facial symptoms with headache combined with shoulder droop implicate the upper trunk. Decreased acuity to pin prick on the radial side of the long finger continuing to the index finger and thumb implicate the lateral cord as well. No change in cervical motion with the cross-arm position combined with the pattern of cervical motion loss implicates the scalenes. As John has full shoulder IR and ER, his limited UE elevation was not likely due to a capsular restriction. RC pathology is unlikely as well since RC strength was 5/5 and he was pain free on testing.

Treatment

Treatment on the first visit consisted of instruction in posture correction exercises, modification of computer placement to encourage proper posture while working, and to limit all overhead activities. John was instructed in nerve gliding exercises to be performed 3 times a day in sets of 3, with his posture correction exercises to be performed hourly in sets of 10.

John's work schedule only allowed for weekly visits, so his treatment program was designed accordingly. On his second visit, John demonstrated excellent technique with his home program. He had avoided all overhead activity and modified his workstation to encourage proper posture. He reported a 50% improvement in symptoms, with no headache for the past week. Brief exam revealed neural mobility at 3+/5, good postural awareness, and less left shoulder drooping.

Treatment consisted of pectoral minor and scalene stretching with nerve glides. Neural mobility improved to 4+/5 by the end of treatment. John's home program was modified to include scalene stretching and pectoralis minor doorway stretches. He could perform nerve glide and stretching exercises as long as his symptoms remained stable in sets of three three times a day. Scapular clock exercises were added to work on proprioception on an hourly basis.

On John's visit 1 week later, he again demonstrated excellent compliance with his home program. He had full neural mobility and his cervical ROM was full. Shoulder position was equal bilaterally. Roos (EAST) test was positive at 45 seconds of testing.

Treatment consisted of home program modification with the addition of scapular strengthening with focus on the upper, middle, lower trapezius, and serratus anterior using resistance bands. All exercises were performed daily in sets of three, once through each exercise before starting the next set. John was instructed to stop exercising if symptoms returned.

On the fourth visit 2 weeks later, John had been symptom free for 1 week. Exam was normal except for a positive Roos test at 1 minute of testing leading to paresthesia into the thumb and index finger. As his condition was stable and he had excellent understanding of his home program, John was discharged from therapy with instruction to call as needed for program progression or if his status changed. He was instructed to avoid surfing.

As John was in excellent shape prior to his injury from surfing, plus he was compliant and motivated, he quickly stabilized and returned to a functional baseline. Many clients have difficulty modifying their lifestyle to avoid further injury to their brachial plexus, resulting in a protracted recovery period.

CASE STUDY 18.2 ■

Fran is a 75-year-old right dominant female who tripped over her cat and sustained a Neer one-part fracture of the proximal humerus. She is 3 weeks postinjury when she presents to therapy in a simple sling for immobilization. Therapy orders are for ROM exercises with no strengthening for the next 3 weeks. Fran is very apprehensive about

moving her arm as she feels that the break is still unstable, since not enough time has passed from her injury date.

Prior to moving Fran's right shoulder, I explained that sound will not travel across an open fracture and used a stethoscope at the humeral head while tapping on the lateral epicondyle to demonstrate to her there is no difference in the sound level. Next, I showed her that the head of her humerus was moving as I rolled her arm from IR to ER, again indicating that she is ready to begin ROM exercise.

Exam revealed severe ecchymosis in the axilla and around the elbow. I explained that when she fractured her arm, there was a lot of bleeding from the bone and that blood has run down her arm along the interior tissue planes to collect around her elbow and distal axilla.

Shoulder elevation was 50 degrees, abduction was 40 degrees, IR was arm across the abdomen and thumb to the iliac crest while attempting arm behind back position. ER was neutral. ROM of the elbow was 20 to 110 degrees with wrist and hand ROM normal. Strength testing was deferred at that time.

I instructed Fran in pendulum and tabletop ROM exercises, which she was to perform hourly in sets of 3 to 10, up to 3 sets each exercise session. She started ROM exercises for her elbow that she was to perform whenever sitting.

Fran's treatment over the next 2 weeks focused on scapulothoracic stabilization via manual resistance applied to the scapula along with scapular mobilization and proprioception scapular clock exercises. PROM of the shoulder was also stressed, focusing on avoidance of substitution patterns of excessive scapular elevation and protraction.

Reevaluation 2 weeks later revealed ROM of elevation at 110 degrees, abduction at 90 degrees, ER to 30 degrees at 75 degrees of abduction and 40 degress at neutral shoulder abduction. IR is at thumb to L5 reaching behind the back.

Treatment continued to focus on ROM, stressing active motion in normal movement patterns as Fran mirrored my UE elevation while I stabilized her shoulder to prevent early scapular elevation. Fran then added wall walking to her program incorporating self-stabilization of the scapula with her left hand.

At 6 weeks postinjury, Fran's shoulder elevation is 150 degrees, abduction is 135 degrees, ER at 90 degrees abduction is 50 degrees, ER at shoulder neutral is 60 degrees, and IR behind the back has progressed little at thumb to L3. Elbow, hand, and wrist ROM are full.

As Fran was then allowed to begin strengthening, isometrics for all planes of shoulder movement and resistance band exercises of the elbow flexors and extensors are added. Behind-the-back stretches with good scapular position and upright posture are stressed as well. At this point, the therapy program included joint mobilization and more aggressive stretching to focus on gaining end ROM.

Fran attended therapy for a total of 6 weeks. She had 160 degrees of elevation, 150 degrees of abduction, and 70 degrees of ER at 90 degrees of abduction and with the shoulder at neutral. IR behind the back remained restricted with the thumb reaching the L2 spinous process. Fran was fully independent in self-care with her right arm and she was pain free. Shoulder strength was 4/5 except for abduction and ER, which were 4–/5. She never regained full IR, as there may have been a rotary component to her fracture as she healed limiting the potential for normal internal rotation.

References

1. Ludewig PM, et al.: Motion of the shoulder complex during multiplanar humeral elevation, *J Bone Joint Surg Am* 91:378–389, 2009.
2. Lugo R, Kung P, Ma CB: Shoulder biomechanics, *Eur J Radio* 68:16–24, 2008.
3. Nam D, et al.: Rotator cuff tear arthropathy: evaluation, diagnosis, and treatment: AAOS exhibit selection, *J Bone Joint Surg Am* 94(6):e34, 2012.
4. Matsumura N, et al.: The function of the clavicle on scapular motion: a cadaveric study, *J Shoulder Elbow Surg* 22(3):333–339, 2013.
5. Mercer SR, Bogduk N: Clinical anatomy of the ligamentum nuchae, *Clin Anat* 16:484–493, 2003.
6. Johnson D, Ellis H: Pectoral girdle, shoulder region and axilla. In Standring S, editor: *Gray's anatomy thirty-ninth edition*, New York, 2005, Elsevier, pp 817–850.
7. Bontempo NA, Mazzocca AD: Biomechanics and treatment of acromioclavicular and sternocoavicular joint injuries, *Br J Sports Med* 44:361–369, 2010.
8. Groh GL, Wirth MA: Management of traumatic sternoclavicular joint injuries, *J Am Acad Orthop Surg* 19:1–7, 2011.
9. Kibler WB, Sciascia A, Wilkes T: Scapular dyskinesis and its relation to shoulder injury, *J Am Acad Orthop Surg* 20:364–372, 2012.
10. Lawrence RL, et al.: Comparison of 3-dimensional shoulder complex kinematics in individuals with and without shoulder pain, part I: sternoclavicular, acromioclavicular, and scapulothoracic joints, *J Orthop Sports Phys Ther* 44(9):636–645, 2014.
11. Ludewig PM, Braman JP: Shoulder impingement: biomechanical considerations in rehabilitation, *Man Ther* 16:33–39, 2011.
12. Mercer SB, Bogduk N: The ligaments and anulus fibrosus of human adult cervical intervertebral discs, *Spine* 24(7):619–626, 1999.
13. Nakashima H, et al.: Abnormal findings on magnetic resonance images of the cervical spine in 1211 asymptomatic subjects, *Spine* 40(5):392–398, 2015.
14. McLain RF: Mechanoreceptor endings in human cervical facet joints, *Spine* 19, 1994. 495–450.
15. Dwyer A, Aprill C, Bogduk N: Cervical zygapophyseal joint pain patterns. I: a study in normal volunteers, *Spine* 15(6):453–457, 1990.
16. Cooper G, Bailey B, Bogduk N: Cervical joint pain maps, *Pain Med* 8(4):344–353, 2007.
17. Travell JG, Simmons DG: *Myofascial pain and dysfunction the trigger point manual*, vol. 1. Baltimore, MD, 1983, Lippincott Williams & Wilkins.
18. Werneke MW, et al.: Clinician's ability to identify neck and low back interventions: an inter-rater chance-corrected agreement study, *J Man Manip Ther* 19(3):172–181, 2011.
19. Salt E, et al.: A systemic review of the literature on the effectiveness of manual therapy for cervicobrachial pain, *Man Ther* 16(1):53–56, 2011.
20. Wainner RS, et al.: Reliability and diagnostic accuracy of the clinical examination and patient self-report measures for cervical radiculopathy, *Spine* 28(1):52–62, 2003.
21. Lemeunier N, et al.: Reliability and validity of clinical tests to assess the anatomical integrity of the cervical spine in adults with neck pain and its associated disorders: part 1 - a systemic review from the Cervical Assessment and Diagnosis Research Evaluation (CADRE) Collaboration, *Eur Spine J* 26:2225–2241, 2017.
22. Tong HC, et al.: The Spurling Test and cervical radiculopathy, *Spine* 27(2):156–159, 2002.
23. Anekstein Y, et al.: What is the best way to apply the Spurling test for cervical radiculopathy? *Clin Orthop Rel Resear* 470:2566–2572, 2012.
24. Spurling RG, Scoville WB: Lateral rupture of the cervical intervertebral discs: a common cause of shoulder and arm pain, *Surg Gynecol Obstetr* 78:350–358, 1944.
25. Takasaki H, et al.: The influence of cervical traction, compression, and Spurling Test on cervical intervertebral foramen size, *Spine* 34(16):1658–1662, 2009.
26. Wilbourn AJ: 10 most commonly asked questions about thoracic outlet syndrome, *Neurologist* 7(5):309–312, 2001.
27. Roos DB: Congenital anomalies associated with thoracic outlet syndrome, *Am J Surg* 132:771–778, 1976.
28. Hooper TL, et al.: Thoracic outlet syndrome: a controversial clinical condition, part 1: anatomy, and clinical examination/diagnosis, *J Man Manip Ther* 18(2):74–83, 2010.
29. Gergoudis R, Barnes R: Thoracic outlet arterial compression: prevalence in normals, *Angiology* 31:538, 1980.
30. Costigan DA, Wilbourn AJ: The elevated arm stress test: specificity in the diagnosis of thoracic outlet syndrome, *Neurology* 35(Suppl 1):74, 1985.
31. Warrens A, Heaton J: Thoracic outlet compression syndrome: the lack of reliability of its clinical assessment, *Ann Royal Col Surg Eng* 69:203–204, 1987.
32. Rayan G, Jensen C: Thoracic outlet syndrome: provocative examination maneuvers in a typical population, *J Shoulder Elbow Surg* 4:113–117, 1995.
33. Nord KM, et al.: False positive rate of thoracic outlet syndrome diagnostic maneuvers, *Electromyogr Clin Neurophysiol* 48(2):67–74, 2008.
34. Leffert RD: Thoracic outlet syndrome, *J Am Acad of Orthop Surg* 2(6):317–325, 1994, Nov.
35. Schwartzman RJ: Brachial plexus traction injuries, *Hand Clinics* 7(3):547–556, 1991.
36. Dilley A, Lynn B, Pang SJ: Pressure and stretch mechanosensitivity of peripheral nerve fibers following local inflammation of the nerve trunk, *Pain* 117:462–472, 2005.
37. Nijs J, et al.: How to explain central sensitization to patients with 'unexplained' chronicmusculoskeletal pain: practice guidelines, *Man Ther* 16(5):413–418, 2011.
38. Degeorges R, et al.: Thoracic outlet syndrome surgery: long-term functional results, *Ann Vasc Surg* 18(5):558–565, 2004.
39. Colli BO, et al.: Neurologic thoracic outlet syndromes: a comparison of true and nonspecific syndromes after surgical treatment, *Surg Neuro* 65:262–272, 2006.
40. Butler MW, et al.: Reliability and accuracy of the Brachial Plexus Neural Dynamic Test, *J Hand Ther* In Press:1–5, 2018.
41. Roos DB, Owens C: The thoracic outlet syndrome, *Arch Surg* 93:71, 1966.
42. Handoll HHG, Ollivere BJ: Interventions for treating proximal humeral fractures in adults (Review), *Cochrane Library* 12:1–76, 2010.
43. Neer 2nd CS: Displaced proximal humeral fractures. Classification and evaluation, *J Bone Joint Surg* 52(6):1077–1089, 1970.
44. Palvanen M, et al.: The injury mechanisms of osteoporotic upper extremity fractures among older adults: a controlled study of 287 consecutive patients and their 108 controls, *Osteoporosis Int* 11(10):822–831, 2000.
45. Gohlke F, Essigkrug B, Schnitz F: The pattern of the collagen fiber bundles of the capsule of the glenohumeral joint, *J Shoulder Elbow Surg* 3:111–128, 1994.
46. Lee MH, et al.: Adhesive capsulitis of the shoulder. Diagnosis using magnetic resonance arthrography as the standard, *J Comput Assist Tomogr* 27:901–906, 2003.
47. Tasto JP, Elias DW: Adhesive capsulitis, *Sports Med Arthros Rev* 15:216–221, 2007.
48. Georgiannos D, et al.: Adhesive capsulitis of the shoulder. Is there a consensus regarding the treatment? A systemic review, *Open Orthop J* 11:65–76, 2017.
49. Jewell DV, Riddle DL, Thacker LR: Interventions associated with and increased or decreased likelihood of pain reduction and improved function in patients with adhesive capsulitis: a retrospective cohort study, *Phys Ther* 89:419–429, 2009.
50. Bunker T: (ii) Frozen shoulder, *Orthop Trauma* 25(1):11–18, 2011.
51. Le HV, et al.: Adhesive capsulitis of the shoulder: review of pathophysiology and current clinical treatments, *Shoulder Elbow* 9(2):75–84, 2017.
52. Milgrom C, et al.: Risk factors for frozen shoulder, *Isr Med Assoc J* 10(5):361–364, 2008.

53. Prodromidis AD, Charalambous CP: Is there a genetic predisposition to frozen shoulder? A systematic review and meta-analysis, *JBJS Reviews* 4, 2016. pii: 01874474-201602000-00004.

54. Smith SP, Devaraj VS, Bunker TD: The association between frozen shoulder and dupuytren's disease, *J Shoulder Elbow Surg* 10(2):149–151, 2001 Mar-Apr.

55. Shaffer B, Tibone JE, Kerlan RK: Frozen shoulder. A long-term follow-up, *J Bone Joint Surg* 74(5):738–746, 1992 Jun.

56. Vastamaki H, Kettunen J, Vastamaki M: The natural history of idiopathic frozen shoulder: a 2- to 27-year followup study, *Clin Orthop Relat Res* 470(4):1133–1143, 2012.

57. Hannafin JA, Chiaia TA: Adhesive capsulitis. A treatment approach, *Clin Orthop Rel Res* 372:95–109, 2000 Mar.

58. Le HV, et al.: Adhesive capsulitis of the shoulder: review of the pathophysiology and current clinical treatments, *Shoulder Elbow* 9(2):75–84, 2017.

59. Wilk KE, Macrina LC, Fleisig GS, et al.: Correlation of glenohumeral internal rotation deficit and total rotational motion to shoulder injuries in professional baseball pitchers, *Am J Sports Med* 39:329–335, 2011.

60. Guerrero P, Busconi B, Deangelus N, Powers G: Congenital instability of the shoulder joint: assessment and treatment options, *J Orthop Sports Phys Ther* 39(2):124–134, 2009.

61. Budoff JE, Nirschl RP, Guidi EJ: Debridement of partial thickness tears of the rotator cuff without acromioplasty, *J Bone Joint Surg* 5:733–748, 1998.

62. Tyler TF, et al.: Correction of posterior shoulder thightness is associated with symptom resolution in patients with internal impingement, *Am J Sports Med* 38:114–118, 2010.

63. Nakamizo H, et al.: Loss of internal rotation in little league pitchers: a biomechanical study, *J Shoulder and Elbow Surg* 17:795–801, 2008.

64. Shanley E, Rauh MJ, Michener LA, et al.: Shoulder range of motion measures as risk factors for shoulder and elbow injuries in high school softball and baseball players, *Am J Sports Med* 39(9):1997–2006, 2011.

65. Burkhart SS, Morgan CD: The peel-back mechanism: its role in producing and extending posterior type II SLAP lesions and its effect on SLAP repair rehabilitation, *Arthroscopy* 14(6):637–640, 1998.

66. Zazzali MS, Vad VB, et al.: Shoulder instability. In Donatelli RA, editor: *Physical therapy of the shoulder fourth edition*, St. Louis, 2004, Churchill Livingstone, pp 483–504.

67. Neer 2nd CS, Foster C: Inferior capsular shift for involuntary inferior and multidirectional instability of the shoulder: a preliminary report, *J Bone Joint Surg* 62A:897–908, 1980.

68. Jacobson ME, Riggenbach M, Woodbridge AN, Bishop JY: Open and arthroscopic treatment of multidirectional instability of the shoulder, *Arthroscopy* 28(7):1010–1017, 2012.

69. Godin J, Sekiya JK: Systemic review of rehabilitation versus operative stabilization for the treatment of first-time anterior shoulder dislocations, *Sports Health* 2(2):156–165, 2010.

70. Cameron KL, et al.: Association of generalized joint hypermobility with a history of glenohumeral joint instability, *J Athl Train* 45(3):253–258, 2010.

71. Johnson SM, Robinson CM: Shoulder instability in patients with joint hyperlaxity, *J Bone Joint Surg Am* 92(6):1545–1557, 2010.

72. Gerber C, Ganz R: Clinical assessment of instability of the shoulder with special preference to anterior and posterior drawer tests, *J Bone Joint Surg Br* 66(4):551–556, 1984.

73. Tzannes A, et al.: An assessment of the interexaminer reliability of tests for shoulder instability, *J Shoulder Elbow Surg* 13(1):18–23, 2004.

74. Farber AJ, et al.: Clinical assessment of three common tests for traumatic anterior shoulder instability, *J Bone Joint Surg Am* 88:1467–1474, 2006.

75. Longo UG, et al.: Epidemiology, genetics and biological factors of rotator cuff tears, *Med Sport Sci* 57:1–9, 2012.

76. Neer 2nd CS: Anterior acromioplasty for the chronic impingement syndrome in the shoulder: a preliminary report, *J Bone Joint Surg Am* 54(1):41–50, 1972.

77. Bigliani LU, Morrison D, et al.: The morphology of the acromion and its relationship to rotator cuff tears, *Orthop Trans* 10:228, 1986.

78. Walch G, Boileau P, et al.: Impingement of the deep surface of the supraspinatus tendon on the glenoid rim, *J Shoulder Elbow Surg* 1:239–245, 1992.

79. Lindblom K: On pathogenesis of ruptures of the tendon aponeurosis of the shoulder joint, *Acta Radiologica* 20:563–567, 1939.

80. Codman EA: *The shoulder*, ed 2, Boston, 1934, Thomas Todd.

81. Finnan RP, Crosby LA: Partial-thickness rotator cuff tears, *J Shoulder Elbow Surg* 19:609–616, 2010.

82. Matsen III FA, Arntz CT: Rotator cuff tendon failure. In Rockwood Jr CA, Matsen III FA, editors: *The shoulder*, vol. II. Philadelphia, 1990, WB Saunders Co, pp 647–677.

83. Kelly SM, Brittle N, Allen GM: The value of physical tests for subacromial impingement syndrome: a study of diagnostic accuracy, *Clin Rehabil* 24(2):149–158, 2010.

84. Mattingly GE, Mackarey PJ: Optimal methods for shoulder tendon palpation: a Cadaver Study, *Phys Ther* 76:166–174, 1996.

85. Park HB, et al.: Diagnostic accuracy of clinical tests for the different degrees of subacromial impingement syndrome, *J Bone Joint Surg Am* 87:1446–1455, 2005.

86. Alqunaee M, Galvin R, Fahey T: Diagnostic accuracy of clinical tests for subacromial impingement syndrome: a systematic review and meta-analysis, *Arch Phys Med Rehabil* 93(2):229–236, 2012.

87. Kijima H, Minagawa H, Nishi T, et al.: Long-term follow-up of cases of rotator cuff tear treated conservatively, *J Shoulder Elbow Surg* 21(4):491–494, 2012.

88. Longo UG, Berton A, Aherns PM: *Sports Med Arthrosc Rev* 19:266–278, 2011.

89. Gerber C, Krushell RJ: Isolated rupture of the tendon of the subscapularis muscle, clinical features in 16 cases, *J Bone Joint Surg Br* 73(3):389–394, 1991.

Elbow Diagnoses

Carol Page

Function of the Elbow

The elbow serves as the essential functional link between the hand and the shoulder, allowing the hand to be brought inward toward the body and outward into the surrounding environment. It also transfers force through the upper extremity (UE) during weight bearing on the hand. The functional range of motion (ROM) required at the elbow is reported to be 30 degrees of extension, 130 degrees of flexion, and 50 degrees each of pronation and supination.[1] However, because functional demands vary, the range required will differ somewhat among individuals. In general, it is easier to compensate for limited extension by moving closer to objects during reach than it is to compensate for limited flexion. Because the most common complication of elbow trauma is stiffness, it is essential that therapists treating individuals with elbow injuries be well versed in effective treatment approaches. To "push harder" or "be more aggressive" is not an effective solution and may instead cause more damage and stiffness. In addition to being mobile, the elbow must also be stable so that it can withstand the forces of daily activities. Maintaining the most effective balance between minimizing stiffness through early motion, preserving stability, and protecting healing structures is a challenge even for experienced therapists.

◎ Clinical Pearl

Elbow stiffness is the most common complication of elbow trauma.

Elbow Anatomy

Three bones contribute to the **elbow joint:** the distal humerus, proximal ulna, and proximal radius (Fig. 19.1). They form the three articulations of the elbow: the ulnohumeral, radiohumeral, and proximal radioulnar joints. The distal humerus has two articular surfaces: the spool-shaped **trochlea** medially and the convex **capitellum** (also known as the *capitulum*) laterally. The **ulnohumeral joint** is the close articulation of the trochlea with the rounded **trochlear notch** formed by the **coronoid** and **olecranon** of the proximal ulna. In full elbow flexion, the **coronoid fossa** on the anterior distal humerus receives the coronoid process of the anterior trochlear notch. In full extension, the **olecranon fossa** on the posterior distal humerus receives the olecranon process of the posterior trochlear notch. The **radiohumeral joint** is the articulation of the capitellum of the distal humerus with the shallow concavity on the proximal aspect of the **radial head.** The radial head and the **radial notch** of the ulna form the **proximal radioulnar joint.**

Due to the oblique orientation of the trochlea of the humerus, in full extension the elbow has a **valgus** angle, known as the **carrying angle.** It has been widely reported that men have a carrying angle of approximately 5 to 10 degrees, while women have a slightly greater carrying angle of approximately 10 to 15 degrees. However, measured radiographically, the normal carrying angle in adults is reported to be 17.8 degrees on average with no significant difference between men and women.[2]

◎ Clinical Pearl

The most reliable way to determine if the carrying angle of an injured elbow is normal is to compare it to the individual's uninjured elbow.

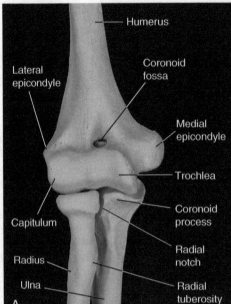
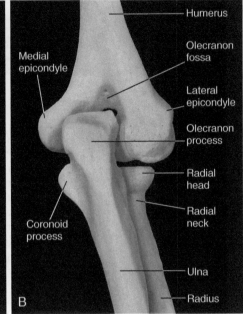

FIG. 19.1 (A) Anterior view of the elbow joint. (B) Posterior view of the elbow joint. (From Thibodeau G, Patton K. eds. *Anatomy & Physiology*. 8th ed. St Louis, MO: Mosby; 2013.)

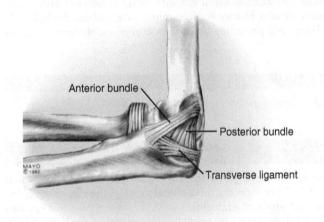
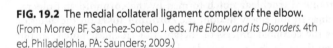

FIG. 19.2 The medial collateral ligament complex of the elbow. (From Morrey BF, Sanchez-Sotelo J. eds. *The Elbow and its Disorders*. 4th ed. Philadelphia, PA: Saunders; 2009.)

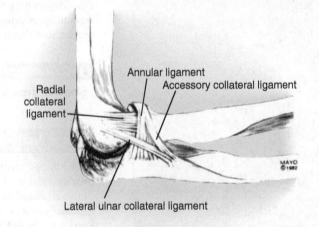

FIG. 19.3 The lateral collateral ligament complex of the elbow. (From Morrey BF, Sanchez-Sotelo J. eds. *The Elbow and its Disorders*. 4th ed. Philadelphia, PA: Saunders; 2009.)

Ligaments

The three elbow articulations share a common joint capsule. The medial and lateral collateral ligament complexes of the elbow are essentially thickenings of the joint capsule. Portions of the collateral ligament complexes remain taut throughout elbow flexion and extension, making an essential contribution to static elbow stability. The **medial collateral ligament complex** (Fig. 19.2) has three components: the anterior bundle, posterior bundle, and the transverse ligament. This ligament complex, particularly the anterior bundle, stabilizes the elbow against valgus (abduction) forces. The **lateral collateral ligament complex** (Fig. 19.3) has four components: the **lateral ulnar collateral ligament (LUCL),** the radial collateral ligament, the annular ligament, and the accessory lateral collateral ligament. The lateral collateral ligament complex is considered to be one of the primary stabilizers of the elbow. It provides restraint from **varus** (adduction) forces. The LUCL, one of the four components of this ligament complex, also provides posterolateral stability to the ulnohumeral joint.

> ⊙ *Clinical Pearl*
>
> Edema often affects all three joints of the elbow because they share a common joint capsule.

The **interosseous ligament**, fibrous tissue lying obliquely between the radius and ulna, transfers forces from the radius to the ulna during weight bearing on the hand. Although not part of the elbow complex, injury to the interosseous ligament can alter the mechanics of the elbow. If the radial head is fractured or excised, the interosseous ligament is critical to load sharing. If it is disrupted, the entire force is shifted to the ulna rather than being shared between the ulna and radius.

Muscles

The muscles that cross the elbow provide it with active power and dynamic stability. Biceps brachii, brachialis, and brachioradialis are the primary elbow flexors. Biceps brachii is the primary supinator of forearm, with supinator acting as an additional, weaker supinator. Triceps is the primary elbow extensor. Pronator teres is the primary forearm pronator with pronator quadratus in the distal forearm acting as another, weaker pronator. The other muscles crossing the elbow joint serve as secondary movers and contribute to dynamic joint stability.

Nerves and Blood Vessels

The muscles that move the elbow are innervated by the musculocutaneous, radial, and median nerves. The musculocutaneous nerve innervates biceps brachii and brachialis. The radial nerve innervates brachioradialis, triceps, and supinator. The median nerve innervates pronator teres. The median, ulnar, and radial nerves and the brachial artery all lie close to the elbow joint and as a result are susceptible to injury in elbow fractures and dislocations. The ulnar nerve is particularly susceptible to injury as it passes posterior to the medial epicondyle through the **cubital tunnel.**

◎ *Clinical Pearl*

Abnormal stress on the ulnar nerve can result from an elbow injury, a direct blow, or prolonged direct pressure (such as when leaning on the elbow or prolonged or repetitive elbow flexion) that stretches the nerve. Numbness and tingling in the small finger and ulnar aspect of the ring finger and grip weakness can be signs and symptoms of ulnar **neuritis** or compression of the ulnar nerve in the cubital tunnel.

Elbow Biomechanics

Motion at the elbow occurs in two axes: flexion-extension and pronation-supination. The elbow acts as a hinge during flexion-extension. However, rather than occurring in a single plane, flexion-extension is accompanied by slight rotation and medial-lateral motion, which results in the carrying angle of the elbow. Normal elbow ROM is approximately 0 degrees extension to 140 degrees flexion. Because flexion is limited by soft-tissue approximation, end-range is variable. Hyperextension of up 10 degrees is observed more commonly in women. During pronation-supination, the radius rotates around the ulna. Normal forearm ROM is approximately 85 degrees pronation and 90 degrees supination. ROM varies among individuals, and a variety of normal values are reported in the literature.

◎ *Clinical Pearl*

Determination of normal elbow and forearm ROM for an individual is best made by comparison to the uninvolved UE rather than to published norms.

Stability at the elbow is provided by both static and dynamic constraints. The osseous structures provide static stability. The highly congruent ulnohumeral joint is the primary stabilizer of the elbow. The radial head also acts as a stabilizing structure.

The joint capsule, medial collateral ligament complex, and lateral collateral ligament complex provide additional static stability. The muscles that cross the elbow, when contracted, contribute dynamic stability to the elbow.

Elbow Fractures

The elbow is a complex joint, vulnerable to fracture from falls on an outstretched hand as well as from direct trauma. Elbow fractures are frequently challenging to treat, often requiring operative intervention. The most common complication of elbow fracture is stiffness. Failure to regain elbow ROM can result in significant functional impairment. To minimize this risk, it is important that mobilization begin early. The necessary stability to safely allow early mobilization of displaced and unstable elbow fractures requires operative management.

Radial Head Fractures

Radial head fractures are the most common elbow fracture in adults. The most common mechanism of injury is falling onto an outstretched hand with the forearm pronated. These fractures can also result from falling directly onto the elbow. The most common complication of both stable, nonoperatively managed radial head fractures and those requiring operative stabilization is **elbow flexion contracture**, the loss of full elbow extension.

◎ *Clinical Pearl*

In the presence of radial head fracture, the forearm and wrist should also be carefully evaluated because there may be associated injuries to the interosseous ligament and the distal radioulnar joint, known as an **Essex-Lopresti lesion**.

Olecranon Fractures

Olecranon fractures are another relatively common elbow fracture in adults. These fractures usually result from a fall onto a bent elbow or a direct blow. The olecranon is particularly vulnerable to direct trauma due to its location just below the skin where it has minimal protective soft-tissue coverage. The majority of olecranon fractures are displaced with a tendency to be widely separated because of the pull of the triceps insertion. Most olecranon fractures require operative management. Severe, unstable olecranon fractures are usually associated with trauma to other structures and can be very complex and challenging to treat.

◎ *Clinical Pearl*

The ulnar nerve is susceptible to injury in olecranon fractures due to its adjacent location.

Distal Humeral Fractures

Fractures of the distal humerus are relatively uncommon in adults. Falling is the most common mechanism of injury. These fractures occur most frequently in children ages 5 to 9 years, with the supracondylar distal humeral fracture being the most common pediatric elbow fracture. In addition, elderly females have an increased risk of distal humeral fractures. The incidence of these fractures is expected to increase as the population ages.[3]

Timelines and Healing

To minimize the risk of elbow stiffness following an isolated elbow fracture, gentle active motion in the stable range is usually initiated within the first week following injury or surgery. While early motion is highly desirable, fracture stability is the prerequisite. Isolated elbow fractures that are stable and nondisplaced are usually referred to therapy several days after injury. Displaced or unstable fractures are treated operatively to restore bony alignment and stability; this is to ideally allow controlled motion within the first week following surgery. Open fractures must be treated operatively to clean the wounds and minimize the risk of deep infection, to restore alignment and stability, and to allow early mobilization.

During the healing process, fractures must be protected from excessive or uncontrolled forces that could disrupt alignment and lead to malunion or nonunion. *Strengthening exercises are not initiated until there is evidence of* ***fracture consolidation***, usually 8 to 12 weeks following the injury or surgery. Return to all previous activities is allowed when the fracture has fully consolidated and normal or near-normal strength has been regained, 3 to 6 months following injury.

Nonoperative Treatment

Elbow fractures that are stable and well aligned are usually referred to therapy within the first few days following injury. Unstable and poorly aligned fractures are treated operatively and then referred to therapy. The initial goal of therapy is to restore motion while protecting the elbow from harmful stresses that could compromise fracture alignment and healing. A removable thermoplastic orthosis is the most common means of protective immobilization. The orthosis is removed, usually within the first week, for initiation of gentle active and active-assisted elbow and forearm motion in the arc that does not compromise stability. Educate your client in precautions, such as any initial restrictions to the arc of motion necessary to protect fracture stability and the avoidance of weight bearing and lifting with the involved UE. Active motion of the digits, wrist, shoulder, and shoulder girdle should be performed to preserve the motion of these uninvolved joints. Elevation, cold packs, light compression wraps, and light massage are useful for the control of pain and edema. In addition to preventing digit stiffness, active digit motion helps minimize edema in the hand and entire UE.

The rate of treatment progression is dependent on fracture healing. *Discuss the degree of fracture stability with the referring physician before proceeding.* Once the physician determines that there is evidence of fracture union and sufficient stability, introduce gentle passive motion, joint mobilization, and soft-tissue mobilization with the goal of restoring full motion. Scar management for operatively managed fractures should begin once the surgical incision is fully healed. As healing progresses, encourage gradual return to use of the involved UE for light functional activities. The protective orthosis is discontinued except for sleep, travel, and other circumstances that might put the elbow at risk.

Following fracture consolidation, instruct your client in resistive exercises to strengthen the involved UE. The ultimate goal

of therapy and best outcome is restoration of the previous level of function with a mobile, stable, and pain-free elbow. If your client reaches a plateau before achieving end-range motion, a static progressive orthosis or serial static orthosis may be required to address joint stiffness (see The Stiff Elbow section later in this chapter).

Operative Treatment

The goal of surgery is to restore alignment and stability to the displaced or unstable elbow fracture. When achieved, elbow motion can be initiated within a few days, minimizing the risk of joint stiffness. *However, stability must never be sacrificed for the sake of mobility.* Motion is initiated once the referring physician has determined that sufficient stability has been restored through surgery or fracture healing.

Complications of elbow fractures are more common when there is articular involvement. In addition to stiffness, the most common postoperative complications of elbow fractures are infection, malunion, nonunion, ulnar **neuropathy**, and **arthrosis.**

While approximately 95% of radial head fractures can be managed nonoperatively,[4] displaced radial head fractures with comminution or mechanical block to forearm rotation require operative treatment. The presence of one or more associated injuries at the elbow, including capitellum fracture, olecranon fracture, ligamentous injuries, and elbow dislocation, is also an indication for operative treatment. Options for the operative treatment of radial head fractures include internal fixation with plate and screws, radial head excision, and radial head replacement. Comminuted fractures are treated with radial head excision or replacement. Displaced fractures with mechanical block to forearm rotation are treated with internal fixation or radial head excision. Note that due to important stabilizing function of the radial head, it must be replaced rather than excised in radial head fractures with associated injuries that compromise elbow stability.

Most olecranon fractures require open reduction and internal fixation. A posterior approach is typically used. The type of internal fixation is chosen depending on the individual characteristics of the fracture. Options include Kirschner wires, tension band wiring, compression screws, and plate fixation. In addition to the complications common to all elbow fractures, hardware on the posterior aspect of the elbow is not always well tolerated and may require excision. In a multicenter study of 182 clients with displaced olecranon fractures treated with plating, 31% had symptomatic hardware resulting in a 15% rate of removal.[5]

Almost all distal humeral fractures are managed operatively with open reduction and internal fixation with plates and screws. A posterior surgical approach is most commonly used for visualization of the fracture and placement of the plates. The triceps is split or elevated and reflected while left in continuity, or an olecranon **osteotomy** is performed. Following an olecranon osteotomy, the olecranon is reattached with plating or tension band wiring with or without screws.[6] In addition to the complications common to all elbow fractures, **heterotopic ossification**, bone in nonosseous tissues, may develop following fractures of the distal humerus.[7] An **anterior ulnar nerve transposition** is sometimes performed during surgery for fracture repair to lessen the likelihood of postoperative ulnar neuropathy.[8] Elderly individuals with complex distal humeral fractures and osteoporotic bone present a particular challenge to the surgeon. **Total elbow arthoplasty,** replacement of the joint surfaces of the distal humerus and proximal ulna, or **elbow hemiarthroplasty**, replacement of the distal humerus only, may be necessary when screws cannot obtain adequate bony purchase for fracture fixation or when traumatic damage to the articular surface is severe.[6,9]

? Questions to Ask the Doctor

- Which bone was fractured and what was the nature of the fracture? Ask for the radiology report.
- Were there any associated injuries?
- Was the fracture treated surgically, and if so, how? Ask for the operative note.
- Is the fracture stable enough to begin active motion?
- Are there any movement limitations or other precautions?
- What are the preferred type, position, and wearing schedule for the protective orthosis?

As the Client Progresses

- When can the protective orthosis be discontinued?
- When can passive motion be initiated?
- When can the use of static progressive orthoses be initiated (if necessary to increase motion)?
- When can resistive exercises be initiated?

( ) What to Say to Clients

About Stable Elbow Fractures

"You may be surprised to start motion exercises so soon after breaking a bone, but elbow stiffness is the most common problem after an injury like yours. Your fracture is stable enough now to safely do the gentle exercises that I'm going to teach you. They will help you maintain and improve your elbow motion."

About the Home Exercise Program

"You'll get more benefit from doing your motion exercises slowly and fully than from doing lots of them quickly. It's best to do the exercises throughout the day. For example, do a set when you first get up in the morning, another at lunch, another after work, and a last set before bed. It's normal to feel tighter in the morning and looser later in the day. When your elbow feels stiff, breathe deeply and relax as you slowly move your elbow as far as it will go. Forceful or quick motions will tend to make all your muscles contract and fight the movement you're trying to do."

Ⓞ Clinical Pearl

When the elbow is viewed from behind in 90 degrees of flexion, the medial and lateral epicondyles of the distal humerus and the tip of the olecranon of the ulna should form an inverted equilateral triangle. With the elbow in full extension, these landmarks should form a straight line.

Evaluation Tips

- When assessing motion, strength, sensibility, and edema, compare the measurements to those of the client's uninvolved UE to determine what is normal for that individual.
- Do not measure passive range of motion (PROM) or strength until cleared by the referring physician.

- Ask your client to complete a client-reported outcome measure at initial evaluation, re-evaluation, and discharge. These questionnaires are useful for tracking and reporting progress as well as for highlighting functional problems that may require attention in therapy. The DASH (Disabilities of Arm, Shoulder, and Hand), its short version the Quick-DASH, and the PREE (Patient-Rated Elbow Evaluation) are commonly used for elbow injuries. The DASH and QuickDASH document UE function, whereas the PREE documents pain and function and is specific to the elbow. Although all are scored from 1 to 100, 100 on the DASH and QuickDASH represents maximum functional disability, whereas 100 on the PREE represents least pain and best function.

Diagnosis-Specific Information That Affects Clinical Reasoning

Radial head fractures that are nondisplaced or minimally displaced are treated non operatively, unless there is a mechanical block to forearm rotation. These fractures have a favorable prognosis as long as motion is begun early. *Be sure to emphasize elbow extension because this motion is most frequently lost after radial head fracture.* Nondisplaced and minimally displaced radial head fractures treated nonoperatively do not require as long a period of protective immobilization as other elbow fractures and radial head fractures treated operatively. The intermittent use of a sling or orthosis as needed for comfort during the first week is usually sufficient. Active motion is ideally initiated within the first several days following injury. A comparison of three mobilization protocols for simple radial head fractures—active elbow motion initiated immediately, after 48 hours and after 7 days—demonstrated that the two early mobilization protocols had better outcomes compared with immobilization for 7 days. Initiation of active elbow flexion and extension 48 hours after injury resulted in the best range of motion and function, with the differences most evident in displaced fractures. In each of the three protocols studied, active pronation and supination were initiated on the eighth day following injury.[10] As long as early motion is initiated, not all individuals with nonoperatively managed radial head fractures require multiple therapy visits to achieve good results. However, to minimize the risk of elbow flexion contracture, it is important to provide a home exercise program to all and an ongoing, structured therapy program to those individuals who are reluctant to move or who are stiff after several weeks of performing a home program.

Some olecranon fractures with minimal or no displacement can be treated nonoperatively. The elbow is immobilized full time in a cast or orthosis at 60 to 90 degrees of flexion and neutral forearm rotation for 1 to 2 weeks. Therapy should then be initiated to minimize the risk of elbow stiffness.

When treating a client referred to you following surgery for a distal humeral fracture, initiate elbow motion exercises with passive or gravity-assisted extension and active flexion. Depending on the type of surgical exposure that was used, either the triceps mechanism or the olecranon osteotomy may require protection for the first 6 weeks or so. *Therefore check with the surgeon before beginning active elbow extension and passive elbow flexion.*

Orthoses

- You will usually fabricate a thermoplastic posterior elbow orthosis to provide protection and support to the recently fractured elbow. Braces, casts, and slings are sometimes used as alternatives to orthoses.
- Most isolated elbow fractures are immobilized with the elbow in 90 degrees of flexion with the forearm in neutral rotation. Olecranon fractures that are managed nonoperatively or have tenuous fracture fixation may require immobilization in more extension to minimize the pull of the triceps at its insertion on the olecranon.
- Instruct your client to remove the orthosis several times daily for active motion exercises unless contraindicated due to instability. Daily removal of the orthosis for hygiene is usually permissible, although initially wearing it covered with a plastic bag or cast cover while showering or bathing offers greater protection.
- Even with optimal treatment, regaining full or at least functional motion following elbow fracture can be challenging. If your client's elbow motion plateaus, fabricate or provide a static progressive or serial static orthosis once the fracture has healed sufficiently (see The Stiff Elbow section).

Motion Exercises

- Unless contraindicated, it is often most comfortable for your client to begin elbow flexion and extension in supine with the upper arm supported on a pillow or folded towel alongside their torso. Progress to other gravity-assisted positions, such as elbow extension while seated and elbow flexion in supine with the shoulder flexed at 90 degrees.
- Instruct your client to gently support the involved UE with their uninvolved hand while performing gentle motion exercises to increase comfort and control.
- It is common to compensate for limited forearm ROM by leaning to the side or substituting shoulder motion. Minimize this by having your client support the upper arm against their torso while they pronate and supinate the forearm. Maintaining erect posture may be easier initially if forearm rotation is performed bilaterally.
- Longer holds at end-range are more effective for increasing motion than performing a greater number of fast repetitions.
- An early means of increasing motion is through active-assisted "place and hold" exercises in which the joint is placed at its end-range position followed by an active holding of the position.
- Precondition soft tissues with moist heat to make active and passive motion exercises more comfortable and effective.

Strengthening Exercises

- When the physician determines that there has been sufficient fracture healing, begin strengthening with isometric exercises and progress to isotonic exercises. In addition to addressing strength deficits of triceps and the elbow flexors, also address any strength deficits of the shoulder girdle, shoulder, wrist, and hand.
- Be sure not to overlook triceps, which tend to be weak following elbow injury. An effective exercise for initiating activation and strengthening of the triceps is elbow extension in supine with the shoulder flexed at 90 degrees.

Most individuals will be more comfortable if you include their wrist when you fabricate the protective orthosis. Make sure that they perform active wrist motion each time they remove the orthosis to prevent loss of wrist motion.

- *Adhere to precautions related to your client's fracture, surgery, and phase of healing, and be sure that your client understands them. Don't sacrifice stability for the sake of mobility.*
- *Progress treatment based on the healing of your client's fracture as determined by their referring physician and on their individual response to therapy.*
- *Passive motion and stretching should be performed slowly and gently. Forceful passive motion may damage rather than lengthen soft tissues.*
- *Be alert for symptoms of ulnar neuritis, such as numbness or tingling in the small finger and ulnar aspect of the ring finger, and if present, report them to the referring physician.*

Elbow Dislocation

Despite its inherent stability, the elbow is the second most commonly dislocated joint, following the shoulder. Mechanisms of injury include falling onto an outstretched hand, motor vehicle accidents, and direct trauma to the elbow. The direction of dislocation is almost always posterior. Severity ranges from **simple elbow dislocation**, joint displacement without associated fractures, to **complex elbow dislocation**, joint displacement with accompanying fracture or fractures. The most common complication of elbow dislocation (as of elbow fracture) is stiffness. While early motion is important for the optimal outcome, mobilization cannot begin without adequate elbow stability.

The approach used in managing an elbow dislocation depends on the structures damaged and the resulting degree of elbow stability. O'Driscoll described a sequential progression of soft-tissue disruption occurring in simple elbow dislocation.[11] Following a fall onto an outstretched hand in shoulder abduction, tissue disruption at the elbow occurs laterally to medially in three stages. The first stage is disruption of the lateral collateral ligament complex. This results in **posterolateral rotatory subluxation** in which the ulna externally rotates on the trochlea of the humerus, causing partial displacement of the ulnohumeral and radiohumeral joints. The subluxation is transient and resolves spontaneously when the elbow is flexed. In the second stage, the anterior and posterior joint capsule is also disrupted, resulting in incomplete posterolateral elbow dislocation. The third, most severe stage of soft-tissue disruption includes disruption of the medial collateral ligament complex in addition to soft tissues injured in the initial two stages. This results in complete posterior elbow dislocation. While many of these injuries appear to follow the sequence described above, more recent evidence suggests that this is not always the case and that some elbow dislocations begin instead with injury to the medial side of the elbow.[12,13]

A discussion of the management of simple elbow dislocations follows. There are additional considerations for managing elbow dislocations with associated fractures. Management of these complex elbow dislocations is discussed in the Elbow Instability section.

Timelines and Healing

Simple elbow dislocations of all stages, despite disruption to the joint capsule and ligaments, can usually be treated nonoperatively. Following closed reduction, support in elbow flexion is initially provided by an orthosis or sling. If there are no associated fractures, active motion in the stable arc can usually begin within the first week of injury without compromising stability and healing. If there is residual instability, elbow extension is initially limited to the stable range and gradually increased as stability is regained through soft-tissue healing. Faster recovery of function is more rapid with shorter periods of immobilization. Return to work following simple elbow dislocation occurred was found to occur twice as rapidly in a group of individuals treated with sling support and early active motion compared to a group initially treated with 2 weeks of cast immobilization. In addition, the rate of redislocation or late instability was not found to be higher in the early mobilization group.[14]

Screening of the UE for associated injuries is essential following elbow dislocation. Fractures of the radial head, coronoid, and/or olecranon commonly accompany elbow dislocation. These complex elbow dislocations, in which both the bony and soft-tissue stabilizers of the elbow are disrupted, are inherently unstable and require operative treatment.

Both simple and complex elbow dislocations carry the risk of neurovascular injuries. The ulnar nerve is most commonly affected. In addition, associated hand, wrist, and shoulder injuries may be present. Late complications of elbow dislocation include flexion contracture, heterotopic bone formation, arthrosis, and recurrent instability.

> ### ◎ Clinical Pearl
>
> The ulnar nerve is susceptible to traction injury during elbow dislocation.

Nonoperative Treatment

Long-term functional outcomes for simple elbow dislocations treated nonoperatively with closed reduction and early active motion are favorable as long as immobilization does not exceed 3 weeks.[15] While some residual elbow stiffness is common, a study of 4878 individuals with simple elbow dislocations managed nonoperatively found that less than 4% required subsequent surgery for either soft-tissue stabilization or contracture release.[16]

Operative Treatment

Operative management of elbow dislocation is required when stability is inadequate to safely allow early active motion in a protected arc. Unstable dislocations usually have associated elbow fractures. Although uncommon, some simple elbow dislocations, although they do not have associated fractures, may also require surgery for restoration of stability. The operative and postoperative management of unstable elbow dislocations is discussed in the Elbow Instability section.

> ### ◎ Clinical Pearl
>
> Fracture of the ulna associated with radial head dislocation is known as a **Monteggia fracture.** This injury requires operative management and careful progression in therapy due to its inherent instability.

> ### ? Questions to Ask the Doctor
>
> - Which structures were injured? Were there associated fractures or nerve injuries?
> - What is the preferred type and position of immobilization?
> - How stable is the elbow?
> - What is the initial safe arc of elbow motion?
> - Are there any other precautions?
>
> ### As the Client Progresses
>
> - When can protective immobilization be discontinued?
> - When can unrestricted motion and resistive exercises be initiated?

> ### ( ) What to Say to Clients
>
> ### After a Simple Elbow Dislocation
>
> "When you dislocated your elbow, you injured the ligaments and other soft tissues that support the joint. Your elbow needs to be protected from stresses that could prevent it from healing properly. This usually requires wearing a sling or orthosis for support for up to 3 weeks. Injured elbows have a tendency to quickly become stiff. So while your elbow is healing, it is also important to move it in a controlled way. I'm going to teach you specific motion exercises to prevent stiffness without putting stress on the structures you injured. After an injury like yours, most people have a good recovery and can go back to their usual activities within 2 or 3 months."

> ### Evaluation Tips
>
> - The evaluation tips listed for elbow fractures also apply for elbow dislocations.
> - If there is residual elbow instability, do not measure ROM in a way that would compromise stability. For example, if the elbow is unstable in end-range extension, delay assessment of extension beyond the prescribed range until the precaution is discontinued by the referring physician.

Diagnosis-Specific Information That Affects Clinical Reasoning

Simple elbow dislocations are usually stable following reduction. There may, however, be some residual instability in elbow extension. Complex elbow dislocations are inherently unstable due to disruption of both the bony and soft-tissue stabilizers, requiring a different management approach than the one described in this section.

> ### ♡ Tips from the Field
>
> ### Orthoses
>
> - For support and comfort following a simple elbow dislocation with minimal or no residual instability, the client initially uses either a sling or a protective orthosis in 90 degrees of flexion.

- The orthosis or sling is removed for controlled motion exercises beginning within the first week following a simple elbow dislocation. It is discontinued within 3 weeks after the injury.

Therapeutic Exercise

- With the exceptions that follow, the exercises for management of stable, simple elbow dislocation are similar to those for isolated elbow fractures.
- Active motion of the elbow and forearm is initially performed in supine with the upper arm supported next to the trunk on a pillow or folded towel. However, if stability is a concern, initiate motion in the supine overhead position as described in the Elbow Instability section.
- Instruct your client to avoid shoulder abduction with internal rotation for the first 3 weeks after injury or longer, as this position places varus stress on the lateral collateral ligament complex.
- It may also be necessary to limit elbow extension to 30 degrees for the first 2 or 3 weeks after injury in simple elbow dislocations with residual instability.
- Stretching and strengthening exercises can usually be safely initiated by 6 weeks following simple elbow dislocations.

▷ Precautions and Concerns

- *Avoid combining end-range elbow extension and supination for the first 6 weeks.*
- *If there is residual elbow instability, some individuals may be required to initially limit end-range extension or to perform the supine overhead exercises described later.*
- *Once permitted, passive motion and stretching should be performed slowly and gently. Excessive force may contribute to the formation of heterotopic ossification, which is a common complication of elbow dislocation.*
- *Unstable, complex elbow dislocations have additional precautions and require different management strategies than simple elbow dislocations (see the Elbow Instability section).*

Elbow Instability

To function effectively, the elbow must be stable as well as mobile. It is subject to varus (adduction) loads during many of our routine daily activities. Gravity imparts this varus load to the elbow as the UE is moved away from the body with the shoulder abducted and internally rotated. Varus forces stress the lateral collateral ligament complex, which is damaged in complex elbow dislocations and essential for elbow stability. **Varus instability**, or lateral collateral ligament insufficiency, usually results from elbow dislocation. It can range from gross instability following acute, complex dislocation to subtle, chronic **posterolateral rotatory instability** due to lateral ligamentous laxity. Posterolateral rotatory instability is recurrent posterolateral rotatory subluxation in which the ulna and radius rotate externally and displace relative to the humerus.

Valgus (abduction) loads on the elbow are far less common in routine daily life than varus loads. Valgus loads occur in activities that stress the medial elbow, such as overhead throwing. **Valgus instability**, or medial collateral ligament insufficiency, tends to be chronic in nature. Repeated valgus stress to the elbows, such as that experienced by ball-throwing athletes, can result in chronic instability.

Timelines and Healing

Before motion can begin following an acute, unstable elbow dislocation, stability must be surgically restored. This allows protected active motion in the stable arc to begin within the first week following surgery. When protected from damaging stresses, ligamentous injuries and fractures of the elbow heal sufficiently for strengthening to begin in approximately 6 to 8 weeks. Return to all previous activities is usually allowed after 4 to 6 months when normal strength has been recovered. Full recovery may take a year or more after severe injuries. Timelines for healing and progression of treatment following reconstruction for recurrent instability are similar to those following surgery for acute instability, but the outcomes are less predictable.

Even with the early initiation of motion, elbow stiffness is a common complication after complex elbow dislocation. *Stability must never be sacrificed in the attempt to gain motion.* If necessary, contracture release and/or excision of heterotopic bone can be performed to address motion deficits once the injured structures have fully healed (see The Stiff Elbow section).

Elbow dislocation with associated fractures of the radial head and coronoid is known as the **terrible triad of the elbow** because it is so challenging to treat. With optimal operative and postoperative management, most have good to excellent outcomes. However, complications are common, and hardware fixation problems, joint stiffness, joint instability, or ulnar neuropathy may require additional surgery.[17]

◎ Clinical Pearl

Isolated coronoid fractures are uncommon. They occur with elbow dislocation and are usually associated with disruption of the lateral collateral ligament complex. In addition to ligament repair, internal fixation of the coronoid fracture fragment is usually necessary to restore sufficient stability for early protected motion.[18]

Nonoperative Treatment

Provision of safe and effective therapy for the unstable elbow requires an understanding of how to protect the injured structures while initiating early, protected motion to avoid stiffness. Treatment progression is dependent on the timing of both soft-tissue and fracture healing, and it requires close communication with the referring physician. Standard edema and scar management techniques should be used as needed.

Therapy for the acute, unstable elbow typically begins postoperatively with fabrication of a thermoplastic orthosis in elbow flexion and pronation. As soon as stability permits, ideally within the first week following surgery, active motion is initiated in the limited arc of motion in which the elbow remains stable. The supine, overhead motion protocol, described in detail by Wolff and Hotchkiss,[19] allows early, protected motion while preserving elbow stability. Elbow and forearm motion are initially performed supine with the shoulder flexed at 90 degrees. This position allows gravity to stabilize the elbow and also positions triceps so that it can act as a joint stabilizer. To protect elbow stability, supination and elbow extension should not be combined until the injured structures have healed for at least 8 weeks following surgery. Elbow extension, performed in pronation, should

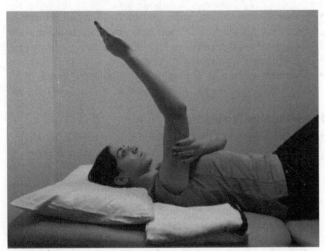

FIG. 19.4 Supine, overhead elbow extension with the forearm pronated, initially limited to 30 degrees.

initially be limited to 30 degrees or the stable end-range (Fig. 19.4). Initiate active ROM of the shoulder girdle, shoulder, wrist, and digits immediately to preserve their motion, but note that *shoulder abduction with internal rotation must be strictly avoided because it places a significant varus stress on the damaged lateral collateral ligaments.*

Joint stability begins improving during the fibroplastic phase of soft-tissue healing, 2 to 6 weeks following surgery. When stability permits, active elbow and forearm motion are progressed to positioning the upper arm next to the torso while sitting or standing. Combined elbow extension and supination must still be avoided. While gentle passive motion can be initiated, avoid both end-range elbow extension and forearm supination. Add gentle strengthening exercises for the wrist and grip.

Motion precautions can be discontinued and progressive strengthening initiated during the scar maturation phase, 8 to 12 weeks following surgery, once stability has been regained.

Operative Treatment

Acute elbow dislocation with fractures of the radial head, coronoid, and/or olecranon is the most common origin of lateral elbow instability. To restore elbow stability following these complex dislocations, the fractures are repaired with open reduction and internal fixation. When associated with dislocation, radial head fractures that are too severe to be repaired are replaced rather than excised to prevent chronic instability. In addition to addressing the fractures, the lateral collateral ligament complex must be repaired due to its critical role in elbow stability and the ubiquity of varus loads in daily activities. The medial collateral ligament complex does not routinely require repair unless the elbow remains unstable following fracture fixation and repair of the lateral collateral ligaments. If the elbow remains unstable despite these procedures, a **hinged external fixator** can be placed in the distal humerus and proximal ulna for approximately 6 to 8 weeks to maintain joint reduction while allowing early elbow motion.

Chronic lateral elbow instability, although uncommon, may be a late complication of elbow trauma. More rarely, it is a complication of overuse or of iatrogenic injury following surgical treatment of lateral epicondylitis, other surgeries to the lateral elbow, or multiple steroid injections. Individuals with this condition report lateral elbow pain and clicking, catching, or locking most frequently in elbow extension and supination against resistance. On examination, it may present as a subtle posterolateral rotatory elbow instability in which the ulna and radius rotate externally relative to the humerus causing a transient posterior subluxation. The operative treatment is reconstruction of lateral ligamentous support with a free tendon graft, most commonly palmaris longus. Hinged external fixation may also be necessary when the treatment of a complex elbow dislocation has been delayed or has failed to restore stability. The hinged external fixator, inserted in the proximal ulna and distal humerus, provides varus and valgus stability while allowing elbow flexion and extension.

For chronic medial instability that does not sufficiently resolve with nonoperative management, a free tendon graft, most commonly palmaris longus, is used for reconstruction of medial ligamentous support.

? Questions to Ask the Doctor

- Which structures were injured? Were there associated fractures or nerve injuries?
- Was surgery performed, and if so, what was done? Ask for the operative notes.
- What is the preferred position of immobilization?
- How stable is the elbow?
- What is the initial safe arc of elbow motion? Should motion be initially performed in the supine overhead motion position or can it be safely performed with the upper arm next to the trunk?
- Are there any other precautions?

As the Client Progresses

- When can protective immobilization be discontinued?
- When can unrestricted motion and resistive exercises be initiated?

( ) What to Say to Clients

About the Condition

"To function properly, your elbow needs to be both flexible and stable. Stability is provided by the bones that make up the elbow joint and the ligaments and other soft tissues that surround it. Because you injured these structures, your elbow has lost stability. It is important to protect these healing structures so that your elbow regains stability."

About the Supine, Overhead Motion Exercises

"I'm going to teach you motion exercises to prevent your elbow from becoming too stiff. As long as you do them correctly, the healing structures in your elbow will be protected. Perform the exercises lying on your back with your upper arm and elbow pointing directly up to the ceiling. Use your other hand to support your injured arm. The specific exercises are forearm rotation with your elbow bent, and elbow bending and straightening with your forearm rotated so that your palm faces toward the ceiling. I'll show you how to do them correctly and how far you can safely straighten your elbow at this time."

- The evaluation tips listed for elbow fractures also apply for unstable elbows.
- If there is residual elbow instability, do not measure ROM in a way that would compromise stability. For example, if elbow and forearm motion must initially be performed in the overhead supine position, perform the motion measurements with the UE in this position, noting it in your documentation.

Diagnosis-Specific Information That Affects Clinical Reasoning

The safest forearm position for immobilization and motion depends on which ligaments were injured and require protection. Pronation with elbow flexion has been demonstrated to stabilize elbows with insufficient lateral collateral ligament support and resultant instability.[20] Therefore the pronated position is recommended for orthoses and motion activities for unstable elbows with lateral collateral ligament disruption. In contrast, elbows with medial collateral ligament damage are more stable in supination. When both the medial and lateral collateral ligaments require protection, neutral forearm rotation with flexion is preferable.

Elbow instability usually requires operative treatment. The exception is chronic medial instability as seen in overhead throwing athletes. If treated early, this condition can be managed nonoperatively with a period of rest from provoking activities and antiinflammatory medication and modalities. This should be followed with a strengthening program for the UE muscles including those of the flexor-pronator mass, especially flexor carpi ulnaris and flexor digitorum superficialis, as they have been shown to provide dynamic support to the medial aspect of the elbow against valgus torque.[21]

Orthoses

- The protective thermoplastic orthosis is fabricated in the position of greatest stability. Because joint reduction and stability is greatest in elbow flexion, the elbow is immobilized in at least 90 degrees of flexion. In many cases, 120 degrees or more of elbow flexion is preferred. Positioning in full pronation protects the lateral collateral ligaments. However, if a medial collateral ligament repair was performed in addition to lateral collateral ligament repair, neutral forearm rotation is indicated. As an alternative to an orthosis, a hinged brace with an extension stop may be ordered.
- When the injured structures have healed and the elbow is stable, approximately 8 weeks after surgery, static progressive orthoses may be necessary to address remaining motion limitations. For individuals making poor progress with elbow extension, use of a serial static night extension orthosis may be initiated 4 to 6 weeks postoperatively if stability permits (see The Stiff Elbow section). Discuss the timing for safely introducing these orthoses with the referring physician.

Supine, Overhead Motion Exercises

- During the supine, overhead exercises for unstable elbows, the shoulder should be maintained at 90 degrees of flexion and not be allowed to abduct.

- Elbow flexion and extension are performed in full pronation. Full flexion is allowed. In most cases extension should initially be limited to 30 degrees (see Fig. 19.4) and then gradually progressed when stability has improved.
- Forearm rotation is performed with the elbow flexed at 90 degrees. Full pronation and supination, within tolerance, are allowed.

Hinged External Fixation

- If a hinged external fixator has been used to stabilize the elbow, it is unlocked for active elbow and forearm motion exercises. Because of the stability provided by the device, exercising in the supine position is not required. In the locked position the fixator is used for passive elbow flexion and extension. Rather than performing multiple repetitions, the elbow is gradually positioned and held for several hours at comfortable end-range flexion and extension.
- Following the removal of the fixator 3 to 6 weeks postoperatively, loss of motion is common. Prompt use of static progressive or serial static orthoses is essential to maintain/gain end-range elbow motion.

Some individuals require several therapy sessions to learn to perform the supine, overhead elbow exercises correctly. The exercises should not be performed as a home program until they can be performed as instructed.

- *Do not combine elbow extension with supination for at least 8 weeks.*
- *Protect lateral collateral ligaments repairs from varus stresses by instructing your client to avoid shoulder abduction with internal rotation for at least 12 weeks. The shoulder should not be allowed to abduct and internally rotate during removal of the protective orthosis and performance of supine, overhead motion exercises.*
- *Be alert for ulnar nerve symptoms and report them to the referring physician.*

Elbow stiffness is so common that therapists treating individuals with UE disorders will inevitably face this challenge. Elbow stiffness is a frequent complication of elbow dislocation, elbow fracture, head injury, and burns. The more severe the trauma and the longer the period of immobilization, the more likely is the loss of elbow motion. Elbow flexion contracture is particularly common.

Multiple factors contribute to the propensity of the elbow to become stiff following injury. Because the elbow is a highly congruent joint, it is not tolerant of disruption of the articular surfaces. There is a tendency for formation of heterotopic ossification in the surrounding soft tissues, such as the medial and lateral collateral ligaments and joint capsule. The thin anterior joint capsule of the elbow is particularly susceptible to injury and **hypertrophy.** The muscle belly of brachialis lies directly over the anterior capsule. Bleeding in brachialis associated with elbow injury can cause it to scar and adhere to the capsule and can contribute to formation of bone in the muscle. Muscle guarding, adaptive soft-tissue shortening, and scarring can also contribute to loss of elbow motion, particularly extension.

> ### ◎ Clinical Pearl
>
> Following injury, the elbow tends to posture at 70 to 80 degrees of elbow flexion, which is the open packed position in which the joint capsule is most lax. Prolonged immobilization in this position of comfort can contribute to the development of an elbow flexion contracture, which is a common complication of elbow trauma.

There are a number of structures lying within and outside of the elbow joint that can limit motion. Elbow stiffness of relatively short duration with extraarticular causes, such as soft-tissue shortening and muscle **cocontraction,** can usually be managed nonoperatively. However, if motion is not regained after optimal nonoperative management, surgical contracture release may be necessary. Heterotopic ossification and intraarticular sources of elbow stiffness, such as joint incongruity, deformity, and impinging hardware from previous surgery, are indications for operative management.

Timelines and Healing

Recovery of a functional ROM following elbow trauma is often challenging, even with good management. If a significant contracture persists beyond 6 months in an individual who has received appropriate therapy including orthoses to increase motion, a contracture release may be required. Without surgical intervention, significant improvement is unlikely after 6 months of nonoperative management, and heterotopic ossification, if present, will have matured sufficiently by this time to be safely removed.[22]

Following elbow contracture release, the importance of therapy cannot be overemphasized. Positive outcomes depend on the coordinated and concerted efforts of the injured individual, therapist and surgeon. Individuals unwilling or unable to actively participate in an extensive postoperative therapy program are not good candidates for this procedure. It is not unusual for therapy to be required for 3 months following this surgery.

While most individuals make significant gains and obtain a functional range of motion following elbow contracture release, complications including recurrent stiffness are not rare. In a study of 103 individuals treated for posttraumatic elbow stiffness with open contracture release followed by physical therapy, a mean increase in elbow extension/flexion arc of 52 degrees and pronation/supination arc of 36 degrees was found at 15 months average follow-up. As reported in previous studies, contractures recurred in some individuals. Greater time from initial injury to initial contracture release was associated with failure to achieve an extension/flexion arc of at least 100 degrees. Approximately 10% of the individuals in this study later had a second contracture release due to recurrence of stiffness. Another 10% had other complications including nerve palsies and postoperative infection. At follow-up there were also reports of recurrent heterotopic ossification. There were no reports of clinically significant elbow instability, possibly related to use of a removable hinged brace worn for 3 weeks when collateral ligament repair was performed.[23]

Nonoperative Treatment

The same techniques for increasing elbow motion are useful for the prevention and treatment of elbow stiffness in non-operatively and operatively managed elbow injuries. Treatment progression following elbow injury must always reflect the phase of soft-tissue healing and degree of joint stability. If stiffness is due to elbow fracture, progression may need to be slower since the phase of bony healing must also be considered.

In the initial, inflammatory phase of healing, effectively controlling edema and pain is crucial for preventing or minimizing stiffness. Edema management techniques include elevation, cold modalities, light compression, active digital motion, and manual edema mobilization techniques. Active motion of the uninvolved joints should be initiated early, and gentle active elbow and forearm motion initiated as soon as healing and stability permits. Passive motion should always be performed slowly and gently to avoid provoking involuntary muscle guarding and damaging healing tissues.

A variety of techniques for increasing motion are useful during the fibroplastic and scar maturation phases of soft-tissue healing. *Avoid aggressive approaches, such as forceful stretching, that may provoke inflammation, damage healing tissues, and increase* **fibrosis** *and stiffness.* Superficial heat prepares soft tissues for motion and is most effective for increasing motion when applied with the elbow positioned at end-range. Ultrasound, used for deeper heating, should be combined or followed with end-range motion. There are a variety of useful manual techniques for increasing motion including gentle stretching, soft-tissue mobilization, joint mobilization, and proprioceptive neurofacilitation techniques, such as contract-relax and hold-relax. Follow the techniques and exercises used to increase passive motion with active motion and functional activities that focus on use of the full available range. Strengthening exercises, which are initiated during the scar maturation phase, should emphasize the end-ranges of motion. Triceps tend to be weaker than the elbow flexors and require greater attention in functional activities and strengthening exercises.

Serial static elbow orthoses, which are molded with the joint at end-range and remolded as motion improves, are generally well tolerated early in the soft-tissue healing process. Static progressive orthoses have been demonstrated to be effective for increasing motion in elbows that are stiff following trauma.[24] Their use is ideally initiated during the fibroplastic phase and is also effective during the scar maturation phase.

Operative Treatment

Elbow contracture release is usually performed as an open procedure through a medial and/or lateral approach. The structures limiting motion are identified and excised. These may include the anterior and posterior joint capsule, **osteophytes**, scarring within the coronoid and olecranon fossas, scarring around the radial head and capitellum, the tip of the olecranon, heterotopic ossification, and hardware from previous surgery. While some parts of the medial collateral ligament complex can be excised without compromising joint stability, the lateral collateral ligaments are preserved whenever possible. The ulnar nerve is often released from scar tissue and heterotopic ossification and transposed to an anterior position to minimize the risk of postoperative irritation.

If there is substantial articular damage, an **interposition arthoplasty**, which is the insertion of soft tissue between the joint surfaces, may be performed. In cases in which the elbow is unstable following contracture release or when distraction is required to protect soft tissue placed between the joint surfaces, a hinged external fixator is applied for approximately 6 to 8 weeks. This device allows maximum gains in motion to be made while stability is regained through soft-tissue healing.

Therapy is essential following elbow contracture release and is typically initiated the day following surgery. The primary goal of therapy is postoperative motion equal to that obtained in the operating room.

? Questions to Ask the Doctor

- What structures were addressed surgically? Ask for the operative notes.
- How much motion was obtained intraoperatively?
- Is the elbow stable postoperatively?
- Was an ulnar nerve transposition performed?

( ) What to Say to Clients

After Contracture Release

"Your surgeon released the structures that were keeping your elbow from moving freely. Right after your surgery your elbow was able to move this far (demonstrate client's intra-operative ROM). Swelling and the gradual formation of scar tissue tend to make your elbow become stiff again. To keep that from happening, it is very important that you come to your therapy sessions and follow your home program. Some swelling is normal but to keep it to a minimum, elevate your arm and apply ice or cold packs as we have discussed. To get the most motion, your elbow will need a lot of your attention for the next several months. Think of doing your exercises and wearing your orthosis (or orthoses) as a full-time job."

About Static Progressive Orthoses

"The purpose of your orthosis is to gradually improve your elbow motion. When you put the orthosis on, adjust it to hold your elbow as straight (or bent) as possible but only to the point that it does not cause pain. After you've had the orthosis on for a while, try to readjust it for more of a stretch. The orthosis works by applying gentle force over long period of time. Using it for a brief, intense stretch will not be as effective. After you take the orthosis off, do your exercises to straighten and bend your elbow as far you can."

Evaluation Tips

- Unless the elbow is unstable following contracture release, it is generally permissible to begin measuring passive and active motion at the first visit.
- While early assessment of strength is not prohibited unless there is postoperative instability, initially pain will be more limiting than weakness. Delay manual muscle testing until after the inflammatory phase when it will be better tolerated.

Diagnosis-Specific Information That Affects Clinical Reasoning

- Biceps brachii and the other elbow flexors have a tendency to cocontract when the injured elbow is extended or positioned in extension.[25] This involuntary muscle guarding is a common

source of limited elbow motion that when not addressed early can contribute to persistent stiffness. Placing a weight on the wrist or in the hand to stretch the elbow into extension is counterproductive if it causes the flexors to contract. While performing passive motion, stretching, and other techniques to increase elbow extension, manually monitor the elbow flexors to make sure they stay relaxed. Avoid rapid and forceful movements. If flexor cocontraction is persistent, biofeedback is a useful tool for increasing awareness and reestablishing normal firing patterns.

- Elbow stiffness that worsens or fails to improve 2 or 3 weeks following contracture release has variable causes and should be reported to the referring physician. Hotchkiss[22] has described a common cause of recurrent elbow stiffness, usually limited flexion, that occurs during this period as "gelling." He states that the usual cause of the loss of flexion gains made in the operating room appears to be pain in the distal triceps against the surface of the posterior humerus. In these cases, gentle manipulation under anesthesia may be necessary to restore motion. Another cause of recurrent stiffness, while no longer as common, is the recurrence of heterotopic ossification that blocks motion.[22]

◎ Clinical Pearl

If a manipulation under anesthesia is performed, it should be followed immediately with therapy, including serial static or static progressive orthoses, to maintain the gains made in end-range motion.

♡ Tips From the Field

End-range Positioning With Thermal Modalities

While using moist heat to precondition soft tissues prior to other treatments, position the elbow at or near its end-range of flexion or extension. When using a cold pack at the end of a therapy session, end-range positioning can help maintain gains made during the session.

Orthoses

- Orthoses that position the elbow at end-range are essential in the treatment of stiffness. Use a custom-made or prefabricated static progressive flexion orthosis to address limited flexion (Fig. 19.5). For a mild limitation of extension, a static orthosis molded at end-range and serially remolded as extension improves can be used (Fig. 19.6). For extension limited by more than 30 degrees, static progressive extension orthoses (Fig. 19.7) are more effective.[26] Wearing schedules vary and depend on individual progress and tolerance to orthotic wear. In general, the more severe the stiffness and limitation into a particular end-range, the more time the elbow will need to be positioned at that end-range. It has been demonstrated in stiff joints that the greater the total end-range time, the greater the improvement in motion.[27] However, always consider individual response to therapy and tissue tolerance to orthotic wear. Extension orthoses are generally better tolerated than flexion orthoses and are therefore commonly worn while sleeping at night. If an ulnar nerve transposition was not performed, carefully monitor for signs and symptoms of ulnar neuritis. If they occur, inform the referring physician and limit wearing time for flexion orthoses.

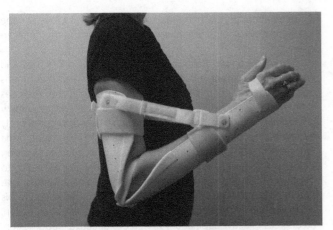

FIG. 19.5 Static progressive elbow flexion orthosis.

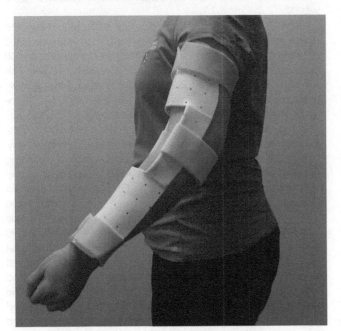

FIG. 19.6 Serial static elbow extension orthosis.

- It may be necessary to use a serial static or static progressive forearm supination orthosis or, less commonly, a pronation orthosis to assist in restoration of limited forearm motion that is not improving with other therapeutic interventions, such as active and passive mobilization techniques.

Therapeutic Exercise

Instruct your client to follow each session of serial static or static progressive orthotic use with active motion exercises and light functional exercises that focus on end-ranges. Doing so will help maintain passive gains made through orthotic wear and will encourage active use of the elbow through the full available range.

Therapy Considerations Following Elbow Contracture Release
Continuous Passive Motion

The effectiveness of continuous passive motion (CPM) machines in the postoperative treatment of elbow contracture release is questionable, with research demonstrating mixed results.[28,29] Hotchkiss[22] has described the use of the CPM machine during the first

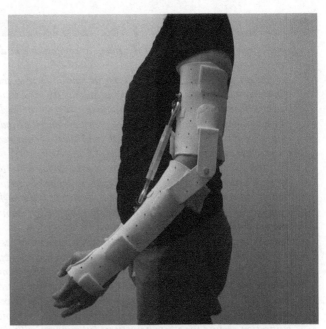

FIG. 19.7 Static progressive elbow extension orthosis.

few weeks following contracture release as a slow, intermittent passive positioning device. He advocates its use to position the elbow in end-range flexion and extension alternating 20 to 30 minutes in each direction.

Orthoses

A static extension orthosis should be fabricated within the first day or two following surgery. It should be worn at night and intermittently during the day. Use of static progressive orthoses for extension and flexion, if necessary, can be initiated as early as the first week following surgery.

Hinged External Fixation

Therapy follows a different course if a hinged external fixator is applied during surgery. Instruct your client in using the device to gradually passively position the elbow at end-range flexion and extension. Initially, flexion and extension may be alternated daily. Within a few days, as comfort improves, they can be alternated several times each day. Within the first week following surgery, instruct your client to unlock the hinge for active ROM exercises and light functional activities with a focus on end-ranges of motion.

◎ *Clinical Pearl*

To capitalize on motion gains made during a therapy session, ask your client to apply their orthosis positioned at the new end-range when the session concludes.

◎ *Clinical Pearl*

Following the removal of a hinged external fixator that was used to treat an elbow contracture, the immediate use of static progressive orthoses is critical to minimize loss of motion gained while using the fixator.

> **Precautions and Concerns**

- *Avoid prolonged positioning of the elbow at comfortable mid-ranges.*
- *Do not use an orthosis to apply a strong or painful force to the elbow in an attempt to gain motion. Instead, use the orthosis to position the joint at end-range. Gradually progress the end-range by applying a low load provided over a prolonged period. Improvements are typically gradual and with continued orthotic use may continue over a period of 6 to 12 months.[30]*
- *The forces applied by the spring or elastic components of dynamic orthoses are not as controlled as those applied by serial static and static progressive orthoses. Therefore, although dynamic orthoses may be as effective for improving elbow motion, they are not always well tolerated.[22,30]*
- *Do not use excessive or uncontrolled force when performing passive motion, stretching, and other mobilization techniques. Forceful attempts to increase elbow motion can inflame or damage healing tissues. Gentle passive motion and orthoses used for end-range prolonged positioning are effective tools for coaxing more motion from a stiff elbow. Recurrence of heterotopic ossification around the elbow has become less common with the use of more controlled methods of applying force.[22]*
- *Be alert for signs and symptoms of ulnar neuritis. Potential causes include irritation related to injury or surgery, repetitive or prolonged stretch of the nerve during flexion activities, and flexion orthotic wear if an anterior ulnar nerve transposition was not performed. Later onset of ulnar neuritis can be caused by compression of the nerve by heterotopic ossification.*
- *Monitor the skin over the tip of the olecranon, where the thin soft tissue that covers it is placed under tension during flexion. The potential for delayed wound healing or necrosis is more of a concern following release of long-standing contractures.*

CASE STUDIES

CASE STUDY 19.1 ■

RM is a 45-year-old, right dominant male who works as an information technologist. His only prior medical history is hypertension controlled with medication. He sustained a right posterior elbow dislocation in a fall from a 3-foot-high wall onto his outstretched hand. His elbow was relocated and subsequently immobilized in the local emergency room. Two days later RM was seen by an orthopedic surgeon who referred him to therapy for nonoperative management with a protective orthosis and protected supine overhead motion with extension initially limited to 30 degrees. The surgeon reported that there were no associated fractures or neurovascular injuries, but due to disruption of the collateral ligaments, the elbow was unstable in full extension.

RM came to therapy following his visit to the surgeon. He reported 7 out of 10 elbow pain at rest. There was moderate localized edema in his elbow. His sensation was intact. I fabricated RM a posterior elbow orthosis in 120 degrees of flexion and full pronation for maximum elbow stability for him to wear. RM was unwilling to begin moving his elbow at this time. I reassured him that I would teach him only exercises that were safe for his elbow. I encouraged him to perform active motion of his digits and to intermittently apply ice or cold packs. I explained the precaution of avoiding

shoulder abduction with internal rotation. He agreed to return the following day to begin protected elbow and forearm motion exercises.

The following day RM appeared less fearful, had less pain, and was willing to fully participate in therapy. I reviewed his precautions and emphasized that he should perform only the exercises instructed, avoiding full elbow extension and combined elbow extension and pronation. The orthosis was to be worn continuously except during his home exercise program, which was to be done four times a day. I taught him protected supine, overhead motion exercises, which were active-assisted elbow flexion and extension to maximum of 30 degrees in full pronation, and supination and pronation in elbow flexion. I also instructed him in active motion of his digits and wrist. At this time RM had 70 degrees of active pronation, 60 degrees of active supination, 95 degrees of active elbow flexion, 40 degrees of active-assisted elbow extension, and normal active motion of his wrist, digits, and shoulder into flexion. His DASH score was 80.

After 3 weeks of attending therapy and performing the supine overhead exercise program, RM's active motion had improved to full pronation, 70 degrees of supination, 120 degrees of flexion, and 30 degrees of extension. His pain and edema were well controlled with superficial heat and cold modalities. He followed up with the referring surgeon who cleared him for motion exercises, including unlimited extension with his upper arm next to his trunk. The orthosis was now required only for protection while sleeping or going outside. RM returned to work and continued attending therapy twice weekly. I instructed him in forearm and elbow motion exercises standing upright next to a wall with a towel roll behind his upper arm to prevent substituting with shoulder motion. I explained that he should continue to avoid shoulder abduction with internal rotation and end-range elbow extension in supination. I instructed him in gentle isometric elbow flexion and extension with his elbow flexed at 90 degrees. At 4 weeks he began using the UE ergometer with minimal resistance. After 6 weeks of therapy, his active motion had improved to 15 degrees of elbow extension and full pronation, supination, and elbow flexion. At this time he returned to the referring surgeon who cleared him for progressive resistance exercises and discontinued the orthosis. After an additional 3 weeks of therapy of motion and progressive resistance exercises, RM had near normal strength throughout his UE and normal UE motion with the exception of 10 degrees of elbow extension. He returned to his prior functional activities and had a final DASH score of 20. I discharged RM from therapy with an independent home exercise program focused on UE strengthening.

CASE STUDY 19.2 ■

AL is a 28-year-old, right dominant, healthy female childcare worker. She came to the surgeon with a chief complaint of a stiff right elbow. Eight months earlier, she had sustained a right olecranon fracture resulting from a fall directly onto the elbow. The fracture was treated 3 days after the injury with open reduction and internal fixation (ORIF). She had attended therapy twice a week for 10 weeks, performed her home exercises regularly, and continued to wear a static progressive extension orthosis at night. Despite appropriate treatment, she had a persistent elbow flexion contracture of 40 degrees. Her flexion had gradually worsened and was now limited to 120 degrees. Her active forearm motion was within normal limits, her forearm and elbow strength good to normal within the available range, and her sensation intact. She reported that limited elbow motion made it difficult to perform her job duties and that she was strongly motivated to participate in whatever intervention was required to improve her elbow motion.

An open contracture release was performed on AL's right elbow. The procedures included anterior and posterior capsulectomies, excision of soft tissue from the olecranon and coronoid fossas, excision of the tip of the olecranon, removal of hardware from the previous surgery, and decompression and anterior transposition of the ulnar nerve. Following surgery while still under anesthesia, her elbow was stable and had a passive range of 10 to 135 degrees.

AL received inpatient therapy for 2 days following surgery prior to discharge home. Her pain was well controlled by the postoperative pain management team. Edema was managed with elevation, light compression wraps, and intermittent use of ice. On postoperative day 1, a therapist instructed AL in active motion exercises for her digits, wrist, and shoulder, and both active and gentle passive motion exercises for her elbow and forearm. The therapist fabricated a custom-molded static elbow extension orthosis at 15 degrees, which was AL's maximum passive elbow extension at that time. AL began using a CPM machine for 6 hours a day, alternating 20 minute holds in end-range flexion and extension and letting the machine cycle for brief periods in between. While hospitalized, she wore the extension orthosis when sleeping and whenever she wasn't performing motion exercises or using the CPM machine. At discharge, she was instructed to continue ice application, elevation, motion exercises, CPM machine use, and the extension orthosis at night.

At her first outpatient session, which was 5 days following the contracture release, AL reported that her elbow was still stiff and that she had constant, localized pain, ranging from 4 to 7 on a scale of 10. She reported that she was using the CPM machine at home for 2 hours, 3 times a day, alternating 20 minute holds at end-range flexion and extension; she was wearing the extension orthosis at night; and she was performing motion exercises as instructed while in the hospital. She had not been consistent with elevation. On examination, AL had an intact surgical incision with no drainage, moderate edema at the elbow, minimal edema in her hand, and normal findings on neurological screening. Her DASH score was 75. Her elbow motion was 30 to 115 degrees actively and 20 to 120 degrees passively. Active pronation was normal, and supination was 10 degrees less than on the left side. ROM of the uninvolved joints was within normal limits. Strength testing was deferred due to pain and recent surgery.

AL attended therapy two times a week. During the first week, we focused on edema and pain control with elevation, light compression wraps, intermittent use of ice and cold packs, and active digit motion. I also educated AL in the correct performance of active and active-assisted "place and hold" elbow and forearm exercises,

emphasizing that she take the time necessary to reach maximum end-ranges rather than simply going through the exercises to get them done. Initially, to minimize biceps brachii cocontraction, I instructed AL to perform her exercises slowly while lying in supine with the upper arm supported next to her trunk on a towel roll.

Two weeks following surgery, AL's pain had decreased, her forearm motion was within normal limits, and her elbow extension had improved to 25 degrees actively and 15 degrees passively. Her elbow flexion had not improved, so I fabricated a static progressive flexion orthosis and instructedAL to wear it for a minimum of 2 hours a day with her elbow flexed to the point of a mild stretch but no increase in pain. By the next session her elbow motion was 120 degrees actively and 125 degrees passively, which was an increase of 5 degrees. Home use of the CPM machine was discontinued, and the importance of continuing use of the flexion and extension orthoses was emphasized. At the start of each therapy session, I applied moist heat with her elbow positioned in either extension or flexion, and I used soft-tissue and joint mobilization and other manual techniques, such as hold-relax and a contract-relax, to decrease muscle guarding and increase passive motion. I encouraged AL to use her right UE for light functional activities and incorporated reaching activities into her therapy sessions. Active elbow extension in supine with the shoulder flexed to 90 degrees and reaching activities were used to target triceps and improve active extension. Overhead pulleys, which later progressed to an upper body ergometer (UBE) with minimal resistance, were used for repetitive elbow motion through the gradually increasing available range. When I applied cold packs to her elbow following treatment, I positioned it in comfortable extension. When AL's surgical incision was fully healed, I instructed her in scar mobilization and the use of a silicone product to minimize scarring.

From 6 to 12 weeks following the contracture release, during the scar maturation phase, AL's elbow motion and function continued to gradually improve, and her pain became mild and less frequent. At 8 weeks, I remolded the extension orthosis to 10 degrees, which was her current passive end-range. In addition to the treatment techniques initiated in the fibroplastic phase, I added resistance exercises with a focus on performing them through the full range of motion and on isolating triceps. Twelve weeks after surgery, AL had active elbow motion from 10 to 135 degrees°, which was equal to her intraoperative motion; she was functionally independent and had good to normal strength throughout her right dominant UE. She had successfully returned to work the previous week. Her DASH score had improved to 15. After discussing the plan with AL and her referring physician, I discharged her from therapy with instructions to continue wearing her orthoses and performing her home exercise program for another 2 to 3 months.

References

1. Morrey BF, Askew LJ, Chao EY: A biomechanical study of normal functional elbow motion, *J Bone Joint Surg Am* 63(6):872–877, 1981.
2. Beals RK: The normal carrying angle of the elbow: a radiographic study of 422 patients, *Clin Orthop Relat Res* 119:194–196, 1976.
3. Kim SH, Szabo RM, Marder RA: Epidemiology of humerus fractures in the United States: nationwide emergency department sample, 2008, *Arthritis Care Res (Hoboken)* 64:407–414, 2012.
4. Kupperman ES, Kupperman AI, Mitchell SA: Treatment of radial head fractures and need for revision procedures at 1 and 2 years, *J Hand Surg Am*, 2017. Epub ahead of print.
5. De Giacomo AF, Tornetta P, Sinicrope BJ, et al.: Outcomes of plating of olecranon fractures: a multicenter evaluation, *Injury* 47(7):1466–1471, 2016.
6. Sanchez-Sotelo J: Distal humeral fractures: role of internal fixation and elbow arthroplasty, *J Bone Joint Surg Am* 94(6):555–568, 2012.
7. Foruria AM, Lawrence TM, Augustin S, et al.: Heterotopic ossification after surgery for distal humeral fractures, *Bone Joint J* 96B(12):1681–1687, 2014.
8. Nauth A, McKee MD, Ristevski B, et al.: Distal humeral fractures in adults, *J Bone Joint Surg Am* 93(7):686–700, 2011.
9. Linn MS, Gardner MJ, McAndrew CM, et al.: Is primary total elbow arthroplasty safe for the treatment of open intra-articular distal humerus fractures? *Injury* 45(11):1747–1751, 2014.
10. Paschos NK, Mitsionis G, Vasiliadis HS, et al.: Comparison of early mobilization protocols in radial head fractures, *J Orthop Trauma* 27(3):134–139, 2013.

11. O'Driscoll SW, Morrey BF, Korinek S, et al.: Elbow subluxation and dislocation. A spectrum of instability, *Clin Orthop Relat Res* 280:186–197, 1992.

12. Rhyou IH, Kim YS: New mechanism of the posterior elbow dislocation, *Knee Surg Sports Traumatol Arthrosc* 20:2535–2541, 2012.

13. Schreiber JJ, Potter HG, Warren RF, et al.: Magnetic resonance imaging findings in acute elbow dislocation: insight into mechanism, *J Hand Surg Am* 39(2):199–205, 2014.

14. Maripuri SN, Debnath UK, Rao P, et al.: Simple elbow dislocation among adults: a comparative study of two different methods of treatment, *Injury* 38(11):1254–1258, 2007.

15. Anakwe RE, Middleton SD, Jenkins PJ, et al.: Patient-reported outcomes after simple dislocation of the elbow, *J Bone Joint Surg* 93(13):1220–1226, 2011.

16. Modi CS, Wasserstein D, Mayne IP, et al.: The frequency and risk factors for subsequent surgery after simple elbow dislocation, *Injury* 46(6):1156–1160, 2015.

17. Chen H, Guo-dong L, Wu L: Complications of treating terrible triad injury of the elbow: a systematic review, *PLoS One* 9(5):e97476, 2014.

18. Chan K, King GJ, Faber KJ: Treatment of complex elbow fracture-dislocations, *Curr Rev Musculoskelet Med* 9(2):185–189, 2016.

19. Wolff AL, Hotchkiss RN: Lateral elbow instability: nonoperative, operative, and postoperative management, *J Hand Ther* 19(2):238–243, 2006.

20. Dunning CE, Zarzour ZD, Patterson SD, et al.: Muscle force and pronation stabilize the lateral ligament deficient elbow, *Clin Orthop Relat Res* 388:118–124, 2001.

21. Park MC, Ahmad CS: Dynamic contributions of the flexor-pronator mass to elbow valgus stability, *J Bone Joint Surg Am* 86(10):2268–2274, 2004.

22. Hotchkiss RN: Treatment of the stiff elbow. In Wolfe SW, Hotchkiss RN, Pederson WC, et al.: *Green's operative hand surgery*, ed 7, Philadephia, 2017, Elsevier, Inc.

23. Haglin JM, Kugelman DN, Christiano A, et al.: Open surgical elbow contracture release after trauma: results and recommendations, *J Shoulder Elbow Surg*, 2017. Epub ahead of print.

24. Veltman ES, Doornberg JN, Eygendaal D, et al.: Static progressive versus dynamic splinting for posttraumatic elbow stiffness: a systematic review of 232 patients, *Arch Orthop Trauma Surg* 135(5):613–617, 2015.

25. Page C, Backus SI, Lenhoff MW: Electromyographic activity in stiff and normal elbows during elbow flexion and extension, *J Hand Ther* 16(1):5–11, 2003.

26. Chinchalkar SJ, Pearce J, Athwal GS: Static progressive versus three-point elbow extension splinting: a mathematical analysis, *J Hand Ther* 22(1):37–41, 2009.

27. Flowers KR, LaStayo P: Effect of total end range time on improving passive range of motion, *J Hand Ther* 7(3):150–157, 1994.

28. Lindenhovius AL, van de Liujtgaarden K, Ring D, et al.: Open elbow contracture release: postoperative management with and without continuous passive motion, *J Hand Surg Am* 34(5):858–865, 2009.

29. Higgs ZC, Danks BA, Sibinski M, et al.: Outcomes of open arthrolysis of the elbow without post-operative passive stretching, *J Bone Joint Surg Br* 94(3):348–352, 2012.

30. Lindenhovius AL, Doornberg JN, Brouwer KM, et al.: A prospective randomized controlled trial of dynamic versus static progressive elbow splinting for posttraumatic elbow stiffness, *J Bone Joint Surg Am* 94(8):694–700, 2012.

20 Peripheral Nerve Problems

Anne Michelle Moscony

Introduction

Functional recovery from a peripheral nerve injury requires the cooperative efforts of the physician, therapist, and client. The potentially severe consequences of these injuries are well known to surgeons and therapists but may not be as obvious to our clients. For example, loss of sensation in the hand can result in difficulties performing such simple tasks as communicating through texting. Clients may inadvertently sustain a burn or laceration to an insensate finger during meal preparation. Muscle weakness or paralysis can result in decreased strength and endurance for household and work tasks, with monetary consequences that include lost work time and/or lost job skills. Pain is usually a sequela of nerve injury, and nerve pain is itself a costly and difficult condition to treat. Inadvertently, clients may further damage their nervous system if they are not properly educated about their injury and relevant precautions. Full client understanding of and participation in their rehabilitation is therefore essential to optimal recovery.

Appreciating the normal static and dynamic aspects of our nervous system is a necessary precursor to understanding how an injury to one part of the nervous system can cause immediate and delayed changes throughout the entire system. Such changes can result in functional problems for our clients. The art of hand therapy is anticipating and assisting our clients in remediation of these functional deficits.

Many of us learned about the nervous system as consisting of the peripheral nervous system (PNS) and the central nervous system (CNS); two segregated systems with similar functions but very different presentations following injury to one or the other.

Clinical Pearl

The nervous system is actually one system that crosses multiple joints and moves through various muscular and fibro-osseous tunnels. It consists of various tissue types interconnected electrically and chemically. All nerve tissue has the same elementary function of continuous electrochemical communication. This system is complex and highly organized. When one part of the system changes there are repercussions throughout the system, even at parts that are metrically distant.

There is an ongoing plasticity within our nervous system. This means the nervous system can change, learn, and adapt or maladapt throughout the individual's life span. Sensory receptors of peripheral nerves will become less sensitive to stimuli that is not harmful to the body if the stimulus is present for a long-enough period of time. For example, if you walk into a room where there is a strong odor, say a baby's diaper, your olfactory sensory receptors will eventually decrease their responsiveness to this smell if you stay in the room for a period of time. This is called **habituation**, and it is defined as a temporary decrease in responsiveness to a benign stimulus. Your PNS has *temporarily* changed its sensitivity to this odor. Still, if you leave the room and come back later, the strength of the stimulus (the bad smell) returns. The intensity of that stimulus is the same as when you entered the room the first time; your habituation to the stimulus was short lived. On the other hand, if your nervous system is exposed to that stimulus for a long-enough time, your nervous system could alter, modulate, or *permanently* change. A gradual and long-lasting change in both the CNS and PNS is called **modulation.** Your sensitivity to a strong odor might permanently decrease (or increase) depending on your nervous system's attempt to maintain **homeostasis.** The capacity of our nervous system to modulate or change either temporarily or permanently is called **neuroplasticity.** This is the cornerstone of neurorehabilitation.[1,2]

Neuroplasticity is predicated on ongoing interactions with our environment. Our nervous system is dynamic; it is continually changing throughout our life span. An injury or change in one part of this system will affect other parts of the system, even to tissue not physically close to the site of injury. Efficient motor coordination (for prehension, for example) is based on a continual stream of sensory input to the brain that is used to guide coordinated motor actions or output. Consider how an injury to the central nervous system (i.e., the brain) can affect both strength and sensation in the contralateral arm and leg (PNS) resulting in gross limb paresis (or weakness) and loss of efficient motor control or coordination. Information in the sensory receptors of the joints of the involved extremity would not be able to supply reliable proprioceptive information that would normally be used to adjust the accuracy of an intended movement. For example, a person with this type of brain injury might find it challenging to accurately reach forward and open and close their fingers just the right amount to efficiently grasp a coffee mug. They would have difficulty recruiting motor units synchronously to pick up the mug and bring it smoothly to their mouth to drink. Following this type of CNS insult, the muscle-tendon units of the involved extremities will atrophy, resulting in further weakness.[1,3] Often, given diminished sensory information from the involved arm, neglect of that body part will develop, further reinforcing this muscle atrophy.[1,3]

Likewise, if there is an injury to a peripheral nerve (for example, let's say the median nerve), there would be ipsilateral muscle paralysis (a PNS symptom) as well as loss of (peripheral) sensory information to the CNS.[4,5] In this case, the client would not be able to actively position their thumb in opposition to grab the cup handle due to paralysis of the opponens pollicis, nor would they be able to feel if the cup was too hot to handle safely. Such deficits in sensorimotor control lead the brain to rapidly adjust to this reduction in sensory input and altered motor output. In fact, the CNS will quickly reorganize its cortical representations of the hand following an alteration of skin sensory inputs induced by a peripheral nerve injury as evidenced by the "smudging" or dampening of the neural connections associated with that body part.[1] Neglect of a body part (for example, following a nerve injury with consequent motor paralysis) will also lead to changes in cortical organization. In fact, how the cortex reorganizes following a peripheral nerve injury has been proposed as a major factor in final functional outcomes, including whether or not our client will develop chronic pain.[1,2]

⊙ *Clinical Pearl*

The therapist must consider how the entire nervous system has been impacted following a PNS or CNS injury during both evaluation and treatment planning.

This chapter reviews normal nerve anatomy and looks at factors that can change or sensitize the nerve and hence the nervous system itself. The chapter explains how the nerve responds to injury and how we as clinicians can assist our clients in modifying the potentially deleterious effects of commonly seen peripheral nerve injuries of the upper extremity (UE). The chapter concludes with a case study using critical reasoning to determine how to treat these clients.

Overview of Neuroanatomy

The **neuron** is the basic unit of the nervous system; it consists of a cell body (the **soma**), some **dendrites**, and usually one **axon.** The dendrites are arbor-like antennae that serve as the primary input sites for the nerve cell. The axon is the primary output unit projecting from the soma to other neurons, muscle cells or glands. An axon can vary in length from 1 mm to up to 1 meter in length. A chain of communicating neurons is called a **pathway.** Within the CNS, a bundle of pathway axons is called a **tract** or a **fasciculus.** Outside the CNS, a bundle of pathway axons is called a **nerve.** In this chapter, the term *axon* is used interchangeably with the term *nerve fiber.*

The CNS is well organized with an intricate system of motor and sensory pathways arranged to reflect and respond to the continual input of information from our interaction in the environment. Cortical information is processed somatotopically with a homunculus or mapping in both the frontal lobe (for the motor pathways) and the parietal lobe (for sensory pathways) to specifically handle compartmental information and assure very quick feedback for movement and sensory integration. This cortical representation or homunculus mapping in the brain is arranged to reflect the amount of neuronal input and output demand; thus the hand is represented as a much bigger part of the homunculus than is the elbow.[3]

All upper motor neurons originate in the frontal lobe and terminate on the anterior horn cells (or lower motor neurons) in the gray matter of the spinal cord. All peripheral motor nerves originate from these lower motor neurons. All peripheral sensory nerves have their cell bodies in the dorsal root ganglia, located adjacent to the intervertebral foramen of the vertebral column. Sensory information arrives here and is initially processed at the spinal cord level. This information must pass upward through the thalamus into the contralateral parietal cortex for further processing or perception. If sensory information does not reach the cortex for processing, the brain will not consciously perceive or recognize the sensory experience (including the sensation of pain). This has implications for pain management.

The sensory and motor roots join together to form a **spinal nerve** (Fig. 20.1). Sympathetic nerve axons from autonomic ganglia also join the spinal nerve by way of the rami communicans. Therefore spinal and somatic peripheral nerves are usually mixed with sensory, autonomic, and motor axons. Shortly after merging, the spinal nerve splits into dorsal and ventral rami. The ventral rami of all spinal nerves, except for T2 to T12, form networks of nerves called **plexuses.** There are four main plexuses; the largest are the brachial plexus and lumbar plexus.

The brachial plexus (Fig. 20.2) is formed by the anterior rami of cervical roots C5 to T1. This plexus emerges from the anterior and middle scalene muscles and passes deep to the clavicle before entering the axilla. In the distal axilla, the sensory, motor, and autonomic axons from the plexus become the radial, median, ulnar, axillary, and musculocutaneous nerves. The entire upper limb is innervated by branches from the brachial plexus.

A peripheral nerve is composed of two types of tissue: one for conducting impulses (the nerve fibers or axons) and the other for supporting and protecting these nerve fibers (the glia). The axons of these nerve cells are very long and very thin; they are braided or bundled together into **fascicles** and are surrounded, separated, and protected by layers of nonconductive connective tissue. These axons are designed to be conduits for transmitting impulses—no matter how or in what position the body moves. We know that

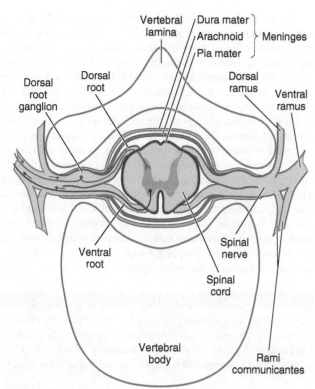

FIG. 20.1 Schematic of a typical spinal nerve formed from the dorsal and ventral roots of the spinal cord. *(From Lundy-Ekman L. Neuroscience: Fundamentals for Rehabilitation. Philadelphia, PA: WB Saunders; 1998.)*

joints move in a matter of degrees, that muscles contract, and that tendons slide. Nerves also move; they move relative to the tissues that surround them. The nerve's axons must stretch and slide within their protective tissue coverings, and the nerve trunk must glide relative to the surrounding external tissues while continuing to perform its essential duty: impulse conduction.

Peripheral nerves are ensheathed, protected, and at times constrained by multiple layers of connective tissue coverings: the **endoneurium, perineurium, epineurium**, and **mesoneurium.** These coverings create a nerve "bed." Within this nerve bed, individual nerve fibers sit gently coiled in a wavy pattern. The nerve fibers change position within the nerve bed as they proceed distally, frequently entwining and separating into different fascicles as they course in an undulating fashion to their final destination. This meshing serves as a protective mechanism, allowing some play in the overall length of the nerve.[5] Thus peripheral nerve fibers are capable of some degree of elastic stretch, allowing the longitudinal length difference needed when a joint moves into an end-range posture. When the shoulder is abducted to 90 degrees and the elbow and wrist are extended (as when you reach out to the side to get something off a shelf) the median nerve is 10 cm longer than when the elbow and wrist are flexed (as when reaching to your mouth).[1] This elongation and slack uptake is distributed evenly throughout a healthy peripheral nerve.[5]

Peripheral nerves are protected from injury to a large extent by their external protective connective tissue coverings (Fig. 20.3). The outermost covering is called the epineurium. It is loose connective tissue that functions to surround the nerve trunk, providing protection from external tensile and compressive forces. The deeper layers of the epineurium function like packing material,

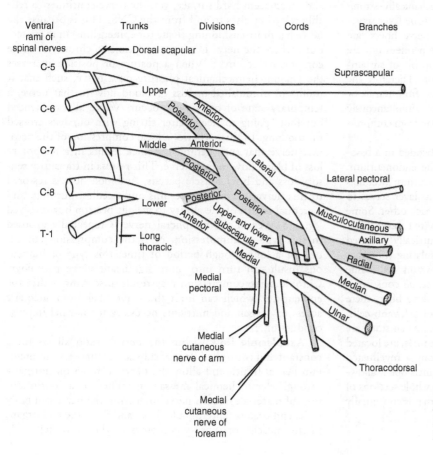

FIG. 20.2 Diagram of the brachial plexus. *(From Jenkins DB. Hollinshead's Functional Anatomy of the Limb and Back. 8th ed. Philadelphia, PA: Saunders; 2002.)*

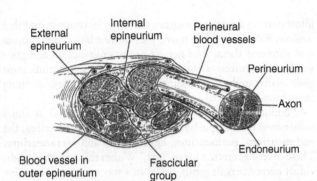

FIG. 20.3 External protective tissue coverings surrounding a segment of a peripheral nerve. *(From Trumble TE, McCallister WV. Physiology and repair of peripheral nerves. In: Trumble TE. ed.* Principles of Hand Surgery and Therapy. *Philadelphia, PA; Saunders; 2000.)*

physically separating the fascicles and facilitating gliding between these bundled groups of nerve fibers. There is a greater percentage of epineural tissue present in areas where the nerve is physically exposed to compressive forces, as when it passes adjacent to a bone or underneath tough fibrous structures, such as the flexor retinaculum of the wrist.[4]

External to the epineurium is a loose areolar tissue that surrounds the peripheral nerve trunk, called the mesoneurium. The role of this tissue is not fully understood; however, it appears to function as added protection against compressive and tensile forces impacting the nerve.[4] It also appears to limit external friction to the nerve trunk by allowing substantial sliding (or side-to-side movement) of the nerve as it passes around and through local structures and tight spaces.[4]

Each nerve fascicle is surrounded by a mechanically strong sheath called the perineurium. This connective tissue layer serves as a molecular diffusion barrier, keeping the nerve fibers safe from neurotoxic compounds.[4] The fibers of the perineurium are predominately composed of elastin, which is capable of sustaining significant stretch without tissue deformation. Therefore the perineurium also serves to protect the nerve fibers from tensile or stretch forces (as experienced when adjacent joints simultaneously move into their end-range of motion) more so than from compressive forces.[6]

The nerve fibers inside the fascicles are embedded in a basement membrane of connective tissue called the endoneurium. Around each nerve fiber (or axon), the endoneurium becomes closely packed, forming a supporting wall. This layer serves to electrically insulate *individual nerve fibers* from each other. Some of these nerve fibers are myelinated. A **myelinated nerve fiber** is one that has a longitudinal chain of concentrically wrapped **Schwann cells** surrounding it, creating an insulating tube that promotes fast impulse conduction. The Schwann cell tissue together with the closely packed endoneurial tissue constitutes the **endoneurial tube.**[6] Along a myelinated nerve fiber, there are discrete areas not covered by the column of Schwann cells, located about 1 mm apart.[6] These nodes or bared sections are called **nodes of Ranvier.** Portals, called **ion channels**, are located at these nodes. Conduction of an impulse along a myelinated nerve fiber can occur very rapidly as these channels open, allowing an infusion of charged ions that depolarize whole sections of the nerve fiber, from node to node, like a fuse that is continually being relit at each node.

Neural tissue has a high metabolic demand. Although the nervous system composes about 2% of the body's mass, nerves may consume up to 20% of the available oxygen in circulating blood[4] to function normally. Within the epineurium is a well-developed, longitudinally oriented vascular system that feeds the peripheral nerve fibers. Nerve fibers are especially vulnerable to vascular changes as a result of altered circulation or blood flow within the epineurium of the nerve.[4,7] The effects vary dependent on the duration, as well as the magnitude, of the trauma. Prolonged or severe stretch or compression with consequent compromised circulation will result in edema within the nerve's connective tissue coverings once circulation is restored. This swelling may lead to intra- and extraneural fibrosis (or scarring), and decreased nerve stretch capability.[4] It is also likely that this fibrosis in and around the epineurial and perineurial tissue will limit oxygen and nutrient uptake, which in turn will compromise impulse propagation potential, and result in a gradual worsening of the nerve injury.[6]

> ### ⊚ *Clinical Pearl*
>
> Do NOT "go for the burn" during stretching exercises. Passive stretching that results in neurological symptoms such as burning pain and/or numbness may compromise neural circulation and cause a temporary or a gradual worsening of nerve injury.

Usually our nervous system is well designed to protect its neurons and their peripheral axons even when the nerve is compressed between a bone and a hard external surface. For example, when we lean on our elbow, the ulnar nerve is trapped between the medial epicondyle of the humeral bone and an adjacent hard surface; yet, the nerve continues to reliably relay impulses to and from the CNS. This is because the nerve has more cushioning tissue (or epineurium) in those sections where the nerve is more susceptible to chronic or acute compressive trauma.[4] When a posture or position increases the amount of mechanical pressure on a nerve, such that it results in diminished or loss of blood flow to that nerve, a temporary state of paresis can occur. We've all experienced our foot "going to sleep" after sitting with our legs crossed for too long. In this scenario, a local compression of the peroneal nerve that runs behind the knee results in a temporary loss of blood flow to that nerve. This results in transitory sensory loss and brief muscle paresis. As blood flow is restored to this nerve, we experience pins and needles, burning, and a gradual return of the ability to weight bear on our involved leg. However, if the peripheral nerve is repeatedly exposed to this type of compression, or if the compression continues for a long-enough period of time, this type of innocuous insult can turn into more significant nerve pathology. Chronic nerve compression may result in scarring within the epineurium, which can limit the nerve fiber from adequate access to oxygen and nutrients necessary for normal impulse conduction.[6]

Axoplasmic flow within the nerve's axon allows for a constant and controlled flow of substances that serve to maintain neural health and allow the nerve to function normally through electrochemical messaging.[8] There is a continuous flow of materials in each nerve fiber from the nerve cell body to its end organs (anterograde flow) and from the end organs in the muscles or sensory receptors to the nerve cell body (retrograde flow). Various substances and organelles are synthesized in the nerve cell body and are transported within the axon to and from its terminal. This requires a continuous energy supply of oxygenated blood flow. The axoplasm thickens and moves more slowly when the nerve is stationary.[5] Impaired axoplasmic flow will lead to compromised neural function, including slowed and/or decreased synaptic activity, and trophic changes in the tissues served by that nerve.[5,8]

> **Clinical Pearl**
>
> Motion is lotion for our nerves. Movement enhances the flow of blood throughout the nerve and improves the axoplasmic flow within the nerve.

Mechanism of Nerve Injuries: Incomplete Versus Complete Injuries

A nerve injury may develop as a result of compression or entrapment of the nerve by an internal source, such as a tumor or scar tissue, or by compression from an external source (such as, crutches or a cast). Nerve injury may occur secondary to traction or stretching of the nerve, by avulsion or laceration, by chemical or electrical burns, or by radiation. A typical peripheral nerve has sensory, motor and autonomic nerve fibers; therefore you can expect that the more severe the trauma to the nerve, the more severe the damage will be to the motor, sensory, and autonomic functions of the nerve. Nerve injuries are classified in various ways in an attempt to estimate the prognosis of, as well as to anticipate the need for and type of medical and/or therapeutic intervention. Seddon classified peripheral nerve injuries (PNI) in 1943 as a neurapraxia, axonotmesis, or neurotmesis,[4] according to the amount of connective tissue and nerve fiber damage. Sunderland expanded on this hierarchy by adding two additional levels in 1951 (Table 20.1).[4]

> **Clinical Pearl**
>
> Although peripheral nerves are injured in various ways, there are only two possible pathological responses: **demyelination** (damage to the myelin around the nerve fiber resulting in a slowing or loss of nerve impulse conduction at that site) and/or injury to the nerve fiber itself.[4,7,9] Segmental demyelination (or **neurapraxia**) results in a transient state of disrupted nerve conduction along the injured segment. If the endoneurial tube remains intact, the nerve fibers have a pathway for regrowth back to the target organs they innervate. More severe degrees of injury to a peripheral nerve in continuity (that is, where the encapsulating connective tissue framework of the nerve remains physically intact) will always involve some amount of nerve fiber disruption. Those with significant nerve fiber disruption and with concomitant and substantial damage to the supporting connective tissues will usually require surgical intervention. Often, an injured peripheral nerve will manifest as a mixed pattern of demyelination and axonal loss. Nerve injuries where the nerve is completely severed or where the nerve shows serious internal disorganization and loss of the endoneurial tube are considered to have the poorest prognosis for functional recovery.[4,6,9] Typically, these cases require surgical intervention to allow for some amount of functional recovery.

Incomplete Injuries (Injuries Where the Nerve Trunk Is Still in Continuity)

Neuropathy is the term used to describe pathological conditions of the peripheral nerve. Incomplete injuries to a nerve are defined as those where the external connective tissue coverings (the nerve's framework) remain to some degree intact. An incomplete injury has important therapeutic implications. **Mononeuropathy** involves damage to a single nerve.[5] An example would be compression of the median nerve at the carpal tunnel, or **carpal tunnel syndrome (CTS)**. **Multiple mononeuropathy** is a multifocal asymmetrical involvement of

Degree	Description	Mechanism of Injury	Prognosis
	TABLE 20.1 Sunderland's Classification		
1	All structures remain intact; local conduction block and demyelination	Acute compression (Seddon's neurapraxia)	Complete recovery (days/months)
2	Axonal disruption with distal (Wallerian) degeneration; however, endoneurial tubes are intact	Mild traction or moderate compression (Seddon's axonotmesis)	Typically, complete recovery (months), limiting factor is distance of regeneration required (viable end organ)
3	Disruption of axons and endoneurial tubes; mild to moderate functional loss; fascicles remain intact	Moderate-severe traction or crush (Seddon's neurotmesis)	Axons may regenerate but in "wrong" endoneurial tube; many result in nerve-target organ mismatch; poor prognosis for proximal injuries
4	Loss of fascicular integrity within the nerve; only epineurium is intact	Severe traction or crush (Seddon's neurotmesis)	Moderate to severe functional loss; may be improved by fascicular repair; neuroma in continuity is common: regenerating axons lost in scar
5	Complete nerve transection	Severe traction or crush; laceration (Seddon's neurotmesis)	Severe functional loss; requires surgery

multiple nerves.[5] Compression of the right median and ulnar nerves as a complication of occupational stresses that require repetitive elbow and wrist flexion is an example of multiple mononeuropathy.

Altered axoplasmic flow in a peripheral nerve that results from diminished blood flow can cause the entire nerve to become sick, and thus to become vulnerable to more than one site of irritation along its axon. Increased susceptibility for a secondary impingement may develop in areas where the nerve must traverse through spaces of increased friction (for example, fibro-osseous tunnels). When the nerve has serial impingements or dual sites of pathologic manifestations that developed without a history of acute trauma, it is called **double** or **multiple crush syndrome.**[10]

Metabolic changes can result in neuropathies as well. Metabolic-induced neuropathy typically presents as **polyneuropathy**, or bilateral extremity damage to two or more peripheral nerves. Peripheral polyneuropathy may involve the feet as well as the hands, and typically presents in a stocking or glove-like distribution. It occurs most frequently in people who smoke, who have nutritional deficiencies secondary to alcoholism, or who have autoimmune disease or diabetes.[5] Neuropathies that develop secondary to pregnancy will usually resolve as the woman's body returns to its prenatal metabolic state.[5] Other polyneuropathies may be stable with medications or may be progressive as the disease advances.

When there is sustained or adequate compression or trauma to the nerve, edema (swelling) will accumulate within the endoneurial sheath or basement membrane that surrounds the nerve fibers. The diffusion barrier created by the perineurium and the lack of lymphatic vessels in the endoneurial space means that once this edema develops, the increased pressure cannot be dissipated. This results in impaired endoneurial microcirculation. The accumulation of edema in the endoneurial space results in increased intraneural pressure and a reduction or cessation of blood flow to the individual nerve fibers, as well as diminished axoplasmic flow within the nerve fibers. This can result in a segmental conduction block (called **neuropraxia**) within the nerve fiber. The nerve can conduct an action potential above and below the injured site, but not across site. The nerve is in continuity, with intact connective tissue coverings, but it does not function because of this blockage. If this conduction block is of long-enough duration and/or intensity, demyelination will occur; affecting the larger myelinated nerve fibers (sensory and motor nerve fibers) first while sparing the thinner, nonmyelinated fibers that conduct pain and autonomic function.[6] This means your client will feel pain but will also experience diminished or loss of light touch sensibility.

Venous blood flow from the peripheral nerves is shown to be reduced with increased vascular pressures of 20 to 30 mm Hg. A classic study by Gelberman et al.[11] demonstrated that with 90 degrees of wrist flexion or extension, carpal tunnel pressure in those persons *without* CTS rose to 30 mm Hg on average. Thus compressive forces on a peripheral nerve can reduce venous blood flow and create a temporary compression neuropathy. When combined with certain provocative postures, such as holding the wrist in end-range of flexion or extension for periods of time, nerve pathology may worsen. If combined with other pathology, such as swelling in the carpal tunnel area following a wrist fracture, a metabolic block (or longer-lasting compression neuropathy) will likely develop.

Timelines and Healing (Incomplete Nerve Injuries)

> **◎ Clinical Pearl**
>
> Compressive neuropathies, of either acute or chronic nature, can often be treated successfully with nonsurgical methods. These include client education about activity modification, rest, nonsteroidal antiinflammatory drugs, corticosteroid injections, and orthotics.[12,13,14]

A typical neuropraxic nerve lesion can resolve within minutes or weeks.[4] A classic example of this level of nerve injury (also classified as a Sunderland type 1 nerve injury) is a **Saturday night palsy**, which is a radial nerve injury at the humeral level that results from compression of the nerve between the humerus bone and some hard external source.

If the compression is of a severe enough nature, the nerve fibers distal to the lesion (and the myelin covering these fibers) would degenerate, but the endoneurial tubes of these axons will remain intact. This type of nerve injury is called an **axonotmesis**, or Sunderland type 2 nerve injury. **Wallerian degeneration** or degeneration of the part of the nerve fiber distal to the injury site (i.e., farther from the neuron's cell body), occurs with this type of nerve lesion. Muscle tissue distal to the injury site will demonstrate fibrillations and sensory loss will be more severe than seen with a neuropraxia.[6] Sensory and motor recovery is dependent on axonal (nerve fiber) regeneration. Generally, there is a good chance of recovery of function (without surgical intervention) because the endoneurial tubes survive. These tubes serve as pathways for the regenerating nerve fiber. The rate of regeneration is predicated on the presence (or absence) of comorbidities, the amount of physical activity that occurs at the injury site, and the distance between the injury site and the final destination of the regenerating nerve fiber.[6] In uncomplicated cases, the rate of recovery ranges from 1.5 to 3 mm per day.[6]

Nerve compression lesions result in sensory, motor, and autonomic dysfunction in the innervated area distal to the injury site. Your nerve-injured client may complain of muscle weakness and/or pain. They may experience autonomic dysfunction, including aberrant changes in blood flow, skin moisture and hair growth, as well as delayed wound healing.[6] Sensory-wise, they will initially experience a loss of proprioception and discriminative touch, followed by a loss of pain and temperature sensation. The loss of proprioception occurs first because compression of a nerve affects the large myelinated fibers (that carry information about proprioception and discriminative touch) prior to affecting the smaller, unmyelinated fibers. If the compression persists or is severe enough, the smaller fibers that carry information about pain and temperature also are lost.[8] When the compression resolves, abnormal sensations called **paresthesia** occur as the blood supply to the nerve resumes. The client may complain of burning, tingling, or pricking sensations. Sensation gradually returns in the reverse order in which it was lost: (1) dull, diffuse aching pain; (2) perception of heat; (3) sharp, stinging sensations; (4) cold perception; (5) conscious proprioception; and finally, (6) discriminative touch.

General Comments Following Nerve Injury

- *If the client has diminished or lost protective sensation, you will need to teach them to protect the insensate part from temperature extremes (including hot bath water) as well as from situations where the insensate part might accidentally be injured (as when they are not visually attending to the injured body part).*
- *Any client with diminished or loss of protective sensation in any part of the UE should be strictly cautioned against exposing this body part to moving machinery because they could further injure that body part without immediately realizing it.*

- What nerve was injured? Where is the injury site?
- What was the mechanism of injury? Was it a stretch injury or a crush injury to the nerve?
- Were electromyogram (EMG) or nerve conduction studies done? What were the results?
- Is surgical decompression indicated at this time?

Complete Nerve Injuries (Injuries Where the Nerve Itself Is Transected and/or There Is Axon Destruction with Significant Loss or Disorganization of the External Connective Tissue Layers)

Neurotmesis is the most severe type of peripheral nerve injury. Grave consequences in terms of motor and/or sensory loss occur following an injury where the peripheral nerve is severed, or where a segment of the nerve is traumatized with serious internal disorganization. Sunderland described three hierarchical levels of neurotmesis[4]; each level demonstrating increased involvement of the eternal connective tissue layers of the nerve. A Sunderland type 3 nerve lesion is defined as loss of continuity of axons and their endoneurial tubes with an intact perineurium.[6] A Sunderland type 4 lesion indicates loss of the continuity of the axons, endoneurium, and perineurium with intact epineurium. In the latter case, significant internal scarring occurs within the nerve trunk that impairs functional recovery. Resection of the fibrotic segment of the nerve trunk followed by nerve repair with a graft would probably be required.

A Sunderland type 5 nerve lesion is defined as a physiological disruption of the entire nerve or a section of a nerve with loss of axons (nerve fibers) and disruption of all of the encapsulating connective tissue layers that surround the axons. Recovery of function is unlikely without surgical intervention as the nerve is unable to repair itself.

When a nerve is severed, an immediate consequence is loss of sensation and muscle paralysis in the area supplied.[5] There will also be a loss of the nerve's vital axoplasmic fluid.[15] Each axon itself contains 90% of the axoplasmic fluid present in that nerve cell. The axoplasmic transport system (with its retrograde and anterograde flows) allows the neuron to maintain its structure and health at its synapses.[6,8] This system also allows the soma (or nerve cell body) to get feedback about the axon's overall health including the health of the (distally located) nerve's synaptic clefts. When this communication and transport system fails, the muscle and sensory receptors associated with that nerve change. There is a loss of, or decrease in, these receptors' ability to receive or generate impulses.[6,8,9] One will also see **trophic changes** in

the target tissues; that is, changes in the tissues served by that nerve that include abnormal hair growth, nail bed changes, cold intolerance, and soft-tissue atrophy.[6,8]

A completely severed peripheral nerve presents as loss of sensation, loss of muscle control, and a loss of reflexes in those structures innervated by the injured nerve and located distal to the injury site.

Another consequence of axonal transection is that the soma (cell body) swells, and the cell's nucleus is displaced peripherally. This reflects a change in the metabolic priority from production of neurotransmitters to production of structural materials needed for axon repair and growth.[9] The proximal axon undergoes traumatic degeneration within the zone of injury (that is, to the next node or nodes of Ranvier). Distal to site of injury, Wallerian degeneration occurs, followed by development of a regenerative fascicle that attempts to join the distal transected segment to complete the process of regeneration.[9] This process begins about 48 to 96 hours after transection and concludes about 3 weeks postinjury.[9] During this time, there is progressive deterioration of the myelin. There is also a proliferation of fibroblasts (cells that produce connective tissue) and Schwann cells. Together, these cells can create internal disorganization, which can result in blockages to nerve fiber regeneration and/or the development of a neuroma (painful thickening of tissue around the nerve fiber stump). This is one of the reasons that the best prognosis for surgical repair of an injured nerve is associated with surgery performed within 48 to 96 hours of the injury.[16]

General Comments Following Nerve Laceration

- *The development of stiff and fibrotic joints and soft tissue in the adjacent areas can occur following a period of immobilization to protect the nerve repair site. Check with the surgeon to insure you are immobilizing the fewest joints and soft tissues possible without compromising the repair.*
- *Be cautious with initial loading of nearby bone and joints once strengthening is permitted if your client has a history of osteopenia or osteoporosis. Either condition may be exacerbated during the postoperative immobilization period.*
- *Muscle tissue atrophy and interstitial fibrosis in the tissue innervated by the involved nerve will occur with an initial weight loss of 30% in the first month and 50% to 60% by 2 months. Muscle atrophy reaches a relatively stable state at 60% to 80% weight loss by approximately 4 months.[17]*
- *Denervated muscle tissue is replaced by fibrotic adipose tissue. Issacs notes that if muscle tissue is not adequately reinnervated by 18 months postinjury, it is unlikely that one will see functional improvements.[18]*

Overview of Postoperative Management—Decompression Versus Nerve Repair

Surgical intervention is always necessary if the nerve is severed and may be necessary if the nerve has enough internal disorganization and scarring. Intervention might include surgical repair, a decompression, and/or a neurolysis. A **primary nerve repair** refers to operative nerve repair performed within the first week after injury. Primary repairs are associated with better results.[19] A **delayed** or **secondary nerve repair** is one performed a week or more after injury. **Nerve grafting** is a type of nerve repair performed when a primary repair cannot be completed without undue tension on the nerve's cut ends.[9] The nerve graft acts to provide a source of empty endoneurial tubes through which the regenerating axon can be directed. A nerve graft can be performed using a commercially available **conduit**, or by using an autograft or allograft. An **autograft** is graft material harvested from typically dispensable sensory nerves and used to repair large mixed nerves. An **allograft** is a tissue graft from another human (harvested from human cadavers, for example). Both allografts and autographs are used to address large nerve gaps, or gaps left following resection of a neuroma.[9,18]

A **neurolysis** is the surgical dissection and exploration of a damaged nerve with the goal of freeing the nerve from local tissue restrictions or adhesions.[19] Peripheral **nerve decompression** surgery is performed when the nerve has become trapped or impinged in some way. This surgical procedure decreases the compressive forces or pressure on a nerve. It may involve cutting tissue that is constricting the nerve, or physically moving the nerve to a different site.

Timelines and Healing Following Complete Nerve Injuries

In general, our nervous system has limited powers of regeneration (the ability to replicate or repair itself after injury).[8] Mature neurons are unable to reproduce; damage to the soma of the peripheral nerve fibers has historically been untreatable. Over the past decade, undifferentiated neural stem cells have been identified in both adult and developing brains.[8] Research into stem cell transplants has concentrated on addressing CNS deficits (e.g., following a spinal cord injury) via implantation of neural stem cells that mature into neurons capable of replacing damaged ones. In the future, it may be possible to address peripheral nerve lesions using neural stem cells to improve the potential for full recovery after a peripheral nerve injury.[8]

Currently, complete peripheral nerve lesions can achieve full or partial recovery following injury *if* certain conditions exist. First, the soma, or nerve cell body, must be viable. Certain severe injuries, such as nerve root avulsions, can kill the motor neurons in the spinal cord and the dorsal root ganglion cells located adjacent to the spinal cord. Damage to the soma results in the death of the entire nerve cell.

Second, the physiological environment in and around the nerve lesion must support axonal sprouting and peripheral growth. Ideally, there is an intact endoneurial tube with undamaged Schwann cells distal to the level of the injury. Schwann cells produce nerve growth factor, which is one of the keys to allowing peripheral nerve damage to resolve.[9] Peripheral growth ceases if the sprouting axons meet scar tissue or bone that blocks access to the empty Schwann sheaths and endoneurial tubes or to the end organ of the axon.

A third condition for recovery is that the regenerated axon must connect to the appropriate end organ, and that end organ still must be viable. The motor nerve fiber must grow to its original motor end plate, and the sensory nerve fiber must connect with its appropriate receptor organ. If a sensory axon is misdirected into a motor distal tubule, the axonal growth will be wasted. Therefore nerve injuries in which the endoneurial tube remains intact have a better prognosis for functional recovery

than does an injury where the endoneurial tube is disrupted. Regenerating nerve fibers will travel down their appropriate neural tube to the correct end organ if the tube is viable and not blocked by scar tissue. Even if the proper nerve fibers get to the correct sensory end organ or motor end plate, the sensory receptors and muscle tissue must be viable. Sensory end organs have no end plate, and therefore they retain the potential for reinnervation for 1 to 3 or more years.[15,17] However, denervated muscle tissue loses the ability to support axonal regeneration as the motor end plate degenerates. The muscle becomes hypersensitive and fasciculates (twitches) clinically. The chances of functional reinnervation diminish if the nerve does not reach the motor end plates within approximately 18 months of denervation.[18]

A final condition for peripheral nerve recovery is that the CNS must perceive and interpret the injured PNS signals appropriately. The CNS will need to reorganize its cortical representations of the hand, for example, following alteration of skin inputs induced by a peripheral nerve injury.

The Medical Research Council (MRC) defines a *good or functional outcome* for nerve recovery following surgical nerve repair as motor: M3 (muscle action against gravity only, or a grade 3/5 muscle strength return) or better, and sensory: S3 (pain and touch perception with 2-point discrimination greater than 15 mm) or better[19]; though it is unlikely that our clients would agree with this opinion. Most major adult peripheral nerve injuries will result in some level of permanent damage,[19] with significant functional limitations that are underidentified, measured and addressed.

❤ Tips From the Field

Nerve Injury

If surgery can be avoided, it should. Typically, there is pain after surgery. In addition, postoperative swelling can exacerbate a compression injury. Thus try conservative management first if possible. For example, compression of the median nerve at the wrist (CTS) may be ameliorated with splinting at night, ergonomic interventions, and client education about provocative positions to avoid.[20]

If surgery is necessary, allow the injured nerve time to recover from the trauma of surgery. The amount of time that is necessary for healing depends on a number of factors, including the severity of the nerve injury before surgery and the type of surgery. An endoscopic **carpal tunnel release (CTR)** is typically less traumatic than the traditional open CTR, for example, allowing for quicker return to work and self-care activities. Other factors that affect the recovery period may include the presence of systemic diseases, such as rheumatoid arthritis or diabetes, which can slow or permanently compromise healing. The existence of concomitant injuries may exaggerate the early phases of tissue healing. Gentle active range of motion (AROM) in the area of the nerve injury usually can begin when the client has moved beyond the inflammatory stage of healing. The typical timeline for this ranges from 2 to 3 days postoperatively to 2 to 3 weeks postoperatively. Avoid strengthening exercises until the remodeling phase of healing, which is typically 3 to 4 weeks (or longer) from surgery. Knowledge about the phases of wound healing enables the therapist to devise an appropriate postoperative program for each client. Again, the reader is cautioned to address each client as an individual, observing that person's tissue response to exercise and adjusting each program accordingly.

? Questions to Ask the Doctor

- What was the date of the repair?
- Was the nerve repair under tension? Was there need for a nerve graft?
- Was there a delay from the time of injury to the time of the nerve repair?
- Are there other structures that were injured and repaired?
- Do you have a particular postoperative therapy protocol you would like to be followed? How long do you want the nerve repair to be protected by immobilization?
- Can we begin range of motion (ROM) of the parts distal and proximal to the repair site to maintain joint suppleness and tissue length and gliding?
- When can we introduce strengthening? Are there any specific limitations in weight and/or activities that you want us to observe?

Diagnosis-Specific Information That Affects Clinical Reasoning

- Repaired peripheral nerves heal at a rate of about a 1 to 3 mm/day after an initial 3- to 4-week latency period.[16] Additional delays may occur as the regenerating axon attempts to cross the injury site and reinnervate the end organ.
- As a nerve regenerates, motor reinnervation occurs from proximal to distal, following the anatomical pathway of the nerve. It is therefore helpful to know the typical order of innervation of those muscles served by the injured nerve.
- Denervated muscle tissue is gradually replaced with fibrotic adipose tissue. If functional reinnervation is not restored to the muscles by 12 to 18 months, it is unlikely that one will see further noticeable improvements.[18]
- Sensory end organs remain viable because there is no end plate like there is in muscles. Thus these organs retain the potential for reinnervation. Nerve grafting a digital sensory nerve defect (in the finger) may provide protective sensation even many years after the initial injury.[15]
- Proximal nerve lesions have a worse prognosis for full sensory and motor recovery than distal nerve lesions. There is a longer latency period between injury and potential reconnection to the motor end plate or sensory end organ. There is also more opportunity for a regenerating nerve fiber to enter the wrong neural tube and end up at the wrong end organ.
- The presence of scar tissue in and around the healing peripheral nerve can significantly impair the surgical and therapeutic goal of accurate and pain-free nerve regeneration.
- Nerve regeneration and functional outcomes are age related. Better functional outcomes in the young may be due to greater cortical plasticity.[17]
- Still, cells that fire together will wire together. Practice strengthens and expands the somatosensory cortical representation of the area that is used.[1,8] Sensory reeducation and cortical retraining may be helpful, even in cases in which the outcome of surgical intervention is poor.

Evaluation Tips

Distinguishing Among Central Nervous System, Spinal Segment, and Peripheral Nerve Lesions

- CNS lesions show motor spasticity/flaccidity and whole limb sensory changes, which are typically on the side of the body contralateral to the injury site.
- Spinal segment lesions show myotomal and dermatomal changes in the corresponding area. Usually, several adjacent spinal levels must be affected before a dermatomal and myotomal pattern can be appreciated.
- Peripheral nerve lesions show sensory or motor loss specific to the involved nerve with symptoms and signs at and distal to the site of injury

Evaluation Tips

General Considerations

Begin by introducing yourself and the purpose of this initial session. Emphasize that your role is to collaborate with your client to facilitate optimal functional recovery and return of independence. Education about nerves, about the specific injury, about the rehabilitation process, and the prognosis for functional recovery should begin at this session.

You will need to gather information about your client's unique social and medical history, as well as the mechanism of their injury. You will also need to ascertain their understanding of the activity limitations imposed by tissue healing timelines and identify the strategies they are using that allow them to function. I make a point of recording the challenges that each of my clients faces. I try to identify the availability of support systems and the strategies that my client is using when faced with challenges (for example, performing toileting tasks).

It is helpful to use an assessment tool that is client centered and looks at the big picture. The Canadian Occupational Performance Measure (COPM)[21] is an assessment tool used to identify our client's roles, environment, and activity performance. Problem areas are identified by the client and then rated in terms of importance. The five most important problems are then the focus of intervention. Intervention may entail the use of adaptive equipment and/or compensatory strategies.)

Observation and Palpation

Observe the posture of the involved extremity. Observe how the client uses (or avoids use of) their extremity in the clinic. Observe for obvious muscle atrophy, skin lesions, edema, color changes (for example, areas of erythema, mottled skin, or skin that has a blanched appearance) and trophic changes.

Precaution. *Make note of and caution the client about vulnerability to blisters and other signs of hand injury that may occur with use of a vulnerable insensate hand. Document areas of edema, **hypersensitivity**, adhesions, and atrophy. Use of a pictorial format in addition to written format may be helpful.*

Precaution. *Always use standard precautions for infection control around any lesions and rashes.*

Assessment of Sensory Function

- Semmes-Weinstein monofilament testing: This is a graded light-touch testing instrument consisting of a kit of 20 nylon monofilament probes. The monofilaments are used by the therapist to map light-touch sensibility in the hand. An abbreviated kit is also available.
- Two-point discrimination testing: According to Moberg, a good indicator of eventual fine motor function following a peripheral nerve injury is the return of two-point discrimination.[22] He asserts that 6mm of two-point discrimination is needed to wind a watch, 6 to 8 mm for sewing, and 12 mm for handling precision tools. Static two-point discrimination and moving two-point discrimination tests assess the client's ability to discriminate between one point and two points of pressure applied randomly to the fingertip. Moving two-point discrimination returns before static two-point discrimination.
- Localization of touch: Neither of the aforementioned tests requires the client to identify the location of the stimulus. Localization requires a more integrated level of perception than simple recognition of a stimulus. Localization is appropriate for testing after a nerve repair because difficulty with localization of a stimulus is a common phenomenon following nerve injury. You can record the client's accuracy in localizing light-touch stimuli by using the lowest Semmes-Weinstein monofilament that can be perceived in the area of dysfunction. Ask your client to close their eyes and indicate verbally if they feels the stimulus. Each time the client answers in the affirmative, ask the client to open their eyes and to point to the exact spot touched. You should record your client's results on a grid-like map of the hand, indicating the actual location of stimulation and the sites of referred touch perception. Draw arrows on the grid to indicate referred perception sites. This test has no formal interpretation or scoring; rather, evidence of poor localization is useful when determining the need for and when planning a sensory reeducation program.
- Moberg pickup test: This is a useful test for assessing median nerve function. The test may be helpful for testing children or adults who have cognitive involvement or who may have secondary agendas that prevent them from full participation in other sensory tests.
- Hoffmann-Tinel's sign: Following trauma, gentle percussion along the course of the injured, regenerating nerve produces a temporary tingling sensation in the distribution of the injured nerve up to the site of regeneration. The tingling persists several seconds. Test from distal to proximal for best accuracy. If this sign is absent or is not progressing distally as is expected with a healing nerve, there is a poor prognosis for continued nerve recovery. Likewise, a progressing Tinel's sign is encouraging but does not necessarily predict complete recovery. Table 20.2 gives a summary of light-touch sensibility testing, standardized tests, and techniques for administration, scoring, and interpretation of scores.

Assessment of Joint Motion and Muscle Function

- Goniometric assessment: Evaluation of articular motion and musculotendinous function is performed with a goniometer. Passive range of motion (PROM) is defined as a measurement of the ability of the joint to be moved by an external source through its normal arc of motion. Limitations indicate problems within the joint or capsular structures surrounding the joint. AROM is defined as a measurement of the individual's own capability for moving a joint through its normal arc of motion. A limitation in AROM when PROM is full may indicate diminished or lost muscle power resulting from a nerve lesion. Therefore assess AROM first, and if limitations exist, then assess PROM.
- Manual muscle testing: Muscle paresis or paralysis can result from a peripheral nerve lesion. Careful documentation of muscle strength, using a manual muscle test (MMT), is an important component of the evaluation following a nerve injury. If possible, compare strength with the uninvolved side to determine what the normal strength is for that client.
- Precaution: Do NOT perform a MMT unless the referring physician has cleared your client for strengthening of that body part.
- When performing a MMT to determine good (4/5) verses normal (5/5) muscle strength, resistance should be applied to the muscle or muscle group in the mid-range of the available ROM arc for that movement. If the client is limited both actively and passively to 50 degrees of shoulder abduction, for example, perform the MMT at 25 degrees of abduction. Tell the client to "hold this position," and say, "Don't let me move you," while exerting a counter-directional force, attempting to move the client's body part out of the test position. Use a grading system that minimizes the number of pluses and minuses because that makes it easier for other health professionals to review the documentation and appreciate what was observed.
- Strength testing—grip and pinch: Once cleared by the referring physician, gross grip and pinch strength can be assessed using standardized tools, the Jamar dynamometer, and the pinch gauge.

Assessment of Autonomic Function

- Sympathetic function: If sweating (sudomotor function) is still present following a nerve lesion, this suggests that the nerve damage is incomplete because peripheral autonomic nerve fibers within the nerve are responsible for sweating. Vasomotor homeostasis is likewise a function of the sympathetic nervous system; therefore abnormal changes in skin temperature and skin color may indicate involvement of these peripheral nerve fibers.
- Trophic changes: The combination of sympathetic and sensory dysfunction results in characteristic trophic changes in all tissues of the involved area. Specifically, one would expect to see nail changes (blemishes, talon-like appearance), abnormal hair growth (may fall out or become longer and finer), cold intolerance, soft-tissue atrophy (most notably in the fingertip pulps), and a slowed rate of tissue healing.
- The O'Riain wrinkle test (1973): This is an objective test that identifies areas of denervation; denervated skin does not wrinkle when soaked in warm water. The denervated hand is placed in warm water (40°C [104°F]) for 30 minutes, and the presence or absence of finger wrinkling is documented. This test is most useful for children or others who may be unable or unwilling to cooperate with sensibility testing.

Assessment of Pain

Pain is usually a consequence of a nerve injury; therefore acknowledging this fact and aiming to quantify and qualify this multidimensional experience is important to the therapist and the client.

TABLE 20.2 Light-Touch Sensibility Testing—Standardized Tests and Techniques

Test/Purpose	Equipment/Instructions to Client	Testing Procedure	Scoring	Interpretation of Scores*
Semmes-Weinstein monofilament: Threshold test for light touch sensibility	Equipment: Quiet test area, colored pencils and map or grid of the hand for recording results, kit of 20 nylon monofilament probes ranging from 1.65 to 6.65. Alternatively: The minikit containing probes: 2.83, 3.61, 4.31, 4.56, and 6.65. Instructions: Introduce test and familiarize client with test expectations by demonstrating in proximal area believed to have normal sensibility. Ask subject to say "yes" if the stimulus is felt. Ask subject to close their eyes during testing. Alternatively, obscure subject's vision with blindfold. The test hand should be securely stabilized on the table.	Begin distally, and progress proximally along the peripheral nerve's receptive field. Start with the probe marked 2.83, apply to skin with enough pressure to bow the filament. Apply in 1.5 seconds, hold 1.5 seconds, and remove in 1.5 seconds. Repeat three times at each site; progress to next thicker filament if prior one is not perceived. Filaments marked ≥4.31 should be applied only once at each site.	One response out of three is considered affirmative. 2.83 = Normal light touch 3.22 to 3.61 = Normal light touch 3.84 to 4.31 = Diminished light touch 4.56 to 6.65 = Loss of protective sensation >6.65 = Absence of all sensation	2.83 = Normal light touch 3.22 to 3.61 = Stereognosis and pain perception intact, close to normal use of hand 3.84 to 4.31 = Mild to moderate impaired stereognosis and pain perception, difficulty manipulating objects 4.56 to 6.65 = Moderate to significant impaired pain and temperature perception, unable to manipulate objects with vision occluded, marked decrease in spontaneous hand use; will need instructions regarding protective care of impaired area >6.65= Unable to identify objects or temperature: with visual guidance, capable of gross coordination only
Static two-point discrimination/functional test: For determining two-point discrimination and ability to use hand for fine motor tasks	Equipment: Hand-held disk-criminator or Boley gauge Instructions: Introduce test and familiarize client with test expectations by demonstrating in the proximal area believed to have normal sensibility. Ask subject to say "one" or "two" in response to perception of one point of pressure or two points of pressure. Ask the subject to close their eyes during testing. Alternatively, obscure the client's vision with a blindfold. The test hand should be securely stabilized on the table.	Typically, only volar fingertips are tested. Begin testing at 5 mm of distance between two points. Apply one or two points randomly with the probes held in a longitudinal orientation to avoid crossover from overlapping digital nerves. Force is applied lightly, just until the skin blanches. If responses are inaccurate, the distance between the ends is increased by increments of 1 to 5 mm. Testing is stopped at 15 mm or sooner if digit length is not adequate.	Score is the smallest distance at which client is able to accurately discriminate between two points of pressure and one point of pressure. Seven out of 10 correct responses are required. Normal ranges: 3 to 5 mm = Normal, ages 18–70 6 to 10 mm = Fair 11 to 15 mm = Poor One point only perceived = Protective sensation only No points perceived = Anesthetic	6 mm = Normal, needed for winding a watch 6 to 8 mm = Fair, needed for sewing 12 mm = Poor, needed for handling precision tools >15 mm = Loss of protective sensation to anesthetic; above this gross tool handling may be possible but only with decreased speed and skill

*Interpretation of scores is based on information in Bell-Krotoski J. Correlating sensory morphology and tests of sensibility with function. In: Hunter JM, Mackin EJ. eds. *Tendon and Nerve Surgery in the Hand: A Third Decade*. St Louis, MO: Mosby; 1997; and in Callahan A. Sensibility assessment for nerve lesions in continuity and nerve lacerations. In: Mackin EJ, Callahan AD, Skirven TM. eds. *Rehabilitation of the Hand and Upper Extremity*. 5th ed. St Louis, MO: Mosby; 2002.

TABLE 20.3   Typical Pain Assessment Tools

Name	Description/Administration	Scoring/Interpretation*
Numeric pain scale	Description: Subjective rating of pain intensity using a 10-point numeric scale Administration: Client is asked to rate his or her current pain on a 0 to 10+ scale, with 0 = no pain and 10 = worst possible pain imaginable. Client may be asked to rate his or her best and worst pain experienced over the past 30 days or since the onset of pain.	Scoring: Record the number identified by the client. Interpretation: 0 to 2 = Low level of pain 3 to 5 = Moderate level of pain 6 to 10+ = High level of pain
Visual analogue scale	Description: Subjective quantitative measure of pain intensity using a 10-cm line with descriptors (no pain at all; pain as bad as it could be) at each end Administration: Clients are asked to make a mark through the line to indicate the pain they are presently experiencing.	Scoring: The distance is measured on the line from the bottom anchor to the client's mark and recorded in centimeters as the client's pain score. Interpretation: 0 to 2.9 cm = Low level of pain 3 to 5.9 cm = Moderate pain level 6 to 10.5 = High pain level
Pain drawing	Description: Subjective drawing of pain diffusion and localization Administration: Clients are given an outline of the body or body part and asked to use symbols (that denote different qualities of pain) to reflect his current distribution of symptoms.	Scoring: No standardized or widely accepted method for scoring exists. Interpretation: Look for patterns of pain diffusion that may indicate radicular symptoms occurring along a specific dermatome. Widespread or nonanatomical pain drawings may indicate chronic pain or poor psychodynamics.

*Interpretations of these scales are based on information in Galper J, Verno V. Pain. In: Palmer ML, Epler ME. *Fundamentals of Musculoskeletal Assessment Techniques.* 2nd ed. Philadelphia, PA: Lippincott-Raven Publishers; 1996.

Many pain assessment tools are one dimensional, attempting to quantify the pain experience numerically. The benefit of such tools is that they are easy and quick to administer and to score, and they produce repeatable results that can be used to assess immediate outcomes following a specific intervention. However, it is challenging to establish an objective long-term goal using these scales, since the multidimensional experience of pain makes it difficult to conclude that pain is a stable state, rather than one that is dynamically influenced by other factors, including social, cultural, cognitive and emotional issues.

Several recent studies have looked at how pain experienced after a PNI can lead to lasting negative consequences including decreased quality of life (QOL), depression, as well as substantial long-term disability with work, education, self-care and avocational tasks.[23-25] It is important that we identify the impact of pain on our clients before we can develop individualized effective coping strategies.

Table 20.3 summarizes typical pain assessment tools with a brief synopsis of administration and scoring instructions. This is not an exhaustive list of pain assessments but rather a list of those that can be used efficiently during an initial evaluation of a client with a peripheral nerve injury.

Other Assessments to Consider

- Reflexes: Complete severance of the efferent or afferent nerve in a reflex arc abolishes that reflex. However, a reflex can be lost even in partial nerve injuries, and so hyporeflexia is not a good guide of injury severity.
- Cold sensitivity: Cold sensitivity or intolerance is a common consequence of peripheral nerve injuries. Cold intolerance is related to functional impairment, and it may adversely affect returning to work and leisure activities in locations where the injured extremity may be exposed to cold. Consider using self-report to document cold intolerance because many of the available test protocols for assessing temperature tolerance lack standardization.
- Edema measurements: The presence of edema compromises the available space for the nerve as it traverses through fibro-osseous tunnels and other tightly confined areas, such as the carpal tunnel. Take edema measurements initially, or once sutures are removed, using a volumeter if there are no wound issues or a tape measure to assess circumference. Establish a baseline before starting therapy. **Precaution.** *A significant increase in edema following treatment along with degradation in sensory status indicates that your treatment program was too aggressive for the healing tissue to tolerate. Adjust your intervention program accordingly.*
- Provocative testing: Testing to provoke symptoms is used to clarify the site of injury and to exclude the possibility that other nonneural tissues may be sources of pain. Provocative nerve testing is predicated on the fact that irritated nerve tissue is sensitized or hyper-responsive to any manual stimulus applied along its length. A manual stimulus is defined as mechanical stimuli acting as percussion along a nerve, or a compressive force to a nerve trunk or a graded force that causes longitudinally directed nerve gliding. In the normal nerve, these forces would not result in an irritated neural response. For example, tapping over a nerve would not normally cause a Tinel's sign unless the nerve was injured. Therefore Tinel testing, or percussion along a nerve that results in an irritated tingling sensation, is considered a positive provocative stress test. Likewise, upper limb tension testing is considered a provocative stress test because the nerves of the brachial plexus are moved passively and longitudinally. A positive upper limb tension test (of symptomatic pain reproduction and limited joint motion when the extremity is placed on full passive stretch) would indicate a pathological response.

TABLE 20.4 Recommendations for Therapist's Evaluation Battery	
Nerve Lesions in Continuity—Nonoperative	**Nerve Lacerations—Postoperative**
• Client history • Observation/palpation of involved tissues • Tinel test at suspected compression site • Semmes-Weinstein monofilament test • Pain assessments (including pain interview) • Provocative stress testing if client reports intermittent symptoms aggravated by certain positions/activities • Moberg pick-up test (for functional assessment with a median nerve injury) • AROM followed by PROM if limitations present with active movement • Strength test: MMT to isolate muscle involvement, grip and pinch testing to assess functional grasp and pinch strength • Modified COPM for goal setting	• Client history • Observation/palpation of involved tissues with special attention to trophic, sudomotor, and vasomotor changes (possible sympathetic dysfunction) • Tinel test to determine distal progression of regenerating axons • Semmes-Weinstein monofilament testing followed by localization (determine light touch sensibility, need for sensory protection techniques and/or sensory reeducation) • Two-point discrimination testing if client is able to perceive ≤4.31 monofilament (predicts functional status, need for sensory reeducation) • Pain assessments (Is there a need for desensitization program?) • AROM followed by PROM (if needed) of involved extremity as permitted by postoperative protocol • Modified COPM for goal setting

AROM, Active range of motion; *COPM,* Canadian Occupational Performance Measure; *MMT,* manual muscle test; *PROM,* passive range of motion.

▷ Precautions and Concerns

About Provocative Testing

- *Neural provocative testing, especially upper limb tension testing, must be done carefully and by a skilled therapist who understands the testing technique and the interpretations and who can manage symptoms once provoked. UE provocative tests are not standardized in terms of precise positioning, how long each position is held, or how much force is applied.*
- *Whenever possible, compare the involved to the uninvolved side to appreciate the client's individual normal response.*

Clinical Reasoning: Determining Which Tests to Use

Table 20.4 contains a list of recommendations for determining which assessment tools to use when evaluating a nerve injury in continuity versus a nerve injury not in continuity.

Radial Nerve

Anatomy and Common Sites of Compression

Table 20.5 provides a summary of radial nerve anatomy, common lesion sites, and typical deficits/deformities associated with radial nerve lesions.

The radial nerve is the most commonly injured of the upper extremity peripheral nerves following humeral fractures.[26] This nerve is particularly vulnerable about mid-humeral level following traumatic mid-shaft fracture as it travels around the spiral groove of the humerus moving medially to laterally (Fig. 20.4). Injury at this level is called a **high radial nerve palsy.** The triceps muscle is spared because nerve fibers innervating this three-headed muscle branch off the main trunk at the level of the axilla (or just distal to this). Thus elbow extension is intact. The supinator and brachioradialis (BR) muscles are paralyzed; however, elbow flexion and forearm supination remain because the musculocutaneous-innervated biceps brachii muscle is a primary elbow flexor and forearm supinator. There is paralysis of all wrist extensors, loss of finger extension at the metacarpophalangeal (MP) joints, and an inability to extend and radially abduct the thumb. This injury is called **wrist drop deformity** (Fig. 20.5), named for its classic dropped or flexed wrist posture.

While the most common cause of a high radial nerve is direct trauma to the nerve, an external compressive force, such as from a crutch in the axilla or along the mid-humeral level where the nerve runs somewhat superficially between the triceps muscle and the humeral shaft, can also result in neuropathy. The latter case is frequently referred to as *Saturday night palsy* or *drunkard's palsy.*[27] Depending on the level of injury, triceps paresis may exist, as well as some posterior arm sensory loss. A therapist will see paralysis of all the wrist and finger extensors and sensory loss along the dorsal lateral aspect of the forearm and hand.

Conservative Management of High Radial Nerve Injuries

Presentations

- Crutch palsy (axilla level, motor and sensory involvement) presents with paresis of triceps function at the elbow (that is, loss of or severe weakness of elbow extension), weakness with supination, loss of digit MP extension, thumb extension, and thumb radial abduction. Gravity can assist with elbow extension for functional tasks, but the therapist should monitor for the development of elbow flexion contractures secondary to the unopposed elbow flexors contracting and adaptively shortening.
- In Saturday night palsy/high radial nerve palsy (mid-humeral compression or shaft fractures) triceps function is typically spared, otherwise motor and sensory involvement is as previously described.

Timelines and Healing

Typically a radial nerve palsy that results from closed injuries represents a neuropraxia, which resolves spontaneously over a period of a few days to 4 to 6 months.[28] Clients who fail to show clinical improvement after 2 to 3 months of conservative management should be considered for electrodiagnostic and ultrasound testing to ascertain the zone of and type of injury.

♡ Tips From the Field

Orthotic Options for High Radial Nerve Palsy

- A wrist immobilization orthosis with the wrist in a functional position of 30-degree extension is an option. An advantage of

TABLE 20.5	Summary of Radial Nerve
Sensation	*Brachial cutaneous branches* supply the posterior region of the arm and lower lateral arm. An *antebrachial branch* supplies the posterior skin of the forearm. The *superficial sensory branch* of the forearm supplies the lateral two-thirds of the dorsum of the hand, the dorsal thumb and the proximal portion of the dorsal index, and long digits and radial half of the proximal ring
Motor	*Innervations, proximal to distal:* Triceps (lateral head), triceps (long head), triceps (medial head), anconeus, BR, ECRL, ECRB, supinator, EDC, extensor digiti minimi, ECU, abductor pollicis longus, extensor pollicis longus, extensor pollicis brevis, and extensor indicis proprius
Function	An intact radial nerve allows for elbow extension and is *essential to the tenodesis action that is fundamental to the grasp-release pattern of normal hand function.* The radial nerve powers all wrist extension, all MP joint extension, and thumb extension and radial abduction
Common sites of entrapment/injury	*Crutch palsy* (axilla level, motor and sensory involvement) *Saturday night palsy/high radial nerve palsy* (mid-humeral compression or shaft fractures—triceps spared, motor and sensory involvement) *PIN palsy* (fracture/dislocations of elbow joint, tendinous edge of ECRB, between two heads of supinator—radial wrist extensors spared, primarily motor involvement) *RTS* (compression between radial head and supinator muscle; primarily a pain syndrome) *Superficial radial sensory nerve palsy* (compression between ECRL and BR tendons or at wrist from tight cast/splint—sensory involvement only)
Results of lesion	*Motor palsy* has significant functional consequences. A lesion to this nerve as it passes medially to laterally across the posterior shaft of the humerus will result in "wrist drop" with a loss of all active wrist, digit, and thumb extension. Supination of the forearm will remain functional because the intact biceps brachii is a powerful supinator of the forearm. Likewise, the triceps is spared because it receives its innervation more proximally. Only high lesions to the radial nerve (as in the axilla) result in loss of all active elbow extension as well as the aforementioned problems. Lesions to the *PIN branch* in the forearm spares the BR and radial wrist extensors, but thumb, digit, and ulnar wrist extension are lost. A *lesion to the superficial radial sensory nerve* results in some loss of sensation on the dorsal lateral hand. This is not typically a debilitating problem for clients. Following radial nerve palsy, clients report an inability to use the hand for grasp or release. The loss of stability at the wrist results in an inability to use the long flexors to make a fist. Clients cannot move their thumb away from their hand to grab hold of a cup or utensil, for example, or skillfully to let go of an object once placed in their hand.

BR, Brachioradialis; *ECRB,* extensor carpi radialis brevis; *ECRL,* extensor carpi radialis longus; *ECU,* extensor carpi ulnaris; *EDC,* extensor digitorum communis; *MP,* metacarpophalangeal; *PIN,* posterior interosseous nerve; *RTS,* radial tunnel syndrome.

using this type of orthotic is cosmesis. A wrist cock-up orthosis is less conspicuous than a dynamic orthosis. It is also more comfortable, without the problems that a bulky outrigger presents, especially when sleeping. Furthermore, this orthosis is less costly and easy to take on and off. This is a reasonable daytime choice when the nerve injury is on the nondominant side, and/or when cosmesis is of greater importance than function for clients.

- A dorsal mobilization orthosis that dynamically holds the MP joints in extension but allows for full digit flexion can be used to substitute for absent muscle power and promote functional use of the injured hand, leaving the palmar surface of the injured hand free for sensory input. There are prefabricated options or you can design a custom-made version. The construction of such a custom orthosis can be tricky, costly and time consuming. It may also be difficult for your client to independently don/doff this orthosis. McKee and Nguyen described a low-profile customized orthosis that provides extension assistance for the wrist, fingers and thumb (Fig. 20.6).[29]

> **Precautions and Concerns**

When fabricating a dynamic radial nerve palsy orthosis, care should be taken to gauge the appropriate force needed to provide adequate digit extension while allowing full flexion. You will need less dynamic extension force for digits four and five. Too much force

can pull the MP joints of these digits into hyperextension, and may impede the normal arch or resting posture of the ulnar aspect of the hand. (Think about how your fingers grab a hammer or golf club. You need digits four and five to allow full flexion at the MP joints, augmented by some flexion at the carpometacarpal (CMC) joints of digits four and five.)

> **Precautions and Concerns**

If using a wrist cock-up orthosis to improve function and stabilize the wrist following a high radial nerve injury, you will need to monitor for decreased full and simultaneous passive extension of the wrist, fingers and thumb. The extensor muscles of the MP joints, as well as the extensors and radial abductor muscle of the thumb, may become overstretched by unopposed flexors. This can result in latent biomechanical issues, such as joint flexion contractures and adaptive shortening of the extrinsic flexor muscles. An alternative is to fabricate a forearm-based wrist orthosis with index through small finger MP joints supported in extension, and thumb in extension and radial abduction.

( ) What to Say to Clients

About Radial Nerve Palsy

"You have an injury to the nerve that powers those muscles that allow you to straighten your wrist and fingers at the same time.

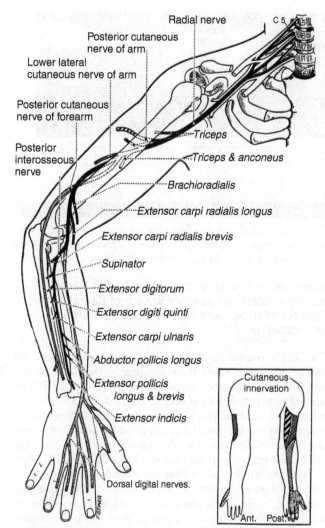

FIG. 20.4 Schematic of the radial nerve. *(From Stanly BG, Tribuzi SM. eds. Concepts in Hand Rehabilitation. Philadelphia, PA: FA Davis; 1992.)*

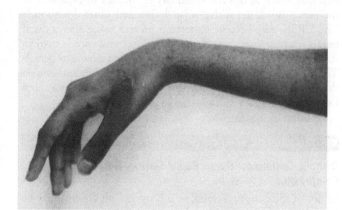

FIG. 20.5 Wrist drop deformity resulting from radial nerve palsy. *(From Stanly BG, Tribuzi SM. eds. Concepts in Hand Rehabilitation. Philadelphia, PA: FA Davis; 1992.)*

Your physician feels that you have an (excellent/good) prognosis for full recovery, but it will take time—perhaps as long as 3 to 4 months. During this time, we must protect your weak muscles from being overpowered or overstretched by those muscles that are working normally. You will need to use a brace to support your

wrist in a functional position, and perhaps to assist with finger and thumb motion. There are a few options available."

Orthoses options should be reviewed with the client using pictures or prototypes. You will need to help guide your client in choosing the best option given their lifestyle, hand dominance and side of injury, financial situation, and ability to return to therapy for occasional orthotic adjustments.

Low Radial Nerve Injuries (Posterior Interosseous Nerve Syndrome, Radial Tunnel Syndrome and Dorsal Radial Sensory Nerve Irritation)

In the proximal forearm, about the level of the radial head, the radial nerve divides into a superficial sensory branch (called the dorsal radial sensory nerve or DRSN) and a motor branch, (called the posterior interosseous nerve or PIN). The motor nerve branch of the radial nerve courses deep beneath the supinator muscle, traveling through the radial tunnel of the forearm. This tunnel is about three to four fingers breadth in length, lying along the anterior aspect of the proximal radius. Injuries to the nerve at this level can occur from compression of the nerve between the humeral and ulnar heads of the supinator muscle (called the *Arcade of Frohse*), from radial head fracture-dislocations, tumors, or from a history of repetitive and strenuous pronation and supination. Entrapment of this deep motor branch can result in two distinct conditions. **Posterior interosseous nerve syndrome** (**PINS**) is a rare nerve palsy involving some of the wrist extensors and all of the finger extensors.[30] The radial wrist extensors, which receive their innervation above the level of the elbow joint, will be spared with this condition. The second syndrome is called **radial tunnel syndrome** (**RTS**), which presents with pain, but no clear palsy or motor loss.[30]

Conservative Management of Low Radial Nerve Injury – PINS

The clinical presentation of PINS is as follows: weakness or paralysis of ulnar wrist extension, digit extension, and extension and radial abduction of the thumb. Often there is pain, described as a "deep ache"[30] with palpation over the proximal lateral forearm. Clients may also complain of vague dorsal wrist pain. Clients with PINS typically present with a gradual onset of weakness or paralysis of the finger and thumb extensor muscles and of the ulnar wrist extensor (extensor carpi ulnaris).[30] PINS occurs more often in the dominant arm and is more symptomatic at night[30] and with activities that engage the extensor muscles of the wrist and fingers, as with typing on a computer. Activities that require forearm pronation with simultaneous engagement of the wrist extensors, such as pulling a suitcase with wheels down a corridor, will also exacerbate the pain.[30] An EMG is usually positive for nerve compression at the radial tunnel.

> ### ◎ Clinical Pearl
>
> Proximal radial nerve lesions can be differentiated from a low or distal motor radial nerve lesion (PIN) through careful manual muscle testing. With a PIN lesion, the triceps brachii and brachioradialis muscles will test with normal strength, and there will be sparing of the extensor carpi radialis longus, allowing for weak radial wrist extension.

> ### ♡ Tips From the Field

Orthotic Options for PINS, Low Radial Nerve Palsy

Combined positioning of elbow flexion, forearm supination, and wrist extension place the least stress and strain on the radial tunnel,

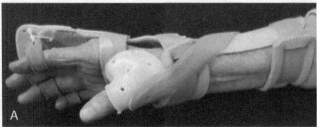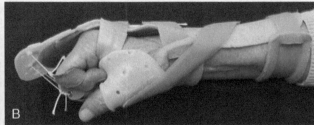

FIG. 20.6 One example of a radial nerve palsy orthosis. *(From McKee P, Nguyen C. Customized dynamic splinting: orthoses that promote optimal function and recovery after radial nerve injury: a case report. J Hand Ther. 2007;20[1]:80.)*

and hence this deep motor branch of the radial nerve.[30] However, maintaining this position is not well tolerated by clients because it seriously limits the tasks or activities that can be done with that arm. Clients may be more comfortable using a wrist brace that positions the wrist in extension (thus avoiding active engagement of those muscles) and avoiding prolonged positions of pronation with elbow extension during daily and work tasks.[30]

Conservative Management of Low Radial Nerve Injuries—Radial Tunnel Syndrome

RTS is a condition caused by compression of the radial nerve in the proximal forearm.[30] The clinical picture is one of dull aching or burning pain along the lateral forearm musculature rather than motor involvement. Etiology is most often compression of the nerve at the fibrous edge of the supinator muscle. This may occur from an external source such as positioning a counterforce brace (used to treat lateral epicondylosis) over the radial tunnel area of the forearm, or from positions that increase the pressure in the radial tunnel, as happens with sustained pronation or repetitive forceful supination.[30]

Symptoms may be confused with, but can coexist with, lateral epicondylosis.[30] With lateral epicondylosis, there is pain localized over, or just distal to, the lateral epicondyle. This pain is provoked by firm palpation over the lateral epicondyle area and/or by resisting wrist extension. With RTS, placing the elbow in extension, forearm in pronation and wrist in flexion along with resisting long finger extension will often provoke symptoms of dull pain or aching and burning in the lateral forearm. Pain associated with RTS is located 3 to 4 cm distal to the lateral epicondyle in the area of the extensor musculature of the forearm (also called the *mobile wad*). Compression and symptoms are aggravated by placing traction on the nerve—extending the elbow, pronating the forearm, and flexing the wrist. There is a negative EMG result with RTS.

♡ Tips From the Field

Orthotic Options for Radial Tunnel Syndrome

As with PIN syndrome, treatment involves rest, splinting, activity modification, gentle stretching of the involved muscles, nerve gliding, and antiinflammatory medications. If splinting the elbow and forearm/wrist, fabricate a long arm orthosis with the wrist in extension, elbow in flexion, and forearm in pronation to neutral rotation. This is the classic position recommended in the literature.[30] However, most people will not wear a long arm orthosis that limits elbow and forearm use during the day; therefore consider recommending a wrist immobilizing orthosis for waking hours, and educating your client about activity modification.

⯈ Precautions and Concerns

If client has RTS, do not use elbow clasp splints or straps, and be cautious with compression sleeves for the elbow. Elbow clasp splints can further compress the radial nerve at the radial tunnel.

Conservative Management of Low Radial Nerve Injuries (Superficial Sensory Branch of Radial Nerve [Dorsal Radial Sensory Nerve] or Wartenberg's Syndrome)

The DRSN courses distally into the forearm deep to the BR muscle. At approximately 9 cm proximal to the radial styloid, the DSRN becomes subcutaneous, traveling between the BR and extensor carpi radialis longus (ECRL) tendons. The DRSN compression can occur at two potential sites. The greatest risk for compression is at the posterior border of the BR because the nerve transitions from a deep to a subcutaneous structure. When the DRSN emerges between the tendons of the BR and ECRL, pronation of the forearm causes these two tendons to come together, thus compressing the nerve. Repetitive pronation-supination results in scissoring of the tendons over the DRSN. Hypertrophy or spasms of the brachioradialis muscle, as can occur with repetitive hammering or use of a computer mouse, can cause DRSN entrapment.[31] The other site of compression is where the DRSN runs in the subcutaneous tissue in the distal forearm. Compression may occur at this site secondary to the lack of excursion of the nerve during repetitive wrist flexion and ulnar deviation.[31] The DRSN may become tethered from scar tissue after a distal radius fracture (especially if an external fixator device is used to stabilize the fracture) or following deQuervain's release surgery.[31] This low radial nerve lesion presents with pain and dysesthesia on the dorsal radial hand emanating to the dorsal thumb, index and long fingers, though it can spread to the forearm.[31]

♡ Tips From the Field

Orthotic Options for Dorsal Radial Sensory Nerve Compression

Although spontaneous resolution is common, an orthosis may be helpful. A volar forearm-based thumb orthosis maintaining the wrist in extension and thumb in retroposition, may minimize tension on the DRSN.

◎ Clinical Pearl

When constructing a thumb spica orthosis to ameliorate DRSN symptoms, monitor the position of the distal forearm strap and consider cutting out the radial styloid area.

Postoperative Management Following Radial Nerve Laceration and Repair Above the Elbow, Below the Axilla

Consider the following guidelines:

- Fit your client with a static long arm elbow orthosis, positioning the forearm in neutral, wrist in extension, and MP joints in 10 to 20 degrees of flexion. (The collateral ligaments of the MP joints are slack when these joints are held in 0-degree extension; therefore it is necessary to place the joints in some degree of flexion to mitigate joint capsule tightness.)
- The initial position of the elbow should be in flexion. You will need to check with the surgeon about the amount of elbow flexion needed to keep the nerve repair tension free.[28] If you are unable to obtain this information in a timely manner, position the elbow in the same degrees of flexion as it was in the postoperative splint.
- The above described position should be maintained for 3 weeks after surgery. After that, the elbow may be extended 30 degrees per week, with the goal of full elbow extension by week six.[28]
- At 6 weeks, discontinue use of the orthosis altogether. Initiate AROM and PROM exercises to the elbow, forearm, wrist, and hand. At this time, you will need to fabricate a radial nerve palsy orthosis to facilitate functional grasp and release and to prevent adverse tissue changes, including wrist joint contractures and soft-tissue adaptive shortening.
- Have the client continue using the radial nerve palsy orthosis until adequate motor return occurs or tendon transfers are done.

Postoperative Management Following Radial Nerve Laceration and Repair at the Elbow or Proximal Forearm

Consider the following guidelines:

- Within the first or second postoperative week, you will need to fabricate an orthosis positioning the wrist in 30 degrees of extension to protect the nerve repair juncture. Inclusion of the elbow is dependent on the surgeon's instructions. Position the digit MP joints in about 10 degrees of flexion, and the thumb in radial abduction and extension. You may leave the interphalangeal (IP) joints of the digits free. Initiate digital IP AROM exercises. (Remember: IP joint extension occurs via the intrinsic interossei muscles, which are innervated by the ulnar nerve).
- At 3 weeks post repair, you may switch to a wrist cock-up splint or to a dynamic extension assist orthosis.[28] The orthosis/splint may be removed for A/AAROM exercises but should not be discontinued until functional active wrist extension has been regained.

Postoperative Management Following Decompression for Radial Nerve Injuries

Compression resulting in motor weakness that does not improve with several months of splinting, antiinflammatory medications, and activity modification is usually treated with surgical decompression. Results after radial nerve decompression are not as favorable as those following CTR or cubital tunnel release.[32]

The optimal duration and efficacy of conservative regimens versus surgical interventions has not been determined. The general consensus at this time is that if there is no improvement in motor function by approximately 3 months, spontaneous recovery is not likely and surgery is recommended.[30] Following decompression of the radial tunnel, the use of an orthosis to support the wrist varies among surgeons. Given the amount of dissection, an over-the-counter wrist cock up splint or a long arm orthosis may be helpful for pain management when used intermittently within the first 10 to 14 days postoperative. Dang and Rodner reviewed current relevant literature and reported that surgical decompression had good results in 86% of clients with a single diagnosis of RTS, but it was only 40% successful in clients with concomitant tennis elbow.[33] Full AROM is encouraged within the first postoperative week; however, in my experience, maximum recovery with pain relief may take 3 to 4 months or longer.

▶ Precautions and Concerns

During the postoperative recovery period, instruct your client to avoid full forearm pronation, elbow extension, and wrist flexion (as when pulling a heavy wheeled suitcase down a hall). This position places excessive tension on the recently decompressed radial nerve and its surrounding soft tissue.

Decompression of the DRSN is performed to free the nerve from any sites of compression or tethering if conservative management is not successful. If an orthosis is ordered, the wrist should be splinted in neutral and the thumb in radial abduction. Cut out the radial border at the distal wrist level to prevent irritation from the rigid material at the scar site. Use soft strap material at the distal wrist. Clients should be encouraged to begin AROM of the fingers, wrist, and elbow immediately after surgery. Desensitization may be necessary to address the typical hypersensitivity that frequently develops at the decompression site.

Median Nerve

Anatomy and Common Sites of Compression

Table 20.6 provides a summary of median nerve anatomy, common lesion sites, and typical deficits/deformities associated with median nerve lesions.

The median nerve arises from the lateral and medial cords of the brachial plexus (Fig. 20.7). It runs distally in the anteromedial compartment of the arm. In the cubital fossa of the anterior elbow and in the forearm, the median nerve lies medial to the brachial artery. Just distal to the elbow joint, the median nerve passes below the bicipital aponeurosis and between the two heads of the pronator teres. The median nerve gives off a purely motor branch, the anterior interosseous nerve (AIN), to the flexor pollicus longus (FPL), to the flexor digitorum profundus (FDP) tendon, to the index finger, and to the pronator quadratus.

The main trunk of the median nerve traverses under the fibrous origin of the flexor digitorum superficialis (FDS) and then emerges to become a more superficial structure in the distal forearm. Just proximal to the wrist, the palmar cutaneous (or sensory) branch arises and runs superficial to the flexor retinaculum to innervate the mid-palm. The terminal portion of this nerve, along with the nine extrinsic digit flexor tendons, runs under the

TABLE 20.6	Summary of Median Nerve
Sensation, includes the palmar cutaneous branch	Volar hand: Thumb, index, long, radial aspect of ring, volar radial palm, dorsal 20% to 35% of terminal dorsal thumb, index, long, and radial ring rays
Motor	*Innervations proximal to distal in this order:* Pronator teres, flexor carpi radialis, palmaris longus, FDS, radial two FDP, FPL, pronator quadratus, abductor pollicis brevis, FPB (superficial head), opponens pollicus, index lumbrical, and middle digit lumbrical
Function	The median nerve allows for forearm pronation; thumb, index, and long digit flexion; and thenar palmar abduction and opposition. These movements combine to position the hand for grasping (as a piece of candy off the table, for example) and allow for precision pinch. The sensory contribution of the median nerve is huge; without intact sensation along the radial volar aspect of the hand, fine motor coordination is not possible.
Common sites of entrapment/ injury	*Pronator syndrome:* Compression at ligament of Struthers, lacertus fibrosis, hypertrophy of pronator teres muscle or at arch of FDS; pain syndrome, sometimes sensory involvement *Anterior interosseous syndrome:* Compression of deep motor branch, paralysis of FPL and FDP to index, sensory symptoms absent, forearm pain present *CTS:* Compression at carpal tunnel resulting from provocative positioning, anatomic anomalies, metabolic conditions, trauma to wrist, space occupying lesions; nocturnal pain and dysesthesia and thenar weakness
Results of lesion	Loss of median nerve integrity at the elbow *(high-level lesion)* results in *ape hand deformity* with loss of precision pinch, loss of thenar opposition, paralysis of FDS and radial two FDP muscles. Forearm pronation is significantly compromised secondary to paralysis of both pronator muscles. Pronation can occur only by abduction of the shoulder and the assistance of gravity. A *lesion to the AIN* results in paralysis of the FPL and index and (sometimes) long digit FDP, making it difficult to make an "O" when attempting to pinch *(Ballentine's sign).* A more distal *(low-level) lesion* of the nerve, as at the *carpal tunnel,* results in loss of thenar opposition with frequently observable thenar muscle wasting. The thumb lies to the side of the radial palm, and a web space contracture may develop secondary to the unopposed pull of the thumb adductor. The *loss or diminution of sensation* in the tips of the thumb, index, and long digits results in significant functional deficits with regard to all fine motor tasks (such as, writing, winding a watch, tying a shoe, or picking up a small object) particularly if vision is occluded. Clients will complain about nocturnal dysesthesia, dropping objects, diminished fine motor coordination, and debilitating numbness.

AIN, Anterior interosseous nerve; *CTS,* carpal tunnel syndrome; *FDP,* flexor digitorum profundus; *FDS,* flexor digitorum superficialis; *FPB,* flexor pollicis brevis; *FPL,* flexor pollicis longus.

flexor retinaculum, and then through the osseous carpal tunnel and under its roof, the volar carpal ligament.

> **Precautions and Concerns**

In the shallow fibro-osseous carpal tunnel, the median nerve sits superficial to the extrinsic flexor tendons as it enters the hand. Here this nerve is particularly vulnerable to compression because it is sandwiched between these nine tendons and the volar carpal ligament.

The distal thenar motor branch of the median nerve innervates the thenar intrinsic muscles; the common digital branches innervate the first two lumbrical muscles to the index and long digits. The nerve continues through the palm as sensory branches that primarily provide sensation to the volar thumb, index, long, and medial half of the ring digits.

Conservative Management of High (Proximal) Median Nerve Palsy (Anterior Interosseous Nerve Palsy and Pronator Syndrome)

Compressive neuropathies of the median nerve in the proximal forearm are unusual lesions.[34] The two major compression neuropathies of the proximal median nerve occur with similar symptoms. Both syndromes involve entrapment of the nerve in the proximal forearm, and both are associated with pain in the proximal (volar) forearm that typically increases with activity.

The more proximal entrapment is called **pronator syndrome.** Compression of the median nerve occurs as it passes between the two heads of the pronator teres muscle or under the proximal edge of the FDS arch. Diffuse pain in the medial forearm or distal volar arm along with dysesthesia in the radial three and one-half digits of the hand (similar to sensory alterations commonly seen with CTS) are hallmarks of this syndrome. Symptoms may be provoked by resisted elbow flexion and are typically exacerbated with concurrent resisted forearm pronation. Hypertrophy of the pronator teres muscle can be a contributing factor. Provocation of symptoms with isolated resistance to the long finger FDS indicates pronator syndrome with the site of compression likely to be at the arch of the FDS.[34] Symptoms have an insidious onset and often are not diagnosed for months to years.[34]

Anterior interosseous syndrome is an entrapment neuropathy of the motor branch of the median nerve. This syndrome presents as nonspecific deep aching pain in the proximal forearm that increases with activity. Usually there are no sensory symptoms. Paralysis of the FPL to the thumb and the FDP to the index and long finger result in collapsed distal IP joints when attempting to pinch or make the "okay" sign. This clinical presentation is called **Ballentine's sign** (Fig. 20.8A). Although paresis of the pronator quadratus may be present, it is difficult to appreciate, given the overlapping action of the stronger pronator teres. Potential sources of compression are the same as with pronator syndrome and include localized forearm edema, and hypertrophy of the pronator teres muscle.

- Both of these syndromes present with a negative Tinel's sign at the carpal tunnel. Symptoms are not provoked with wrist flexion. Nocturnal symptoms, as seen with CTS, do not occur.

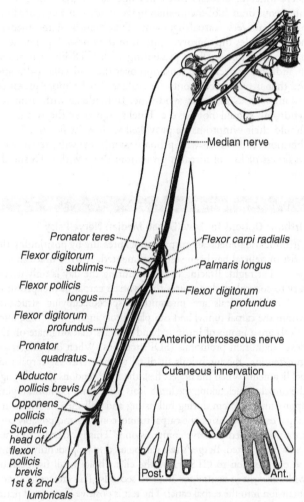

FIG. 20.7 Schematic of median nerve. *(From Stanly BG, Tribuzi SM. eds.* Concepts in Hand Rehabilitation. *Philadelphia, PA: FA Davis; 1992.)*

- Pronator syndrome typically occurs with diffuse forearm pain aggravated by resisted elbow flexion and forearm pronation and sensory changes along the volar radial three and one-half digits of the hand.
- Anterior interosseous syndrome (AIS) typically presents with diffuse forearm pain, a positive Ballentine's sign with loss of true tip pinch, and no sensory changes.

Timelines and Healing

Many clients have vague symptoms for months or years before a diagnosis is made. This is frustrating for the client and may require serial clinical examinations and repeat electrodiagnostic studies to confirm anterior interosseous syndrome or pronator syndrome. Furthermore, prolonged compression of the median nerve indicates a poor prognosis for full recovery, even following surgical decompression.[34,35]

Ideally, clients with a proximal median nerve entrapment neuropathy are evaluated and educated. Teach your client strategies to compensate for sensory and/or motor loss. Persons with AIS will have a difficult time activating an aerosol can, for example, given the loss of index distal interphalangeal (DIP) joint flexion. Consider introducing ergonomic strategies such using a split keyboard that minimizes the amount of forearm pronation needed for keyboarding. Provide a home exercise program that includes gentle stretching and nerve gliding. Caution your client to restrain from gym exercises that contribute to pronator teres hypertrophy. A short course of in-clinic pain management may be helpful, followed by interim therapy visits every 2 to 4 weeks to assess symptom abatement and to continue providing assistance in using strategies that enhance function until resolution of symptoms occurs.

Orthotic Options for High (Proximal) Median Nerve Injuries

Most clients with anterior interosseous syndrome or pronator syndrome improve with conservative management of client education, rest from provocative activities, splinting, and antiinflammatory medications.[34,35]

- Orthotics for anterior interosseous syndrome involve stabilizing the IP joint of the thumb, and often the index finger, in a position of flexion, using custom tip orthoses or commercially

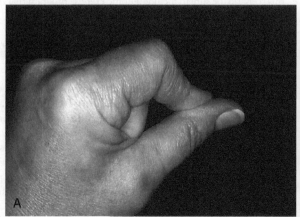
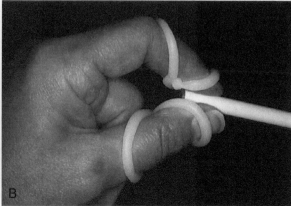

FIG. 20.8 (A) Positive Ballentine's sign indicating anterior interosseous nerve palsy. Note that the client is unable to oppose the index finger tip with the thumb tip. (B) Tip splinting for anterior interosseous palsy. *(From Mackin EJ, Callahan AD, Skirven TM. eds.* Rehabilitation of the Hand and Upper Extremity. *5th ed. St Louis, MO: Mosby; 2002.)*

available figure-eight splints to enhance function/tip pinch with activities, such as holding a pen for writing (Fig. 20.8B).

- Conservative management for pronator syndrome includes fabricating an orthosis to rest the irritated tissues with instructions to use the orthotic as much as possible over the initial 2 to 3 weeks, removing it for hygiene, and gentle AROM and nerve gliding only.
- If compression is at the fibrous arch of the heads of the FDS (resistance to FDS of the long finger aggravates symptoms), consider fabricating a forearm-based orthosis with the hand included.
- If compression is at the pronator teres, pain/paresthesia will be aggravated by resistance to forearm pronation and will be enhanced as the elbow is extended. In this case, fabricate a long arm orthosis with the forearm in neutral, the wrist in neutral, and the elbow in about 90 degrees of flexion.
- If symptoms are aggravated by resisted flexion of elbow with forearm in full supination, compression is likely at the lacertus fibrosus, and the orthosis should limit elbow flexion and forearm supination. Consider an anterior long arm orthosis with the forearm neutral rotation, using the lightest thermoplastic material option possible.

Conservative Management of Low (Distal) Median Nerve Palsy (Carpal Tunnel Syndrome)

CTS, or compression of the median nerve at the carpal tunnel space of the wrist, is the most common type of peripheral nerve entrapment syndrome.[20,36,37] Hallmark symptoms of CTS include paresis of the thenar muscles with consequent weakness or loss of thumb opposition, and sensory loss in the tips of the thumb, index, and long fingers. Clients with CTS complain of dropping things, and difficulty with fine motor coordination activities. Complaints of numbness or tingling and pain are typically worse at night. Nocturnal symptoms are associated with positions of the wrist that increase mechanical pressure on the nerve, such as bending the wrists.

Estimates concerning the prevalence of CTS range from 1% to 10% of the population.[20,36,37] CTS can develop in any individual; however, it presents more frequently in women over the age of 30.[36] Occupations such as meat packing or automobile parts assembly that require repetitive forceful wrist movements have been associated with increased incidence of CTS.[20,36] The prolonged positioning of the wrist in a flexed or hyperextended posture, as while on a computer keyboard, has also been associated with an increase in CTS occurrence.[37] Trauma, infection, and pregnancy can temporarily increase swelling at the carpal tunnel of the wrist, causing compression of the median nerve at the carpal canal.[36,37] Other factors that have been associated with the development of CTS include diabetes, hypothyroidism, gout, and rheumatoid arthritis.[20,37]

CTR surgery is the most common type of hand surgery in the United States.[38] CTR and endoscopic carpal tunnel release (E-CTR) are associated with few post-operative complications. However, surgical complications do occur, including injury to the median nerve, scar tenderness, and/or development of complex regional pain syndrome.[37,38] Research has compared the efficacy of surgical intervention verses nonsurgical management of CTS and found that CTR has a superior benefit over conservative management. However, conservative management provides sufficient relief in those with mild to moderate CTS such that a trial before surgery is warrented.[20]

Discriminating between CTS and pronator syndrome can be difficult because both syndromes present with pain in the volar wrist and forearm, and numbness or paresthesia in the median nerve-innervated radial three and one-half digits. The palmar cutaneous branch of the median nerve arises 4 to 5 cm proximal to the transverse carpal ligament. This branch of the median nerve provides the sensory input from the mid-volar and radial palm. Therefore a client presenting with CTS-like symptoms in addition to decreased sensation over the mid-volar palm and the thenar eminence should be evaluated for a more proximal lesion, such as pronator syndrome. Individuals with pronator syndrome should not have a Tinel's sign over the wrist, nor should their symptoms be provoked with wrist flexion.[34] Furthermore, individuals with pronator syndrome will present with weakness or loss of forearm pronation; those with CTS should not.

♡ Tips From the Field

Orthotic Options for Low (Distal) Median Nerve Palsy

Orthotic use to decrease carpal tunnel pressure by positioning the wrist in neutral has been well documented. A wrist brace should be used at night. Bracing the wrist during the day is only necessary to control work postures that worsen carpal tunnel pressure.

The lumbricals are intermittent space-occupying structures within the carpal tunnel and can play a role in CTS.[39,40] The lumbricals are a group of intrinsic hand muscles that originate on the flexor digitorum profundus (FDP) tendons. When our fingers are in extension, the lumbricals sit distal to the transverse carpal tunnel ligament. When the fingers flex, the FDP tendons glide through the carpal tunnel, taking the lumbricals with them. Lumbricals glide approximately 3 cm during full fisting and will then lie within the carpal canal, increasing the carpal tunnel contents and possibly contributing to median nerve compression.[39] This is exacerbated when the wrist is flexed. **Berger's test** can be used to help identify lumbrical contribution to CTS. Have the client hold a full fist position with the wrist in neutral for 30 to 40 seconds. This creates lumbrical incursion into the carpal canal. The test is positive if pain and paresthesia occur within 30 to 40 seconds. If Berger's test is positive, add an MP flexion block (MPs at 20 to 40 degree flexion) to the traditional wrist orthosis to prevent lumbrical migration during grasp. In this scenario, be sure to include a home exercise program that focuses on stretching the lumbrical muscles (Fig. 20.9).

⟨⟩ What to Say to Clients

About Carpal Tunnel Syndrome

"You have an injury to the median nerve. As this nerve travels down your arm and enters your hand, it travels through a tight space called the *carpal tunnel*. There are other structures that also run through this space. If the space becomes congested (as by swelling), or if the space becomes smaller (as from bony changes from arthritis), your nerve may get pinched. If you bend or straighten your wrist frequently, or if you position your wrist for a period of time in a stretched extended or bent posture, you may further irritate this nerve."

- Try to keep your wrist in a neutral position during daily activities.
- Avoid sustained pinch or gripping, particularly prolonged pinching when your wrist is in a flexed posture.

- Avoid repetitive overuse of the wrist.
- Avoid positioning your wrist in a flexed posture (the fetal position) when sleeping. Use your orthosis at night to keep your wrist from bending.
- Whenever possible, use tools (kitchen, workplace, garden) that have larger grips contoured to your hand. Your hand should easily close around the handle. The grip handle can be adjusted with dense foam to increase the diameter (if necessary) and to pad the surface so that it is easier on the structures, like your nerve, that lie underneath the skin of your hand.
- Look at a workstation design handout to figure out how to set up your office at home or work. This information is free on the Internet.

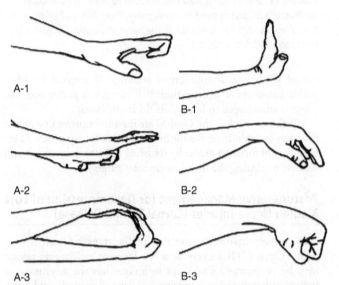

FIG. 20.9 Lumbrical stretches (A-1) Rest the hand, palm down on the thigh with the proximal interphalangeal (PIP) and distal interphalangeal (DIP) joints fully flexed. (A-2) The opposite hand then presses downward over the metacarpophalangeal (MCP) joints. (A-3) The wrist, MCP, PIP and DIP joints are then pulled into maximal extension with the opposite hand. (B-1) Hold a position of composite wrist and finger extension (B-2) followed by a 5-second rest period, (B-3) then place hand into composite wrist and digit flexion, followed by another 5-second rest period. *(From Baker NA, Moehling KK, Rubinstein EN, et al. The comparative effectiveness of combined lumbrical muscle splints and stretches on symptoms and function in carpal tunnel syndrome. Arch Phys Med Rehabil. 2012;93(1):1-10.* https://doi.org/10.1016/j.apmr .2011.08.013.*)*

Postoperative Management Following High (Proximal) Median Nerve Lacerations and Repairs—Elbow to Wrist Level

Severance of the median nerve in the forearm typically occurs from knife or glass lacerations. The clinical presentation is one of sensory and motor involvement with specific deficits depending on the site of injury. Loss of median nerve integrity at the elbow or proximal forearm (high-level lesion) results in an **ape hand deformity** with loss of precision pinch, loss of thenar opposition, and paralysis of the FDS and radial two FDP muscles and their corresponding two lumbrical muscles. The thenar eminence is atrophied with the thumb lying to the side of the palm. Loss of ability to oppose and palmarly abduct the thumb occurs. Index finger metacarpal (MP) and proximal interphalangeal (PIP) joint flexion is lost, as is thumb IP joint flexion. Forearm pronation is significantly compromised. Some forearm pronation can occur, however, with the assistance of gravity when the shoulder is abducted slightly. Sensory loss typically includes the radial three and one-half digits and the volar palm.

Timelines and Healing Following Surgical Repair

Consider the following guidelines:
- Apply a light compressive dressing for edema control.
- Fabricate a dorsal wrist blocking orthosis with the wrist in palmar flexion (no more than 45 degrees). The amount of wrist flexion is predicated on the amount of tension at the nerve repair site. Replicate the wrist position of the postoperative cast if the surgeon is not immediately available to give you guidelines.
- Include a dorsal block over the MP joints to limit median nerve excursion at the carpal tunnel.
- Have the client wear the orthosis continuously for 4 to 6 weeks (as dictated by the surgeon) except for protective skin care. Hygiene should occur with the orthosis on.
- Begin AROM and PROM of the digits and thumb; do 10 repetitions every waking hour within the brace. Instruct the client in active tendon glide exercises so that the extrinsic flexor tendons glide separately and do not become adherent at the area of surgical repair (Fig. 20.10).
- Begin gentle scar massage/mobilization techniques 24 to 48 hours after sutures are removed.
- At 4 weeks postoperatively, adjust the dorsal wrist blocking orthosis to 20 degrees of palmar flexion.
- At 5 weeks postoperatively, adjust the dorsal wrist blocking orthosis to 0 to 10 degrees of palmar flexion.

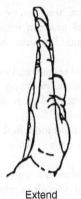
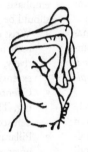
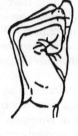

Extend   Hook   Straight   Fist

FIG. 20.10 Tendon glide exercises. *(From Mackin EJ, Callahan AD. eds. Hand Clinics: Frontiers in Hand Rehab. Philadelphia, PA: WB Saunders; 1991.)*

- By 6 weeks postoperatively, discontinue use of the dorsal wrist blocking orthosis and initiate progressive strengthening. Begin by having the client incorporate the postoperative hand into daily activity use. Strengthening can be as simple as setting a table, tying a shoe, or writing a grocery list.
- By 8 weeks postoperatively, the client can typically begin a rehabilitation program designed to address residual strength and coordination deficits that adversely affect return to work.

Postoperative Management Following Laceration of the Median Nerve at the Wrist

Typically, an isolated median nerve repair at the wrist will require a dorsal-block wrist splint for a period of 3 to 6 weeks. Isolated median nerve laceration is rare. More commonly, concurrent flexor tendon injuries occur. In this situation, you will need to address postoperative protocols for flexor tendon repairs as well as for the nerve repair.

An isolated laceration of the median nerve at the wrist presents with paralysis of the intrinsic thenar muscles that oppose and palmarly abduct the thumb. Wasting of the thenar eminence may develop, and the thumb will lie to the side of the palm because of the unopposed pull of the thenar adductor pollicus. Loss of sensation to the volar thumb, index, and long tips (and radial half of the ring finger) results in loss of fine motor coordination and an increased risk for soft tissue injuries in this area, such as burns or lacerations, especially during prehension tasks where vision is occluded.

Client education is critical regarding sensory impairment. Teach the client protective sensation techniques, including visually monitoring all activities performed with the insensate hand until there is adequate protective sensory return.

> ### Precautions and Concerns
>
> *With a high or low median nerve injury, thenar web space contractures are the most common and preventable deformity that should be addressed by proactive orthotic use.*

A rigid hand-based web spacer orthotic that positions the thumb in palmar abduction and opposition should be fabricated for night wear (Fig. 20.11). An orthosis made of neoprene or leather can be used to hold the thumb in a stable and opposed, if not fully abducted, position during the day if function is retarded with a rigid orthosis.

Postoperative Management for Decompression of High Median Nerve Injuries (Anterior Interosseous Nerve or Posterior Interosseous Nerve Syndrome)

Surgical decompression of the median nerve to address pronator syndrome is uncommon and occurs only after 2 to 3 months of conservative measures have failed to provide relief.[34] When surgery is necessary, the success rate in the treatment of pronator syndrome approaches 90%.[34] Early active motion is recommended after this surgery. **Precaution.** *If the pronator teres is released and reattached, avoid active pronation and end range supination for 4 to 6 weeks.*

Surgical decompression for AIN syndrome is also rarely performed. Spontaneous full recovery has been reported even as long as 12 to 18 months after onset of symptoms.[34] Etiology and pathophysiology for AIN palsy is not clearly understood. Compression is a theory based on analogy with carpal and cubital

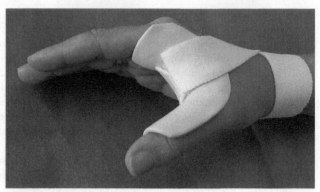

FIG. 20.11 Static thenar web spacer splint to prevent adduction contracture following median nerve palsy. *(From Mackin EJ, Callahan AD, Skirven TM. eds. Rehabilitation of the Hand and Upper Extremity. 5th ed. St Louis, MO: Mosby; 2002.)*

tunnel syndrome. Resolution of weakness is atypical for idiopathic compressive neuropathies.[34] If surgery is performed, the client is encouraged to begin AROM immediately.

Orthoses (such as the Oval-8) are used to improve fine motor function by stabilizing the thumb and index for tip pinch. Exercises should focus on gradually restoring full elbow extension and supination during the first 2 weeks after surgery.

Postoperative Management for Decompression of Low Median Nerve Injuries (Carpal Tunnel Release)

CTR surgery involves transection of the transverse carpal ligament. Open CTR surgery or a less invasive endoscopic release may be performed. The latter technique has the advantage of less postoperative pain, a quicker recovery of strength, and faster return-to-work time.[37] However, endoscopic release is associated with increased complications including incomplete release of the transverse carpal ligament with consequent reoccurrence of CTS.

Open CTR is always performed if the surgeon suspects that a flexor tenosynovectomy or a neurolysis may be needed. The goal of the tenosynovectomy is to remove the diseased synovial tissue so that there will be better gliding between the tendons and the nerve and to decompress the nerve further. A neurolysis is performed to resect constricting scar tissue that is affecting circulation within the nerve.

> ### Tips From the Field
>
> #### Postoperative Management of Carpal Tunnel Release
>
> After a simple CTR surgery, many clients do not need therapy. When therapy is needed, it is often a minimal program with emphasis on the home program. Skilled therapeutic intervention should be considered for the following:
> - Wrist control positioning to decrease incisional tension and to prevent overuse and inflammation for 2 to 3 weeks postoperatively. The wrist should be positioned in about 25 degrees of extension because this prevents wound site tension.[39]
> - Clients with diabetes may need wound care to promote healing. These clients are at a higher risk for infections or wound dehiscence.
> - Pillar pain (pain on either side of the CTR incision) is a normal postoperative occurrence. The pain can make it difficult to grip or perform palmar weight-bearing activities; and return to

TABLE 20.7 Summary of Ulnar Nerve	
Sensation: Dorsal cutaneous branch and superficial sensory branch	Ulnar/medial side of palm (both volar and dorsal); entire fifth digit and ulnar aspect of fourth digit (both volar and dorsal)
Motor	*Innervations, proximal to distal:* FCU, FDP to digits 4 and 5, abductor digiti minimi, opponens digiti minimi, FDM, fourth and third lumbrical muscles, three palmar interossei muscles and four dorsal interossei muscles, deep head of the FPB, and adductor pollicis
Function	The ulnar nerve allows for simultaneous strong wrist flexion and ulnar deviation, as well as power grip via full flexion of the ulnar two digits. This is necessary for tasks such as swinging a golf club or a hammer. Ulnar nerve integrity is necessary to allow for powerful tip and lateral or key pinch because the adductor pollicis and first dorsal interossei assist in stabilizing the thumb and index during pinching. The hypothenar muscles and the interossei muscles allow the hand to powerfully cup an object, such as a doorknob or a basketball.
Common sites of entrapment/injury	*Cubital tunnel syndrome:* Causes include direct compressive trauma, repetitive or sustained elbow flexion, cubitus valgus deformities, second-degree supracondylar fractures, disease processes; symptoms include pain, dysesthesia, and motor weakness *Guyon's canal compression:* Causes include pisiform or hook of hamate fractures, arthritis, thrombus, and mass/ganglion; symptoms include pain, intrinsic muscle weakness, and dysesthesia
Results of lesion	Motor ulnar palsy has significant functional consequences. The balance between extrinsic and intrinsic muscles is lost, secondary to paresis of most of the intrinsic muscles of the hand. This results in a flattening of the normal arches of the hand. Low-level lesions, as at the wrist, produce the *classic claw deformity* of the digits with hyperextension of the MP joints and flexion of the IP joints. (This posture is less noticeable in the index and long digits because the lateral two lumbrical muscles, which serve to flex the MP joints, remain innervated by the median nerve.) There is wasting of the interosseous muscles, of the thenar adductor, and of the hypothenar eminence. Paralysis of the thenar adductor causes *significant loss of pinch strength*. If the client attempts to pinch, the distal phalanx typically assumes a position of flexion *(Froment's sign)*, and the proximal phalanx may hyperextend *(Jeanne's sign)* as the unimpaired FPL and the extensor pollicis brevis attempt to stabilize the thumb. High-level lesions, for example lesions to the nerve proximal to the innervation of the FCU, result in all of the aforementioned deficits and loss of simultaneous wrist flexion and ulnar deviation. Typically a client complains about significant loss of grip strength (that is, for swinging a golf club or a hammer), difficulty with gross grasp (that is, unable to effectively grasp a doorknob), and loss of ability to perform such in-hand manipulation tasks as shaking dice or moving coins into position to place into a slot. The client may report difficulty with lateral pinch (that is, unable to turn a key in the ignition) and difficulty donning gloves and typing (resulting from paresis of the interossei). Sensory loss, although problematic, is not as severely disabling as with the median nerve. Clients tend to complain of difficulty gauging the force needed to hold an object (such as a glass).

FCU, Flexor carpi ulnaris; *FDM,* flexor digiti minimi; *FDP,* flexor digitorum profundus; *FPB,* flexor pollicis brevis; *FPL,* flexor pollicis longus; *IP,* interphalangeal, *MP,* metacarpophalangeal.

work is often delayed due to this.[39] The exact cause of pillar pain is unknown. The various theories suggest that it is ligamentous or muscular in origin or a result of an alteration of the carpal arch. Typically, this pain decreases in about a year. Intervention strategies include gel pads positioned across the irritated site, education about the etiology and prognosis for pain resolution, and manual therapy/scar massage.

Ulnar Nerve

Anatomy and Common Sites of Compression

Table 20.7 gives a summary of ulnar nerve anatomy, common lesion sites, and typical deficits/deformities associated with ulnar nerve lesions. The ulnar nerve (Fig. 20.12) arises from medial cord of the brachial plexus (C7 to T1 roots). The nerve runs down the humerus and passes superficially between the medial epicondyle and the olecranon. The ulnar nerve enters the forearm between the two heads of the flexor carpi ulnaris (FCU) and descends within the anteromedial forearm under the cover of the FCU. In the lower third of the forearm, the ulnar nerve gives off

a dorsal cutaneous branch, which supplies the skin of the ulnar half of the dorsum of the hand. At the wrist, the ulnar nerve runs with the ulnar artery through the **Guyon's canal.** This is a superficial passageway between the pisiform and hamate bones of the carpus. Just distal to the pisiform, the ulnar nerve divides into two terminal branches: the superficial (palmar) cutaneous branch and the deep motor branch. The motor branch winds around the hook of the hamate and innervates the three intrinsic hypothenar muscles (opponens digiti minimi, abductor digiti minimi and flexor digiti minimi), the ulnar two lumbrical muscles, and the interossei muscles (three palmar adductors and four dorsal abductors). The ulnar nerve terminates at the adductor pollicis and the deep head of the flexor pollicis brevis (FPB). The sensory branch supplies the skin of the ulnar half of the volar hand and the fifth digit and the medial half of the fourth digits.

Conservative Management of High (Proximal) Ulnar Nerve Compression (Cubital Tunnel Syndrome)

The cubital tunnel is bound by the medial epicondyle anteriorly, the ulnohumeral ligament laterally, and the two heads of the occur with elbow flexion greater than 100 to 110 degrees,[41] and increasing pressure and traction develops in the ulnar nerve with concomitant shoulder abduction.[42] The development of cubital tunnel syndrome will depend on the severity and duration of the compression.

Cubital tunnel syndrome may present with sensory symptoms and/or motor dysfunction. Pain can be sharp or aching. Pain may be located on the medial side of the proximal forearm, or it can be diffuse and radiate proximally and distally. Paresthesia presents as decreased sensation in the ulnar digits and often, a feeling of coldness. Motor weakness and wasting of the ulnar-innervated intrinsic muscles are present in more severe cases. This muscle paresis results in decreased power grip. In advanced cases, one sees clawing of the ring and small fingers as a result of paralysis of the ulnar-innervated interossei and lumbrical muscles. When the balance between extrinsic and intrinsic muscles is lost, you can expect to see a flattening of the normal arches of the hand. The ability to cup the hand around an object or to hold water in one's hand to wash one's face is lost. The unopposed extensor digitorum communis (EDC) pulls the MP joints into hyperextension, and the IP joints assume a position of flexion. This is called a **claw hand deformity** (Fig. 20.13A). (This posture is less noticeable in the index and long digits because the lateral two lumbrical muscles, which serve to flex the MP joints, remain innervated by the median nerve.) If the MP joints are passively held in flexion, the EDC force will be shunted distally, allowing IP joint extension (Fig. 20.13B).

Wasting of the interosseous muscles, thenar adductor, and hypothenar eminence occurs. The client will lose the ability to abduct and adduct the digits, which are needed for typing or playing the piano. Paralysis of the thenar adductor causes significant loss of lateral or key pinch strength. If the client attempts to perform this type of pinch, the thumb's distal phalanx typically flexes (**Froment's sign**) and the proximal phalanx may hyperextend (**Jeanne's sign**) as the unimpaired flexor pollicus longus (FPL) and the extensor pollicis brevis attempt to stabilize the thumb.

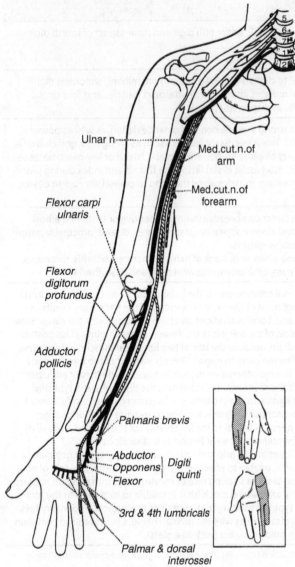

FIG. 20.12 Schematic of the ulnar nerve. *(From Stanly BG, Tribuzi SM. eds.* Concepts in Hand Rehabilitation. *Philadelphia, PA: FA Davis; 1992.)*

FCU posteromedially. A fibrous band extending from the olecranon to the medial epicondyle forms the roof of this tunnel. The ulnar nerve can be palpated easily here. Compression of the ulnar nerve within this tunnel is called **cubital tunnel syndrome.** It is the second most common peripheral compression neuropathy in the UE.[41]

There are a variety of causes for ulnar nerve compression at the elbow.[41] Systemic disease (such as, diabetes or chronic alcoholism) may predispose one to compression neuropathies. External sources of compression include tourniquets or pressure from a hard surface when leaning on the elbow. Work activities that require repetitive or sustained elbow flexion can induce compression. Fractures and dislocations of the elbow may lead to acute or chronic nerve compression. Congenital or posttraumatic deformities can result in ulnar nerve compression.

The cubital tunnel is at its roomiest when the elbow is in extension; this space becomes increasingly smaller as the elbow is flexed.[41] The most significant ulnar nerve pressure increases

Evaluation Tips

- Froment's sign: When the client attempts powerful lateral pinch the thumb's IP joint flexes as the FPL attempts to compensate for the paralyzed or weak adductor pollicis and flexor pollicus brevis.
- Wartenberg's sign: This sign is present if the fifth finger is postured in an abducted position from the fourth finger. This indicates interosseous muscle weakness (specifically paresis of the palmar adductor interossei).
- Elbow flexion test: This provocative maneuver is designed to reproduce the symptoms of ulnar nerve compression. The elbow is flexed fully, and the wrist is held in neutral for up to 5 minutes. A positive test is the reproduction of paresthesia and pain symptoms.

Clinical Pearl

The muscle strength of the ring and small finger flexor digitorum profundi can be an important diagnostic tool to help determine the level of compression along the ulnar nerve. Normal strength of these muscles indicates a distal or low-level entrapment, most likely at Guyon's canal.

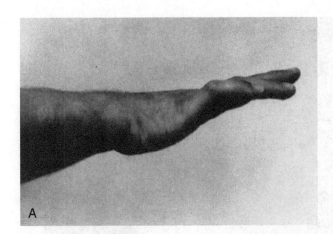

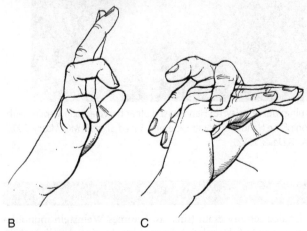

FIG. 20.13 (A) Claw hand deformity secondary to ulnar nerve palsy. (B) Drawing of the clawing posture of the fourth and fifth digits following ulnar nerve palsy, which results from paralysis of the lumbrical muscles and the unopposed pull of the antagonist muscle, the extensor digitorum communis (EDC). (C) If the metacarpophalangeal joints are passively blocked in flexion, the force of the EDC will translate distally, allowing interphalangeal joint extension. *(A From Stanly BG, Tribuzi SM. eds.* Concepts in Hand Rehabilitation. *Philadelphia, PA: FA Davis; 1992.)*

Orthotic Interventions for Cubital Tunnel Syndrome

- Nocturnal elbow splinting to restrict the elbow from flexion is a common intervention.[43] The literature recommends a long arm orthosis with the elbow positioned at 30- to 70-degree flexion, forearm and wrist in neutral, and digits free. However, clients have a difficult time tolerating this orthotic. If necessary, make a long arm orthosis with the lightest material possible, positioned on the anterior aspect of the arm/forearm. If the cubital tunnel is particularly sensitive to external compression, such as pressure from the mattress of the bed, consider fabricating this night orthosis over a padded elbow pad or Heelbo.
- There are commercially available prefabricated splints that clients can purchase to limit elbow flexion if a custom-made orthosis is not an option.
- One economic solution to prevent flexion of the elbow while sleeping is to use a large bath towel fastened circumferentially around the elbow and secured with duct tape. This towel splint

has been shown to decrease symptoms of cubital tunnel as effectively as some commercially available splints.[43]

- Using a padded elbow sleeve during the day helps prevent external compression at the cubital tunnel (as when one leans on the elbow at a table). If your clinic does not have elbow pads, small pillows lightly ace-wrapped to the elbow may substitute.
- Corrective orthotics for intrinsic weakness/claw deformity may be necessary. Also consider an orthotic to stabilize the thumb during lateral pinch tasks, especially if the compression is on the client's dominant side.

When making an anticlaw orthosis for a hand with ulnar nerve palsy, take care to fabricate the splint so that the MP joints do not buckle or pop out of the splint inadvertently when the client attempts digital extension. Make sure that the palmar bar is form fitting and wide enough to cover the entire MP joint. Also, make sure the carefully molded dorsal hood of the orthosis extends all the way to the PIP joints, ending at the axis for PIP joint movement. At the same time, the splint should allow full finger flexion of all digits (Fig. 20.14).

Those who prefer to sleep on their stomach with their hand above their head may be exacerbating cubital tunnel issues. Since we cannot comfortably (or easily) control the position of the shoulder when sleeping, look to modify the position of the elbow, forearm, and wrist. Try to avoid elbow flexion while sleeping by using some type of splint or orthosis.

To prevent a fixed claw deformity of the ring and small fingers, a dorsal MP joint blocking orthotic with the MP joints in flexion should be fabricated. This helps redistribute force *from the EDC to the IP joints* to allow full IP joint extension.

About Cubital Tunnel Syndrome

"You have an injury to the nerve at your elbow. You know when you hit your funny bone? You're actually hitting your nerve, which is like a live wire close to the surface. You need to protect that nerve, especially right now when it's so sensitive. One way to protect the nerve is to avoid what I call the 'phone position.' That is the elbow position you assume when you're holding your phone up to your ear. Your nerve doesn't like this posture. If you have to use the phone a lot, consider using a headset or the hands-free option to avoid that position. Also, you'll need to avoid that bent elbow position when you sleep. We can talk about some brace options for this."

Conservative Management of Low (Distal) Ulnar Nerve Injuries (Ulnar Tunnel Syndrome or Entrapment at Guyon's Canal)

The ulnar tunnel at the wrist, called *Guyon's canal*, contains the ulnar nerve and artery. The canal is bounded by the pisiform and

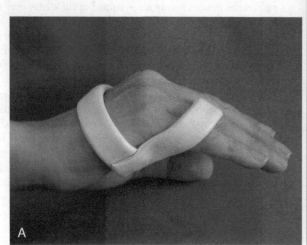

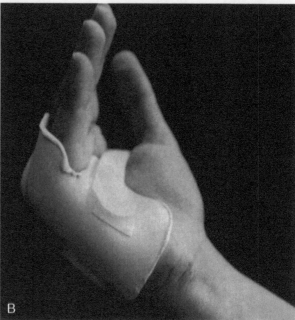

FIG. 20.14 (A) Hand-based splint designed to prevent clawing secondary to ulnar nerve palsy. (B) Hand-based ulnar nerve anticlaw splint with good volar support. *(A, From Mackin EJ, Callahan AD, Skirven TM. eds.* Rehabilitation of the Hand and Upper Extremity. *5th ed. St Louis, MO: Mosby; 2002; B, From Stanly BG, Tribuzi SM. eds.* Concepts in Hand Rehabilitation. *Philadelphia, PA: FA Davis; 1992.)*

insertion of the FCU ulnarly and the hook of the hamate radially. The roof of the canal is the flexor retinaculum. After giving off the dorsal cutaneous branch about 5 to 6 cm proximal to the wrist, the ulnar nerve enters Guyon's canal. Within the canal, the ulnar nerve divides into two branches: the superficial sensory branch and the deep motor branch.

The most common cause of ulnar nerve compression at the wrist is a space-occupying lesion (such as, a tumor, lipoma, or ganglion) followed by neuritis. Other causes include a pisiform or hook of hamate fracture, pisotriquetral arthritis, thrombus, or vessel anomalies. Smoking or the use of a pneumatic drill can predispose clients to ulnar artery thrombosis. Prolonged compression of the hypothenar eminence from activities (such as holding on to a handlebar of a bike) can contribute to symptoms.[41,42]

The clinical picture is one of sensory loss and motor paresis affecting the intrinsic ulnar-innervated muscles, including the interossei and the adductor pollicis. Occasionally, the hypothenar opponens, abductor, and flexor digiti minimi (FDM) muscles are spared. The sensory deficit involves the palmar ulnar aspect of the hand, the little finger, and the ulnar border of the ring finger. The dorsal ulnar aspect of the hand is spared because it is supplied by the more proximal dorsal cutaneous branch. Pain and paresthesia are usually worse at night and exacerbated by prolonged wrist flexion or extension.

Motor ulnar palsy has significant functional consequences. The balance between extrinsic and intrinsic muscles is lost, a consequence of paralysis of most of the intrinsic muscles of the hand. This produces a flattening of the normal arches of the hand, with loss of the ability to cup the hand around an object, such as a door knob. The unopposed extensor digitorum produces the classic claw hand deformity with hyperextension of the MP joints and flexion of the IP joints. As with high ulnar nerve lesions, there will be wasting of the interosseous muscles, thenar adductor, and hypothenar eminence.

Evaluation Tips

A detailed sensory exam (such as, Semmes-Weinstein monofilament testing) of the volar and dorsal hand assists the clinician in detecting the site of compression.

◎ Clinical Pearl

Sensory loss on the dorsal and volar hand would indicate a lesion proximal to Guyon's canal, whereas intact dorsal hand sensation with diminished sensation of the volar hand, small digit, and ulnar half of the ring digit would indicate compression within or just distal to Guyon's canal.

♡ Tips From the Field

Orthotic Options for Low (Distal) Ulnar Nerve Palsy (Ulnar Tunnel Syndrome)

Design an ulnar nerve palsy orthosis, also called an *anticlaw orthosis*, to prevent overstretching of the denervated lumbrical muscles and interossei of the ring and small fingers (see Fig. 20.14). Instruct the client to remove the orthosis for hygiene only. Continue use of the brace until the muscle imbalance resolves or until tendon transfers are performed. If proximal interphalangeal (PIP) flexion contractures of the involved digits have developed, a dynamic PIP extension orthosis will be needed to address joint contractures before using the static anticlaw orthosis. I have found commercially available spring coil splints effective for mild contractures (30 degrees or less).

A padded antivibration glove, a bicycle glove that has a gel pad that crosses the wrist crease, or a custom-made padded glove can be used to protect Guyon's canal from external irritation during activities, such as riding a mountain bike, using a push lawn mower, or grasping hand bike brakes.

Ergonomic tools designed to minimize stress on the ulnar wrist are good choices for clients with **ulnar tunnel syndrome**. An ergonomic hammer, for example, has a shaft that is designed to conform to the arches of the hand and has the tool head angled so that hammering can occur with the wrist in neutral. Educate the client about provocative postures and activities. Tell the client to avoid prolonged positions of simultaneous ulnar deviation and wrist flexion. For the biking enthusiast, suggest foot brakes or having the hand brakes repositioned to avoid this posture. Have the client avoid vibratory input as much as possible, or at least use dampening gel pads or padding on the handles of the equipment.

Postoperative Management Following Ulnar Nerve Laceration and Surgical Repair—Elbow to Wrist Level

Lacerations to the ulnar nerve can occur from a knife or glass. Typically, these injuries occur with concurrent flexor tendon injuries or ulnar artery injuries. Postoperative protocols need to consider all injured structures.

Consider the following guidelines:

- Fabricate a dorsal blocking orthosis with the wrist in 20 to 30 degrees of flexion, depending on the amount of tension at the nerve repair junction. If in doubt, position the wrist in the same amount of flexion as in the postoperative cast. Incorporate into the splint an MP dorsal block that limits MP joint extension to 45 degrees. This further minimizes tension on the nerve repair by limiting nerve excursion during digit extension and simultaneously blocks clawing or hyperextension at the MP joints of the ring and little digits.
- If there is no concurrent tendon injury and repair, AROM and PROM can begin immediately within the orthosis.
- Desensitization of hypersensitive scar tissue may begin after sutures are removed and wounds are healed.
- Between weeks 3 and 6 postoperatively, gradually adjust the dorsal blocking splint at the wrist, bringing it closer to neutral. Progression is dictated by the surgeon.
- By week 6 the dorsal blocking splint is discharged. A hand-based anticlaw splint may be needed until intrinsic muscle function returns.
- AROM of the wrist and hand outside the orthosis can begin by week 6. Progressive strengthening exercises and resumption of self-care activities can usually be added over the next 2 weeks.
- By week 8, you should be able to address residual strength issues that limit return to work.

Postoperative Management Following Decompression for High Ulnar Nerve Lesions (Cubital Tunnel Syndrome)

Cubital Tunnel Release in Situ

An in situ cubital tunnel decompression consists of releasing the fascial roof of the cubital tunnel to decompress the nerve, thus opening up the cubital tunnel space at the elbow. All restricting fibrous bands are excised. This eliminates the restriction and pressure that has occurred along the ulnar nerve at the elbow. This procedure is done if the symptoms do not respond to conservative management and if the ulnar nerve does not dislocate around the medial epicondyle groove of the humerus.[42] Therapy

postoperatively will focus on addressing pain or hypersensitivity. There are typically no ROM restrictions.

An **endoscopic release** may be utilized. This is an option for clients with mild to moderate preoperative symptoms. Postoperative splinting is usually not ordered, and the client is encouraged to begin AROM and nerve gliding within the symptom-free range.[42]

Anterior Transposition of the Ulnar Nerve: Subcutaneous Versus Submuscular

There are a number of surgical options for persistent cubital tunnel syndrome aggravated by painful subluxation of the ulnar nerve. Typically, the nerve is exposed, elevated from its bed, and transferred anterior to the medial epicondyle. With a **subcutaneous ulnar nerve transposition**, the nerve is then positioned below the subcutaneous fascia of the anterior forearm, medial to the median nerve. In a **submuscular ulnar nerve transposition**, the nerve is placed in a well-vascularized muscular bed. Traditionally, the flexor-pronator muscle origin was separated and then reattached to its origin on the medial epicondyle. However, a musculofascial lengthening technique for submuscular transposition of the ulnar nerve at the elbow is an alternative surgical option that avoids cutting the flexor-pronator muscle origin.

> **Precautions and Concerns**

Know which surgical technique for ulnar nerve transposition was performed. The need for orthotics, activity restrictions, and the postoperative therapy program are based on the type of surgery. Ultimately, the surgeon will dictate the course of rehabilitation.

- *If the flexor-pronator muscle origin was reflected and reattached in surgery, AROM of the elbow, forearm, and wrist is typically delayed for 3 to 4 weeks to allow the reattachment to heal.*
- *If the flexor-pronator muscle origin was reattached, passive forearm supination with elbow, wrist, and finger extension is contraindicated because this will stress the repair site.*
- *Premature stretching and strengthening activities can result in avulsion of the flexor/pronator origin. Regarding initiation of strengthening, it is always best to err on the cautious side with clients who have had a submuscular transposition.*
- *Following any of these procedures, strong gripping and lifting are contraindicated for 3 to 8 weeks.*

> **Tips From the Field**

Subcutaneous and Submuscular Transposition

- Subcutaneous transposition: Use of a long arm orthotic is surgeon-specific. If the surgeon requests a long arm orthotic, fabricate one on the posterior aspect of the arm with the elbow in 90 degrees of flexion. Carefully pad the incision site to prevent irritation from the rigid material. Inclusion of the wrist in this orthotic depends on client comfort. Typically, clients may remove their orthotics to begin exercise immediately. Full active elbow extension is expected by 4 weeks.
- Submuscular transposition: A long arm orthotic is typically used for 4 to 6 weeks postsurgery to protect the flexor-pronator mass. Place the elbow in 90 degrees of flexion, forearm in neutral to slight pronation, and wrist in neutral to slight flexion. Passive ROM may be initiated for the elbow, forearm, and

wrist; but aggressive end-range stretching should be avoided. Initiation of AROM is typically allowed at 4 to 6 weeks post-surgery.

- Submuscular transposition utilizing a musculofascial lengthening: This z-lengthening technique of the flexor-pronator fascia allows for full AROM immediately postoperatively. Proponents of this technique report that only intermittent use of a sling for comfort is necessary. For the rest of the time, the arm may be placed on a pillow in a comfortable position. Nonetheless, it is my experience that some surgeons continue to prescribe intermittent use of a long arm orthosis for 4 to 6 weeks post this procedure to provide protection of the soft-tissue structures affected by the surgery.

◎ Clinical Pearl

In the adult client with a high (proximal) median or ulnar nerve injury, complete return of motor and sensory function is rare. Therapists should provide honest and realistic information about what to expect, without eliminating hope. Address your client's emotional reaction to their trauma while promoting appropriate coping mechanisms that facilitate safe return to independent living.[44]

Postoperative Management Following Decompression of Low (Distal) Ulnar Nerve Palsy (Ulnar Tunnel Syndrome)

Surgery involves decompressing the ulnar nerve at the wrist. Postoperative therapy involves use of orthotics as described before, wound/scar management, and activity modification as described before. A postsurgical wrist orthosis is not typically needed following decompression; rather a bulky dressing serves the purpose of resting the tissues for the first 3 to 10 days postoperatively. Full ROM is usually allowed immediately postoperative.

♡ Tips From the Field

Severe Ulnar Nerve Compression With Intrinsic Muscle Paralysis

Intrinsic muscle function does not commonly return in adults following severe ulnar nerve compression with intrinsic muscle paralysis. Tendon transfers are typically needed to correct the muscle balance. In this scenario, the use of an orthosis to prevent joint contractures will be necessary until tendon transfers have been performed.

Postoperative Management Following Digital Nerve Repairs

Digital nerves are the most frequently injured upper limb nerve. Ideally, surgical repair of acute digital nerve lacerations is performed with a primary tension-free repair. Cast immobilization for 3 weeks has been the standard of care for almost a century.[45] Following digital nerve injury and repair, common functional impairments include poor two-point discrimination, cold intolerance, and hyperesthesias.[45] Evidence indicates that immobilization of a limb or joint will lead to joint stiffness, impaired tendon gliding, and muscle-tendon shortening.

Use of a hand-based dorsal block orthosis for 3 weeks versus free AROM following primary tensionless repair of a digital nerve injury has been studied.[45,46] Results indicate that immobilization

does not improve the integrity of the repair from a sensibility standpoint or in self-reported function/limitation. Certainly, not requiring immobilization with a cast or orthosis would be an advantage for clients. However, you should follow the conservative protocol of 3 weeks of immobilization following digital nerve surgery unless the surgeon states otherwise.

Precaution. *All clients undergoing a digital nerve repair, whether treated with a traditional cast/orthosis or allowed early AROM, should avoid full passive wrist and digit extension during the initial 3 weeks after surgery.*

After digital nerve repair, hand therapy focuses on three areas: (1) protection of the repair site; (2) short arc motion to encourage excursion of the nerve and prevent joint contracture; and (3) sensory reeducation.[46] Traditionally, this requires fabrication of a dorsal block orthosis with the involved MP joint(s) at 70 to 90 degress of flexion and IPs in extension. If the thumb is involved, position the CMC joint at 15-degrees flexion, MP at 30-degrees flexion, and IP in extension. AROM is allowed within the orthosis. The orthosis is discontinued at 3 weeks postsurgery

Therapy should include edema control, scar massage, and desensitization once sutures are removed. Use of the involved hand for activities of daily living should be encouraged at 3 weeks following tension-free digital nerve repairs.

◎ Clinical Pearl

There is a correlation between client's reports of hyperesthesia (or hypersensitivity) and their own estimation of recovery. There is also a high degree of correlation between reported quality of life and perceived disability following a peripheral nerve injury. Issues that predict disability include difficulty sleeping following the injury; pain; onset of depression following the injury; and limited ability to participate in work, household, sexual and social activities. Therefore the socioemotional impact of the client's injury should be addressed throughout the course of therapy.[44-46]

Conservative Management of Double Crush Syndrome

An injured nerve could conceivably have two (or more) sites of compression, each being insufficient in itself to cause clinical symptoms, but with the effects of each summating to create symptomatology.[47] Mononeuorpathy may predispose the rest of the nerve trunk to an increased susceptibility to irritation along the nerve and thus secondary neuropathies.[47] Since the peripheral nerve is one long continuous cell, injury in one part of the cell will likely have consequences in other areas of the cell, especially at those more vulnerable sites, such as where the nerve must traverse through spaces of increased friction (for example, fibroosseous tunnels). The presence of a distinct compression at two or more locations along the course of one peripheral nerve is called **double crush syndrome (DCS)**. The proposed pathophysiology of DCS is the disruption of the axoplasmic flow within the nerve cells.[47] Clients with this condition present with diffuse upper extremity complaints and two or more sites of minor peripheral nerve irritations or entrapments.

Typically, electrodiagnostic testing will objectively quantify abnormal peripheral nerve function. However, minor changes in the nerve fibers may not register as abnormal on electrodiagnostic tests, or these tests may not be specific enough to identify the presence of multiple sites of (mild) nerve irritation.[47] The most commonly studied double crush syndrome is the CTS-cervical spine injury,[47] followed by cubital tunnel syndrome and thoracic outlet syndrome

Commonly, clients will report intermittent and varying-intensity diffuse UE pain with a spread of symptoms from one area to another (for example, from the wrist to the elbow). Pain and paresthesia may be induced with specific postures of the arm that place tension on the involved neural structures. As the nerve irritation progresses, the client may assume a protective posture of the involved extremity that minimizes tension on the irritated nerve(s) and/or may develop a disuse atrophy as a means of coping with a chronic pain that seems to "have a mind all of its own."[48]

Conservative and Postoperative Management of Double Crush Syndrome

There isn't much written about the treatment of double crush syndrome. As with any peripheral nerve irritation, the therapist must follow protocols for tissue tolerances and wound care. If surgical decompression is performed, the postoperative protocols should follow those specific for that surgery. For example, if a CTR is done, follow the postoperative protocols for this surgery, and augment with interventions aimed at addressing the other, more proximal "crush" site(s).[49] If multiple sites of entrapment are decompressed, then the timeline for healing is lengthened. Below are some additional tips.

- Early compression stage: clients in this stage will have intermittent and position-dependent symptoms with slight provocation of symptoms upon examination. There may be a hypersensitive response to vibratory stimuli. Surgery is not recommended unless symptoms fail to improve after at least 3 months of conservative management. Splinting and instructions to decrease activities that cause repetitive compression of the nerve are helpful. Oral steroids and/or injections at the site(s) of compression may also be helpful.[47]
- Moderate compression stage: Clients in this stage will have intermittent symptoms, though more pronounced than in the earlier stage. Motor weakness is evident and measurable. Sensory threshold testing will indicate changes from normal sensibility perception. Symptoms may interfere with daily activities.
- Severe compression stage: Clients in this stage have persistent symptoms with muscle wasting, finger numbness, abnormal two-point discrimination, and significant limitations in role performance secondary to pain. These clients will not improve without surgical intervention. Following surgery, it is important that the decompressed nerve not be immobilized for more than 1 week. ROM exercise at the joint crossed by the released nerve and nerve gliding exercises should be introduced early. The postoperative client may not be able to return certain previous repetitive activities nor to using vibratory or pneumatic impact tools.

♥ Tips From the Field

Double Crush Syndrome

- Client education and cooperation are keys to successful management. Educate the client about the underlying pathology and about conditions that can further pervert the already irritable nervous system. Encourage the client to find a safe and comfortable imaginary "zone" in which they can move their arms without pain/increased symptoms. Have them practice "staying within this zone or box" when performing self-care and work tasks. Reinforce concepts by reviewing the client's

responses to "staying within the box." Later, as the nerve irritation diminishes, the boundaries of the "box" can be increased.
- Ergonomics can help lessen the external stresses on the irritable nerve. Teach your client to avoid repetitive UE movements in the ranges and postures that aggravate the nerve. For example, instead of bending the elbow to hold the receiver to the ear, use a headset. Avoid using vibratory or pneumatic impact tools; if they are necessary, use an antivibration glove with a palmar gel pad to absorb some of the shock. Educate clients about their syndrome and about modifications needed for sleep and work. An ergonomic assessment of the work place may be helpful in identifying those tasks that contribute to perpetuation of symptoms. Good posture and frequent stretch breaks are key components to managing symptoms.
- Nerve gliding should never be painful; find a way to encourage movement without irritating the nerve further. Even a little bit of movement at a joint where the nerve crosses is better than none. If, for example, the client is unable to perform the entire brachial plexus glide without pain, adapt the glide so that the proximal joints remain still, minimizing some of the tension on the nerve, while the distal joints move, creating nerve glide in the distal extremity. Then hold the distal joints still, in a position that minimizes tension on that nerve, as the proximal joints move to create proximal nerve gliding.
- Sometimes incomplete symptom resolution is the best that it gets. Not all clients will recover completely from double crush syndrome. In fact, many will not. Help the client make the psychological adjustment necessary to living with a chronic and painful condition by teaching the client pain management strategies and by allowing the client to verbalize their grief. Listen, acknowledge their grief, and when necessary, refer the client to mental health services.

? Questions to Ask the Doctor

- Does electrodiagnostic testing support the diagnosis of double crush syndrome? Is there radiological evidence of cervical degenerative changes that suggest cervical radiculopathy is a contributing factor? (If so, consider requesting a course of physical therapy to address cervical compression).
- Where are the proximal and distal sites of entrapment?
- Is the client a candidate for decompression surgery? What is the likely outcome of surgical intervention?

Treating Nerve Injuries—Conservative and Postoperative

The artistry of excellent therapeutic intervention for a peripheral nerve injury lies in addressing more than the resulting physical impairment.[50] Consideration of the psychological, social, and behavioral aspects of your client's injury will facilitate a more complete picture of your client's illness experience. Infusing a client-centered approach into traditional biomechanical treatment protocols begins with a comprehensive assessment coupled with empathetic listening. Research supports patient participation in decision-making about goals and intervention options, as it results in greater patient satisfaction, improved outcomes and adherence to treatments.[51] The collaborative goal-setting process should be predicated on educating our clients about their injury, their prognosis, and the rationale for each suggested intervention. I've frequently received the feedback from clients that "No one ever explained (the injury/surgery/reason for this exercise/splint, etc.) before!" The following interventions may be useful.

Nerve Gliding

The definition of nerve gliding has changed over the past 20 years (1997–2017), resulting in a disparity in the literature about what this intervention is and how it should be delivered. An early concept of nerve gliding was popularized in 1991 by Butler and Jones,[48] who proposed that movements that fostered the gliding of nerves through tight spaces might enhance nerve health. Totten and Hunter[52] performed cadaver studies to demonstrate the physiological movements necessary to create optimum median nerve excursion at the thoracic outlet and the carpal tunnel. Since this time, there have been numerous books, articles, and research studies on the use of nerve gliding to facilitate nerve homeostasis, to minimize neural adhesions, and to decrease nerve pain.[53-56]

We know that nerve health is predicated on motion.[5] Motion is lotion to the nerves! There are mechanisms inherent in a healthy peripheral nerve that allow its nerve fibers to accommodate to changes in length during normal joint motion. For example, your nerves must be able to continue to function whether your arm is stretched into end-range abduction and external rotation (as when throwing a football), or if your arm is tucked under you, with your elbow, wrist and fingers curled into a flexed posture (as when you sleep). The connective tissue coverings absorb much of the compressive or tensile forces; and in addition, the individual nerve fibers will fold or unfold within their fascicles to accommodate length changes. As the stretching or shortening continues, the nerve itself will glide relative to its neighboring structures.[5] However, if normal nerve movement is restricted at one location, you would expect to see an increase in neural tension at and distal to the site of this restriction during extremity motion. In this scenario, nerve function would be (temporarily) compromised. Nerve strain greater than 5% to 10% impairs nerve conduction, axoplasmic flow, and intraneural blood flow[55] and may trigger the development of abnormal impulse-generating sites along the nerve, exacerbating pain symptoms.[56] A burning sensation, indicating increased neural tension with concomitant decreased vascular flow would be experienced. Therefore care must be taken when designing a nerve gliding program to facilitate the health of an entrapped peripheral nerve. We need to ensure that the prescribed exercise fosters gentle nerve longitudinal sliding, not nerve tensioning or stretching. The goal of a nerve gliding program for an entrapped peripheral nerve is to enhance blood flow to the nerve and to facilitate axoplasmic flow. Such a nerve gliding program attempts to maximize the excursion of the nerve while minimizing the strain on the nerve.

If a nerve is significantly constrained or compressed, surgery may be necessary. Once the nerve is decompressed, therapeutic exercises should be introduced as soon as possible to restore and maintain the normal excursion of the nerve. Thus an important goal of a nerve gliding program *following decompression* is to restrict the formation of motion-limiting adhesions between the nerve and its surrounding tissue.[52]

Researchers[56, 57] have coined the terms *tensioner* to indicate a mobilization technique that increases strain on the nerve; and *slider* to indicate a mobilization technique that allows for maximum elongation of the nerve while minimizing strain. These researchers recommend the use of sliders with median nerve mobilization for CTS. Nerve sliding involves encouraging gliding of the nerve while decreasing the tension at the proximal or distal ends of the range. A slider is more likely to reduce neural symptoms and protective muscle guarding while facilitating nerve health. The concept of nerve slides as a treatment technique

may be visualized as sliding a piece of floss through teeth. When one end (of the floss) is pulled, the other end is free from tension. Likewise, as the peripheral nerve is pulled across a joint or through a tunnel, tension must be eased at one end or the other so as not to create or increase adverse nerve tension. Nerve sliding should be done slowly, moving the extremity as if one was a dancer. Advise the client to pay attention to how these exercises feel and to stop at any point in the sequence if numbness, discomfort, or pain increases.

Precaution. *It is important to instruct the client that nerve gliding can increase symptoms and nerve irritability if not done carefully and correctly. Creating nerve tension by simultaneously pulling on both ends of a nerve to complete an exercise or activity will surely increase symptoms.*

> ### ◉ Clinical Pearl
>
> Incorporating the movements of the nerve slide into a functional activity makes the nerve glide easier to remember. For example, the carpal tunnel median nerve glide begins with the involved hand in a gentle fist and wrist and forearm in neutral, and ends with the hand open with forearm supinated and wrist in some extension, as if the hand is showing what's in the palm. I call this the "Show me the money" nerve glide. Remember that the goal of these exercises is to gently slide the nerve through its available range to promote axoplasmic flow and general nerve health. These exercises should *never* be painful.
>
> **Precaution.** *Median nerve glide has historically been taught ending with the opposite hand pulling the thumb into extension and abduction. DO NOT pull on the thumb at the end of a median nerve glide. This turns the slider into a tensioner and can increase both nerve pain and joint pain at the CMC joint of the thumb.*

Sensory Reeducation

An important part of rehab for clients with sensory loss from peripheral nerve damage is sensory reeducation. Peripheral nerve lesions can result in a shuffling of skin "addresses" or end organ sites with respect to CNS addresses. In other words, individual regenerating axons may not end up reinnervating the exact same end organs as prior to the injury. This will result in an altered, and likely diminished, pattern of input coming from this area of the periphery to the somatosensory cortex. The cortex will reorganize in response to this altered pattern or picture.[57] Thus the goal of sensory reeducation is to improve the client's perception of sensory information arising from receptors in the hand so that the client can correctly interpret the (altered) pattern of incoming sensory signals.

Sensory reeducation may be divided into two stages—a protective and a discriminative stage. The goal of protective sensory reeducation is to educate the client to compensate for loss of sensory protection. These clients are unable to evaluate the potential harmfulness of hot/cold or of sharp objects. They are at significant risk for unknowingly injuring their insensate hand, especially when vision is occluded. Education about risk for reinjury and compensation strategies can typically be performed in one or two sessions. Tell the client to avoid working around machinery and to avoid situations where the environmental temperature is below 60°F (16°C). The client should be advised to use vision to compensate for sensory loss. Reaching into a pocket becomes a potentially harmful situation for a client without protective sensation.

The goal of discriminative sensory reeducation is the recovery of stereognosis (that is, the ability to recognize the form of an object without using visual or auditory cues). Following a nerve injury, there is a predictable pattern of sensory recovery, beginning with pain perception and progressing to vibration of 30 cps (cycles per second), moving touch, and constant touch. The return proceeds from proximal to distal. This phase of sensory reeducation will incorporate graded training tasks involving localization and discrimination of textures, shapes and objects. A visual-tactile matching process can be used; the client attempts to correctly identify the stimulus location or modality type, first with eyes closed. If the client is wrong, then the stimulation is repeated with eyes open, and the client concentrates on matching what he/she feels with what he/she sees.

For successful carryover of newly developed discriminative sensory skills, the client must have the motor skills for object manipulation. The client must ultimately be able to hold and manipulate an object for a short time without the object slipping through the fingers, even with vision occluded.

Cortical plasticity is dependent on tactile experiences with the environment. Specific cortical and subcortical reorganization can occur within minutes of a peripheral nerve injury and can be long-standing, if not permanent. Initially, visual and auditory cues can be used to minimize synaptic reorganization of the somatosensory mapping of the insensate aspect of the hand. Functional magnetic resonance images[58] have confirmed that there is a continuous cortical interplay within the brain, with polymodal association areas 'lighting up' during a single modal sensory or motor task. For example, when a blind person reads Braille, the primary visual cortex is activated along with the somatosensory cortex. Imagining a movement will activate the premotor cortex. When imagining music, the auditory cortical areas are recruited. While there is need for further research, current work in this area suggests that we can minimize adverse cortical mapping by asking clients to visualize movement of the wrist and hand; and to imagine how it feels to touch and massage the involved area. Observing movement and/or touch of the uninvolved hand in a mirror while thinking about both hands performing the same movement or feeling the massage may 'fool' the brain and minimize early synaptic disorganization.[58]

Using the injured hand/limb in functional and familiar tasks, as opposed to exercises only, facilitates faster return of function and discourages learned nonuse.[57] Sensory relearning, combined with desensitization can influence sensory recovery as well as the development of pain after injury. Cortical changes are facilitated or modulated by the strength of the behavioral reinforcement. Behavioral reinforcement is predicated on what our client perceives as interesting and motivating to them.

> **◎ Clinical Pearl**
>
> Sensory reeducation is more successful if the exercise or reeducation program is functionally oriented, client-centered, and appropriately challenging to that individual.[58]

Both protective and discriminative sensory reeducation should begin as soon as possible after a nerve injury in order to encourage the client to use the affected extremity before abnormal use patterns can develop. This minimizes compensatory use of the uninvolved arm with resultant neglect of the involved extremity. A sensory reeducation program can begin within 3 weeks of digital nerve repair.[57]

Pain Management

Pain is almost always a sequela of nerve injury. After injury to a peripheral nerve, the nervous system responds by temporarily enhancing responsiveness to pain and by increasing inflammation to protect the injured body part. If exposed to continual noxious input, the CNS can trigger an ongoing heightened sensitivity to pain perception with an increase in responsiveness to both painful and nonpainful stimuli.[59] Functional imaging studies of the brain following exposure to severe and/or chronic pain from a peripheral nerve injury have demonstrated adverse cortical reorganization of the motor and somatosensory cortexes, with decreased representation of the affected limb and smudging of the neural pathways for dexterous finger movement.[59] This pathological response is called complex regional pain syndrome II (CRPS).

It is important that we identify those clients *at risk* for CRPS and address their pain aggressively through education, desensitization, and inclusion of the injured body part in normal functional and familiar activities as soon as possible. Clients are often fearful about their injury, about life changes that have occurred or may still occur secondary to their injury, about reinjury, and/or about expectations for recovery. Pain associated with a peripheral nerve injury often can be diminished if the client understands the cause of their pain and loses fear associated with such unknown variables as healing expectations and timelines. Therapists are in the best position to address many of these concerns simply because we spend more time with the client than the physician. The following may also be helpful in mitigating the client's pain experience.

Precaution. *Clients may think they are supposed to tolerate painful activities/stretches because they have been indoctrinated to think this way. Therapists must instruct clients that pain is an indication of tissue injury and is to be avoided. Clearly and regularly state to your clients that the mantra, "no pain, no gain," is not true.*

Desensitization

Immediately after injury, the local neural tissue will lower its sensory stimulus threshold in response to the sensitizing effects of inflammatory mediators. In other words, it is easier for the sensory nerve to achieve an action potential. Sensory input that is nonnoxious, such as palpation or percussion along the nerve, may be perceived as irritating or painful. Prolonged irritation to the neural tissue can result in a state of **hyperalgesia**, or hypersensitivity, with local sensitivity changes that will be reflected in the way the central somatosensory system processes sensory inputs. Clients with hyperalgesia may complain of extreme discomfort with tactile stimulation to their involved body part. For example, hypersensitivity of the skin around the radial styloid and proximal thumb is a fairly common phenomenon occurring with radial sensory nerve irritation. Interestingly, even when the source of irritation (such as, a tight cast or splint) is removed, the hypersensitivity may remain.

Desensitization is the systematic process of applying nonnoxious stimuli to peripheral tissues to retrain the nervous system. The ideal client must be motivated to participate in a home program. For desensitization to be successful, frequent sessions with various tactile stimulations must occur throughout the day. The more sessions, the quicker the results. Initially, clients may need to apply the stimulus around the irritated tissues rather than directly on the tissues. The client applies their own stimulus, so the amount of pressure is under the client's control.

( ) What to Say to Clients

About Hypersensitivity and Desensitization

"Your nerve is irritable, and that's why things that shouldn't be painful feel painful. To decrease this hypersensitivity, you will need to reeducate your nerve. To help it recover, you will need to touch the irritated skin regularly. Try short sessions at first, say 5 to 10 minutes. Try to touch the irritated skin every waking hour. Try to relax when you do this. You can put on nice music, watch a favorite TV show, or go into a quiet room—whatever works for you. Try touching or tapping your skin with a towel or a piece of cotton or massaging the area with cream. Or, you could use a soft toothbrush and gently brush over the irritated area—always moving in the same direction (that is, fingertip to elbow or elbow to fingertip). The key to getting better is to do this often and every day. If you wait, your brain will learn that this pain is normal and the pain message may become permanently fixed, like a memory."

Modalities

Modalities can be a helpful adjunct when treating a client with a peripheral nerve injury. Commonly used modalities include ultrasound,[59] iontophoresis,[60] transcutaneous electrical nerve stimulation (TENS),[60] hot packs, fluidotherapy,[60] paraffin baths, and cryotherapy.[60] Please see Chapter 9 for a more in-depth discussion of modality use.

▷ Precautions and Concerns

- *Scar massage and ultrasound should not be performed over a nerve conduit.[61]*
- **Precaution.** *Do not use superficial heat or cold modalities if your client has loss of protective sensation, as there is a much greater risk of burning the tissue. Without normal sympathetic function of the peripheral nerve, the overlying skin will not be able to sweat to cool down the tissue before it burns. Be cautious if your client has diminished light touch sensation.*

Manual Techniques

Manual therapy techniques, designed to increase blood flow and reduce pain, are also helpful. Therapeutic touch can be augmented by discussions about stress management, relaxation, visualization, and activity pacing. Incorporating these cognitive-behavioral techniques with manual therapies, in my experience, facilitates pain reduction by acknowledging the presence of pain and by gently and supportively instructing the client in self-management strategies for pain reduction. Discussion of soft-tissue mobilization and myofascial release techniques are beyond the scope of this chapter. The reader is encouraged to seek out courses in these areas to develop appropriate knowledge and skills before applying these techniques.

( ) What to Say to Clients

Typical Concerns

- Why is my hand/wrist/forearm/elbow still swollen?
  - Typical Answer: "Swelling is a normal part of healing. Your body is producing the cells that are needed for healing. Following an injury or surgery, you will see swelling, but we will reduce it with hand therapy as quickly as possible. Try to keep your injured arm elevated above your heart as much as you can during the first week after surgery. Use pillows to

help maintain this position. Ultimately, though, you may experience some amount of swelling for up to 1 year from your injury or surgery."
- Will my scar open up if I massage over it?
  - Typical Answer (once sutures are out and the wound is showing adequate tensile strength): "No, your wound won't break open if you apply cream and massage your scar. Begin gently, using any kind of lotion. I prefer something with an oily feel because while the nerve is healing, it's not as efficient at maintaining the skin's normal healthy elasticity. Massage the whole hand, not just the scar."
- Why do I have pain? Or why do I still have pain? Should I keep exercising if I have pain?
  - Typical Answer: "Pain is your body's normal mechanism for telling you that something is wrong. Usually that's a good thing, letting you know that you're doing too much or that something is amiss. Sometimes this warning mechanism continues to alert you, even when you've taken care of the initial problem. Your brain comes to expect pain, even when what you're doing should not be painful. When that happens, you need to learn how to self-manage your symptoms. Knowing the difference between pain that is a 'good' warning pain and pain that needs to be self-managed is difficult. I can help you with this. You should always tell me if you have pain with anything I give you in therapy (or with anything you are trying to do at home). Do not work through pain unless we discussed that this is to be expected. You can actually injure yourself further if you push through pain."

♡ Tips From the Field

Orthoses

Orthotics are used in the treatment of peripheral nerve injuries for three reasons: (1) protection, (2) prevention, and (3) functional enhancement. The rationale for choosing and providing an orthosis is where clinical reasoning comes into play: Why choose one orthotic over another over another?

- For protection: To diminish neural tension to create a healing environment. It is used to abate acute symptoms or symptoms that are observed at rest and increased with activity.
- For prevention: To prevent motions that result in additional compression to the nerve, reducing potential inflammation that could lead to worsening of symptoms. To prevent contractures secondary to muscle imbalance. Myoplasticity is the principle that muscle tissue will adapt structurally and functionally to changes in activity level and/or to prolonged positioning. Overstretched muscles result in an increase in sarcomeres (the functional unit of the muscle). An increase or decrease in sarcomeres means that the muscle adapts to its new resting length. Muscles can only generate optimal force at their resting length. Furthermore, muscles will contract about 50% of their resting length to generate this optimal force.[62] Thus overstretched reinnervated muscles to the wrist/hand will demonstrate a decreased ability to generate optimum strength during functional activities/use.
- For functional enhancement: To substitute for or enhance impaired function. When we stabilize an arthritic joint, as with the CMC joint of the thumb, we expect improved stability and strength at that joint and a decrease in joint pain during activity. When we develop a static progressive orthotic that provides

a slow and steady stretch to the tissues, we expect to see improved tissue extensibility and thus improved motion and function at that joint. When we provide our client with a dynamic radial nerve palsy brace that provides passive MP joint extension, but allows digit flexion, we intend to improve the client's functional grasp following a radial nerve palsy. We must educate clients about how orthoses will improve their function. If possible, give clients options and allow them input into the process.

CASE STUDY

PR is a 32-year-old, right hand dominant female executive who sustained puncture injuries to her right third and fourth digits, volar surface, from her cat's claws. She was seen by her family physician, who prescribed antibiotic medication to prevent infection. She continued to complain of pain, numbness, stiffness, and swelling at her follow-up appointment. Her physician referred her for a course of hand therapy to address her complaints.

At her initial visit, which was approximately 1-month post injury, PR had significantly swollen and stiff long, ring, and small digits per circumference measures. The volar puncture wounds had healed with minimal observable scar tissue, although PR reported some hypersensitivity with gentle palpation to these areas. AROM measurements were taken; isolated joint motion indicated that all extrinsic flexor tendons were intact. Active flexion-to-the-distal palmar crease ranged from 2.2 cm (small digit) to 4.5 cm (long digit). Semmes-Weinstein monofilament testing indicated normal light touch (2.83) at the tip of the fifth digit, tip of the index, and along the ulnar aspect of the fourth digit. The radial aspect of the ring finger responded with diminished light touch (3.61) at the base of the digit to diminished protective sensation (3.84) at the tip. The ulnar aspect of the long finger responded with diminished protective sensation (3.84 to 4.31). The radial aspect of the long finger responded with diminished light touch (3.22 to 3.61). PR reported tingling radiating to the tips of both her ring and long fingers with percussion to the digital nerves about 1 cm distal to the puncture sites. PR reported that her finger "numbness" had not improved since the date of injury. She reported concerns about the integrity of her nerves and voiced concern that she might need surgery to "fix them." The sensory findings were explained to PR as consistent with the physician's diagnosis of a nerve injury in continuity. Persistent sensory symptoms were likely aggravated by venous stasis.

During goal setting with PR at this first visit, it became clear that she was avoiding normal use of her right hand during work and at home because "it hurts." She was typing one-handed and utilizing her left hand to cook and clean whenever possible. She was observed being hesitant to grip her briefcase with a hook fist, preferring to use a modified grasp (between the index and thumb) to secure the handle.

PR was instructed in tendon glide exercises and blocking exercises for the digits to encourage better pull through and gliding of the extrinsic flexor tendons. She was also instructed in edema control measures, including use of 1-inch Coban, retrograde massage and in active fisting to assist the overwhelmed venous system. She was educated about the likely repercussions of continuing to avoid using her right hand, and she was encouraged to begin to incorporate her hand in such activities as holding onto the toothbrush while brushing her teeth. Cylindrical foam was provided, and PR was instructed in application of the foam to her toothbrush, her eating utensils, and even her briefcase handle so that she could comfortably and securely grip these items during use. She was also instructed to use her right hand once or twice daily when she was grooming her cat with her cat hair brush. Finally, PR was educated about how nerves respond to trauma and was given an expected timeline and guideline for what she could expect as the nerves continued to heal. Protective sensory education strategies were discussed and appropriate cautions (such as not reaching into a suds-filled basin for a knife) were reviewed.

PR returned to therapy 1 week later. Although she did not have a complete fist, she was now able to touch her palm with each fingertip after a few warm up exercises. Her swelling was less noticeable, and she demonstrated correct application of Coban. She requested another roll, indicating consistent use of it. She continued to complain of some scar hypersensitivity and of intermittent "zinging" up to the tips of her involved fingers. She was assured that this was a normal response as the nerves healed, and she was told to continue with scar massage and normal hand usage. She also reported some cold intolerance with marked change in the fingers' ability to tolerate the air conditioner blowing on them. This would appear to indicate a concomitant digital vascular injury. She was instructed to continue her tendon glide exercises even after full digit motion was achieved to encourage nerve gliding within the digits.

PR was seen once a week for short sessions over the next 3 weeks. She was now approximately 9 weeks from her injury. Digit motion was full. She reported that she had resumed all preinjury work and home activities using her right hand. Sensory testing showed moderate improvements in light touch sensibility with both the ring and long neurologically impaired areas responding with diminished light touch (3.61). Since it was likely that the digital nerves would continue to heal at a rate of about 1 mm/day, and since she had successfully returned to all preinjury activities and had achieved the goals she had set for herself, a final but optional visit was offered (1 month later) to document continued nerve healing. PR reported that she would call if she had further issues; she was satisfied that her hand would continue to heal as she had been instructed.

References

1. Siengsukon C: Neuroplasticity. In Lundy-Ekman L, editor: *Neuroscience: fundamentals for rehabilitation*, ed 5, St Louis, 2018, Elsevier.
2. Lundy-Ekman L: Pain as a disease: neuropathic pain, central sensitivity syndromes, and pain syndromes. In Lundy-Ekman L, editor: *Neuroscience: fundamentals for rehabilitation*, ed 5, St Louis, 2018, Elsevier.
3. Lundy-Ekman L: Central somatosensory system. In Lundy-Ekman L, editor: *Neuroscience: fundamentals for rehabilitation*, ed 5, St Louis, 2018, Elsevier.
4. Carp SJ: The anatomy and physiology of the peripheral nerve. In Carp SJ, editor: *Peripheral nerve injury: an anatomical and physiological approach for physical therapy intervention*, Philadelphia, 2015, F. A. Davis. Available from eBook Collection (EBSCOhost), Ipswich, MA.
5. Lundy-Ekman L: Peripheral region. In Lundy-Ekman L, editor: *Neuroscience: fundamentals for rehabilitation*, ed 5, St Louis, 2018, Elsevier.
6. Carp SJ: The biomechanics of peripheral nerve injury. In Carp SJ, editor: *Peripheral nerve injury: an anatomical and physiological approach for physical therapy intervention*, Philadelphia, 2015, F. A. Davis. Available from eBook Collection (EBSCOhost), Ipswich, MA.
7. Smith KL: Nerve response to injury and repair. In Skirven T, Osterman L, Fedorcyzk J, et al.: *Rehabilitation of the hand and upper extremity*, ed 6, St Louis, 2011, Elsevier.

8. Lundy-Ekman L: Physical and electrical properties of cells in the nervous system. In Lundy-Ekman L, editor: *Neuroscience: fundamentals for rehabilitation*, ed 5, St Louis, 2018, Elsevier.

9. Houdek MT, Shin Y: Management and complications of traumatic peripheral nerve injuries, *Hand Clinic* 31:151–163, 2015.

10. Kane PM, Daniels AH, Akelman E: Double crush syndrome, *J Am Acad Orthop Surg* 23(9):558–562, 2015.

11. Gelberman RH, Hergenroeder PT, Hargens AR, et al.: The carpal tunnel syndrome: a study of carpal canal pressures, *J Bone Joint Surg Am* 63(3):380–383, 1981.

12. Karl HW, Tick H, Sasaki KA: Non-pharmacologic treatment of peripheral nerve entrapment. In Trescot AM, editor: *Peripheral nerve entrapments: clinical diagnosis and management*, Switzerland, 2016, Springer, https://doi.org/10.1007/978-3-319-27482-9-1.

13. Duff SV, Estilow T: Therapist's management of peripheral nerve injury. In Skirven T, Osterman L, Fedorcyzyk J, et al.: *Rehabilitation of the hand and upper extremity*, ed 6, St Louis, 2011, Elsevier, pp 619–633.

14. Porretto-Loerke A, Soika E: Therapist's management of other nerve compressions about the elbow and wrist. In Skirven T, Osterman L, Fedorcyzyk J, et al.: *Rehabilitation of the hand and upper extremity*, ed 6, St Louis, 2011, Elsevier, pp 695–712.

15. Slutsky DJ: A practical approach to nerve grafting in the upper extremity, *Hand Clin* 10:73–92, 2005.

16. Slutsky DJ: New advances in nerve repair. In Skirven T, Osterman L, Fedorcyzyk J, et al.: *Rehabilitation of the hand and upper extremity*, ed 6, St Louis, 2011, Elsevier, pp 611–618.

17. Lee SK, Wolfe SW: Peripheral nerve injury and repair, *J Am Acad Orthop Surg* (8)243–252, 2000.

18. Isaacs J: Major peripheral nerve injuries, *Hand Clin* 29:371–382, 2013.

19. Isaacs J: Treatment of acute peripheral nerve injuries: current concepts, *J Hand Surg Am* 35(3):491–497, 2010.

20. Shi Q, MacDermid JC: Is surgical intervention more effective than non-surgical treatment for carpal tunnel syndrome? A systematic review, *J Orthop Surg Res* 6(1):17, 2011.

21. Law M, et al.: *Canadian occupational performance measure manual*, Toronto, 1991, CAOT Publications ACE.

22. Callahan AD: Sensibility assessment for nerve lesions in continuity and nerve lacerations. In Skirven T, Osterman L, Fedorcyzyk J, et al.: *Rehabilitation of the hand and upper extremity*, ed 5, St Louis, 2002, Mosby, pp 214–239.

23. Novak CB, Anastakis DJ, Bearton DE, Katz J: Patient-reported outcome after peripheral nerve injury, *J Hand Surg* 34:281–287, 2009.

24. Stonner MM, Mackinnon SE, Kaskutas V: Predictors of disability and quality of life with an upper extremity peripheral nerve disorder, *Am J of Occ Ther* 71(1), 7101190050p1–8, 2017.

25. Chemnitz A, Dahlin LB, Carlsson IK: Consequences and adaptation in daily life – patients' experiences three decades after a nerve injury sustained in adolescence, *BMC Musculoskeletal Disorders* 14(1):252, 2013.

26. Nachef N, Bariatinsky V, Sulimovic S, Fontaine C, Chantelot C: Predictors of radial nerve palsy recovery in humeral shaft fractures: a retrospective review of 17 patients, *Orthop Traumatol: Surg Res* 103:177–182, 2017.

27. Jacoby SM, Eichenbaum MD, Osterman AL: Basic science of nerve compression. In Skirven T, Osterman L, Fedorcyzyk J, et al.: *Rehabilitation of the hand and upper extremity*, ed 5, St Louis, 2002, Mosby, pp 649–656.

28. Ljungquist KL, Martineau P, Allan C: Radial nerve injuries, *J Hand Surg Am* 40(1):166–172, 2015.

29. McKee P, Nguyen C: Customized dynamic splinting: Orthoses that promote optimal function and recovery after radial nerve injury: a case report, *J Hand Ther* 20(1):73–88, 2007.

30. Seroussi RE, Singh V, Karl HW: Deep branch of the radial nerve entrapment. In Trescot AM, editor: *Peripheral nerve entrapments: clinical diagnosis and management*, Switzerland, 2016, Springer, https://doi.org/10.1007/978-3-319-27482-9-1.

31. Trescot AM, Karl WK: Superficial radial nerve entrapment. In Trescot AM, editor: *Peripheral nerve entrapments: clinical diagnosis and management*, Switzerland, 2016, Springer, https://doi.org/10.1007/978-3-319-27482-9-1.

32. Abzug J, Martyak GG, Culp RW: Other nerve compression syndromes of the wrist and elbow. In Skirven T, Osterman L, Fedorcyzyk J, et al.: *Rehabilitation of the hand and upper extremity*, ed 5, St Louis, 2002, Mosby, pp 686–694.

33. Dang AC, Rodner CM: Unusual compression neuropathies of the forearm, part I: radial nerve, *J Hand Surg Am* 34(10):1906–1914, 2009.

34. Dang AC, Rodner CM: Unusual compression neuropathies of the forearm, part II: median nerve, *J Hand Surg Am* 1915–1920, 2009.

35. Chi Y, Harness N: Anterior interosseous nerve syndrome, *J Hand Surg Am* 35(12):2078–2080, 2010.

36. Cole O: Carpal tunnel syndrome: a review of current best practice, *The Dissector* 43(4):24–28, 2016.

37. Padua L, Coraci D, Erra C, et al.: Carpal tunnel syndrome: clinical features, diagnosis and management, *Lancet Neurol* 15(12):1273–1284, 2016.

38. Karl JW, Gancarczyk SM, Strauch RJ: Complications of carpal tunnel release, *Orthop Clini N Am* 47(2):425–433, 2016.

39. Evans RB: Therapist's management of carpal tunnel syndrome: a practical approach. In Skirven T, Osterman L, Fedorcyzyk J, et al.: *Rehabilitation of the hand and upper extremity*, ed 6, St Louis, 2011, Elsevier, pp 666–677.

40. Baker NA, Moehling KK, Rubinstein EN, et al.: The comparative effectiveness of combined lumbrical muscle splints and stretches on symptoms and function in carpal tunnel syndrome, *Arch Phys Med Rehabil* 93:1–10, 2012.

41. Singh V, Trescot AM: Ulnar nerve entrapment. In Trescot AM, editor: *Peripheral nerve entrapments: clinical diagnosis and management*, Switzerland, 2016, Springer, https://doi.org/10.1007/978-3-319-27482-9-1.

42. Rekant MS: Diagnosis and surgical management of cubital tunnel syndrome. In Skirven T, Osterman L, Fedorcyzyk J, et al.: *Rehabilitation of the hand and upper extremity*, ed 6, St Louis, 2011, Elsevier, pp 678–685.

43. Apfel E, Sigafoos GT: Comparison of range of motion constraints provided by splints used in the treatment of cubital tunnel syndrome-a pilot study, *J Hand Ther* 19:384–392, 2006.

44. Chemnitz A, Dahlin LB, Carlsson IK: Consequences and adaptation in daily life – patients' experiences three decades after a nerve injury sustained in adolescence, *BMC Musculoskeletal Disorders* 14(1):252, 2013.

45. Vipond N, Taylor W, Rider MR: Postoperative splinting for isolated digital nerve injuries in the hand, *J Hand Ther* 20:222–231, 2007.

46. Stonner MM, Mackinnon SE, Kaskutas V: Predictors of disability and quality of life with an upper extremity peripheral nerve disorder, *Am J of Occ Ther* 71(1), 7101190050p1–8, 2017.

47. Kane PM, Daniels AH, Akelman E: Double crush syndrome, *J Am Acad Orthop Surg* 23(9):558–562, 2015.

48. Butler DS: *Mobilisation of the nervous system*, Melbourne, 1991, Churchill Livingstone.

49. Vaught MS, Brismée JM, Dedrick GS, et al.: Association of disturbances in the thoracic outlet in subjects with carpal tunnel syndrome: a case-control study, *J Hand Ther* 24(1):44–52, 2011.

50. Colaianni DJ, Provident I, DiBartola LM, Wheeler S: A phenomenology of occupation-based hand therapy, *Aus Occ Ther J* 62:177–186, 2015.

51. Vranceanu A, Cooper C, Ring D: Integrating client values into evidence-based practice: effective communication for shared decision-making, *Hand Clini* 25:83–96, 2009.

52. Totten PA, Hunter JM: Therapeutic techniques to enhance nerve gliding in thoracic outlet syndrome and carpal tunnel syndrome, *Hand Clini* 7(3):505–520, 1991.

53. Lim YH, Chee DY, Girdler S, Lee HC: Median nerve mobilization techniques in the treatment of carpal tunnel syndrome: a systematic review, *J Hand Therapy* 30(4):397–406, 2017.

54. Ballestero-Perez R, Plaza-Manzano G, Urraca-Gesto A, et al.: Effectiveness of nerve gliding exercises on carpal tunnel syndrome: a systematic review, *J Manipulative Physiol Ther* 40(1):50–59, 2017.

55. Coppieters MW, Alshami AM: Longitudinal excursion and strain in the median nerve during novel nerve gliding exercises for carpal tunnel syndrome, *J Orthop Res* 25(7):972–980, 2007.

56. Coppieters MW, Butler DS: Do 'slides' slide and 'tensioners' tension? An analysis of neurodynamic techniques and considerations regarding their application, *Manual Therapy* 13:213–221, 2008.
57. Priya BA: Effectiveness of sensory re-education after nerve repair (median or ulnar nerve) at the wrist level, *Indian J Physiotherapy & Occ Ther* 6(3):62–68, 2012.
58. Rosen B, Lundborg G: Sensory reeducation. In Skirven T, Osterman L, Fedorcyzyk J, et al.: *Rehabilitation of the hand and upper extremity*, ed 6, St Louis, 2011, Elsevier, pp 634–648.

59. Pollard C: Physiotherapy management of complex regional pain syndrome, *Aust N Z J Psychiatry* 41(2):65–72, 2013.
60. Bracciano AG: *Physical agent modalities: theory and application for the occupational therapist*, ed 2, Thorofare, NJ, 2008, Slack, Inc.
61. Michlovitz SL: Is there a role for ultrasound and electrical stimulation following injury to tendon and nerve? *J Hand Ther* 18:292–296, 2005.
62. Lundy-Ekman L, Peterson C: Motor system: motor neurons and spinal motor function. In Lundy-Ekman L, editor: *Neuroscience: fundamentals for rehabilitation*, ed 5, St Louis, 2018, Elsevier.

21 Wrist Fractures

Emily Seeley
Sarah Baier
Mike Szekeres

Introduction

Fractures of the wrist are very common. A wrist fracture can have devastating and long-term effects on an individual's ability to resume normal functional activities, including employment. Fractures of the radius, ulna, and carpal bones present in a variety of ways, dependent on the features of the fracture and concomitant soft-tissue trauma. This chapter reviews the pieces of this complex puzzle with an emphasis on clinical reasoning for the beginning hand therapist.

Osteology

Whether labeled as a break, crack, crush, or fracture, all terms synonymously refer to a disruption in the continuity of the skeletal structure.[1] Bones of the upper extremity vary greatly in their form and function. They range from long bones in the forearm that act as load-bearing levers, to short bones in the carpus that provide stability and movement. Despite these differences, they share a common anatomy. Their thick, well-organized outer cortex (**cortical** or **lamellar bone**) provides the stiff scaffolding that supports their less dense, sponge-like inner core (**trabecular** or **cancellous bone**). While cortical bone makes up about 80% of the human skeleton and trabecular bone makes up the remaining 20%, the relative quantity of each of these varies within each bone according to its functional requirements.[2] Cancellous bone has a richer blood supply than cortical bone, thus decreasing healing time when a bone is fractured in a location where the ratio of cancellous bone to cortical bone is higher.[3] The origin and quantity of blood supply to the wrist bones varies greatly and accounts for various healing times following fracture.

Fractures occur when a force is exerted against a bone that is greater than the bone can withstand. This occurs during high-force trauma with sudden loading; with long-term repeated stress that eventually weakens the bone; or due to pathological reasons such as osteoporosis, cancer, or osteogenesis imperfecta.[2] Fortunately, bones have the ability to heal without forming fibrous scar tissue. That is, bone heals through regeneration, restoring the damaged tissue to its preinjury cellular composition, structure, and biomechanical function.[4] Understanding the biological processes involved in bone healing is crucial for managing wrist fractures, as this will guide hand therapy interventions.

Bone Healing and Timeline

Fracture healing is a continuous process that is divided into three overlapping phases: inflammatory, repair, and remodeling. When a bone breaks, the body initiates a highly organized, physiological response, referred to as *secondary healing* (also called callus healing or indirect healing) (Fig. 21.1). The initial **inflammatory phase** begins when the fracture ruptures blood vessels within the **periosteum** (a highly vascular tissue that envelopes the nonarticular surfaces of bone), **endosteum** (medullary cavity of mature bone), and surrounding soft tissues. This leads to the formation of a *hematoma*.[5] The hematoma serves as a scaffolding for early fracture stabilization and is gradually replaced with granulation tissue. The **reparative phase** involves removal of damaged cells (via osteoclasts), including the hematoma, while endosteal **chondrocytes** (cartilage-forming cells) and periosteal **osteoblasts** (bone-forming cells) form a soft callus in and around the fracture defect. At this point, 2 to 3 weeks post fracture, stability is adequate to prevent shortening, but fracture angulation is still possible. The soft callus is then gradually converted to a hard callus, or **woven bone**, starting peripherally and progressively moving toward

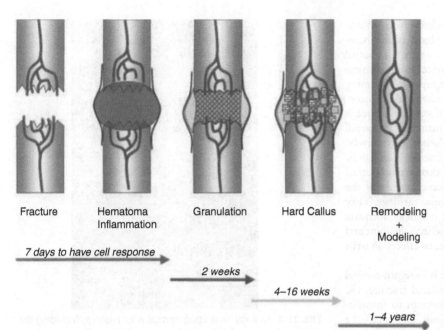

Fracture

Hematoma
Inflammation

Granulation

Hard Callus

Remodeling
+
Modeling

7 days to have cell response

2 weeks

4–16 weeks

1–4 years

FIG. 21.1 Secondary fracture healing. A hematoma develops at the fracture site during the initial *inflammatory phase* (day 1–7). Inflammation triggers the growth of new blood vessels forming granulation tissue and, in the presence of micromotion, a fibrocartilaginous *soft callus* is observed around 2 weeks postinjury. In the *reparative phase*, soft callus converts to hard callus or woven bone through enchondral ossification. The final *remodeling phase* restores the bone's preinjury structure with gradual change of woven to lamellar bone over the course of months to years. *(From Baroli B. From natural bone grafts to tissue engineering therapeutics: brainstorming on pharmaceutical formulative requirements and challenges. J of Pharm Sci. 2009;98[4]:1317-1375.)*

the center of the fracture gap.[6] This process of mineralization, or **enchondral ossification,** is usually completed by 6 weeks post fracture; however, it can continue up to 4 months.

The final **remodeling phase** actually begins in the middle of the repair phase and can continue for months to years.[6] In this phase, woven bone remodels to lamellar bone as a result of osteoclastic/osteoblastic activity and mechanical loading. This final phase helps restore a bone's preinjury strength and structure.[4]

Fracture stability dictates the type of healing that will take place. Fractures require stability in order to heal and to prevent a **nonunion.** When a fracture is stabilized by nonrigid fixation, the bone heals via the **secondary healing** process. With this process, healing is enhanced by micromotion at the fracture site.[6] Examples of nonrigid fixation include casting, immobilization in an orthosis, external fixation, and intermedullary fixation.

Alternatively, when a fracture is stabilized by rigid fixation (held in place with a plate that allows less than 1 mm of motion at the fracture site), the bone will heal via a process called **primary healing**[5] (Fig. 21.2). During the primary healing process, the three phases outlined above are bypassed and direct regrowth of bone occurs across the fracture defect. The rigid internal stabilization and compression offered by plates and screws acts as a substitute soft callus. This type of fracture management eliminates the need for prolonged cast immobilization and is stable enough to allow early wrist motion. However, new osteon construction under the plate at the fracture site takes approximately 5 to 6 weeks to complete.

Factors Affecting Healing

A number of factors contribute to the rate and degree of healing.[1] Systemic variables that can negatively influence healing include old age, vitamin D and calcium deficiency, systemic disease (osteoporosis, osteogenesis imperfecta, diabetes), nicotine use, immunosuppression, long-term drug use (nonsteroidal antiinflammatories, corticosteroids), and delayed time to initial diagnosis/treatment. Local factors that can influence healing include blood supply to the bone, mechanical factors of the fracture

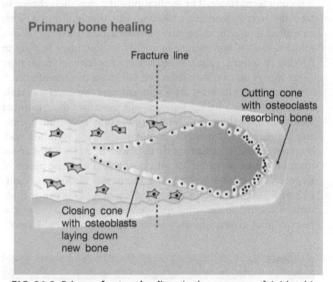

Primary bone healing

Fracture line

Cutting cone with osteoclasts resorbing bone

Closing cone with osteoblasts laying down new bone

FIG. 21.2 Primary fracture healing. In the presence of rigid stabilization, osteoclasts from intact bone create cutting cones (moving left to right) that resorb dead bone as they tunnel across the fracture line. Osteoblasts trail behind and lay down osteocytes (new bone) to repair the fracture defect. *(From Nyary T. Principles of bone and joint injuries and their healing. Surgery. 2018;36(1):7-14.)*

(location and pattern, degree of trauma, articular involvement), inadequate reduction/immobilization, infection, and pathology. It is imperative to determine if any of these factors are present at the initial assessment because they can contribute to delayed healing or nonunion.

Medical Management

When a fracture is suspected, prompt medical evaluation is required to determine the care needed to support proper healing. The medical provider will examine the patient both clinically and radiographically. Standard posteroanterior (PA)-, lateral-, and oblique-view radiographs are typically relied on to investigate bony integrity. However, due to the complexity of the three-dimensional relationship between the distal forearm and carpal bones, certain fractures may be difficult to detect using conventional X-rays and require computed tomography (CT) scanning or magnetic resonance imaging (MRI) to visualize and diagnose.

Wrist fractures can present in a variety of ways. If a bone is fractured, either partially or completely, but maintains its overall anatomical alignment, it is said to be **nondisplaced**. Alternatively, if a bone breaks and is no longer aligned, the fracture is said to be **displaced**. Fractures can also be described as **extraarticular** and/ or **intraarticular**. Extraarticular fractures occur outside of the joint and therefore do not interrupt the articular cartilage. They often require little intervention, and casting is usually adequate to allow healing. Intraarticular fractures extend into the joint and can alter joint surfaces. This can have detrimental effects on wrist motion and potentially lead to osteoarthritis.

One of the goals of medical management is to regain normal anatomy of the wrist. In the event of a displaced fracture, the medical provider (usually a physician) will attempt to manipulate and realign the bone fragments in the clinic. This is called a **closed reduction**. If the fracture remains appropriately aligned, it is considered stable. The medical provider may then choose to treat the fracture conservatively with cast immobilization. This treatment approach, using external stabilization (cast) that allows micromotion at the fracture site, relies on secondary healing to develop an internal callus. When a fracture is casted, it must have X-ray follow-up to ensure reduction (alignment) is maintained.

If the fracture loses its alignment and becomes unstable after casting, the medical provider will reevaluate the treatment approach. Sometimes, if the displaced fracture falls within acceptable limits of malalignment, immobilization is continued with the cast. However, significantly displaced fractures that cannot maintain adequate reduction with casting and have the potential to go on to **malunion** (heals in an abnormal position) or nonunion, require some type of surgical fixation. This can include various internal and external approaches such as the use of percutaneous pins, external fixators, bone grafts, or plates and screws.

The Distal Radius

Normal Anatomy

The wrist is comprised of the distal radius, ulna, eight carpal bones, associated joint capsule, and several ligaments (Fig. 21.3). The distal end of the radius is contoured with the scaphoid and lunate fossae (ellipsoid in shape) that allow a perfect fit of the scaphoid and lunate (condylar in shape) when articulating with the radius. This articulation forms the **radiocarpal joint.** The radiocarpal joint has two axes of motion, allowing the motions of wrist flexion/extension and radial/ulnar deviation. The distal end of the radius is oriented in a precise manner. When the radius is observed from the posterior/anterior view, radial inclination is approximately 23 degrees.[7] On the lateral view, the distal end tilts in a volar direction with an angle of approximately 12 degrees[7] (Fig. 21.4). Restoring this anatomical alignment in the fractured distal radius is important with respect to long-term outcomes.[8]

The distal ulna does not directly articulate with the proximal carpus. The **triangular fibrocartilage complex (TFCC)** is interposed between the triquetrum and distal ulna, acting as a

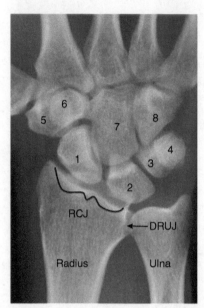

FIG. 21.3 An X-ray illustrating normal wrist anatomy including the distal radius, ulna, distal radioulnar joint *(DRUJ)*, radiocarpal joint *(RCJ)*, scaphoid *(1)*, lunate *(2)*, triquetrum *(3)*, pisiform *(4)*, trapezium *(5)*, trapezoid *(6)*, capitate *(7)*, hamate *(8)*, Courtesy of Sarah Baier.

ligamentous sling and cushion between these two bones. The TFCC also stabilizes the **distal radioulnar joint (DRUJ)** via the dorsal and volar radioulnar ligaments. The TFCC has a central disc portion that allows gliding of the ulnar carpus. This central portion is avascular and, because of this, does not heal well if torn. More peripheral ligamentous attachments are responsible for bearing the tensile loads of this joint during gripping and weight bearing. Normally the radius will bear about 80% of the axial load from the carpus and the ulna will bear 20%.

The DRUJ allows forearm rotation (pronation/supination). The hand and carpus move in conjunction with the DRUJ resulting in "palm up" in supination and "palm down" in pronation. Movement at the DRUJ occurs with the radius rotating over a fixed ulna; the ulna does not move during forearm rotation. As the radius rotates over the ulna into pronation, the radius shortens in relation to the ulna. This movement is referred to as *proximal-distal translation.*[9] Even though the ulna does not move, this translation is described as the ulna sliding up to 2 mm distally in relation to the radius during pronation. As a result of this translation, there is increased load on the ulnar side of the wrist in pronation. In supination, the same translation results in the ulna sliding proximally in relation to the radius and this position decreases load on the ulnar wrist. Translation becomes important following fracture of the distal radius and ulna, which can change the length of these bones and alter the ideal relationship between the two.

◉ Clinical Pearl

If the distal radius does not maintain its length following fracture (heals in a shortened position), the relationship between the radius and ulna is altered, resulting in a change in the 80/20 force distribution between the two bones. Since the ulna is now relatively too long, clients may present with increased pain on the ulnar side of the wrist and difficulty with ulnar deviation.

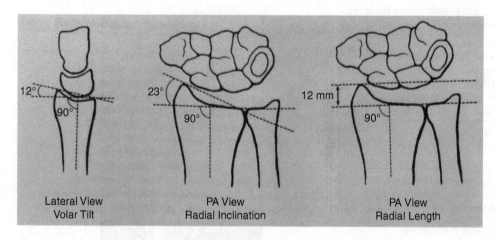

FIG. 21.4 A schematic diagram illustrating average anatomical parameters of the distal radius including volar tilt, radial inclination, and radial length. *PA, Posteroanterior. (From Smith DW, Brou KE, Henry MH. Early active rehabilitation for operatively stabilized distal radius fractures.* J Hand Ther. *2004;17(1):43-49.)*

Distal Radius Fractures

In the United States, distal radius fractures are the most common fracture of the upper extremity.[10] Fractures of the distal radius usually result from a fall on outstretched hand (**FOOSH**) injury. The fracture tends to occur in two main groups: (1) individuals less than 18 years of age (usually a result of high-energy forces); and (2) those older than 50 years of age (usually a result of lower-energy forces). The fracture is seen on the distal 2 cm of the radius where the bone is more porous, making it is easier for fractures to occur in this area. Fortunately, this area of the radius also houses a good blood supply, making these fractures fairly easy to heal.[11]

The most common form of distal radius fracture (DRF) is the **Colles' fracture**, which is an extraarticular fracture of the distal metaphysis. It results from the scaphoid and lunate placing a dorsal force through the distal radius with subsequent dorsal displacement. Colles' fracture is often used as a blanket term to refer to all fractures of the distal radius (Fig. 21.5A). Other common fracture patterns and eponyms are outlined in Table 21.1.

Nonoperative Treatment of Distal Radius Fractures

Closed reduction with casting is the most common treatment for DRFs. Extraarticular and stable fractures, as well as nondisplaced intraarticular fractures, are casted for 2 to 8 weeks. Casting may also be considered for more unstable intraarticular fractures in individuals with low functional demands and high surgical risk given their medical history. In these situations, the client needs to be informed that there will likely be a resultant deformity with reduced available wrist motion.[12]

There has been some debate in the literature as to the optimal wrist position for closed reduction casting,[13] but the wrist is usually casted in slight flexion and ulnar deviation based on the theory that this position uses the supporting soft tissues surrounding the joint to stabilize the fracture.

Surgical Treatment of Distal Radius Fractures

Unstable DRFs will require surgery to ensure proper alignment and healing. There is considerable debate in the surgical community over the best method of surgical intervention.[14] Surgical options include **percutaneous pinning**, **open reduction and internal fixation** (ORIF), open reduction with volar or dorsal plates, and **external fixation**.

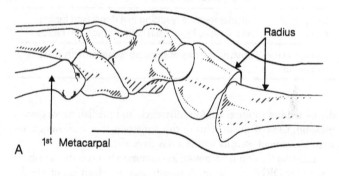

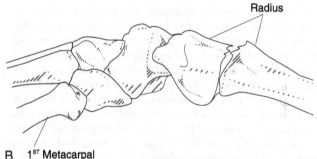

FIG. 21.5 Schematic of two types of distal radius fractures. (A) Colles' fracture showing classic dorsal displacement of the distal fragment. (B) Volar displacement of the distal fragment is indicative of a Smith's fracture. *(From Moscony AMB, Shank T. Wrist fractures. In: Cooper C. ed.* Fundamentals of Hand Therapy. *2nd ed. St. Louis, Elsevier;2014, pp. 317.)*

Percutaneous pinning involves driving pins/wires into the reduced fracture to secure the fragments. This can often be seen in the treatment of radial styloid fractures. Following pinning, the individual is placed in a cast or custom wrist orthosis to prevent wrist motion. The pin site provides a direct path to the bone, which increases the risk for **osteomyelitis** (bone infection). Therefore pin sites need to be kept clean, and the client should be taught how to perform pin care.

Complex intraarticular fractures, comminuted extraarticular fractures, and fractures with open soft tissues will usually be treated with an ORIF using volar or dorsal plate and screws to rigidly fix the fracture pieces. There has been a definite trend toward volar plating over dorsal plating the past 10 years. Using volar locking plates for open reduction of unstable fractures is now a common surgical practice[15] (Fig. 21.6). Complications of plating include

TABLE 21.1	Common Distal Radius Fracture Patterns
Colles Fracture	Distal fragment of radius displaced dorsally. Often extraarticular. Results from hyperextension of the wrist. Managed with closed reduction or if unstable, open reduction internal fixation (ORIF) with volar plating (see Fig. 21.6).
Smith's Fracture	A fracture of the distal radius with volar angulation. Results from a fall on flexed wrist (see Fig. 21.5B).
Barton's Fracture	Fracture of dorsal or volar rim of radius, with dislocation from carpus. Surgical intervention will be needed to realign carpus and fixate the radius.
Chauffeur Fracture	Radial styloid fracture. Surgical management involves pinning. May not need therapy as the fracture is extraarticular.
Die-punch Fracture	Articular fracture resulting in a depressed lunate facet. Caused by an axial load through the radius.
Salter-Harris Fracture	Pediatric fracture of the epiphyseal growth plate.

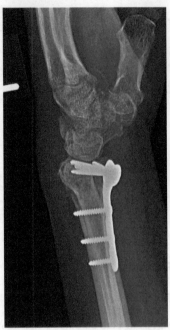

FIG. 21.6 Lateral view of an open reduction internal fixation with volar plating of an intraarticular fracture. Courtesy of Emily Seeley.

digital tendon rupture, tendon adherence, and median nerve compression. One of the benefits of this surgery is that it allows early wrist movement, usually within a few days of surgery.

External fixation is becoming less common but remains a viable option for DRFs. It relies on ligamentotaxis, in which longitudinal traction is placed across the radiocarpal joint to optimize the length of the radius and alignment of the fracture. The distal pins of the fixator are placed in the second or third metacarpals, and the proximal pins are placed along the shaft of the radius. These pins are attached to the fixator that act as an external scaffolding. Risks are pin site infection, dorsal sensory branch irritation, and median nerve neuropathy. Early finger motion is encouraged immediately following surgery, but the wrist cannot move while the external fixation device is in place. Supination and pronation are allowed but will be very limited. The device is usually worn for 4 to 6 weeks and the wrist is then placed in a supportive orthosis upon removal of the fixator.

? Questions to Ask the Doctor

Following Distal Radius Surgery
- Was there a secondary ulnar fracture?
- Was there any loss of radial height?
- How soon can we perform passive range of motion exercises?
- What is the preferred pin care/wound care routine?

Potential Complications Following Distal Radius Fracture

Unfortunately, complications do occur following DRF. Early detection is important, and communication with the treating physician will assist in managing these complications, either therapeutically or surgically. Outcomes following wrist fracture will vary among individuals, and residual pain, loss of motion, ongoing sensory loss or paresthesia, and changes in the cosmetic appearance of the wrist can leave some clients disappointed. When hand therapy, adaptation of the environment, and acceptance of the change/loss does not resolve the client's concerns, surgical consultation may be considered in some cases.

Complex Regional Pain Syndrome (CRPS)

The exact incidence of CRPS following DRFs is not known, but recent studies have reported rates as high as 8.3%[16] and 32.2%.[17] The cause of CRPS remains unclear. The pain is neuropathic in nature and is extreme during attempted movement of the affected limb. There is fluctuation in vasomotor function including skin color, temperature, and sweating. CRPS can lead to extreme stiffness, loss of function, and significant disability. Early detection and treatment are key to resolving this condition. Evidence suggests that a pain level of 5 or greater on the pain numerical rating scale during the first 3 postoperative days is linked with increased incidence of CRPS.[18]

Individuals presenting with CRPS are best managed with a multidisciplinary approach including hand therapy (see Chapter 37), psychiatry, and pain management.[19] Various medications may be prescribed, and clients are often referred to a pain clinic for sympathetic blocks. There has been a special interest in the relationship between early supplementation of vitamin C after DRF and the prevention of CRPS, but more studies are needed to validate this relationship.[20] The American Association of Orthopedic Surgeons recommends that physicians routinely prescribe vitamin C following DRF.[8]

Precaution. *Clients should be closely monitored following DRF for signs of CRPS including pain, discoloration of the hand, temperature changes, mottling, sweating, increased hair growth, and edema. Observing a cluster of these symptoms could indicate early CRPS, and concerns need to be communicated to the physician for possible medical management.*

Malunion

Malunion results when a fracture loses reduction, resulting in malalignment upon healing. This can lead to significant pain at the radiocarpal joint, distal ulna, and DRUJ, and post-traumatic arthritis can develop in these areas. Pain with movement and loss of motion are primary complaints. Resolving these problems will usually require corrective surgery to restore the height and angles of the distal radius anatomy.[21] Several procedures exist to correct pain and dysfunction related to malunion—corrective osteotomy of the radius and/or ulna, distal ulna resection, and radiocarpal fusion. Wrist fusion is always a last option and considered a salvage procedure, but an immobile, pain free, and stable wrist is more functional than a painful wrist with limited strength. Functional orthoses can sometimes provide symptom management when surgery is not an option.

When malunion results in ulnar-sided wrist pain, it can be attributed to increased load on the ulna following loss of radial height from the fracture. Change in radial height, even by a few millimeters, can result in an increase in the relative height of the ulna as compared to the radius. This is known as **ulnar positive variance**. This change may alter force distribution through the distal radius, distal ulna, and interposed TFCC. For example, the typical force distribution of 80/20 might become 70/30. Alteration in the load taken through the ulnar side of the wrist may contribute to increased pain, especially if there is also damage to the TFCC. Ulnar positive changes can further progress to **ulnar abutment** (also known as *ulnar impaction syndrome*). Ulnar abutment presents as a continuum of changes including decreased grip strength, limited ulnar deviation, degeneration and impingement of the TFCC, and finally osteoarthritis of the ulnar wrist.[22] Ulnar positive variance can be resolved surgically by correcting the distal radius anatomy or by shortening the ulna. The aim of surgery is to create "ulnar neutral" and proper realignment of the DRUJ.[23]

Soft-Tissue Injury

Considerable force is required to break a bone, so some amount of soft-tissue injury (STI) in conjunction with the fracture is always present. Measures performed to reduce the fracture can result in further compromise to the soft tissue. While fractures are often easily identifiable on X-ray and heal in a relatively short period of time, STIs can be more challenging to manage. The literature reports an incidence of associated carpal ligament injuries at 50% for scapholunate (SL) ligament tears and 15% for lunotriquetral (LT) ligament tears.[24,25] Radiographic review will reveal a greater than normal separation between the scaphoid and lunate in the presence of a SL ligament disruption. Carpal ligaments that are compromised during DRF can lead to wrist instability requiring prolonged therapy or surgery to resolve (see Chapter 22).

Tendon Irritation or Rupture

Tendon irritation following DRF can be caused by general overuse, adherence of tendon to underlying scar, or friction between tendon and sharp bone or internal hardware. Tendons can rupture from repeated movement and friction over volar and dorsal plates. A recent systematic review[26] reported a 1.5% incidence of tendon ruptures with volar plating and a 1.7% incidence with dorsal plating. If hardware must be removed due to these complications, it is generally not performed until at least 6 months postsurgery to ensure bone has matured and plate removal won't compromise bony integrity. Tendon ruptures must be repaired, but the timing of the repair depends on when the tendon ruptures. Some tendons rupture shortly after the fracture occurs, while other ruptures happen months or years after the fracture has healed. Tendons can be repaired directly, grafted, or addressed with tendon transfer.[27]

Nerve Compression or Irritation

The median nerve, dorsal radial sensory nerve (DRSN), and ulnar nerve can be affected by a DRF. The median nerve is the most commonly involved. Nerve compression can result from edema, the development of flexor tenosynovitis, trauma to the carpal tunnel during a FOOSH injury, repeat reductions, or fracture fragments compressing the nerve. It can be seen acutely at the time of fracture or can develop over time.[28] Acute carpal tunnel syndrome (CTS) presents in 5.4% of distal radius fractures treated surgically,[29] and can be treated with a carpal tunnel release at the time of ORIF. If CTS develops later, surgical release is an option in the subacute stage.

The DRSN provides sensation over the dorsal radial hand. It can become damaged or irritated from pin placement or from compression in a cast. This can be aggravating to the client but usually resolves over time. Less frequently, ulnar nerve symptoms may be reported due to swelling in the area of Guyon's canal at the wrist or from irritation at the elbow due to the propensity to hold the elbow in flexion during immobilization. Edema control efforts and alterations in positioning often assist in managing these symptoms.

Distal Ulna Fractures

Fractures of the distal ulna usually occur in conjunction with DRFs, and it is uncommon to see them in isolation. Distal ulnar fractures (DUF) are important because if they are not treated correctly, persistent ulnar-sided wrist pain, DRUJ instability, and loss of forearm rotation can result. DUFs include injuries to the ulnar styloid, ulnar head, or ulnar metaphysis. Ulnar styloid fractures accompany DRFs in 50% of the cases.[30] Nonunion is the end result for 50% to 70% of ulnar styloid fractures, conservative treatment is the norm, and few remain symptomatic.[31] Those DUFs at risk for affecting function of the DRUJ are stabilized using Kirschner-wires (also called *K-wires*), plate and screws, cannulated screws, and tension band wiring.

Carpal Fractures

The wrist, or carpus, is composed of eight uniquely shaped bones (see Fig. 21.3) bound by ligaments that provide a fine balance between stability and mobility. Coordinated movement of these highly mobile carpal bones allow a variety of motions while tolerating stress and strain in order to perform life's daily tasks. These carpal bones are susceptible to fracture following a FOOSH injury, a direct blow to the wrist, or with repeated trauma. Carpal fractures have the potential to disrupt the ligamentous stability of the wrist and lead to more disabling sequelae.

Scaphoid Fractures

The scaphoid is the most frequently fractured carpal bone in adults, accounting for 80% of all carpal fractures. Scaphoid fractures typically occur in young males averaging 25 years of age who are often involved in sports and manual labor.[32] The scaphoid is the second largest carpal bone and is shaped like a kidney bean. It has a proximal pole (20% of fractures), waist (70%), and distal tubercle (10%)[33] (Fig. 21.7). As part of the proximal carpal row and radiocarpal joint, the scaphoid also spans the midcarpal

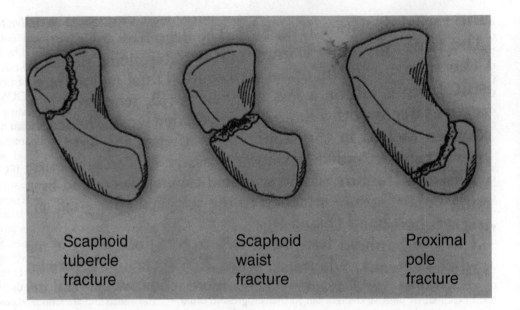

FIG. 21.7 Scaphoid fractures can be divided into three main types: fractures of the scaphoid tubercle, scaphoid waist fractures, and proximal pole fractures. *(From Trumble TE, Rayan GM, Budoff JE eds. Principles of Hand Surgery and Therapy. 3rd ed. St. Louis, Elsevier. p101, Fig. 5.2.)*

Scaphoid tubercle fracture

Scaphoid waist fracture

Proximal pole fracture

joint. As a result, it plays an integral role in overall wrist kinematics. These fractures can greatly impact function if managed improperly.

Diagnoses and Pathology of Scaphoid Fractures

Scaphoid fractures typically result from a fall on a hyperextended and radially deviated wrist. It is not uncommon for scaphoid fractures to go undiagnosed for a prolonged period of time because they can be hard to see on the initial X-ray. Clients will present with radial-sided wrist pain, swelling, and reduced wrist extension and grip strength. Axial compression of the thumb (known as the *scaphoid compression test*) and tenderness within the anatomical snuff-box and over the distal pole help diagnose a scaphoid fracture.[34] As many as 30% of scaphoid fractures go undiagnosed upon initial radiograph.[35] Untreated scaphoid fractures have a high rate of nonunion and progression to disabling arthritis. Therefore if primary X-rays are negative but a scaphoid fracture is suspected, individuals are immobilized and X-rays are repeated within 1 to 2 weeks. This delay allows for bony resorption adjacent to the fracture site, making the fracture more visible on X-ray.

Treatment of Scaphoid Fractures

Scaphoid fracture healing times rely greatly on the fracture location and blood supply. With 80% of its articulating surfaces lined with cartilage, a majority of scaphoid vascularity enters at the distal pole. Therefore injuries that disrupt the blood supply render the proximal pole susceptible to fragment death or avascular necrosis (AVN).[36] While blood supply improves as you move distally through the scaphoid, highly comminuted or largely displaced fractures can leave other parts of the scaphoid susceptible to delayed or nonunion.

> ### ◎ *Clinical Pearl*
>
> Based on fracture location, you can expect the following scaphoid fracture healing times with conservative treatment (casting): distal pole 6 to 8 weeks, waist 8 to 12 weeks, and proximal pole 12 to 24 weeks.[37]

Distal pole and waist fractures that are nondisplaced, stable, and without associated ligamentous injuries are typically managed with cast immobilization for approximately 6 to 10 weeks. The type of cast remains controversial. Many continue to include the thumb in the cast; however, some research suggests that immobilization of the thumb is unnecessary for CT- or MRI-monitored fractures.[38] Nondisplaced proximal pole fractures require 6 weeks in a long arm thumb spica cast (to prevent forearm rotation) followed by at least 6 weeks in a short arm thumb spica cast.[39] Although conservative treatment avoids potential surgical complications, prolonged periods of immobilization are associated with increased stiffness, muscle atrophy, and a delay in the resumption of activities of daily living.[40] As a result, percutaneous fixation using cannulated screws has been utilized for some nondisplaced fractures, allowing for faster healing, earlier mobilization, and faster return to function.[41]

Fractures that are displaced, comminuted, and associated with soft-tissue injuries are reduced and surgically stabilized to prevent malunion and nonunion. Various surgical techniques exist, but ORIF with compression screw is the most common approach.[42] Surgery is followed by 2 weeks of cast immobilization, then initiation of active range of motion (AROM) using a thumb spica orthosis for support between exercises. Bone graft is reserved for fractures that are significantly displaced, sclerotic, or have not united as expected.[43] Longer periods of postoperative immobilization are required when bone grafting is involved.

> ### ❓ *Questions to Ask the Doctor*
>
> **Scaphoid Fractures**
>
> - What is the location of the scaphoid fracture – proximal, waist, or distal pole?
> - Should the thumb be included in the postcast orthosis? If so, should the interphalangeal (IP) joint be free?
> - Were there any known concomitant ligamentous injuries?
> - For the postoperative client, what type of fixation was used? Was a bone graft used?
> - What precautions are there for initiating exercise/strengthening following conservative/surgical management?

Other Carpal Fractures

Diagnosis and Pathology

Fractures sustained to the remaining seven carpal bones are exceedingly rare in comparison to scaphoid fractures.

The **triquetrum** is a small pyramid-shaped bone found adjacent to the lunate in the proximal carpal row. Triquetrum fractures can occur with compression between the hamate and ulnar styloid, avulsion from numerous ligament attachments, or perilunate fracture dislocations involving significant injury to the lunotriquetral interval ligament.[44]

The **trapezium** is located between the scaphoid and the base of the first metacarpal. This highly mobile carpal bone plays an integral role in thumb movement, so fracture detection and treatment is paramount in restoring pinch and grip function. Fractures usually occur due to a direct blow to the hand or from a FOOSH injury, and clients typically complain of point tenderness at the base of the thumb and pain with pinching.[45]

Fractures to the hook of the **hamate** occur more frequently than fractures to the body of the hamate.[45] Sudden axial loads, such as with a direct blow to the palm, can fracture the hamate body. Hook of hamate fractures are frequently associated with the forceful swing of a hammer, bat, or golf club resulting in an avulsion fracture.[44] In addition to acute tenderness over the hook, clients may report discomfort with resisted motion of the fourth and fifth digits and paresthesia in the ulnar nerve distribution.[46] Hook of hamate fractures may be complicated by symptomatic nonunion or avascular necrosis due to its tenuous blood supply.[47]

The crescent-shaped **lunate** is an integral component of wrist motion. Fractures typically occur from a FOOSH injury where the capitate is driven into the lunate. Careful assessment of the attaching scapholunate (SL) and lunotriquetral (LT) ligaments is crucial as their integrity can affect carpal stability (see Chapter 22). When fractured, the lunate is susceptible to avascular necrosis due to its limited blood supply at the palmar pole.[48] Lunate fractures are associated with **Kienbock's disease.** While the actual cause remains unclear, Kienbock's disease is a pathological process whereby blood flow to the lunate is compromised, progressing to bone death and carpal collapse.[49]

Volar to the triquetrum is the pea-sized **pisiform** bone. Comminuted fractures typically result from a direct blow to the hypothenar eminence, while an avulsion fracture may occur with forceful contraction of the flexor carpi ulnaris.[46] Acute pain over the pisiform is the primary symptom. The pisiform also forms the ulnar border of Guyon's canal, so clients may also present with ulnar nerve dysfunction.

Isolated fractures to the **trapezoid** and **capitate** are infrequent and usually the result of a FOOSH injury or high-velocity axial load through the second and third metacarpals. These fractures are often associated with perilunate dislocations, carpometacarpal (CMC) joint dislocation, or fractures to nearby carpals.[45] The capitate presents with a tenuous blood supply, leaving it vulnerable to avascular necrosis.[47]

Treatment Options for Other Carpal Fractures

The degree of fracture displacement, blood supply, and the presence of concomitant injuries are factors that help determine the management of carpal fractures. Due to ligament injuries commonly associated with carpal fractures, the primary goal of treatment is not only to restore bony alignment but to also ensure ligamentous stability. Conservative management of small avulsion or minimally displaced carpal fractures with good blood supply includes short arm cast immobilization for 4 to 6 weeks. This typically applies to trapezium, trapezoid, pisiform, lunate, and triquetral fractures.[44,46,47,50] Due to their tenuous blood supply, fractures of the capitate and hamate may be casted for periods ranging from 6 to 12 weeks or longer.[46,47] Surgical stabilization with percutaneous pins, ORIF, or compression screws is an option for displaced and unstable fractures. Repair or reconstruction of the surrounding ligaments is sometimes required to restore carpal stability. In the event of severe comminution and chronic pain, bone grafting, partial fusion, or proximal row carpectomy may be necessary.[44]

Potential Complications Following ALL Carpal Fractures

Carpal fractures are vulnerable to numerous complications. Individuals who seek treatment within 4 weeks have improved union rates and outcomes.[39] If proper treatment is delayed, disastrous complications can result. Displaced fractures with associated ligamentous injury can progress from malalignment to carpal instability to posttraumatic arthritis. For example, a malaligned scaphoid fracture demonstrating a *humpback deformity* (volar angulation of the distal fragment) with an associated scapholunate (SL) ligament injury can develop **scapholunate advanced collapse (SLAC).** A scaphoid fracture nonunion will place stress on the radioscaphoid articulation and progress to **scaphoid nonunion advanced collapse (SNAC)** arthritis[51] In advanced cases of posttraumatic arthritis, distal scaphoid excision, pisiform excision, proximal row carpectomy, or total wrist fusion may be necessary to reduce pain and restore function.[52]

Due to the close proximity of the ulnar and median nerves to the pisiform, hamate, and trapezium, paresthesia can occur with acute fractures or following surgery. Symptoms usually resolve over time, but if marked intrinsic weakness or chronic sensory deficit develops, a pisiformectomy and carpal tunnel release are indicated.[44,46]

Tendinopathy of the flexor digitorum profundus and flexor carpi radialis and potential attritional rupture of these tendons due to rubbing on fracture fragments can result following hook of hamate and trapezial fractures, respectively.[44,53]

Assessment of Wrist Fractures

Indications for referral to hand therapy at the acute phase of healing (0 to 6 weeks following injury or surgery) are the presence of moderate to severe edema, poor finger motion, concerns regarding elbow or shoulder motion, initiation of early wrist range of motion (ROM) following rigid fixation, and/or management of function while in the cast. If an individual is managing quite well in the acute phase, they will usually be referred in the subacute period once the cast has been removed (at approximately 6 weeks).

A thorough evaluation is crucial to treatment planning and provides a baseline for comparison when using outcome measures. Client-specific information such as age, hand dominance, occupation, and avocational activities should be noted. Injury-specific information should be obtained, such as the date and mechanism of injury and the date and details of surgery. A review of the medical record, including radiographs, will detail bony alignment, type of reduction, stability, and soft-tissue involvement. Note the client's current health and medication use as well as previous injuries to the upper extremity. Assess the client's psychosocial status to gain an understanding of how they are coping. Observe for challenges with cognition or preexisting diagnoses that will alter the individual's ability to follow through with instruction. The evaluation tips below outline factors to consider and suggests areas to evaluate upon initial assessment of an individual with a wrist fracture.

Client-rated outcome measurement tools are an essential component of the evaluation process. They provide objective data to evaluate return to normal function, help validate what we do as therapists, and assist the client in judging their progress. Chapter 5 provides an overview of functional outcomes measures appropriate for use with wrist fractures.

Evaluation Tips

- Observe how the client holds their injured extremity throughout the interview. Do they appear comfortable, willing to participate, and relaxed, or do they appear in pain, guarded, and protective of their extremity? Some may arrive with a sling or pillow that keeps their injured arm in an internally rotated and flexed position. How they carry or rest their injured arm may contribute to assessment findings and recommendations.
- Observe and compare sympathetic changes with the noninjured wrist/hand including vasomotor (temperature, color, swelling), sudomotor (decreased or excessive sweating), pilomotor (absence of "goosebumps"), and trophic (skin texture, nail and hair growth) differences. Also note any muscle wasting, incisions, scars, rashes and bruising. If needed, draw pictures or take photographs to document findings.
- Rate pain at rest and with activity using a simple client-reported single-dimensional scale such as Visual Analog Scale, Numeric Rating Scale,[54] or Faces Pain Scale-Revised,[55] or a multidimensional scale such as the McGill Pain Questionnaire.[56]
- Perform a global ROM assessment of the client's shoulder and elbow to highlight any areas of limitation. Occasionally, less significant proximal injuries or secondary complications can be overlooked during the assessment of distal upper extremity injuries. Measure AROM and passive range of motion (PROM) goniometrically as needed.
- If edema is present while in the cast, descriptive terms such as mild, moderate, and severe, or pitting versus brawny, can be used subjectively. Circumferential finger girth measurements provide for objective measurements, if needed. Once the cast is removed, the American Society of Hand Therapists recommends measuring with the figure-of-eight method.[57] This technique measures hand size using a tape measure wrapped circumferentially in a prescribed method around the wrist and hand. Alternatively, perform volumetric measurements if no cast/pins/external fixation devices are present. As therapy progresses, measure edema both pre- and postexercise to help guide rehab progression.
- Perform sensory testing if indicated. The Semmes-Weinstein monofilaments can screen for a nerve compression. However, this test is often time consuming. Alternatively, the Ten Test,

as first described by Strauch,[58] is quick to administer, requires no equipment, and demonstrates excellent validity.
- Assess/describe the wound and scar following an open injury or postsurgical case. Wound and scar presentation is typically assessed using a therapist's description of properties including: size, depth, profile, discharge, color, adherence, and sensitivity. Validated wound and scar scales exist to evaluate parameters; however, assessment time is often limited so therapist descriptions are often relied on for efficiency purposes.
- Measure isolated finger A/PROM as pain, surgery, edema, and lack of exercise while immobilized can contribute to reduced motion. Inadequate casting techniques can also poorly position the digits and limit ROM (e.g., volar portion of the cast extends to far distally, limiting full metacarpophalangeal flexion). Assess composite finger motion as well as the presence of intrinsic or capsular tightness. A quick method of documenting finger ROM is to measure the distance from the tip of the flexed finger to the distal palmar crease and opposition of the thumb across the hand.
- Evaluate the integrity of the extensor pollicis longus tendon by placing the client's hand palm down on the table. Ask them to raise and hold their extended thumb off the tabletop. If they are unable to do this, determine whether adhesions limit this action or query rupture of the tendon.
- If able, measure isolated wrist and forearm AROM (flexion, extension, radial and ulnar deviation, pronation, supination) as well as combined wrist/digit AROM in both extension and flexion to determine the presence of extrinsic tightness.
- Once the physician has noted sufficient bone healing and the client's swelling and pain allows, evaluate grip and pinch strength using a Jamar dynamometer and pinch gauge. In addition, the push-off test is a valid and reliable test used to quantify weight-bearing ability through the palm.[59]

Rehabilitation of Distal Radius and Carpal Fractures

The goal of rehabilitation following any wrist fracture is to maximize functional recovery of the upper extremity. However, some debate exists surrounding the efficacy of supervised hand therapy involvement versus the performance of a home exercise program (HEP) following wrist fracture. Some studies have indicated that it is possible for most clients to do just as well on their own without the ongoing guidance of a hand therapist.[60-62] Other studies have found that a supervised therapy program is more effective for improving function and pain when compared to a HEP.[63] Despite controversy in the literature, need for formal therapy exists. The client's experience with therapy support throughout the entire process cannot be discounted.

One of the most important roles the hand therapist has is teaching the client that they are a partner in the rehabilitation process. Clients must understand the importance of adhering to the prescribed HEP. This program will be performed by the client between therapy visits. It should be modified on a regular basis as the client progresses. The initial HEP often includes ROM exercises, edema control techniques, pain management strategies, use of orthoses, and guidelines for participation in functional activities. Therapists should ensure the client understands the instructions. Return demonstration, use of instruction sheets, and video (on the client's own cellphone) recording the client performing their exercises may help with performance and adherence to the HEP.[64]

Treatment Guidelines

The following therapy treatment guidelines are divided into acute and subacute phases to assist in clinical reasoning during rehabilitation of distal radius and carpal fractures. Clinical decision making for each client is individualized and many variables will influence the progression through the stages.

Acute Phase (0–6 weeks)

Immobilization is common following wrist fracture. The period of immobilization can lead to deleterious effects such as loss of muscle strength, decreased motion, impairment of fine motor function, and eventual representational loss in the motor and sensory cortex.[65] Unfortunately, less than 10% of clients are referred to therapy in the acute phase.[66] This low referral rate may contribute to the development of complications that could otherwise be avoided. Ideally, clients treated with casts, external fixators, or ORIFs will be referred to hand therapy within the first week of casting or surgery.

Cast/Orthotic Use

A primary goal during the acute phase is protection of the healing fracture. The client should have a properly fitting cast. A cast that is too tight may contribute to edema or other complications such as complex regional pain syndrome.[67] The client with an ORIF of the distal radius will need a wrist orthosis for protection following surgery. It is important that any orthosis be well fitting and comfortable or it will contribute to further pain and swelling.

Edema Management

Stiffness starts with edema. Edema is a natural by-product of trauma, and the development of some edema following injury and surgery is normal and expected. However, moderate to severe swelling that persists is the silent enemy, as it will infiltrate every tissue and alter the normal gliding of joints and tendons. Over time, there can be increased collagen formation and progression from moveable edema to more fibrous protein-rich edema that ultimately turns to scar tissue. This dense edema can take months to resolve and is the foundation of all stiffness. Adaptive shortening also plays a role in stiffness. Tissues that are not allowed to move to length will naturally shorten.

Early management of edema is essential. Edema is constantly laying the groundwork for scar, and time spent managing edema in this early phase will save the client and therapist several hours of work and frustration down the road. AROM, elevation, cold application, compression, and lymphatic drainage are all used to manage edema[68] (see Chapter 8).

♡ **Tips From the Field**

Edema Management

The following tips will assist with edema reduction in the acute phase.

Active range of motion (AROM): AROM of all available joints while in the cast, orthosis, or external fixator is vital to edema control and to maintaining tissue length. AROM acts as a pump mobilizing edema through the lymphatic system.

Elevation: Elevation uses gravity to assist venous and lymphatic return from the extremity to the heart, and can be effective in the early stages of healing. Ensure the elbow and hand are held at a level higher than the heart. Positioning the arm across the chest does not allow the proper gradient for edema reduction, and the flexed elbow position blocks venous and lymphatic return. The shoulder needs to be placed in a slightly elevated/abducted position to allow drainage of the full extremity.

Precaution. *If upper extremity arterial insufficiency is a concern, elevation should not be used, as this position will compromise blood flow to the affected limb.*

Cold: Cold application causes local vasoconstriction of vessels and can be beneficial to edema control during the acute phase. Cold also helps with pain management for many clients.

Compression: Low-grade compression in the form of edema gloves, Coban wraps, elasticized compression bandages, or other compressive wraps can be used to limit the space available for swelling in the acute phase.[68]

Manual edema mobilization (MEM): These techniques promote drainage and can be very beneficial for individuals following wrist fractures.[69] MEM is a specialized skill that requires formal training, but therapists who learn the techniques have another tool to aid in the reduction of edema.

Range of Motion

Clients should be instructed in a program of active (and passive, if needed) ROM exercise to all noninjured joints in the affected upper extremity, including the shoulder, elbow, and fingers. Many individuals avoid finger motion for fear of disrupting healing at the wrist level. Educate the client that finger ROM helps reduce edema, encourages tendon excursion, promotes the maintenance of tissue length, and improves overall outcomes following wrist fracture.[70] Clients should be encouraged to move the fingers through their full available range for maximum benefit in preventing finger stiffness. Simply "wiggling" the fingers does very little to preserve tissue length.

Active wrist ROM following stable distal radius ORIF can be initiated as early as 7 to 10 days postsurgery, whereas wrist motion must be delayed until the cast is removed (at approximately 6 weeks) in the case of closed treatment.[71] Gentle passive ROM of the wrist can be added with ORIF if the client is particularly stiff, the reduction is solid, the surgeon is consulted, and pain and swelling are under control.

Individual finger blocking exercises at the interphalangeal (IP) joints will promote differential gliding of the flexor digitorum superficialis (FDS), flexor digitorum profundus (FDP), and flexor pollicus longus. These exercises are particularly important in the case of volar plating. Exercises to promote gliding of extensor tendons are important following dorsal plating. Isolated extensor digitorum communis excursion can be performed by going from a full composite fist in flexion to a hook fist. Hook fist will also allow FDS and FDP excursion and work on intrinsic tightness.

External fixation presents its own set of challenges for ROM. The points of contact of the external fixator on the metacarpals can cause pain with motion exercises. This pain needs to be respected, but ROM exercises are encouraged. In all wrist immobilization scenarios gentle PROM to the digits can be gradually progressed if pain and swelling allow.

ROM exercises may cause a mild increase in discomfort and swelling when performed, but this should resolve within an hour.

The client should be encouraged to work at their exercises using a slow and steady approach rather than an aggressive painful approach. Exercise dosing is dependent on the complexities of the injury as well as external and internal factors that vary across clients.[72] However, most clients do well with 5 to 10 repetitions of each exercise performed 5 times per day. Instruct the client to hold stretches for at least 5 seconds to give tissues time to stretch.

Pain Management

Pain control is essential at all stages of rehabilitation, but it is crucial during the acute phase when proper management can reduce the client's long-term disability level[73] and risk for CRPS. Clients participate better in their therapy program if pain is controlled. Use of pain medication (as prescribed by the physician), ice, heat (if edema is resolving), contrast baths, and graded motor imagery (GMI)[74,75] can assist with pain management.

Wound Management and Scar Desensitization

Wounds and pin sites must be properly managed to prevent infection (see Chapters 17 and 31).

Scar massage should be initiated when pink scar tissue is present. Scar tissue can feel thick and may cause decreased mobility by adhering to underlying tissues. Scars may be numb, hypersensitive to touch, or painful. Clients should massage scar with unscented lotion using circular motions and enough pressure to challenge the tissue. This will mobilize the scar tissue and desensitize the area. Scar massage can be performed 2 to 3 times per day for approximately 5 minutes. Graded desensitization techniques can be used if scar is hypersensitive.

Use of Orthoses to Address Adherence and Tissue Shortening

Volar plate fixation can lead to extrinsic flexor tightness, as the application of the plate involves separation of flexor tendons. Teaching the client to actively glide flexor tendons and passively stretch the flexors helps reduce this tightness. Also, progressive thermoplastic volar hand orthosis use with the fingers in comfortable extension helps (Fig. 21.8). The orthosis can be used at night when fingers would normally sit in flexion and further contribute to tightness. Dorsal plating can cause the extrinsic extensor tendons to become tethered as a result of scar tissue from the surgical procedure. This presents as decreased ability to actively extend the digits, resulting in the fingers resting in a flexed position. A volar orthosis can also be used in this situation to support the digits in extension and decrease the development of flexor tightness.

Functional Use

During the acute phase, lifting and carrying is usually limited to 1 to 2 pounds (0.5–1 kg), and no weight bearing is allowed on the extremity. Light functional use of the arm and hand is permitted and encouraged, but overuse may cause increased pain and swelling, which may interfere with the client's ability to perform ROM exercises.

Strengthening

Strengthening is not initiated in the acute phase, as bony healing has not progressed to allow force through the bone. Strengthening during this phase can cause mechanical failure of plates and/or loss of fracture alignment.

Precaution. *Bone healing following an ORIF does not progress any faster than with other forms of fracture management. The presence of a plate does not allow heavier function or strengthening in the*

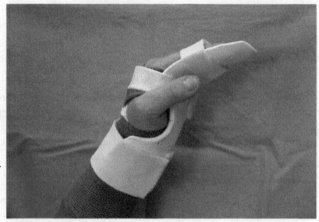

FIG. 21.8 A thermoplastic volar orthosis can be molded over a forearm cast in an effort to treat extrinsic digital flexor tightness. Courtesy of Emily Seeley.

acute phase. The bone beneath the plate needs time to strengthen. Too much stress in the early phase of healing can cause the metal plate to bend or break.

Subacute Phase: 6 Weeks and Beyond
Cast/Orthotic Use

During the subacute phase, the client may be fitted with a wrist orthosis. The primary goal of the orthosis is to support the soft tissues and encourage the wrist to remain in extension to facilitate finger motion. The orthosis is typically worn during the performance of heavier tasks, at night, and when out in public. A custom thermoplastic orthosis can be remolded into increasing wrist extension as a method of serial static splinting, if needed. Gradual decrease in orthosis utilization is progressed over time as pain decreases and motion and strength improve.

Edema Management

Persistent edema past 6 weeks is generally fibrotic and will take weeks to resolve. Edema can be treated as outlined in the acute phase, but elevation will not be as beneficial for more fibrotic, high-protein edema. Manual edema mobilization can be beneficial for this type of chronic edema. Compression can be used to soften fibrotic edema and is often helpful for edema management in this phase.

Range of Motion

In the case of ORIF, wrist ROM will likely have started as early as the first week post surgery. Clients with a cast, pin(s), or external fixator will usually be allowed to begin wrist ROM upon removal of these devices. Wrist ROM should be added to the home program progressing through flexion/extension, radial and ulnar deviation, and forearm rotation. More powerful wrist flexors will try to override extensors during grip. Focusing on isolated wrist extension and maintaining extension while gripping is important.

◎ Clinical Pearl

Upon starting wrist ROM, clients often compensate for weak wrist extensors by using the finger extensors (extensor digitorum communis) to perform active wrist extension. Instruct clients to isolate the primary wrist extensors by making a fist when performing active wrist extension exercises.

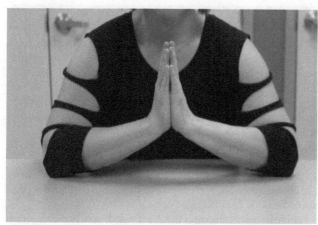

FIG. 21.9 This prayer stretch can be performed to address extrinsic flexor tightness and stretch the wrist joint. Palms of the hands are placed together, and the elbows are slowly moved apart from each other order to increase the stretch. Courtesy of Emily Seeley and Lesley Von Dehn.

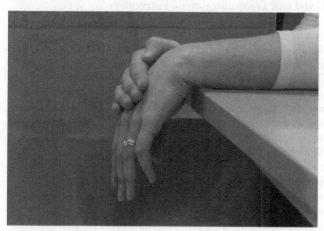

FIG. 21.10 Passive wrist flexion. The forearm of the affected wrist is placed on the table for stability while the other hand passively flexes the wrist over the edge Courtesy of Emily Seeley and Lesley Von Dehn.

PROM exercises can be added to the program when pain and swelling are controlled and X-ray confirms adequate bone healing. If in doubt, confirm with the physician. Teach clients to stretch gently and to hold the stretch for 30 seconds. Prolonged gentle stretching promotes scar remodeling and elongation of tissues. Aggressive stretching will cause further microtears and lead to increased stiffness.

Many passive stretch exercises exist. The prayer position (Fig. 21.9) promotes wrist extension and the stretching of the long flexors. Wrist flexion can be stretched by placing the forearm over a table and manually flexing the wrist with the other hand (Fig. 21.10). Supination and pronation can be stretched using a towel (Fig. 21.11) or hammer held in the hand, as long as ulnar wrist pain does not increase. Additionally, therapists trained in manual joint mobilization techniques can perform these in therapy sessions, as manual mobilization can be beneficial in restoring ROM to the challenging wrist.

Preconditioning tissues with moist heat prior to ROM exercises can be beneficial, as this promotes tissue extensibility and helps make stretching more comfortable for the client. The use of heat can be initiated if edema is resolving.[76]

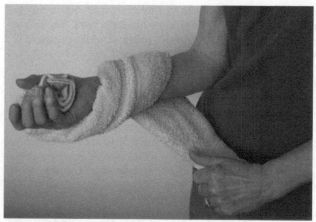

FIG. 21.11 Supination can be stretched using a towel. Pronation can be stretched by reversing the direction. *(From Moscony AMB, Shank T. Wrist fractures. In: Cooper C. ed.* Fundamentals of Hand Therapy. *2nd ed. St. Louis, Elsevier; 2014, p. 329.)*

Pain Management

A mild increase in pain may occur as new exercises are introduced and as function increases, but this pain should be easily managed with activity modification and rest. More intense pain that persists into the subacute phase is concerning and may indicate CRPS. Therapeutic strategies used for pain management at this stage include ice, moist heat application, contrast baths, graded motor imagery, and electrical modalities such as transcutaneous electrical nerve stimulation (TENS).

Scar Management and Desensitization

Scar massage and desensitization should continue as outlined in the acute phase. Occasionally, painful neuromas can develop in this phase and will need to be addressed by the physician.

Use of Orthoses to Address Adherence and Tissue Shortening

Some motions can be difficult to achieve following a wrist fracture. Supination and wrist extension are often the most limited motions, but this varies among clients. When the traditional methods of stretching do not improve range to a functional level and progress has plateaued, dynamic and static progressive splinting should be considered. These mobilization orthoses use the concept of total end-range time (TERT) to elongate tissues. This concept is based on the principle that the longer a tissue is held at its maximum tolerable end-range ("low-load prolonged stretch"), the more the range will improve over time.[77] Chapter 7 presents information on orthoses.

Functional Use

Encourage clients to progress upper extremity functional use, as tolerated, in the subacute stage and provide functional adaptation as required. Most clients require guidance to avoid overuse and the risk of persistent joint pain and tendonitis during this phase.

What to Say to Clients

About Returning to Activity

"Now that the bone is healing and you are moving your wrist, you can gradually resume normal activities. Start with tasks that are important to you, because your tolerance for function may be limited in the beginning. Gradually add heavier tasks. Any activity that causes significant and persistent pain and swelling needs to be avoided until you are better able to tolerate it."

Strengthening

Strengthening is usually started around 8 to 10 weeks dependent on pain, swelling, and progression of bony healing. If in doubt, confirm with the physician. Isometric exercises should be introduced first, followed by open kinetic chain exercises, and then closed chain exercises. Open chain exercises are those that allow the distal part to move (grip strengthening, wrist curls, and forearm rotation with a weight). Grip strengthening is often started with a sponge ball or therapy putty. Wrist curls are started using a one-pound (0.5-kg) weight. Home programs for strengthening are usually carried out every other day using sets with enough repetition to fatigue muscles. Closed kinetic chain exercises where the distal extremity remains fixed (such as wall push-ups and pull-ups) can be added as strength improves; however, these strengthening exercises may not be appropriate for all clients.

For the elderly client with low functional demands, functional daily activities will gradually improve strength without the need for any formal strengthening program at all.

Precaution. *Grip strengthening should be performed with caution when there is a known/suspected SL ligament tear or TFCC injury. Gripping, especially in pronation, places increased load on both the SL ligament and TFCC, which can contribute to further aggravation of these structures.*

Wrist Sensorimotor Impairment and Rehabilitation

Grip strength and AROM are two of the most frequently reported deficits following distal radius fractures (DRF).[78] However, a growing field of research is attempting to understand how wrist sensorimotor (SM) dysfunction following trauma can also impact functional outcomes.[79] The SM system integrates peripheral afferent signals (from receptors in skin, ligaments, and muscles) within the central nervous system (CNS) to provide proprioceptive information about the wrist joint during functional use.[80] Soft tissue trauma and pain following DRF can disrupt the generation and transmission of proprioceptive information and can lead to neuroplastic changes in the CNS.[81] This can alter processing of input and may result in SM dysfunction.[82] This deficit can be observed in the clinic as sensation and joint coordination problems, muscle strength or recruitment difficulty, and delayed functional return.

The active wrist joint position sense test is currently the most meaningful measure to assess conscious sensorimotor control after DRF.[83] However, strong evidence to support interventions is limited. Some promising methods for proprioception and joint sense training following DRF include manual techniques, mirror therapy, closed and open chain active wrist ROM exercises, isometric and isotonic exercises, perturbation training, and smartphone applications such as Tilt Maze and Labyrinth.[64,79] Further research is needed to substantiate the efficacy of SM training methods in order to guide future wrist rehabilitation paradigms.

Pediatric Wrist Fractures

The forearm is the most commonly fractured structure in children aged 0 to 19 years, and boys are twice as likely as girls to experience a fracture.[84,85] The bone of children is different from adult bone in many ways. One primary difference is the presence of the growth plate (also called the epiphyseal plate or physis). The growth plate allows longitudinal growth of long bones, and fractures in this area can lead to disruption of this process. Secondary ossification centers (areas in long bones where bone is being deposited) are also present, making it difficult to identify fractures.[86] A child's bone has a thicker periosteum and forms more abundant callus, and the younger the child, the greater propensity for bone remodeling.

Pediatric radius fractures can be divided into two categories dependent on location: physeal or extraphyseal. A Salter-Harris fracture is a **physeal fracture** (involves the epiphyseal plate). Type I and type II Salter-Harris fractures are less severe and are usually treated without complication using casting. Unstable complete fractures and intraarticular fractures (Salter-Harris type III and type IV) require surgical intervention.[87]

Extraphyseal fractures usually occur on the metaphysis and are categorized based on the amount of cortex involved. These include buckle, greenstick, and complete fractures.[87] **Buckle fractures** result from compression without cortical disruption. These fractures are stable and are usually casted or splinted for 3 weeks with good results.[88] **Greenstick fractures** result in disruption of the cortex on one side of the bone. They are managed with a cast for 4 to 6 weeks. These injuries can present with angulation and rotation and need to be monitored weekly to ensure alignment is maintained and that the fracture does not advance through both cortices. **Complete fractures** involve disruption of both cortices. Fractures of this nature are more complex and may require reduction with casting for 4 to 6 weeks. Fractures that cannot maintain reduction may require surgery.

The most commonly performed procedure for pediatric fractures is percutaneous pinning with avoidance of the physis (when possible). ORIF is rarely indicated for pediatric fractures, and the benefits must outweigh the risk of further physeal damage.[88] The ability of children's bone to remodel is remarkable. Pediatric fractures tolerate higher amounts of angulation, and malunions usually resolve over a period of 2 years in children who are at least 2 years from skeletal maturity.

Carpal fractures cannot occur until children reach adolescence because prior to this, carpal bones have their ossification centers surrounded by a spherical growth plate.[89] This growth plate protects the carpal bone from fracture until around puberty when the bone ratio is higher than cartilage.[90] Scaphoid fractures are the most common pediatric carpal fracture. Fractures of the other carpals are rare. Carpal fractures are typically casted for 4 to 6 weeks without complication. Unstable and comminuted carpal fractures can require surgical intervention.

The rehabilitation of pediatric distal radius and carpal fractures follows the same principles as the adult population. However, children recover much more quickly than their adult counterparts. Younger children may not even require therapy, as loss of range and function are typically minimal following casting. Because children are active and unpredictable, they risk reinjury immediately following cast removal and may come to hand therapy for a protective orthosis to wear for a few weeks.

Conclusion

The treatment of wrist fractures involves an understanding of normal anatomy, bone healing, and the methods used to restore the wrist and surrounding structures to acceptable anatomical congruency. New guidelines, surgical methods, and hardware are continually being developed with the goal of attaining improved alignment. These methods will continue to change the rehabilitation of wrist fractures. Therapy can be beneficial in the treatment of wrist fractures, especially where complications arise, but randomized studies evaluating the effectiveness of our strategies are needed.

CASE STUDY

Marie is a 53-year-old left hand dominant teacher who sustained a FOOSH injury while standing on a chair to hang a picture in her classroom. She immediately knew she had sustained a significant injury when she felt pain and saw the odd appearance of her wrist. She was taken to the hospital by her friend and assessed by the emergency room physician. She was diagnosed with a comminuted intraarticular fracture of the distal radius with radial shortening and extension into the radiocarpal and DRUJ. She was placed in plaster slab and wrap and referred to the local orthopedic surgeon. Upon seeing the surgeon a week later, she was told her forearm was too swollen to cast. She was placed in a second plaster slab and told to return for reassessment in 2 weeks.

Marie was concerned about her wrist position and the amount of time before the next appointment. She went to visit family in a larger city and had her family physician refer her to another hand surgeon there. The fracture was reevaluated and surgery was recommended. The surgeon stated the fracture had lost all normal alignment and without surgery she would have a malformed joint, significant pain, and loss of rotation. She underwent surgery 4 days later (now 11 days since her fall). A volar plate was placed and the alignment was restored as adequately as possible. She was casted and booked for follow-up with the surgeon 10 days later. She was referred to hand therapy due to concerns regarding swelling and stiffness.

At her hand therapy evaluation she presented with moderate edema, flexor tightness, and inability to extend the digits fully. She was unable to make a full composite fist; distance of the fingertips to the distal palmar crease with active motion was 2 to 3 cm in all fingers. Pain was reported as 4 out of 10 using the visual analog scale. Marie was very anxious as she was an artist and a flute player. She was eager to learn her home exercises and start her recovery. She was instructed in active and passive finger flexion and extension exercises. Passively, she was focusing on long flexor stretch holding fingers back in extension at all finger joints. She was completing passive composite finger flexion stretches along with individual FDP and FDS gliding exercises to allow pull through of digital flexors.

Active composite flexion was very challenging at this point due to adherence of flexors along the surgical path. Marie was encouraged to perform her exercises every 2 hours, with 10 repetitions, and end-range positions held for 5 seconds. The goal was to increase range without the negative effects of pain and swelling. A thermoplastic nighttime volar wrist/hand extension orthosis was molded over Marie's cast. This extension orthosis placed a stretch on the long flexors at night. Elevation was encouraged for edema control.

Marie attended her second therapy visit 10 days later following her visit with the surgeon. Cast and sutures had been removed and she was fitted with a removable wrist orthosis. New orders were sent to begin gentle wrist ROM. Wrist ROM was very limited with 5 degrees of flexion and 10 degrees of extension. Supination of the forearm was only to neutral. Marie was instructed to add gentle wrist AROM to her home program and to use ice for edema and pain control. She was also fitted with an edema glove to wear intermittently during the day. Her incision was well healed but moderately sensitive. Marie was told to begin scar massage for 5 minutes, 2 to 3 times a day. When she was sitting, Marie was to remove the orthosis and rub the scar with her fingers or on clothing to help decrease scar sensitivity.

On the next therapy visit, 2.5 weeks postsurgery, finger range was improving, edema was decreasing, but forearm rotation remained limited and wrist extension was poor. The surgeon was consulted to determine if gentle passive exercises could be initiated. The surgeon was pleased with fixation and allowed gentle PROM to the wrist and forearm (rotation). The volar wrist/hand orthosis was remolded to increase finger extension at each visit. Use of heat in the form of warm water soaks was also encouraged because edema was decreasing and even small increases in edema following heat would likely outweigh the benefits of increased extensibility and pain reduction.

As Marie progressed through the weeks, she continued to gain in all areas of motion and function; however, she continued to be limited in wrist extension. She started handling her flute and attempting to play simple notes. At the 6-week physician follow-up, an X-ray showed excellent progression of bony union. The surgeon sent orders to therapy stating he wanted more aggressive passive stretching. Marie was taught more aggressive passive stretches for wrist extension, flexion, supination, and pronation. She was instructed to perform stretches 4 times a day and to complete 5 repetitions, holding each stretch at a comfortable place for 30 seconds. She was told it was better to hold the stretch for 30 seconds comfortably than to stretch with pain for a few seconds.

Marie was instructed to remove the orthosis in the home for light activity, but to keep it on for heavier tasks. Gradually, range progressed to wrist flexion 45 degrees and extension 50 degrees. Full finger ROM was achieved and supination increased to 70 degrees. She was given the hammer stretch to use gravity to stretch into supination. Marie returned to work as a teacher at 8 weeks postsurgery with modified duties including no lifting or carrying greater than 5 lbs. At 10 weeks postsurgery Marie was not using her orthosis at all except at night. She was performing all her light daily tasks without difficulty, and swelling was resolved. Grip strength using the Jamar Dynamometer measured 10 lbs on the left and 40 lbs on the right. She was given grip strengthening using a foam ball and wrist extension curls using a 1-lb weight. She was told to complete 3 sets of 10 repetitions of each exercise every other day to fatigue. At this point, she also began simple painting and playing the flute for 20 to 30 minutes daily. Dexterity was improving.

At 15 weeks postsurgery, Marie was managing well with her home program and completing all duties at work with some wrist fatigue. She had increased to 2 lbs with the wrist curls. Grip strength measured 20 lbs on the left. There was no pain. ROM had increased to 55 degrees for flexion, 60 degrees extension, supination 80 degrees and pronation full. She continued to report morning stiffness so she was continuing her stretches three times daily. She was satisfied with her overall progress and planned to continue her home program and return to therapy for reassessment and discharge in 1 month.

References

1. Mirhadi S, et al.: Factors influencing fracture healing, *Trauma1* 5(2):140–155, 2013.
2. Clark B: Normal bone anatomy and physiology, *Clin J Am Soc Nephrol* 3(Suppl 3):S131–S139, 2008.
3. Thompson J: *Netter's concise orthopaedic anatomy*, Philadelphia, 2010, Saunders/Elsevier, pp 142–149.
4. Einhorn TA, Gerstenfeld LC: Fracture healing: mechanisms and interventions, *Nat Rev Rheumatol* 11(1):45–54, 2015.
5. Marsell R, Einhorn TA: The biology of fracture healing, *Injury* 42(6):551–555, 2011.
6. Loi F, et al.: Inflammation, fracture and bone repair, *Bone* 86:119–130, 2016.
7. Smith DW, et al.: Early active rehabilitation for operatively stabilized distal radius fractures, *J Hand Ther* 17(1):43–49, 2004.
8. Lichtman DM, et al.: Treatment of distal radius fractures, *J Am Acad Orthop Surg* 18:180–189, 2010.
9. Altman E: The ulnar side of the wrist: clinically relevant anatomy and biomechanics, *J Hand Ther* 29(2):111–122, 2016.
10. MacIntyre NJ, Dewan N: Epidemiology of distal radius fractures and factors predicting risk and prognosis, *J Hand Ther*(29)136–145, 2016.
11. Maheshwari J: Chapter 15: injuries of the forearm and wrist. In Maheshwari J, editor: *essential orthopedics*, ed 4, New Delhi: India, 2011, Jaypee Brothers Medical Publishers Ltd, pp 108–116.
12. Medoff RJ: Distal radius fractures classification and management. In Skirven T, et al.: *Rehabilitation of the hand and upper extremity*, ed 6, Philadelphia, 2011, Elsevier, pp 941–948.
13. Baruah RK: Immobilisation of extra-articular distal radius fractures (Colles type) in dorsiflexion. The functional and anatomical outcome, *J Clin Orthop Trauma* 6(3):167–172, 2015.
14. Abe Y, et al.: Management of intra-articular distal radius fractures: volar or dorsal locking plate—which has fewer complications? *Hand* 12(6):561–567, 2017.
15. Imatani J, Akita K: Volar distal radius anatomy applied to the treatment of distal radius fracture, *J Wrist Surg* 6(3):174–177, 2017.
16. Beerthuizen A, et al.: Demographic and medical parameters in the development of complex regional pain syndrome type 1(CRPS 1): prospective study on 596 patients with a fracture, *Pain* 153:1187–1192, 2012.
17. Jellad A, et al.: Complex regional pain syndrome type I: incidence and risk factors in patients with fracture of the distal radius, *Arch Phys Med Rehabil* 95(3):487–492, 2014.
18. Savas, et al.: Risk factors for complex regional pain syndrome in patients with surgically treated traumatic injuries attending hand therapy, *J Hand Ther* 31(2):250–254, 2018.
19. Patterson RW, et al.: Complex regional pain syndrome of the upper extremity, *J Hand Surg Am* 36(9):155–162, 2011.
20. Mauck BM, Swigler CW: Evidence-based review of distal radius fractures, *Orthop Clin N Am* 49(2):211–222, 2018.
21. Mulders MA: Corrective osteotomy is an effective method of treating distal radius malunions with good long-term functional results, *Injury* 48(3):731–737, 2017.
22. Sammer DM, Rizzo M: Ulnar impaction, *Hand Clin* 26:549, 2010.
23. Barbaric, et al.: Ulnar shortening osteotomy after distal radius malunion: review of literature, *Open Orthop J* 15(9):98–106, 2015.
24. Lindau T, et al.: Intraarticular lesions in distal fractures of the radius in young adults. A descriptive arthroscopic study in 50 patients, *J Hand Surg Br* 22:638–643, 1997.
25. Forward DP, et al.: Intercarpal ligament injuries associated with fractures of the distal part of the radius, *J Bone Jt Surg* 89(11):2334–2340, 2007.
26. Azzi AJ: Tendon rupture and tenosynovitis following internal fixation of distal radius fractures: a systematic review, *Plast Reconstr Surg* 139(3):717e–724e, 2017.
27. Rhee PC, et al.: Avoiding and treating perioperative complications of distal radius fractures, *Hand Clin* 28(2):185–198, 2012.
28. Patel VP, Paksima N: Complications of distal radius fracture fixation, *Bull NYU Hosp Jt Dis* 68(2):112–118, 2012.
29. Dyer G, et al.: Predictors of acute carpal tunnel syndrome associated with fracture of the distal radius, *J Hand Surg Am* 33(8):1309–1313, 2008.
30. Sammer DM, Chung KC: Management of distal radioulnar joint and ulnar styloid fracture, *Hand Clin* 28(2):199–206, 2012.
31. Logan AJ, Lindau TR: Management of distal ulnar fractures—a review of the literature and recommendations for treatment, *Strat Traum Limb Recon* 3:49–56, 2008.
32. Rettig AC, Kollias SC: Internal fixation of acute stable scaphoid fractures in the athlete, *Am J Sports Med* 24(2):182–186, 1996.
33. Dell PC, et al.: Management of carpal fractures and dislocations. In Skirven T, et al.: *Rehabilitation of the hand and upper extremity*, ed 6, Philadelphia, 2011, Elsevier, pp 988–1001.
34. Grover R: Clinical assessment of scaphoid injuries and the detection of fractures, *J Hand Surg Br* 21(3):324–327, 1996.
35. Bhat M, et al.: MRI and plain radiography in the assessment of displaced fractures of the waist of the carpal scaphoid, *J Bone Jt Surg* 86:705–713, 2004.
36. Adams JE, Steinmann SP: Acute scaphoid fractures, *Hand Clin* 26(1):97–103, 2010.
37. Brach P, Goitz R: An update on the management of carpal fractures, *J Hand Ther* 16(2):152–160, 2003.
38. Buijze G, et al.: Cast Immobilization with and without immobilization of the thumb for nondisplaced and minimally displaced scaphoid waist fractures: a multicenter randomized, controlled trial, *J Hand Surg Am* 39(4):621–627, 2014.
39. Gelberman RH, Menon J: The vascularity of the scaphoid bone, *J Hand Surg Am* 5:508–513, 1980.
40. Arsalan-Werner A, et al.: Current concepts for the treatment of acute scaphoid fractures, *Eur J Trauma Emerg Surg* 42:3–10, 2016.
41. McQueen MM, et al.: Percutaneous screw fixation versus conservative treatment for fractures of the waist of the scaphoid: A prospective randomised study, *J Bone Jt Surg* 90B:66–71, 2008.
42. Dias JJ, et al.: Clinical and radiological outcome of cast immobilization versus surgical treatment of acute scaphoid fractures at a mean follow up of 93 months, *J Bone Joint Surg Br* 90(7):899–905, 2008.
43. Hirche C, et al.: Vascularized versus non-vascularized bone grafts in the treatment of scaphoid non-union: a clinical outcome study with therapeutic algorithm, *J Ortho Surg* 25(1):1–6, 2017.
44. Pan T, et al.: Uncommon carpal fractures, *Eur J Trauma Emerg Surg* 42:15–27, 2016.
45. Suh N, et al.: Carpal fractures, *J Hand Surg Am* 39(4):785–791, 2014.
46. O'Shea K, Weiland AJ: Fractures of the hamate and pisiform bones, *Hand Clin* 28(3):287–300, 2012.
47. Urch EY, Lee SK: Carpal fractures other than scaphoid, *Clin Sports Med* 34:51–67, 2015.
48. Beckenbaugh RD, et al.: Keinbock's disease: The natural history of Kienbock's disease and consideration of lunate fractures, *Clin Orthop Relat Res* 149:98–106, 1980.
49. Wollstein R et al: A therapy protocol for the treatment of lunate overload or early Kienbock's disease, *J Hand Ther* 26(3):255–260.
50. Sin CH, et al.: Non-union of the triquetrum with pseudoarthrosis: a case report, *J Orthop Surg* 20(1):105–107, 2012.
51. Shah CM, Stern PJ: Scapholunate advanced collapse (SLAC) and scaphoid nonunion advanced collapse (SNAC) wrist arthritis, *Curr Rev Musculoskelet Med* 6:9–17, 2013.
52. Gupta V, et al.: Managing scaphoid fractures. How we do it? *J Clin Orthop Trauma* 4:3–10, 2013.
53. Milek MA, Boulas HJ: Flexor tendon ruptures secondary to hamate hook fractures, *J Hand Surg Am* 15(5):740–744, 1990.
54. Scudds RA: Pain outcome measures, *J Hand Ther* 14(2):86–90, 2001.
55. Hicks CL, et al.: The faces pain scale-revised: toward a common metric in pediatric pain measurement, *Pain* 93(2):173–183, 2001.
56. Melzack R: The McGill pain questionnaire: major properties and scoring methods, *Pain* 1(3):277–299, 1975.

57. Maihafer GC, et al.: A comparison of the figure-of-eight-method and water volumetry in measurement of the hand and wrist size, *J Hand Ther* 16(4):305–310, 2003.
58. Strauch B, et al.: The ten test, *Plast Reconstr Surg* 99(4):1074–1078, 1997.
59. Vincent JI, et al.: The push-off test: Development of a simple, reliable test of upper extremity weight-bearing capability, *J Hand Ther* 27(3):185–191, 2014.
60. Krischak GD, et al.: Physiotherapy after volar plating of wrist fractures is effective using a home exercise program, *Arch Phys Med Rehabil* 90(4):537–544, 2009.
61. Souer JS, et al.: A prospective randomized controlled trial comparing occupational therapy with independent exercises after volar plate fixation of a fracture of the distal part of the radius, *Bone Joint Surg Am* 93(19):1761–1766, 2011.
62. Valdes K, et al.: Therapist supervised clinic-based therapy versus instruction in a home program following distal radius fracture: a systematic review, *J Hand Ther* 27(3):165–173, 2014.
63. Gutierrez-Espinoza H, et al.: Supervised physical therapy vs home exercise program for patients with distal radius fracture: a single-blind randomized clinical study, *J Hand Ther* 30(3):242–252, 2017.
64. Algar L, Valdes K: Using smartphone applications as hand therapy interventions, *J Hand Ther* 27:254–257, 2014.
65. Schott N, Korbus H: Preventing functional loss during immobilization after osteoporotic wrist fractures in elderly patients: a randomized clinical trial, *BMC Musculoskelet Disord* 15:287, 2014.
66. Michlovitz SL, et al.: Distal radius fractures: therapy practice patterns, *J Hand Ther* 14(4):249–257, 2001.
67. Li Z, et al.: Complex regional pain syndrome after hand surgery, *Hand Clin* 26(2):281–289, 2010.
68. Villeco JP: Edema: a silent but important factor, *J Hand Ther* 25(2):153–161, 2012.
69. Artzberger SM, Prignanc VW: Manual edema mobilization. In Skirven T, et al.: *Rehabilitation of the hand and upper extremity*, ed 6, Philadelphia, 2011, Elsevier, pp 868–881.
70. Kuo LC, et al.: Is progressive early digit mobilization intervention beneficial for patients with external fixation of distal radius fracture? A pilot randomized controlled trial, *Clin Rehabil* 27(11):983–993, 2013.
71. Valdes K: A retrospective pilot study comparing the number of therapy visits required to regain functional wrist and forearm range of motion following volar plating of a distal radius fracture, *J Hand Ther* 22(4):312–319, 2009.
72. Brody LT: Effective therapeutic exercise prescription: the right exercise at the right dose, *J Hand Ther* 25(2):220–231, 2012.
73. MacDermid JC, et al.: Pain and disability reported in the year following distal radius fracture: a cohort study, *BMC Musculoskelet Disord* 4:24, 2003.
74. Dilek B, et al.: Effectiveness of graded motor imagery to improve hand function in patients with distal radius fracture: a randomized controlled trial, *J Hand Ther* 31(1):2–9, 2018.
75. Priganc V, Stralka SW: Graded motor imagery, *J Hand Ther* 24(2):164–168, 2011.
76. Szekeres M: The short-term effects of hot packs vs therapeutic whirlpool on active wrist range of motion for patients with distal radius fracture: a randomized controlled trial, *J Hand Ther* 1–5, 2017.
77. Flowers KR, LaStayo P: Effect of total end range time on improving passive range of motion, *J Hand Ther* 150–157, 1994.
78. Harris JE, et al.: The international classification of functioning as an explanatory model of health after distal radius fracture: a cohort study, *Health Qual Life Outcomes* 3:73, 2005.
79. Hagert E: Proprioception of the wrist joint: a review of current concepts and possible implications on the rehabilitation of the wrist, *J Hand Ther* 23(1):2–16, 2010.
80. Karagiannopoulos C, Michlovitz S: Rehabilitation strategies for wrist sensorimotor control impairment: from theory to practice, *J Hand Ther* 29(2):154–165, 2016.
81. May A: Chronic pain may change the structure of the brain, *Pain* 137(1):7–15, 2008.
82. Karagiannopoulos C, et al.: A descriptive study on wrist and hand sensorimotor impairment and function following distal radius fracture intervention, *J Hand Ther* 26(3):204–215, 2013.
83. Karagiannopoulos C, et al.: Responsiveness of the active wrist joint position sense test after distal radius fracture intervention, *J Hand Ther* 29(4):474–482, 2016.
84. Naranje SM, et al.: Epidemiology of pediatric fractures presenting to emergency departments in the United States, *J Pediatr Orthop* 36(4):e45–e48, 2016.
85. Ryan LM, et al.: Epidemiology of pediatric forearm fractures in Washington, DC, *J Trauma* 69(Suppl 4):S200–S205, 2010.
86. Kozin SC: Pediatric distal radius fractures. In Slutsky DJ, Osterman AL, editors: *fractures and injuries of the distal radius and carpus*, ed 1, Philadelphia, 2009, Saunders, pp 165–173.
87. Bae DS, Howard AW: Distal radius fractures: what is the evidence? *J Pediatr Orthop* 32(Suppl 2):S128–S130, 2012.
88. Dua, et al.: Pediatric distal radius fractures, *AAOS Instr Course Lect* 66:447–460, 2017.
89. Dwek JR: The periosteum: what is it, where is it, and what mimics it in its absence? *Skeletal Radiol* 39:319–323, 2010.
90. Little JT, et al.: Pediatric distal Forearm and Wrist Injury: an imaging review, *Radiographics* 34(2):472–490, 2014.

22 Wrist Instabilities

Sarah Mee

Introduction

The wrist is a complex and intricate joint. Its many articulations are formed by bones with varying degrees of curvatures and congruencies supported by ligaments and controlled by muscles. A wrist is considered stable when it is able to maintain normal carpal positions with loading as well as through a full range of motion (ROM). Wrist stability is maintained by a balance of tensile and compressive forces at the joints (known as tensegrity).[1] A fully stable wrist is only achieved with normal bony congruency, innervated and intact ligaments, an effective sensorimotor process, and strong active stabilizing muscles.[2]

Carpal dislocations and instabilities are common injuries. Most carpal disruptions are caused by trauma. However, they can also be caused by conditions such as congenital laxity, infection, inflammatory processes (rheumatoid arthritis), or congenital defects. Delayed identification and inadequate management of carpal instabilities will cause abnormal intercarpal and radiocarpal loading, ultimately leading to degeneration of the articular surfaces.

Carpal instability is defined as dislocation or loss of contact of bones within the same row or between the distal and proximal carpal rows. Clients commonly report wrist pain, weakness, sudden loss of control, or clunking. In order to understand carpal instability, an appreciation of the anatomy of the wrist joint and the kinematics of the carpal bones is imperative.

Osseous Anatomy

The wrist consists of the distal radius, ulna, and carpus – forming the distal radioulnar joint (DRUJ), radiocarpal joint (RCJ), midcarpal joint (MCJ), and the carpometacarpal joints (CMCJs). The distal radioulnar joint consists of the ulna head fitting into the sigmoid notch of the radius, allowing rotation of the forearm. Rotation is only possible with the involvement of the proximal radioulnar joint (PRUJ), which incorporates the proximal ulna and the radial head.[3] The distal radius is typically tilted 12 degrees in the anterior-posterior (A-P) plane (Fig. 22.1A) and 23 degrees in the radioulnar plane (Fig. 22.1B).[4] The distal surface of the ulna is covered by the triangular fibrocartilage.

The proximal carpal row is formed by the scaphoid, lunate, triquetrum, and pisiform; and the distal row by the trapezium, trapezoid, capitate, and hamate. The joint formed between these rows is the midcarpal joint. The midcarpal joint has three articulations: lateral, central, and medial. This joint is highly synovial, allowing for maximal motion in all the planes. The scaphoid bridges both proximal and distal carpal rows. The proximal carpal row has been termed an intercalated segment between the distal carpal row and the radius. The bones of the proximal carpal row move directly in response to the muscular force regulated by the ligaments that connect to the forearm and the distal carpal rows.[3,4]

Ligamentous Anatomy

The ligamentous structures are divided into extrinsic and intrinsic, palmar and dorsal.[3] The shape and attachments of the carpal ligaments are designed to become taut when acting as constraints, and/or to relax when allowing movement. This is particularly important in controlling intercarpal rotation motion.[2]

A key function of the wrist ligaments is providing afferent feedback for proprioception and sensorimotor control via the mechanoreceptors.[5]

Palmar Ligaments

The palmar extrinsic ligaments arise from the distal radius and ulna and connect to proximal and distal carpal rows. They are key ligaments in maintaining midcarpal joint and carpal stability (Fig. 22.2A). The radioscaphocapitate ligament (RSCL) is

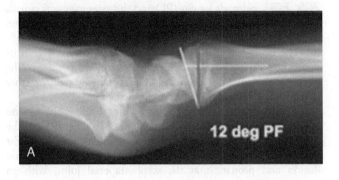

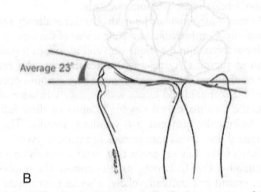

FIG. 22.1 (A) The distal radius is typically tilted an average of 12 degrees of palmar tilt in the anterior-posterior plane. (B) The distal radius is tilted an average of 23 degrees of radial inclination in the radial-ulnar plane.

the most radial ligament and is important for volar carpus and midcarpal joint stability. It is a primary radial stabilizer of the wrist and resists ulnar translation of the carpus across the radius. It is also a strong scapholunate joint volar stabilizer.[2] This ligament blends into the ulnocapitate ligament arising from the ulnar side.

Lateral to the RSCL, the radioscapholunate ligament (RSLL) provides stability to these joints. Lateral to the RSLL, the long radiolunate (LRL) and short radiolunate (SRL) ligaments offer primary resistance to lunate displacement.

The triangular fibrocartilage complex (TFCC) is the key stabilizer of the ulnar wrist and is comprised of the extensor carpi ulnaris subsheath, the palmar radioulnar ligament (PRUL), dorsal radioulnar ligament (DRUL), the meniscus homologue, the ulnolunate ligament (ULL), and the ulnotriquetral ligament (UTL). On the palmar aspect of the TFCC, the UTL and ULL arise from the PRUL and attach to lunate and triquetrum.[6]

The proximal carpal bones are stabilized by the scapholunate ligament (SLL) on the radial side, the lunotriquetral ligament (LTL) on the ulnar side, and the scaphotriquetral ligament (STL) across the row. The SLL has three components: (1) the dorsal portion stabilizes traction and torsion forces between the scaphoid and lunate, (2) the volar portion controls the rotational stability of these two bones, and (3) the proximal portion is a shock absorber.[7] The LTL prevents ulnar translation of the lunate. The scaphocapitate and palmar triquetrumcapitatehamate ligaments help stabilize the midcarpal joint. Trapeziotrapezoid, trapeziocapitate, and capitohamate ligaments connect the bones of the distal carpal row.

Dorsal Ligaments

The dorsal intrinsic wrist ligaments are not as well defined or as strong as the volar intrinsic ligaments, but they provide the most sensorimotor input.[8] The most important dorsal extrinsic wrist ligaments are the dorsal radiocarpal (DRC) and dorsal interosseous (DI) ligaments (Fig. 22.2B). The DRC ligament prevents ulnar translation of the carpus. The DI ligament provides

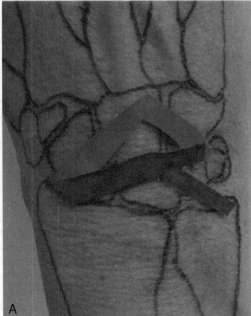
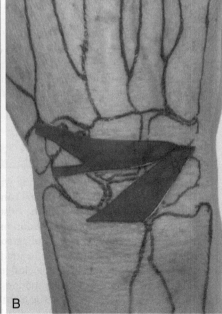

FIG. 22.2 (A) Important palmar stabilizing carpal ligaments: long radiolunate ligament and ulnar ligament, palmar triquetrumhamate-capitate ligament, and radioscaphocapitate ligament. (B) Important dorsal stabilizing carpal ligaments: dorsal interosseous ligament and radiocarpal ligaments

stability to the midcarpal joint, preventing dorsal dislocation of the capitate. The dorsal radiotriquetral ligament (DRTL) supports the radiocarpal joint and midcarpal joint and controls supination forces, while laterally, the dorsoradial scaphotrapeziotrapezoidal ligament (DRSTTL) maintains dorsal and supination stability.[2]

Radioulnar Joint Ligaments

The palmar and dorsal radioulnar ligaments originate from the margin of the sigmoid notch of the distal radius. These ligaments control the distal radius in its arc of rotation around the ulna head, enabling dynamic control at all points of the range and allowing stable dorsal/volar translation of the ulna.[6,9]

Retinacular Ligaments

Other attachments to the carpus include fascial layers of extensor and flexor retinaculum. The extensor retinaculum inserts on the lateral margin of the distal radius, triquetrum, and pisiform. In between two layers of extensor retinaculum, vertical septii divide the extensor tendons into six compartments.[3] The extensor carpi ulnaris (ECU) is firmly stabilized in the groove of the ulna head by deep circumferential fascia. This allows controlled slide of the ECU during rotation, changing its mechanical advantage for two different movements. In pronation, the ECU lies on the ulnar side of the ulna head and acts as an ulnar deviator and stabilizer. In supination, the ECU lies on the dorsal aspect of the ulna head close to the radius and acts as an extensor and a dorsal carpal stabilizer.[3] The distal radioulnar joint is dynamically stabilized by the ECU and the pronator quadratus (PQ).[1]

Palmarly, the flexor retinaculum attaches ulnarly to the hamate and pisiform and radially to the scaphoid and trapezium. This encloses the carpal canal containing the median nerve and nine flexor tendons. The flexor carpi radialis (FCR) inserts on the base of the second and third metacarpals (MCs), whereas the flexor carpi ulnaris (FCU) inserts on the pisiform with ligament extensions to the hamate and base of the fifth MC. The abductor pollicis longus (APL) insertions are variable but inserts (in 90% of people)[3] on the trapezoid, trapezium, and/or scaphoid before the base of the first MC. The APL stabilizes the first MC and is a wrist radial deviator.[2]

The interosseous membrane stabilizes the forearm bones through rotation, particularly with loading, connecting along the length of the radius and ulna.[6] The distal oblique band travels from the distal ulna shaft and inserts into the sigmoid notch and the palmar and dorsal radioulnar ligaments – augmenting distal radioulnar joint and ulnar stability.[6]

Normal Kinematics of the Wrist Joint

The motion of the carpal bones during wrist flexion/extension and radial/ulnar deviation is extremely complex. The literature identifies that in neutral position of the wrist, the scaphoid maintains approximately 47 degrees of flexion orientation in relation to the lunate and radius on lateral radiograph. The scapholunate ligament plays an important role in neutralizing the flexion tendency of the scaphoid under physiological loads.[10] The proximal carpal row's behavior during wrist motion is dependent on the compressive loads placed by the distal carpal row. The musculotendinous units inserting distal to the distal carpal row produce

this physiological load on the carpus.[11] Having normal anatomical relationship of the proximal carpal row structures along with the radius is critical for normal functioning of the wrist joint.

Flexion/Extension Motion

Flexion/extension movements are initiated and controlled by the FCR, FCU, palmaris longus (PL) and the extensor carpi radialis longus (ECRL), extensor carpi radialis brevis (ECRB), ECU, and APL, respectively. These muscles produce axial loading for stability. The distal carpal row moves initially at the CMCJ with its strong attachment to the base of the metacarpals that define the plane of movement of the hand. The distal row will therefore always move in the same direction as the hand.[12]

In normal wrists, the scaphoid and lunate follow the motion of the capitate across the midcarpal joint.[13] In wrist flexion, the scaphoid flexes and pronates while doing the opposite in wrist extension. Compressive forces in grip and loading will increase flexion and pronation at the scaphotrapezial joint, with an increase in further pronation at the trapezoid and across the distal carpal row. The lunate moves similarly but with a smaller motion, while the capitate rotates volarly.

At the triquetrohamate joint, the hamate is already resting in a dorsal tilt. Compression on the ulnar side of the wrist increases the dorsal force onto the triquetrum and it extends further. Pronation at the distal carpal row further increases the extension force on the hamate and triquetrum. These actions oppose flexion of the scaphoid and lunate and produce a balance of forces across the proximal carpal row.[2,11] In order to allow full ROM into flexion, the proximal row translates dorsally. The dorsal radiocarpal and dorsal interosseous ligaments prevent excessive rotation of the lunate, preventing volar intercalated segmental instability (VISI). During wrist extension, the scaphoid and lunate extend and translate volarly, whereas the capitate rotates dorsally. The palmar radiolunate ligament prevents excessive rotation of the lunate, preventing dorsal intercalated segmental instability (DISI).

Radial and Ulnar Deviation Motion

Radioulnar motion of the wrist is more complex than flexion/extension. The radioulnar motion of the wrist causes the carpal rows to move in a ring-type motion. The distal carpal row rotates in a radial direction, whereas the proximal row slides in an ulnar direction when radial deviation is performed; a reversal mechanism occurs when the wrist is brought into an ulnar deviation posture. During radioulnar motion, the magnitude of the movement at the midcarpal joint is 1.5 times greater than at the radiocarpal joint.[12]

Upon radial deviation of the wrist, the scaphoid is compressed between the radial styloid proximally and the trapezium-trapezoid distally, forcing the scaphoid to flex in an almost perpendicular direction to the radius. As the scaphoid flexes, the entire proximal carpal row also assumes a flexed position via intact scapholunate and lunotriquetral ligaments. During radial deviation the ulnar ligaments stretch, whereas the ligaments on the radial side become lax. Tensioning of the ulnotriquetral ligament influences the triquetrum, causing it to slide or disengage off the hamate. Radial direction produces a translatory effect on the proximal carpal row, which then slides in an ulnar direction. The synchronous motion that occurs with radial deviation involves execution of the proximal row in pronation and flexion, whereas the distal carpal row moves in the opposite direction of supination and extension.

As the wrist is moved into ulnar deviation, a compressive force is produced by the hamate over the triquetrum, which forces it into extension, and subsequently the entire proximal carpal row is pushed into extension. The entire proximal row slides radially because of tensioning of the RSCLs, LRLs, and SRLs. In addition, as the extension of the proximal carpal row increases with the increment of the deviation, the scaphoid is pulled into extension with the lunate and triquetrum. The proximal row executes supination and extension, whereas the distal row moves in pronation and flexion.[11]

Dart-Throwing Motion

Physiological motions of the wrist in an oblique plane are commonly used in activities of daily living (ADLs). ADLs such as combing hair or hammering a nail are performed in a manner incorporating radial extension and ulnar flexion. This motion has been coined *dart-throwing motion.*[14,15] In healthy wrists with intact scapholunate ligaments, there is little scapholunate joint movement during dart-throwing motion in comparison to flexion/extension movement.[16] However, in injured wrists with scapholunate ligament disruption, there is obvious gapping of the scapholunate joint through this oblique motion.[17]

Forearm Rotation

Forearm rotation requires both the distal and proximal radioulnar joints to produce full movement. The ulna is fixed, and the radius moves around it up to 180 degrees. There are three planes of movement: (1) rotation along the longitudinal axis, (2) volar/dorsal translation of the ulna, and (3) proximal/distal pistoning of the ulna. At the distal radioulnar joint, the distal radius rotates around the fixed head of the ulna; while at the proximal radioulnar joint, the radial head spins within the annular ligament.[6] Distally the ulna head translates in volar/dorsal and distal/proximal planes to enable full ROM. In extreme supination, the ulna head sits on the volar and proximal edge of the sigmoid notch, while in pronation it translates to the dorsal and distal edge of the notch.[18] There is little bony stability as the sigmoid notch is shallow, and motion/loading is controlled via the palmar and dorsal radioulnar ligaments and the TFCC.[9]

Motion of the Carpus during Gripping

During axial loading in grip, the extrinsic muscles act across the metacarpal base, through the distal carpal row, to the midcarpal joint, across the proximal carpal row, to the radiocarpal joint. There is a distinct parallelism between the curvatures of the proximal and distal carpal rows.[19] In neutral axial loading 78% of the axial load is via the radius, 46% via the radioscaphoid joint, and 32% via the radiolunate joint. Only 14% is across the ulnolunate joint and 8% via the ulnotriquetral joint. This loading will change with different hand positions.[12] The load variation changes proportionately, either negative or positive, if ulnar variance is present. In neutral ulnar variance, the forces produced by the flexors and extensors are transmitted from the digits to the distal carpal row upon gripping. During gripping the scaphoid tends to rotate into flexion and pronation, while the lunate rotates dorsally. The rotatory tendency of the carpus

during gripping activities suggests that the proximal carpal row moves together because of intact scapholunate and lunotriquetral ligaments.[20]

Forces applied axially along the third MC to a normal and neutral wrist result in distal carpal row pronation and proximal migration. This increases the force on the midcarpal joint increasing the pronating movement. At the scaphotrapeziotrapezoidal joint level, the forces push the scaphoid into flexion and pronation. At the triquetrohamate joint level the hamate (already sitting pointing dorsally) induces triquetral extension as the volar triquetrohamate ligament tightens. If all ligaments are intact, the extension moment of the triquetrum balances the flexion of the scaphoid resulting in stability at the proximal carpal row.[2]

Muscular Contributions to the Motion of the Wrist and their Effect on Carpal Stabilization

The wrist muscles control the force and direction of carpal movement through loading and pull. In particular, they produce a pronating and supinating force at the midcarpal joint. When all wrist muscles isometrically load across the wrist together, the distal carpal row supinates.[2] A passive axial load to the wrist causes distal row pronaton.[11] Muscles with oblique pull produce the most rotation. Loading of the dorsal muscles induces midcarpal joint supination. Loading of ECU generates midcarpal joint pronation. On the volar surface, loaded FCU produces supination.[11,21,22] These dynamic motions produce tension on ligaments.

Coordinated action of these ligaments and muscles, along with proprioception, provide stability to a normal wrist. Injury to any of these ligaments will alter sensorimotor control of the wrist, transforming a muscle from a "friendly" controller to an "unfriendly" deforming force. Additionally, ligament injury at the wrist alters proprioceptive feedback, so proprioceptive training should be part of a comprehensive rehabilitation program following these types of wrist injuries.[2,20,23]

Proprioceptive Input during Wrist Motion

The term *proprioception* describes our body's regulation of posture, balance, joint stability, and audiovisual-motor coordination.[24] The term *sensorimotor function* describes the sensory, motor, and central integration and processing components involved with maintaining joint homeostasis during movement.[25] Wrist stability during motion is maintained by mechanoreceptors and proprioceptors embedded in the joint capsule and ligaments. These structures are continuously sending feedback to the central nervous system (CNS) about the position of the joint and the speed of motion being performed. In addition, the information about pressure, torsion, and pain sent to the CNS regulates muscular contraction to maintain the joint stability. The process of maintaining joint control and stability is accomplished through the relationship between the static and dynamic joint stabilizers.

Fast monosynaptic reflexes are sent to produce action or inhibition in muscles, as needed, for stability.[2,11,13] Ligaments, joint capsule, cartilage and joint articulation with bony geometry comprise the static stabilizers.[2] Dynamic contributions to joint stability arise from the muscles that cross the joint structures. If there is a disruption in the static stabilizers of a joint, the dynamic joint stabilizers must work harder to provide joint stability.[11] There is increased awareness that instability following wrist injury is extremely complicated because it involves disruption of this proprioceptive feedback loop.

Classification of Carpal Instability

Carpal instabilities are common and may result from various conditions including ligament injuries, inflammatory synovitis, scaphoid nonunion/malunion, or Kienböck disease. These instability patterns result from ligamentous disruption between the bones of the same carpal row or between rows. Perhaps the most widely adopted classification system for these instabilities is the Mayo Classification,[26] which classifies carpal instability into four major categories:

- Carpal instability dissociative (CID)
- Carpal instability nondissociative (CIND)
- Carpal instability complex (CIC)
- Carpal instability adaptive (CIA)

Carpal Instability Dissociative

CID is caused by fracture or ligament disruption within the same carpal row – usually the proximal row. This form of instability involves pathology to the intrinsic ligaments and includes injuries to the scapholunate or lunotriquetral ligaments.

Scapholunate Ligament Tears

Scapholunate instability occurs most commonly in young to middle-aged individuals. It is typically a result of a fall on outstretched hand (FOOSH) causing wrist hyperextension, ulnar deviation, and midcarpal supination. Clients with acute injury often present with a painful and swollen wrist, which may be diffusely tender. With time, pain becomes more localized over the scapholunate ligament dorsally.

Lunotriquetral Instability

Lunotriquetral instability is far less common than scapholunate instability. For an isolated tear of the lunotriquetral ligament, the method of injury is usually a FOOSH causing wrist extension and radial deviation. Force is generated through the ulnar side of the hand leading to carpal hyperpronation and damage to the lunotriquetral ligament.

Carpal Instability Nondissociative

CIND often results in abnormal motion of the entire proximal carpal row at the radiocarpal and/or midcarpal joint. Thus it is not specific to a carpal row. CIND involves a large array of disorders, which include midcarpal instability, ulnar translation of the carpus, capitolunate instability, triquetrohamate instability, and ulnar carpal instability. Clients may have underlying hypermobility spectrum disorder or hypermobility Ehlers-Danlos.[27] Clients often present with wrist pain that is not well defined or localized.

Carpal Instability Complex

With the CIC category both CID and CIND may be present simultaneously. Common findings in this category of instability are perilunate dislocation along with radiocarpal ligament injuries, resulting in scapholunate and lunotriquetral dissociation with ulnar translation of the lunate.

Carpal Instability Adaptive

This category of instability presents as an adaptive change of the carpus in relation to the radius following malunited distal radius fractures or untreated carpal instabilities.

Rehabilitation of Carpal Instabilities

Evidence to support rehabilitation of carpal instability has been limited. Many therapists choose their methods based on their own preference and clinical experience.[28] However, there is recent literature proposing specific rehabilitation methods – mainly for scapholunate instabilities.[2,29,30,31,32] These programs are based on sound clinical reasoning; however, they are not yet established as best practice and investigation is ongoing.

In general, rehabilitation following operative or nonoperative management of wrist ligament injury should include the following:
- Managing edema and pain
- Maintaining ROM of uninvolved joints
- Initiating controlled, protected mobilization to the involved structures based on tissue healing, potential tension to repaired structures, and symptomology of the client
- Avoiding exercise or activity that could compromise tissue healing or place undue load to the healing structures
- Initiating individualized, clinically reasoned wrist ROM and strengthening exercises
- Avoiding painful end-range or excessive active ROM (AROM) exercises

The goal for treatment and rehabilitation of wrist injuries is to achieve a stable wrist with functional ROM. There is some agreement in the literature that functional wrist ROM is around 40 degrees of wrist flexion, 40 degrees of extension, 40 degrees of combined deviation, and 75% rotation both pronation and supination.[15]

Innovative and Emerging Approaches to Carpal Instability Rehabilitation

Following injury, the body's sensorimotor system is often altered, reducing the intensity and frequency of proprioceptive input from the mechanoreceptors in and around the wrist joint. This alters processing and response from the CNS, often resulting in an imbalance of motor control and a "switching off" of painful (often stabilizing) muscles. Over time, this produces a dynamically unstable wrist. Research has elucidated the importance of proprioception rehabilitation for unstable wrists.

Hagert[5] proposed a proprioceptive rehabilitation program for the unstable wrist based on identifying muscles that serve a protective function for the specific ligament deficiency and training those muscles to respond more efficiently to prevent further deterioration (Table 22.1).[5] Clinical research on its validity is yet to be confirmed, but it is based on sound clinical reasoning and early research.

Ligamentous and Muscular Reflexes, Proprioception, and the Wrist

The sensorimotor system in the wrist includes three actions that are constantly rebalancing and correcting: (1) sensory afferent feedback from intact peripheral joints, ligaments, musculoskeletal

TABLE 22.1   Rehabilitation Strategies in Wrist Proprioceptive Reeducation (Hagert[5])

Stages of Proprioception Rehabilitation	Rehabilitation Plan	Purpose	Techniques	Assessment of Outcome
1	Basic rehabilitation	Edema and pain control; Promote motion	Basic hand therapy techniques	VAS; Degree of motion (ROM)
2	Proprioception awareness	Promote conscious joint control	Mirror therapy	VAS and ROM
3	Joint position sense	Ability to replicate a predetermined joint angle	Blinded passive and active reproduction of joint angle	Accuracy of joint motion measured with goniometer or exercise machine
4	Kinesthesia (threshold to detection of passive movement)	Ability to sense joint motion without audiovisual cues	Motion detection using an exercise machine (preferable) or manual passive motion	Degree of joint angle at which motion was sensed, measured with goniometer or exercise machine
5	Conscious neuromuscular rehabilitation	Strengthening of specific muscles to enhance joint stability	Isometric training Eccentric training Isokinetic training Co-activation	Evaluation of specific muscle strength, wrist stability during co-activation, joint stability during isometric exercises
6	Unconscious neuromuscular rehabilitation	Reactive muscle activation	Powerball exercises; Plyometric training	Muscle activation patterns using EMG

EMG, electromyography; *ROM*, range of motion; *VAS*, visual analog scale.

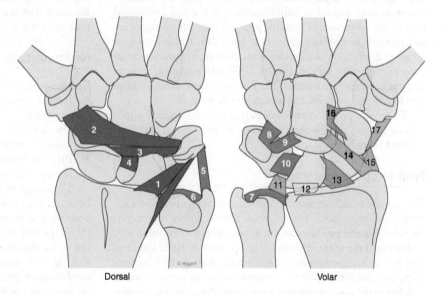

FIG: 22.3 Mechanoreceptor and nerve distribution in the wrist ligaments including the triangular fibrocartilage complex. Ligaments: *(1)* dorsal radiocarpal, *(2)* dorsal intercarpal, *(3)* scaphotriquetral, *(4)* scapholunate interosseous, *(5)* ulnar collateral, *(6)* dorsal radioulnar, *(7)* volar radioulnar, *(8)* triquetrohamate, *(9)* triquetrocapitate, *(10)* palmar lunotriquetral, *(11)* ulnolunate, *(12)* short radiolunate, *(13)* long radiolunate, *(14)* radioscaphocapitate, *(15)* radioscaphoid, *(16)* scaphocapitate, *(17)* scaphotrapeziotrapezoid. (Courtesy Hagert E, Wrist ligaments: Innervation patterns and ligamento-muscular reflexes. Karolinska Institute, 2008.)

neuroreceptors, and skin – reacting to joint pressure, motion, and velocity; (2) CNS processing of afferent input, which is interpreted as joint position sense, kinesthesia, sense of resistance, motion threshold, and velocity; and (3) motor feedforward output sending efferent neuromuscular messaging to joints and muscles for stability and movement. Motor signals are generated as specific sequencing of muscle activation to control force, direction, and velocity.[33]

We have known about the specialization of mechanoreceptors in wrist ligaments since 1997.[34] Since that discovery, studies have found that nerve endings in many wrist ligaments are located close to the ligament insertion into bone.[7,4,35] This ensures that mechanoreceptors in these ligaments fire particularly at the extremes of joint motion.[36] Mechanoreceptors found in other ligaments are located in the pliant epifascicular regions where they

are able to provide information throughout the range of wrist motions.[23,35] The mechanically important ligaments designed to withstand axial loads are mainly located in the radial column of the wrist. The key sensory ligaments are the dorsal and ulnar wrist ligaments emerging from the triquetrum and should be regarded as key elements in the generation of proprioceptive information required for adequate neuromuscular wrist control (Fig. 22.3).[8]

Assessment of the Unstable Wrist

Assessing wrist instability can be challenging, as stability is a complex mix of mechanical, sensorimotor, and CNS processes. Standard hand and wrist assessment techniques should be used to evaluate pain, ROM (including dart-throwing motion), accessory movements, and grip strength. Imaging, provocative tests, and palpation of individual ligaments, joints, and wrist movements will add to the overall understanding of the instability. A useful method for assessing the surface anatomy and differential diagnosis of the wrist was described by Brown and Lichtman.[37]

An assessment for hypermobility spectrum disorder and hypermobility Ehlers-Danlos may be downloaded from the website (https://www.ehlers-danlos.com/medical-professionals). New criteria and assessment was published in 2017. The **TFCC Tear Weightbearing test**[38] can be used to assess the ability of the client to maintain static weight bearing and loading on the wrist. As part of this test (in an effort to aid treatment choices), tape may be placed around the distal radioulnar joint to add compression. Sometimes, taping reduces pain and improves loading potential. The **Push–off test**[39] uses the Jamar dynamometer to assess load potential and pain as well as static wrist balance. A client-related observed functional upper limb assessment may help with assessing aspects of sensorimotor processing including laterality, body image, motor imagery, speed, accuracy, close and distant placement, and sudden wrist angle changes with anticipatory movements and coactivation. It is important to consider all aspects that make up proprioception conscious and unconscious neuromuscular control.

Proprioceptive Reeducation of the Wrist

Although proprioceptive reeducation is a relatively new rehabilitation concept applied to wrist instability, it is a well-established part of the treatment of unstable joints.[40] Pain following injury can produce neuroplastic changes in the CNS, which may have an adverse effect on the sensorimotor system. Appropriate early pain management will reorganize CNS processing via sensory and proprioception awareness, and prevent these changes from developing and contributing to an unstable wrist.[41]

The major proprioceptive senses that have therapeutic implications include proprioceptive awareness, kinesthesia, and joint position sense.[5]

Proprioceptive Awareness

Proprioceptive reflexes exist between the wrist ligaments and the wrist forearm muscles. For example, stimulation of the scapholunate ligament produces an immediate excitatory or inhibitory activation of the antagonist muscle as a protective initial stabilization just before the agonist initiates actual movement.[35] Secondarily, coactivations of the wrist muscles occur to provide overall stability to the static position or movement. Awareness of the sensorimotor and neuromuscular systems that control muscle activation sequence may be encouraged in the early stages of recovery by using illusionary sensory feedback interventions such as mirror therapy [42,43] and motor imagery training,[44] including laterality, visualization, and imagined movements to improve awareness of joint position. Additionally, proprioceptive awareness of the wrist and upper limb can be trained with exercises such as rolling a ball on the table, circumducting the wrist resting on an air cushion, and wiping a cloth around a surface. These activities increase tactile sensory feedback.[41]

Kinesthesia

Kinesthesia is the ability to sense motion of a joint or limb. It is primarily influenced by muscle spindles and secondarily influenced by skin receptors and joint receptors.[5] In clinical practice, kinesthesia is measured as the smallest change in joint angle

required to elicit conscious awareness of joint motion.[36,40] To evaluate kinesthesia at the wrist, some suggest placing the wrist at a certain angle and then passively moving it at a slow speed of 0.5 degrees to 2 degrees per second until the client signals that motion is occuring.[5] The client should be blinded during initial kinesthesia testing because limb movement is greatly influenced by visual cues.

Joint Position Sense

Joint position sense is a separate entity from kinesthesia.[45] Describing the differences between joint position sense and kinesthesia is beyond the scope of this chapter. However, they do differ due to their central processing and interpretation in the brain.[40] In the context of proprioceptive retraining, joint position sense is defined as the ability to accurately reproduce a specific joint angle.[5] This form of retraining can be done with visual cues or blinded, as well as with active muscle contraction or through passive motion. Client progress and accuracy of joint position sense can easily be recorded using a goniometer. The client is instructed to move the involved wrist to a predetermined joint angle established by goniometry. This can be performed actively by the client or passively by the therapist slowly moving the wrist until the client identifies when the target position is reached.[41] Adding weight or load to a joint may help improve joint position sense.[46] Some suggest beginning joint position sense training with visual cues and progressing to vision-occluded exercises.[5] Be aware that muscle fatigue adversely affects awareness of joint position sense and sensorimotor control.

Neuromuscular Rehabilitation

The purpose of neuromuscular wrist rehabilitation is to[5]:
- Regain synchronous and balanced wrist motion following instability
- Use dynamic muscular compression to compensate for ligamentous insufficiency
- Promote ligamentous-friendly muscle contractions to provide joint protection and stability

The design of a neuromuscular rehabilitation program should be custom tailored for each client based on which structures have been injured or repaired. The hand therapist must work within the range and loading limits safe for that injury while promoting wrist stability and monitoring the client's pain, swelling, and signs of instability. The components of a neuromuscular rehabilitation program include conscious isometric, concentric, eccentric, and isokinetic exercise; coactivation rehabilitation; and unconscious neuromuscular control with reactive muscle activation and plyometric/perturbation exercises.[5]

Conscious Neuromuscular Rehabilitation

Isometric Exercise

Isometric strengthening is a static form of exercise in which a muscle contracts with a fixed joint angle and a maintained muscle length.[5] The purpose is to increase CNS awareness of muscles at specific joint angles, as well as improve strength and endurance. This form of exercise can be applied early following ligamentous injury or repair because, done correctly, it places no tension on the healing ligaments. Isometric exercise increases conscious neuromuscular control for agonist and antagonist muscle groups, encouraging cocontraction in neutral or static wrist positions.[47]

The therapist must clinically reason the effects of the compressive forces produced by specific muscle activations because this may place excessive stress on the recently repaired or healing structures.

Eccentric and Concentric Exercise

Eccentric strengthening is designed to increase strength by applying load while physically lengthening the activated muscle. This form of muscle activation is often initiated following a period of isometric strengthening and proprioception training. The goal of this form of resistance training is to enhance proprioception; reduce pain[48]; and increase strength, endurance, and coactivation of wrist muscles without placing excessive tension on the healing ligamentous structures. The main benefit of eccentric exercise and activity to wrist stability is in the concurrent shortening on the antagonist muscle(s) working toward balance of coactivation and control.[35]

In concentric contractions, where the muscle shortens, the force generated by the muscle is always less than the muscle's maximum. As the load on the muscle that is required to lift decreases, contraction velocity increases. This occurs until the muscle finally reaches its maximum contraction velocity. By performing a series of constant velocity shortening and lengthening contractions, a concentric and eccentric relationship is established.

Coactivation Exercise

Coactivation exercises (using slow balance and control activities) utilize isometric, eccentric, and concentric contractions to increase proprioception and CNS awareness – thereby improving wrist stability.[35] A simple method of coactivation training is to perform balance ball exercises (Fig. 22.4). The client's hand(s) are placed on a weighted ball. The client is instructed to slowly move the ball around the table, which allows for simultaneous activation of extensors, flexors, and deviators of the wrist. Coactivation retraining with vision and vision occluded improves wrist stability by increasing proprioceptive awareness during motion, with greater control of the muscles. Exercises through range and with resistance using free weights or elastic bands will increase sensorimotor feedback and reciprocal and recurrent muscle action. Limited plane and range activities (e.g., toy hammer or miming a dart throw) will activate stabilizers with graded loading.[49]

Isokinetic Exercise

Isokinetic exercise is when the velocity of limb movement is held consistent by a rate-controlled device. This form of exercise is most frequently performed by high-level athletes and requires specialized equipment not typically found in hand therapy clinics. Clients who place extreme demands on the wrist joint (such as professional athletes, gymnasts, or musicians) may benefit from this form of exercise as it may enhance overall proprioceptive function and allow earlier return to activity-specific training.[5]

Unconscious Neuromuscular Rehabilitation

Reactive Muscle Activation Exercise

Clients need to achieve good conscious neuromuscular control, a relatively pain-free wrist, and good proprioception and coactivation prior to starting a reactive muscle activation (RMA) program. The purpose of RMA activity is to improve the neuromuscular reflex activation patterns that are altered in joints with injured ligaments.[5,30,31] Activities incorporating plyometrics, balance, reaction to change in wrist/hand positions, speed and endurance of muscles,

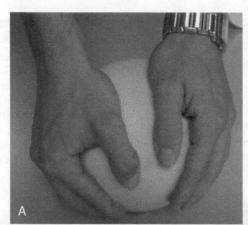
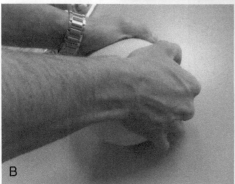
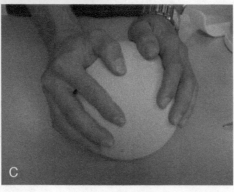

FIG. 22.4 Demonstration of balance ball exercises. For example, the client may perform flexion and ulnar deviation, extension and radial deviation with simultaneous coactivation of the muscles needed to control these actions. (A) Demonstrates the hand and wrist position at the beginning of this exercise. (B) and (C), Demonstrates movement pattern on the ball.

change in upper limb position, and stability with open chain tasks are all part of this rehabilitation program. RMA exercises increase anticipatory muscle control, which is the ability to sense potentially harmful or unstable motion during function.[5]

Closed chain reactive tasks (hand/upper limb in constant fixed position) with vision and vision occluded should be graded to open chain (upper limb free to move) tasks with increasing speed, loads, and reaction times.[30,32] Proprioception may be increased by using a ball, wobble board, or air cushion to increase the balance and anticipatory requirements of the tasks. Activation of wrist muscles can be encouraged with resisted grip (e.g., using tweezers to pick up objects), which often results in static cocontraction of all wrist muscles.

Open chain activities require greater wrist stability and incorporate control of the upper limb. Exercises such as oscillating a flexible bar (Fig. 22.5), rotating a container of marbles (Fig. 22.6A), directing a wand around a wire shape (Fig. 22.6B), using a wrist maze, and controlling water in a slosh pipe encourages high levels of sensorimotor feedback and random, rapid muscle control activation. More complex and higher velocity upper limb control exercises will encourage multiple muscle activations for

the entire upper limb.[50] Examples include use of a powerball (Fig. 22.7A), balancing a ball on a racquet, catching and throwing a ball, and press-ups on a wobble board (Fig. 22.7B).

RMA is likely the most beneficial and important wrist proprioceptive activity[5] but may be challenging to provide in the hand therapy clinic. Home programs incorporating gym and exercise circuits can be set up to incorporate activities requiring more space or equipment.

Rehabilitation Concepts Based on Specific Carpal Instability Patterns

Consideration should be given to nonoperative management of partial ligament injuries with predynamic or dynamic instability. If nonoperative management of carpal instability is unsuccessful, or more severe symptoms develop, surgical reconstruction may be indicated to provide stability. Following such procedures clients are typically immobilized for 6 to 12 weeks in a cast followed by a referral to hand therapy. This long immobilization period often results in significant wrist stiffness, requiring lengthy rehabilitation programs with an emphasis on regaining extension and radial/ulnar deviation.

Consideration should also be given to implementing a postoperative early controlled mobilization program following ligament repairs. This requires close collaboration between the surgeon and hand therapist. The surgeon must communicate the details of the surgical procedure, especially the amount of intraoperative tension placed on the repaired ligament, in order for the therapist to safely apply mobilization that will not compromise the reconstruction. It is very important to reduce the adverse changes to the sensorimotor process and CNS recognition of the limb during a period of immobilization.

Scapholunate Instability Patterns

Scapholunate dissociation is the most common carpal instability pattern and may appear as an isolated injury or in conjunction with other injuries, such as scaphoid or distal radius fractures. The precipitating injury is typically a FOOSH that causes wrist hyperextension, ulnar deviation, and midcarpal supination. A spectrum of scapholunate injuries that range from minor ligament sprains to complete perilunar dislocations are possible.[51] This spectrum produces alterations to carpal kinematics, which result in varying levels of dysfunction.

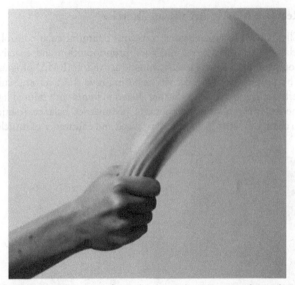

FIG. 22.5 Reactive muscular activation to increase proprioception and challenge anticipatory reactions with control: oscillating elastic bar for perturbation sense.

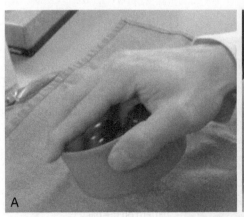
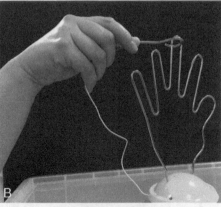

FIG. 22.6 Reactive muscle activation (A) controlling continuous movement of marbles in a rotating container (B) moving a wand around a wire shape without touching the wire.

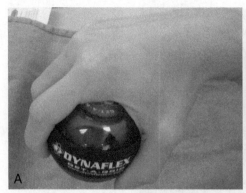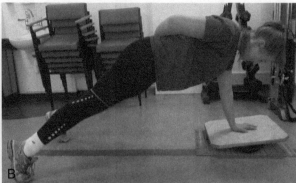

FIG. 22.7 Reactive muscle activation training by using (A) the Dynaflex Powerball. This is a gyroscope. The central sphere of this device produces random multidirectional forces stimulating proprioceptive end-organs enabling reactive muscle activation for joint stability. (B) Wobbleboard to balance in plank position bilateral or unilateral for high-level proprioceptive and muscle coactivation control.

Clients usually present with central or radial side wrist pain and complain that the wrist gives way during heavy activities. There may be some edema over the scapholunate interval with the wrist in flexion. There is likely to be good range of motion, but with pain on end-range of flexion and extension. Power grip may be weak.

Clinical assessment should include palpation, and areas of maximal tenderness should be noted. If sharp pain is elicited by pressing on the area just distal to Lister's tubercle, a scapholunate ligament tear should be suspected. Palpation should include ballottement of the scapholunate joint directly and a **Watson's Scaphoid Shift Test.**[52] Start with the wrist in ulnar deviation. Apply pressure over the volar prominence of the scaphoid tuberosity as the wrist is passively moved into radial deviation. Normally, the scaphoid flexes as the wrist radially deviates. With scapholunate dissociation or ligament laxity, the pressure on the scaphoid forces it under the dorsal rim of the radius. When the pressure is removed, the scaphoid returns to position with a painful clunk. A positive test reproduces the client's symptoms with this clunk. This test has been found to have 66% specificity and 69% sensitivity.[53]

Evaluation of the wrist should include review of radiographs. Static and dynamic radiographs will often demonstrate the following in the presence of complete scapholunate ligament tears[26,54]:

- P-A views may demonstrate a scapholunate gap of greater than 2 to 3 mm (Fig. 22.8A). This has been termed the Terry Thomas sign. Visualization may require a "clenched fist" view for dynamic instabilities.
- The scaphoid may be palmarly flexed, giving the appearance of a ring on the P/A neutral film (Fig. 22.8B).
- Lateral views of the wrist may demonstrate the lunate dorsiflexed 15 degrees or greater in relation to the capitate, and an abnormal scapholunate angle of more than 60 degrees. This deformity is called a DISI (Fig. 22.8C and D).
- Long-standing instability may show degenerative changes to the radial styloid and at the capitolunate joint.

Predynamic Instability

The predynamic instability stage is the earliest sign of scapholunate pathology.[50] In this stage, the scapholunate membrane is attenuated or partially torn, producing mild abnormal motion between the scaphoid and the lunate. This kinematic change

produces wrist synovitis and pain. If this injury is left untreated in clients with repetitive stress or recurring wrist trauma, there is attenuation of the secondary stabilizers of the wrist and further degeneration of the scapholunate ligament, which may lead to dynamic and static instability.[55] In this stage of injury, plain radiographs are normal. Stress radiographs are typically normal as well.

Dynamic Instability

This stage of instability includes ligamentous tears of either the palmar and/or dorsal portions of the scapholunate ligament. Complete disruption of the scapholunate membrane and ligaments results in substantial kinematic and force transmission change but does not necessarily demonstrate carpal malalignment. Static radiographs are most often normal. However, special stress radiographs will often demonstrate instability.

Static Instability

Static carpal malalignment occurs when there is failure of the scapholunate membrane and ligaments as well as the secondary scaphoid stabilizers. The scaphoid is further pulled into flexion, as the lunate extends. The scaphoid becomes a distal carpal row bone with its attachments to the trapezial bones. The lunate and triquetrum may then sublux dorsally, altering the angle of the lunocapitate joint. This is known as a DISI deformity, which has an increase in the scapholunate angle of greater than 60 degrees. The normal scapholunate angle is 30 to 60 degrees.

This form of instability may occur acutely because of a FOOSH injury or secondarily as a result of progressive attenuation of the secondary stabilizers. Clients often present with swelling in the wrist, pain, limited ROM, decreased grip strength, and limited functional use of the hand.

Scapholunate Advanced Collapse (SLAC) Wrist

Long-standing DISI deformities result in altered kinetics and radiocarpal load, which causes a sequential deterioration of the carpus leading to degenerative arthritis. This form of arthritis is predictable and begins at the radioscaphoid articulation, particularly at the tip of the styloid. Later advances include capitolunate changes. Further progression results in degeneration throughout the entire carpus.

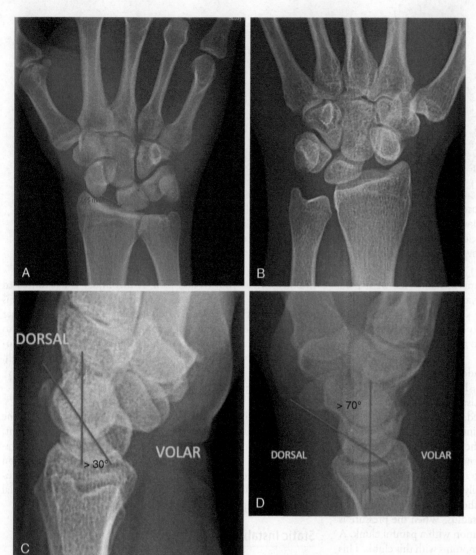

FIG. 22.8 (A) Posterior-anterior (P-A) radiograph of the wrist demonstrating a scapholunate gap of greater than 2 to 3 mm. (B) Scaphoid is palmarly flexed giving the appearance of a ring on P-A neutral radiograph. (C) Lateral views of the wrist may demonstrate the lunate dorsiflexed 15 degrees or greater in relation to the capitate. This deformity is called dorsal intercalated segment instability. (D) Lateral radiograph of the wrist demonstrating abnormal scapholunate angle of more 70 degrees.

Rehabilitation of Scapholunate Injury

Management of scapholunate injuries is quite challenging for both the surgeon and the hand therapist. The best treatment approach, where a diagnosis of static instability has been confirmed, is early surgical intervention. This allows for the restoration of normal carpal alignment while preventing attritional changes to the secondary wrist stabilizers. The management of predynamic and dynamic instabilities is controversial. Recently it has been suggested that stage 1 partial scapholunate injury[51] (predynamic or dynamic) should be managed by therapy and splinting.[56,57] Each client and injury should be discussed with the physician and an individualized program developed for them.[17]

Studies have shown that, in scapholunate dissociation, forces act across the scapholunate joint and produce gapping.[16,17] The implication for hand therapists is to consider implementing early controlled motion utilizing the dart-throwing motion pattern following surgical repair of scapholunate ligaments or acute dynamic scapholunate injuries.[56] However, early use of dart-throwing motion for partial or dynamic scapholunate injuries needs careful consideration as it may risk increasing forces to the injured ligaments.[17] An orthotic can be utilized to ensure that

wrist motion is within the arc of the dart-throwing motion pattern of movement. There is no clinical research determining the optimal time to introduce the dart-throwing motion, nor the safe range, nor the length of time to restrict motion following injury or surgery.

Predynamic and Dynamic Instability Rehabilitation

In acute injury with predynamic instability, clients may be casted for 7 to 10 days for pain and edema. Then the cast may be discontinued and the client given an orthosis to use during symptom-producing activities for an additional 2 to 6 weeks. The orthosis should hold the wrist in slight extension and ulnar deviation, with the distal carpal row in supination (hand in slight supination will achieve this) to reduce the ECU deforming action.[2] The purpose of the orthosis is for symptom control and to protect the wrist from inadvertent stresses during ADLs.

The client is encouraged to perform pain-free controlled AROM exercises to reduce wrist stiffness that may have occurred from immobilization. AROM exercises should be performed in the dart-throwing motion pattern, initially into radial extension to midrange (to reduce increasing forces on the scapholunate into

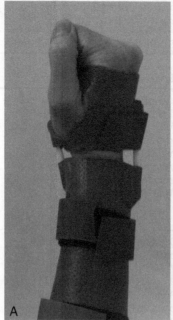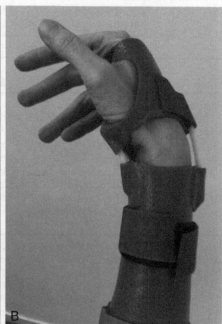

FIG. 22.9 Custom-made dart-throwing motion orthosis. (A) Demonstrating radial deviation with slight extension. (B) Demonstrating ulnar deviation with slight flexion. Bars volar and dorsal restrict flexion and extension and extremes of the desired movements.

ulnar flexion).[16,21,22] Most ADL tasks are performed in a plane from 40-degree wrist extension and 20-degree radial deviation to 0-degrees flexion and 20-degree ulnar deviation (similar to the dart-throwing motion).[15] Once the client can perform this motion pain free, they can be progressed to AROM in all planes. However, the client must be instructed not to perform rigorous passive ROM (PROM) or end-range ulnar deviation because this may place too much stress on the carpal ligaments and disrupt healing.

Once nearly full pain-free wrist AROM is achieved, the client can progress to strengthening and resistance exercises, which increase coactivation for stability.[5] Strong compressive grips during functional activity or therapy should be avoided as they may increase scapholunate ligament strain. Grip strength has been shown to improve with neuromuscular training alone.[32] In painful wrists, gentle isometric exercises in midrange can be started immediately to provide neuromuscular feedback with no tension to scapholunate ligaments.

Therapists should consider an early motion program in a dart-throwing motion–controlled orthosis for wrists with dynamic instability and complete rupture of scapholunate ligaments (but intact secondary stabilizers). This allows for healing of ligaments without surgical intervention and alongside a sensorimotor program.[56] A dart-throwing motion orthosis allows a controlled range through radial extension into ulnar flexion as the ligament heals, while restricting pure flexion/extension and deviation (Fig. 22.9A and B). Some therapists try to further protect scapholunate ligaments by placing the forearm in supination with above-elbow splinting. This may reduce carpal loading and strain at the scapholunate joint.[58] However, this practice needs careful consideration, as it inconveniences the client, causes stiffness at the distal and proximal radioulnar joints, and reduces proprioceptive awareness and neuromuscular feedback.

Most clients with symptomatic predynamic or dynamic instability resolve within 6 months without surgical intervention. However, in unresolved chronic cases, scapholunate surgery may be required.[54]

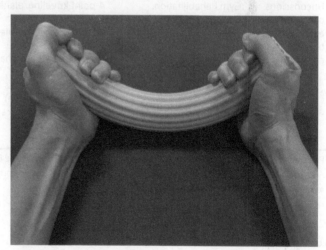

FIG. 22.10 Use of an elastic bar for coactivation of wrist muscles.

Proprioceptive Reeducation in the Presence of Predynamic and Dynamic Scapholunate Instability

Stability exercises need to be specific. Work on FCR, APL, and ECRL to stabilize and protect the scaphoid.[2,5] The ECRB may act as a lunate stabilizer by promoting extension of the capitate, which increases pressure on the palmar portion of the lunocapitate joint, which then counteracts the extension tendency of the lunate.[26] FCR is a "friendly" muscle in partial scapholunate ligament injuries and will support the scaphoid volarly.[5,26] Coactivation of ECU is beneficial but overactivity is not, so avoid strong or end-range FCU exercise, as this tends to pronate the scaphoid, strain the scapholunate ligament, and gap the scapholunate joint.[2] This deforming force is worst in end-range supination, so this position may be avoided during exercise and activity. Co-activation exercises focusing on radial muscles will increase stability—most easily carried out by bending an elastic bar into "smile" and "frown" shapes (Fig. 22.10).

TABLE 22.2   **The Birmingham Wrist Instability Programme for the Therapeutic Management of Stage 1 Scapholunate Instability – A Guideline**

THE BIRMINGHAM WRIST INSTABILITY PROGRAMME – TREATMENT GUIDELINES

Rehab Stage	Suggested Exercises	Exercise Examples/Plan	Aims/Reasoning	Criteria for Progression
Conscious control and isometric loading	Pain-free isometric strengthening with resistance bands (3 sets 8 reps, alternate days) Start in supination, progress to neutral and then pronated position Pain-free strengthening through range, resistance bands	In supination: 30-degree wrist ext., digits relaxed, isometric ECRL, FCR, APL In pronation: ECRL, FCR, APL isometric holds through 30 degrees incremental wrist positions Isometric loading ECRL, FCR, APL through wrist AROM	Overcome fear/avoidance and reduce pain Activate/strengthen scaphoid supinators in safe/functional position and range Work on kinesthesia/JPS Early perturbation exercises through ROM as wrist must be maintained in neutral deviation	Able to maintain neutral position during exercise Reducing pain at rest Able to maintain control though ROM, particularly at end of range extension
Unconscious control: "wrist balance"	Early weight bearing and RMA/perturbation	Bilateral hands on ball – neutral, pro/sup, rolling/circles Work to fatigue Progress to one hand Progress to standing e.g., wall press up Progress to load/surface Powerball	Early weight acceptance and proprioceptive challenge	No pain at end of extension ROM with overpressure
Unconscious control: higher load "wrist balance" and conditioning	Gym Rehabilitation. Return to sport	4-point kneeling/plank weightbearing. Bosu/gym ball Wobble board/sit fit Upper limb kinetic chain conditioning Low-load plyometrics (e.g., ball drop /catch) High-load plyometrics (e.g., clap press up). Sport-specific rehab	Increased load and complexity to challenge proprioception Start of power / plyometric exercises High-level activities, as required	Pain-free weight bearing with low load Return to normal level of competitive sport

Proposed Treatment Guidelines for stage one scapholunate ligament injuries – The Birmingham Wrist Instability Programme[30]

AROM, Active range of motion; *ECRL*, extensor carpi radialis longus; *FCR*, flexor carpi radialis; *APL*, abductor pollicis longus; *ext.* extension; *JPS*, joint position sense; *RMA*, reactive muscle activation; *pro/sup* pronation/supination.

The **Birmingham Wrist Instability Programme**[30] is a recently proposed treatment guideline (Table 22.2). It offers suggestions for exercises based on clinical reasoning and criteria for progression.[30] The guidelines suggest starting with isometric elastic band resistive exercise to activate the "friendly" muscles, reduce pain and fear avoidance, and help with early perturbation sensory feedback. Once isometrics are stable and pain free, co-activation exercise may be initiated with weight bearing onto soft and then hard surfaces. Finally, once the wrist is pain free with weight bearing and end-range extension, RMA, and more challenging activities, such as low-load plyometrics, upper-limb open chain, and sport/activity specific activities can be included.

Flexor Carpi Radialis Strengthening – or Not?

Instability of the scapholunate interval is one example of ligament injury where isometric training may be either beneficial or harmful, depending on the degree of ligament injury. If the scapholunate ligament is intact, the FCR is thought to be an important dynamic stabilizer of the scaphoid.[2] After a complete scapholunate ligament disruption with widening of the scapholunate interval; however, there is increased load distribution through the radial carpus with further displacement of the scaphoid when

the FCR is contracted.[54] Hence in a client with partial scapholunate ligament injury or laxity, isometric FCR exercise is beneficial through its stabilizing action on the scapholunate interval. In a complete, untreated scapholunate ligament injury, however, FCR strengthening exercises are detrimental and only serve to enhance scapholunate instability.

Surgical Management of Static Scapholunate Dissociation and Acute Rupture of Scapholunate Ligament

Acute static scapholunate instability can present with disruption of the scapholunate ligament; however, there is also significant trauma to the secondary stabilizing ligaments. The ideal timeframe for acute surgical repair has not yet been defined, but attaining a successful repair is difficult after 2 to 6 weeks post injury, as the intrinsic ligaments tend to undergo rapid degeneration.[54] Thus early repair is preferred. There are numerous surgical procedures to achieve successful repair.[54] Some of the options include:

• *Arthroscopic repair*
• *Percutaneous and Arthroscopic Kirschner Wire (K-wire) Fixation*

Typically, this is completed through a dorsal approach repairing the dorsal scapholunate ligament plus percutaneous K-wire fixation left in situ for 3 to 6 weeks.

Tendon reconstruction of the scaphoid stabilizers

Various surgical techniques using a tendon graft to reconstruct the scaphoid-stabilizing ligaments. Typically, a strip of FCR is used.

Reduction association of the scapholunate joint (RASL procedure)

This method consists of an open reduction, repair of the scapholunate ligament, and stabilization of the repair by internally fixating the scapholunate joint with one headless screw. The screw fixation is often maintained for 12 months or more.[26]

Open reduction and internal fixation (ORIF)

Capsulodesis and secondary ligament repair

Dorsal capsulodesis: The most commonly used technique is the Blatt capsulodesis. This procedure consists of tightening the radioscaphoid capsule to prevent excessive scaphoid rotation into flexion and pronation. This is done by creating a capsular checkrein from the dorsal capsule that limits scaphoid rotation. However, there is also a permanent loss of wrist flexion. Typically, individuals are limited to approximately 20 degrees of flexion.

Partial carpal fusion

The most common partial fusions in clinical practice are the scaphoid-trapezium-trapezoid, scaphoid-lunate, scaphoid-capitate, and radius-scaphoid-lunate fusions with distal scaphoidectomy.

Four corner fusions with scaphoidectomy is a common procedure for a SLAC wrist.

The overall results of ligament repair are acceptable in the acute phase when no degeneration is present. Clients often report minimal pain with return of more than 80% grip strength and 75% wrist motion. Less than one-third of clients develop degenerative changes within the carpus.[54]

Postsurgical Rehabilitation

Following primary scapholunate ligament repair or secondary reconstruction, the wrist is typically immobilized in a cast for 6 to 12 weeks. During this time, the client is instructed in a home exercise program consisting of finger, forearm, elbow, and shoulder ROM, and edema control techniques. Consideration should be given to immediate sensorimotor training in the cast using mirror therapy,[59] motor imagery,[44] unloaded isometric exercises of "friendly" muscles, and contralateral strengthening exercises. This has been shown to reduce pain by producing a CNS laterality effect activating the opposite sensorimotor cortex.[60]

Once the cast is removed, the client may need a wrist orthosis for intermittent protection, support, and pain control as symptoms dictate. Upon cast removal, the client should be instructed in the dart-throwing motion and midrange ROM exercises, avoiding ECU/FCU primary actions in order to prevent excessive tension on the repaired scapholunate ligament. There may be variations to the safe range of motion, loading, and strengthening resistance for specific types of surgery and this must be taken into consideration during the instruction of ROM and activity modification. Rehabilitation then continues as for dynamic scapholunate ligament injury as discussed earlier.

If significant limitations in wrist flexion or extension persist, the client may benefit from dynamic or static progressive post-through lever orthotic application following principles of low-load prolonged stretch and total end-range time[61] (Fig. 22.11A and B). Additionally, joint mobilization and heat modalities combined with prolonged stretch may be of benefit to gain range.

Early Controlled Protected Motion Following Surgical Repair

Dorsal capsulodesis procedures are sometimes performed to treat static scapholunate instability, as well as to treat dynamic scapholunate instability; and a modified capsulodesis can be used to correct capitolunate instability.[62] With scapholunate dissociation, the purpose of the capsulodesis procedures is to prevent volar rotation of the scaphoid with a capsular tether from the dorsum of the radius. This tether limits wrist flexion, usually aiming for approximately 45 degrees of flexion; thus the hand therapist must not be overzealous with attempts to regain postoperative wrist flexion after these procedures. A capsulodesis produces marked secondary wrist stiffness, particularly into flexion as well as tendon tethering. Tight or scarred repaired ligaments will alter the mechanics of the carpal bones and may produce ulnar pain with strain on the lunotriquetral ligament and TFCC.

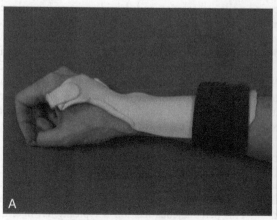
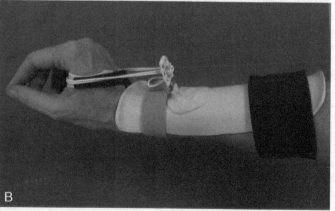

FIG. 22.11 Custom fabricated orthoses. (A) Serial static wrist extension orthosis. (B) Dynamic wrist extension orthosis.

To try to avoid these issues after capsulodesis, it has been proposed that instead of immobilizing the wrist for 6 to 10 weeks postoperatively, we might (based on sound clinical decision making and collaboration with the surgeon) place clients in a hinged wrist orthosis within the first few days or weeks of surgery. The hinged orthotic allows for controlled dart-throwing motion and wrist flexion/extension.[63] There is limited evidence for the efficiency of this treatment approach, but the clinical reasoning is that this approach reduces stress placed on the repair to prevent attenuation; preserves radial wrist extension, midrange, and other movements; and reduces lengthy immobilization. End-range flexion and ulnar deviation should be slowly gained. This rehabilitation approach should be reserved for reliable and motivated clients to ensure adherence to the program.

Specific Considerations: Intercarpal Fusion—Four Corner Fusion with Scaphoidectomy

Four corner fusion is often performed to manage static scapholunate dissociation with degenerative changes within the carpus. Following such procedures clients are immobilized in a cast for 8 to 16 weeks until bony consolidation is observed either through radiography or computed tomography scan. The purpose of such procedures is to provide pain relief and wrist stability. At final outcome, clients typically achieve approximately 50% wrist flexion-extension compared to the contralateral wrist.[64] Once bony consolidation is confirmed, the cast is removed and the client begins AROM and gentle PROM of the wrist and forearm in all planes. A wrist orthosis can be provided and worn as needed for support and pain control. The range of flexion/extension may need to be controlled with an orthotic for some weeks. Sensorimotor and neuromuscular rehabilitation is a priority, as these are often clients with chronic pain who will have altered CNS processing with reduced awareness and activation of "friendly" stabilizing muscles.[41]

Lunotriquetral Instability

Lunotriquetral instability is the second most common form of carpal instability and would be classified as a CID type.[26] Typically, lunotriquetral instabilities occur from either a traumatic or a degenerative cause. Clients will often present with ulnar-sided wrist pain, swelling over the ulnar dorsal area, pain with palpation of the joint, and pain in pronation. The pain is worse on deviation or rotation of the wrist. There may be ulnar nerve paresthesia from edema, and the wrist may give way with heavy loads. An audible click/clunk may be provoked on the ulnar side of the wrist, which may be worse with ulnar deviation. There may be a weak grip or a loss of ROM at the wrist.

Radiographs will often demonstrate the following:
- Lateral radiographs may demonstrate a VISI deformity, which is a capitolunate angle of greater than 30 degrees.
- Lateral radiographs will demonstrate that the lunate is more palmarly flexed.
- Lateral radiographs will demonstrate a normal scapholunate angle.

Most isolated injuries to the lunotriquetral supporting ligaments occur as a result of a backward FOOSH with the arm being in external rotation, forearm in supination, and the wrist in extension and radially deviated. With this, most of the impact is concentrated over the hypothenar eminence. However,

lunotriquetral instability can also be a result of a chronic condition, such as ulnocarpal abutment syndrome where increased load and pressure crosses through the lunotriquetral joint causing strain and attenuation of the ligaments. Either way, these injuries can be managed either operatively or nonoperatively.

Acute Lunotriquetral Injuries

If acute lunotriquetral injuries are diagnosed early, nonoperative management may be attempted. Typically, clients with predynamic or dynamic instability are immobilized for 2 to 6 weeks in a short arm cast or orthosis. The optimum orthosis needs to reduce the action of the "unfriendly" muscles (ECRL, APL, FCR) and enhance ECU. FCU may be "friendly" or "unfriendly" depending on the degree of instability. The orthosis should aim for a slightly pronated hand and neutral wrist extension/radial deviation. A pad beneath the pisiform and over the dorsum of the ulna may help maintain optimal alignment.

In complete rupture of lunotriquetral ligaments, unless pronation and supination is blocked, the amount of motion that occurs in the lunotriquetral joint during forearm rotation is substantial owing to the "pistonage" effect of the ulna against the carpus through the TFCC.[54] This micromotion can prevent proper healing of lunotriquetral ligaments. Thus, in the early stages, an above-elbow cast is recommended in cases where conservative management is attempted in the treatment of acute complete lunotriquetral injuries.[54]

Sensorimotor and neuromuscular rehabilitation is vital for recovery.[2] The muscles to focus on are ECU (+/– FCU) with reduced activation of ECRL, APL, FCR. Controlled co-activation exercises/activities provide dynamic balance and stability.

Static Instability: Postsurgical Management

When conservative management has failed to provide the client with symptom control or the injury is severe and acute, surgical intervention may be considered. Surgical options include reconstruction of the lunotriquetral ligaments; lunotriquetral partial arthrosis; and in advanced cases, a proximal row carpectomy. However, proximal row carpectomies are often reserved for clients who have a static VISI pattern of carpal alignment and/or lunotriquetral joint degeneration.

Wrist Arthroscopy

Following wrist arthroscopy and debridement of lunotriquetral ligament injury, a removable orthosis may be worn for 1 to 3 weeks postoperatively to provide pain control and prevent overzealous hand usage. The orthosis can be removed within the first 2 to 5 days postoperatively to initiate gentle active wrist ROM in all planes, with care taken in radial extension. The client is progressed to light loading and increased hand usage during functional activities, as tolerated. Incorporate sensorimotor and neuromuscular rehabilitation throughout.

Percutaneous Fixation of the Lunotriquetral Joint

It has been suggested that acute lunotriquetral ligament tears are best treated by percutaneous fixation of the lunotriquetral joint.[26,54] This percutaneous fixation is typically left in situ for a duration of 3 to 6 weeks while the client is immobilized in a short arm cast or orthosis. Consideration for an above-elbow cast

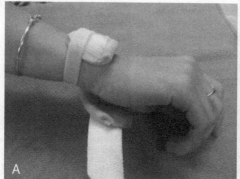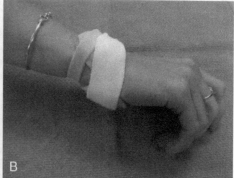

FIG. 22.12 Custom fabricated ulnar boost orthosis utilizing elastic strapping to reduce ulnar volar carpal sag.

should be given.[54] The client should be referred to hand therapy within the first week postoperatively to be instructed in finger, forearm, elbow, and shoulder ROM exercises and edema control techniques. Sensorimotor processing should be initiated immediately along with isometric exercises of the ECU.

Once the fixation is removed, gentle and controlled AROM of the wrist should be started in all planes, with care to minimize radial extension. At approximately 10 weeks post-surgery, PROM can be implemented as needed. The client is then progressed to a strengthening and RMA program.

Proprioceptive reeducation should be continued post initial healing with the focus on the FCU and hypothenar muscles to enhance dynamic stability of the lunotriquetral joint and ulnar wrist. Isometric contraction of the FCU and hypothenar eminence muscles produces a dorsally directed force on the triquetrum through the pisiform that helps assist with wrist stability.[5,54] The client is instructed to avoid impact loading and forceful forearm rotation for as long as 4 to 6 months, depending on pain and stability of the ulnar wrist.

Chronic Lunotriquetral Instability

In clients with chronic lunotriquetral instability who are not surgical candidates, symptom management and joint protection are the focus of hand therapy intervention. Orthoses are used to provide joint protection and symptom control during aggravating activities. The goal of hand therapy is to prevent further discomfort and to prevent the progression of lunotriquetral instability and secondary degenerative changes within the carpus. Typically, the chief complaint is ulnar-sided wrist pain with near full wrist ROM and strength. A home program is often sufficient for such clients and should consist of AROM of the wrist in all planes performed in a pain-free manner and isometric exercise of the FCU and hypothenar muscles. A custom-made ulnar boost orthosis may also prove to be useful for symptom control (Fig. 22.12).[65] As symptoms improve, the client may also attempt ulnar boost taping during work- or sports-related tasks. The therapist should instruct the client to avoid activities, wrist movements, and exercises that increase abutment, such as gripping with the forearm pronated. This increases ulnar variance and contributes to the symptoms of ulnar-sided wrist pain[54] RMA training exercises will increase proprioception to the lunotriquetral joint.

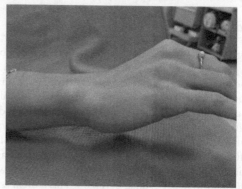

FIG. 22.13 This wrist demonstrates an ulnar volar sag of the carpus in relation to the distal ulna joint.

or intrinsic factors. Intrinsic midcarpal instability is characterized by generalized wrist ligament laxity, whereas extrinsic forms are secondary to bone abnormalities outside the carpus. Examples of extrinsic forms are distal radius fracture malunions and extrinsic ligament injuries found in association with ulnar minus variance. Intrinsic forms may be dorsal, palmar, or combined dorsal/palmar.

Midcarpal instability often results in a sense of wrist instability; significant wrist pain (either volar or dorsal); an abrupt painful click, clunk, or snap during ulnar deviation of the wrist; and weakness with gripping. The client often reports a painful clunk that occurs during ADLs, work, and sporting endeavors. This injury may be a result of trauma to the wrist or could have occurred more gradually with no traumatic history. Many clients who have symptoms of midcarpal instability often have generalized ligamentous laxity in other joints, so a screening for hypermobility spectrum disorder is useful.

The capitate can often be subluxated on the lunate when a dorsally-directed force is applied to the hand with the forearm held in neutral position. The reverse maneuver with a palmar-directed force on the hand can cause volar subluxation at the midcarpal area. The ligaments are likely to be partially torn or attenuated, keeping the carpal orientation intact. Radiologically, the carpal bones appear in normal orientation, thus making diagnosis difficult.

Clinical Examination

Observation of a client's wrist with midcarpal instability often reveals a volar sag over the ulnar carpus due to ligament laxity. This is best observed from the ulnar or axial view of the wrist (Fig. 22.13). Clients with generalized laxity will commonly have

Midcarpal Instability

Midcarpal instability is a common cause of wrist pain and is classified as a CIND pattern. Midcarpal instability refers to instability between the proximal and distal carpal rows.[26] It can be a result of extrinsic bilateral ulnar volar sag of the wrists but often have only unilateral symptoms. Physical examination often reveals tenderness over the triquetrohamate joint. A painful clunk over the midcarpal joint as the wrist is actively moved from radial to ulnar deviation may be felt and observed. Passive radioulnar motion with the forearm positioned in pronation or neutral rotation often reveals a click or clunk within the midcarpal joint.[54]

The **midcarpal shift test** is described by Lichtman and colleagues[66] and shows good sensitivity and specificity. This test is performed by placing the client's wrist in neutral and the forearm in pronation. A P-A force is applied at the level of the capitate and ulnar carpus. The wrist is then passively ulnarly deviated. This test is considered positive if a painful clunk occurs that reproduces the client's symptoms.

Diagnostic Imaging

Imaging the client with midcarpal instability often demonstrates normal plain radiographs including normal radiolunate, capitolunate and scapholunate angles.[61] A lateral radiograph in neutral deviation and magnetic resonance imagining may reveal a VISI or less often a DISI resting stance. However, it often does not identify any ligamentous disruption. The most helpful evaluation is videofluoroscopy combined with a physical examination.[54] The lateral fluoroscopic view in palmar often demonstrates a sudden dramatic shift of the position of the proximal carpal row when the wrist moves from radial to ulnar deviation. This is often associated with a clunk. This clunk occurs because the proximal carpal row is not moving synchronously from palmar flexion to dorsal flexion while moving from radial to ulnar deviation. The proximal carpal row gets behind and catches up, which leads to a dramatic clunk back into place. This is termed a **catch-up clunk.** Also, a **reverse catch-up clunk** is often demonstrated under fluoroscopy as the wrist moves from ulnar deviation back to neutral. This clunk pattern represents the wrist returning to its original subluxated position. On the P-A fluoroscopic view, a similar clunk can be seen within the proximal carpal as the wrist moves into ulnar deviation.

Rehabilitation of Midcarpal Instabilities

Nonoperative management of midcarpal instability can be challenging for the client and hand therapist. Therapy should begin with education and activity modification. The client should be instructed to avoid activities that require repetitive radial-ulnar motion. The aim of therapy is to support the volar sag and try to relocate the ulnar carpus with taping, splinting, improved muscle action and cocontraction. Prioritize sensorimotor proprioceptive awareness, mirror therapy, joint position sense, kinesthesia, and isometric exercises. Exercises should be initially performed in supination, which decreases ulna variance. The midcarpal clunk often reduces in supination.

Make sure that the early sensorimotor awareness, conscious control, and coactivation is pain free and stable before progressing to RMA. Consider then working the "friendly" ECU muscle for the dorsal ulnar carpus, and the FCU/ADM (abductor digiti minimi) for volar ulnar carpus.[54] Co-activation of the ECU and FCU muscles is important to support the ulnar carpus and TFCC through range.[5,54] Include FCR action, as this also pronates the carpus and may help stabilize the ulnar wrist. Perform

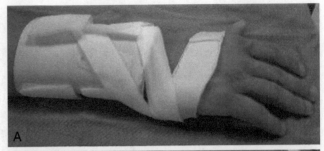
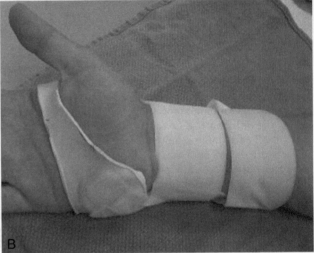

FIG. 22.14 (A) Dorsal view of custom-fabricated forearm-based ulnar-boost orthosis. (B) Volar view of custom-fabricated, forearm-based ulnar-boost orthosis.

reverse dart-throwing motion concentrating on radial flexion and ulnar extension movements.[2] Exercises with resistance bands, water bottles, ball rolling, and soft weight bearing will increase proprioceptive awareness.

The client should also be instructed how to properly contract the FCU, ECU, and hypothenar eminence muscles during ADLs and aggravating activities in order to provide dynamic stability to the midcarpal joint. Cocontraction of the FCU, ECU, and hypothenar eminence during ulnar deviation may provide sufficient dynamic muscle stabilization during the activities that produce the symptoms of a painful clunk.[5] Taping, either mechanical tape or elastic tape, may be used to add ulnar support and proprioceptive sensory feedback.[67]

Orthotic Application for Midcarpal Instability

If activity modification does not result in symptom reduction or resolution, clients may be placed in a midcarpal stabilization orthosis (Fig. 22.14A and B). This orthosis should provide a dorsally directed pressure on the pisiform with volar counterpressure over the head of the distal ulna to reduce the volar sag of the carpus and achieve a near neutral carpal alignment.[28] The orthotic may be worn full time for a period if pain/injury demands, but sensorimotor and isometric rehabilitation must be used alongside. Otherwise, it may be worn as needed for loaded or sustained function.

If the midcarpal instability is profound, or acute with marked pain, consideration should be given to a short period of above-elbow orthotic application with the forearm/wrist positioned in supination, and with an ulnar boost component in a Meunster type orthosis/sugar tong splint. However, this reduces all sensorimotor input, produces stiffness, is difficult to wear, and should be used with caution. Ideally, the orthosis should be forearm based.

If the pain is mild or resolves within the first few weeks, the client can be transitioned to a less cumbersome hand-based ulnar boost orthosis that allows for increased motion at the wrist. The orthosis aims to support the volar sag, reduce radial-to-ulnar movement, and prevent end-range pronation.[28] There are a variety of options and each client must be carefully assessed in pronation, neutral, and supination before a design is chosen. Care must be taken to avoid painful pressure over the pisiform or irritation of the ulnar nerve.

If the client plans to return to high-impact or forceful hand use and sports, consideration should be given to either continued use of the ulnar boost orthotic or ulnar boost taping techniques. This provides added wrist stability and protection during such activities. It is advised to delay return to aggressive hand use until the wrist is pain free and unconscious neuromuscular rehabilitation and strengthening have been completed.

Surgical Management of Midcarpal Instability

When all conservative measures fail to control symptoms, surgery is an option. Surgery is considered a salvage procedure as the kinematics of the wrist will be altered and the client needs to adapt in function. The surgical options have two categories consisting of soft-tissue procedures or limited midcarpal arthrodesis. During the rehabilitation phase, the surgeon and therapist must collaborate to ensure that the timing and progression of stress to the carpus will be appropriate and not compromise the surgery. A common soft-tissue procedure is DRTL reefing with K-wire. The DRTL is a major midcarpal joint stabilizer. Limited midcarpal arthrodesis has also been recommended in the literature for management of midcarpal instability.[6]

The client is casted for 8 to 12 weeks following surgery. Postoperative hand therapy should include proprioceptive awareness training, isometric exercises, and contralateral strengthening.[58] Postimmobilization, splinting may be worn for pain relief, avoidance of loading, and end-range radial-to-ulnar movements.

Distal radioulnar joint and TFCC instability can occur with trauma following distal radius fracture. TFCC injury occurs with 40% to 85% of unstable distal radius fractures.[68] Instability can also occur with radial head or Galeazzi fractures (fracture of the distal third of the radius with dislocation of the distal radioulnar joint), Essex-Lopresti lesions (interosseous ligament disruption between the radial and ulnar shafts occurring in combination with other trauma such as a radial head fracture), ulna impaction/abutment syndrome, ECU subluxation or tendinopathy, chronic distal radioulnar joint instability from missed ligament injury, and hypermobility spectrum disorder.[27] Clients complain of ulnar-sided pain, worse with rotation, loss of rotation range, clicking in rotation with decreased strength, and a feeling of the wrist "giving way." There may be an obvious dorsal displacement of the ulna most easily observed in pronation.[6] The **Ulna Fovea Test**[69] is indicative of foveal disruption of the distal radioulnar joint ligaments or of ulnotriquetral ligament injury. The **TFCC Press Test**[70] will reproduce ulnar-sided wrist pain with this injury.

Rehabilitation for Distal Radioulnar Joint and TFCC Instability

As previously discussed in lunotriquetral and midcarpal instability, rehabilitation should focus on sensorimotor processing prior to RMA and strengthening. Most proprioceptive sensory feedback is provided by the dorsal-ulnar mechanoreceptors, particularly those attaching to the triquetrum. Priority should therefore be given to proprioceptive awareness training and conscious neuromuscular rehabilitation focusing on PQ, FCU, ADM. Positioning in supination encourages tightening of the dorsal radioulnar ligament deep fibers and palmar radioulnar ligament volar fibers[6,11,54]. PQ is isolated in action with full elbow flexion (Fig. 22.15A). FCU contraction will produce pisiform compression onto the triquetrum and volar support to the ulnar wrist. Also work on the stabilizers of the proximal radioulnar joint (supinator, biceps, pronator teres). Exercises for ECU need to be assessed as its dorsal action on the ulna may be a deforming force in more severe instabilities. Coactivation

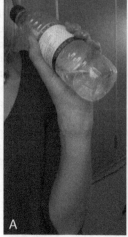
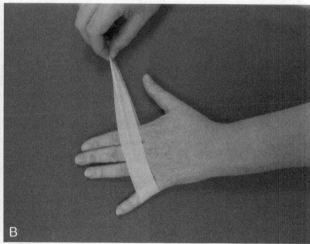

FIG. 22.15 (A) Gaining proprioception with oscillating water in a bottle during the isolating PQ rotation exercises. (B) Concentric and eccentric neuromuscular exercises for abductor digiti minimi to encourage ulnar and mid-carpal stability.

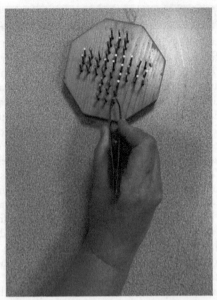

FIG. 22.16 Use of resisted grip with tweezers for coactivation of wrist muscles, particularly radial and intracarpal supination control muscles (extensor carpi radialis longus, abductor pollicis longus, flexor carpi radialis).

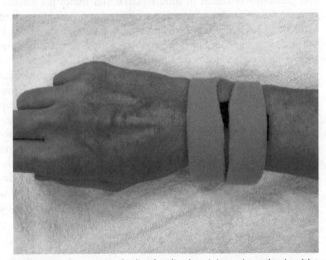

FIG. 22.17 Custom-made distal radioulnar joint wrist orthosis with ulnar support proximal and distal to ulna head, and compression at the distal radioulnar joint.

should be encouraged once conscious muscle control has improved. Isometric or concentric ADM will fire ulnar wrist stabilizers (Fig. 22.15B). Pinch grips with resistance will encourage radial muscle cocontraction[5] (Fig. 22.16).

Circumferential taping and orthoses may be beneficial (Fig. 22.17). Each client's degree of instability, pain, and functional requirements need to be considered when making these decisions. Orthoses should increase proprioceptive awareness and not reduce sensorimotor feedback or muscle function.

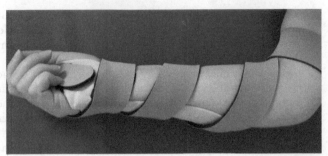

FIG. 22.18 Custom-made wrist extension post-through splint with neoprene rotation strap above elbow to gain rotation force at the distal and proximal radioulnar joints.

Surgical Management of Distal Radioulnar Joint/TFCC Instabilities

The underlying cause of the instability will guide surgical choices. For example, chronic distal radioulnar joint instability without degenerative change at the joint may be managed with ligament reconstruction.[6] Postoperatively, rotation may need to be initially restricted in an above-elbow cast or orthosis to allow ligament healing. An ulnar forearm-based orthosis may then be made to restrict end-range rotation and reduce loading across the TFCC and distal radioulnar joint.[6] Flexion/extension in neutral rotation will produce less force across the distal radioulnar joint than in end rotation. It is vital to work though conscious and unconscious neuromuscular rehabilitation to gain stability. Weight bearing should be avoided for some time.

A common complication of distal radioulnar joint/TFCC surgery is stiffness in rotation. A dynamic orthosis may be used to gain range both at the proximal and distal radioulnar joints. This should follow both total end-range time and low-load prolonged stretch [61] principles with a minimum of 6 hours of stretch per day (Fig. 22.18).

Summary

Rehabilitation following carpal ligament injury and reconstruction requires an in-depth understanding of the various instability patterns and their associated patho-anatomy. Close collaboration between the surgeon and hand therapist is essential, especially following reconstruction.

Rehabilitation must take into consideration many factors—the activity demands of the client; the specific injury pattern; phases of healing; and "friendly and unfriendly" muscle contributions and coactivation in stability and loading, alongside their effect on carpal alignment. The importance of maintaining and rehabilitating sensorimotor and neuromuscular processes while maximizing proprioceptive awareness is now well understood and must be integrated into the therapy program.

References

1. Hagert E, Hagert CG: Understanding stability of the distal radioulnar joint through understanding of its anatomy, *Hand Clin* 26:459–466, 2010.
2. Esplugas M, et al.: Role of muscles in the stabilisation of ligament-deficient wrists, *J Hand Ther* 29:166–174, 2016.
3. Huang JL, Hanel DP: Anatomy and Biomechanics of the distal radioulnar joint, *Hand Clin* 28:157–163, 2012.
4. Lichtman DM, Martin RA: Introduction to the carpal instabilities. In Lichtman DM, editor: *The wrist and its disorders*, Philadelphia, 1988, WB Saunders, pp 245–250.
5. Hagert E: Proprioception of the wrist joint: a review of current concepts and possible implications on the rehabilitation of the wrist, *J Hand Ther* 23(1):2–16, 2010.
6. Altman E: The ulnar side of the wrist: clinically relevant anatomy and biomechanics, *J Hand Ther* 29:111–122, 2016.
7. Mataliotakis G, et al.: Sensory innervation of the sub regions of the scapholunate interosseous ligament in relation to their structural composition, *J Hand Surg* 34(8):1413–1421, 2009.
8. Hagert E: *Wrist ligaments –innervation patterns and ligamento-muscular reflexes*, Stockholm, Sweden, 2008, Karolinska Instititet, p p51.
9. Kleinman WB: Stability of the distal radioulnar joint: biomechanics, pathophysiology, physical diagnosis and restoration of function. What we have learnt in 25 years, *J Hand Surg* 32(7):1086–1106, 2007.
10. Linscheid RL, et al.: Traumatic instability of the wrist: diagnosis, classification, and pathomechanics, *J Bone Joint Surg Am* 54:1612–1632, 1972.
11. Salva-Coll G, et al.: Effects of forearm muscles on carpal stability, *J Hand Surg Eur* 36(7):553–559, 2011.
12. Berger R: Anatomy and kinesiology of the wrist. In Mackin EJ, Callahan AD, Skirven TM, et al.: *Rehabilitation of the hand and upper extremity*, ed 6, St Louis, 2011, Mosby, pp Pp18–27.
13. Kamal RN, et al.: Carpal kinematics and kinetics, *J Hand Surg Am* 41(101):1–1018, 2016.
14. Patterson R, et al.: Scaphoid anatomy and mechanics: update and review, *Atlas Hand Clin* 9:129–140, 2004.
15. Palmer AK, et al.: Functional wrist motion: a biomechanical study, *J Hand Surg Am* 10:39–46, 1985.
16. Tang JB, et al.: In vivo length changes of carpal ligaments of the wrist during dart-throwing motion, *J Hand Surg Am* 36(2):284–290, 2011.
17. Garcia-Elias M, et al.: Dart-throwing motion in patients with scapholunate instability: a dynamic four dimensional computed tomography study, *J Hand Surgery Eur* 39(4):346–352, 2014.
18. Huang JL, Hanel DP: Anatomy and Biomechanics of the distal radioulnar joint, *Hand Clin* 28:157–163, 2012.
19. Gillula LA, Weeks PM: Post-traumatic ligamentous instabilities of the wrist, *Radiology* 129(3):641–651, 1978.
20. Garcia-Elias M: Kinetic analysis of carpal stability during grip, *Hand Clin* 13(1):151–158, 1997.
21. Salva-Coll G, et al.: Scapholunate instability: proprioception and neuromuscular control, *J Wrist Surg* 2:136–140, 2013.
22. Salva-Coll G, et al.: Role of the extensor carpi ulnaris and its sheath on dynamic carpal stability, *J Hand Surgery Eur* 27(6):544–548, 2012.
23. Hagert E, et al.: Differences in the presence of mechanoreceptors and nerve structures between wrist ligaments may imply differential roles in wrist stabilization, *J Orthop Res* 23(4):757–763, 2005.
24. Jeter E, et al.: Conservative rehabilitation. In Lichtman DM, Alexander AH, editors: *The wrist and its disorders*, ed 2, Philadelphia, 1997, WB Saunders, pp 699–708.
25. Clayman CB: *The American Medical Association encyclopedia of medicine*, New York, 1989, Random House.
26. Dobyns JH, Cooney WP: Classification of carpal instability. In Cooney RL, Linscheid RL, Dobyns JH, editors: *The wrist: diagnosis and operative treatment*, vol 1. St Louis, 1998, Mosby, pp 490–500.
27. Tinkle BT, et al.: *The ehlers-danlos syndromes: reports from the international consortium on the ehlers-danlos syndromes*, March 2017, pp 5–237. 175C:1.
28. Skirven TM: Rehabilitation for carpal ligament injury and instability. In Mackin EJ, Callahan AD, Skirven TM, et al.: *Rehabilitation of the hand and upper extremity*, ed 6, St Louis, 2011, Mosby, pp 1013–1023.
29. Wolff AL, Wolfe SW: Rehabilitation for scapholunate injury: application of scientific and clinical evidence to practice, *J Hand Ther* 29:146–153, 2016.
30. Holmes M, et al.: Early outcomes of 'The Birmingham Wrist Instability Porgramme": a pragmatic intervention for stage one scapholunate instability, *Hand Therapy* 22(3):90–100, 2017.
31. Karagiannopoulos C, et al.: A descriptive study on wrist and hand sensorimotor impairment and function following distal radius fracture intervention, *J Hand Ther* 23(3):204–214, 2013.
32. Hincapie OL, et al.: Proprioceptive retraining for a patient with chronic wrist pain secondary to ligament injury with no structural instability, *J Hand Ther* 29:183–190, 2016.
33. Braun C, et al.: Dynamic organisation of the somatosensory cortex induced by motor activity, *Brain* 124:2259–2267, 2001.
34. Petrie S, et al.: Mechanoreceptors in the palmar wrist ligaments, *J Bone Joint Surg Br* 79(3):494–496, 1997.
35. Hagert E, et al.: Evidence of wrist proprioceptive reflexes elicited after stimulation of the scapholunate interosseous ligament, *J Hand Surg Am* 34:642–651, 2009.
36. Solomonow M: Sensory-motor control of ligaments and associated neuromuscular disorders, *J Electromyogr Kinesiol* 16:549–567, 2006.
37. Brown DE, Lichtman DM: The evaluation of chronic wrist pain, *Orthop Clin North Am Apr* 15(2):183–192, 1984.
38. TFCC Tear Weight-bearing test –transcript at www.wrist widget.com.
39. Vincent JL, et al.: The push-off test: development of a simple, reliable test of upper extremity weight-bearing capacity, *J of Hand Ther* 27:185–191, 2014.
40. Riemann BL, Lephart SM: The sensorimotor system. Part II: The role of proprioception in motor control and functional joint stability, *J Athl Train* 37(1):80–84, 2002.
41. Karagiannopoulos C, Michlovitz S: Rehabilitation strategies for wrist sensorimotor control impairment: from theory to practice, *J Hand Ther* 29:154–165, 2016.
42. Altschulwe EJ, Hu J: Mirror therapy in a patient with a fractured wrist and no active wrist extension, *Scand J Plast Reconstr Surg Hand* 42:110–111, 2008.
43. Rosen B, Lundborg G: Training with a mirror in rehabilitation of the hand, *Scand J Plast Reconstr Surg Hand* 39:104–108, 2005.
44. Sabate M, et al.: Brain lateralisation of motor imagery: motor planning asymmetry as a cause of movement lateralisation, *Neuropsychologia* 8:1041–1049, 2004.
45. Proske U, Gandevia SC: The kinaesthetic senses, *J Physiol* 587:4139–4146, 2009.
46. Salles JI, et al.: Effect of strength training on shoulder proprioception, *J Athlet Train* 50(3):277–280, 2015.
47. Prosser R, et al.: Current Practice in the diagnosis and treatment of carpal instability –results of a survey of Australian 100 hand therapists, *J hand Ther* 20:239–242, 2007.
48. Woodley BL, et al.: chronic tendinopathy: effectiveness of eccentric exercise, *Br J Sports Med* 41:188–198, 2007.
49. Rainbow MJ, et al.: Functional Kinematics of the wrist, *J of Hand Surgery Eur* 41(1):7–21, 2016.
50. Balan SA, Garcia-Elias M: Utility of the Powerball in the invigoration of the musculature of the forearm, *Hand Surg* 13:79–83, 2008.
51. Garcia-Elias M, et al.: Three ligament tenodesis for the treatment of scapholunate dissociation: indications and surgical technique, *J Hand Surg Am* 31:125–134, 2006.
52. Watson HK, et al.: Examination of the scaphoid, *J Hand Surgery* 13A:657–660, 1988.
53. LaStayo P, Howell J: Clinical provocative tests used in evaluating wrist pain: a descriptive study, *J Hand Ther* 3:10–17, 1995.

54. Garcia-Elias M: Carpal instability. In Mackin EJ, Callahan AD, Skirven TM, et al.: *Rehabilitation of the hand and upper extremity*, ed 6, St Louis, 2011, Mosby, pp Pp1002–1012.

55. Tang JB, et al.: Wrist kinetics after scapholunate dissociation: the effect of scapholunate interosseous ligament injury and persistent scapholunate gaps, *J Orthop Res* 20:215–221, 2002.

56. Sorensen AA, et al.: Minimally clinically important differences of 3 patient rated outcome instruments, *J Hand Surg Am* 38:641–649, 2013.

57. Chennagiri RJR, Lindau TR: assessment of scapholunate instability and review of evidence for management in the absence of arthritis, *J Hand Surg Eur* 38:727–738, 2013.

58. Farr, et al.: Wrist tendon forces with respect to forearm rotation, *J Hand Surg Am* 38:35–39, 2013.

59. Leon-Lopez MT, et al.: Role of the extensor carpi ulnaris in the stabilisation of the lunotriquetral joint. An experimental study, *J Hand Ther* 26:312–316, 2013.

60. Lee M, et al.: Unilateral strength training increases voluntary activation of the opposite untrained limb, *Clin Neurophysiol* 120:802–808, 2009.

61. Flowers K, LaStayo P: Effect of Total End range time on improving passive range of motion, *J Hand Therapy* 7(3):150–157, 1994.

62. Blatt G: Capsulodesis in reconstructive hand surgery. Dorsal capsulodesis for the unstable scaphoid and volar capsulodesis following excision of the distal ulna, *Hand Clin* 3:81–102, 1987.

63. Chinchalkar SJ, et al.: Controlled active mobilization after dorsal capsulodesis to corret capitolunate dissociation, *J Hand Ther* 23(4):404–410, 2010.

64. Bednar JM, et al.: Wrist reconstruction: salvage procedures. In Mackin EJ, Callahan AD, Skirven TM, et al.: *Rehabilitation of the hand and upper extremity*, ed 6, St Louis, 2011, Mosby, pp 1024–1033.

65. Chinchalkar S, Yong SA: An ulnar boost splint for midcarpal instability, *J Hand Ther* 17:377–379, 2004.

66. Lichtman DM, Wroten ES: Understanding midcarpal instability, *J Hand Surg Am* 31:491–498, 2006.

67. Porretto-Loehrke A: Taping techniques for the wrist, *J Hand Ther* 29:213–216, 2016.

68. Sammer DM, Chung KC: Management of the distal radioulnar joint and ulnar styloid fracture, *Hand Clin* 28:199–206, 2012.

69. Tay SC, et al.: The "ulnar fovea sign" for defining ulnar wrist pain: an analysis of sensitivity and specificity, *J Hand Surg Am* 32:438–444, 2007.

70. Lester B, et al.: "Press Test" for office diagnosis of triangular fibrocartilage complex tears of the wrist, *Ann Plast Surg* 35(1):41–45, 1995.

23

Hand Fractures

Melissa J. Hirth
Angela C. Chu
Julianne Wright Howell

Introduction

Our hands take part in nearly every vocational and avocational human activity, which makes them vulnerable to injury. As a result, 20% of all fractures in adults and children involve the hand.[1] Half of all hand fractures involve the metacarpals, with phalangeal fractures of the distal, proximal, and middle phalanx in that order, composing the other half. When a fracture disrupts the skeletal foundation of the hand, concomitant soft-tissue injury is likely. Fracture management necessitates skillful and timely intervention so not to permanently affect the complex biomechanics of the hand and digits. Hand fractures vary in severity, so are often managed by a team of healthcare professionals that may include a physician, hand therapist, and hand surgeon. While some hand fractures require surgery, most do not, though all require time for the bone to heal and strengthen. Hand trauma can give way to psychosocial issues, dependence on others for assistance with self-care, and the inability to participate in usual work and leisure activities.

After metacarpal and phalangeal fracture, skeletal stability is lost. The once useful dynamics of the extrinsic and intrinsic muscles potentially convert to forces of deformity that can interfere with bone healing. To achieve the primary objectives of fracture management, hand therapists must understand bone repair, fracture patterns and muscle dynamics effect on fracture stability, surgical and nonsurgical methods of management, and techniques for safe implementation of early controlled mobilization. With these essentials, fractures will heal and strengthen, and joint stiffness, tendon adhesion, and loss of muscle function will be minimized.

Anatomy for Hand Fracture Management

Fracture management starts with an appreciation of the normal architecture of the hand; fluency with the names and locations of the bones; and comprehension of how the normal extrinsic and intrinsic muscle forces, after fracture, challenge a less than stable skeleton. The dorsally convex metacarpal bones act as skeletal arches to provide a gliding surface for the long extensor tendons and a concavity in which the long flexors and lumbrical muscles tuck away into the palm. The convex shape of the metacarpal **shaft** makes it structurally strong, with the denser cortical bone on the volar rather than dorsal surface.[2] Each metacarpal (MC) varies in length and width. The longest is the **index finger** or **second MC**, followed by the **long finger** or **third MC**, **ring finger** or **fourth MC**, **small finger** or **fifth MC**, and the **thumb** or **first MC** (Fig. 23.1). The **base** of each metacarpal is twice as wide as its shaft, and articulates with the carpal bones to form the **carpometacarpal** (CMC) joints. Mobility of each CMC joint varies indirectly with the length of the MC shaft. The thumb, with the shortest MC, is the most mobile, followed by the CMC joints of the ring and small fingers that have 15 to 25 degrees of motion. The index finger CMC joint is the least mobile.

There are three bony arches of the hand, the **longitudinal arch** is best seen by looking at the lateral view of the long metacarpal shaft. There are two **transverse arches**. The **proximal** transverse arch at the carpal tunnel is formed by the articulation of the metacarpal bases with the carpal bones (CMC). The **deep intermetacarpal ligaments** create the **distal** transverse arch by linking finger metacarpal **heads** (Fig. 23.2). These archways create the frame on which the extrinsic and intrinsic hand muscles coordinate to perform gross and fine motor functions, such as grasping a cellular phone and cupping the hand to hold pills or coins. These stable arch systems are potentially at risk following metacarpal fracture or CMC joint fracture/dislocation when the intrinsic and extrinsic muscle forces are not sufficiently controlled and/or immobilized improperly.

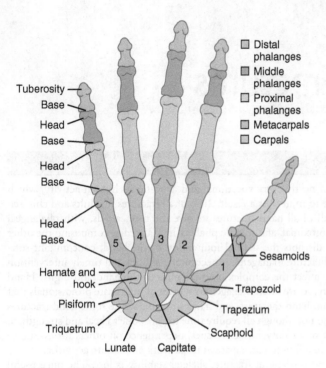

Distal phalanges
Middle phalanges
Proximal phalanges
Metacarpals
Carpals

Tuberosity
Base
Head
Base
Head
Base
Head
Base

5 4 3 2
1

Sesamoids

Hamate and hook
Pisiform
Triquetrum
Lunate   Capitate

Trapezoid
Trapezium
Scaphoid

Bones of right wrist and hand (palmar view)

FIG. 23.1 Volar view of the bones of the hand and wrist. *From Pratt NE. Anatomy and kinesiology of the hand. In: Skirven TM, Osterman AL, Fedorczyk JM, et al. eds. Rehabilitation of the Hand and Upper Extremity. 6th ed. Philadelphia, PA: Mosby Elsevier; 2011.*

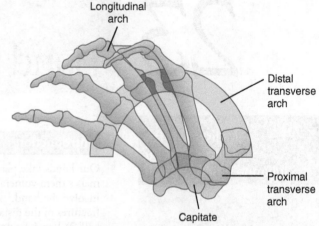

Longitudinal arch

Distal transverse arch

Proximal transverse arch

Capitate

FIG. 23.2 The longitudinal and transverse arches of the hand. *From Pratt NE. Anatomy and kinesiology of the hand. In: Skirven TM, Osterman AL, Fedorczyk JM, et al. eds. Rehabilitation of the Hand and Upper Extremity. 6th ed. Philadelphia, PA: Mosby Elsevier; 2011.*

The extrinsic **extensor carpi radial longus** (ECRL) and **extensor carpi radials brevis** (ECRB) attach respectively into the dorsal base of the second MC and third MC. Opposite to these muscles is the **flexor carpi radialis** (FCR) insertion into the second and third MC. The **extensor carpi ulnaris** (ECU) inserts into the dorsal base of the small or fifth MC opposite the **flexor carpi ulnaris** (FCU) insertion into the volar fifth MC base. Three **palmar interossei** muscles insert proximally along the MC shafts facing the axis of the hand on the second, fourth, and fifth MCs. The four **dorsal interossei** muscles have double origins from neighboring first to fifth MC shafts.[3] The pisiform and hook of the hamate serve as origins for the **abductor digiti minimi** (ADM) and the distal insertions are into the capsule of the fifth MC periarticular structures and the extensor hood. The hook of the hamate and the flexor retinaculum proximally anchor the **opponens digiti minimi** (ODM) while the distal insertion is along the entirety of the ulnar/volar fifth MC shaft.

Similar to the metacarpals, all 14 **phalanges** have volar facing concave shafts, proximal epiphysis or base; and all except the distal phalanx have a distal epiphysis or head connected to the MC shaft by a neck. The terminal end of the distal phalanx is the **tuft**. The thumb has only two phalanges, proximal and distal.

The long tendon of the **flexor digitorum profundus** (FDP) and **terminal tendon** of the extensor mechanism insert respectively into the volar and dorsal base of the finger's distal phalanx or **P3**. The nailbed stabilizes the highly innervated and mobile volar fat pad of the distal phalanx, to aid sensibility and prehensile dexterity of the digits (explaining why distal phalangeal injuries can be so painful). The **extensor pollicis longus** (EPL) dorsally, and **flexor pollicis longus** (FPL)

volarly, are extrinsic muscles that move the distal phalanx of the thumb. The extrinsic **flexor digitorum superficialis** (FDS) inserts into the volar base of the middle phalanx or **P2** of the finger, while the **central slip** or extensor digitorum communis (EDC) tendon of the extensor mechanism and the superficial attachments of the interosseous muscles insert to the dorsal base of P2.

The **extensor hood** covers two-thirds of the proximal phalanx (**P1**) with contributions from the common extensor, lumbrical, and interosseous muscles. Only the dorsal section of the dorsal interossei insert into the base of P1 at the radial tubercle (second to third) and ulnar tubercle (fourth).[3] The pisiform and radial MC base of the small finger serve as the proximal insertion for the **flexor digiti minimi** (FDM), and the distal insertion is to the ulnar base of the fifth digit's proximal phalanx.[3]

The thumb or **thenar** intrinsic muscles, the **abductor pollicis brevis** (APB), **flexor pollicis brevis** (FPB) and **opponens pollicis** (OP) muscles originate primarily from the flexor retinaculum. The APB inserts distally into the extensor hood of the thumb, which covers the dorsal surface of P1. The superficial head of the FPB inserts into the metacarpophalangeal (MCP) joint capsule and base of P1 with the deep head attaching to the radial sesamoid. The OP inserts into the radial shaft and neck of the first MC. The **adductor pollicis** (AP) has two heads, oblique and transverse, the former originating from the carpals and second and third MC bases, and the latter from the volar MC shaft of the long finger. Distal insertion of the AP oblique is the ulnar sesamoid and transverse AP inserts into the extensor hood of the thumb.[4]

Joint or **intraarticular fractures/dislocations** may involve the bone, cartilage, and the soft-tissue structures. Joint stability is dependent on the congruity of the bone articular surfaces and soft-tissue structures such as the volar plate, collateral ligaments, and the joint capsule. Healthy articular surfaces and intact soft-tissue restraints are necessary to control excessive extension and lateral or rotational forces encountered by the hand. The proximal interphalangeal (PIP) joint is a bicondylar hinge joint reinforced volarly by a fibrocartilage volar plate, attached to the central volar base of the P2 laterally by the proper and accessory collateral ligaments attaching to the lateral head of P1 and

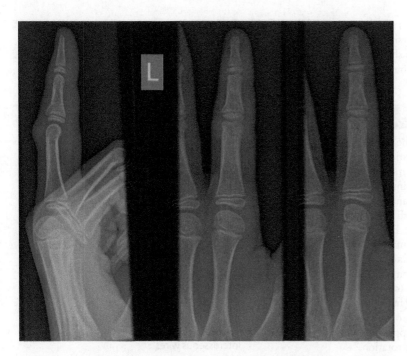

FIG. 23.3 X-rays of left index finger middle phalanx Salter-Harris type II fracture.

lateral base of P2 and into the volar plate. The potentially harmful dynamics following PIP joint fracture/dislocation come from the extensor forces delivered by the central slip tendon anchored to the dorsal tubercle at the base of P2 and the opposing FDS attachment to the base of P2 just beyond that of the volar plate.

The articular contact between the wide cam-shaped MC heads and the shallow P1 bases enable radial to ulnar deviation of the MCP joint. The collateral ligaments stabilize the MCP joints most in flexion not MCP joint extension. The suspension composed of the sagittal band, volar plate, collateral ligaments, and the intermetacarpal ligament provide for MCP joint stability. The intermetacarpal ligament is a key stabilizer after MC fracture, preventing metacarpal proximal migration and rotation. After MCP joint fracture/dislocation, it is evident how the interossei muscles, the EDC, and extrinsic long flexors become potential destabilizers.

The interlocking carpal bones of the proximal transverse arch have strong interosseous ligaments securing them to each other and to the stout MC bases. High-impact forces are required to fracture/dislocate the CMC joints, with the more mobile thumb, ring, and small finger CMC joints most often involved. Stability of the contoured saddle-shaped thumb CMC joint or **trapeziometacarpal joint** is dependent on the strong **palmar oblique** or **beak ligament** and intrinsic thenar muscles. When this joint is fracture/dislocated, the extrinsic abductor pollicis longus (APL) and AP are the key dynamic destabilizers. Also joined by interosseous ligaments, the highly mobile ring and small finger CMC joints become vulnerable to the destabilizing forces of the ECU and FCU after fracture/dislocation.

Assessment and Classification of Hand Fractures

Diagnosis of hand fractures requires a thorough assessment including interview, physical examination, and radiographs (X-rays). The client's description of the incident may be helpful to better understand the mechanism of injury.[5] The client's hand dominance, vocation, and hobbies directly affect the plan of care.

Physical examination should include observation for skin abrasions, edema, and angular or rotational deformity of the digits during active motion. The hallmark of fracture examination is tenderness or pain with palpation of the suspected fracture site. Closed fractures allow palpation; however, soft-tissue wounds associated with open or exposed fractures will prohibit it. A brief neurovascular exam may be indicated dependent on the mechanism of injury (e.g., crush and gunshot), presence of skin punctures/cuts, or client report of sensation loss. X-rays are necessary to complete the actual diagnosis of fracture. X-ray **views** are taken in one plane or combination of planes such as **lateral, posterior-anterior** (P-A) or **anterior-posterior** (A-P), and **oblique**. At least three hand series views are standard, with other views such as Brewerton views for MC head fractures taken to better assess the fracture configuration.[6]

Fractures are either **extraarticular** (away from the joint) or **intraarticular** (involving the joint). A global classification system for fractures and dislocations has been developed and recommended by the Orthopaedic Trauma Association (OTA) in conjunction with the AO Foundation.[7] This classification system assigns numbers to each carpal, metacarpal, and phalanx. Areas of fracture location are diaphyseal versus shaft, and proximal or distal end segments as opposed to neck or head and base, respectively.[7] Fracture types for the end segments are assigned A for extraarticular, B for partial articular, and C for complete articular.[7] Diaphyseal fracture types are A for simple, B for wedge, and C for multifragmentary.[7] Most hand surgeons, hand therapists, physicians, and radiologists continue to use the traditional fracture nomenclature in daily communications (as written in this chapter). However, awareness of the OTA/AO classification system is important when reviewing and publishing in professional literature.

The most widely used classification for **pediatric** fractures is the Salter-Harris system. There are five types of **physeal** or **growth plate** fractures dependent on the involvement of the metaphysis, physis, or epiphysis.[8] The X-ray in Fig. 23.3 shows the fractured left index finger of a 9-year-old girl following a basketball injury. This is a SH-II fracture of the metaphysis of the proximal middle phalanx. The lateral X-ray best shows the fracture extending from the dorsal cortex to the metaphysis. There is no significant displacement or angulation, and the shadowed outline is representative of local edema expected after fracture.

Pathology of Hand Fractures

When a bone fractures, the outer wrapping around the bone or **periosteum** is injured, the amount of periosteal disruption coincides with the degree of bone displacement. For the most part, when a bone remains (aligned) **nondisplaced** or minimally displaced, the periosteum stays intact. Conservative management is generally the choice for nondisplaced fractures with a stable fracture patterns such as transverse or short oblique. Fractures that are less stable but non-displaced may require splinting with Kirschner-wires (K-wires) for added protection. **A displaced** fracture causes variable periosteal disruption, which in conjunction with fracture pattern may require manual re-alignment (**closed** or **open reduction**) and potentially, fixation with surgical hardware. The decision to declare a fracture displaced includes observing one or more of the following factors on X-ray review: appropriate volar angulation, dorsal angulation, shortening, and/or rotation.[9]

Table 23.1 provides an overview of surgical and nonsurgical methods used to control fracture alignment to be discussed later in this chapter.

Second to Fifth Metacarpal Fracture Pathology

The highly mobile first to fifth metacarpals are the most commonly fractured followed by the fourth MC, which has the most narrow shaft diameter.[10] The most common concerns with MC shaft fractures involve issues with fracture shortening (displacement and angulation) and rotation, which may require surgical intervention to correct. **Transverse** and **oblique** MC fractures usually result from direct impact or longitudinal compression.[11] Transverse fractures are generally more stable than oblique, with the oblique fracture more likely to have additional concerns such as fragment rotation and loss of relative bone height.[11]

Most metacarpal fractures have a **dorsal apex** (angulate dorsally), a direct influence of the deforming forces from the palmar interossei muscles.[11] Although aesthetically displeasing for some, these fractures are more forgiving and do not always require surgery to improve function. Surgical intervention of MC fractures depends on the digit and the extent of angulation. Surgery is considered when the angulation is greater than 40 to 50 degrees in the fifth MC, 30 degrees in the fourth MC, 20 degrees in the third MC, and 15 degrees in the second MC.[6] Angulation results in shortening of the digit, more common in the ring and small finger, less in the index and long finger, all of which are constrained by the intermetacarpal ligament. Every 2 mm of metacarpal shortening can result in 7 degrees of PIP joint extensor lag. However, some surgeons will accept 6 mm of shortening and do no surgery. MC fracture fragments that are dorsally extended have the potential to cause traumatic rupture of the EDC tendon and thus require surgical review.[11] Rotation in any finger fracture creates scissoring upon flexion of the fingers. The extent of rotation is not often appreciated until the fingers actively flex. Normally, when flexed, all fingers should point toward the scaphoid tubercle. Each degree of metacarpal rotation results in 5 degrees or 1.5 cm of finger overlap. The surgeon determines which metacarpal fractures are manageable by

TABLE 23.1   Fracture Relative Stability, Method of Reduction and Healing

Relative Fracture Stability	Method of Reduction	Method of Healing
Least Stable/ Unstable	**Closed Reduction (CR)**	**Secondary**
	Cast	
	Fracture brace/orthosis	
	Percutaneous pins (PCP) or Kirschner wire (K-wire)	
	External fixator	
	Traction with PCP	
	Open Reduction with Internal Fixation (ORIF)	
Less Stable	Percutaneous pins (PCP) or K-wires	Secondary/ Primary
	Interosseous wires	
	Intramedullary pins	
Stable	Interfragmentary screw	Primary*
	Tension band wire	
	Tension band plate	
Rigid	Lag screws	
	Plates and screws	
	90-90 interosseous wires	

*Probably also includes secondary healing.

immobilization and which require surgical stabilization with closed reduction and fixation (CRF), or open reduction internal fixation (ORIF) to insert plates, screws, tension band wires or K-wires.[11]

Metacarpal base fractures are the least common owing to their anatomical stability, and most are likely to occur because of a heavy direct blow or crushing injury. MC base fractures often are intraarticular and displaced, therefore requiring surgical ORIF to restore the stable load-bearing function of the CMC joint.[11]

Metacarpal neck fractures are the most common metacarpal fracture seen in the hand clinic. These are caused by a compressive force that travels proximally from the metacarpal head toward the base. The common scenario for a fifth MC and sometimes a fourth MC neck fracture is a fisted hand striking a solid object, recognized as a **boxer's fracture** (although rarely seen in skilled boxers).[10,11] Surgery is considered for displaced and/or comminuted MC neck fractures when the dorsal angulation exceeds 15 degrees in the ring or small fingers and 10 degrees in the index or long fingers.[11] Some surgeons, however, prefer not to do surgery when angulation is less than 30 degrees in the small finger, and less than 20 degrees in the ring finger.[12] Consequences of not following these guidelines are the late clinical effects of lost active MCP joint flexion, pseudoclaw deformity with PIP joint extension lag, and tenderness in the palm during grip due to the volar displacement of the metacarpal head.[11] In Fig. 23.4 are the X-rays of a

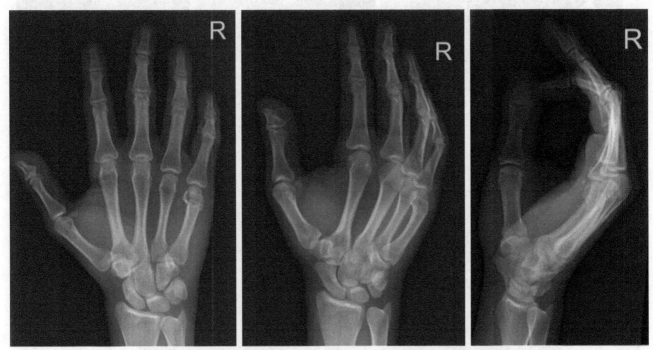

FIG. 23.4 X-rays of right fifth metacarpal head/neck minimally displaced fracture.

boxer's fracture in an 18-year-old who punched a wall with his right hand. Notice three X-ray views were required to appreciate the fracture pattern. During physical examination, active motion produced no digital rotation or PIP joint extension lag. Conservative management with immobilization was chosen for his minimally angulated/displaced fifth metacarpal head/neck fracture.

Metacarpal head fractures are uncommon, but serious in nature due to intraarticular involvement. The mechanism of injury is often an axial load.[11] Nonsurgical management is considered only when less than 25% of the metacarpal head is involved and displacement is less than 1 mm.[6]

Thumb (First Metacarpal) Fracture Pathology

Most extraarticular metacarpal base fractures of the thumb are stable after reduction; however this is not true of intraarticular fractures that involve the thumb CMC joint.[11] A **Bennett's fracture**

is an intraarticular **comminuted** (two-part) fracture of the CMC joint. An axial load on the metacarpal is the mechanism of injury forcing the thumb into abduction.[11] The strong stabilizing **palmar oblique** or **beak ligament** remains attached to the trapezium causing an ulnar-sided MC base avulsion fracture. Bennett's fractures often result in trapeziometacarpal subluxation due to competing forces between the APL still attached to the MC base distracting the fragment proximally, while the AP still attached to the metacarpal rotates the other fragment into supination. Closed reduction and stabilization with K-wires is preferred for most Bennett's fractures. However, if the joint remains unstable and reduction cannot be achieved by closed technique, or more than 25% of the joint surface is involved, ORIF is pursued.[12]

A more forceful axial load than a Bennett's fracture causes **Rolando's fracture**. This is also an intraarticular comminuted fracture of the thumb CMC joint with three or more fragments, in a "T" or a "Y" configuration.[11,13] Associated concerns are loss of MC length and the destabilizing regional forces of the palmar oblique ligament, the APL, and AP muscles. In the majority of cases, surgical stabilization is required to restore the articular surface of this mobile load-bearing joint.

Fractures of the thumb metacarpal shaft are rare because the forces are absorbed by the stable MC base.[11] Shaft fractures are generally transverse or oblique, although those caused by high velocity forces may be comminuted.[11] As in finger metacarpal shaft fractures, the fracture apex is dorsal with the distal fragment pulled into adduction and flexion by the FPB, AP, and APB, while the APL pulls the proximal fragment dorsal. Dorsal angulation of more than 30 degrees is an indication to consider fracture reduction.[11]

X-ray views in Fig. 23.5 show a right thumb extraarticular proximal metacarpal shaft fracture with comminution and mild displacement. Notice that the APL muscle has destabilized the distal fragment, thus creating a dorsal apex in this thumb fracture. Interestingly, a healed fourth metacarpal shaft fracture can also be seen on this X-ray.

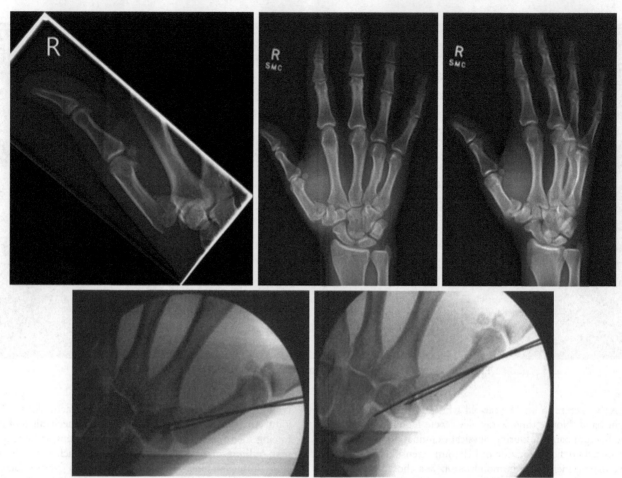

FIG. 23.5 X-rays of right thumb extraarticular proximal metacarpal shaft fracture with comminution and mild displacement (top row). Image of K-wire reduction (bottom row).

The most common mechanism in a fracture of the metacarpal head comes from radially directed forces, which either strain the thumb's MCP joint ulnar collateral ligament (UCL) or cause an avulsion/fracture of the UCL from the metacarpal head.[11] This fracture has been called **skier's thumb** as the ski pole forces the thumb radially to challenge the UCL. Protected immobilization may be sufficient if the avulsion fracture is nondisplaced, otherwise when displaced, surgery is required to restore a stable pain-free thumb.

Phalangeal Fracture Pathology

Proximal Phalanx (P1) Fracture of the Fingers

Fractures of the proximal phalanx occur often in the 10 to 29 years age group. The leading cause is injury during sport involving the fifth digit. These fractures have a volar apex due to the destabilizing forces of the intrinsic muscles that flex the proximal fragment and the opposing central slip insertion into the base of P2, extending the distal fragment (Fig. 23.6). Extrinsic long flexor regional forces also contribute to gap the apex volarly.[1] Volar angulation results in shortening of the proximal phalanx to upset the balanced forces of extension, causing extensor lag of the PIP joint. The most common problem encountered in P1 fractures is extensor lag, caused by too much volar angulation and/or adhesion of the extensor hood that covers two-thirds the surface of P1. Scar of the fracture (soft callus) coupled with surgical insertion of plates, screws, tension band wires, or K-wires increase the

likelihood of adhesion formation resulting in PIP joint extensor lag. A noncorrected volar apex of the proximal phalanx exceeding 25 degrees, impacts long flexor biomechanics shown by a loss of finger flexion. Oblique fractures of the proximal phalanx may cause similar problems to those previously describe plus an element of digital rotation or scissoring with active flexion of the fingers if not reduced and stabilized.

X-rays in Fig. 23.7 show before and after ORIF views of a right small finger extraarticular oblique P1 base fracture with radial angulation and mild dorsal displacement. X-rays in Fig. 23.8 show before and after ORIF using crossed K-wires management of a right ring finger extra-articular oblique P1 shaft fracture. The lateral X-ray view confirms the volar apex of the fracture.

Middle Phalanx (P2) Fracture of the Fingers

Extraarticular middle phalanx or P2 fractures are rare, perhaps because P2 is broader and shorter than the other phalanges. High-impact forces are the mechanism of injury such as those associated with sports or machinery. These are often accompanied by soft-tissue trauma because the ligaments of the PIP joint fail before P2 fractures.[14] A fracture of the proximal third of P2 produces a dorsal apex fracture owing to the dorsal pull of the central slip P2 base insertion and the opposing FDS, which flexes the distal fragment.[1] When the fracture is at the distal third of P2 the fracture apex then goes volar because the strong FDS flexes the proximal fragment, then the opposing force of the extensor terminal tendon extends the digit.[1]

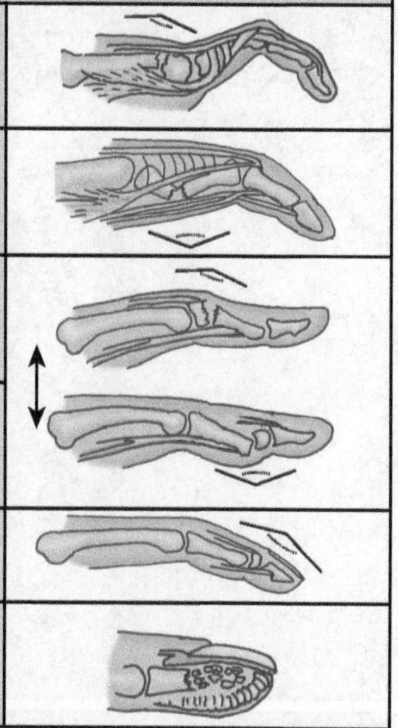

Bone	Region	Regional deforming forces	Pattern of malunion	
Metacarpal (MC)		**Intrinsic muscle:** distal flexes	Apex dorsal	
Proximal phalanx (P1)		**Intrinsic muscle:** proximal flexes **Extensor mechanism:** distal extends	Apex volar	
Middle phalanx (P2)	Proximal 1/3	**Central tendon:** proximal extends **FDS:** distal flexes	Apex dorsal	
	Distal 1/3	**FDS:** proximal flexes **Extensor tendon:** distal extends	Apex volar	
Distal phalanx (P3)	Shaft	**Extensor tendon:** N/A (nail bed injury) **FDP:** distal flexes	Apex dorsal	
	Tuft	N/A: no tendon insertions	N/A	

Note: All malunions - functional bone shortening +/– digital rotation or lateral angulation distal to fracture

FIG. 23.6 Regional dynamic deforming forces and common patterns of fracture displacement. *From Feehan LM. Extra-articular hand fractures part II: therapist's management. In: Skirven TM, Osterman AL, Fedorczyk JM, et al. eds. Rehabilitation of the Hand and Upper Extremity. 6th ed. Philadelphia, PA: Mosby Elsevier; 2011.*

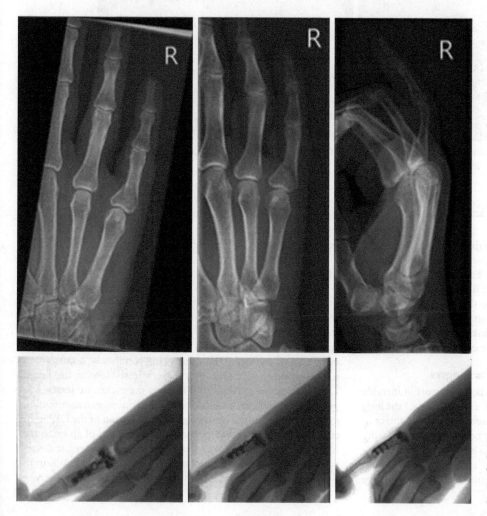

FIG. 23.7 X-rays of right small finger extraarticular oblique P1 base fracture with radial angulation and mild dorsal (top row). Images after ORIF with plate and screws (bottom row).

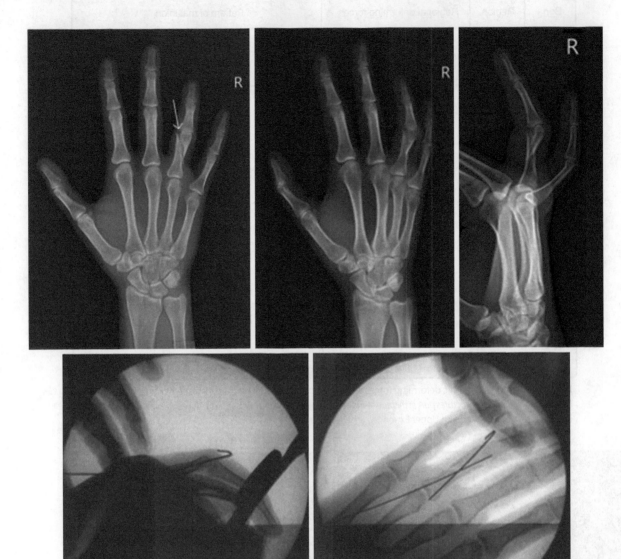

FIG. 23.8 X-rays of right ring finger extraarticular oblique P1 shaft fracture (top row). Image after fracture reduction with crossed K-wires (bottom row).

Proximal Interphalangeal Joint Fracture/Dislocation of the Fingers

Intraarticular and fracture/dislocations of the PIP joint are typically caused by axial compression forces. A dorsal dislocation is more common and refers to the direction that the middle phalanx travels relative to the proximal phalanx. A volar dislocation in which the middle phalanx moves volarly relative to the proximal phalanx is much less frequent. Volar dislocations often result in a **boutonniere deformity** (PIP joint flexion and distal interphalangeal [DIP] joint hyperextension) due to injury of the extensor central slip.

Distal Phalanx (P3) Fracture of the Fingers

The distal phalanx is most exposed and therefore more vulnerable to fracture than other bones of the hand, especially P3 of the long finger. Crush is the usual mechanism, such as shutting a finger in a door, getting it stuck in machinery, or being stepped on during sports.[14] Soft-tissue injuries may include nail bed trauma, hematoma formation, digital nerve damage, and/or dorsal skin and extensor tendon lacerations. Distal phalanx fractures may involve

the tuft or the shaft of the phalanx. If the shaft of P3 is fractured, the apex goes dorsal because of the opposing volar compressive pull from the FDP.[1] Fig. 23.9 shows a long finger intraarticular distal phalanx base fracture with dorsal angulation created by the FDP destabilizing forces opposing those of the terminal tendon.

A distal phalanx avulsion fracture identifies that a fragment of bone has been pulled off by either the FDP volarly or the terminal extensor tendon, dorsally. These usually are intraarticular fractures. Generally, avulsion of the FDP requires surgical management. The mechanism for an FDP avulsion fracture is forced extension of a flexed DIP joint. This commonly occurs when a football player grabs another player's jersey forcing the flexed DIP joint into extension, thus earning the nickname **jersey finger.** The mechanism for avulsion of the terminal extensor tendon or **bony mallet finger** results from forced flexion of the DIP joint such as when a basketball or baseball hits the end of an extended DIP joint. The percentage of articular surface involved and success of fracture reduction dictates management after avulsion of the extensor terminal tendon, but most do not require surgery.

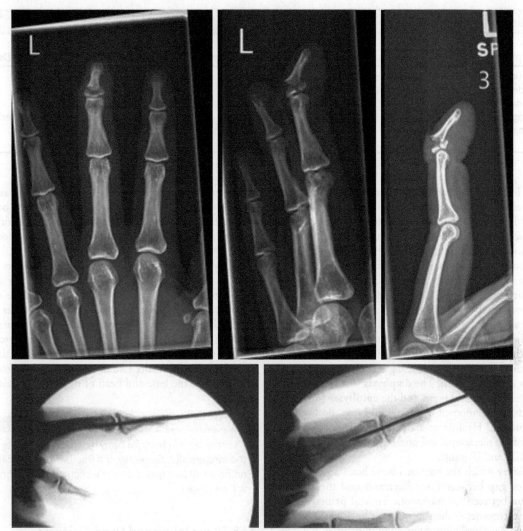

FIG. 23.9 X-rays of long finger intraarticular distal phalanx base fracture with dorsal angulation (top row). Images after longitudinal K-wire reduction (bottom row).

Fracture of the Thumb Phalanges

In frequency of occurrence, distal phalanx (P2) thumb fractures are second to long finger P3 fractures. The EPL is avulsed dorsally or the FPL is avulsed volarly, which creates either a droopy interphalangeal (IP) joint (EPL) or loss of functional IP joint flexion (FPL). Most likely, these fractures will have an intraarticular component. Stability of the IP joint depends on the amount of joint surface involved and bony displacement. More FPL avulsion/fractures undergo surgery than EPL avulsion /fractures, which are managed nonsurgically as a bony mallet.

The proximal phalanx (P1) of the thumb, similar to the finger proximal phalanx, is covered with an extensor hood and intrinsic muscle contributions. Dynamic regional anatomy affects P1 thumb fractures in that the FPL is a strong flexor pulling the distal component volar, and the extensor hood pulls into extension to create a dorsal apex. Scar of the fracture (soft callus) is prone to adhere to the extensor hood, limiting excursion and resulting in extensor lag. This same scar may cause adhesions of the FPL limiting IP joint flexion. Managed similarly to finger fractures of the proximal phalanx, decisions depend on the fracture type, ability to keep the fracture reduced, and associated soft-tissue injury.

Clinical Pearl

To improve communication with colleagues, first provide pertinent client demographics, mechanism of injury, and days post fracture/surgery. Then describe the fracture as organized in Table 23.2.

Timelines and Bone Healing

Bone Healing Fundamentals

After a hand fracture, bones heal at a faster pace in children than in adults, and healing timeframes vary between bones. Fractures are said to regenerate or heal **primarily** (directly, by contact or with minimal gap) or **secondarily** (indirectly or with gap). Bone is a living biological structure made of metabolically active cells that assimilate into a rigid framework. The bone is in a constant state of deposition, resorption, and remodeling.[15] The desired outcome of fracture healing is regeneration of bone and restoration of bone strength. Regeneration of bone involves the **periosteum** (outer bone covering) and the **endosteum** (the

TABLE 23.2	Describing the Fracture				
1 Hand	2 Digit	3 Location	4 Bone and Bone Location	5 Fracture Pattern*	6 Additional Descriptors*
Right Left	Thumb (1st) Index finger (2nd) Long finger (3rd) Ring finger (4th) Small finger (5th)	Intra-articular Extra-articular	Carpal # Metacarpal # Phalanx # Head or distal segment Base or proximal segment Shaft or diaphysis	Transverse Oblique Comminuted Spiral	Open Closed Displaced Non-displaced Dorsal apex Volar apex

*Partial list of terms that could be applied.

thin vascular lining of the medullary canals). The endosteum produces the enchondral or **soft bone callus**. In the skeletally immature child, the periosteum and endosteum are thicker and have more vascularity to allow a more robust response in bone regeneration and soft bone callus production.

Bone structure varies within a bone, and applied stress determines the type of bone: cortical, cancellous or woven bone. **Cortical bone** (compact or lamellar) is well-organized dense bone. **Cancellous bone** (trabecular bone) is a loose network of bone organized like a honeycomb. **Woven bone** is found in embryonic tissue and in the soft bone or callus of early fracture healing. With skeletal maturity and successful fracture healing, woven bone remodels and is replaced with the stronger and more organized cortical and/or cancellous bone. The **diaphysis** (shaft) of a metacarpal or phalange is cortical bone, and the **epiphyses** (proximal and distal ends) are composed of cancellous bone, both enveloped by periosteum. Hyaline or **articular cartilage** covers the joint surfaces of the metacarpal and phalangeal bones to compose the CMC, MCP, and IP joints.

The process by which the fractured bone heals is dependent on the space or **gap** between bone fragments and the amount of micromotion between the fragments. To heal **primarily** (by direct contact osteogenesis) the gap must be less than 0.2 mm, compressed, and have negligible micro-motion between the fragments. The process of healing **secondarily** occurs when the fracture gap is greater than 0.2 mm and no more than 1 mm wide. Indirect healing begins in early repair with soft callus remodeling to woven bone callus, then later in the repair phase maturing to bone.

It is unlikely that fractures outside a controlled laboratory environment heal entirely by primarily intention; nor is it realistic to believe that bone fixation methods, which use the most rigid hardware, apply perfect compression. Even with 100% client compliance, inter-fragment micromotion will happen![16] If our primary intention is to heal the fracture, it is wise to understand the clinical implications of the three overlapping phases of indirect fracture healing. During the early inflammatory phase, many types of "clean up" cells flood the repair area joined by fibroblasts. There is vascular ingrowth, and osteoblasts and chondrocytes migrate to the area of injury. Nourishment and oxygen for this healing activity is sustained by exposed cancellous bone and muscle.[15] With the onset of the repair phase there is formation of a collagen matrix, and osteoblasts form a soft callus at the repair site. At this point, the repair site remains very weak for 4 to 6 weeks until the soft callus ossifies to form a bridge of woven bone between the fracture fragments. Too much motion or stress at the repair site during this stage will result in either a nonunion or an unstable fibrous union. During the remodeling phase, the healing bone begins

to resemble the former bone in shape, structure, and mechanical strength. It takes 3 to 6 months for this new bone to reach full restoration. Axial loading supports this process and the extent of applied stress thus determines deposition or resorption of new bone.[15]

No pain or tenderness at the fracture site defines when a fracture is **clinically healed**. X-rays at this time may show cloudiness about the fracture site, indicating the phase of soft bone formation, until sufficient bone remodeling occurs the fracture line will remain visible. Many variables affect fracture **clinical healing times**. In general, middle phalanx shaft fractures are the slowest to heal (10 and 14 weeks); compared to shaft fractures of the proximal phalanx (5 and 7 weeks); and metacarpal, distal phalanx, and the base and head of the middle phalanx (3 and 5 weeks).[17]

◎ Clinical Pearl

A simple test to check for bony healing is to palpate firmly over the fracture site. Generally, if a fracture has **clinically healed**, no pain will be reported by the client. If still healing, the area will be tender.

Soft-Tissue Injury and Hand Fractures

The most common fracture complications involve the soft tissue, not the failure of bone to heal.[1] Because the bone and soft tissue are cohesive, the force that fractures a bone wounds the dense connective tissue of the periosteum, joint capsule, volar plate, ligament, tendon, intrinsic muscle, fascial interfaces, tendon sheaths, and peripheral and digital nerve sleeves.[9,18] Soft-tissue injury associated with a nondisplaced fracture may be subtle with local periosteal edema, or very obvious as seen in an open fracture with complex multitissue trauma. In both examples, mechanisms within the injured soft tissue also trigger the wound repair response, which opens the door to the "one wound–one scar" phenomenon responsible for adhesions.[19] Although necessary to address some fractures, surgery creates another injury, which can amplify the repair response.

The best treatment for any fracture is early intervention, anticipation, and controlled motion. **Early intervention** means getting the client to therapy within the first week after fracture or surgery. Localized swelling and abnormal posturing of the injured hand/digit are normal responses after bone and soft-tissue trauma. The key is to anticipate which joints are likely to get stiff and which tendons may adhere, and to remember the noninjured digits. Introduce active **controlled motion** when and where it is safe, so not to destabilize the fracture in support of joint mobility, tendon excursion, and muscle function. Often a comprehensive set of range of motion measurements lacks efficiency; instead measure the digits or joints anticipated as problems while keeping a close watch over the entire picture. Timely intervention during the initial 3 weeks consisting of a well thought out management plan communicated with the client and surgeon is vital to the outcome!

Nonoperative Treatment of Hand Fractures

Conservative (nonoperative) management of any hand fracture requires a coordinated effort from all team members to communicate the details of the fracture and the subsequent plan of management. Although not implied in the term *conservative*, the responsibility of the therapist increases when asked to provide early fracture management and a protective orthosis. Informed conservative management requires knowing fracture details such as mechanism of injury, the bone and location, type of fracture pattern and stability, and the regional forces that will negatively affect fracture healing. Therapists must anticipate for joint and tendon problems, and have a broad familiarity of available programs and orthoses. Combining these key details with client factors that influence outcome supports an individualized plan of care. The decisions around timing the movement of joints nearest the fracture; when to commence protected functional hand use for leisure, work or sport activities; and when bone strength is sufficient to begin strengthening exercises, are all at the core of an individualized management plan.

Fracture Orthoses Fundamentals

Use thermoplastic materials found in the hand therapy clinic much in the same way as plaster, fiberglass, or synthetic polyester casting materials to protect the hand after fracture. Distinct advantages to having the hand therapist fabricate a fracture orthoses include early entry into hand therapy, and a custom-made thermoplastic orthosis to support the specific needs of the

fracture, soft tissue, and client. The outcomes of nonsurgical fracture management improves with early entry to hand therapy, which allows anticipation rather than correction of the complications of stiff joints, tendon adhesions, and muscle fibrosis.

A fracture orthosis supports the healing bone by providing a conforming exterior shell molded to hug the fracture. In the early weeks of healing, the orthosis design controls motion of the joints proximal and distal to the fracture. As healing progresses, remove the fracture orthosis to permit controlled motion exercises of the joints proximal and distal to the fracture, which applies gentle stresses to the soft tissue and bone. Once achieving clinical healing, the orthosis can be further modified to permit the joints on either side of the fracture to move. Use of the protective orthosis in this final phase lets the client participate in functional hand use and continues the controlled application of stress for bone strengthening.

Controlled Motion and Functional Hand Use Fundamentals

Use controlled mobilization with extraarticular hand fractures when (1) the fracture is closed, stable, and minimally to non-displaced, or (2) after reduction and surgical stabilization of an unstable displaced fracture. Between these two categories, fractures fall into a "gray-zone," with use of early controlled motion done with careful consideration so not to displace the gray-zone fracture.[1] Feehan recommends grading early controlled motion directly with fracture stability and configuration, stressing that both stability and bone strength fall along a continuum.[1] Factors that influence relative bone stability and structural strength are outlined in Table 23.3.[1] These "factor questions" are a useful guide to establish any fracture management program. There is a menu of suggested options to select from to customize each controlled motion program (Table 23.4). These options include arc of motion, type of motion, direction of motion, frequency of motion, and number

TABLE 23.3 Factors That Influence Relative Bone Stability and Structural Strength

Factor	Description
Which bone and where in the bone?	Knowing fracture location and the regional dynamic anatomy help anticipate potential destabilizing forces that may compromise fracture stability.
Number and nature of fracture line(s)	The fracture pattern helps gain an understanding of the structural strength of the bone, and helps determine what types of forces and in what direction the fragments are likely to displace.
Initial displacement and alignment	The fracture pattern helps gain an understanding of the structural strength of the bone, and helps determine what types of forces and in what direction the fragments are likely to displace.
Type of reduction and fixation	Vascular and soft-tissue disruption is relates to the type of fracture reduction method used, which also influences how the bone repairs (primarily or secondarily).
Post-reduction and fixation alignment	The method and stability of surgical reduction and fixation guides selection of the protective orthosis, controlled motion exercises and functional use.
Nature of additional soft-tissue injury	Anticipating associated soft-tissue injury, as result of the injury or surgery helps develop a comprehensive therapy plan.
Time since fracture or surgery	Generally, fractures gain structural strength the longer the time from time of fracture or surgery.
Normal daily functional demands and patient priorities	Obtaining this information assists the therapist to determine the extent of fracture orthosis protection required for early hand function, and set patient-centered goals.

From Feehan LM. Extra-articular hand fractures part II: therapist's management. In: Skirven TM, Osterman AL, Fedorczyk JM, et al. eds. *Rehabilitation of the Hand and Upper Extremity*, 6th ed. Philadelphia, PA: Elsevier Mosby; 2011, pp 386-401.

TABLE 23.4 Controlled Motion Exercise Options and Description for Customizing Each Client's Exercise Program

Controlled Motion Exercise Options	Descriptions
Arc of motion	No motion, range of motion controlled, or limited or full motion
Type of motion	Passive: one joint/periarticular tissue stretch composite joint/extraarticular tissue stretch Active-Assisted: place & hold or tenodesis-assisted Active: tendon gliding and muscle performance Passive end-range: one/periarticular tissues stretch composite joints/extraarticular tissue stretch Resisted active: tendon gliding, muscle strengthening
Direction of motion	Flexion, extension, or both
Number of joints moving	Isolated (one joint) Composite (two or more joints)
Frequency of motion	Number of repetitions Frequency/day

Adapted from Feehan LM. Extra-articular hand fractures part II: therapist's management. In: Skirven TM, Osterman AL, Fedorczyk JM. et al. *Rehabilitation of the Hand and Upper Extremity*. 6th ed. Philadelphia, PA: Elsevier Mosby; 2011, pp 386–401.

of joints moving with motion. Choices within these options are dependent on fracture stability and structural strength of the healing bone.[1]

The time to resume functional use of the fractured hand is also on a continuum that takes into account fracture stability and strength of the healing bone. In the early phases of bone repair, the protection of a fracture orthosis will be required. Use of the involved hand while wearing the fracture orthosis during the initial 3 weeks post fracture should be pain free and consist of light activity. At this time the fracture may still be tender to palpation; however, introducing stability and strength-appropriate hand function should not increase this tenderness. If so, reduce the demand on the healing bone.

In general, fracture palpation tenderness should be absent between 3 to 6 weeks postinjury (signaling "clinically healed"). At this time, the stability of the bone is increasing because of soft callus formation but the strength of the bone is at the low end of the continuum. For example, for a client with a fifth MC fracture, removing the orthosis for very light activities such as to shower may be appropriate. However, playing video games or riding a bike is not. Moving toward 6 weeks post fracture, light activities like video games match bone stability and add controlled stresses necessary for bone strengthening. At this time, the orthosis continues to protect the fracture during heavy activities like riding a bike or lifting a loaded backpack. Between 6 and 8 weeks, X-ray and surgeon consultation determine if bone strength is functionally ready for sport and higher demand hand use (with or without the fracture brace). Usually by 12 to 16 weeks, bone strength is functionally ready for unrestricted use.

Bone-Specific Nonoperative Management

Metacarpal Fracture

Most finger metacarpal shaft and neck fractures, especially those of the fifth digit are stable.[6] Current opinion varies about nonoperative management of metacarpal fractures. Analysis of a group of MC fracture patients 1 year post injury, showed better patient satisfaction scores in those managed surgically. However, in the nonsurgical groups, functional and aesthetic scores were better.[20]

As a result of varied opinion and evidence, a typical clinical discussion between the hand surgeon and the client will range from: (a) expect to heal with some deformity but function will be good, to (b) discussion about the risk of surgery and a scar.[21]

To date there is no one metacarpal fracture management program or orthosis that has proven superior to another. There is however, consensus that the orthosis position of the MCP joints for digits second to fifth be in at least 60 degrees of flexion. This functional position preserves the length of the collateral ligaments and provides added stability for the distal end of the metacarpal. Therapist preference or client factors may determine when the wrist is included or not in the design of the orthosis. This decision should consider the location of the fracture(s) and relative stability of the fracture pattern and the time from injury.

Including the wrist provides for greater proximal stability, necessary for fractures of the MC base. Immobilization of the wrist is not required for MC shaft, neck, or head fractures. However, for active clients or precarious fracture patterns involving the fourth or fifth digits, temporary inclusion of the wrist eliminates torsional forces applied to the ulnar metacarpals during wrist motion. The design decision when making a fourth or fifth MC fracture ulnar gutter style or radial second or third MC gutter style orthosis should take into consideration how inclusion of the adjacent finger stabilizes the linking intermetacarpal ligament and better controls regional destabilizing forces of the intrinsic and extrinsic muscles. Not only is this adjacent digit design more comfortable, but two fingers are left accessible to assist with light functional tasks such as dressing. When the fracture involves more than two metacarpals consider including all four digits in the orthosis design for stability. Early in fracture healing, including the IP joint in the design of the orthosis will better stabilize the MCP joint; however, this does not require full-time immobilization of the IP joint. Fabricating a clamshell style radial or ulnar gutter with an open volar surface will allow the desired amount of IP joint motion for exercise and protection. Early in fracture management, if the design is not clamshell, leaving the digits out from the PIP joint distally or buddy taping adjacent digits adds stability while allowing routine motion. Fig. 23.10 shows a hand-based orthosis option for MC shaft, neck, and head fractures.

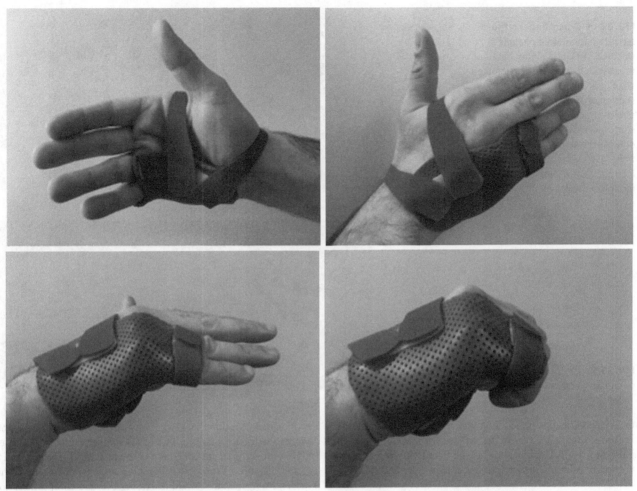

FIG. 23.10 Hand-finger-based orthosis option for metacarpal shaft, neck, and head fractures.

Design considerations for an orthosis used in the conservative management of thumb metacarpal fractures include how active is the client, how much thumb IP joint motion is safe, fracture stability, and how many days post fracture. In general, thumb MC fractures do not require the wrist to be included. Immediate unrestricted thumb IP joint motion is allowable provided the fracture is stable and the client is adherent. If the client is too active, there is a strong inflammatory response, or the fracture has tenuous stability, design the orthosis to control motion of the IP joint. The design lengthens the thumb post to semi-block full motion of the distal joint. Another idea is to extend the orthosis to the end of the thumb, cut out the volar aspect for IP joint motion, strap up the distal phalanx at rest, inserting controlled motion for home exercises until client adherence and fracture stability warrant.

Proximal Phalanx Fracture of the Fingers

A proximal phalanx fracture at any location is prone to IP joint stiffness, adhesion of the extensor mechanism, and secondary PIP joint extensor lag. Immobilization for 4 weeks has shown to reduce IP joint motion more than 60%, impairing function.[22] Manage closed non-displaced or minimally displaced P1 shaft fractures with a hand-based orthosis that includes both the injured finger and an adjacent finger. Allow controlled active motion of the IP joints with the MCP joints flexed to 70 to 90 degrees (the intrinsic-plus position). Active movement of the IP joints in this position (1) tightens

the extensor mechanism around the proximal two-thirds of the proximal phalanx to add to the relative stability of the fracture by applying compression, and (2) reduces the soft-tissue problems associated with proximal phalangeal fractures. Fabrication requires the orthosis cover the dorsal aspect of the fingers at least to the PIP joint, but can include the DIP joint without compromise of the concept. Actively move the IP joints or strap them up for more protection, releasing the straps to perform controlled motion exercises. There is usually no need to include the wrist. Involvement of multiple digits requires inclusion of more digits, following the idea of incorporating the adjacent digit for lateral stability of the injured finger.

Middle Phalanx Fracture of the Fingers

Many middle phalanx fractures are amenable to closed reduction followed by casting or a fracture orthosis. In this region the concern is for loss of extensor mechanism excursion resulting in IP joint stiffness or extensor lag. A dorsal finger-based orthosis will hold the IP joints in extension at rest (Fig. 23.11). Note that the dorsal orthosis has a thermoplastic reinforced volar strap to provide circumferential stabilization at the fracture for safe active IP joint motion An option for active clients is a volar finger-based orthosis, which blocks the forces of the long flexor tendons; removing the orthosis for manual stabilized controlled exercises of the IP joints. When additional fracture protection is needed and/ or multiple fingers are involved, make a hand-based orthosis with

FIG. 23.11 Dorsal finger orthosis option for middle phalanx fracture. **(A)** Dorsal finger-based orthosis with thermoplastic reinforced strap to provide circumferential support of an index finger middle phalanx fracture. **(B)** Reinforced strap released. Not shown, release of only the distal strap allows for controlled isolated motion of the distal interphalangeal joint or composite motion of the IP joints.

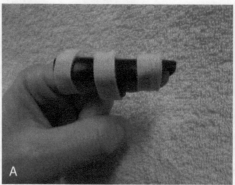
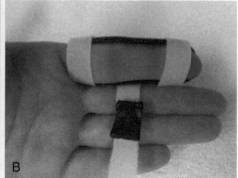

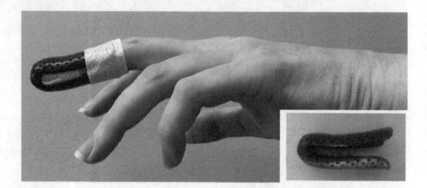

FIG. 23.12 Clamshell or cap finger-based orthosis option for distal phalanx fracture.

the MCP joints positioned in at least 70-degrees flexion and the IP joints extended. Remove the orthosis for motion of the MCP joint and manual stabilization of the fracture during controlled motion IP joint exercises to avoid scar adherence and stiffness.

Proximal Interphalangeal Joint Fracture/Dislocation of the Fingers

Conservative management for fracture/dislocation of the finger PIP joint works when 25% to 30% or less of the articular surface is involved. PIP joint fracture/dislocations, defined as **simple dislocation** require the condyles of the proximal phalanx head to remain in contact with the base of the middle phalanx. A **complex dislocation** indicates loss of contact. Since a fracture/dislocation challenges the restraining structures of the PIP joint, anticipate soft-tissue involvement. Depending on the direction of fracture/dislocation (dorsal or volar), key structures to monitor include the volar plate, collateral ligaments, extensor central slip, or the FDS/FDP tendons.

Depending on the extent of volar plate/collateral ligamentous injury, use a protective finger-based fracture orthosis with the PIP joint safely positioned between 0 and 25-degrees flexion. The orthosis secured with straps to the dorsal finger surface counteracts harmful external extension forces and leaves the volar IP joint surfaces open. As edema subsides, adjustment to the orthosis will be required, particularly if applied within the first week post fracture. Adherent pressure wrap applied over the entire fracture orthosis to control motion and edema as needed. The design of this orthosis allows early controlled flexion of the IP joints followed by extension without removal of the orthosis.

For example, protected controlled motion exercises beginning within the first week would include release of the DIP joint strap for active DIP joint motion followed by partial-release of the PIP joint strap, which limits PIP joint motion to approximately 45 to

60degrees. Motion that is respectful of the inflammatory response and is without pain dutifully addresses the anticipated problems of IP joint stiffness and adherence of the tendons. Depending on the fracture, direct the controlled motion progression between 2 and 4 weeks post fracture toward increasing PIP and composite IP joint flexion, and adjusting the orthosis into neutral PIP joint extension. Once clinically healed (4–6 weeks), the decision to reduce orthosis wear and increase functional use depend on the client's activity level. After 6 to 8 weeks most often the orthosis or the finger is buddy taped to an adjacent digit for sport or rigorous hand use.

Distal Phalanx Fracture of the Fingers

A closed articular avulsion fracture of the dorsal distal phalanx with the dorsal fragment attached to the extensor terminal tendon is a **bony mallet finger.** Nonsurgical management is typical for those injuries that involve less than 30% of the joint surface. The concern for avulsion/fractures and shaft fractures are failure to heal and DIP extension lag. Orthoses are used routinely to manage shaft and tuft fractures. A "clamshell" or "cap" finger-based orthosis (Fig. 23.12) used to conservatively manage nondisplaced fractures of the distal phalanx base, shaft, or tuft is easily adjusted for fluctuations in edema. The orthosis shown in the figure is longer on the dorsal surface and designed to allow for full PIP joint motion. The FDP flexion forces are a strong nemesis, pulling the unstable distal phalanx fracture into flexion. To control for FDP forces an alternative clamshell design covers the dorsum of the whole finger and the volar surface is open from the PIP joint proximally then secured with straps around the proximal and distal phalanges. Release of the proximal strap permits controlled motion of the PIP joint for designated exercise times. Either version of this orthosis requires full-time wear during clinical healing (at least 4–6 weeks). Thereafter, especially with an avulsion/fracture of the extensor terminal tendon, orthosis wear full time can be as long as 8 weeks to avoid an extensor lag. All fractures of the distal phalanx will demonstrate flexion stiffness that will resolve over time given gentle exercise and functional use. Tuft fractures or crush type injuries of the distal phalanx may require desensitization as the nerves repair.

Fractures of the Thumb Phalanges

Conservative management is appropriate for either proximal or distal phalanx fractures of the thumb that have stable configuration with minimal displacement. Anticipation of IP joint stiffness or loss of extensor hood or FPL excursion is a good idea. Fractures of the distal phalanx with a crush component are likely to have digital nerve pain or a nailbed injury. Management of a proximal phalanx thumb fracture depends on the time post injury and fracture stability and location. There is the option of either a hand-based or a thumb-based orthosis. Consideration of a thumb-based orthosis for a stable non-displaced fracture of the proximal phalanx head is reasonable. A hand-based orthosis provides more protection, especially for the very active thumb. The basic design allows the CMC joint freedom while circumferentially securing the MCP joint and phalanges. As the fracture stabilizes, start controlled or free IP joint motion by cutting out the volar surface of the orthosis; maintaining the dorsal surface to protect bumping the thumb. Between 3 and 4 weeks, as clinical healing indicates, expose the IP joint or substitute a thumb-based clamshell orthosis. A clamshell-type, or cap, orthosis similar to that applied for nonsurgical management of distal phalangeal finger fractures works well for the thumb's distal phalanx fracture. If necessary, make the orthosis longer to extend across the MCP joint dorsally for more protection. As there is less fracture palpation tenderness, trim the volar aspect of orthosis to allow MCP or IP joint controlled motion and function.

◎ *Clinical Pearl*

Timing and amount of mobilization and functional hand use require consideration for both the relative stability and the structural strength of the fracture. Nonsurgical fracture management *usually* indicates the fracture configuration is relatively more stable than a fracture that requires K-wire fixation. K-wires improve on the original fracture stability so that controlled motion and protected hand function is now an option. For both, a protective orthosis is required, and the decision to start early controlled motion of the joints on either side of the fracture is client specific. In contrast, a fracture pattern that requires ORIF with internal hardware is stable after surgery because rigid hardware now buttresses the fracture. After ORIF, a protective orthosis is still required to minimize fracture micromotion; however, it is imperative to move the joints immediately proximal and distal to the fracture to offset the biological response that accompanies surgery.

Operative Treatment and Rehabilitation Considerations

Metacarpal Fracture

Indications for surgical management of metacarpal fractures include an open or unstable fracture with angulation and/or rotational displacement beyond the guidelines outlined previously. Surgical management techniques vary and are at the discretion of the surgeon.

These include applications using bones grafts, K-wires, pins, plates, screws, and external fixation devices. K-wires hold bone fragments in place so that healing can occur. Crossed K-wires control rotation of the bone fragment(s). Fig. 23.5 demonstrates crossed K-wires in a thumb metacarpal fracture as viewed on X-ray. An **external fixator** device looks like scaffolding and restores the length of the metacarpal bone. This may be used after multitissue trauma such as gunshot injury, and grafting of bone may accompany this procedure. **ORIF** involves surgical stabilization after reduction with plates, screws, or wires. Although it is rarely required, internal hardware may be removed at a later date if there is loose or prominent hardware that causes pain or tendon irritation. ORIF is more common in second to fifth MC shaft and neck fractures, and K-wire fixation more likely with metacarpal head and base fractures. Thumb metacarpal head fractures are considered for ORIF or K-wire fixation if more than 20% of the articular surface is involved.[11] Thumb MC base fracture/ CMC dislocations, such as Bennett's and Rolando's, are managed with surgical reduction and K-wire fixation.

Surgical access to metacarpal head fractures requires a longitudinal split of the EDC tendon, so early motion of adjacent joints is important to avoid tendon adherence.[11] Exposed K-wires may limit or "skewer" soft tissue, limiting excursion over the underlying bone and limiting full finger flexion and/or extension. Anticipate too, that the surgical scar will limit motion if not addressed. In both situations, to minimize MCP joint capsular restrictions and maximize extensor tendon excursion, instruct the client to flex the MCP joints while flexing and extending the IP joints for controlled motion exercise. Initiate scar massage 1 to 2 days following suture removal. Most clients will have their sutures removed between 10 and 14 days following surgery. Some early scar management techniques include silicone gel or elastomer pads placed under the orthosis, paper tape, or gentle scar mobilization techniques.[11-13]

Considerations for design of the postsurgical protective orthosis are similar to those discussed in the conservative management section, such as hand-based or forearm-based specifics, and number of digits to include. The design of the orthosis after surgery requires accommodation of the exposed hardware (described in Tips from the Field) to permit easy removal for K-wire cleaning and controlled exercise. To avoid compression and vascular compromise of fracture fragments post ORIF, flexion of the involved metacarpal MCP joint(s) beyond 70-degree flexion is not advised.[11]

Proximal Phalanx Fracture of the Fingers

The extent of angulation or rotation determines the K-wire technique used in displaced fractures of the proximal phalanx. Figure 23.8 is an example of the crossed K-wire method. ORIF is considered when the fracture pattern is comminuted, oblique (Fig. 23.7), or the fracture is open requiring **irrigation and debridement**. Early controlled motion after surgery is essential to minimize adherence of the extensor mechanism and flexor tendons. Close supervision by the hand therapist is important to insure proper support of the fracture with an orthosis or the client's contralateral hand during exercise involving the joints adjacent to the fracture. Selection of controlled motion should match fracture stability and healing. Exercises tips include: (1) position the MCP joints in moderate flexion for AROM of the IPs for added stability and maximum tendon excursion, and (2) isolate the IPs during AROM for FDS or FDP excursion or to address capsular restrictions.

A hand-based orthosis including the digit(s) with the MCP joints flexed to 70 to 90 degrees and IP joints extended provides three-points of pressure if made to fit circumferentially. This is

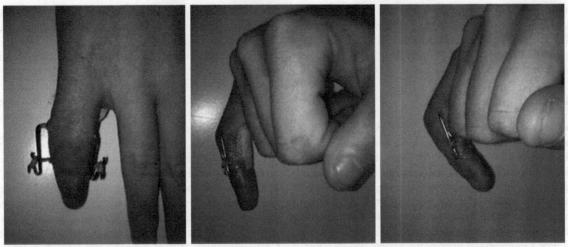

FIG. 23.13 Pins and rubber band traction system for intraarticular proximal interphalangeal joint fracture.

easily removed for controlled exercises and/or the volar splint can be cut away to allow controlled IP joint motion by releasing the distal strap. For comfort and lateral fracture support, an adjacent digit can be included in the design.

> **Clinical Pearl**
>
> There are two major reasons for **PIP joint extensor lag** after proximal phalanx fracture: (1) adhesions between the extensor mechanism and the fracture site, and (2) shortening of the proximal phalanx secondary to fracture angulation.[23] Keep in mind that extensor lag caused by disproportionate length between the bone and tendon will not respond to therapy.

Middle Phalanx Fracture of the Fingers

Operative management of middle phalanx fractures may include any of the methods outlined in Table 23.1. If a K-wire crosses the PIP joint, early controlled motion of that PIP joint will not be possible; however, early controlled motion of neighboring joints is necessary. A finger-based orthosis that positions the IP joints in extension is usually adequate for a single digit injury. If multiple digits are involved, especially if there are protruding K-wires, a hand-based orthotic may be more comfortable. Fabricate both orthoses to be easy to remove or modify to allow for controlled PIP and DIP joint motion.

The tendency for extensor tendon lag and PIP joint flexion contracture is high, so anticipation steps include ensuring full IP extension in the orthosis, which may require serial splint modifications as edema and soft tissue allow. Avoidance of extensor tendon lag requires regular controlled motion exercise of the IP joints and scar management techniques. Contractures of the PIP joint do occur, so as strength of the bone allows, use of a dorsal static-progressive hand and finger-based orthosis or dynamic Capener orthosis may be helpful.

Proximal Interphalangeal Joint Fracture/Dislocation of the Fingers

The PIP joint is unstable when more than 30% of the articular surface is involved and this condition requires surgical intervention.[24] Intraarticular fractures pose a difficult surgical challenge to reconstruct the congruity of the articular and bony alignment.

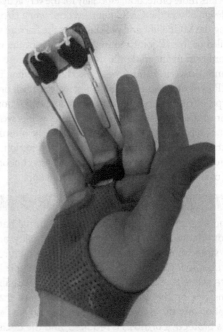

FIG. 23.14 Hand-based swing traction for intraarticular proximal interphalangeal joint fracture.

As such, many are not amenable to ORIF methods or K-wire fixation. Often the best solution to optimize outcome of PIP joint function is the application of traction using the principle of **ligamentotaxis**. This principle applies the use of a continuous distraction force distal to fracture comminution to re-align the fracture fragments.[25] This externally applied traction can be achieved by use of one of two common methods, either surgical application of a pins and rubber bands system (Fig. 23.13) or a traction system. Skin taping is one method used to apply the traction; however, use of a transverse K-wire is more common. Transverse K-wires drilled by the surgeon into the bone away from the fracture leave the ends of the K-wire exposed for attachment of an elastic band or spring to a custom-made orthosis (Fig. 23.14). Intervention methods that provide for both traction and joint motion have resulted in superior outcomes to those providing for one or the other.

A hand-based orthosis is needed for some clients managed with a pins and rubber band traction system to protect from knocking and damaging the system. Others do well with a thin dorsal finger-based orthosis to hold the PIP joint in extension overnight for prevention of PIP joint flexion contractures. Orthoses designs that require attachment of a transverse K-wire are divided into three types: static traction, dynamic arcuate, and dynamic swing hinge.[26] A dynamic swing hinge traction orthosis design can be hand-based as shown in Fig. 23.14 or forearm-hand-based. In general, the transverse K-wire remains in for 6 weeks and the client is seen weekly for X-rays to check the position of the fracture. To prevent PIP joint instability, extension is limited as per surgeon, and at least 50 degrees of active PIP joint flexion is the initial aim.

Postoperative management of a volar plate arthroplasty requires a dorsal blocking finger-based orthosis similar to that used for conservative management for a period of 4 to 6 weeks. Place the PIP joint in as much extension as comfortable (no less than 30-degrees flexion), then serially straightened over subsequent therapy sessions guided by tenderness about the fracture. For stubborn flexion contractures, a dynamic extension orthosis can be applied in accordance with joint stability no earlier than 6 to 8 weeks after surgery.

Distal Phalanx Fracture of the Fingers

Surgical fixation is required in cases where the angulation of the distal phalanx fracture is too great to reduce by manipulation alone, or the joint is subluxed, or more than 50% of the articular surface is involved. Fig. 23.9 shows an axial K-wire to reduce the joint and align the fracture. The K-wire can be buried so not to protrude from the skin, *and then* removed in *the* surgical theatre or the outpatient setting. Buried axial K-wires do not always require orthotic protection unless there is concomitant soft-tissue damage such as open wounds, nailbed, or digital nerve irritation, which require protection. In the case of K-wires that extend beyond the tip of the finger, a protective orthosis can help prevent knocking or catching the K-wire.

Clinical Pearl

During fabrication of a hand-based orthosis, place an oversize rubber glove over the dressing; or for fingertip injuries, simply cut the "finger" off a rubber glove to keep the thermoplastic material from sticking to the underlying dressing.

Fractures of the Thumb Phalanges

Thumb phalanx fractures that are not reducible and remain unstable may require surgery. ORIF intervention for the proximal phalanx can be with internal or K-wire fixation. Distal phalanx fractures include fracture/avulsion of either the EPL or FPL. Insertion of a single axial K-wire for displaced distal phalanx shaft or tuft fractures is the usual choice. For a proximal phalanx fracture use a hand-based thumb orthosis design that includes the IP joint. A distal phalanx fracture stabilized with an axial K-wire may require a "cap" orthosis that includes the thumb's IP joint to protect from overuse and bumping.

Clinical Pearl

Adhesion formation is not limited to the surgically managed fracture. Bleeding and edema with any hand fracture set the stage for adhesion formation, especially on the dorsum of the hand and fingers. Early controlled motion and edema control are effective antidotes.

? Questions to Ask the Doctor

Developing a dependable line of communication with the referring physician for management of clients with hand fractures includes having access to view X-rays and the surgical report before the client arrives. To facilitate attending physician communication, we have developed a list of common questions to consider during the initial 3 weeks postfracture management:

- How long ago was the fracture and/or surgery, and what was the mechanism of injury?
- What bone and what location within the bone?
- What is the fracture pattern?
- Was fracture reduction required?
- Was fixation required? If yes, by what method of fixation?
- Does the fixation hardware interfere with any joint movement?
- How confident is the surgeon in fracture stability?
- Will fracture stability permit early controlled motion?
- Are there associated soft-tissue injuries? If yes, are there any precautions?
- When is removal of the external hardware or subcutaneous K-wires planned?
- When is the next follow-up X-ray?
- What are your thoughts about timelines for return to sport, work, or hobbies with or without the protective orthosis?

( ) What to Say to Clients

Clients who understand their injury and the rationale behind restrictions are likely to be more involved and participate in their own care.

About the Injury

- Use a diagram or anatomical model to show the fractured bone and explain the process of fracture healing and recovery of bone strength.
- A personalized timeline calendar that plots bone healing/strengthening and return to functional use is helpful.
- When there is hardware, show the client their X-ray or a picture to explain the hardware's role and timeframes for healing and hardware removal.
- Review wound dressing application and pin site care/precautions.
- For success, set appropriate/attainable short-term goals, and reassure with positive feedback.

About the Orthosis

- To improve client adherence, share with them the benefits of a fracture orthosis over those of a cast, such as preventative versus corrective care, reduced therapy visits, and the opportunity to do regular hand hygiene.

- Verbal and written orthosis instructions are equally important. Include details about wear, hand use, and how to remove/replace the orthosis.
- Review how to cover the orthosis with a plastic bag/glove and tape the proximal end, or advise the client to buy a commercially made shower guard for bathing.
- Instruct in cleaning the orthosis and the properties of low temperature thermoplastics.
- Ask the client to monitor for areas of skin tenderness or redness that indicate too much pressure. Clients with compromised sensation are at risk of skin breakdown.
- Remind clients not to self-adjust the orthosis! They should contact the hand therapist when concerned.

About Exercises

- Clients can be hesitant to move or touch their injured hand, fearing harm or pain. Take time to explain the exercise benefits/precautions. To build confidence, start exercise on the uninjured digits and safe joints.
- Encourage bilateral ROM when possible and be sure not to overlook the shoulder and elbow.
- Explain the difference between the correct response to exercise, which may feel tight but subsides quickly, compared to an incorrect feeling of sharp or stabbing pain that lasts longer.
- Instill the concept of using pain as a guide. Exercises should produce steady gains in motion with minimal discomfort.
- Encourage pacing of activities and exercise. Suggest several short frequent exercise sessions throughout the day rather than a couple long sessions.
- Introduce the injured hand to early functional use to stimulate the sensorimotor cortex. These activities include brushing teeth, eating, holding cellphone, or computer use.
- To improve client understanding, try using written instructions, diagrams, or the client's cellphone to video/photograph proper exercises performance for later reference.

Evaluation Tips

- Begin formulating a comprehensive management plan prior to hands-on examination to assemble the clinical picture with available client information. Examples include mechanism of injury, fracture details and soft-tissue involvement, method of fracture reduction/fixation, and managing physician insights.
- Take into consideration the client's previous injuries or illness, occupation and interests, and social supports that may affect the rehabilitation process.
- Use ROM measurements of the uninjured hand as a comparison and for establishing goals.
- Recognize limited digital motion may be a result of scar adhesion and/or external hardware tagging soft-tissue excursion.
- Uncharacteristic pain, swelling, and stiffness that develops after the first week of injury may be sympathetically mediated, which requires immediate attention and communication with the attending physician to avoid complications like complex regional pain syndrome (CRPS).
- Use evidence-based self-reported questionnaires such as the Disabilities of the Arm, Shoulder, Hand (DASH); SF-36; Michigan Hand Questionnaire (MHQ); or the Patient-Specific Functional Scale (PSFS)[27] to assess general impairment and function.

Diagnosis-Specific Information That Affects Clinical Reasoning

Early Clinical Reasoning (0–3 Weeks Post Fracture/Surgery)

- Use information regarding fracture pattern, time since injury, and method of fixation as a guide to select the most appropriate therapy management program.
- Soon after ORIF with rigid hardware, move the joints proximal and distal to the fracture while using the opposite hand to support the fracture from the volar and dorsal aspects. Follow similar guidelines for the stable nonsurgical fracture.
- "Gray Zone" fractures are less stable, so delay controlled active motion of the joints proximal and distal to the fracture. Consult Table 23.1 for relative fracture stability.

Later Clinical Reasoning (3–8 Weeks Post Fracture/Surgery)

- Distinguish between intrinsic versus extrinsic tightness, joint/capsular restrictions, and tendon adhesion to develop a specific treatment plan to remedy ROM limitations.
- As the client's function increases, any unusual numbness/tingling of the fingers and/or pain with active motion may indicate the client is doing too much too soon; these red flags require activity reduction to calm the signs and symptoms of flexor tenosynovitis.

♥ Tips From the Field

- To protect K-wires, open a 2 x 2 gauze pad, fluff it up to form a pillow over the end of the wire then mold the thermoplastic orthosis. On removal of the gauze, there will be an air bubble for the K-wire within the orthosis.
- Pediatric orthoses require extra coverings or taping to prevent removal. A figure-of-eight tape wrap adheres to the orthosis and becomes secure when passed around the wrist; or place a stockinet glove over the orthosis and tape into place. A sling will also deter hand use at school or during rigorous activity.
- Use light compression wrap from distal to proximal to manage edema. Remove the wrap for controlled exercises to reduce resistance and allow for full joint motion.

➤ Precautions and Concerns

- *Any exposed surgical hardware is a potential site for infection. Minimize the risk by keeping these sites dry, clean, and pressure/snag free. Each surgeon will have preferences for cleaning the hardware and site. Infection risk increases when K-wires remain in beyond 3 weeks.*
- *K-wires will loosen and occasionally start to back out. Do not attempt to push the K-wire in. Subcutaneous K-wires may also back out, causing pain due to pressure from the overlying orthosis, make an air bubble modification (see Tips from the Field above). In both instances, notify the surgeon.*
- *Injury to the nailbed can result in nail deformity as the nail grows out; instruct the client how to massage the cuticle and to tape over irregular nails to prevent snagging.*
- *Hematomas under the fingernail are generally acute and seen after a crush injury, and pain is relieved by drainage. Contact the attending physician.*

- *Digital nerves injured in crush injuries of the distal phalanx often become painful and hypersensitive 10–14 days post injury. Intervene by reassuring the client and initiate desensitization techniques.*
- *Intraarticular fractures tend to be stiffer and remain swollen longer. Forced mobilization of these fractured joints should not be painful as symptoms may be prolonged. Long term, these joints may develop traumatic arthritis.*
- *Nonunion, fibrous union, and delayed healing can indicate too much micromotion; inadequate fracture reduction (gap); interruption of bone repair secondary to health factors, medication, or tobacco use; and/or poor client compliance.*

Conclusion

Hand fractures are commonly seen in hand therapy practice. Fractures do not occur without involvement of the soft tissue, which often results in functionally debilitating stiffness and deformity when not managed correctly. Protective stabilization of the fracture for healing does not imply prolonged immobilization. Therapist understanding of factors that positively and negatively influence bone healing, surgical and nonsurgical management methods, and fracture orthoses designs are the underpinnings of successful outcome. A well-developed line of communication with the attending physician about X-ray and operative notes, the fracture management plan, and projected result is helpful. However, if the client's cooperation is not engaged through open communication and sharing of educational information, success will be limited. Methods for managing hand fractures surgically and nonsurgically is ever evolving, and staying current will advance therapy outcomes.

CASE STUDY

MM is a right-handed 2-year-old boy, who crushed his finger in a door hinge and attended the physician 3 days postinjury. X-ray (Fig. 23.15) shows a right long finger extraarticular distal phalanx tuft transverse displaced fracture; a nailbed hematoma and a dorsal skin laceration, with no tendon involvement. The physician sent MM and his mother to hand therapy for fabrication of a custom, protective clamshell type orthosis and for instruction in AROM exercises to all but the DIP joint of the injured digit. After removal of the bandages and alumifoam splint MM was teary and reluctant to have his hand touched. Evaluation noted limited ROM of the uninjured secondary to edema and reluctance to use his hand for grasp activities.

Fabrication of an orthosis on a 2-year-old is a challenge, tactics used to distract MM included placing a bandage over his teddy bear's hand to mimic his own, and playing with the warmed thermoplastic with him to improve his comfort level. The critical first step in fabrication of the orthosis was to stretch the finger part of an examination glove over the dressing to keep it dry and to prevent the warmed thermoplastics from sticking. Once cooled, removal of the exam glove finger and orthosis was quick and pain free. The clamshell finger-based orthosis design immobilized the DIP joint and allowed PIP joint motion. The application of an adjustable strap eliminated the need to return to therapy for orthosis adjustment secondary to changes in edema or bandage size, which his mother could snug up for a better fit. Use of a figure-of-eight tape wrapped from finger to wrist insured that MM did not wiggle out of his orthosis. To keep the orthosis dry during bath time, a rubber sleeve covered the orthosis.

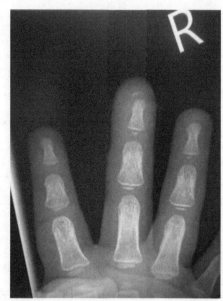

FIG. 23.15 Right long finger distal phalanx tuft fracture in 2-year-old child.

At 2 weeks postsurgery, as edema had decreased, the orthosis required adjustment for a better fit. Instructions advised full-time orthosis wear except for bath time and change of bandages. Understandably, MM with the orthosis on, avoided use of his injured hand and was not spontaneously using it for bilateral play. A favorite toy, soft exercise putty, and slime were favored over traditional AROM therapy exercises to encourage use of the right hand.

At week 4, although MM still did not allow the therapist to touch his finger, the timeframe for clinical healing of the tuft fracture indicated that it was time to encourage time out of the orthosis for safe play. Because MM avoided use of his hand and did not like to touch his injured finger, desensitization techniques consisting of tapping/touching different textures and massage of the fingertip with lotion. Singing songs accompanied by finger motions encouraged active use of the injured hand. The orthosis was worn for comfort and protection when at childcare and for robust play.

By week 6, there was no need to wear the orthosis, since the fingertip was no longer hypersensitive, and MM was using his hand. Tape over the fingertip to prevent snagging the irregular nail during play helped. At this time, MM required prompting to include the long finger for grasp tasks. Hand therapy consisted of PROM for DIP joint stiffness, active flexion for functional use, and desensitization of the injured fingertip. To improve DIP joint stiffness, the therapist filled a basin with warm water in which he played games such as bursting soap bubbles and squeezing a soft sponge toy. Adding textures to his favorite slime exercises accomplished both desensitization and active grasp and pinch.

On discharge, MM used his hand for most play activities including holding his crayons and eating utensils, and gripping the swing chains. There was no fingernail deformity and he had full range of motion.

Acknowledgments

Many clinicians have enhanced our basic understanding and management of hand fractures. We encourage the reader to seek out the primary source acknowledged within each reference we have cited in this chapter.

References

1. Feehan LM: Extra-articular hand fractures part II: therapist's management. In Skirven TM, Osterman AL, Fedorczyk JM, et al.: *Rehabilitation of the hand and upper extremity*, ed 6, Philadelphia, 2011, Elsevier Mosby, pp 386–401.
2. Jones WW: Biomechanics of small bone fixation, *Clini Orthop* 214:11–18, 1987.
3. Valentin P: The interossei and lumbricals. In Tubiana R: *The hand volume 1*. Philadelphia PA, 1981, WB Saunders Co., pp 244–246.
4. Fahrer M: The thenar eminence: an introduction. In Tubiana R: *The hand volume 1*. Philadelphia PA, 1981, WB Saunders Co., pp 255–256.
5. Meals C, Meals R: Hand fractures: a review of current treatment strategies, *J Hand Surg [Am]* 38A:1021–1031, 2013.
6. Kollitz KM, et al.: Metacarpal fractures: treatment and complications, *Hand* 9:16–23, 2014.
7. Meinberg E, Agel J, Roberts C, et al.: Fracture and dislocation classification compendium–2018, *J Orthop Trauma* 32(1) Supplement, 2018.
8. Cepela DJ, Tartaglione JP, Dooley TP, Patel PN: Classifications in brief: salter-harris classification of pediatric physeal fractures, *Clin Orthop* 474:2531–2537, 2016.
9. Hardy M, Wegener EE: Hand fracture management, *J Hand Ther* 16(2):79–80, 2003.
10. Soong M, Got C, Katarincic J: Ring and little finger metacarpal fractures: mechanisms, locations, and radiographic parameters, *J Hand Surg [Am]* 35(8):1256–1259, 2010.
11. McNemar TB, Howell JW, Chang E: Management of metacarpal fractures, *J Hand Ther* 16(2):143–151, 2003.
12. Weinstein LP, Hanel DP: Metacarpal fractures, *J Am Soc Surg Hand* 2(4):168–180, 2002.
13. Lehman T, Hildenbrand J: Fractures and ligament injuries of the thumb and metacarpals. In Trumble TE, Rayan GM, Budoff JE, et al.: *Principles of hand surgery and therapy*, ed 2, Philadelphia, 2010, Saunders Elsevier, pp 35–59.
14. Cannon NM: Rehabilitation approaches for distal and middle phalanx fractures of the hand, *J Hand Ther* 16:105–116, 2003.
15. Kalfas IH: Principles of bone healing, *Neurosurg Focus* 10(4):1–4, 2001.
16. Feehan L: *Personal communication with J Howell*, May 2018.
17. Moberg E: The Use of traction treatment for fractures of the phalanges and metacarpals, *Acta Chir Scand* 99:341–352, 1950.
18. Feehan LM: Early controlled mobilization of potentially unstable extra-articular hand fractures, *J Hand Ther* 16(2):161–170, 2003.
19. Peacock EE, Van Winkle W: *Surgery and biology of wound repair*, Philadelphia, 1970, W. B. Saunders Company, pp 332.
20. Westbrook AP, et al.: The clinical significance of malunion of fractures of the neck and shaft of the little finger metacarpal, *J Hand Surg* 33E(6):732–739, 2008.
21. Giddins G: The non-operative management of hand fractures: a review, *J Trauma and Orthop* 4(4):48–51, 2016.
22. Strickland J, et al.: Phalangeal fractures: factors influencing digital performance, *Orthop Rev* 39–50, 1982.
23. Freeland AE, Hardy MA, Singletary S: Rehabilitation for proximal phalangeal fractures, *J Hand Ther* 16(2):129–142, 2003.
24. Shuler MS, Slade JF: Fractures of the phalanx. In Trumble TE, Rayan GM, Budoff JE, et al.: *Principles of hand surgery and therapy*, ed 2, Philadelphia, 2010, Saunders Elsevier, pp 60–80.
25. Goldman SB, Amaker RJ, Espinosa RA: James traction splinting for PIP fractures, *J Hand Ther* 21(2):209–215, 2008.
26. Packham TL, et al.: A scoping review of applications and outcomes of traction orthoses and constructs for the management of intra-articular fractures and fracture dislocations in the hand, *J Hand Ther* 29(3):246–268, 2016.
27. Novak CB, Williams MM, Conaty K: Evaluation of the patient-specific functional scale, *Hand* 10:85–87, 2015.

24 Elbow, Wrist, and Hand Tendinopathies

Kathryn S. McQueen
Tim Pemberton

Introduction

Clients with tendinitis/tendinosis experience pain that can significantly limit their daily activities. Simply picking up a coffee cup may be a painful task. Stirring food, putting away groceries, or using a keyboard may provoke pain, and exercise routines can be interrupted. These clients may not seek medical assistance hoping that the symptoms will pass. Unfortunately, those who wait may develop chronic changes, which can be more difficult to treat. Symptoms associated with tendinitis/tendinosis include pain with active range of motion (AROM), resistance, or stretching of the involved structures.

Anatomy

Tendons are viscoelastic structures with unique mechanical properties that allow muscles to transmit forces, which create motion at joints. They are composed of connective tissues made of collagen, tenocytes, and ground substance, and are poorly vascularized.[1] The factors that most affect a tendon's biomechanical properties are aging, pregnancy, and mobilization (or immobilization). Up to the age of 20, the collagen cross-links in tendons increase in number and improve in quality, resulting in increased tensile strength. With aging, tensile strength decreases.[2]

General Pathology

Previously, tendinitides were considered inflammatory conditions, with interventions largely focused on reducing inflammation.[3] The histological research reveals that inflammation is rarely present in clients with tendinitis and symptoms are more likely the result of degenerative changes of the tendon due to aging and overuse.[3,4] Therefore names for tendinopathies such as epicondylitis are a misnomer, as these are not inflammatory pathologies. Based on this information, intervention should be focused on treating tendinitis as a **tendinosis** (breakdown of collagen) rather than a **tendinitis** (inflammatory process characterized by heat, swelling and pain), as traditional approaches to addressing inflammation may prove unsuccessful over time.[3,4,5]

◎ Clinical Pearl

To achieve the best possible therapeutic outcome, it is very important to help your client identify activities contributing to tendinopathy and to make as many ergonomic changes and activity modifications as possible.

◎ Clinical Pearl

Tendons remodel in response to imposed mechanical stress. They become stronger by being exposed to increased stress (e.g., movement), and they weaken when stress is reduced or eliminated (e.g., immobilization, such as when wearing an orthosis). Thus participation in regular activities of daily living in conjunction with exercise that targets the specific symptomatic tendon(s) is important for tendon remodeling after injury. However, with tendinopathies, clients need to initially curtail activities that increase symptoms to allow tendon healing to occur.

Lateral Epicondylosis

One of the most common upper extremity conditions is **lateral epicondylosis**, also known as tennis elbow, lateral epicondylitis, lateral epicondylalgia, and tendinitis of the forearm extensor muscles.[6,7] Currently, this condition affects 1% to 3% of the general population, with males and females equally affected. The condition occurs most frequently in 40- to 60-year-olds.[8,9,10] Lateral epicondylosis is characterized as an overuse or force overload injury due to the degeneration of the tendon as the structure ages. Lateral epicondylosis affects the common extensor tendon at its point of origin on the lateral epicondyle of the humerus. The extensor carpi radialis brevis (ECRB) is the extensor tendon most commonly affected.[11,12,13] A common example of an individual that would present with this condition is a 50-year-old female experiencing sudden onset of lateral elbow pain after a day of gardening.

Diagnosis

Clients typically present with complaints of pain over the lateral portion of the elbow and with decreased grip strength. These symptoms can affect a client's ability to participate in sports, work tasks, and basic activities of daily living (ADLs).[14,15]

In addition to tenderness to palpation over the lateral epicondyle, three main clinical tests exist to support a diagnosis of lateral epicondylosis: Cozen's test, Mills' test, and Maudsley's test. All three tests are considered positive if they reproduce pain. Cozen's test is performed by placing the client's forearm in pronation, full elbow extension, and resisted wrist extension.[16] Mills' test places the client's forearm in pronation, wrist in a flexed position, and the elbow is then moved into extension.[17] Maudsley's test is similar to Cozen's test except resistance is placed at the third finger instead of the wrist.[18] With grip strength, the ECRB must work to counteract the flexors of the wrist and digits and this causes pain at the lateral epicondyle. Due to the mechanical necessity of the ECRB, another potential test to support the diagnosis of lateral epicondylosis is a grip strength test. The test is positive for lateral epicondylosis if grip strength is stronger with the elbow in 90 degrees of flexion and weaker when the elbow is fully extended. In a healthy elbow, the reverse would be true in which grip strength would increase with full elbow extension.[19]

◎ Clinical Pearl

It is important to ensure that the client does not have radial tunnel syndrome (See Table 24.1 for details on assessing for radial tunnel). If radial tunnel syndrome is suspected, do not use a counterforce strap, and add radial nerve glides to the treatment program.

Nonoperative Treatment

Mainstay conservative treatments for lateral epicondylosis include rest, ice, activity modifications, orthoses, corticosteroid injection, and strengthening. Although strong evidence for one optimal treatment approach does not currently exist,[20] many therapists use a two-phase approach when treating tendinosis. Phase one of treatment focuses on reducing pain and restoration of tendon length that has been reduced due to scarring of the tendon that is characteristic of tendinosis. Phase two of treatment introduces gentle progressive strengthening. While various types of strengthening (eccentric, eccentric-concentric, and isometric) are supported in the literature, the general consensus among therapists at this time is eccentric strengthening is considered the most critical to the treatment of lateral epicondylosis.[6,20,21] Furthermore, it is important to educate the client that full resolution of pain may take several months.[6,20,22] A typical two-phase program for lateral epicondylosis might progress as follows.

Phase I: Pain Relief and Tendon Lengthening[23]
Education
Education consists of the pathoanatomy of tendinosis, activity modification to avoid activities that cause pain, and body mechanics training to avoid lifting objects with the forearm in pronation. It is also important to educate clients that a positive therapeutic outcome may be hindered if the client is unable or unwilling to modify activities that cause pain.

Orthosis
A wrist cock-up orthosis (Fig. 24.1) or counterforce strap is issued, and the client is educated on wear and care. The wrist cock-up orthosis is placed on the volar portion of the wrist to unload the ECRB thereby reducing pain. The counterforce strap is placed over the proximal end of the forearm extensor muscle bellies to decrease the tension on the common tendon insertion. While both are considered appropriate options, the wrist cock-up orthosis has proven more effective than the counterforce strap for providing long-term pain relief.[22,24] A counterforce strap should be tightened to a snug position, but not worn too tightly. A too-tight counterforce strap can irritate the radial nerve.

Pain Management
The client may be instructed in the use of ice over the origin of the problematic tendon to decrease pain. Take care to avoid applying ice directly over the radial and ulnar nerves.

Regain Tendon Length
Because of the degeneration of the tendon, scarring results in tendon length insufficiency. In order to restore normal tendon dynamics, the structures will need to be lengthened. From onset of therapy, the client should begin stretching the forearm extensor muscles. Instruct the client to use the unaffected hand to passively flex and ulnarly deviate the wrist gently with the elbow in full extension (Fig. 24.2). The stretch should be held in a pain-free range for 20 to 30 seconds.[20] The right dose for stretches to be effective is debated;[5,6,20] however, the more frequently the client performs the stretch in a pain-free range the sooner tendon length will be restored and pain resolved. A typical home exercise program includes stretching every 2 to 3 hours: 3 to 5 repetitions with 20- to 30-second holds.

Phase II: Strengthening
Currently, no strong evidence yet supports the need for strengthening. However, from a clinical reasoning standpoint, strengthening may be beneficial. Eccentric strengthening of the forearm extensors loads the tendon in a lengthened position and can be done without causing pain. Concentric exercises tend to be painful and contradict instructions to avoid palm down lifting and should therefore be avoided in the early stage of strengthening. Strengthening exercises should be performed 1 to 2 times per day: 10 repetitions using a 1lb (0.5kg) weight. Slowly increase to 30 repetitions as this is an endurance exercise. Once this becomes easy, increase to a 2lb (1kg) weight. Always instruct the client to stretch before and after completing strengthening exercises.

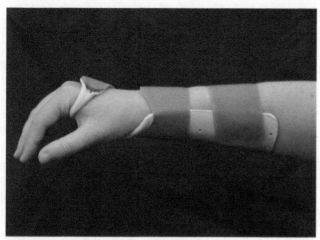

FIG. 24.1 Typical design for a wrist cock-up orthosis that can be used for either lateral or medial epicondylosis.

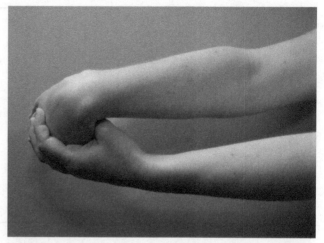

FIG. 24.2 Full stretch position for lateral epicondylosis. If there is pain in the full stretch position, the client can gradually progress to this end position.

Strengthening can be added to a home exercise program as early as the second visit if the client can tolerate. Once the client is able to complete strengthening with a 2lb (1kg) weight, the client should begin to slowly reintroduce activities that were avoided due to pain as long as the activities remain pain free.

Corticosteroid Injection by a Physician

If the client continues to report consistent pain and has followed the prescribed home exercise program, the client may benefit from a corticosteroid injection administered by the physician. Corticosteroid injections have shown good results in the short term to decrease pain (within 1 to 4 weeks); however, long-term results have proven less favorable. Thus, completion of a conservative management program should be attempted first.[25] If a client receives a corticosteroid injection, they should resume therapy to ensure length is restored to the tendon. Once pain is decreased and stretching is tolerated, the client should progress to strengthening.

Surgical Intervention

Surgical intervention is suggested for clients that continue to experience decreased function due to debilitating pain despite 6 to 12 months of conservative management.[23] The postoperative home exercise program is the same as that prescribed for conservative management with the exception of the addition of scar management and edema control techniques. Stretches can begin 6 weeks postsurgery.[23,26,27,28]

> **Clinical Pearl**
>
> Stretches are the cornerstone for decreasing pain. Until more flexibility is achieved, pain will continue.

> **Clinical Pearl**
>
> Full recovery may be less likely for clients who experienced prolonged symptoms prior to seeking treatment,[29] for clients with a prior diagnosis of lateral epicondylosis, or for those clients who have received a previous cortisone injection.

Medial Epicondylosis

Medial epicondylosis, more commonly known as Golfer's Elbow, is characterized by pain, swelling, and tenderness to palpation over the medial aspect of the elbow.[26,27] Symptoms of medial epicondylosis occur with activities such as gripping a golf club or heavy lifting that leads to damage of the common flexor tendon at its point of origin on the medial epicondyle of the humerus.[26,27,28] Pathological changes are most often found in the pronator teres and flexor carpi radialis muscle tendons, although the palmaris longus, flexor digitorum superficialis, and flexor carpi ulnaris may also be impacted.[26,28,30] Medial epicondylosis is much less common than lateral epicondylosis, accounting for no more than 20% of total epicondylosis diagnoses.[26,27] As with lateral epicondylosis, people between the ages of 40 and 60 are most likely to be impacted by the syndrome, and instances of medial epicondylosis are distributed equally among men and women.[27]

Diagnosis

Clients with medial epicondylosis typically report pain of insidious onset centered over the medial epicondyle that is exacerbated by activities requiring resisted pronation and wrist flexion.[26,27,30] While range of motion is not always impacted, clients often report severely diminished functional task performance secondary to increased pain when engaging in desired or required activities.[26,27]

Nonoperative Treatment

Nonsurgical treatment is generally effective and is considered the mainstay for treating medial epicondylosis.[26,27,28] Common treatment techniques include rest, ice, activity modifications, orthoses (see Fig. 24.1), corticosteroid injection, and strengthening. A typical conservative management program would progress in the same manner as the previously described lateral epicondylosis program with the exception that stretches and strengthening are focused on the wrist flexors. Stretches are performed in supination with the elbow extended and wrist passively stretched into extension to lengthen the flexor pronator tendon group (Fig. 24.3).

TABLE 24.1   Overview of Tendinopathies of the Upper Extremity

Diagnosis	Structures Most Involved	Provocative Tests	Differential Diagnoses	Orthotic Considerations
Lateral epicondylosis	ECRB, EDC	• Cozen's test • Mills' test • Maudsley's test • Palpation of lateral epicondyle • Resisted wrist extension • Gripping with elbow extended	• Cervical radiculopathy • Proximal neurovascular entrapment • Radial tunnel syndrome	• Volar wrist cock-up orthosis at 35 degrees wrist extension • Counterforce brace on extensor wad • Soft four-finger buddy strap
Radial tunnel syndrome	Superficial radial nerve	• Middle finger test • Percussion of superficial radial nerve (distal to proximal)	• Lateral epicondylitis	• No counterforce brace
Medial epicondylosis	Pronator teres, FCR, PL	• Palpation of medial epicondyle • Resisted elbow extension with supination and wrist extension • Repetitive or forceful pronation • Resisted wrist flexion • Passive composite extension (elbow, wrist, digits)	• Cervical radiculopathy • Proximal neurovascular entrapment • Ulnar neuropathy • Elbow ulnar collateral ligament problem	• Volar wrist cock-up orthosis with wrist in neutral • Counterforce brace on flexor wad • Soft four-finger buddy strap
de Quervain's tenosynovitis	APL and EPB at first dorsal compartment	• Finkelstein's test • Resisted thumb extension or abduction • Pain/thickening at first dorsal compartment	• Osteoarthritis of thumb CMC joint or wrist • Scaphoid fracture • Intersection syndrome • Radial nerve neuritis	• Forearm-based thumb spica orthosis with IP joint free
Digital stenosing tenosynovitis	Digital flexor tendon at the A1 pulley	• Tenderness at A1 pulley • Possible palpable nodule • Crepitus with active digital flexion	• Flexor tendon tumors, ganglia, lipoma	• Hand-based orthosis with MP joint in neutral • Digital volar gutter orthosis with PIP joint in neutral. MP and DIP joints free

Diagnosis	Structures Most Involved	Provocative Tests	Differential Diagnoses	Orthotic Considerations
Intersection syndrome	APL and EPB muscle bellies, approximately 4 cm proximal to wrist where they intersect with ECRB and ECRL	• Snapping or locking with active composite digital flexion • Swelling locally at muscle bellies	• De Quervain's tenosynovitis	• Same as for de Quervain's tenosynovitis
EPL tendinitis	EPL at Lister's tubercle	• Pain with resisted wrist extension • Similar provocative tests as for de Quervain's tenosynovitis • Pain at Lister's tubercle • Resisted composite thumb extension • Passive composite thumb flexion	• De Quervain's tenosynovitis • Intersection syndrome	• Forearm-based thumb spica orthosis with composite thumb extension, IP joint included
ECU tendinitis	ECU	• Forearm supination with wrist ulnar deviation • Pain at ulnar wrist	• DRUJ instability • TFCC tear	• Forearm-based ulnar gutter orthosis • Ulnar head padded as needed for comfort
FCR tendinitis	FCR	• Resisted wrist flexion and radial deviation • Pain with passive wrist extension • Pain over proximal wrist crease and at scaphoid tubercle	• Ulnocarpal abutment • Ganglion cysts • Thumb CMC osteoarthritis • Scaphoid fracture • De Quervain's tenosynovitis	• Volar wrist cock-up orthosis with wrist in neutral or position of comfort
FCU tendinitis	FCU	• Pain with palpation over pisiform • Resisted wrist flexion and ulnar deviation • Passive wrist extension and radial deviation	• Pisiform fracture • Pisotriquetral arthritis	• Forearm-based ulnar gutter orthosis

APL, Abductor pollicis longus; *CMC*, carpometacarpal; *DIP*, distal interphalangeal; *DRUJ*, distal radioulnar joint; *ECRB*, extensor carpi radialis brevis; *ECRL*, extensor carpi radialis longus; *ECU*, extensor carpi ulnaris; *EDC*, extensor digitorum communis; *EPB*, extensor pollicis brevis; *EPL*, extensor pollicis longus; *FCR*, flexor carpi radialis; *FCU*, flexor carpi ulnaris; *IP*, interphalangeal; *MP*, metacarpophalangeal; *PIP*, proximal interphalangeal; *PL*, palmaris longus; *TFCC*, triangular fibrocartilage complex.

Modified from Lee MP, Biafora SJ, Zelouf DS. Management of hand and wrist tendinopathies. In: Skirven TM, Osterman AL, Fedorczyk JM. eds. *Rehabilitation of the Hand and Upper Extremity.* 6th ed. Philadelphia, PA: Mosby; 2011; Evans RB, Hunter JM, Burkhalter WE. Conservative management of the trigger finger: a new approach. *J Hand Ther.* 1988;1:59–68; Trumble TE. Tendinitis and epicondylitis. In: Trumble TE. ed. Principles of Hand Surgery. Philadelphia, PA: WB Saunders; 2000; Lindner-Ions S, Ingell K. An alternative splint design for trigger finger. *J Hand Ther.* 1998;11:206–208; and Verdon ME. Overuse syndromes of the hand and wrist. *Prim Care.* 1996;23:305–319.

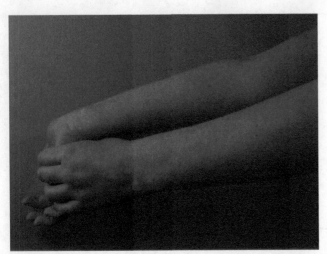

FIG. 24.3 Full stretch position for medial epicondylosis. If there is pain in the full stretch position, the client can gradually progress to this end position.

Surgical Intervention

If the client undergoes surgical debridement of the tendon, stretching and strengthening should be initiated 6 weeks postsurgery and follow a progression that matches conservative management with the addition of scar and edema management.

> ### ⊙ *Clinical Pearl*
>
> Prior to initiating treatment for medial epicondylosis, ulnar neuritis and ulnar collateral ligament instability should be ruled out.[26,27,28]

> ### ⟫ *Precautions and Concerns*

Although a counterforce strap may assist clients with returning to desired activities after a diagnosis of medial epicondylosis, anterior interosseous nerve compression and posterior interosseous nerve entrapment have been noted with use of counterforce straps. Clients should be instructed to report any new onset of shooting or burning pain, and use of the strap should be discontinued immediately if new pain is reported.[26,28] When applying ice to the medial aspect of the elbow, the client should avoid placing ice directly over the ulnar nerve to prevent irritation of the nerve.

De Quervain's Tenosynovitis

De Quervain's tenosynovitis, also known as stenosing tenovaginitis or stenosing tenosynovitis, is an overuse pathology involving impaired gliding of the abductor pollicis longus (APL) and extensor pollicis brevis (EPB) tendons as they pass through the first dorsal compartment on the radial side of the wrist.[4,31,32] Diminished smooth motion of the APL and EPB tendons is caused by a thickening of the extensor retinaculum over the first dorsal compartment.[4] Actions that may contribute to thickening of the extensor retinaculum include forceful or repetitive grasp combined with wrist ulnar deviation, repetitive thumb abduction, and/or repetitive thumb metacarpophalangeal (MP) joint flexion.[31,32,33] De Quervain's is most commonly seen in females

between the ages of 35 and 55 and is typically associated with the dominant hand.[4,31]

Diagnosis

Clients diagnosed with de Quervain's typically report pain of insidious onset over the radial styloid that may radiate distally to the thumb or proximally to the shoulder.[3,31,32] To identify presence of de Quervain's, provocative testing may include palpation over the first dorsal compartment, Finkelstein's test, and resisted APL.[4,32,33,34] To perform Finkelstein's test instruct the client to flex the thumb into the palm of the hand, then ulnarly deviate the wrist.[4,34] The test is considered positive if symptoms are reproduced.

Nonoperative Treatment

Orthosis

Decreasing repetitive load on the APL and EPB tendons is the primary goal of utilizing an orthosis to manage de Quervain's. A forearm-based thumb spica orthosis (Fig. 24.4) that places the wrist in neutral and thumb in opposition is recommended to assist with pain management by preventing thumb MP joint flexion and wrist ulnar deviation.[4] The thumb interphalangeal joint should be left free, as the extensor pollicis longus tendon is located in the third dorsal compartment, and typically not problematic for individuals with de Quervain's.[4,33] The orthosis should be worn during the day as much as possible and always worn at night for 4 to 6 weeks. Ice and cessation of all exacerbating activities should be coupled with orthosis wear to manage symptoms during the acute treatment phase.[4,33] Although physical agent modalities are frequently used in the nonoperative management of de Quervain's, there is no consensus in the literature that supports their efficacy.[1]

> ### ⊙ *Clinical Pearl*
>
> To avoid irritation of the superficial radial nerve when wearing the thumb spica orthosis, care should be taken to create a bubble around the radial styloid during fabrication.

Activity Modification

Clients should avoid all motions and activities that exacerbate pain. Activity modifications should focus on avoidance of repetitive or sustained loading of the APL and EPB tendons.[35] Task division, pacing of activities, and use of the unaffected extremity to perform problematic ADLs are all effective strategies for alleviating pain.[35]

Progressive Stretching and Strengthening

Once pain and swelling are addressed through orthosis wear and activity modification, active and passive range of motion and stretching should be introduced to promote APL and EPB tendon gliding through the first dorsal compartment.[33] If stretching and ROM do not exacerbate symptoms, the client's program should be advanced to include progressive strengthening exercises beginning with isometrics, advancing to light weight (1–2lbs) (0.5–1kg), and ending with full weight bearing.[33]

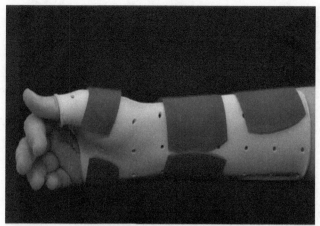

FIG. 24.4 Volar forearm-based thumb spica orthosis that can be used for de Quervain's tenosynovitis.

Corticosteroid Injection by a Physician

A corticosteroid injection administered by a physician to the first dorsal compartment is considered one of the most common and effective methods for treating de Quervain's, with many clients reporting relief of symptoms after one injection.[4] The literature supports the use of a thumb spica orthosis in conjunction with injection for optimal outcomes. No significant improvements in client outcomes were noted when either technique was administered independently.[36] The timeline for relief of symptoms is 1 to 4 weeks.

Operative Treatment

Surgical intervention is recommended if two corticosteroid injections combined with 6 months of conservative management fail to relieve symptoms.[4] Surgical outcomes are generally excellent, with as many as 91% of clients reporting complete relief of symptoms after surgery.[4]

Postoperative therapy may be initiated approximately 10 to 14 days after surgery. Edema and scar management techniques should be added to the client's home program.[32,33] Active and active assisted range of motion exercises may be introduced 2 weeks after surgery, and a progressive strengthening program may be initiated 4 weeks postsurgery.[32] Timeline for recovery after surgical intervention is 6 to 8 weeks.

> **Clinical Pearl**
>
> Pregnant women in their third trimester and mothers with small children are at increased risk for de Quervain's.[4] To avoid interference during infant feeding, a radial-side forearm-based thumb spica orthosis may be best for new moms.

Trigger Finger

Trigger finger also known as digital stenosing tenosynovitis or flexor tenosynovitis is "snapping," "popping," or "catching" of the flexor tendon during finger movement.[37] The triggering is caused by "a mismatch between the volume of the flexor tendon sheath and its contents,"[38] which prevents smooth motion of the digits during flexion and extension. The A1 pulley is most often affected. Women in their 50 and 60s are most often impacted, and people who are diabetic are also at increased risk.[39]

Diagnosis

On examination, clients primarily complain of pain with palpation at the A1 pulley. Locking in flexion (particularly in the morning) and pain with gripping are additional cardinal signs of trigger finger. Assess for proximal interphalangeal (PIP) joint flexion contracture, inability to make a full fist, and swelling over the distal palmar crease. It is not uncommon to have symptoms affecting more than one finger; thumb, long, and ring fingers are most often affected followed by index and small fingers.[37,38,40] Infants may demonstrate a trigger finger (typically of the thumb), which is usually addressed with surgical release if not resolved by 10 to 12 months of age.

> **Clinical Pearl**
>
> When evaluating for a PIP joint flexion contracture, distinguish between extrinsic tightness and joint contracture by placing the wrist in flexion when testing PIP extension lag.

Nonoperative Treatment

Orthosis

The goal of the orthosis is to reduce tendon gliding and thus decrease friction forces through the A1 pulley and ultimately resolve inflammation.[41] Several studies have addressed the efficacy of orthoses as well as the effectiveness of different orthosis designs. An MP joint orthosis (Fig. 24.5A) at 0 to 15 degrees has a success rate ranging from 70% to 93%.[37,40,41,42] Distal interphalangeal (DIP) joint extension orthoses (Fig. 24.5B) demonstrate a wide range of success from 47% to 83%.[43,44] One study demonstrated an 87% success rate at 1-year follow-up after wearing a PIP joint extension orthosis for 6 to 10 weeks (Fig. 24.5B). In summary, an MP orthosis at 0 to 15 degrees seems to have more support in the literature to decrease trigger finger symptoms.[37,40,43,44] However, PIP or DIP orthoses may also decrease symptoms. Therapists and clients should be aware that 6 to 10 weeks of wear are necessary to assess the success of a trigger finger orthoses. As with corticosteroid injections, if trigger finger symptoms were present for less than 6 months, treatment with an orthosis is more successful.[37]

The need to use our hands for everyday life tasks can make wearing orthoses difficult for clients. Consider fabricating two orthoses such as a MP and a DIP extension orthosis that the client can alternate depending on task demands. Check to make sure that each orthosis limits triggering of the involved digit.

Activity Modification

Instruct clients to avoid activities that cause pain and triggering.

Home Exercise Program

A typical home exercise program should include passive PIP and DIP joint flexion, active composite full-finger flexion, both active and passive full-finger extension, and active hook fisting. Clients should remove their orthosis and complete five repetitions of each exercise three times a day.[41] It is important that the therapist ensures the exercises do not cause snapping or popping. If these symptoms do occur, modify exercises to eliminate the issue. Try instructing the client in a half fist versus full fist, or only passive flexion and active extension. Progress the home exercise program as symptoms allow.

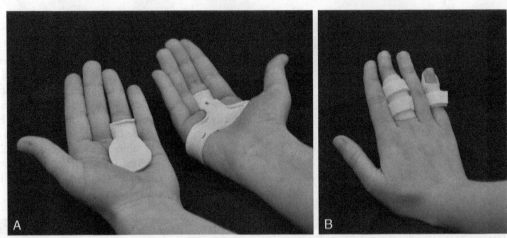

FIG. 24.5 There are several orthosis design options to treat trigger finger. **(A)** These designs block MP joint flexion. **(B)** The orthosis on the middle finger prevents PIP joint flexion, and the stax orthosis on the small finger prevents DIP joint flexion.

> ⊙ **Clinical Pearl**
>
> Trigger finger symptoms should improve after just a few sessions of formal therapy. If symptoms do not improve after 6 – 8 weeks of conservative management with use of an orthosis, refer your client back to the physician for possible corticosteroid injection or surgical release.

Corticosteroid Injection by a Physician

A corticosteroid injection consists of a subcutaneous or intrasheath injection into the area of the A1 pulley.[45] Clients may complain of tenderness or soreness for a couple of days; however, most will notice a decrease in symptoms within 1 week of the injection. Some clients may require up to 4 weeks to notice symptom improvement.[46] Corticosteroid injections are shown to be a fairly effective course of treatment with success rates ranging from 67% to 94%.[42]

Operative Treatment

Open release of the A1 pulley has been the surgical technique of choice for the last 100 years.[38] However, percutaneous release is gaining popularity because it can be completed in the physician's office using local anesthetic. Typically, only a supportive dressing is needed after surgery and clients will be able to return to normal activities 1 to 4 weeks postsurgery. Most clients do not require therapy services after an A1 pulley release. If therapy is required, it is typically due to decreased motion from a PIP joint flexion contracture, scar tenderness, or generalized limited hand motion. Treatment would mirror the conservative management home exercise program with the addition of scar management.

CASE STUDY

Case Study 24.1

Jane is a 56-year-old female who presents to your clinic after seeing a hand surgeon. The referral from the physician states, "OT/PT evaluate and treat right lateral epicondylosis." During the subjective interview, the client states that her pain started about 4 weeks ago in her elbow after raking leaves. She reports that she is a retired teacher who currently enjoys exercising and caring for her 1-year-old grandson. During your evaluation, the client has tenderness to palpation over the lateral elbow and forearm extensor muscle bellies. Provocative testing is positive for Cozen's, Mills', and grip tests. Her right composite wrist flexion is 35 degrees versus 55 degrees for noncomposite wrist flexion, indicating forearm extensor tightness. The client reports a 2/10 pain at rest and 7/10 with activity. Evaluation results indicate lateral epicondylosis. During the first session, you educate the client to avoid activities in the palm down position, particularly when lifting objects such as purse or grocery bag. The client is advised against any upper extremity exercises that increase pain for the next several weeks. You instruct the client to wear the prescribed wrist cock-up orthosis at night and as needed to manage pain during the day. Finally, you discuss and demonstrate a home exercise program consisting of stretches in a pain-free range to decrease tightness of the forearm extensor muscles. You also stress that it is important to try to complete the stretches every 2 to 3 hours, 3 to 5 repetitions, with 30-second holds.

Jane returns in 2 weeks and is doing very well. She reports she has 0/10 pain at rest and notices the most pain with caring for her grandson. You review the stretches and instruct the client to continue stretching consistently throughout the day. You decide to discontinue the wrist cock-up orthosis since the client's pain is improving and she is independent with her exercises. Jane schedules a second follow-up appointment in 4 weeks.

At 6 weeks the client returns. She reports that she has had no pain and is able to appropriately demonstrate all stretches. Based on her progress you add eccentric strengthening for the forearm extensors and flexors. The client is instructed to perform strengthening exercises 1 to 2 times/day starting with 10 repetitions and 1lb (0.5kg) weight and progressing to 30 repetitions with 2lb (1kg) weight if pain free.

At 10 weeks, Jane returns very happy because she watched her grandson all weekend and had no pain while picking him up. Your reassessment yields no tenderness at the lateral elbow or extensor muscle bellies, and Cozen's and Mills' tests are also negative. Her composite wrist flexion is comparable on her left and right. Jane is completing all exercises correctly using 2lb

(1kg) weights. Jane reports she is still completing the stretches approximately every 3 hours. Since she is doing so well, you discuss transitioning to a maintenance level with her home program, which involves completing stretches and strengthening 2 to 3 times per week. If she experiences return of pain at the elbow, Jane is instructed to return to consistently doing the stretches and strengthening until the pain resolves. The client is then discharged from your care.

References

1. Fedorczyk JM: Tendinopathies of the elbow, wrist, and hand: histopathology and clinical considerations, *J Hand Ther* 25:191–201, 2012.
2. Nordin M, Frankel VH: *Basic biomechanics of the musculoskeletal system*, ed 3, Baltimore, 2001, Lippincott Williams & Wilkins.
3. Ashe MC, McCauley T, Khan KM: Tendinopathies in the upper extremity: a paradigm shift, *J Hand Ther* 17:329–334, 2004.
4. Ilyas AM, Ast M, Schaffer AA: Thoder J: de Quervain's Tenosynovitis of the Wrist, *J Am Acad Orthop Surg* 15(12):757–764, 2007.
5. Oken O, Kahraman Y, Ayhan F, et al.: The short-term efficacy of laser, brace and ultrasound treatment in lateral epicondylosis: a prospective, randomized, controlled trial, *J Hand Ther* 21:63–68, 2008.
6. Martinez-Silvestrini JA, Newcomer KL, Gay RE, et al.: Chronic lateral epicondylosis: comparative effectiveness of a home exercise program including stretching alone versus stretching supplemented with eccentric or concentric strengthening, *J Hand Ther* 18:411–420, 2005.
7. Bisset L, Smidt N, Van der Windt DA, Bouter LM, Jull G, Brooks P, et al.: Conservative treatments for tennis elbow do subgroups of patients respond differently? *Rheumatology* 46:1601–1605, 2007.
8. Allander E: Prevalence, incidence and remission rates of some common rheumatic disease and syndromes, *Scand J Rheumatol* 3:145–153, 1974.
9. Putnam MD, Cohen M: Painful conditions around the elbow, *Orthop Clin North Am* 30:109–118, 1999.
10. Thurston AJ: Conservative and surgical treatment of tennis elbow: a study outcome, *Aust N Z J Surg* 68:568–572, 1998.
11. Nirschl RP: Tennis elbow, *Orthop Clin North Am* 4:787–800, 1973.
12. Nirschl RP: Soft tissue injuries about the elbow, *Clin Sports Med* 5:637–640, 1986.
13. Kraushaar B, Nirschl R: Current concepts review – tendinosis of the elbow (tennis elbow). Clinical features and findings of histological immunohistochemical and electron microscopy studies, *J Bone Joint Surg Am* 81:259–285, 1999.
14. Bisset LM, Vicenzino B: Physiotherapy management of lateral epicondylalgia, *J Physiother* 61:174–181, 2015.
15. Coombes BK, Bisset L, Vicenzino B: Management of lateral elbow tendinopathy: one size does not fit all, *J Orthop Sports Phys Ther* 45:938–949, 2015.
16. Valdes K, LaStayo P: The value of provocative tests for the wrist and elbow: a literature review, *J Hand Ther* 26:32–43, 2013.
17. Mills GP: Treatment of tennis elbow. *Br Med J* 212, 1937.
18. Walz DM, Newman JS, Konin GP, Ross G: Epicondylosis: pathogenesis, imaging, and treatment, *RadioGraphics* 30:167–184, 2010.
19. Dorf ER, Chhabra AB, Golish SR, McGinty JL, Pannunzio ME: Effect of elbow position on grip strength in the evaluation of lateral epicondylitis, *Hand Surg Am* 32(6):882–886, 2007.
20. Stasinopoulos D, Stasinopoulos I: Comparison of effects of eccentric training, eccentric-concentric training, and eccentric-concentric training combined with isometric contraction in the treatment of lateral elbow tendinopathy, *J Hand Ther* xx,1–6, 2016.
21. Ramen J, MacDermid JC, Grewal R: Effectiveness of different methods of resistance exercises in lateral epicondylosis – a systematic review, *J Hand Ther* 25:5–25, 2012.
22. Wuori JL, Overend TJ, Kramer JF, et al.: Strength and pain measures associated with lateral epicondylosis bracing, *Arch Phys Rehabil* 79:832–837, 1998.
23. Fedorczyk JM: Elbow tendinopathies: clinical presentation and therapist's management of tennis elbow. In Skirven TM, Osterman AL, Fedorczyk JM, et al.: *Rehabilitation of the hand and upper extremity*, ed 6, Philadelphia, 2011, Mosby, pp 1098–1108.
24. Garg R, Adamson GJ, Dawson PA, et al.: A prospective randomized study comparing a forearm strap brace versus a wrist splint for the treatment of lateral epicondylosis, *J Shoulder Elbow Surg* 19:508–512, 2010.
25. Smidt N, van der Windt DAWM, Assendelft WJJ: Corticosteroid injections, physiotherapy, or wait and see policy for lateral epicondylosis: a randomised controlled trial, *Lancet* 359:657–662, 2002.
26. Ciccotti MC, Schwartz MA, Ciccotti MG: Diagnosis and treatment of medial epicondylosis of the elbow, *Clin Sport Med* 23:693–705, 2004.
27. Amin NH, Kumar NS, Schickendantz MS: Medial epicondylosis: evaluation and management, *J Am Acad Orthop Surg* 23:348–355, 2015.
28. Van Hofwegen C, Baker III CL, Baker Jr CL: Epicondylosis in the Athlete's Elbow, *Clin Sport Med* 29:577–597, 2010.
29. MacDermid JC, Wojkowski S, Kargus C, et al.: Hand therapist management of the lateral epicondylosis: a survey of expert opinion and practice patterns, *J Hand Ther* 23:18–30, 2010.
30. Vinod AV, Ross M: An effective approach to diagnosis and surgical repair of refractory medial epicondylosis, *J Shoulder Elbow Surg* 24:1172–1177, 2015.
31. Moore JS: De Quervain's tenosynovitis: stenosing tenosynovitis of the first dorsal compartment, *J Occup Environ Med* 39(10):990–1002, 1997.
32. Goel R, Abzug JM: de Quervain's tenosynovitis: a review of the rehabilitative options, *Hand* 10:1–5, 2015.
33. Jaworski CA, Krause M, Brown J: Rehabilitation of the wrist and hand following sports injury, *Clin Sport Med* 29:61–80, 2010.
34. Rettig AC: Athletic injuries of the wrist and hand part ii: overuse injuries of the wrist and traumatic injuries to the hand, *Am J Sports Med* 32(1):262–273, 2004.
35. Papa JA: Conservative Management of De Quervain's Stenosing Tenosynovitis: a case report, *J Can Chiropr Assoc* 56(2):111–120, 2012.
36. Cavaleri R, et al.: Hand therapy versus corticosteroid injections in the treatment of de Quervain's disease: a systematic review and meta-analysis, *J Hand Ther* 29:3–11, 2016.
37. Colbourn J, Heath N, Manary S, et al.: Effectiveness of splinting for the treatment of trigger finger, *J Hand Ther* 21:336–343, 2008.
38. Ryzewicz M, Wolf JM: Trigger digits: principles, management, and complications, *J Hand Surg* 31A:135–146, 2006.
39. Makkouk AL, Oetgen ME, Swigart CR, et al.: Trigger finger: etiology, evaluation, and treatment, *Curr Rev Musculoskelet Med* 2:92–96, 2008.
40. Evans RB, Hunter JM, Burkhalter WE: conservative management of the trigger finger: a new approach, *J Hand Ther* 1(2):59–68, 1988.
41. Valdes K: A retrospective review to determine the long-term efficacy of orthotic devices for trigger finger, *J Hand Ther* 25:89–96, 2012.
42. Patel MR, Bassini L: Trigger fingers and thumb: when to splint, inject or operate, *J Hand Surg* 17A:110–113, 1992.
43. Rogers JA, McCarthy JA, Tiedman JJ: Functional distal interphalangeal joint splinting for trigger finger in laborers: a review and cadaver investigation, *Orthopedics* 21:305–310, 1998.
44. Tarbhai K, Hannah S, von Schroeder HP: Trigger finger treatment: a comparison of 2 splint designs, *J Hand Surg* 37A:243–249, 2012.
45. Taras JS, Raphael JS, Pan WT, et al.: Corticosteroid injections for trigger digits: is intrasheath injection necessary? *J Hand Surg Am* 23:717–722, 1998.
46. Peters-Veluthamaningal C, Winters JC, Groenier KH, et al.: Corticosteroid injections effective for trigger finger in adults in general practice: a double-blinded randomised placebo controlled trial, *Ann Rheum Dis* 67:1262–1266, 2008.

25 Finger Sprains and Deformities

Gary Solomon

Digital injuries and deformities are common reasons for clients to be referred to hand therapy. Many clients expect digital injuries to heal on their own, and sometimes do not recognize that the injury can lead to permanent deformity. Clients may be referred to therapy with the diagnosis of "sprain/strain" for a finger or thumb but may actually have unidentified serious injuries, such as a collateral ligament injury or a **volar plate (VP)** injury. This is especially likely when the referral comes from a physician who is not a hand surgeon. In this situation, the hand therapist has an opportunity to identify the clinical findings and facilitate appropriate treatment.

Injuries to the digits occur often during athletic activities. Individuals participating in volleyball, basketball, and football have a high incidence of proximal interphalangeal (PIP) joint injuries. Dorsal dislocations are more common than volar dislocations in these sports-related injuries. Boutonniere deformities frequently occur in basketball players. Mallet injuries may occur when the player's fingertip strikes a helmet or ball.[1] Therapists whose clients participate in athletic activities can expect to see these common sprains and finger injuries as part of their caseload.

Many digit injuries initially go untreated. Clients who seek medical attention later may have chronic pain, edema, and stiffness. Long-term problems such as persistent residual pain and swelling can be very challenging to treat.

Mallet fingers, boutonniere deformities, and swan neck deformities are common digit injuries that have distinct characteristics. They can be treated successfully by precise management. The trauma and disease processes that cause these deformities vary, but regardless of the cause, the hand therapist's detailed knowledge of pathomechanics and therapy guidelines helps manage and direct the course of treatment.

Mallet Finger

A finger with drooping of the distal interphalangeal (DIP) joint is called a **mallet finger** (Fig. 25.1).[2] Typically the DIP can be passively extended to neutral but the client is unable to *actively* extend it. This condition is called a **DIP extensor lag.** If the DIP joint cannot be passively extended to neutral, the condition is called a **DIP flexion contracture.** A DIP flexion contracture is seldom present early after injury; however, if the injury goes untreated, this problem may develop.

Anatomy

The DIP joint of the finger is a **ginglymus joint** (hinge joint). It is **bicondylar** (a joint in which two rounded surfaces of one bone articulate with shallow depressions on another bone) and is similar to the PIP joint in its capsular ligaments. The terminal extensor tendon and terminal flexor tendon attach to the most proximal edge of the distal phalanx. This insertion contributes to the joint's dynamic stability.[3]

Diagnosis and Pathology

A mallet injury is frequently caused by a blow to the fingertip with flexion force or by axial loading while the DIP is extended.[4] The terminal extensor tendon is avulsed. An avulsion fracture also may occur and should be ruled out. Laceration injuries (extensor zone I) are another cause of this deformity. Anterior-posterior (A-P) and true lateral X-rays are typically obtained. In addition, the PIP joint should be examined for possible injury.[5]

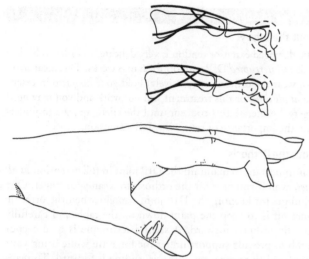

FIG. 25.1 Mallet finger deformity. A fracture may also occur with this injury. *(From American Society for Surgery of the Hand:* The Hand: Examination and Diagnosis. *2nd ed. Edinburgh, UK: Churchill Livingstone; 1983.)*

Timelines and Healing

The DIP joint is immobilized by an orthosis in full extension for 6 to 8 weeks to allow the delicate terminal extensor tendon to heal. **Precaution:** *The joint should not be allowed to flex even briefly during this period of immobilization.* After the period of immobilization, the client is weaned off the orthosis while the hand therapist observes for DIP extensor lag.[6]

Nonoperative Treatment

An orthosis is fabricated to hold the DIP joint in extension to slight hyperextension. If hyperextension is prescribed by the physician, the therapist should make sure the position of hyperextension is less than that which causes skin blanching. **Precaution.** *Exceeding tissue tolerance in DIP hyperextension can compromise circulation and nutrition to the healing tissues.*[7]

Many types of DIP orthosis designs are available (Fig. 25.2). If PIP joint hyperextension is noted, consider a dorsal-based design with the proximal end blocking end-range PIP extension while permitting full flexion. Clients may also need a second orthosis for showering; the client can remove the shower othosis after showering, taking care to hold the DIP joint in full extension at all times, and replace it with a dry orthosis. In this way, the skin is protected against maceration, which occurs if a wet orthosis is left on a digit. Casting can also be used when a client's adherence to the plan of care is a concern. Casts, of course, must be protected from water. Instruct clients to cover casts with plastic for showering.

Perforated orthotic material is recommended to allow airflow. The PIP should be allowed to fully flex without disturbing the position of DIP extension. If multiple orthoses are provided, consider one dorsally based and one volarly based so that the client can switch to protect skin integrity.

If the DIP joint cannot initially be passively extended to neutral, serial adjustments of the orthosis can be performed. If necessary, a small static progressive DIP extension orthosis can be used.[8] Dorsal edema and tenderness over the DIP are common and can interfere with full DIP extension. Edema is treated (as

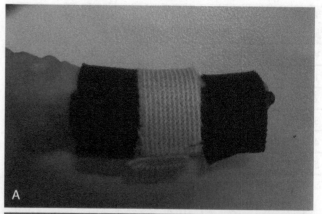

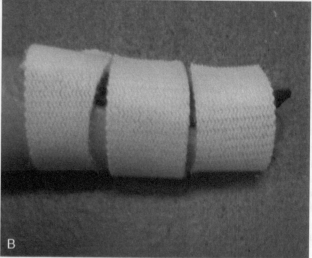

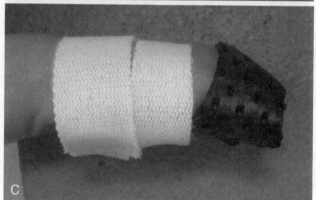

FIG. 25.2 Mallet orthoses. (A) Custom thermoplastic volar. **(B)** Dorsal. **(C)** Combination dorsal/volar. *(Reproduced with permission, Gary Solomon, MS, OTR/L, CHT.)*

needed) and the client is instructed in full PIP active range of motion (AROM) with the DIP immobilized in the orthotic.

After 6 to 8 weeks of continuous orthosis use, if no DIP extensor lag is present and the physician approves, start gentle AROM of the DIP joint. Gentle half-fist motion and limited DIP blocking can be safely initiated. For DIP blocking, an AlumaFoam template can be provided to allow the client to actively flex and extend the DIP from 0 degrees to 25 degrees flexion for 1 week; the template is then adjusted to allow 35 degrees of flexion the next week. Emphasis of AROM should be in the direction of *extension*. If no lag is present, gentle composite AROM should then be permitted.

TABLE 25.1   Mallet Orthosis Weaning Schedule Example After Immobilization Period

Week	Daytime	Nighttime
1	remove 1 hour 2x/day	Continuous
2	Remove 2 hours 2x/day	Continuous
3	Use 2 hours during day	Continuous
4	Use only if lag occurs	Continuous
5	Discontinue	Discontinue

The therapist should instruct the client to avoid forceful or quick grasping or forceful DIP flexion in the early phase of therapy, and emphasis during exercise should be on DIP *extension*. It is very important to watch for DIP extensor lag. If DIP extensor lag occurs, the orthosis use and exercise progression must be adjusted. **Precaution.** *Passive motion to restore DIP flexion should not be used except in cases of extreme stiffness with limited progress performing AROM. Passive flexion will significantly increase the risk of extensor lag especially in the early rehabilitation process.*

The DIP extension orthosis is initially continued between AROM sessions, and then gradually weaned during the day over a 2- to 3-week period. Night orthosis use continues for an additional 2 to 3 weeks. If DIP extensor lag recurs, daytime use should be reinstituted. Table 25.1 outlines a typical progression for weaning from the mallet finger orthosis. If orthotic use does not correct the DIP extensor lag, surgery may be required for correction of the deformity.

If there is a mild extensor lag, the hand therapist should monitor closely for the development of a secondary swan neck deformity. If PIP hyperextension is noted, then an orthosis that blocks end-range PIP extension while allowing full flexion is recommended.

Although the use of an orthosis is best initiated as soon as possible after injury, even a delayed regimen can be effective.[9] Surgical intervention can produce complications; therefore nonoperative solutions are often well worth the effort.

Operative Treatment

If the mallet injury has associated large fracture fragments (greater than 30% of the joint surface) or the client asserts that they cannot adhere to the orthotic wearing schedule, surgery may be necessary. A variety of procedures can be performed to treat a mallet finger.[4,10,11] Surgical complications include the possibility of infection and nail deformities.

Postoperatively, the client may be sent to hand therapy for edema control, a protective orthosis, and instruction in pin site care if Kirschner wire was used and protrudes through the skin. When the fracture demonstrates appropriate healing, the pin will be removed and AROM can be initiated. The DIP extension orthosis is continued after the pin is removed and then is gradually weaned. As with nonoperative treatment, the therapist should observe for DIP extensor lag.

?   Questions to Ask the Doctor

- Is there a fracture (bony mallet)?
- Does the physician prefer the DIP in neutral position or in hyperextension?
- If the DIP is pinned, how long will the pin remain in place?

◖◗   What to Say to Clients

About the Injury

"The damaged extensor tendon is very delicate. In order to heal, it needs *uninterrupted* DIP support for 6 to 8 weeks. This means you must wear the orthosis or (passively) hold your fingertip in extension *at all times* or this treatment will not work and you may need surgery." Reiterate this concept until the client appears to understand the importance of *continuous* DIP extension.

About the Orthosis

"It is important to maintain the DIP joint in full extension *at all times*, even if you take off the orthosis to clean your finger. One technique for keeping the DIP joint straight when the orthotic comes off is to keep the palm down on the table and carefully slide the orthosis forward. A second technique is to use your thumb to provide support under the fingertip while using your other hand to remove the orthosis, sliding it forward. To reapply, maintain DIP extension with your other hand as you put the orthosis back on." Work with the client to devise a schedule for removing the orthosis one or two times daily to clean the orthosis and check the skin. Make sure the client knows the proper techniques for keeping the DIP supported in extension *at all times*.

Emphasize the importance of skin care: "Moisture that is trapped inside the orthotic may lead to skin problems such as maceration, which must be avoided." Teach the client what skin maceration looks like.

About Exercise (after 6 to 8 weeks continuous orthosis wear)

"Initially, remove the orthosis four times a day and gently bend the tip down to the template followed by fully straightening the tip. In 1 week, we will increase the amount of bending permitted; and the following week, you will begin making a full fist."

"Avoiding powerful gripping and forceful bending of the injured fingers to prevent any strain on the healing extensor tendon."

Instruct the client in AROM of the uninvolved digits and PIP flexion of the injured digit: "Achieving full PIP active flexion is very important. The injured finger could stiffen at the PIP joint if it is not exercised gently while you are wearing the DIP orthosis. It is also very important to prevent the uninjured digits from stiffening." Demonstrate and practice gentle PIP blocking exercises, isolated flexor digitorum superficialis, and "straight fist" motions with the DIP orthosis in place (Fig. 25.3).

Evaluation Tips

- The client's finger is likely to be tender and swollen over the dorsal DIP area. Use a gentle touch around this area.
- Assess the client for digital hypermobility. Observe for DIP extensor lag or PIP hyperextension of other digits and treat accordingly (see description of swan neck deformity).
- Gently check isolated DIP flexion of the other digits while the injured DIP is immobilized in the orthotic. If the client can isolate this without stressing the terminal tendon of the injured digit, it helps prevent development of adhesions that could lead to a quadriga effect (an active flexion lag in fingers adjacent to the injured finger).

Precaution. Avoid volumetric measurement of edema because this would leave the DIP unsupported, which is contraindicated.

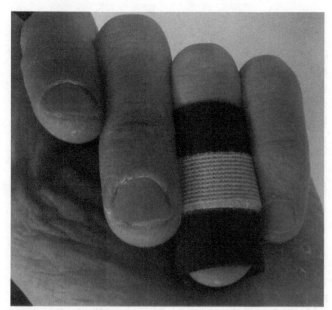

FIG. 25.3 Straight fist with mallet orthosis permitting full PIP flexion. *(Reproduced with permission, Gary Solomon, MS, OTR/L, CHT.)*

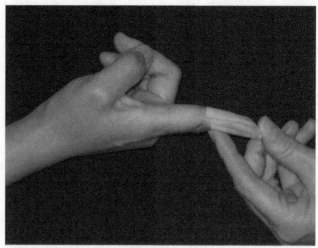

FIG. 25.4 Taping distal interphalangeal joint into position for use of mallet orthosis. *(Reproduced with permission, Gary Solomon, MS, OTR/L, CHT.)*

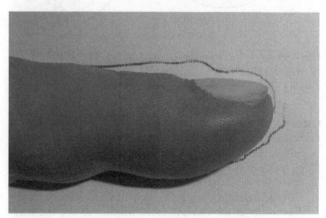

FIG. 25.5 Tracing lateral view of distal interphalangeal joint position on card for client to use as reference during home exercise program. *(Reproduced with permission, Gary Solomon, MS, OTR/L, CHT.)*

Diagnosis-Specific Information That Affects Clinical Reasoning

Individualize treatment based on your observations and evaluation. If DIP hyperextension has been ordered but the client cannot tolerate it, support the DIP in a tolerable position and see the client every few days for orthosis modification until the desired position is achieved. Notify the physician if full DIP extension or hyperextension cannot be achieved in the orthosis.

If edema is significant, assume that you will need to readjust the orthosis as edema resolves and schedule recheck visits accordingly. Upgrade interventions as appropriate for edema management.

A client who is hypermobile and has laxity of the uninjured digits is at greater risk for developing a secondary swan neck deformity. This client needs an orthosis that prevents PIP hyperextension and supports the DIP in extension. Teach clients isolated flexor digitorum superficialis (FDS) exercise with the DIP orthosis in place.

Precaution. *Make sure clients are well trained in monitoring skin condition inside the orthosis. Instruct clients to call the hand therapy clinic for a recheck if any skin problems occur.* Using more than one style of orthosis can help prevent skin problems.

♡ Tips From the Field

Orthoses
- Show the client pictures or samples of DIP orthoses. Explain your recommendation in terms of comfort, effectiveness, and adjustability. Ask clients about their preferences. Advise the client to tape (or use Coban) the orthosis in place at night to decrease the risk of the orthosis sliding off during sleep.
- Consider taping the DIP in extension underneath the orthosis for additional protection (Fig. 25.4).[7]
- Ask the client about their daily activities. If they perform a lot of fine motor tasks, consider a dorsal mallet orthosis.

- Keeping the PIP joint in flexion while fabricating the orthosis decreases the flexion tension on the flexor digitorum profundus (FDP) and makes it easier to fully extend the DIP joint.
- For a volar orthosis, it is critical that the lateral and medial borders are no greater than half the thickness of the digit in order for the straps to contour and hold securely.
- Use a soft strap directly over the DIP joint where the skin is typically sensitive.
- Small orthoses are not always quick to make. Allow time to fine-tune and readjust it.
- Clients often appreciate having a separate orthosis to use in the shower. They can change into the dry orthosis after the shower, which helps prevent maceration of skin.
- When starting active flexion of the DIP joint, trace the DIP in full extension from a lateral view onto a business card. This allows the client to self-monitor for any developing extensor lag between therapy sessions (Fig. 25.5).

Exercise Template
- AlumaFoam makes an excellent template to use as a guide when clients begin active DIP flexion. The AlumaFoam template is also easy to adjust on subsequent visits as increased flexion is permitted.

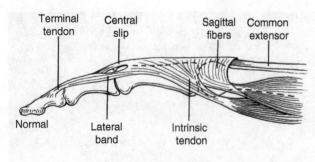

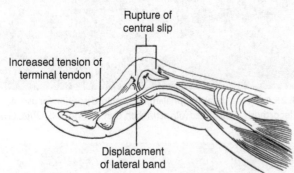

FIG. 25.6 Boutonniere deformity. *(From Burke SL. Hand and Upper Extremity Rehabilitation: A Practical Guide. 3rd ed. St Louis, MO: Churchill Livingstone; 2005.)*

Client Adherence to Program

- Some clients need more supervision and follow-up than do others. Reasons to recheck the client more often include: (1) resolving or fluctuating edema, (2) wound care, (3) PIP stiffness, (4) risk of swan neck deformity developing, and (5) questionable technique for putting on and taking off the orthosis. Document in the therapy record whether or not the client demonstrates good technique.

> **Precautions and Concerns**

- *Check for skin maceration.*
- *Emphasize the importance of avoiding forceful gripping and quick flexion motions.*
- *Monitor for the development of PIP hyperextension, especially if the client demonstrates laxity of the digits.*
- *If the orthosis is taped on at night, caution the client to avoid circumferential taping because this could produce a tourniquet effect.*

Boutonniere Deformity

Anatomy

With a **boutonniere deformity**, the finger postures in PIP flexion and DIP hyperextension (Fig. 25.6). The injury may be open or closed. With a closed injury, the boutonniere deformity may not develop immediately and might become noticeable within 2 or 3 weeks after the injury.[9] The client may have a PIP extensor lag or, with an older injury, a PIP flexion contracture. This distinction affects therapy decisions.

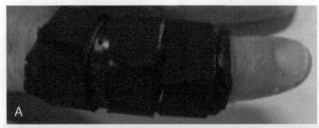

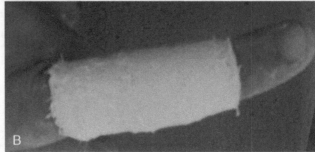

FIG. 25.7 **(A)** Circumferential boutonniere orthosis. **(B)** Circumferential cast for boutonniere deformity. *(Reproduced with permission, Gary Solomon, MS, OTR/L, CHT.)*

Diagnosis and Pathology

A boutonniere deformity involves disruption of the central slip of the extensor tendon, which normally inserts into the dorsal base of the middle phalanx. The disruption of the central slip causes the **lateral bands** to slip volar to the PIP joint axis of motion, creating flexor forces on the PIP joint.[12] The imbalance results in hyperextension of the DIP joint.[13] With this DIP posture, the **oblique retinacular ligament (ORL)**, which is located at the dorsal DIP joint, is at risk for becoming tight. A **pseudoboutonniere deformity** is an injury to the PIP volar plate and is usually the result of a PIP hyperextension injury.

> ⊙ **Clinical Pearl**
>
> With a boutonniere deformity, the damage occurs at the *dorsal* surface. With a pseudoboutonniere deformity, the damage occurs at the *volar* surface.[3]

Timelines and Healing

A PIP extension thermoplastic orthosis or circumferential cast with the DIP joint free[14] is typically used day and night for up to 6 weeks (Fig. 25.7A and B). When range of motion (ROM) of the PIP is initiated, flexion to 30 to 45 degrees is typically permitted and advanced 15 degrees per week as long as no extension lag is present. This is followed by 3 weeks of nighttime and intermittent daytime orthosis use. The orthosis is used during the time needed for the central slip to reestablish tissue continuity and for correction of the deformity.[9]

A variation from complete immobilization for 6 weeks is early short arc motion[6] that combines immobilization with intermittent controlled PIP motion to 30 to 40 degrees of flexion and active DIP flexion with the PIP in full extension. The client is provided a template for PIP ROM at home (Fig. 25.8) and after approximately 3 weeks, if no extension lag is present, the template is advanced into more flexion 10 to 15 degrees per week.

A relative motion extension orthosis (Fig. 25.9) can also allow PIP flexion while restoring PIP extension.[15] While there is emerging evidence for the use of relative motion in the management of acute boutonniere injury, it may also be used after the period of immobilization to facilitate active PIP extension. By keeping the involved digit in flexion at the metacarpophalangeal (MP) joint relative to the other digits, forces will transfer during active extension from the MP to the PIP and facilitate the restoration of PIP extension.

Nonoperative Treatment

The ability to passively extend the PIP is an indicator for nonoperative treatment with PIP immobilization in extension. Different types of orthoses can be used for this purpose. The MP and DIP are not included in the orthosis. Serial adjustments to the orthosis may have to be made to achieve full PIP extension.

It is very important for the client to perform isolated DIP flexion exercises while the PIP is immobilized. This helps to recover normal length of the ORL. These exercises are done actively and passively in a gentle fashion (Fig. 25.10). The therapist should watch for any deviation from normal MP motion and should exercise this as needed.

Precaution. *After the client has been medically cleared to begin PIP active flexion, initiate restricted amounts of flexion at first and watch for PIP extensor lag.*

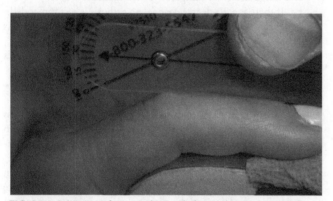

FIG. 25.8 Initiation of proximal interphalangeal joint protected flexion to 30 degrees using an AlumaFoam template. *(Reproduced with permission, Gary Solomon, MS, OTR/L, CHT.)*

It is important to emphasize PIP active extension, which is facilitated by positioning the digit in MP flexion. Continuous orthosis use is reinstituted if a PIP extensor lag develops.

If exercise fails to recover DIP flexion with the PIP extended, **ORL tightness** (limited passive DIP flexion with the PIP extended) may need to be addressed with an orthosis. Various small, custom-made orthoses can be used for dynamic or static progressive DIP flexion with the PIP in full extension.[16]

Operative Treatment

Boutonniere deformity is caused by injury to zone III of the extensor tendons. Various surgical techniques are used to treat these injuries.[9] The therapy management is determined in collaboration with the hand surgeon. The short arc of motion protocol for zone III extensor tendon repairs is often used.

Nonoperative Clients

- Is the client a candidate for early controlled active motion, or would continuous immobilization be preferred?
- Six weeks of immobilization is typical. Is that when active PIP flexion should be started?

Operative Clients

- Was a strong repair achieved (ask to see the operative report)?
- Would this particular client benefit from early active motion or more conservative therapy such as immobilization?
- Are there any additional precautions?

( ) **What to Say to Clients**

About the Injury

(Show diagram to client)
"Notice how, as a result of injury to the central slip, the lateral bands have slipped forward (volar) and how they now contribute to the bent posture of the PIP joint. The PIP joint needs to be supported in extension for the injured tendon to heal in proper alignment. Also note how the tip of the finger is tipped upward (hyperextended). As the injury at the PIP is corrected, the fingertip position will also improve. In addition, specific exercises can help correct this."

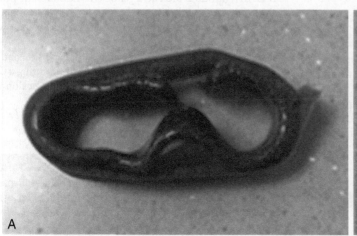
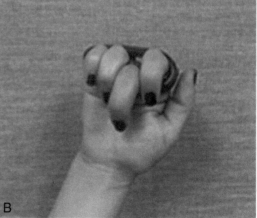

FIG. 25.9 (A) Relative motion orthosis designed to flex a right hand middle finger MP joint relative to the adjacent digits. **(B)** The same relative motion orthosis in place on a right hand. Note how the middle finger MP joint is more flexed than the MP joints of the other fingers. This position helps promote PIP joint extension of the middle finger. *(Reproduced with permission, Gary Solomon, MS, OTR/L, CHT.)*

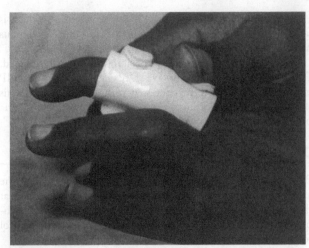

FIG. 25.10 Oblique retinacular ligament stretch entails isolated distal interphalangeal flexion with proximal interphalangeal supported in extension. This is done actively and passively. *(From Clark GL. Hand Rehabilitation: A Practical Guide. 2nd ed. New York, NY: Churchill Livingstone; 1998.)*

About Exercises

"With this diagnosis, improving DIP flexion while the PIP is extended actually helps improve PIP extension. Therefore flexing just the DIP helps correct the lack of extension at the PIP. It is very important to exercise by bending the tip gently while the PIP is immobilized because this is corrective for your injury."

- Check for hypermobility of the other digits. Do the uninjured digits have a boutonniere-like posture?
- Determine whether the PIP joint can be passively corrected to neutral and whether the DIP joint can be passively corrected to normal flexion with the PIP in extension (that is, check for ORL tightness).
- Check and practice isolated DIP flexion of the other digits. Think ahead about preventing a quadriga effect.
- Check composite flexion of the other digits, as you are able.

Diagnosis-Specific Information That Affects Clinical Reasoning

In nonoperative clients, determine whether the injury involves a PIP extensor lag (the PIP can be passively extended to neutral position, but the client cannot actively extend it) or a PIP flexion contracture (the PIP cannot be passively extended to neutral position). This distinction affects orthosis decisions (see later).

Determine whether the client has ORL tightness. With this condition, both active and passive DIP flexion with PIP extension are limited.

♡ *Tips From the Field*

Clinical Picture

- Edema over the area of injury (dorsal PIP) worsens the deforming forces of a boutonniere position. Treat the edema as a high priority because this helps recover PIP joint passive extension

and promotes normalization throughout. Light compression wrapping can help reduce the edema.

- Isolating and exercising DIP active flexion of the uninjured digits while protecting the injured finger is a good measure for preventing a quadriga effect.
- PIP cylindrical thermoplastic or plaster orthoses may be helpful for performing isolated blocking exercises for DIP flexion. These can be used on all digits to isolate DIP active flexion with varying MP positions.

Orthosis

- If the client has a PIP flexion contracture, a corrective serial cast or orthosis may be necessary. Choices for recovering PIP extension include serial static orthoses, serial casts, static progressive orthoses, and dynamic orthoses. These may be prefabricated or custom made and either digit based or hand based. The goal of the orthosis is to maximize the total end-range time in extension and achieve contracture correction without causing increased inflammation of the soft tissues around the PIP joint. Ken Flowers proposes using a **Modified Weeks Test** to determine the best orthosis to address PIP joint stiffness.[17] The orthosis selection process is based on how much contracture resolution is achieved after the joint is heated and stretched. Passive range of motion (PROM) measurement is initially taken cold and prior to intervention. After ROM in a thermal modality and 10 minutes of end-range stretch, a comparative measurement is taken:
  - If there is a 20-degree change, no orthosis is recommended.
  - If there is a 15-degree change, an end-range static orthosis should be effective.
  - If there is a 10-degree change, a dynamic orthosis is recommended.
  - If change is less than 5 degrees, a static progressive orthosis is recommended.
- The client should participate in the orthosis selection process because activates of daily living (ADLs) and work needs can influence adherence to the orthotic wearing schedule. Comfort, fit, and skin tolerance also influence these choices.
- If full passive PIP extension is possible, a small PIP extension orthosis or cast may be used. Adjust it as needed to accommodate resolution of edema and the client's comfort. It is very important to keep the DIP free and to perform frequent DIP active and passive flexion exercises while the PIP is immobilized in extension.
- If ORL tightness is present, a gentle DIP flexion static progressive or dynamic orthosis may be appropriate. Ease of application and adjustability are criteria that help determine which type should be used.
- If the client has been cleared for active PIP extension and flexion exercises and if ORL tightness is present, try using a dorsal DIP extension block orthosis that maintains DIP flexion while actively exercising PIP extension.

Precaution. *If ORL tightness is present, the client may be at risk of losing FDP excursion, and a quadriga effect could develop.*

After the client has been medically cleared for active PIP extension exercises, position the MP in flexion for the exercises. A relative motion extension orthosis can be beneficial to achieving this goal.[15]

Check for intrinsic versus extrinsic tightness if composite flexion is limited and prioritize the MP position accordingly for PIP exercise.

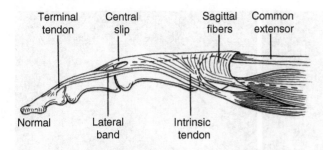

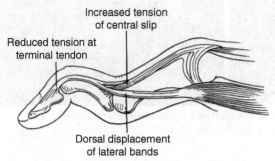

FIG. 25.11 Swan neck deformity. *(From Burke SL. Hand and Upper Extremity Rehabilitation: A Practical Guide. 3rd ed. St Louis, MO: Churchill Livingstone; 2005.)*

Precaution. *As PIP flexion improves, watch closely for PIP extensor lag.*

> **Precautions and Concerns**

- *Avoid PIP flexion during the immobilization phase.*
- *If the client has had surgery, follow the guidelines presented in Chapter 26. Instruct the client in techniques for supporting the digit while putting on and taking off the orthosis for skin care needs. If surgery was not required, instruct the client in ways to manage orthosis and skin care while avoiding PIP flexion. If a cast has been applied, change it at least weekly.*
- *ORL tightness contributes to the boutonniere-deforming forces. Monitor this condition throughout the program and continue exercising active and passive DIP flexion with the PIP extended.*
- *Monitor for loss of FDP excursion and difficulty isolating the FDS, particularly in the involved digit.*
- *If the client has had surgery, adhesions may occur at the incision sites.*

Swan Neck Deformity

Anatomy

In a **swan neck deformity,** the finger postures with PIP hyperextension and DIP flexion (Fig. 25.11).[5] The MP tends to be flexed, and the finger appears to zigzag when observed from the side. The interphalangeal (IP) joints may be passively correctable or they may be fixed in their deformity positions. The IP positions in the swan neck deformity are the opposite of their positions in the boutonniere deformity.

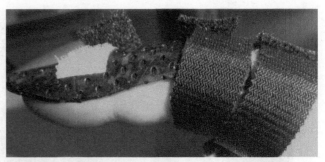

FIG. 25.12 Proximal interphalangeal joint dorsal block orthosis. The distal strap may be released to allow the client to perform flexion exercises with extension limited to the orthosis level. *(Reproduced with permission, Gary Solomon, MS, OTR/L, CHT.)*

Diagnosis and Pathology

The swan neck deformity can be caused by injuries at the level of the DIP, PIP, or MP joint. At the DIP level, a mallet injury can lead to swan neck deformity. In this case, the terminal extensor tendon is disrupted (stretched or ruptured). This allows the extensor force to be more powerful proximally at the PIP joint, leading to PIP hyperextension.[13,18]

If the cause is primarily at the PIP level, the volar plate/joint capsule is involved with hyperextension of the PIP joint. The lateral bands are dorsally displaced, contributing to PIP hyperextension. This minimizes the pull on the terminal extensor tendon; therefore the DIP joint assumes a flexed posture. Normally the FDS helps deter PIP hyperextension. However, if the FDS has been ruptured or lengthened, PIP hyperextension forces are less restricted or controlled. Intrinsic muscle tightness compounds the problem.[13] Painful snapping may be noticed with active flexion. This snapping is caused by the lateral bands at the proximal phalanx condyles.[19]

If the cause of the swan neck deformity is primarily at the MP level, MP volar subluxation and ulnar drift may be the initiating factors, as is seen in rheumatoid arthritis (RA). The MP joint disturbance leads to intrinsic muscle imbalance and tightness with resulting PIP hyperextension forces.[13]

Timelines and Healing

Swan neck deformity is a challenging diagnosis. In conservative management of this condition, an orthosis may be used indefinitely if it promotes improved function and eliminates painful snapping with active flexion.

Nonoperative Treatment

An orthosis that positions the PIP in slight flexion may be very helpful functionally. Many different kinds of orthoses can be used for this type of deformity, including dorsal blocking (Fig. 25.12) and commercially available orthoses such as the Silver Ring (Fig. 25.13) and Oval 8 splints. The purpose of the orthosis is to prevent hyperextension at the PIP joint and to promote active PIP flexion.

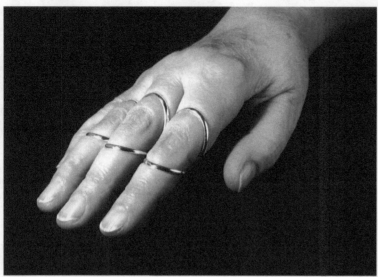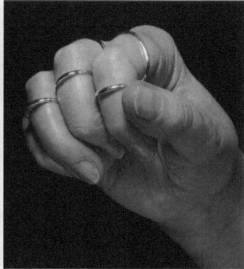

FIG. 25.13 SIRIS (silver ring) orthosis prevents proximal interphalangeal joint hyperextension and allows proximal interphalangeal joint flexion. *(Courtesy Silver Ring Splint Co., Charlottesville, VA.)*

Operative Treatment

Surgery to correct swan neck deformity may be done in conjunction with other reconstructive procedures for clients with RA. Surgical techniques include FDS tenodesis or volar plate advancement procedures.[18,19] Some researchers have found that capsulodesis and tenodesis techniques for restoring balance lose effectiveness as a result of attenuation if these tissues are stressed over time.[20]

After the surgery, clients may be referred to hand therapy for a protective dorsal PIP extension block orthoses (in approximately 30 degrees flexion) or for pin site care, wound care, and/or edema control. After the client has been medically cleared, active DIP extension exercises may be started. Positioning the digit in PIP flexion helps promote DIP active extension excursion.

Pins/Kirschner wires are often used postoperatively to maintain PIP flexion. When the pins are removed, digit-based dorsal PIP orthoses are used and fabricated in 20 to 30 degrees of flexion. This is done to prevent recurrence of PIP hyperextension and imbalance. Active PIP flexion exercises are started when ordered by the surgeon. The PIP dorsal orthosis can remain in place during PIP AROM. The Velcro straps are removed distally to allow PIP flexion while full extension is blocked (Fig. 25.12).

The therapist should focus on balancing digit and hand function while avoiding stress or PIP hyperextension. DIP orthoses may be helpful exercise tools to promote ease of PIP flexion. As a result of the imbalance associated with swan neck deformities, clients habitually initiate flexion motions with the PIP in hyperextension by visibly initiating motion with DIP flexion. Their flexion motions look awkward and difficult to achieve. The therapist should try practicing gentle arcs of motion with smooth congruent flexion of the PIP and DIP joints. It may be helpful to use a hand-over-hand technique, facilitating flexion with gentle tactile input from the therapist to facilitate normal functional movement mechanics.

? Questions to Ask the Doctor

Nonoperative Clients
- What do you believe was the primary cause of the deformity (RA, volar plate laxity, untreated mallet)?

- Is the client planning to have surgery or do we need more permanent orthoses such as an Oval 8 or silver ring type?

Operative Clients
- What structures were repaired (ask to see the operative report)?
- When will the pins be removed?
- When can active PIP flexion be started?
- What specific precautions are in order?

( ) What to Say to Clients

About the Injury

(Show diagram to client)
"Notice how the lateral bands have slipped upward (dorsally) and how they now contribute to the overextended posture of the PIP joint. The PIP joint needs to be supported in flexion for balance and proper alignment to be restored."

About Exercises

"With this diagnosis, it is very important to avoid extending the PIP joint beyond its newly pinned or corrected position until the physician upgrades the program. For this reason, we will use a protective dorsal orthosis. When the soft tissues heal adequately to allow protected motion, it is important to practice gentle bending movements at the PIP joint in a comfortable range."

Evaluation Tips

- Check for hypermobility or swan neck posture of uninjured digits. Document this condition if present.
- Determine whether PIP hyperextension is passively correctable or fixed. Does it affect function?
- In a nonoperative client, distinguish between primary injury to the DIP or the PIP: stabilize the PIP in neutral position. If the client cannot actively extend the DIP, the injury is primarily a DIP extensor injury. If the client can actively extend the DIP, the injury is primarily a volar PIP injury.

- When the client is cleared to begin active movement, observe the quality of active flexion and promote practice of motions that do not elicit snapping.

Diagnosis-Specific Information That Affects Clinical Reasoning

Focus treatment on the primary cause of the deformity. If the client has RA, are other digits involved or at risk? Have any tendons ruptured? Consider antideformity orthoses for other digits, if appropriate. Is MP involvement present? Is intrinsic tightness of other digits a factor? Nighttime orthotic use or intrinsic stretching (or both) to counteract deforming forces may be valuable. Is PIP extension block orthotic use likely to be long term? If so, consider a low-profile, long-lasting style, such as a silver ring or Oval 8.

♡ Tips From the Field

- Observe the balance of the digit and the hand and address uninvolved digits unless this is contraindicated. Promote normal ROM throughout the extremity as appropriate.
- If the client's joints are hypermobile, instruct the person in hand use patterns for ADLs that do not encourage PIP hyperextension. For example, teach the client not to put stress on the digits in PIP hyperextension.
- Avoid "intrinsic plus" exercises or positioning during ADL tasks.

⮞ Precautions and Concerns

- *If you are treating a mallet injury, watch closely for signs of PIP hyperextension (see the Mallet Finger section).*
- *Clients do not need to be hypermobile to develop a swan neck deformity after distal digital injury.*
- *Mallet injury is not the only diagnosis that can lead to PIP hyperextension. A distal crush or fracture requiring DIP splinting may also result in PIP hyperextension. Be alert for this and treat it accordingly with PIP splinting in slight flexion to normalize the balance of the digit.*

Proximal Interphalangeal Joint Injuries

Digital PIP injuries occur frequently, yet they can be extremely challenging to treat. Proper therapy helps prevent the situation from becoming frustrating.

PIP joint dislocation is a common injury.[20,21,22] Clients may initially ignore sprains of the small joints of the hand, not realizing the significance of the injury, and may not seek medical attention for days or weeks after the injury. By this time, significant edema, fibrosis, and stiffness may be established. Joint enlargement and flexion contractures are common residual problems.[3,18]

◎ Clinical Pearl

Therapists see clients with digital sprains or dislocations quite often. Because clients may not understand the serious clinical implications of this seemingly simple diagnosis, they can become frustrated with the progression of treatment. Early communication with the client about the nature of PIP joint injury and the likelihood of a prolonged recovery are important.

Anatomy

Proximal Interphalangeal Joint Architecture

The PIP joint is a hinge joint with 100 to 110 degrees of motion. At the proximal phalanx are two condyles and between the condyles is the intercondylar notch. Because of the slight asymmetry of the condyles, about 9 degrees of supination occurs with PIP flexion.[3] At the base of the middle phalanx are two concave fossae and a ridge that separates the phalanx's flat, broad base. Stability is enhanced by the amount of congruence of this joint and by its tongue-and-groove contour. The IP joint of the thumb is architecturally similar to the PIP joints of the other digits.[20]

Proximal Interphalangeal Joint Stability

The architecture of the PIP joint, along with its ligamentous support, provides joint stability. The **collateral ligaments** are the main restraints on deviation forces at the PIP joint. These ligaments are 2 to 3 mm thick and are extremely important to the joint's stability. The collateral ligaments have two components: the **proper collateral ligament (PCL)** and the **accessory collateral ligament (ACL)**, which are differentiated by their areas of insertion.

The PCL originates on the lateral aspect of the proximal phalanx. The fibers of this ligament insert volarly and distally on the lateral tubercles of the middle phalanx. The fibers of the ACL insert in a more volar direction on the VP. The VP is fibrocartilaginous and is situated between the collateral ligaments on the volar aspect of the PIP joint. The convergence of the PCL, ACL, and VP at the middle phalanx is known as the *critical corner*, a term that reflects its importance to PIP joint stability.[3]

The anatomic arrangement of the VP functions to prevent PIP hyperextension. The VP also acts as a secondary PIP joint stabilizer laterally when the collateral ligaments have been injured.[3,20]

The dynamic stability of the PIP joint is enhanced by the tendons and ligaments that cross the joint. These are the **central extensor tendon** (central slip), the lateral bands, the **transverse retinacular ligament (TRL)**, and the ORL. The central slip is part of the dorsal capsule of the PIP joint and attaches to the middle phalanx at the dorsal tubercle. The lateral bands have intrinsic muscle contributions and lie volar to the MP joint axis; they join dorsal to the PIP joint axis to form the terminal extensor tendon. The TRL originates from the volar surface of the lateral bands and envelops the collateral ligaments and PIP joint, thereby preventing dorsal displacement of the lateral bands. The ORL originates from the flexor sheath, progresses volar to the PIP joint axis, and inserts at the terminal extensor tendon dorsally. The ORL tightens when the PIP joint extends. It provides concomitant PIP and DIP extension and helps prevent hyperextension of the PIP joint (Fig. 25.14).[3]

Diagnosis and Pathology

Physical examination of ligament injuries at the PIP joint requires assessment of joint stability. A-P and true lateral X-rays can identify articular involvement, but X-rays alone may not reveal subtle injuries. The critical issue is whether joint stability exists with active motion.[20]

The **functional stability** of the PIP joint is tested actively and passively. If the client demonstrates normal AROM with

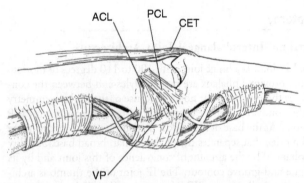

FIG. 25.14 Structures that provide proximal interphalangeal joint stability include the accessory collateral ligament *(ACL)*, the proper collateral ligament *(PCL)*, the dorsal capsule with the central extensor tendon *(CET)*, and the volar plate *(VP)*. *(From Mackin EJ, Callinan N, Skirven TM, et al. Rehabilitation of the Hand and Upper Extremity. 5th ed. St Louis, MO: Mosby; 2002.)*

BOX 25.1   Grades of Ligament Sprain Injuries

Mild Grade I Sprain
- Definition: No instability with AROM or PROM; macroscopic continuity with microscopic tears. The ligament is intact, but individual fibers are damaged.
- Treatment: Immobilize the joint in full extension if comfortable and available; otherwise, immobilize in a small amount of flexion. When pain has subsided, begin AROM and protect with buddy taping.

Grade II Sprain
- Definition: Abnormal laxity with stress; the collateral ligament is disrupted. AROM is stable, but passive testing reveals instability.
- Treatment: Orthosis for 2 to 4 weeks. The physician may recommend early ROM. Avoid any lateral stress.

Grade III Sprain
- Definition: Complete tearing of the collateral ligament along with injury to the dorsal capsule or VP. The finger is usually dislocated by the injury.
- Treatment: Early surgical intervention is often recommended.

AROM, Active range of motion; PROM, passive range of motion: ROM, range of motion; VP, volar plate.
Modified from Campbell PJ, Wilson RL. Management of joint injuries and intraarticular fractures. In Mackin EJ, Callahan AD, Skirven TM, et al. eds. *Rehabilitation of the Hand and Upper Extremity.* 5th ed. St Louis, MO: Mosby; 2002; and Glickel SZ, Barron A, Eaton RG. Dislocations and ligament injuries in the digits. In Green DP, Hotchkiss RN, Pederson WC. eds. *Green's Operative Hand Surgery.* 4th ed. Philadelphia, PA: Churchill Livingstone; 1999.

no PIP joint displacement, joint stability is adequate despite the injury. A brief period of immobilization can be followed by protected ROM exercises. If the joint is displaced with AROM, major disruption of the ligaments has probably occurred. In these cases, the position of immobilization is determined by the physician—partly by identifying the range at which the displacement occurs (Box 25.1). In grade I and mild grade II injuries, the joints are swollen; they also are painful on palpation and with lateral stress.

BOX 25.2   Directional Types of Proximal Interphalangeal Joint Dislocation

Dorsal PIP Dislocations
Dorsal PIP dislocations are classified according to three subcategories:
- Type I (hyperextension): Volar plate (VP) avulsion and minor split in collateral ligaments longitudinally. If left untreated, this type of dislocation can lead to a swan neck deformity.
- Type II (dorsal dislocation): Dorsal dislocation of proximal interphalangeal (PIP) joint and VP avulsion with major split in collateral ligaments bilaterally.
- Type III (fracture-dislocation): Dorsal dislocation of the PIP with fracture of the volar articular surface of the middle phalanx. Stability:
  - Fracture less than 30% of middle phalanx articular surface = Stable/non-surgical
  - 30% to 50% = Tenuous; surgical stabilization typically indicated
  - More than 50% = Unstable

Lateral PIP Dislocations
Lateral stability is tested with the PIP joint in extension so that the collateral ligaments and secondary stabilizers, including the VP, can be assessed. Complete collateral ligament disruption is suggested by deformity that exceeds 20 degrees with gentle stress.

Volar PIP Dislocations
Volar PIP dislocations are rare. The injury may have a rotational component and the central slip may be ruptured.

Modified from Glickel SZ, Barron A, Eaton RG. Dislocations and ligament injuries in the digits. In Green DP, Hotchkiss RN, Pederson WC. eds. *Green's Operative Hand Surgery.* 4th ed. Philadelphia, PA: Churchill Livingstone, 1999.

Direction of Proximal Interphalangeal Joint Dislocation

The direction of dislocation is determined by the position of the middle phalanx at the time of joint injury (Box 25.2). The direction of dislocation typically determines the type of orthosis needed as well as the progression of treatment.[13,18,21,22] Dorsal dislocations involve injury to the distal portion of the volar plate, so PIP extension should be limited to prevent further stress on that structure. Volar dislocations involve injury to the central slip, so PIP flexion should be limited. Lateral dislocations involve the collateral ligaments, and so stress must be avoided on those structures during healing.

> **Clinical Pearl**
>
> PIP joint sprains often require immobilization or restricted motion to heal, and clients are at risk for long-standing edema. Permanent limitations in ROM and function are not uncommon.

Timelines and Healing

PIP joint sprains initially have **fusiform swelling** (swelling that is fuller at the PIP joint and tapers at both ends), and ligament fibrosis can progress for over a year after injury resulting in limitations in ROM and function. Uninjured digits may become stiff, and a quadriga effect can occur.

Nonoperative Treatment

Dorsal Dislocation[4,19,21,22,23]

Dorsal dislocation of a PIP joint is typically caused by trauma from a force that pushes the PIP joint into hyperextension causing failure of the volar plate.[3] Grade I injuries are treated with edema control and PIP immobilization in slight flexion while acute pain is present for approximately 1 week.

Grade II injuries are treated with a PIP dorsal block orthosis for approximately 6 weeks. PIP extension is typically blocked at 30 degrees for the first 3 weeks, then extension is increased 10 degrees per week for 4 to 6 weeks. If early AROM is prescribed, the therapist instructs the client to perform gentle flexion exercises but to extend only to the orthosis level. Edema is treated as it is possible. Gentle compression wrapping may be performed. Compressive sleeves may be difficult for the client to don without compromising the safe positioning of the PIP joint.

Grade III injuries frequently require surgical correction if the fracture involves more than 30% of the joint surface of the middle phalanx.[19,23] If joint congruence is present within a safe range, conservative treatment may be attempted. AROM with specific extension limitations should be provided and based on X-ray or fluoroscopy. The amount of PIP flexion in the PIP dorsal block orthosis is usually 20 to 30 degrees; however, this can vary depending on the stability of the joint. The therapist must know how much to limit extension to ensure safe ROM parameters.

Operative Treatment

When 30% to 50% of the articular surface of the middle phalanx is involved in the fracture, Kirschner wire PIP extension block, open reduction internal fixation, external fixation, traction splinting, or volar plate arthroplasty may be performed for grade III dorsal dislocations.[3,19,21,22,23,24] For fractures of more than 50%, a Hemi-Hamate[24] arthroplasty procedure may be indicated, which involves using a portion of the hamate bone to recreate the shape of the articular surface. In general, motion is initiated in flexion with extension permitted to a designated point of stability – typically determined intraoperatively.

A PIP dorsal block orthosis should be fabricated postoperatively at approximately 30 degrees° flexion. Active flexion exercises are permitted with extension limited to the orthosis level. At 3 weeks postoperative, it is usually appropriate to gradually advance extension with unrestricted ROM typically allowed by 6 weeks postsurgery.

◎ Clinical Pearl

When measuring the position of a digit in an orthosis, measure laterally, as dorsal edema may make the PIP joint appear more flexed than the actual position of the joint. X-Ray or fluoroscopy is beneficial in making sure the joint is properly reduced in the orthosis.

While flexion contracture is a common complication, corrective measures to increase extension should focus on total end-range time positioning.[17] Aggressive extension interventions

(such as forceful PROM), over long periods of time, will lead to increased inflammation, edema, and thickening/fibrosis of the joint capsule.[25] A combination of low-tension dynamic or static progressive orthoses as well as static nighttime orthoses can be used to successfully overcome flexion contractures. Serial casting should also be considered for clients with good PIP flexion but limited extension.[26]

? Questions to Ask the Doctor

Nonoperative Clients

- Does extension need to be blocked, and at what degree is the joint stable?
- It is typical to allow the client to perform flexion/extension exercises to the orthotic level. Is that appropriate in this case?
- Would you like to gradually increase permitted extension 10 to 15 degrees per week after 3 weeks, or wait until after the client is reexamined at the next physician appointment?

Operative Clients

- What structures were repaired (ask to see operative report)?
- Is PIP extension to be restricted? If so, to what degree?
- Typical advancement of extension is 10 to 15 degrees per week after 3 weeks. Is that progression appropriate in this case?
- What ROM does the physician expect the client to ultimately achieve?

( ) What to Say to Clients

About the Injury

"This diagnosis heals slowly and swelling persists for much longer than you might expect. It helps to be aware of this so you won't be discouraged by persistent swelling or stiffness. Sometimes clients need their rings resized, but time will tell whether this will be necessary. It may be helpful to use sleeves or wraps for the swelling."

"Because the injury involved tearing the tissue on the palm side of your finger, we need to protect that tissue by avoiding overstretching it while it heals. You can safely bend your finger, but you need to avoid straightening the injured joint all the way.

"While the tissue is healing over weeks and months, it is very important not to stress the finger with forceful or high-demand gripping activity. If you do something with your hand and the finger swells or becomes painful, this is a sign that your tissues can't tolerate that much stress yet. It is best to avoid this response so that swelling and flexibility can continue to improve."

About the Orthosis

"The purpose of the orthosis is to stop you from straightening your finger past the level that could cause you to re-dislocate, re-injure, or delay the healing of the finger. Focus on frequently bending the finger and straightening only up to the orthotic limit."

About Dynamic or Static Progressive Extension Orthoses

"Now that it is safe to work on straightening the finger, the purpose of the orthosis is to position your joint at the end of the range and add light tension to help increase your motion. It is extremely important to understand that more force will not result in a better outcome; however, more time at the end of the range will help."

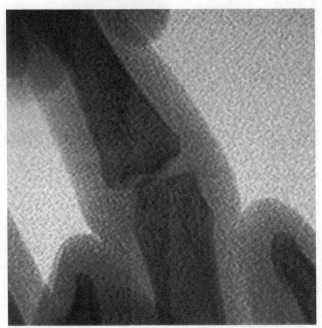

FIG. 25.15 X-ray of lateral proximal interphalangeal dislocation. *(Reproduced with permission, Gary Solomon, MS, OTR/L, CHT.)*

Lateral Dislocation

Lateral dislocation involves failure of either the medial or lateral collateral ligaments of the PIP joint. This is often caused by the finger sustaining a trauma pushing the joint in a sideways direction (Fig. 25.15).

Nonoperative Treatment

Grade I injuries may be managed by edema control and a brief period of resting orthotic use during the acute phase followed by AROM. Buddy straps or a hinged PIP orthosis may be used to support the PIP joint to avoid lateral stress during motion and functional use (Fig. 25.16A and B). Exercises should include DIP blocking and gentle ORL stretches to keep the lateral bands gliding properly.

During the acute phase of grade II injuries, a digital gutter orthosis is typically used and compression wrapping is recommended for edema control. The PIP joint may be in slight flexion because grade II tears can extend down to the volar plate. Orthosis use may continue for up to 2 weeks; however, gentle early active motion may be initiated with the ligament supported by buddy straps to the adjacent digit on the injured side. For an index finger radial collateral ligament (RCL) injury or small finger collateral ligament injury, a hinged PIP orthosis is recommended. (The small finger PIP joint often does not line up well with the adjacent finger for use of a buddy strap.)

If the joint can be reduced with closed treatment in a grade III injury, the PIP is typically protected with a digital dorsal block orthosis and short arc motion may be initiated within a stable range. Grade III injuries may require open surgical reduction. While the variety and complexity of surgical interventions is beyond the scope of this discussion, treatment progression is dependent on the stability of fixation and the ability to restore motion gradually without causing further stress to repaired structures.

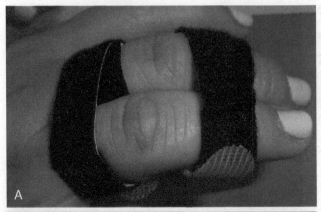
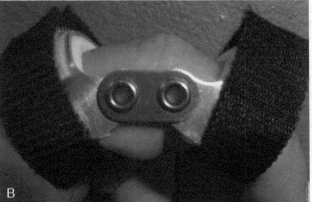

FIG. 25.16 **(A)** Buddy straps support the injured digit to facilitate motion. **(B)** Hinged proximal interphalangeal (PIP) orthosis supporting PIP during motion. A hinged orthosis is especially useful for index radial collateral ligament injury and small finger injury. *(Reproduced with permission, Gary Solomon, MS, OTR/L, CHT.)*

() *What to Say to Clients*

About the Orthoses

"As you begin moving your finger, wearing either a buddy strap or protective hinge orthosis will support the injured ligament as you begin to regain motion in your finger."

About Exercise

"Each time your tissue is stimulated by pain-free movement favorable clinical responses occur, including lubrication and circulation to promote healing. The more this happens, the better the finger will be. However, exercises that result in swelling or pain are not helpful and are actually detrimental."

Evaluation Tips

- Ask about previous injuries to this or other digits because preexisting stiffness may affect the client's prognosis.
- Be very gentle when evaluating the digit; the client's finger may be quite sore.
- Distinguish between fusiform swelling (swelling localized around the PIP joint) and uniform swelling (edema throughout the digit).
- When the client is cleared for AROM exercises, check isolated FDS and FDP function. Also check for ORL tightness (that is, check for DIP flexion with PIP extension).

- Distinguish between intrinsic, extrinsic, and joint tightness.
- Inquire about ADLs to determine whether some may be detrimental to the healing process.

Diagnosis-Specific Information That Affects Clinical Reasoning

The mechanics of the injury and whether the VP is involved are important pieces of information. If the VP was involved, the PIP should be protected in 20 to 30 degrees of flexion to promote VP healing. Also, keep in mind that collateral ligaments are at risk for tightening if full extension is not achieved in a timely fashion.

Edema management is paramount with PIP joint injuries, which are notorious for persistent swelling. Swelling contributes to pain, shortening, or tightening of the collateral ligaments, and loss of joint motion and tendon excursion. Therefore the treatment of swelling should be a priority. AROM and all exercises should be limited to the amount of stimulation that does not cause increased swelling.

Clinical Pearl

Aggressive interventions resulting in a temporary increase in motion but causing an increase in pain and edema are contraindicated. Aggressive treatment like this will not improve motion. In fact, it is possible to lose motion due to pain and edema caused by overworking the joint.

Devise exercises that are tissue specific. Distinguish between intrinsic and extrinsic tightness and position the finger for exercises accordingly. Check FDS and FDP excursion in the uninjured digits and perform isolated FDS exercises because these promote PIP flexion and prevent the insidious development of limitations.

Tips From the Field

Tissue Tolerances and Client Education
Monitor tissue tolerances. These dictate hand therapy interventions. Explain to clients that with this type of injury they cannot force motion to improve, and strenuous hand movements will only worsen the condition. Despite this instruction, clients may be inclined to perform forceful exercises to recover flexion and this is actually injurious to the tissues. Reinforce the concept of tissue tolerances with clients and teach them how to perform pain-free exercises. Friends may have recommended forceful gripping exercises (such as squeezing a tennis ball or a resistive gripper). Explain that tissues need to be ready for this much stimulation, negative tissue responses are manifested by swelling and pain after exercise, and these responses can slow recovery.

Buddy Taping
Normally, the finger that supports the injured side is selected for buddy taping with the injured finger. If the middle finger sustained an injury to the PIP RCL, it needs protection to avoid ulnar stress. In this instance, buddy tape the middle finger to the index finger to promote neutral alignment.

Buddy tapes may be most helpful when used at two levels (for example, proximal phalanx and middle phalanx). The important features are support, comfort, and ease of use. Monitor the tightness of the buddy tapes because tapes that are too tight can worsen edema by creating a tourniquet effect.

Volar Dislocation[19,21,22,23]

Volar dislocation is significantly less common than other PIP dislocations.[23] Central slip avulsion, collateral ligament injury, and fracture of the dorsal lip of the middle phalanx may be involved.

Conservative Treatment

If the joint is stable after reduction and the central slip is intact, gentle ROM may be initiated.

If the central slip is avulsed, the PIP is immobilized in a gutter orthosis with the DIP joint free for 4 to 6 weeks. The client is instructed to perform isolated DIP blocking exercises to maintain the positioning and integrity of the lateral bands and spiral ORL.

When the client is cleared to begin AROM, short arc motion is initiated. It is also important to support any associated collateral ligament injury with either buddy straps or a hinged PIP orthosis as described in the previous section.

Operative Treatment

If the PIP joint remains unstable after reduction, the joint may be pinned with a Kirschner wire in extension.

Exercise Guidelines

Brief, frequent, pain-free exercises are more effective than infrequent sessions. Explain to the client that tissue tolerance dictates the exercise regimen.

Precautions and Concerns

- *Avoid exercises that cause increased pain or stiffness. With PIP joint injuries, the importance of tissue tolerance cannot be overstated.*
- *Uncontrolled persistent edema can lead to serious clinical and functional consequences.*
- *The long healing timeline for this type of injury makes therapy challenging. Therapists must be creative in providing factual information about steady progress while trying to prevent the client from becoming discouraged.*

Thumb Metacarpophalangeal Joint Injury

Clients with thumb MP joint injuries, particularly ulnar collateral ligament (UCL) injuries, are frequently referred for hand therapy. Proper therapy can facilitate recovery of stable pain-free function.

Injury to the thumb MP joint may involve either the UCL or the RCL. The UCL is injured much more frequently than the RCL. The treatment guidelines described for UCL injury also apply to the RCL.

Anatomy

The MP joint of the thumb is primarily a hinge joint. Flexion and extension comprise the primary arc of motion. Pronation-supination and abduction-adduction are considered secondary arcs of motion at this joint. Pronation occurs as the thumb MP joint flexes because the radial condyle of the metacarpal head is wider than the ulnar condyle.[3,20]

The thumb MP joint's ROM is unique; it has the most variation in the amount of movement of all the body's joints. ROM at the thumb MP joint ranges from 55 to 85 degrees of flexion. People with flatter metacarpal heads tend to have less motion, and those with more spherical metacarpal heads have more motion. Lateral motion at the thumb MP joint ranges from 0 to 20 degrees when the MP is in extension. The stability of this joint comes primarily from ligamentous, capsular, and musculotendinous support.[20]

Laterally, the thumb MP joint displays strong PCLs that arise from the metacarpal lateral condyles and progress volarly and obliquely to their insertion on the proximal phalanx. The ACL originates volar to the PCL and inserts on the volar plate and the sesamoid bones.[19] The sesamoid bones have been described as the convergence point of the thumb MP joint's periarticular structures.[27,28] The PCLs are tightest with MP flexion.

The thumb MP joint receives stability from thenar intrinsic muscles, specifically the adductor pollicis (AP), the flexor pollicis brevis (FPB), and the abductor pollicis brevis (APB). The FPB and the APB insert on the radial sesamoid, and the adductor pollicis inserts on the ulnar sesamoid.[20,28]

Diagnosis and Pathology

A UCL injury is called **skier's thumb** because a fall on outstretched hand with the thumb in abduction is a common skiing injury. The ski pole handle may cause the thumb to abduct. Historically, this injury has also been called **gamekeeper's thumb** because the term describes an injury that occurs as a result of killing rabbits with a technique that stresses the thumb MP joint radially. Currently, the term *gamekeeper's thumb* refers to chronic UCL instability at the thumb MP joint.[3]

Acute UCL injuries of the thumb MP joint usually involve detachment of the ligament from its proximal phalanx insertion. Concomitant injury of the ACL, the volar plate, or the dorsal capsule can also occur. If complete disruption occurs along with forceful radial deviation at the thumb MP joint, displacement of the ligament superficially with interposition of the adductor aponeurosis may result; this condition is called **Stener's lesion** (Fig. 25.17). **Precaution.** *Stener's lesion requires surgical correction because the interposition prevents healing of the ligament.*[3]

RCL injuries to the MP of the thumb are less common. The mechanism of injury is usually trauma causing forced adduction of the thumb. Treatment progression follows a similar course to UCL injury with care to avoid lateral stress ulnarly.

The thumb MP joint is clinically assessed for MP instability injury by providing gentle stress in radial deviation (to assess UCL) or ulnar deviation (to assess RCL) to the thumb with the MP joint in both extension and flexion at 30 degrees. This result is compared with that on the contralateral side. Physicians may use an injection of anesthetic if pain prohibits testing. Varying criteria are used to describe a complete ligament tear: (1) instability greater than 35 degrees, or (2) instability 15 degrees greater than on the uninjured side.

> **Clinical Pearl**
> Stress testing may be more painful on a partial tear than on a complete tear.

X-rays in the A-P, lateral, and oblique views are taken to ruleout the possibility of an avulsion fracture. Stress X-rays may also be helpful.[27] Additional imaging techniques, such as ultrasound

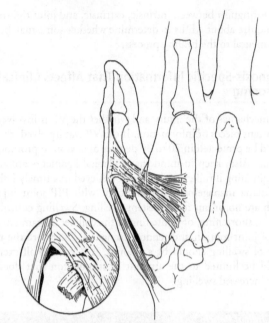

FIG. 25.17 Stener's lesion. The ulnar collateral ligament is displaced with interposition of the adductor aponeurosis. Surgery is required for this type of injury because interposition of the adductor aponeurosis prevents healing. (*From Mackin EJ, Callinan N, Skirven TM. et al.* Rehabilitation of the Hand and Upper Extremity. *5th ed. St Louis, MO: Mosby; 2002*).

studies, magnetic resonance imaging, and arthrograms, may be performed. An overlooked and untreated injury can lead to pain and instability.

Timelines and Healing

The thumb MP joint is immobilized for 4 to 6 weeks to allow healing. Thumb IP joint ROM should be encouraged throughout the immobilization stage. It can take a few months after injury for resistive pinch or axial loading of the thumb to be comfortable and safe to perform.

Nonoperative Treatment

If the ligament injury is a partial tear, the thumb is immobilized in a hand- or forearm-based thumb spica orthosis (with the IP joint left free) for 2 to 4 weeks. After this, AROM exercises are initiated with medical clearance and the orthosis is continued between exercises.[29,30] For UCL injury, flexion, extension, and radial abduction are initiated; AROM is then progressed to gentle palmar abduction and opposition. Progression to active-assistive range of motion occurs at approximately 6 weeks. Light lateral pinch exercises may be started early, but tip pinch and thumb tip loading exercises are not performed until medically approved, which may be 8 weeks or longer after injury. This restriction is necessary to prevent stress on the ligament.[3] *For a RCL injury, the progression of treatment is similar; however, lateral pinch is avoided for up to 8 weeks.*

Operative Treatment

Surgical procedures may include open reduction and internal fixation to reduce fracture fragments. The UCL may be reattached to its insertion. The MP joint may be pinned and this is often done with a slight overcorrection ulnarly to prevent stress on the repaired ligament. A thumb spica cast or thermoplastic orthosis is used for 4 weeks, at which time the pin is usually removed.[3]

If Kirschner-wire fixation is used, AROM of the thumb carpometacarpal and MP joints is initiated after pin removal. Scar management and edema control are helpful for minimizing the risk for adherence of the extensor pollicis longus (EPL) tendon at the incision scar. As in the nonoperative program, lateral pinch may be initiated sooner than tip pinch, which should be avoided for about 8 weeks after surgery to prevent stress on the repair. A protective thumb spica orthosis is used for 6 to 8 weeks after surgery. The therapist should inform the client that some tenderness at the ulnar MP joint is normal for a few months after this surgery.[3]

? Questions to Ask the Doctor

Nonoperative Clients

- We typically begin motion for the thumb with flexion/extension and radial abduction. Is this client also clear for palmar abduction and opposition?
- Should we wait 8 weeks before allowing resistive tip pinch with this client?

Operative Clients

- Was there a Stener's lesion?
- How much ROM does the physician expect the client to achieve at the MP joint?
- Should activities requiring resistive tip pinch or axial loading be avoided for 8 weeks?
- Should any other precautions be taken?
- How long should the protective orthosis be used?

( ) What to Say to Clients

About the Injury

"With this diagnosis, it is more important to achieve a pain-free stable thumb MP joint than it is to achieve full MP motion. You may not recover full MP motion but achieving functional pain-free motion for pinching and resistive hand use is a successful result."

About the Orthosis

"You will need to wear your protective orthosis (Fig. 25.18) to prevent forceful use of or stress on the injured thumb. It may also help signal others to be careful when shaking your hand or interacting with you in public."

About Exercises

"It is important to focus on the motion at the last joint (the IP joint) to prevent stiffness at this site. However, be careful not to put pressure on the end of the thumb tip and do not use a powerful pinching motion against the tip of the thumb until the doctor permits this."

Evaluation Tips

- Observe the client's contralateral thumb for laxity (including laterally).
- Assess the contralateral thumb for MP and IP AROM.
- Is tightness of the injured thumb's web space present?

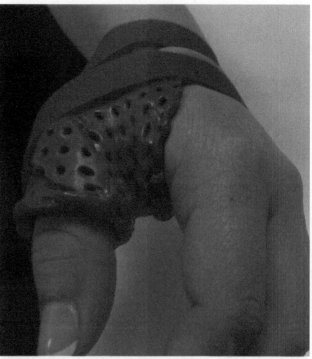

FIG. 25.18 Short thumb spica orthosis with interphalangeal joint free. Care is taken to provide good lateral support to MP joint. (*Reproduced with permission, Gary Solomon, MS, OTR/L, CHT.*)

- In clients who have had surgery, observe for scar adherence and test for full excursion of the EPL.
- Explore the client's ADL needs and any adaptations needed to protect the injured tissue.

Diagnosis-Specific Information That Affects Clinical Reasoning

Fabricate the orthosis with a good web space opening and with the thumb positioned to prevent loading of the tip. Make sure there is good lateral support to the proximal phalanx of the thumb to protect against lateral stress. Adjust the orthosis as edema decreases to maintain good lateral stability.

♡ Tips From the Field

- The flexor pollicis longus is easier to isolate than the FPB. Because of this and because immobilization contributes to MP stiffness, clients often have difficulty isolating active flexion at the thumb MP. If they override with IP flexion, try using a volar IP extension gutter orthosis to isolate for active MP flexion exercises. Simultaneous proximal support of the metacarpal may also help.

⊳ Precautions and Concerns

- *Be alert for and take steps to prevent a thumb web-space contracture. Although a typical approach is to position the thumb in overcorrection (slight ulnar deviation), don't allow tightness of the thumb web space.*
- *Avoid tip loading and resistive pinching.*
- *Assess and problem-solve ADLs to protect injured structures.*

> *Try building up the girth of implements (for example, construct padded pens) to reduce the load on the thumb MP joint.*
> • *Instruct clients to avoid painful use of the thumb.*

CASE STUDIES

Case Study 25.1

Oliver, a 34-year-old airport transportation van driver, jammed his right small finger while lifting a passenger's suitcase. He was treated initially at an urgent care center and placed in an Aluma-Foam full-finger orthosis, which he was removing for hygiene.

Oliver was referred for a mallet orthosis for his small finger. Options of volar, dorsal, and combination styles were discussed, and it was determined that the combination of a dorsal base with volar support under the distal phalanx would provide the best support and protection for work tasks. The client was also instructed in isolated PIP ROM in the orthosis.

At 6 weeks, he was cleared to begin AROM of the DIP. Oliver demonstrated DIP ROM from 0 to 20 degrees. A template was made with AlumaFoam at a 25-degree angle, and the client was assigned a home exercise program to gradually work toward DIP flexion to the template while emphasizing DIP extension.

At follow-up the next week (7 weeks post injury), he had achieved his 0 to 25-degree goal. The template was then adjusted to 40 degrees, and the client was again instructed to gradually work toward that goal. He was also instructed to remove the mallet orthosis for 1 to 2 hours 2 times per day during sedentary activity.

At 8 weeks post injury, Oliver was permitted to perform composite fist, hook, and unrestricted DIP active blocking exercises.

The orthosis was to be worn 2 hours in the middle of the day and at night. He was permitted to return to work with restrictions of no forceful gripping/heavy lifting, and at 10 weeks post injury had achieved ROM of 0 to 55 degrees, at which time activity restrictions were lifted.

Case Study 25.2

Trudi, a 14-year-old female, came to therapy with a right ring finger PIP dorsal dislocation. The joint was examined under fluoroscan by her hand surgeon who determined that the joint became unstable when extended more than 50 degrees. Surgical options were explained. However, the client and parents opted to attempt conservative treatment.

After joint reduction and several attempts of thermoplastic orthosis fabrication under the fluoroscan, the joint reduction could not be adequately maintained. At that time, a digital plaster cast was attempted and the joint was reduced and immobilized at 60 degrees flexion.

After 3 weeks the joint was reexamined and was stable enough to increase extension to 45 degrees and was recast for one additional week.

At 4 weeks, a thermoplastic dorsal block was fabricated at 30 degrees flexion, and the client started active flexion and extension exercises to the orthosis level. The orthosis was serially adjusted to allow 10 degrees additional extension per week.

At 8 weeks, her PIP motion was 15 to 90 degrees and a low-tension PIP extension orthosis was initiated as well as a night gutter orthosis for PIP extension.

By 10 weeks, she had achieved full PIP ROM and resumed unrestricted activities including sports.

References

1. Bertini TH, Laidig TJ, Pettit NM, et al.: Treatment of the injured athlete. In Skirven TM, Osterman AL, Fedorczyk J, et al, editors: *Rehabilitation of the hand and upper extremity*, ed 6, Philadelphia, 2011, Elsevier Mosby.
2. Brzezienski MA, Schneider LH: Extensor tendon injuries at the distal interphalangeal joint, *Hand Clin* 11:373–386, 1995.
3. Little KJ, Jacoby SM: Intra-articular hand fractures and joint injuries: part I-surgeon's management. In Skirven TM, Osterman AL, Fedorczyk J, et al, editors: *Rehabilitation of the hand and upper extremity*, ed 6, Philadelphia, 2011, Elsevier Mosby.
4. Hofmeister EP, Mazurek MT, Shin AY, et al.: Extension block pinning for large mallet fractures, *J Hand Surg Am* 28A:453–459, 2003.
5. American Society for Surgery of the Hand: *The hand: examination and diagnosis*, ed 2, Edinburgh, 1983, Churchill Livingstone.
6. Valdes K, Naughton N, Algar L: Conservative treatment of mallet finger: a systematic review, *J Hand Ther* 28:237–246, 2015.
7. Evans RB: Clinical management of extensor tendon injuries: the therapist's perspective. In Skirven TM, Osterman AL, Fedorczyk J, et al, editors: *Rehabilitation of the hand and upper extremity*, ed 6, Philadelphia, 2011, Elsevier Mosby.
8. Biernacki SD: A flexion contracture splint for the distal interphalangeal joint, *J Hand Ther* 14:302–303, 2001.
9. Doyle JR: Extensor tendons: acute injuries. In Green DP, Hotchkiss RN, Pederson WC, editors: *Green's operative hand surgery*, ed 4, Philadelphia, 1999, Churchill Livingstone.
10. Tetik C, Gudemez E: Modification of the extension block kirschner wire technique for mallet fractures, *Clin Orthop Relat Res* 404:284–290, 2002.
11. Lin JS, Samora JB: Surgical and nonsurgical management of mallet finger: a systematic review, *J Hand Surg* 43:146–163.e2, 2018.
12. Grau L, Baydoun H, Chen K, et al.: Biomechanics of the acute boutonniere deformity, *J Hand Surg* 43:80.e1–80.e6, 2017.
13. Alter S, Feldon P, Terrono AL: Pathomechanics of deformities in the arthritic hand and wrist. In Skirven TM, Osterman AL, Fedorczyk J, et al, editors: *Rehabilitation of the hand and upper extremity*, ed 6, Philadelphia, 2011, Elsevier Mosby.
14. Colditz J: Plaster of paris: the forgotten hand splinting material, *J Hand Ther* 15:144–157, 2002.
15. Hirth MJ, Howell JW, O'Brien L, et al.: Relative motion orthoses in the management of various hand conditions: a scoping review, *J Hand Ther* 29:405–432, 2016.
16. Saleeba EC: Dynamic flexion splint for the distal interphalangeal joint, *J Hand Ther* 16:249–250, 2003.
17. Flowers KR: A proposed decision hierarchy for splinting the stiff joint, with an emphasis on force application parameters, *J Hand Ther* 15:158–162, 2002.
18. Catalano LW, Skarparis AC, Glickel SZ, et al.: Treatment of chronic, traumatic hyperextension deformities of the proximal interphalangeal joint with flexor digitorum superficialis tenodesis, *J Hand Surg* 28A:448–452, 2003.
19. Chinchalkar S, Lanting B, Ross D: Swan neck deformity after distal interphalangeal joint flexion contractures: a biomechanical analysis, *J Hand Ther* 19:420–425, 2009.
20. Glickel SZ, Barron A, Eaton RG: Dislocations and ligament injuries in the digits. In Green DP, Hotchkiss RN, Pederson WC, editors: *Green's operative hand surgery*, ed 4, Philadelphia, 1999, Churchill Livingstone.
21. Chinchalkar SJ, Gan BS: Management of proximal interphalangeal joint fractures and dislocations, *J Hand Ther* 16:117–128, 2003.

22. Katsoulis E, Rees K, Warwick DJ: Hand therapist led management of mallet finger, *J Hand Ther* 10:10–17, 2005.

23. Dennerllein J: Finger flexor tendon forces are a complex function of finger joint motions and fingertip forces, *J Hand Ther* 18:120–127, 2005.

24. Calfee RP, Keifhaber R, Sommercamp TG, Stern PJ: Hemi-hamate arthroplasty provides functional reconstruction of acute and chronic proximal interphalangeal fracture-dislocations, *J Hand Surg* 34A:1232–1241, 2009.

25. Waris E, Mattila S, Sillat T, Karjalainen T: Extension block pinning for unstable proximal interphalangeal joint dorsal fracture dislocations, *J Hand Surg* 41:196–202, 2016.

26. Glasgow C, Tooth LR, Fleming J: Mobilizing the stiff hand: combining theory and evidence to improve clinical outcomes, *J Hand Ther* 23:392–401, 2010.

27. Gallagher KG, Blackmore SM: Intra-articular hand fractures and joint injuries: part II therapist's management. In Skirven TM, Osterman AL, Fedorczyk J, et al, editors: *Rehabilitation of the hand and upper extremity*, ed 6, Philadelphia, 2011, Elsevier Mosby.

28. Mohler LR, Trumble TE: Disorders of the thumb sesamoids, *Hand Clin* 17:291–301, 2001.

29. Rotella JM, Urpi J: A new method of diagnosing metacarpophalangeal instabilities of the thumb, *Hand Clin* 17:45–60, 2001.

30. Galindo A, Suet L: A metacarpophalangeal joint stabilization splint, *J Hand Ther* 15:83–84, 2002.

26 Extensor Tendon Injury

Linda J. Klein

Extensor tendon injuries have long been considered to be less complex than flexor tendon injuries, with fewer complications and better results. Numerous authors reflect that complications caused by extensor tendon injuries can be just as frustrating and result in significant loss of motion and function of the injured digit and hand.[1-3] According to Rosenthal and Elhassan, "The extensor muscles to the digits are weaker, their capacity for work and their amplitude of glide are less than their flexor antagonists, yet they require a latitude of motion that is not necessary for flexor function."[1] Extensor tendons are thinner and broader than flexor tendons. They are superficial in comparison with the flexor tendons, allowing adhesion to the fascial layers and skin. Over the proximal phalanx, the extensor tendon has a broad tendon-to-bone interface that can result in dense adhesions. Shortening of the extensor tendon because of surgery may result in difficulty regaining full flexion. Dorsal swelling may prevent the tendons from gliding. Recreating the normal balance between the intrinsic and extrinsic muscle/tendon units can be a difficult task for the surgeon and therapist following extensor tendon injury. Common functional complications include loss of flexion, extensor lag, and decreased grip strength.[2] To prevent these complications, extensor tendon approaches, similar to flexor tendon approaches, have evolved to include controlled passive and active mobilization immediately following surgery. Results, especially in the first 12 weeks, show improved outcome over immobilization.[3-11] The goal of this chapter is for the reader to understand the anatomy, pathology, healing process, and rehabilitation approaches for the differing zones of the extensor tendons to achieve maximal function with minimal complications for the client following extensor tendon repair.

Diagnosis and Pathology

Traumatic injury to the extensor tendons may be by open or closed means. Open lacerations most often occur from a sharp object lacerating the extensor tendon. Open injuries are diagnosed at the time of injury as the wound is explored for tendon, nerve, and ligament damage. Injury to the tendon can vary from partial to complete laceration, from clean to dirty, and from a straight to jagged cut. Associated injury to the extensor retinaculum, sagittal bands, bone, ligament, nerve, or vessel may occur, and a crushing force will increase the complexity of injury. Repair of the tendon and associated structures is performed as soon after the injury as possible, often in the emergency room.

Closed traumatic injuries of the extensor tendon may occur as a rupture of the tendon from its attachment, from friction of the tendon across a rough bony prominence, or from disease that weakens the tendon, such as rheumatoid arthritis. Closed extensor tendon injuries in the digit include mallet and boutonniere injuries. Rheumatoid arthritis can cause synovial invasion of an extensor tendon, often at the level of the wrist, eventually resulting in tendon rupture. Closed extensor tendon ruptures also occur at the wrist by friction of the tendon over a bony prominence, such as an extensor pollicis longus (EPL) rupture over Lister's tubercle, or extensor digiti minimi (EDM) rupture over a rough edge of the distal ulna.

This chapter focuses on surgical repair, postoperative healing, and rehabilitation approaches following extensor tendon repair. Closed injuries to the tendon that do not require surgical repair (such as mallet and boutonniere injuries) are discussed in Chapter 25.

Surgical Repair of Extensor Tendons

Less attention has been given to the types of surgical repair for extensor tendons than flexor tendons. However, the strength of repair of an extensor tendon is important in preventing gapping or rupture when motion is initiated. A number of suture techniques for extensor tendons exist.[1,2,12,13] Newport notes that because extensor tendons are smaller and flatter than flexor tendons and have less cross-linking, performing a stronger, multistrand repair in the extensor tendon is more difficult. The same repair technique performed in an extensor tendon is approximately 50% as strong as if it was performed in a flexor tendon due to the smaller size of the tendon and lack of collagen cross linking.[1,13] The type of suture performed on the lacerated extensor tendon is largely dependent on the area the tendon was injured. A thinner area of extensor tendon (such as in the digit) will not tolerate multiple strands required for stronger repair.[1] The therapy protocols discussed in this chapter for extensor tendon injury are not dependent on the type of surgical technique used.

Timelines and Healing

Tendon healing relies on direct blood supply and synovial diffusion. The blood supply to the extensor tendons is through vascular mesenteries, which travel through the fascia to the tendons from the radial and ulnar arteries and deep palmar arch. Nutrition from synovial diffusion to the extensor tendons occurs from the deep fascial layer in the dorsum of the hand and the extensor retinaculum.[1]

Three basic approaches to rehabilitation of repaired tendons in the hand are (1) immobilization, (2) immediate passive motion in the direction of the repaired tendon, and (3) immediate active motion in the direction of the repaired tendon. The main difference in these approaches is within the early phase, or first month, of tendon healing.

Precaution. *Before using an immediate motion protocol, the therapist must know whether or not the surgeon considers the repair to be sufficiently strong to tolerate this type of rehabilitation approach.*

The early phase of tendon healing consists of the **inflammatory phase** and early **fibroplasia phase** of tendon healing when the tendon is at its weakest and collagen is just beginning to be laid down at the repair site. The intermediate phase of tendon healing is when the tendon repair gains tensile strength. During the late phase of tendon healing, the tendon repair continues to gain tensile strength and begins to remodel in alignment with the tension placed on it. The repaired tendon is considered to have adequate tensile strength at 12 weeks after the repair to tolerate almost any activity. Tissue remodeling continues for a number of months.

Most clients who have had an extensor tendon repair are allowed to use their hand for light activities by 6 to 8 weeks following the repair. This is because although normal use of the hands consistently offers resistance to the flexor tendons, it rarely offers resistance to the extensor tendons.

Knowledge of tendon healing is the basis for determining when it is safe to advance a repaired tendon to resistive exercise. This is an important concept to understand. Guidelines based on this knowledge affect clinical decisions about strengthening of grip or pinch following a flexor tendon repair, or about applying resistance to digital extension following an extensor tendon repair. It is appropriate to introduce resistance to tendon motion when adhesions limit active motion more than passive motion. Resistance places tension on scar tissue to improve proximal gliding of the tendon. However, this same resistance can overcome the tensile strength of the repair and result in a rupture. Good

active motion of a repaired tendon indicates lack of adhesions. Without the support and restriction of surrounding adhesions, a great amount of tension is transferred directly through the tendon when the muscle pulls against resistance. This increases the risk of tendon rupture. Therefore all timelines in this chapter must be individualized. Introducing resistance to a repaired tendon that is showing good to excellent gliding should be done later in the timeline or deferred until the surgeon determines the tendon is near or at full tensile strength.

Precautions for Minimizing Tension on a Repaired Extensor Tendon

Tendon repairs are never at their full strength when motion is initiated. Therapists should be cautious to avoid gapping or potential rupture of a tendon until 12 weeks after repair. Two things cause gapping or rupture of a repaired tendon. The first of these is overstretching of the extensor tendon repair by moving too far into flexion (pulling the tendon repair apart) before the tendon is strong enough to tolerate that amount of tension. The second is an excessive internal pull on the tendon by the muscle during active or resisted motion in the same direction as the repaired tendon. This would include active or resisted extension following an extensor tendon repair before the tendon is strong enough to tolerate that amount of internal tension on the tendon.

Precaution. When initiating active motion, do it gently with a gradual increase in tension applied to the tendon as healing advances.

As we encourage tendon gliding for active motion, we must consider the amount of tension the muscle is placing on the repaired tendon to achieve the active motion. Our goal in tendon rehabilitation is to achieve tendon gliding while minimizing tension on the repair during the healing process. We can minimize resistance or tension on the tendon when mobilizing the tendon by decreasing edema and joint stiffness, performing motion slowly and gently, and using optimal positions of proximal joints during active motion. When we mobilize stiff joints associated with the tendon repair in the first 6 weeks after repair, we must do it with the tendon in a protected position.

> ◎ *Clinical Pearl*
>
> To place an extensor tendon in a protected position during exercise, support all joints (except the one you are moving during the exercise) in extension, *especially the joints proximal to the one being moved.* This will reduce tension on the extensor tendon repair.

For instance, if the PIP joint is stiff at 3 weeks after repair of an extensor tendon injury over the dorsum of the hand, support the wrist and metacarpophalangeal (MP) joint in extension while applying gentle joint mobilization or passive proximal interphalangeal (PIP) flexion. This will prevent overstretch of the repaired extensor tendon while improving flexion of the individual joint.

> ？ **Questions to Ask the Doctor**

There are a large number of variables that exist in the type and complexity of injuries to tendons, so having a good understanding of each injury and surgery before beginning treatment is important. Questions to ask the physician may include the following:

- Which tendons were lacerated and at what level/zone? (Note: This does not necessarily correlate with the location of the skin laceration.)
- What other structures were injured (sagittal band, ligament, vessel, nerve, bone)?
- Were all structures viable for a strong repair, or are there concerns with strength or healing of certain structures?
- Does the surgeon prefer any particular tendon repair protocol: Immobilization? Immediate passive motion? Immediate active motion? Clarify the approach you are planning to use for your shared client. This may require some discussion and negotiation.
- Which joints should be included in the orthosis?
- Is a separate night-resting orthosis indicated?
- If the client was not referred to hand therapy immediately following surgical repair: How was the client positioned following surgery? Was any motion allowed before the client presented for therapy?
- Clarify the exercise and activity level that is currently allowed. Is passive flexion and/or resistive exercise contraindicated at the time of referral? Are there any restrictions, or is the client to be advanced as tolerated?

( ) *What to Say to Clients*

"An extensor tendon connects the muscle to the bone, and it is what makes your finger/thumb straighten" (illustrate with your hand). Use a picture or diagram to show the client how the injured extensor muscle becomes tendon, and how the tendon must be pulled by the muscle to glide proximally to result in active extension, and glide distally to allow flexion.

"When your extensor tendon was injured, it could no longer straighten at this (these) joint(s) (illustrate with your hand). Now that the surgeon has repaired it, it needs time to heal. A tendon takes 12 weeks to fully heal, but you will be allowed to use your hand for light activities after 6 to 8 weeks. We will increase what you do with your repaired tendon gradually, but if you do too

much too soon, it will tear apart. The two things that will cause your tendon to tear apart, or rupture, are a stretch on the tendon into a bent position (illustrate on your hand how a stretch into flexion would place excessive stretch on a repaired extensor tendon) or a pull from the muscle on the inside that is too strong for the tendon repair to tolerate. For this reason, you must follow the directions for use of your protective brace (orthosis) closely. It will prevent the tendon from overstretching or overuse. Under no circumstances should you do more than we instruct you to do with your hand during this healing process, or the tendon may rupture. If it ruptures, it may not be able to be repaired again, or if further surgery is done, the results are not likely to be as good."

Anatomy

Extrinsic extensor tendons to the digits include the extensor digitorum communis (EDC), extensor indicis proprius (EIP), extensor digiti minimi (EDM), extensor pollicis longus (EPL), extensor pollicis brevis (EPB), and abductor pollicis longus (APL). Each of these tendons crosses the wrist dorsally, passing under the extensor retinaculum, which is separated into six compartments to maximize mechanical efficiency of the extensor tendons as they cross the wrist, preventing **bowstringing** (Fig. 26.1).

Proximal to the MP joints, the **juncturae tendinum** fibers separate from the EDC tendon, providing a cross-connection to the adjacent EDC tendon. This cross-connection of fibers exists to a variable extent in each individual but most consistently occurs between the EDC to the ring finger and the EDC tendons to the small and middle fingers. The juncturae tendinum fibers assist in extension of the neighboring finger and help maintain the EDC in midline over the metacarpal head during finger flexion.

The extrinsic extensor tendons serve the primary purpose of extending the MP joints of the fingers and the thumb MP and IP joints. The EDC also assists in extension of the finger PIP joints by its anatomical contribution to the lateral bands and weakly by its attachment on the proximal portion of the middle phalanx.

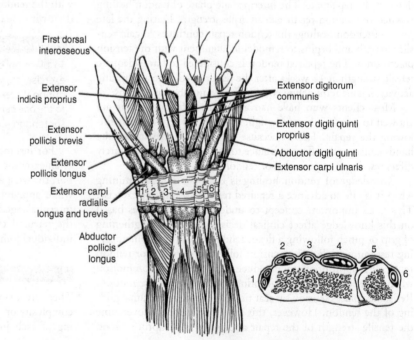

FIG. 26.1 Extensor tendon anatomy in zones VI and VII. The extensor retinaculum acts as a pulley to maintain the mechanical efficiency of the extrinsic extensor tendons and prevent bowstringing. It also assists in extensor tendon nutrition via synovial diffusion. *(From Fess EE. Hand and Upper Extremity Splinting: Principles and Methods. 3rd ed. St Louis, MO: Mosby; 2005.)*

First dorsal interosseous
Extensor indicis proprius
Extensor pollicis brevis
Extensor pollicis longus
Extensor carpi radialis longus and brevis
Abductor pollicis longus
Extensor digitorum communis
Extensor digiti quinti proprius
Abductor digiti quinti
Extensor carpi ulnaris

Extension of the finger PIP and distal interphalangeal (DIP) joints is performed primarily by the lateral bands, which consist of portions of the lumbrical and interossei tendons with contributions from the EDC (Fig. 26.2). The lateral bands on both sides of the fingers pass dorsal to the axis of motion at the PIP and DIP joints and merge over the DIP joint to form the terminal extensor tendon. Extension at the PIP and DIP joints is delicately balanced by a combination of tendon fibers and ligamentous support in an uninjured finger to prevent excessive dorsal or volar migration (subluxation) of the lateral bands. The transverse retinacular ligament supports the lateral bands volarly, and the triangular ligament supports the lateral bands dorsally. The oblique retinacular ligaments (ORLs) run along the sides of the finger and cross the PIP and DIP joints volar to the PIP axis of motion and dorsal to the DIP axis of motion. Thus when the PIP joint extends, it places tension on, or stretches, the ORL. This causes the ligament to tighten across the DIP joint, placing a passive extension assist on the DIP joint by this tenodesis effect.

The IP joint of the thumb is extended primarily by the EPL tendon, and the MP joint is extended by a combination of the EPL and the EPB. The APL, EPB, and EPL tendons extend the carpometacarpal (CMC) joint.

Injuries to the extensor tendon are discussed in relation to the zone of injury, for there are different protocols following repair of the extensor tendon for each set of zones. Extensor tendon zones are illustrated in Fig. 26.3. Orthoses used for extensor tendon repairs in the early phase of tendon healing are reviewed in Table 26.1.

Zones I and II Extensor Tendon Injuries

Diagnosis and Pathology

Injuries to the extensor tendon in zone I and distal zone II result in a mallet finger. Closed injuries may be caused by a tendon rupture or avulsion, resulting in a drooped (flexed) distal phalanx of the digit. Treatment of the closed mallet finger is covered in

FIG. 26.2 (A) The extensor tendon at the metacarpophalangeal *(MP)* joint level is held in place by the transverse lamina or sagittal band, which tethers and centers the extensor tendons over the joint. This sagittal band arises from the volar plate and the intermetacarpal ligaments at the neck of the metacarpals. Any injury to this extensor hood or expansion may result in subluxation or dislocation of the extensor tendon. **B,** The intrinsic tendons from the lumbrical and interosseous muscles join the extensor mechanism at about the level of the proximal and midportion of the proximal phalanx and continue distally to the distal interphalangeal *(DIP)* joint of the finger. The extensor mechanism at the proximal interphalangeal *(PIP)* joint is best described as a trifurcation of the extensor tendon into the central slip, which attaches to the dorsal base of the middle phalanx, and two lateral bands. The lateral bands continue distally to insert at the dorsal base of the distal phalanx. The extensor mechanism is maintained in place over the PIP joint by the transverse retinacular ligaments. *cent.,* central; *Lat.* lateral; *ORL.,* oblique retinacular ligament; *Trans ret. LIG.,* transverse retinacular ligament. *(From Doyle JR. Extensor tendons: acute injuries. In Green DP, Hotchkiss RN, Pederson WC. eds.* Green's Operative Hand Surgery *4th ed. New York, NY: Churchill Livingstone; 1999.)*

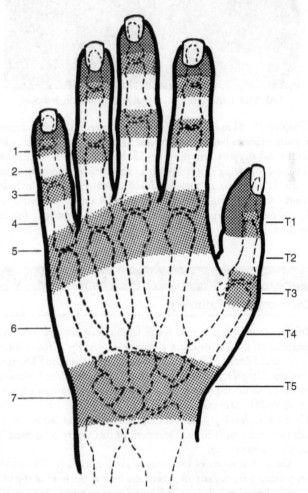

FIG. 26.3 Extensor tendon zones as defined by the Committee on Tendon Injuries for the International Federation of the Society for Surgery of the Hand. *(From Kleinert HE, Schepel S, Gill T. Flexor tendon injuries.* Surg Clin North Am. *1981;61:267.)*

TABLE 26.1   Overview of Orthoses Used for Extensor Tendon Repairs in the Early Phase of Tendon Healing

Zone of Injury	Immobilization	Immediate Passive Extension	Immediate Active Extension
I and II	DIP extension orthosis (see Fig. 26.4)	None available	None available
III and IV	Finger gutter, full IP extension, taped in place (see Fig. 26.5)	Hand-based outrigger allowing 30 degrees of PIP flexion (see Fig. 26.6)	Finger gutter, taped in place between exercises (see Fig. 26.5) Exercise template with 30 degrees of PIP flexion, 20 degrees of DIP flexion (see Fig. 26.7)
V, VI, and VII	Full-length resting pan in partial wrist extension and full digit extension or slight MP flexion (see Fig. 26.8)	Dynamic MP extension outrigger allowing 30 degrees of MP flexion (see Fig. 26.9, A and B)	Immediate active extension orthosis using wrist support and yoke (see Fig. 26.10) *Or* dynamic outrigger removed for active extension component

DIP, Distal interphalangeal; *IP*, interphalangeal; *MP*, metacarpophalangeal; *PIP*, proximal interphalangeal.

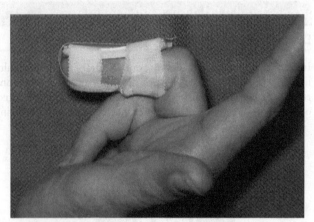

FIG. 26.4 Distal interphalangeal joint extension orthosis.

Chapter 25. Management of an open laceration of an extensor tendon in zones I and II is managed by surgical repair, often with additional support of a pin to hold the DIP joint in extension. Therapy following surgical repair of an extensor tendon in zones I and II is similar to that for closed treatment, which includes immobilization (Fig. 26.4) for a number of weeks as determined by the referring surgeon, followed by a gradual increase in flexion of the DIP joint.

Zones III and IV Extensor Tendon Injuries

Diagnosis and Pathology

Injuries in this region may result from closed ruptures or open lacerations. Closed ruptures are often caused by a direct blunt force to the dorsal PIP joint, resulting in rupture of the EDC tendon from its attachment on the middle phalanx. Closed ruptures result in weakened active PIP extension with a limited amount of active PIP extension still present from the intact lateral bands. Over time, development of a larger PIP extension lag results in a boutonniere deformity. Treatment of this injury is covered in detail in Chapter 25.

Open lacerations of the extensor tendon in zones III and IV are common from sharp objects of any kind at the level of the PIP joint and proximal phalanx. Following primary repair of the extensor tendon in this zone, three types of protocols are available in the early phase of tendon healing: immobilization, immediate passive, and immediate active extension. Immobilization is often

applied, but as advances in surgical management progress, immediate passive and active motion are being used more commonly, especially in the presence of a complex injury. The three types of protocols vary in application of orthoses and exercises in the first 4 weeks following tendon repair during the early phase of tendon healing. After that time, the client is advanced according to the amount of limitation present. Traditionally, the physician determined the postoperative protocol and guided the advancement of rehabilitation. However, as our education, skill level, and visibility has advanced over the years, hand therapists are now taking a more collaborative role in this process. Factors to consider when choosing a protocol or advancing a program include the type, level, and complexity of injury, the strength of the repair, and client compliance, motivation, and health factors. Before reviewing the specific protocols for extensor tendon rehabilitation, it is important to understand the ways in which evaluation of range of motion (ROM) following extensor tendon repair is modified to protect the healing tendon throughout its stages of healing (Box 26.1), and the important concepts to remember when treating a repaired hand tendon (Box 26.2).

Rehabilitation: Early Phase

The early phase of tendon healing begins immediately upon repair and commences through the first 3 to 4 weeks following repair.

Immobilization Protocol

- Orthosis: When the repaired extensor tendon is treated with immobilization in the initial phase of tendon healing, a postoperative splint applied by the physician, a finger length cast, or a thermoplastic orthosis made in therapy is applied to hold the PIP joint in full extension. If the lateral bands were injured in addition to the EDC tendon, the DIP is held in full extension as well. The orthosis is worn full time until 3 to 4 weeks postoperatively (Fig. 26.5).
- Exercises: In an immobilization protocol, the repaired tendon is protected in extension at all times during the first 3 to 4 weeks. In the early phase of tendon healing, the client moves only the joints that are not restricted within the orthosis.

Immediate Passive Extension Protocol

- Indications: When dense adhesions are expected to limit gliding of the tendon, an immediate passive extension approach to rehabilitation may be prescribed. The goal of this approach is to achieve 5 mm of extensor tendon glide distally.

BOX 26.1 **Evaluation of Range of Motion Following Extensor Tendon Repair**

Extensor Tendon Repair
1. When initiating therapy in the early phase of healing after an extensor tendon repair, assess passive extension to 0 degrees at all finger joints and wrist extension passively as tolerated.
2. Do not assess active extension immediately following an extensor tendon repair unless an immediate active extension protocol is being used.
3. Do not assess finger flexion in the early phase of tendon healing, with the exception of 30-degree flexion when an immediate passive or active extension protocol is used. Awareness of the position that protects the tendon is essential when allowing controlled motion in the direction that will place tension on the repair.
4. In the intermediate phase of tendon healing, first evaluate the extensor tendon for flexion at each individual finger joint while supporting the other joints in extension. One to two weeks later, evaluate composite flexion of the fingers with the wrist in extension, and evaluate the wrist for flexion with the fingers relaxed.
5. At the completion of treatment, composite flexion of the fingers, subtracting any loss of active extension, gives the total active motion results for the injured digits.

BOX 26.2 **Concepts to Remember When Treating the Repaired Tendon in the Hand**

- Initial orthoses are designed to protect the repaired tendon by preventing tension of the tendon.
- Repaired tendons rupture from stretch or from active contraction by the muscle of the repaired tendon that is too strong for the repair to withstand.
- Three types of protocols are designed for all tendon repairs with the exception of extensor tendon zones I and II. These are, from the most conservative to least conservative: immobilization, immediate passive motion, and immediate active motion protocols.
- Motion, when initiated, is done gently. Motion is begun when the surgeon determines the repair and tensile strength of the tendon can withstand gentle motion.
- The better the active motion in the early to intermediate phase of tendon healing, the fewer adhesions are present. The fewer adhesions present, the longer resistance to the repaired tendon is delayed.
- Passive motion in the direction that would stretch the tendon repair is done for joint stiffness only with the tendon supported on slack in a protected position.
- Advancement from one phase of exercises to the next is done with the awareness of the referring surgeon.
- Resistance to the repaired tendon is deferred unless active motion is limited by adhesions in the intermediate phase of tendon healing.

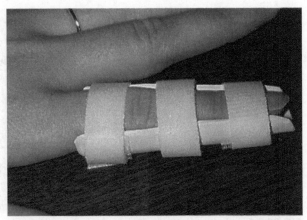

FIG. 26.5 Finger gutter, taped in place, used for immobilization following zone III to IV extensor tendon repairs, or between exercises in an immediate controlled active motion program.

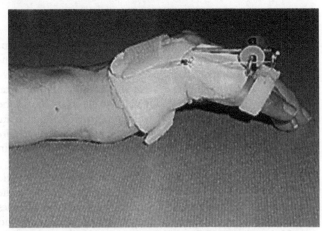

FIG. 26.6 Hand-based outrigger allowing 30 degrees of proximal interphalangeal joint flexion used in immediate controlled passive program for zone III to IV extensor tendon repairs.

- Orthosis: Within the first 3 days following repair, the therapist fabricates a hand-based extension outrigger orthosis that supports the MP joint and provides passive extension of the PIP joint (Fig. 26.6). The PIP joint is allowed to actively flex to only 30 degrees, with an elastic extension sling then bringing the PIP joint passively back to 0 degrees.[7] The outrigger holds the finger in full PIP extension at rest, between exercises.
- Exercises: Instruct the client to exercise hourly with the orthosis on at all times. The client performs 10 repetitions of active 30-degree PIP flexion followed by passive extension achieved by relaxing in the sling attachment. Flexion is limited to 30 degrees by a block on the outrigger line. The outrigger orthosis is left in place for the first 3 to 4 weeks. Some protocols allow a gradual increase in the number of degrees that the PIP is flexed during the 3- to 4-week period.[8] After 3 to 4 weeks, the orthosis is removed, and the client is allowed to flex to tolerance as discussed in the intermediate phase exercises that follow.

Precaution. *It is important to educate the client not to override the orthosis flexion block. Flexing further than instructed could rupture the extensor tendon repair.*

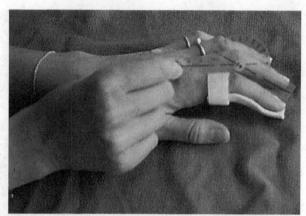

FIG. 26.7 Exercise template with 30 degrees of proximal interphalangeal joint flexion and 20 degrees of distal interphalangeal joint flexion used in an immediate controlled active motion program for zone III to IV repaired extensor tendon.

Immediate Active Extension Protocol

- Indications: An immediate active extension protocol is appropriate in the same situations as an immediate passive extension protocol and has the added benefit of more definitive proximal tendon gliding. This approach also promotes distal tendon gliding, as found in the passive approach. Begin the protocol within the first 3 days after repair. One immediate controlled active extension approach is known as the *short arc motion protocol (SAM protocol)*. It is described by Evans,[3,9] in the following paragraph.
- Orthoses: The SAM protocol calls for three thermoplastic gutter-style finger orthoses. The first orthosis supports the finger in full (0 degrees) PIP and DIP extension at all times except exercise. A second orthosis with 30 degrees of PIP and 20 degrees of DIP flexion is used as an exercise template (Fig. 26.7). A third, shorter orthosis holds the PIP joint in full extension and allows the DIP to flex to tolerance.
- Exercises: Hourly, the exercise template that allows 30-degree PIP and 20-degree DIP flexion is placed on the finger. The wrist is placed in 30-degree flexion to give slack to the flexor tendons, resulting in less resistance to active extension of the IP joints. With the finger gutter exercise template in place, the finger actively flexes to the exercise template and then actively extends at the IP joints. If the lateral bands are uninjured, the third shorter exercise orthosis is applied, and while holding the PIP joint in full extension, the DIP is actively flexed to tolerance. If the lateral bands were injured and repaired, the DIP joint is limited to 30-degree flexion during this exercise, which the client visually monitors. Brief but frequent exercises (10 to 20 repetitions hourly) are performed. At 2 weeks after repair, the exercise template is increased to 40-degree PIP flexion. At 3 weeks after repair, the exercise template is increased to allow 50-degree PIP flexion, and at 4 weeks, 70-degree PIP flexion. The exercises then progress into the intermediate phase of exercises.

Rehabilitation: Intermediate Phase

At 4 weeks, discontinue use of orthoses, and begin active flexion with individual joint flexion. Active finger flexion is likely to be most limited in the client who has been using an immobilization

protocol in the early phase of tendon healing. At 5 weeks, advance to gentle composite flexion. Heat may be used to warm the tissues before active exercises if swelling is not a significant issue.

Precaution. *Client education about exercise technique is very important. Early overly-aggressive flexion of the PIP joint may result in reinjury of the extensor tendon.*

> **◎ Clinical Pearl**
>
> The tendon that has been immobilized in the early phase of tendon healing is often limited by adhesions when it is time to move the finger. The temptation is to immediately apply force to help it move. However, motion must be initiated gradually, maintaining the ability to extend the finger while gradually regaining flexion.
>
> At 6 weeks, if active flexion is not showing steady, gradual progress, therapy may advance to use of passive flexion. Heat with support in flexion may assist in regaining composite flexion. Also, initiate grip strengthening at this time. A gentle dynamic or static progressive flexion orthosis may be used after 6 weeks following repair if flexion remains significantly limited. It is important to consult with the referring surgeon before applying an orthosis that applies force to the repair.

> **( ) What to Say to Clients**
>
> "We are now going to start moving the finger in a way that places a little stress on the repaired tendon. Because the tendon is not at full strength yet, it is important to do the motions slowly and to aim for a gradual increase in ability to bend the middle and tip joints. You don't want to force the finger down using an outside force (such as your other hand), or you may reinjure your tendon. We hope to see about 30 degrees of improvement each week, and make sure that you can keep straightening your finger. It is easier to get better at bending the finger but harder to regain the ability to straighten the finger once it is lost."

Diagnosis-Specific Information That Affects Clinical Reasoning

When an immediate passive or active extension protocol is used in the initial phase of healing, we expect fewer problems with achieving flexion in the intermediate phase of tendon healing.

Precaution. *If steady, gradual progress is being made with active flexion, defer passive flexion exercise or use of dynamic flexion orthoses until a plateau occurs to prevent excessive force to the healing extensor tendon that could result in rupture.*

Limited extension of the IP joints caused by **extensor tendon adhesion** (indicated by passive extension measuring more than active extension) is treated with use of a night extension orthosis, an emphasis on active extension exercises during the day, and less emphasis on strong flexion.

Because IP joint extension is performed most strongly by the lateral bands, it increases efficiency of the extensors to hold the MP joint in flexion while performing active IP extension. This is called *reverse blocking*. MP hyperextension should be avoided when performing IP extension exercises because MP hyperextension limits the ability of the EDC to assist in IP extension and decreases efficiency of the lateral bands.

The individual with an extensor tendon repair is often allowed to return to full use of the hand without restriction after 6 weeks postsurgery and may be discharged from therapy at this time if motion is functional and the client is advancing with a home exercise program (HEP). However, when strong adhesions are present, the finger may not achieve an acceptable level of motion during the intermediate phase of healing. When limited motion interferes with function, additional therapy is indicated.

Rehabilitation: Late Phase

From 8 to 12 weeks following extensor tendon repair, the client is usually allowed full normal use of the injured hand. In therapy, limited flexion should be treated with heat combined with stretch, passive and active flexion of individual joints, blocking exercises, composite flexion exercises, and grip strengthening. Static progressive or dynamic flexion orthoses can be used to supplement the HEP to increase flexion. Limited *active* IP extension should be treated with **reverse blocking exercises**, night IP extension gutter, and the addition of resistance to the repaired tendon. Resistance to extension facilitates a stronger proximal pull on the adherent extensor tendon to improve active extension. This is performed by applying reverse blocking with light manual resistance, or the client may extend the fingers against a loop of putty, resistive band strip, or rubber band. However, these exercises are only effective in improving gliding of the extensor tendon in zones III and IV if MP hyperextension is blocked during the exercise.

> ### ◎ Clinical Pearl
>
> Blocking the MP by use of a relative motion orthosis that holds the MP of the injured finger in slightly more flexion than adjacent fingers assists the force of the extensor tendon in transferring to the PIP joint. This position improves the effectiveness of PIP extension exercises.

If *passive* IP extension is limited, use of a dynamic IP extension orthosis intermittently during the day, and use of a night static extension orthosis is indicated.

Zones V, VI, and VII Extensor Tendon Injuries

Diagnosis and Pathology

Injuries in zones V, VI, and VII are most often due to lacerations. Another cause of injury to extensor tendons in zone VII is rupture from an inflammatory condition (such as rheumatoid arthritis) or fraying and rupture from a tendon repeatedly rubbing against a bony abnormality. Tendon injuries in these zones require surgical repair. Following repair, there are protocols for immobilization, immediate passive extension, and immediate active extension approaches from which to choose.

Rehabilitation: Early Phase

Immobilization Protocol

- Orthosis: Immobilization of extensor tendon repairs at and proximal to the MP joints requires a full-length resting cast or thermoplastic orthosis (Fig. 26.8). Some surgeons keep the client in a postoperative slab for the full 4 weeks; others have a thermoplastic orthosis fabricated in the therapy clinic. The

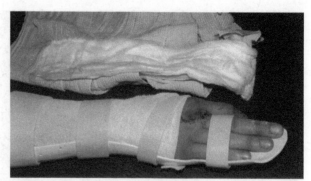

FIG. 26.8 Full-length resting pan extension orthosis used in an immobilization approach following repair in zone V to VII.

orthosis holds the wrist in slight extension and the digits in full extension. Some surgeons prefer slight MP flexion (20 degrees) in the orthosis; however, this may result in an MP extension lag.[3] When the repair is proximal to the juncturae tendinum on the dorsum of the hand, the tendons on either side of the injured tendon must be supported in extension along with the injured tendon. If the repair is over the MP joint, distal to the juncturae tendinum, the finger with the repaired tendon should be held in full extension, but the adjacent MPs may be positioned in 30-degree flexion or allowed to flex to tolerance. Flexion of the adjacent fingers, when the repair is distal to the juncturae tendinum, pulls the proximal portion of the repaired tendon distally, reducing tension on the repair.

- Exercises: When using an immobilization protocol, hand and wrist exercises begin in the intermediate phase of tendon healing at approximately 4 weeks after repair.

Immediate Passive Extension Protocol

- Indications: Immediate passive extension may be used for complex injuries, multiple tendon injuries, injuries under the extensor retinaculum at the wrist, or when preferred by the surgeon and therapist. The most frequently used immediate controlled passive extension program was developed by Evans, who recommends immediate motion for all extensor tendon repairs proximal to zones I and II.[3,10] Because finger extensor tendons in zone VII and thumb extensor tendons in zone V are in the area of the extensor retinaculum, repairs here are prone to problematic adhesion formation. Evans recommends a rehabilitation approach using immediate passive or active motion to minimize adhesions. Results comparing immobilization to the immediate passive and active extension approaches show a significant improvement in tendon gliding using the immediate motion programs.[3,10]

The immediate passive extension protocol is initiated within 3 days following surgical repair.[3,10]

- Orthosis: The orthosis for immediate passive extension supports the wrist in slight extension and consists of an extension outrigger that holds the injured fingers in full extension at rest, while allowing only 30 degrees of MP flexion at the index and long and up to 40 degrees of MP flexion at the ring and small fingers during exercise (Fig. 26.9). MP flexion may be blocked by a volar orthosis or by a stop bead placed on the outrigger line. The orthosis is worn full time for the first 3 weeks after repair. It is removed in the therapy clinic only for cleansing the orthosis and skin. Many clients note that it is difficult to sleep and get dressed with the dorsal

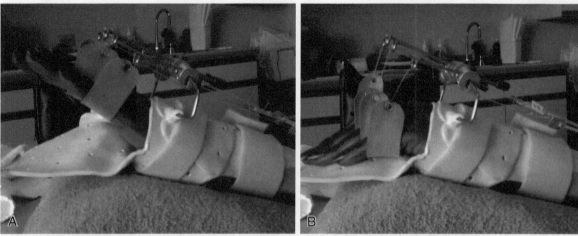

FIG. 26.9 (A) Dynamic metacarpophalangeal (MP) extension outrigger allowing 30-degree MP joint flexion. **(B)** Active flexion within the immediate passive extension orthosis is blocked at 30 degrees by a volar portion of the orthosis base. Used in an immediate passive program following extensor tendon repair in zones V to VII.

outrigger in place. In these cases a night resting pan extension orthosis may also be fabricated, allowing the dorsal outrigger orthosis to be removed for sleeping and getting dressed.[3]

Precaution. *The client must understand the potential risk of rupture if the orthosis is removed and the finger is allowed to flex too far.*

- Exercises: Instruct the client to actively move the fingers, using only MP flexion, to the orthosis stop (30–40 degrees) and then to relax the fingers. When the fingers are relaxed, the sling attachments on the outrigger move the fingers passively back to full (0 degrees) extension. MP flexion of 30 to 40 degrees results in 5 mm of extensor tendon distal glide, which reduces the risk for dense adhesions like those that occur with immobilization. The IP joints of the fingers can also be flexed gently through their full available range with the MP and wrist joints supported in full extension. Ten to twenty repetitions of these exercises are performed every hour. At 3 weeks following repair, remove the flexion block from the orthosis and allow the client to flex fingers to tolerance. The client should continue to perform only passive extension for another 2 to 3 weeks, allowing the outrigger slings to move the fingers back to full extension.
- Passive wrist tenodesis exercises are only performed with the therapist in the clinic, as follows: The therapist passively extends the client's wrist fully while allowing the MPs to relax to 40-degree flexion (therapist supports the fingers manually to prevent too much flexion); then the therapist passively lifts the fingers to full extension while allowing the wrist to flex to 20 degrees.
- This protocol can be applied to a lacerated EPL tendon following repair in thumb extensor zone V.[3] The orthosis holds the wrist and the thumb MP and CMC joints in extension while an outrigger and sling support to the IP joint. The IP joint is allowed to flex 60 degrees to attain 5 mm of tendon gliding in thumb extensor zone V (under the retinaculum). The passive wrist tenodesis exercise following thumb extensor tendon repair in zone V is performed by the therapist as follows: Support the wrist at 0 degrees, and hold all joints of the thumb in full extension. Then, relax the thumb and passively extend the wrist to full extension.
- At 3 to 4 weeks following repair, exercises are advanced to allow removal of the orthosis and gradual active flexion at

each individual joint of the thumb and wrist while all other joints are held in extension. The orthosis can be removed for careful showering and exercises, but is worn at all other times until 5 to 6 weeks following repair.

Immediate Active Extension Protocol

- Indications: Evans[3,10] has described an immediate active extension program for repairs in zones V to VII that is performed only in the clinic with the therapist. She states that the program can be used for any extensor tendon repair, but is especially suited for repairs that are considered complex, and those under the extensor retinaculum at the wrist. Howell, Merritt, and Robinson[11] describe another immediate active extension protocol for repairs in zones IV to VII that controls motion using a relative motion orthosis. This protocol has received positive reviews in recent publications and has been used to treat other extensor tendon conditions such as sagittal band injury and boutonniere deformity.[14,15,16]
- Orthoses and exercise using these two protocols:

Immediate Controlled Active Motion Program designed by Evans: The immediate active rehabilitation approach described by Evans and Thompson[3,10] is appropriate for extensor tendon repairs in zones V to VII. It uses the same outrigger orthosis as described in the immediate passive extension program. The client wears the orthosis at all times except during exercise sessions with the therapist. The orthosis is removed only in the therapy clinic for the active motion portion of the exercise program, as follows. The therapist performs slow, repetitive wrist/MP tenodesis motion on the client, as described in the passive motion protocol, until passive motion offers minimal resistance (decreases stiffness and effects of edema). The active hold portion of the exercise is then performed by supporting the client's fingers in full extension and allowing the wrist to flex 20 degrees. The client is then asked to hold the fingers actively in this position of extension for a few seconds. The MP joints are then allowed to flex to 30 degrees and actively extend back to 0 degrees with the wrist supported in 20-degree flexion. This is performed for 20 repetitions.

Immediate Controlled Active Motion using Relative Motion Orthotic Positioning: This program described by Howell, Merritt, and Robinson[3,11] is appropriate for repairs in zones IV to

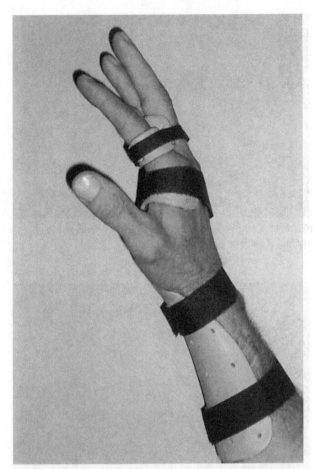

FIG. 26.10 Immediate controlled active motion orthosis using wrist support and yoke. Also referred to as a relative motion orthosis. *(From Howell JW, Merritt WH, Robinson SJ. Immediate controlled active motion following zone 4-7 extensor tendon repair. J Hand Ther. 2005;18[2]:182.)*

VII. Within the first 5 to 10 days after surgical repair, a two-piece orthosis is fabricated. One component of the orthosis is a volar wrist support that holds the wrist in 20- to 25-degree extension. The second component of the orthosis is a yoke that is made from a long, thin piece of thermoplastic material, which is the width of the proximal phalanx and 1.5 times the length of the dorsum of the hand across the metacarpals. This yoke is wrapped under the injured fingers and over the uninjured fingers to support the injured fingers in 15 to 20 degrees of relative MP hyperextension compared with the adjacent fingers. This is called a *relative motion orthosis* (Fig. 26.10). When multiple digits are injured, there are specific recommended methods of supporting the injured fingers in the reference.

Full active composite flexion and extension as available within the orthosis are performed the first 3 weeks following extensor tendon repair. The client wears the orthosis full time during these 3 weeks. At 3 weeks following surgery, the client removes the wrist component of the orthosis to allow gentle wrist ROM with only the yoke component of the orthosis in place. However, the client continues to wear the wrist and yoke combination for moderate to heavy activities until 5 weeks after repair. Between 5 and 7 weeks, the client wears only the yoke component of the orthosis. Most clients were discharged from therapy at 7 weeks postoperatively, with more than 90% of clients reporting good to excellent results.[3,10,11]

Rehabilitation: Intermediate Phase

Orthoses

At 4 weeks following repair and immobilization, the protective orthosis is used only intermittently during work and heavy activities, and is gradually discontinued. If extension is limited, a night resting pan orthosis in full extension is indicated.

When extensor tendon repair is followed by an immediate active or passive extension protocol, the orthosis described under those protocols may be continued until week 6 to 7 (as described earlier).

Exercises

At 4 weeks following repair of extensor tendons in zones V, VI, and VII, a gradual increase in active flexion for individual joints is allowed as follows:
- MP flexion with IP joints extended
- IP flexion with MP joints extended
- Wrist flexion with fingers extended

Modalities may include heat of choice to decrease stiffness if not otherwise contraindicated.

At week 5 or 6, begin composite flexion of fingers. Gentle passive flexion may be added if flexion is significantly limited. Support the fingers in a flexion wrap to tolerance, and apply heat as appropriate. At 6 to 7 weeks, composite flexion of wrist/fingers may be added.

Diagnosis-Specific Information That Affects Clinical Reasoning

When active MP extension is limited because of adhesions in zone V, VI, or VII, an extensor lag results in which passive extension exceeds active extension. In addition to an extension orthosis at night, active extension exercises are important to place proximal tension on the adhesion to improve proximal gliding of the adherent tendon.

Regaining full composite digital extension, which requires a balance of EDC and intrinsic muscle function, may be even more challenging. Supporting the finger in full passive extension, such as on a table, and attempting to actively lift the limited finger up from the table can facilitate this motion. When the repaired EDC is adherent, clients may be unsuccessful in lifting the finger up from the table, but they can often feel the proximal tugging of the extensor tendon on the dorsal hand. This facilitates proximal gliding of the tendon and provides feedback to clients that they are using the correct muscle/tendon. If clients flex the MP joints during this exercise rather than use the EDC to attempt to lift the MP joint, they will feel increased pressure on the table at the fingertip, providing feedback that they are using the wrong muscles.

> **Ⓒ Clinical Pearl**
>
> The most effective way to improve active MP extension is to work on this motion with the IP joints flexed or relaxed. When the MP joint is limited in active extension and the client attempts to extend the entire finger actively, the intrinsic muscles often work first, for they are not limited by adhesions. Because the intrinsic muscles perform IP extension with MP flexion, they will be ineffective in performing MP extension, defeating the purpose of the exercise. Isolated MP extension is achieved with the IP joints relaxed in flexion. It is the most successful way to improve proximal gliding of adherent EDC tendons proximal to the MP joint.

Rehabilitation: Late Phase

Continue with exercises to maximize proximal and distal gliding of the extensor tendon as described for the intermediate phase exercises. Add grip strengthening and progressive functional upper extremity exercise at 6 weeks following repair. For flexion deficits, add a dynamic or static progressive flexion orthosis used intermittently during the day beginning at 6 to 8 weeks after repair, and as approved by the surgeon.

CASE STUDIES

Case Study 26.1

EE, a 53-year-old meat cutter, sustained a work-related saw injury of the dorsal right small finger while cutting meat. He was seen at an emergency room at a workmen's compensation clinic associated with the workplace. He developed an infection, was treated with intravenously administered antibiotics, and was referred to the hand surgeon 8 days after injury. Surgery was performed 9 days after injury, and exploration showed a ragged laceration extending into the extensor mechanism, including the central slip. The saw also had removed part of the dorsal condyle and articular surface of the PIP joint. The central slip was repaired, and the PIP joint was pinned in almost full extension (Fig. 26.11).

EE was referred to therapy 10 days after repair for fabrication of a thermoplastic orthosis to support the wrist in neutral and the ring and small fingers in extension and to protect the pin (Fig. 26.12). The surgeon chose full support and immobilization because of the combination of bone and tendon injury, history of infection, and questionable level of understanding and compliance by the client.

The pin was removed 4 weeks after surgery, and active therapy was initiated three times per week. For the first week, use of the orthosis was continued between bathing and exercises. Beginning the second week (5 weeks postoperatively), the orthosis was used only when EE was out of the house until 6 weeks after surgery. Initial ROM of individual joints was 0 to 50 degrees for MP joints, –15 to 20 degrees for PIP joints, and 0 to 5 degrees for DIP joints. Wrist motion was present through 75% of normal range. EE was instructed in a HEP for active individual joint flexion, reverse blocking extension exercises, and passive extension. Because of extreme limitations in motion, exercises were advanced to include active composite flexion and gentle passive flexion of individual joints within a week of starting therapy. After 1 week, active ROM was 0 to 60 degrees for MP joints, –25 to 40 degrees for PIP joints, and 0 to 10 degrees for DIP joints. Passive extension was to –5 degrees at the PIP joint.

The client returned to light duty wrapping meat at 5 weeks after surgery while wearing the protective orthosis. Therapy consisted of wrapping the fingers in flexion to tolerance with a heat application, followed by active and passive flexion and extension exercises, reverse blocking exercises, and functional grasp and release activities. Buddy straps from small to ring finger were provided in an attempt to improve motion of the small finger. ROM at 6 weeks after repair was 0 to 75 degrees for MP joints, –30 to 55 degrees for PIP joints, and 0 to 10 degrees for DIP joints. Passive extension was available to –5 degrees at the PIP joint, indicating extensor tendon adhesions. Active motion improvements stalled at this time. Improvements of 10 degrees of flexion at each

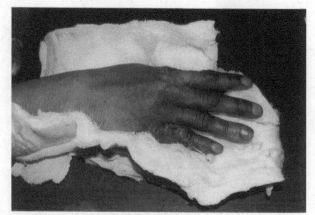

FIG. 26.11 Complex extensor tendon injury in zones III and IV requiring repair and pin support.

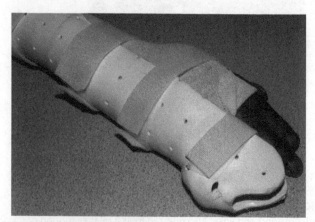

FIG. 26.12 Full-length extension ulnar gutter orthosis for protection of pin and tendon repair.

joint would be made in therapy; however, the client would arrive in therapy with the same limitations in motion as the previous session. At 8 weeks after injury, functional strengthening was initiated, and putty was provided for resistance exercises at home in addition to active and passive home exercises.

The diagnosis of posttraumatic arthritis of the PIP joint was made by radiographic evaluation 11 weeks after surgery. Therapy was discontinued at this time with ROM of 0 to 90 degrees for MP joints, –25 to 60 degrees for PIP joints, and 0 to 25 degrees for DIP joints at the end of a session. The surgeon will continue to follow the client for motion and function of the small finger and hand and will make a determination in the future regarding the potential benefit of further surgery, including extensor tenolysis to remove tendinous adhesions.

This case demonstrates the difficulty of regaining flexion and extension of the IP joints with a complex injury when dense adhesions form between the extensor tendon, surrounding tissue, and bone in zones III and IV. An immediate motion protocol, which may have prevented the limiting adhesions, was not considered because of the involvement of injury to the bone at the articular surface and because of client understanding and compliance issues. This case shows that when this combination of factors exists, it may be necessary to immobilize the digit and accept an intact tendon with adhesions, recognizing the potential need for further surgery to improve motion and function.

References

1. Rosenthal EA, Elhassan BT: The extensor tendons: evaluation and surgical management. In Skirven TM, Osterman AL, Fedorczyk JM, et al.: *Rehabilitation of the hand and upper extremity*, ed 6, Philadelphia, 2011, Elsevier Mosby, pp 487–520.
2. Newport ML, Tucker RL: New perspectives on extensor tendon repair and implications for rehabilitation, *J Hand Ther* 18(2):175–181, 2005.
3. Evans RB: Clinical management of extensor tendon injuries: the therapist's perspective. In Skirven TM, Osterman AL, Fedorczyk JM, et al.: *Rehabilitation of the hand and upper extremity*, ed 6, Philadelphia, 2011, Elsevier Mosby, pp 521–554.
4. Mowlavi A, Burns M, Brown RE: Dynamic vs. static splinting of simple zone V and zone VI extensor tendon repairs: a prospective, randomized, controlled study, *Plast and Recon Surg* 115(2):482–487, 2005.
5. Talsma E, de Haart M, Beelen A, et al.: The effect of mobilization on repaired extensor tendon injuries of the hand: a systematic review, *Arch Phys Med Rehabil* 89:2366–2372, 2008.
6. Hall B, Lee H, Page R, et al.: Comparing three postoperative treatment protocols for extensor tendon repairs in zones V and VI of the hand, *Am J Occup Ther* 64(5):682–688, 2010.
7. Walsh MT, Rinehimer W, Muntzer E, et al.: Early controlled motion with dynamic splinting versus static splinting for zones III and IV extensor tendon lacerations: a preliminary report, *J Hand Ther* 7(4):232–236, 1994.
8. Thomes LJ: Early mobilization method for surgically repaired zone III extensor tendons, *J Hand Ther* 8(3):195–198, 1995.
9. Evans RE: An analysis of factors that support early active short arc motion of the repaired central slip, *J Hand Ther* 5(4):187–201, 1992.
10. Evans RE, Thompson DE: The application of force to the healing tendon, *J Hand Ther* 6(4):266–284, 1993.
11. Howell JW, Merritt WH, Robinson SJ: Immediate controlled active motion following zone 4-7 extensor tendon repair, *J Hand Ther* 18(2):182–190, 2005.
12. Lee SK, Dubey A, Kim BY, et al.: A biomechanical study of extensor tendon repair methods: introduction to the running-interlocking horizontal mattress extensor tendon repair technique, *J Hand Surg Am* 35:19–23, 2010.
13. Newport ML, Williams CD: Biomechanical characteristics of extensor tendon suture techniques, *J Hand Surg Am* 17(6):1117–1123, 1992.
14. Merritt WH: Relative motion splint; active motion after extensor tendon injury and repair, *J Hand Surg Am* 39(6):1187–1194, 2014.
15. Burns MC, Derby B, Neumeister MW: Wyndell merritt immediate controlled active motion (ICAM) protocol following extensor tendon repairs in zone IV-VII: review of literature, orthosis design, and case study – a multimedia article, *Hand (N Y)*. 8(1):17–22, 2013.
16. Hirth MJ, Howell JW, O'Brien L: Relative motion orthoses in the management of various hand conditions: a scoping review, *J Hand Ther* 29(4):405–432, 2016.

27

Flexor Tendon Injury

Linda J. Klein

Flexor tendon repair and rehabilitation have posed challenges to surgeons and therapists for decades. Flexor tendons are required to glide large distances to allow the digits full composite flexion and extension, running within a tight pulley system to maximize their efficiency (Fig. 27.1). Following repair, **flexor tendon adhesions** develop quickly because the tendon becomes adherent to surrounding tissue due to scar formation, especially when repaired within the pulley system. Once adherent, the flexor tendon does not glide as needed to perform active flexion, functionally limiting active range of motion (AROM) more than passive range of motion (PROM). Fewer adhesions would occur if the tendon were allowed to glide immediately after surgery, but this approach historically resulted in rupture of the tendon repair. A large number of solutions have been attempted over the past 50 years, resulting in numerous approaches to flexor tendon repair and rehabilitation. The challenging goal has been to improve flexor tendon gliding by minimizing adhesion formation to the tendon while avoiding rupture of the repaired tendon.

This chapter helps the therapist gain an understanding of the rationale behind the various approaches to flexor tendon management. Physician and therapist communication is necessary to determine the most appropriate approach for each client. Close supervision by an experienced hand therapist is essential.

Anatomy

The extrinsic flexor tendons to the digits enter the hand through the carpal tunnel. They are comprised of the flexor digitorum superficialis (FDS) for each finger, flexor digitorum profundus (FDP) for each finger, and flexor pollicis longus (FPL) to the thumb. The FDP tendons are deep to the FDS tendons in the forearm, wrist, and hand. At the level of the proximal phalanx, the FDS tendon separates, becoming two separate slips, which then re-converge just before attachment on the middle phalanx (Fig. 27.2). The FDS flexes the metacarpophalangeal (MP) and proximal interphalangeal (PIP) joints. The FDP tendon emerges through the separation of the FDS tendon at the level of the proximal phalanx and continues distally to insert on the distal phalanx. The FDP tendon is the sole tendon responsible for distal interphalangeal (DIP) flexion of the finger. In the thumb, the FPL tendon inserts on the distal phalanx and is the sole flexor of the thumb interphalangeal (IP) joint.

As the flexor tendons run under the retinaculum and transverse carpal ligament at the wrist and palm, they are surrounded by a **synovial bursa**, which is a sheath filled with synovial fluid that allows tendon gliding without excess friction (see Fig. 27.1). A synovial sheath also surrounds the flexor tendons in the digit, where they run under a series of pulleys that prevent the flexors from bowstringing as active flexion occurs (see Fig. 27.1). Bowstringing occurs when the pulleys are not intact and the flexor tendon is pulled away from the bone with a muscle contraction, rather than being efficiently pulled proximally. Pulleys hold the flexor tendon snugly to the bone and allow efficient proximal glide of the flexor tendon when the muscle contracts.

Diagnosis and Pathology

Pathology of the flexor tendon occurs most often by traumatic injury, either by open laceration or closed rupture. The open laceration may be complete or partial; it may include loss of tendon length; and it may be a clean laceration, jagged tear, or cut with frayed ends. The wound may be clean or dirty. Associated pulley injuries and ligament, nerve, bone, or vessel injuries may have occurred, increasing the complexity of repair. Ideally,

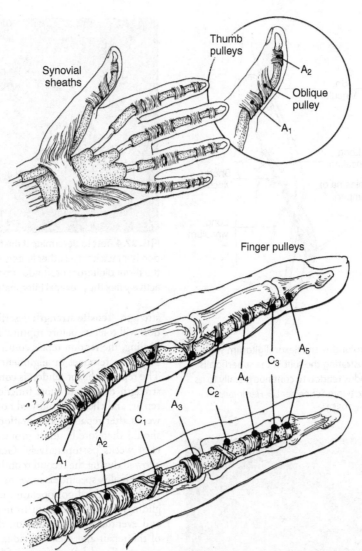

FIG. 27.1 Flexor tendon anatomy illustrating the synovial lining around the tendons within the pulley systems at the wrist and within the digits. Fingers have five annular pulleys (designated A in the image) and three cruciate pulleys (C in the image). The thumb has two annular pulleys and one oblique pulley. (From Chase RA. *Atlas of Hand Surgery.* Vol 2. Philadelphia, PA: WB Saunders; 1984.)

repair of the tendon and associated structures is performed as soon after the injury as possible, often in the emergency room. Occasionally, a client presents to the physician's office indicating that their "finger doesn't work" due to a previous injury in which the flexor tendon injury may have been missed or because the client did not seek medical care at the time of the injury. Flexor tendon injuries that are repaired late must often be treated with a flexor tendon graft or with a salvage procedure.

Closed traumatic injuries of the flexor tendon occur most often to the FDP tendon, due to a rupture from its attachment on the volar surface of the distal phalanx. This injury occurs as the flexed fingertip is extended forcefully, causing rupture of the FDP from the bone or an avulsion fracture. It is also known as **"jersey finger"** because it is seen in football players holding the jersey of a player attempting to break the grasp by pulling away.

To diagnose if the FDP tendon is intact, hold the finger below the DIP joint and ask the client to bend the tip of the finger (Fig. 27.3). Because the FDP is the only flexor tendon to cross the DIP joint, active DIP flexion indicates that the FDP tendon is intact.

To diagnose whether the FDS tendon is intact, the action of the FDP must be eliminated so that it does not assist with flexion at the PIP joint. To eliminate the action of the FDP at the PIP joint and isolate the FDS, manually hold all the other fingers completely straight and ask the client to flex the PIP joint of the finger being tested (Fig. 27.4). The DIP joint of the finger being tested should be relaxed and without tension if the FDP action is successfully eliminated.

Timelines and Healing

Flexor tendons retract after laceration or rupture, and surgical repair is necessary to regain active motion. The tendon gradually heals after repair by both intrinsic and extrinsic means. The blood supply to the tendon enters from the dorsal surface of the tendon through vinculae supplied by the digital arteries (see Fig. 27.2). Flexor tendons are relatively avascular between these vinculae and on the volar surface of the tendon. The vinculae may be damaged during the injury or repair. Lacerated flexor tendons in the digit

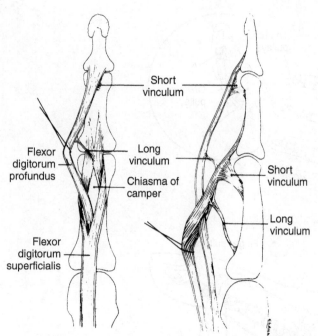

FIG. 27.2 Flexor digitorum profundus and flexor digitorum superficialis anatomy in the digit illustrating the split in the superficialis tendon that allows the profundus tendon to continue distally to its insertion on the distal phalanx. (From Schneider LH. *Flexor Tendon Injuries.* Boston, MA: Little Brown; 1985.)

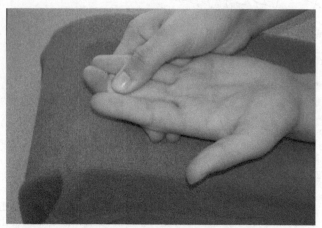

FIG. 27.3 Test to determine if flexor digitorum profundus is intact: hold below the distal interphalangeal (DIP) joint, and ask the client to actively flex the DIP joint.

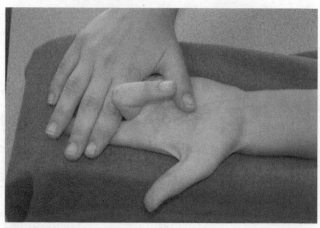

FIG. 27.4 Test to determine if the flexor digitorum superficialis tendon is intact: hold all other fingers in complete extension to prevent the flexor digitorum profundus from assisting, and ask the client to actively flex the proximal interphalangeal joint.

were initially thought to require blood supply from adhesions in order to heal following repair (extrinsic healing). Research has since shown that repaired flexor tendons have the ability to heal by nutrition from direct blood supply and from diffusion of nutrients in the synovial fluid that surrounds the tendons within the pulley system (intrinsic healing).[1]

Tendon phases of healing overlap and include the **inflammatory phase** (0–1 week following repair); the **fibroplasia phase**, or reparative phase (1–6 weeks following repair); and the remodeling phase (more than 6 weeks following repair).[2] During the inflammatory phase, the tendon is at its weakest and collagen is just beginning to be laid down at the repair site. The intermediate phase of tendon healing is when the tendon repair gains tensile strength. **Tensile strength** describes the amount of force the tendon will tolerate before rupture. During the late phase of tendon healing, the tendon repair continues to gain tensile strength and begins to remodel in alignment with the tension placed on it. The repaired flexor tendon is considered to have adequate tensile strength to tolerate most functional activities at 12 weeks after repair, and clients are allowed normal use of the hand at 12 to 14 weeks after repair. Rehabilitation following flexor tendon repair should therefore be most protective of the repair for the first 3 to 4 weeks postoperatively. Gradual increase of force may be allowed during the second month if active motion is initially limited. Finally, specific exercises to assist the remodeling process are used in the third postoperative month if adhesions limit tendon gliding. The advancement from passive flexion to active flexion and eventually resisted flexion depends on the tensile strength of the repair and each individual's tissue response to injury and surgery. See the Progression of Exercises section of this chapter for specific guidelines.

Operative Treatment

Flexor tendon repair techniques have been changing for the past few decades. Historically, outcomes of flexor tendon repairs in the digit have been plagued by poor results because of adhesions or, if early active motion was attempted, rupture. Numerous studies have investigated suture materials and techniques to determine the best way to create a repair strong enough to tolerate immediate stress on the flexor tendon and obtain gliding while minimizing adhesions, without rupture.[3-10] When lacerated, the flexor tendon ends are approximated (brought together) and sutured with the technique of choice while attempting to maintain as much of the pulley system as possible. The A2 and A4 pulleys are the most important to preserve to prevent bowstringing.

When the FDP has ruptured from its distal phalanx attachment or is lacerated within 1 cm of its distal attachment, the surgeon performs advancement and reinsertion of the tendon.[9] In this situation, the FDP tendon is sewn back to the bone using a suture that extends through the tendon into the distal phalanx. This suture is attached to the bone with an anchor, or the suture is brought dorsally all the way through the bone and

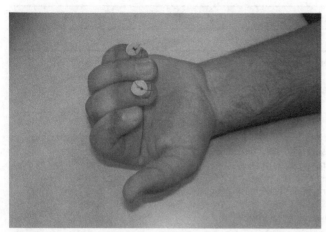

FIG. 27.5 Suture over a button placed on the nail of a client that has undergone advancement and reinsertion of the flexor digitorum profundus to the bone in multiple fingers.

nail, where it is knotted over a button placed on the nail (Fig. 27.5). Repair of the FPL to the thumb is performed in a similar manner.

Digital nerve injuries occur frequently when a flexor tendon is lacerated. When a digital nerve repair has been performed, talk to the surgeon about the possible need to block the IP joint in slight flexion within the orthosis for the first 2 to 3 weeks postoperatively to prevent tension on the nerve repair.

Research shows that, in general, the more strands of suture material that cross the tendon repair, the stronger the repair.[3,10] The traditional suture repair technique consists of a two-strand repair, meaning that two strands of suture material cross the repair site. This type of repair tolerates application of an immobilization protocol or **immediate passive motion protocol** in the early phase of tendon healing, but it is not shown to be sufficiently strong enough to consistently tolerate **immediate active motion protocols** following a flexor tendon repair. A four-strand repair has been shown to tolerate immediate gentle active motion.[3] Repairs of six or more strands certainly will tolerate immediate gentle active motion; however, these repairs are technically demanding and may become so bulky as to prevent gliding under the pulleys and create friction, possible wearing, and potential rupture. Thus a four-strand suture technique is commonly used for flexor tendon repair in which an immediate active motion protocol is applied, although some surgeons are electing to perform repairs with six or more strands.[11] **Precaution.** *The hand therapist must know the number of suture strands used in the repair of a flexor tendon before determining what type of motion protocol may be appropriate for rehabilitation.*

Postoperatively, flexor tendon rehabilitation poses a challenge due to dense flexor tendon adhesions that occur within the flexor pulley system of the digit in zones 1 and 2. Flexor tendon zones of the hand are shown in Fig. 27.6. Three basic approaches to rehabilitation of the repaired flexor tendon in the hand are: (1) immobilization; (2) immediate passive motion in the direction of the repaired tendon; and (3) immediate active motion in the direction of the repaired tendon. The main difference in these approaches occurs in the early phase (first month) of tendon rehabilitation. All flexor tendon approaches protect the flexor tendon repair with some version of a dorsal blocking orthosis that flexes the wrist and/or MP joints to protect the repaired tendon from excessive stretch

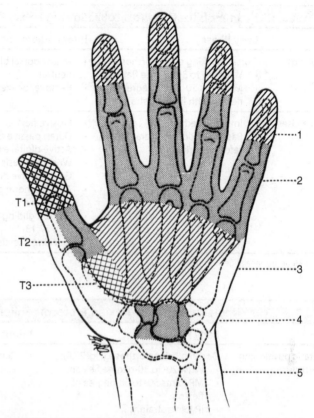

FIG. 27.6 Flexor tendon zones in the hand. (From Kleinert HE, Schepel S, Gill T. Flexor tendon injuries. *Surg Clin North Am.* 1981;61:267.)

BOX 27.1   Overview of Orthoses Used for Flexor Tendon Repairs in the Early Phase of Tendon Healing

Immobilization
- Dorsal blocking orthosis or cast

Immediate Passive Flexion
- Dorsal blocking orthosis with static interphalangeal positioning (Fig. 27.8)
- Dorsal blocking orthosis with elastic traction (Fig. 27.9)

Immediate Active Flexion
- Dorsal blocking orthosis with metacarpophalangeal (MP) and wrist flexion, static for protection at rest (Fig. 27.10B)
- Wrist hinge orthosis for exercise (Indiana protocol, Fig. 27.10A)
- Dorsal blocking orthosis with elastic traction, wrist neutral, for protection and home exercises (Klein protocol, Fig. 27.11)
- Dorsal blocking orthosis with MP and wrist flexion, with elastic traction, removed in therapy only for active component of exercise (Evans protocol)

until approximately 6 weeks postoperatively. Box 27.1 summarizes the orthoses used in the early phase of rehabilitation for various approaches following flexor tendon repair. The orthoses and exercises for each phase of healing are presented in Table 27.1 through Table 27.3.

TABLE 27.1   Immobilization Protocol Following Flexor Tendon Repair

	Early Phase	Intermediate Phase	Late Phase
Orthosis	Dorsal blocking cast or orthosis • Wrist 20- to 30-degree flexion • MP joints 50- to 60-degree flexion with IP joints straight	• Adjust dorsal blocking orthosis to wrist neutral • Remove for exercises	• No protective orthosis • Orthosis for extension at night, if needed
Exercises	• Immobilized • Passive flexion by therapist if referred early	• Passive flexion • Duran passive exercises (Fig. 27.7) • Active digital extension with wrist flexed • Wrist tenodesis exercise • Gentle active digital flexion • Assess tendon gliding at 3 weeks; if adherent, add: • Tendon gliding with straight and hook fist (Fig. 27.13) • Blocking exercises	Add the following: • Full active flexion and extension • Blocking • Light resistance

MP, Metacarpophalangeal; *IP*, interphalangeal.

TABLE 27.2   Immediate Passive Flexion Protocols Following Flexor Tendon Repair

	Early Phase	Intermediate Phase	Late Phase
Static positioning orthosis	Dorsal blocking orthosis (Fig. 27.8): • Wrist 20- to 30-degree flexion • MP joints 50- to 60-degree of flexion • IP joints straight	• Remove orthosis for bathing and exercises	• No protective orthosis • Add night extension orthotic if loss of extension
Elastic traction orthosis	• Same as static positioning orthosis, but add the following: • Elastic traction to fingertips during day (Fig. 27.9)	• Remove elastic traction from fingertips • Remove orthosis for bathing and exercises	• No protective orthosis • Add night extension orthosis if loss of extension
Exercises	• Passive flexion • Duran passive exercises (Fig. 27.7) • Active IP extension in orthosis	Remove orthosis, and add the following: • Wrist tenodesis • Place and active hold digital flexion • Gentle active digital flexion • Finger extension with wrist flexed, gradually bring wrist to neutral • Assess tendon gliding • If adherent, add gentle blocking and tendon gliding	Add the following: • Finger extension with wrist neutral, gradually extend wrist • Light resistance if adherent; if minimal adhesions, delay resistance until 8–12 weeks • Passive IP extension if needed

MP, Metacarpophalangeal; *IP*, interphalangeal.

TABLE 27.3   Immediate Active Flexion Protocols Following Flexor Tendon Repair

	Early Phase	Intermediate Phase	Late Phase
Orthosis options	• Wrist tenodesis orthosis and static dorsal blocking orthosis (Fig. 27.10) • Dorsal blocking orthosis wrist neutral, with or without elastic traction (Fig. 27.11)	• Continue orthosis wear to 6 weeks; if elastic traction was used, discontinue at 4 weeks	• No orthosis, or hand-based dorsal blocking orthosis during heavy activities, work • Dynamic IP extension orthosis after 8–10 weeks if IP flexion contracture exists
Exercises	• Wrist tenodesis • Passive digital flexion • Active IP extension with MP joints flexed • Place and active hold in flexion	• Continue with early-phase exercises, add the following: • Gentle active flexion • Straight fist (Fig. 27.13) • Composite fist • Blocking if adhesions present • Passive IP extension if needed	• Continue with intermediate phase exercises, and add the following: • Hook fist (Fig. 27.13) • Light gripping at 8 weeks if adhesions present, delay if good to excellent tendon gliding

MP, Metacarpophalangeal; *IP*, interphalangeal.

Rehabilitation of Flexor Tendon Repairs

Immobilization Approach

An immobilization approach[12,13] is rarely applied following flexor tendon repair in the digit, but there are certain situations in which it is appropriate. Children younger than age 12 are most often placed in immobilization for the first 3 to 4 weeks, but the therapist and surgeon should evaluate each child's maturity level and ability to comply with the exercises and precautions of alternative approaches. An immobilization approach might be used with other clients unlikely to adhere to the plan of care and with people who have cognitive limitations such as dementia.

When there is a concomitant fracture or significant loss of skin requiring a skin graft, a period of immobilization may be necessary to allow the bone or skin graft to heal adequately before beginning motion.

> **◎ Clinical Pearl**
>
> In the early phase of rehabilitation using an immobilization approach, no active contraction of the repaired flexor musculotendinous unit is allowed. Therefore limited, if any, gliding of the flexor tendon occurs.

Flexor tendon adhesions and joint stiffness are common complications following immobilization in the early phase of flexor tendon rehabilitation. General guidelines for orthoses and exercises within an immobilization approach are summarized in Table 27.1.

Immediate Passive Flexion Approach

Immediate passive flexion protocols,[13-16] developed in the 1960s and 1970s, were the treatment of choice for decades in an attempt to minimize dense adhesions that develop within zone 2. In a study of practice patterns published in 2005,[17] 74% of therapists utilized some type of immediate passive flexion approach for flexor tendon repair rehabilitation. The therapist should initiate an immediate passive flexion protocol within 3 to 4 days following a traditional two-strand flexor tendon repair. Sometimes, stronger (four or more strands) repairs are performed, and the client is placed in a passive flexion approach program due to healing factors or client adherence issues that prohibit placement in an immediate active flexion approach.

The therapist should fabricate a dorsal blocking orthosis that holds the wrist and MP joints in flexion and IP joints in extension to prevent excessive tension on the repaired tendon(s). Instruct the client to passively flex the fingers using Duran and Houser's technique designed to improve tendon gliding (Fig. 27.7) and active IP extension within the dorsal blocking orthosis. Orthotics and exercise guidelines for immediate passive flexion protocols are summarized in Table 27.2.

The benefits of an immediate passive flexion approach over immobilization are improved circulation for tendon healing, decreased joint stiffness, partial distal gliding of the flexor tendon, and, in some cases, a limited amount of proximal gliding of the repaired tendon.

While many variations of immediate passive flexion protocols exist, they fall into two main categories. These two categories include: (1) approaches that use an orthosis that holds the IP joints statically between exercises (Fig. 27.8) during the early phase of

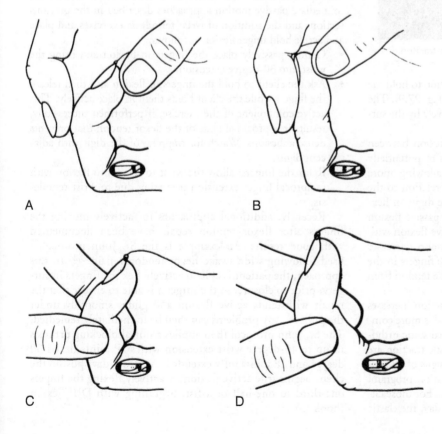

A   B   C   D

FIG. 27.7 Duran and Houser's exercises for passive flexor tendon gliding. (A) and (B) With the metacarpophalangeal (MP) and proximal interphalangeal (PIP) joints flexed, the distal interphalangeal (DIP) joint is passively extended. This moves the flexor digitorum profundus repair distally, away from the flexor digitorum superficialis repair. (C) and (D) Then, with the DIP and MP flexed, the PIP joint is extended passively. This moves both repairs distally away from the site of repair and any surrounding tissues to which they might otherwise form adhesions. (From Duran RJ, Coleman CR, Nappi JF, et al. Management of flexor tendon lacerations in zone 2 using controlled passive motion postoperatively. In Hunter JM, Schneider LH, Mackin EJ, et al., eds. *Rehabilitation of the Hand.* 3rd ed. St Louis, MO: Mosby; 1990.)

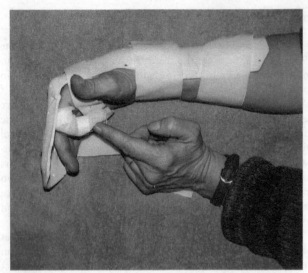

FIG. 27.8 Dorsal blocking orthosis with static interphalangeal positioning.

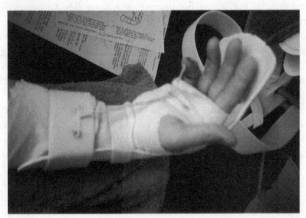

FIG. 27.9 Dorsal blocking orthosis with elastic traction.

tendon healing, or (2) an orthosis with elastic traction to hold the fingers in flexion dynamically between exercises (Fig. 27.9). The type of orthosis used is usually decided collaboratively by the surgeon and the hand therapist.

The rationale for holding the IP joints in flexion between exercises in the early phase of tendon healing is to potentially increase proximal tendon gliding, in part by allowing more time for the tendon to be resting proximally in relation to the repair site and to the pulley system. Holding the digits in flexion decreases stiffness of the digits by applying passive flexion for a greater portion of time. Placement in passive flexion with elastic traction to the fingers between exercises also decreases the potential for inadvertent active flexion of the fingers in the early phase of flexor tendon healing, protecting the tendon from rupture.

Holding the fingers in flexion with elastic traction increases the potential to develop IP flexion contractures and is more complicated for the client than using a less complicated static orthosis. Immediate passive flexion protocols with elastic traction are an option for those clients who are not showing signs of IP flexion contracture, who can adhere to the rehabilitation program, and who have no soft-tissue healing complications. For those clients using a dynamic flexion orthosis during the day, the elastic

traction is detached at night and the fingers are usually strapped to the hood of the dorsal blocking orthosis. If a client tends to clench their fists at night, the fingers may be left free of strapping to avoid resistance against the straps.

Reports indicate a wide variety of results with use of immediate passive flexion approaches. Limited gliding of the FDP with passive flexion of the digit[18] has been demonstrated, and research continues to develop improved surgical techniques for improved outcomes.

Immediate Active Flexion Approach

Immediate active flexion approaches following flexor tendon repair began in the 1990s and are the result of surgical advancements with stronger repair techniques (four or more strand repairs). The benefit of an immediate active flexion approach following tendon repair is to achieve flexor tendon gliding prior to the formation of dense adhesions. Numerous researchers[7,19-22] have found significantly improved outcomes, including improved flexor tendon gliding, with use of an immediate active flexion approach in the early phase of healing. There are multiple protocols in the literature that use immediate active flexion following an adequately strong flexor tendon repair. Orthoses and exercise guidelines for some of the commonly applied immediate active flexion protocols are outlined in Table 27.3.

The therapist should protect the client in a dorsal blocking orthosis at rest and instruct in **place and active hold** exercise of the fingers in flexion. The exercises are done within an appropriate orthosis at home or in therapy without an orthosis while the therapist assists with wrist tenodesis positioning.

Exercises consist of preparing the digit with slow gradual passive flexion to decrease edema and stiffness, followed by the same passive flexion and active IP extension exercises used for immediate passive motion approaches described in the previous section, and the addition of **wrist tenodesis exercises** and place and active hold finger flexion as follows:

- Gently, passively place the fingers in flexion and bring the wrist into 30-degree extension.
- Ask the client to hold the fingers in flexion and then release the fingers while the client holds them in place actively. This active component of the exercise, if performed successfully, results in a proximal glide of the flexor tendon that prevents dense adhesions. Watch for trapping of the digit with adjacent digits.
- Relax the fingers; allow the wrist to relax into flexion with reciprocal finger extension occurring due to wrist tenodesis.

Recently, additional approaches for actively moving the fingers after flexor tendon repair have been documented with good results. An example is the St. John protocol,[23] used following wide-awake flexor tendon repair.[23,24] In this approach, the patient is able to actively flex the fingers in surgery, prior to closure, so the surgeon is able to ensure that the repair withstands active flexion and glides smoothly under the pulleys. Any problems can then be immediately remedied. The St. John protocol then applies a dorsal blocking orthosis in up to 45-degree wrist extension with MP joints flexed 30 degree and IP joints fully extended. At 3 to 5 days postop the client begins true active flexion by actively flexing the fingers one-third to one-half of a fist, beginning with DIP flexion (hook fist).[23]

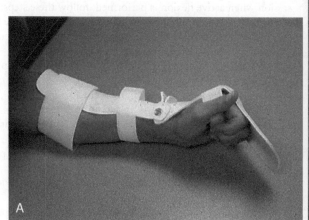
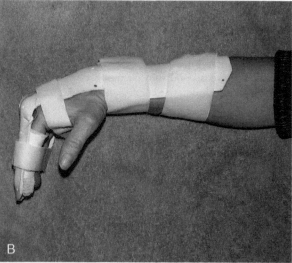

FIG. 27.10 (A) Wrist hinge orthosis for exercise in an immediate active flexion approach to rehabilitation. (B) Dorsal blocking orthosis with static positioning for protection.

Orthoses Used With an Immediate Active Flexion Approach

- Wrist hinge orthosis (Fig. 27.10A): Used in the Indiana protocol[19] for exercise. Fabricate forearm and hand portions of the orthosis with the edges that meet at the wrist formed to block wrist extension at 30 degrees. The MPs of the hand portion are flexed 60 degrees with full IP extension. Also, fabricate a dorsal blocking orthosis (Fig. 27.10B) with the wrist and MPs flexed and the IPs in extension for use between exercises. Benefits include optimal wrist positioning to decrease tension on the repair during active flexion in the early phase of tendon rehabilitation. The client must be trusted to change the orthoses for exercises without using or positioning the injured hand in any other way during the changing of orthoses.
- Dorsal blocking orthosis with wrist neutral (Fig. 27.11): Used in the Klein protocol[20] for both protection and place and active hold exercises at home, removed in therapy for wrist tenodesis with the active hold component of exercise. In this protocol, orthosis wrist position is based on work by Silfverskiold and May,[7] which used a wrist-neutral cast following repair with no increase in rupture rate and had 95% good and excellent results. A wrist-neutral position results in significantly less tension during active digital flexion than wrist flexion, but it is not as ideal of a position as partial wrist extension. Current application is used either with or without four-finger elastic traction, depending on the client's tissue response and surgeon preference. Benefits include simple orthotic fabrication and the ability to wear the orthosis at all times, which enables use with clients who are not able to safely change the orthosis between exercises.
- Dorsal blocking orthosis with wrist and MPs flexed and IPs extended: Used in the Evans protocol[21] with elastic traction to all four fingers, this traditional dorsal blocking orthosis is removed for wrist tenodesis and place and active hold exercises in therapy only. The client performs exercises as in the passive flexion approach described in the previous section at home with no active component except in therapy in the early phase of rehabilitation.

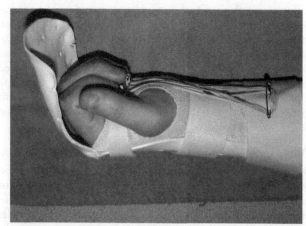

FIG. 27.11 Dorsal blocking orthosis with elastic traction, wrist neutral. Used in an immediate active flexion approach to rehabilitation.

Considerations for Using an Immediate Active Flexion Approach With Clients

- The type of suture repair: When a four or more strand flexor tendon repair has been performed, it is appropriate to consider use of an immediate controlled active flexion protocol with surgeon approval. Although a protocol exists for use of active flexion following a two-strand repair,[21] it was originally designed and applied by a very experienced therapist.
- The level of swelling and joint stiffness should be considered, as these factors increase the work of flexion and, if excessive, may prevent a client from being placed into an immediate active flexion approach. *Work of flexion* is a term that describes the amount of tension created within the tendon during active flexion to overcome resistive forces including joint stiffness, edema, friction caused by bulk of repair, tight pulleys, or swelling of the tendon.[25]
- Client healing factors: The presence of disease, such as diabetes, may result in slower healing.
- The client's ability to adhere to the plan of care: Poor compliance increases the probability that the client will do more than prescribed, or remove the orthosis, increasing potential

for rupture. Compliance concerns should preclude a client from being placed into an immediate active flexion approach, and might even justify an immobilization approach to protect the tendon from rupture.

- The therapist's level of experience: It is recommended that the therapist have a good understanding of flexor tendon healing, suture technique strengths, risks, and precautions before applying an immediate active flexion protocol.

> **Clinical Pearl**
>
> It can be difficult to know a client's ability to adhere to the plan of care at the first therapy session. If a client demonstrates inability to adhere appropriately with the precautions and exercises using a certain approach, a rehabilitation approach allowing less motion may become necessary, or a cast may be needed instead of a removable orthosis in the first 3 to 4 weeks postoperatively.

Diagnosis-Specific Information That Affects Clinical Reasoning When Using an Immediate Active Flexion Approach

Minimize stress on the tendon during active flexion, especially in the early phase of tendon healing, to prevent rupture. Edema, stiffness, and any internal friction encountered by the tendon because of bulk of repair, tight pulleys, or swelling of the tendon increases work of flexion with active flexion. Our goal as therapists is to minimize the work of flexion, thereby minimizing stress on the repaired tendon, especially when active motion is initiated immediately following repair. This is achieved by minimizing edema and joint stiffness and by using optimal joint positions that reduce the amount of tension developed within the tendon during active flexion.

Optimal Wrist Position

Research shows that the position that results in the least tension within the flexor tendon during active flexion is partial wrist extension and MP flexion.[26] When the wrist is flexed, a significantly increased amount of work is required by the flexor muscles to flex the fingers. By placing the wrist in slight extension, the extensor tendons are given slack at the wrist, allowing the fingers to relax into partial flexion. It requires only a slight pull by the muscle to flex the digits further and actively into a light fist. Thus most immediate active flexion protocols use a position of wrist neutral or slight wrist extension during the active flexion exercises and avoid active digit flexion with the wrist flexed.

Avoid tight end-ranges of active flexion in the early phase of flexor tendon healing because this significantly increases tension within the flexor tendon.[21] **Precaution.** *Our goal in the early phase of flexor tendon healing in an active flexion protocol is to attain a light fist that includes DIP flexion (to ensure FDP gliding), not a tight fist that is made with force. Education of the client in using this approach is important, for those clients who attempt to do more than allowed are much more likely rupture the repair.*

Clinical Reasoning Considerations for all Flexor Tendon Repairs

Initiating Active Flexion

While active flexion is initiated right after surgery in the immediate active flexion approach, the immobilization and immediate passive flexion approaches do not begin *active* flexion until 3 to

4 weeks postoperatively. Adjust the dorsal blocking orthosis to bring the wrist to neutral at this time, and allow the client to perform active flexion with or without the orthosis. At the first session when active flexion is performed, follow these steps:

- Maximize joint mobility with passive flexion and while holding the wrist and MPs in flexion, perform active IP extension.
- Perform passive wrist tenodesis exercises:
  - Passively flex the fingers, and bring the wrist into approximately 30-degrees extension.
  - Bring the wrist to neutral; relax the fingers.
  - Flex the wrist, and actively extend the fingers.
- Perform place and active hold of fingers in flexion with the wrist in partial extension.
- Perform active flexion of the fingers with the wrist in partial extension.
- Assess flexor tendon gliding by comparing passive flexion to active flexion.

When active flexion is significantly more limited than passive flexion, this indicates the presence of adhesions preventing proximal gliding of the flexor tendon. In this situation, it is appropriate to consider progressing the client to exercises that add more tension on the tendon in a proximal direction if not improved by the next therapy session.

> **Clinical Pearl**
>
> When initiating active motion, do it gently with a gradual increase in tension applied to the tendon as healing progresses. Grasp or pinch of objects greatly increases tension within the flexor tendons and must be avoided in the early phase of flexor tendon rehabilitation and in the intermediate phase unless adhesions limit gliding.

Progression of Exercises

Progression of exercises following flexor tendon repair should begin with the exercises that result in the least force to the tendon repair, and should increase to those exercises that gradually introduce more tension when gliding is limited. Groth[27] researched the amount of force created by typical flexor tendon exercises and provided a "pyramid of progressive forces" to guide therapists in the advancement of exercises when adhesions limit active flexion. The force in exercises advances in this order, from least force to most force: Passive flexion and protected extension, place and active hold in flexion (Fig. 27.12), active composite fist, hook and straight fist (Fig. 27.13), isolated joint motion (blocking), resisted composite fist, resisted blocking. When adhesions limit active flexion more than passive flexion, advance to the next level of exercises. Allow the client to perform these at home for one to two sessions, and advance to the next level only when there is no improvement within the current level of exercise. Consider the following points when upgrading flexor force with exercise:

- The degree of adhesions that justify increasing tension on a flexor tendon repair is not clearly identified in the literature; therefore, this decision relies on judgment, experience, and communication with experienced therapists and the referring surgeon. While one reference in the literature suggests that a 50-degree difference between passive and active flexion justifies the use of greater flexor force,[12] another[28] suggests 15 degrees, and yet another defines an active lag as more than 5 degrees difference between active and passive flexion.[27] I con-

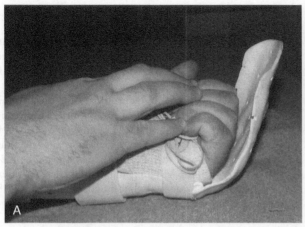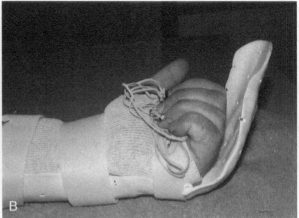

FIG. 27.12 Place and active hold in flexion following a four-strand flexor tendon repair begins with gentle passive placement of the fingers in flexion using the client's other hand (A), followed by release of the fingers while they are held in place actively (B).

There are three ways of making a fist:

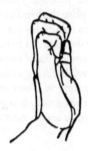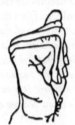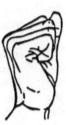

Hook Fist   Straight Fist   Full Fist

FIG. 27.13 The three different positions of tendon gliding exercises: hook fist, straight fist, and full fist. (From Stewart Pettengill K, van Strien G. Postoperative management of flexor tendon injuries. In: Mackin EJ, Callahan AD, Skirven TM, et al., eds. *Rehabilitation of the Hand and Upper Extremity.* 5th ed. St Louis, MO: Mosby; 2002.)

sider a 10 to 15 degrees difference or more between passive and active flexion at the PIP and/or DIP joint an indication of adhesions limiting active flexion. I am most concerned about active DIP flexion, as the FDP tendon tends to become the most densely adherent, limiting composite flexion, fine dexterity, and grip strength. Using an appropriate amount of tension on adhesions facilitates remodeling over time in the direction of the tension, allowing improved gliding of the tendon.

- **Precaution.** *Adding too much force can overpower the adhesions and repair and result in rupture of the repaired flexor tendon.*
- If a client has good early active motion, delay resistive exercises because there are fewer adhesions. If a client lacks motion due to adhesions, resistive exercises can be initiated sooner. Resistance is introduced appropriately when adhesions limit active motion more than passive motion, in an effort to place tension on the scar to improve proximal gliding of the tendon. This same resistance, however, may overpower the tensile strength of the repair and result in a rupture. Good active motion of the repaired tendon indicates lack of adhesions that would prevent proximal gliding of the repaired tendon. Tension develops in the flexor tendon when the muscle pulls against added resistance. Without the support and restriction of surrounding adhesions, all this tension is transferred directly through the repaired tendon, and the risk of tendon rupture greatly increases when resistance is introduced. Thus all timelines in this chapter must be indi-

vidualized, and progression to resistance of a repaired flexor tendon that has good to excellent glide is postponed until the referring surgeon determines the tendon is near or at full tensile strength.

- **Precaution.** *Resistance is initiated in the intermediate phase of healing only in the presence of significant flexor tendon adhesions that prevent active flexion more than passive flexion. If active flexion is not limited significantly, resistance is deferred until the late phase of tendon healing or until the surgeon has determined the tendon is near or at full tensile strength. Tendon repairs are never at their full strength when motion is initiated. The risk exists for gapping or potential rupture of a tendon throughout the healing process.*

Knowledge of tendon healing, the relative strength of the tendon repair over time, and the restricting effect of tendon adhesions forms the basis for determining safe upgrades to resistive exercises of the repaired tendon.

Interphalangeal Flexion Contractures

A frequent complication following flexor tendon repair is development of PIP flexion contracture, where the PIP joint is unable to be passively extended due to joint capsule and ligament tightening. To minimize flexion contractures, the dorsal blocking orthosis should be properly fabricated initially with the IPs strapped in extension at night. It is important to attempt to attain full active IP extension with the MP flexed as soon as possible after repair to prevent a flexion contracture from occurring. There are safe and appropriate techniques to prevent/correct IP flexion contractures. These should be done only with the supervision of an experienced hand therapist, very gently, with maximal MP flexion of the involved digit to minimize stress on the repaired tendon. This is potentially dangerous and requires caution.

> ### ⊙ Clinical Pearl
>
> A flexor tendon is in a protected position when it is on slack (passively flexed) at the other joints it crosses. In this protected position, the contracted joint can be gently and more safely encouraged into extension.

For instance, following a flexor tendon repair, when a PIP joint flexion contracture exists at 4 weeks after repair, support the wrist and MP joint in flexion while applying gentle joint mobilization or passive PIP extension. This will prevent excessive stretch of the repaired flexor tendon while providing assistance to improve extension of the joint. Perform the passive extension slowly and respect any guarding. Guarding may indicate end-range, and the client may protect by engaging the flexor tendon, eliciting resistance, which is unsafe to the repair.

A volar extension gutter orthosis to improve PIP extension may be used at night beginning at 5 to 6 weeks postoperatively, or as approved by the surgeon.

Regardless of the goals, especially following use of an immobilization or an immediate passive flexion protocol, active flexion of a repaired flexor tendon may be limited because of adhesion formation. Limited active flexion of the repaired digit, especially the DIP joint, frequently occurs due to adhesions, and there may be difficulty actively flexing the adjacent digits because of the common muscle belly of the FDP (**quadriga effect**). Grip strength is diminished because of loss of active flexion. Flexor tendons with adhesions commonly require a more prolonged period of rehabilitation with a strong emphasis on a home exercise program (HEP). The HEP should include blocking exercises and resistance even longer than the 12-week healing period, to continue to facilitate tendon gliding during the long remodeling process. Further surgical procedures are available for the repaired flexor tendon with significant adhesions that limit hand function. If needed, these procedures are often performed 4 to 6 months after repair.[2]

Outcomes for the flexor tendon that is allowed immediate passive flexion are improved over those that have been immobilized.[14-16] Outcomes using immediate active flexion protocols are even better,[7,19-21] but these protocols require a strong repair, an experienced hand therapist, and a responsible client who can reliably adhere to the prescribed plan of care.

Zone-Specific Approaches

There are numerous protocols in the literature for flexor tendon repairs in zone 2. Repairs in other areas of the hand receive less attention. Evans[29] has designed a specific protocol for flexor tendon repairs in zone 1. Flexor tendon repairs proximal to zone 2 result in less limiting adhesions and respond better to exercises to improve gliding. The author uses the same orthoses and general time guidelines for repairs in all zones of the repaired flexor tendon unless the surgeon decides to advance the exercises earlier for a client with a strong repair proximal to zone 2.

FPL repair requires a dorsal blocking orthosis for the thumb, holding the carpometacarpal in a relaxed position avoiding extension, MP at 30-degrees flexion, and full IP extension unless a digital nerve has been repaired and needs protection. The wrist can be positioned in 20- to 30-degrees flexion for a passive flexion protocol, or neutral for immediate active flexion protocol. While some include the fingers in the orthosis,[30] the author allows fingers to be free. A specific exercise recommended to attain FPL tendon gliding is to stabilize the MP joint while passively flexing and extending the IP joint. A study by Brown and McGrouther[31] showed that gliding of the FPL occurred at the level of the proximal phalanx with the MP joint stabilized while performing passive IP flexion and extension, but no gliding occurred if the MP was flexed during the passive IP motion.

> ### ♡ Tips From the Field
>
> **Orthoses Tips**
>
> When applying an orthosis within a few days following tendon repair, therapists often need to remove postsurgical dressings and apply a light dressing to the surgical incision. During dressing application and orthotic fabrication, place the hand in the tendon-protected position. For a flexor tendon repair, this is attained easily by relaxing the wrist and fingers over the edge of a bolster. **Precaution.** *Clients may want to stretch or move the hand when the postoperative dressings and orthosis are removed, and it is essential to instruct clients to stay in the position you place them in.* **Precaution.** *As you fabricate the orthosis, it is essential that you avoid placing a stretch on the repaired tendon because this could cause tendon rupture.*

> ### Evaluation Tips
>
> The first therapy session with a client following tendon repair includes removal of the postoperative dressings/splint, fabrication of an orthosis, instruction in a HEP, and an abbreviated evaluation. The evaluation portion of the session consists of observation of the wound or surgical incision for drainage, bleeding, or signs of infection, and observation of the amount of swelling in the digits and upper extremity. A verbal description of pain is obtained. Sensation is discussed, and because of the need to fabricate an orthosis at the first appointment, specific sensory testing may be deferred to a later session. **Precaution.** *When sensory testing is done, it is important that the hand and digits be maintained in a tendon-protected position.*
>
> ROM is not assessed in the usual manner immediately following a tendon repair. The healing tendon cannot safely be moved through its full excursion in the early phase without rupture. Limited evaluation of ROM is appropriate as indicated in Box 27.2. Box 27.3 describes the method of final assessment of motion following a flexor tendon repair using the Strickland-Glogovac formula.[32]
>
> No strength assessment is appropriate during an evaluation immediately following a tendon potential repair. Assessment of grip and pinch strength is deferred until after the full 12- to 14-week healing period following surgery. Because it is a maximal force activity, the author recommends that grip and pinch strength testing be done only with approval of the referring surgeon.
>
> Treatment of tendon repairs in the hand is challenging. It requires hand therapists to stay abreast of current changes and

gain the experience necessary to understand the process of tendon healing. Box 27.4 summarizes the important concepts to remember when treating a client with a repaired tendon. **Precaution.** *It is strongly recommended that you have supervision when beginning to treat tendon repairs to ensure proper hands-on management and a good understanding of these important concepts.*

? Questions to Ask the Doctor

Because of the large number of variables that exist in the type and complexity of injuries to tendons, the therapist must have a good understanding of the injury and surgery before beginning treatment. Questions to ask the doctor may include the following:

- Which tendons were lacerated? (This is not always obvious from the laceration.)
- What other structures were included in the injury (nerve, ligament, vessel, bone)?
- Were all structures able to be repaired strongly, or are there concerns with strength or healing of certain structures?
- What type of repair was done (that is, how many strands were used in the flexor tendon repair)?
- If referred immediately after repair, is the client being placed into an immobilization protocol or immediate passive or immediate active motion protocol? Clarify the approach you are planning to use for your client.

( ) *What to Say to Clients*

"A tendon connects muscle to bone and is what makes your finger/thumb move in this direction" (illustrate with your hand). Use a picture or diagram to show the client how the flexor muscle becomes tendon and how the tendon must be pulled proximally to achieve active flexion.

"When your tendon was injured, it could no longer bend your finger/thumb. Now that the surgeon has repaired it, it needs time to heal. A flexor tendon takes 12 weeks to heal. We will increase what you do with your repaired tendon gradually, but if you do too much too soon, it will tear apart. There are two things that will cause your tendon repair to rupture. One is a stretch that pulls the repair apart (illustrate on your hand how a stretch into extension would place excessive stretch on a repaired flexor tendon). The other is a contraction of the muscle that is too strong for the tendon repair to tolerate. For this reason, you must keep your orthosis on at all times for the first month. It will prevent the tendon from overstretching and will protect from injurious muscle use at this early stage. We will take the orthosis off only in therapy to clean your hand and the orthosis, and to do some additional exercises. If you follow the directions carefully, you will avoid having the muscle contract or pull too hard on the tendon."

"Under no circumstances should you do more than we instruct you to do with your hand through this healing process, or the tendon may rupture. If it ruptures, it may not be able to be repaired again, or if further surgery is done, the results are not likely to be as good."

CASE STUDIES

CASE STUDY 27.1

John is a 23-year-old man employed as a bartender. He suffered an injury to the volar surface of the small finger, lacerating the FDP and FDS tendons in zone 2 when a glass that he was washing broke in his hand. The surgeon performed a four-strand repair to the tendons and requested an immediate active flexion protocol.

Three days after repair, a dorsal blocking orthosis with the wrist in neutral, MP joints flexed, and IP joints in full extension was fabricated with elastic traction to all four fingers (Fig. 27.11). John was instructed in a HEP of passive flexion, place and active hold in flexion (Fig. 27.12), and IP extension within the orthosis. He was instructed to keep the orthosis on at all times at home. The orthosis was removed in therapy for cleansing of skin and the orthosis, dressing changes, and wrist tenodesis exercises of 30 degrees wrist extension with gentle passive finger flexion and wrist flexion as tolerated with fingers relaxed. Passive finger flexion and place and active hold finger flexion with the wrist in 20- to 30-degree extension were performed in therapy, and the client did the same

at home within the orthosis, keeping the wrist in neutral. IP extension was performed to 0 degrees with the MP joints supported in flexion.

Initial evaluation revealed moderate swelling in the small finger, mild swelling in the hand, and no drainage from the incisional line. Pain was moderate with ROM on the date the orthosis was fabricated. ROM was evaluated for passive finger flexion, IP extension, and place and active hold in flexion gently. Passive small finger flexion was 70 degrees for the MP joint, 70 degrees for the PIP joint, and 50 degrees for the DIP joint. Place and active hold in flexion was evaluated with 70 degrees for the MP joint, 65 degrees for the PIP joint, and 45 degrees for the DIP joint. IP extension was evaluated as −10 degrees for the PIP joint and −5 degrees for the DIP joint with the MP joints supported in flexion. The client attended therapy two times per week. Gradual gains were made in passive and place and active hold flexion.

At 4 weeks after surgery John was able to attain equal passive and place and hold flexion of 75 degrees for the MP joint, 85 degrees for the PIP joint, and 55 degrees for the DIP joint with IP extension to −5 degrees for the PIP joint and −5 degrees for the DIP joint. At 5 weeks postoperative, the elastic traction was removed from the orthosis. John was allowed to remove the orthosis for active flexion and extension of the fingers with wrist tenodesis and for bathing. At 8 weeks, the orthosis was modified to a hand-based orthosis to allow wrist motion, and John was instructed to use the orthosis at work or during heavy activities to prevent resistance to DIP flexion. Small finger ROM at 12 weeks after surgery was 0 to 90 degrees for the MP joint, 0 to 90 degrees for the PIP joint, and 0 to 70 degrees for the DIP joint (Fig. 27.14). John returned to regular duty and unrestricted use of the hand at 12 weeks after repair with instructions to avoid resisted fingertip resistance (such as, a hook grasp with weight) for another 1 to 2 weeks. The motion results were calculated as $[(90 + 70) − 0] \div 175 = 92\%$, which falls into the excellent result category according to the Strickland-Glogovac formula.[32]

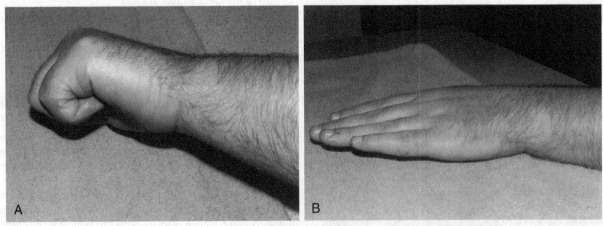

FIG. 27.14 Case study results at 8 weeks after flexor tendon repair for (A) flexion and (B) extension.

This case study is an example of a client with minimal flexor tendon adhesions and good tendon gliding in the early phase of rehabilitation that did not require advancement beyond the place and active hold and active exercises through the entire course of rehabilitation.

CASE STUDY 27.2

Sarah, a 28-year-old female, lacerated the FDP and FDS tendons of the left ring finger when attempting to separate frozen meat patties with a knife. She came to therapy 3 days after four-strand repairs to the tendons with a request for immediate active flexion approach without elastic traction. A dorsal-blocking orthosis with wrist neutral, MPs flexed to 50 degrees, IPs straight is fabricated. Initial evaluation shows mild to moderate edema, minimal drainage from the incisional site with pain reported as 8/10, and significant anxiety verbalized about her injury and the need to move her finger so soon after surgery. Passive flexion is attained to 70 degrees for the MP, 70 degrees for the PIP, and 30 degrees for the DIP. Place and active hold in flexion is 60 degrees for the MP, 45 degrees for the PIP, and 20 degrees for the DIP. Extension of the IP joints with the MPs supported in flexion is −15 degrees for the PIP and −10 degrees for the DIP. Extensive time is spent in client education and reassurance that the pain level will decrease from the current level by performing the exercises prescribed and that she is in control of the effort and pain level that results from her exercises.

Sarah is scheduled to attend therapy two times per week, but she missed two sessions in the first 3 weeks. At 2 weeks postoperatively, passive flexion is 75 degrees for the MP, 75 degrees for the PIP, and 35 degrees for the DIP at the end of the session with place and active hold in flexion of 70 degrees for the MP, 55 degrees for the PIP, and 20 degrees for the DIP. The difference between place and active hold and passive flexion is 40 degrees, and the patient is advanced to active flexion. At 3 weeks postoperatively, Sarah has made slight gains to 70 degrees for the MP, 65 degrees for the PIP, and 25 degrees for the DIP; however, there is a 50-degree difference between passive and active flexion, and gentle blocking exercises are initiated after discussion with the referring surgeon.

The following week, a hook and straight fist is added to the exercise program (Fig. 27.13). At 6 weeks, gentle gripping with light putty is initiated. Gains are made very gradually, and the result at 12 weeks postoperatively are 0 to 80 degrees for the MP, −10 to 90 degrees for the PIP, and −10 to 30 degrees for the DIP motion. The results according to the Strickland-Glogovac formula[32] are $[(90 + 30) − (10 + 10)] \div 175 = .57 \times 100\% = 57\%$ of normal, which falls into a fair result category (Box 27.3).

This case study demonstrates the advancement of exercises for a client with significant flexor tendon adhesions that limit active flexion more than passive flexion throughout the rehabilitation process. It is also an example of how client response may limit outcome related to attendance and anxiety.

References

1. Lundborg G, Rank F: Experimental intrinsic healing of flexor tendons based upon synovial fluid nutrition, *J Hand Surg* 3(1):21, 1978.
2. Seiler III JG: Flexor tendon repair, *J Am Soc Surg Hand* 1(3):177–191, 2001.
3. Strickland JW: The scientific basis for advances in flexor tendon surgery, *J Hand Ther* 18(2):94, 2005.
4. Tang J, Gu YT, Rice K, et al.: Evaluation of four methods of flexor tendon repair for postoperative active mobilization, *Plast Reconstr Surg* 107:742–749, 2001.
5. Taras JS, Raphael JS, Marczyk S, et al.: Evaluation of suture caliber in flexor tendon repair, *J Hand Surg Am* 26A:1100–1104, 2001.
6. AlavanjaG Dailey E: Mass DP: Repair of zone II flexor digitorum profundus lacerations using varying suture sizes: a comparative biomechanical study, *J Hand Surg Am* 30(3):44–54, 2005.
7. Silfverskiold KL, May EJ: Flexor tendon repair in zone II with a new suture technique and an early mobilization program combining passive and active flexion, *J Hand Surg Am* 19:53, 1994.
8. Trail IA, Powell ES, Noble J: The mechanical strength of various suture techniques, *J Hand Surg Br* 17:89–91, 1992.
9. Seiler III JG: Flexor tendon injury. In Wolfe SW, Hotchkiss RN, Pederson WC, et al.: *Green's operative hand surgery*, ed 7, Philadelphia, 2017, Elsevier.
10. Momose T, Amadio PC, Zhao C, et al.: Suture techniques with high breaking strength and low gliding resistance: experiments in the dog flexor digitorum profundus tendon, *Acta Orthop Scand* 72(6):635–641, 2001.
11. Taras JS, Martyak GG, Steelman PJ: Primary care of flexor tendon injuries. In Skirven TM, Osterman AL, Fedorczyk J, et al.: *Rehabilitation of the hand and upper extremity*, ed 6, St Louis, 2011, Elsevier.
12. Cifaldi Collins D, Schwarze L: Early progressive resistance following immobilization of flexor tendon repairs, *J Hand Ther* 4:111, 1991.
13. Pettengill KM, van Strien G: Postoperative management of flexor tendon injuries. In Skirven TM, Osterman AL, Fedorczyk J, et al.: *Rehabilitation of the hand and upper extremity*, ed 6, St Louis, 2011, Elsevier.
14. Duran RJ, Coleman CR, Nappi JF, et al.: Management of flexor tendon lacerations in zone 2 using controlled passive motion postoperatively. In Hunter JM, Mackin EJ, Callahan AD, editors: *Rehabilitation of the hand*, ed 3, St Louis, 1990, Mosby.
15. Kleinert HE, Ashbell TS, Martinez T: Primary repair of lacerated flexor tendons in "no man's land," *J Bone Joint Surg* 49:577, 1967.
16. Dovelle S, Kulis Heeter P: The Washington regimen: rehabilitation of the hand following flexor tendon injuries, *Phys Ther* 69:1034, 1989.
17. Groth GN: Current practice patterns of flexor tendon rehabilitation, *J Hand Ther* 18(2):169–174, 2005.
18. Silfverskiold KL, May EJ, Tornvall AH: Flexor digitorum profundus tendon excursions during controlled motion after flexor tendon repair in zone II: a prospective clinical study, *J Hand Surg Am* 17:122–133, 1992.
19. Strickland JW, Gettle KH: Flexor tendon repair. In Hunter JM, Schneider LH, Mackin EJ, editors: *Tendon and nerve surgery in the hand—a third decade*, St Louis, 1997, Mosby.
20. Klein L: Early active motion flexor tendon protocol using one splint, *J Hand Ther* 16(3):199, 2003.
21. Evans RE, Thompson DE: The application of force to the healing tendon, *J Hand Ther* 6:262, 1993.
22. Trumble TF, Vedder NB, Seiler JG, et al.: Zone II flexor tendon repair: a randomized prospective trial of active place-and-hold therapy compared with passive motion therapy, *J Bone Joint Surg* 92(6):1381–1389, 2010.
23. Lalonde D: How the wide awake approach is changing hand surgery and hand therapy: inaugural AAHS sponsored lecture at the ASHT meeting, San Diego, *J Hand T her* 26(2):175–178, 2013. 2012.
24. Higgins A, Lalonde D: Flexor tendon repair postoperative rehabilitation: the saint john protocol, *Plast Reconstr Surg Glog Open* 4(11), 2016.
25. Halikis MN, Manske PR, Kubota H, et al.: Effect of immobilization, immediate mobilization, and delayed mobilization on the resistance to digital flexion using a tendon injury model, *J Hand Surg Am* 22:464, 1997.
26. Savage R: The influence of wrist position on the minimum force required for active movement of the interphalangeal joints, *J Hand Surg Br* 13:262, 1988.

27. Groth GN: Pyramid of progressive force exercises to the injured flexor tendon, *J Hand Ther* 17(1):31–42, 2004.

28. Sueoka SS, Lastayo PC: Zone II flexor tendon rehabilitation: a proposed algorithm, *J Hand Ther* 21(4):410–413, 2008.

29. Evans RB: Zone I flexor tendon rehabilitation with limited extension and active flexion, *J Hand Ther* 18(2):128, 2005.

30. Elliot D, Southgate C: New concepts in managing the long tendons of the thumb after primary repair, *J Hand Ther* 18(2):141–156, 2005.

31. Brown C, McGrouther D: The excursion of the tendon of flexor pollicis longus and its relation to dynamic splintage, *J Hand Surg Am* 9:787–791, 1984.

32. Strickland JW, Glogovac SV: Digital function following flexor tendon repair in zone II: a comparison of immobilization and controlled passive motion techniques, *J Hand Surg* 5:537, 1980.

28 Tendon and Nerve Transfers

Deborah A. Schwartz

Working with clients undergoing major reconstructive surgeries, such as tendon and/or nerve transfers, is an incredibly exciting and rewarding process. These individuals have sustained major trauma and/or injuries, resulting in compromised functional abilities. Their trauma may have been a life-changing event and will require tremendous support and understanding on your part. Perhaps your client has never experienced great hand function due to congenital deformities. Transfer surgeries offer clients the possibility of improved or enhanced function and, hopefully, a more independent lifestyle. The approach to both tendon and nerve transfer surgery should be that of a team effort, involving the surgeon, client, you as therapist, and psychological support from social workers or psychologists as needed.[1] You have an important role to play from the beginning and throughout the entire course of rehabilitation. During the pre-surgery assessment, you evaluate and record accurately all of the client's functional abilities and progress. You are the major source of information regarding what your client can and cannot do and what he or she clearly hopes to accomplish via the surgery. You can educate the client and their family about the planned surgical procedures and the course of rehabilitation, including what to expect at every stage. You are an active advocate for your client, working with the surgeon to help clarify what is most important in terms of recovery of functional activities. You should arrange for counseling as needed with a social worker or psychologist, and help prepare the client for support services and postoperative employment opportunities. Do not hesitate to refer the client to their case manager (if this is a workman's compensation case) or to their health insurance company to seek out these additional support services. Preoperative therapy sessions are devoted to conditioning, stretching the tissues and tight joints to regain full passive motion, preventing deformities, and strengthening and/or activation of the selected donor muscles. This will help to establish improved motor retraining and reeducation postoperatively. During this preoperative period, you may have the most one-on-one contact with your client. Consider your work together as a partnership to maximize your client's progress toward his or her functional goals.

Indications for Tendon Transfers

Tendon transfer surgery involves the operative repositioning of a tendon of a working muscle unit to take over the function of an absent or nonfunctioning muscle.[2,3] Tendon transfer surgery is, above all, an attempt to rebalance an imbalanced hand (Fig. 28.1). Indications for tendon transfer surgery include imbalance in the hand caused by central neurological deficits, such as seen in spinal cord injuries or cerebral palsy, or trauma to the upper extremity where nerves and tendons are lacerated or crushed and cannot be repaired. Prolonged nerve compression can also lead to irreversible damage of muscle. Other causes for muscle imbalance are disease processes, such as poliomyelitis, rheumatoid arthritis, or Charcot Marie Tooth syndrome (which affects the intrinsic muscles of the hand causing wasting of the muscle fibers); and congenital deformities, such as those occurring with brachial plexus palsy or thumb hypoplasia.[1-4]

Indications for Nerve Transfers

Nerve transfers involve taking the proximal portion of an expendable healthy nerve and transferring it to the distal part of the denervated nerve to the target muscle.[5-7] This procedure has revolutionized peripheral nerve surgeries with very good functional outcomes.[8] The indications for this procedure are most commonly brachial plexus injuries where nerve grafting is not possible, and/or peripheral nerve injuries with long distances between injured

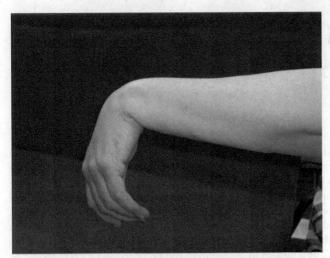

FIG. 28.1 Imbalanced hand due to radial nerve palsy.

structures and muscles. Nerve transfers are a treatment option for clients with proximal nerve root avulsions, significant scarring at the site of nerve injury, and/or clients with multilevel nerve injuries.[8,9] Nerve transfers can help to limit the degree of motor end plate degradation, and speed up the reinnervation of target muscles before they are completely atrophied. The commonly accepted goal is to reinnervate the target muscle by 12 to 18 months.[8] Additional advantages of nerve transfers over tendon transfers are the ability to restore sensation, the ability to reinnervate multiple muscles with a single transferred nerve, and the elimination of extensive dissection required to harness tendons for transfer.[5,7-9] Donor nerves are commonly referred to by the muscles they innervate, even though the nerve itself is being transferred.

General Considerations for Tendon and Nerve Transfer Surgery

Alternative procedures may have been performed prior to tendon transfer surgery, such as nerve decompression, nerve repair, and muscle and/or tendon repair. Tendon transfers may be considered as a restorative option when there is no further recovery or nerve regeneration from the precipitating event. Surgeons typically wait 3 to 4 months from the time of injury before proceeding, when it is unlikely that spontaneous motor recovery will occur.[2]

The prerequisites for surgery should include the following [2-9]:
- Analysis of client's needs
- Bony stability
- Edema or inflammation have subsided
- Adequate soft-tissue bed
- Mobile joints
- Expendable donor muscles and/or nerves

Muscles perform specific functions, but alternate muscles may also perform the same function. The transfer of the expendable muscle must not in itself cause another deficit of motor function. Nerves also perform certain functions, and suitable donor nerves are those nerves that innervate expendable muscles or nerves to muscles with duplicate innervations.

The selection of a donor nerve is similar to the selection of a donor muscle—using synergistic muscles and their nerves makes it easier to recruit the desired action postoperatively, although it is possible to work with antagonistic muscle/nerve transfers.[5-9]

The selection of the donor tendons must take into consideration the following[2,3]:
- A muscle that has sufficient strength to overcome the strength and passive tension of the antagonist muscle
- A muscle that lies in an appropriate direction of the desired action
- A muscle that travels a straight route and performs a single function
- Potential excursion of the muscle once it is freed from all connective tissue attachments

The muscle should contract through a distance about equal to the resting length of individual muscle fibers. The required **excursion** is the excursion needed to move a joint through its full range of motion (ROM), but the available excursion is limited by the surrounding connective tissue.[2,3] Additional considerations that come into play are the staging of multiple procedures on both the flexor and the extensor sides of the extremity, and the selection of alternative procedures, such as nerve transfers, **arthrodesis** (joint fusion), and/or tenodesis. (Surgery can create or enhance a tenodesis effect by rerouting the transected tendon across a more proximal joint and attaching it there.)[1-3]

A key component for the success of these reconstructive surgeries lies in the motivation and understanding of the client. Without clearly defined functional goals and a willingness to work toward the outcome, the surgical procedure by itself will not lead to improved outcomes. The client should demonstrate active participation in the process.[1,2]

> ◎ **Clinical Pearl**
>
> The client needs to have an appreciation of the surgical expectations and limitations offered by tendon or nerve transfer surgery. Carefully explain to your client that the concept of "normal" hand function and/or appearance is unrealistic. Reinforce the key point that the goals of these procedures are to improve functional outcomes and independence.

Preoperative Treatment

Clients with peripheral nerve injuries can benefit from therapeutic intervention while awaiting either nerve regeneration or restorative surgery. The fabrication of well-designed orthoses can greatly increase the functional capabilities of clients diagnosed with radial, median, and/or ulnar nerve palsies. Left unsupported, these nerve injuries can lead to significant joint contractures and overstretching of muscle tendon units.[1,10,11] At a minimum, peripheral nerve injuries cause joint stiffness and discomfort, as well as awkward posturing. A variety of immobilization or mobilization orthoses can be fabricated for this purpose.
- Clients with radial nerve palsy require support of the wrist and metacarpophalangeal (MP) joints in extension (Fig. 28.2).
- Clients with median nerve palsy require support and positioning of the thumb in opposition and abduction for fine motor tasks (Figs. 28.3 and 28.4).
- Clients with ulnar nerve palsy require that the MP joints be positioned in flexion to prevent clawing of the ulnar digits and to substitute for lack of intrinsic function. If the median nerve is also involved, clients may require additional support for the thumb in abduction (Figs. 28.5 and 28.6).

If the client has elected to proceed with transfer surgery, therapeutic management includes the preoperative evaluation,

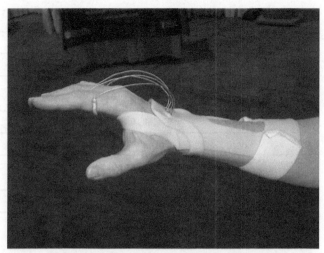

FIG. 28.2 Dynamic orthosis for radial nerve palsy.

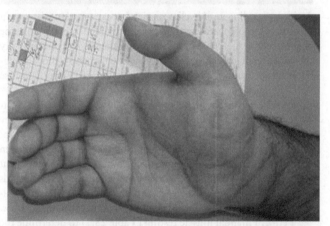

FIG. 28.3 Client with adducted thumb due to median nerve palsy.

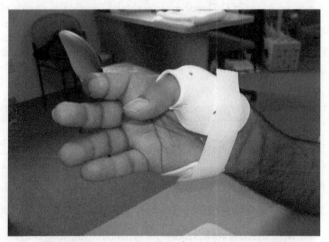

FIG. 28.4 Functional orthosis for median nerve palsy.

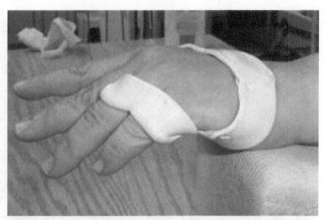

FIG. 28.5 Static anticlaw orthosis (figure-eight) for ulnar nerve palsy.

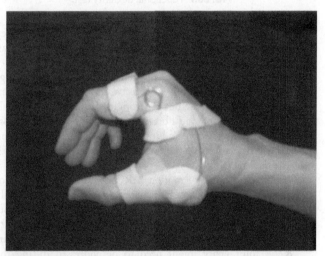

FIG. 28.6 Dynamic orthosis for ulnar nerve palsy/median nerve palsy.

conditioning, and client education.[1,10,11] Working together for this extended time period reinforces the rapport between you and your client. Unfortunately, many clients requiring hand therapy may not have been seen by you prior to their surgery. If this is the case with your client, you must work quickly and effectively to gain the client's confidence and trust.

The Evaluation

Initiate your evaluation with an interview to determine the client's expectations of the outcomes from the planned surgery. When working with a child, meet and discuss this with the family as well. During your evaluation:

- Assess the client's ability to comply with the postoperative rehabilitative protocol. It is helpful if you have already worked with the client through their posttrauma rehabilitation, but you can still develop a rapport with the client at any point by explaining concepts; developing a working relationship as coach, educator, and partner; and forming a treatment plan geared toward function.
- Record a detailed history of the injury, all surgical procedures, and therapy that has taken place up to this point, leading to the decision for tendon and/or nerve transfer surgery.
- Examine the affected extremity; observe and record the skin appearance and the placement of scars, adhesions, atrophy of muscles, prominent bony landmarks, and skin coloring.
- Determine sensory status using the Ten Test, Semmes-Weinstein monofilament test, two-point discrimination testing, and/or stereognosis testing.[1,10-12] When working

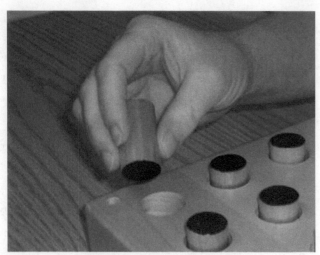

FIG. 28.7 Functional dexterity test.

TABLE 28.1	Manual Muscle Testing	
Grade	Terminology	Description
5	Normal	Full ROM and full strength
4	Good	Full ROM against gravity with some resistance
3	Fair	Full ROM against gravity
2	Poor	Full ROM with gravity eliminated
1	Trace	Slight contraction without joint movement
0	None	No evidence of contraction

ROM, Range of motion.

with children, you will need to closely observe how they integrate the use of their involved hand into play. You can incorporate a game of stereognosis to determine their ability to interpret sensory input in their involved hand. **Stereognosis** refers to the ability to perceive and recognize the form of an object using tactile cues from its size and texture. Evaluating a child may be a bit more challenging, but it is possible through creative and interactive play and by discussing your observations of the use of the affected extremity with the parents.[1]

- Take active range of motion (AROM) and passive range of motion (PROM) measurements. Evaluate each joint carefully to ascertain whether it has a hard or soft end feel, and note whether a contracture is present or if there is ligament laxity in the joint. Contractures should be addressed prior to surgery. Joint laxity might need to be addressed during the tendon transfer surgery so that the proper amount of tension can be applied.

- Evaluate the current use of the hand through functional testing, such as the Jebsen Hand Function Test, the functional dexterity test (Fig. 28.7), or the Moberg's pickup test.[1,13]

- Include one of the following client self-report outcome measures: the Canadian Occupational Performance Measure, Disabilities of the Arm, Shoulder, and Hand (DASH) or Quick DASH, or the Michigan Hand Outcomes Questionnaire.[14] These self-assessments contribute crucial information to an overall picture of how the client rates their own independent functioning, and they help determine how your client views progress toward achievement of functional goals throughout the rehabilitation process.[14]

In addition to the above assessments, observe the client's movement patterns, and note the presence of substitution or **compensatory movement patterns.**[1] These are patterns of movement that your client may have begun to use to make up for the lack of normally functioning muscles. These movement patterns can lead to overstretching and weakening of muscles that are not yet injured. You will need to retrain your client not to use these patterns of movement after surgery. It is best to point these patterns out early and teach your client to recognize and avoid them.

Tips From the Field

A video recording and/or clinical pictures can greatly assist you in recording the preoperative functional level. You can even use the client's cell phone. This is a great tool for assessing compensatory movement patterns, checking progress, and comparing how the client was functioning prior to surgery and after surgery in the course of rehabilitation.

At the conclusion of the assessments, record a list of the greatest functional needs of the client in their own words. Ask what they would most like to do with their involved hand. Hold a hairbrush? Drink from a soda bottle? Hold a water bottle so that they can open the cap independently? Do not make the mistake of telling the client what these goals should be. Let the client define in their own words what would they would like to accomplish. In the case of young children, let the parents step in and describe what they would like to see.

Perform manual muscle testing (Table 28.1) to determine the status of the involved muscles. It is important to ensure that all possible donor muscles are strong enough to be transferred to new positions.[1-4,15] Donor muscles should function at a grade of full ROM against gravity or higher. We do not select muscles that are typically described in textbooks as available donor muscles without verifying that these muscles are present and active in our client. Not everyone has a palmaris longus (PL) tendon available for transfer!

Clinical Pearl

It is helpful to create a list of four muscle groups as follows:
- What muscles are working? All muscles detected by manual muscle testing.
- What muscles are not working? All muscles not detected by manual muscle testing.
- What functions are needed? All motions needed to improve function.
- What muscles are available? All expendable muscles with full ROM against gravity and some resistance (Fig. 28.8).[2]

During the course of your evaluation, you can utilize an orthosis to simulate the proposed function of the tendon transfer. This can help a client see right away if changing the position of a specific joint can indeed improve function. For example, prior to **opponensplasty** (tendon transfers to restore thumb opposition), fabricate a short opponens thumb orthosis and observe the

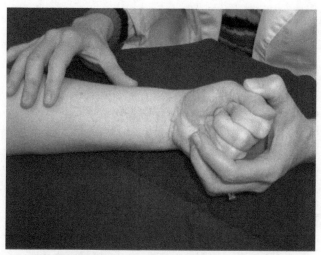

FIG. 28.8 Manual muscle testing of flexor carpi ulnaris.

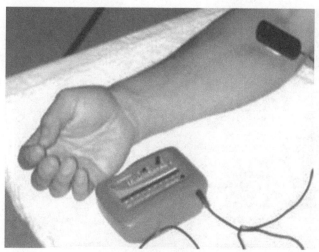

FIG. 28.9 Neuromuscular electrical stimulation.

client's ability to hold and/or pinch while wearing this orthosis.[1] You may note that your client displays an improved pinch or an increased ability to hold a tool. Or you might try fabricating a wrist orthosis for a client contemplating tendon transfers for wrist extension. The ability to keep the wrist in extension greatly improves grasp and release patterns of the digits. Wearing a wrist orthosis might enable your client to demonstrate improved hand functioning. In addition, wrist support helps prevent shortening of the wrist flexors.[1,10]

◎ Clinical Pearl

Help your client create realistic expectations and functional goals. Make sure they understand what the possible outcomes may be.
- Explain terms and procedures in a manner your client can easily understand.

Once the donor muscles and/or nerves have been selected and a plan for surgical intervention is set, help the client prepare for the procedure both physically and emotionally.

Ask the surgeon if you, as the consulting therapist, can attend the transfer surgery. This is a unique opportunity to gather information and make observations. It also allows you to see firsthand the status of the involved tendons/nerves, the strength of the repair, and what specific tendons/nerves were used (which might not be what was planned in advance).

❨ ❩ What to Say to Clients

"The surgeon is going to reroute one of your 'working muscles to the joint where the muscle does not work' (or 'working nerve to the muscle where the nerve does not work.') The therapy before the surgery is very important to get you ready and help make the surgery more successful. We need to make sure that your joints are nice and loose with passive motion exercises and stretching. We need to stretch the joint to full range of motion. An orthosis can help to maintain the stretch over time. Wear the orthosis at night so that it doesn't affect your ability to use your hand during the day. If your joint is tight, the donor tendon will not be able to move your joint through the full range of motion. We are going to try and exercise the donor muscle before the surgery to help it get stronger so that it will be ready to work in its new position."

Donor muscle strengthening can be performed through progressive resistive exercises and/or through biofeedback and/or neuromuscular electrical stimulation (Fig. 28.9).[1] An example of this would be strengthening of the pronator teres (PT) muscle prior to transferring this tendon to the insertion of extensor carpi radialis brevis (ECRB) for wrist extension after radial nerve palsy.

◎ Clinical Pearl

It is extremely beneficial to help your client gain awareness of the donor muscle contraction and learn how to recruit it independently prior to surgery. Have your client place their noninvolved hand on the donor muscle belly during activity to feel the contraction. For example, let your client feel the PT muscle contracting during active pronation. If they cannot feel it easily, you can make their contraction stronger and more palpable by offering some resistance to their forearm in the direction of supination, and ask them not to let go. Let your client practice contracting this muscle first with self-applied resistance and gradually learn how to contract independently without resistance.

Make sure to inform clients of the loss of sensory input along the distribution of the injured peripheral nerve and the potential for burns and/or skin breakdown. It may be very obvious to your client when they have no feeling in the fingertips due to a median nerve or ulnar nerve injury. However, even the radial nerve has a sensory terminal branch: the dorsal sensory branch of the radial nerve. This area of insensate skin can be injured when the client begins to use their hand in activities of daily living (ADLs). Note the bandage over dorsal first web in Fig. 28.10 showing where the client burned herself removing items from a hot oven.

Throughout the course of the preoperative therapy program, engage your client in a discussion of realistic functional outcomes. Include the perspective of the surgeon in this dialogue, and the perspective of the parents if young children are involved. Discuss the time frame of surgery, postoperative immobilization, and postoperative course of therapy visits. Avoid surprises regarding the time and commitment expected for rehabilitation after surgery. Outline the schedule of follow-up visits with the surgeon as well because many clients and their parents expect to see the surgeon at every therapy visit if therapy occurs in the physician's office. Always strive to establish a genuine rapport with your client and create a solid working and trusting relationship.

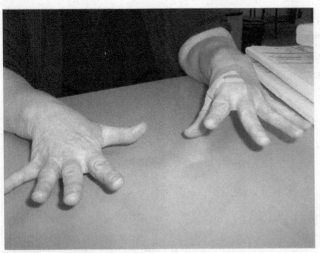

FIG. 28.10 Client after tendon transfers for radial nerve palsy.

BOX 28.1   Common Tendon Transfer Procedures for Median Nerve Palsy[2,3,16,25]

Camitz: Palmaris longus is transferred for palmar abduction (not true opposition)

Royle, Bunnell, and Thompson: Flexor digitorum superficialis of the ring finger transferred for opposition with different distal attachment techniques

Huber: Abductor digiti minimi transferred to abductor pollicis brevis for opposition

Richter and Peimer: Transfer of the flexor digitorum superficialis of the ring or little to abductor pollicis brevis for opposition

---

Operative Treatment: General Guidelines

Based on the requirements of each client and the results of the manual muscle testing, the surgeon selects the donor muscles and/or nerves for transfer.

Common Tendon Transfer Procedures

Various names have been assigned to specific sets of transferred tendons for each of the three main nerve palsies of the upper extremity. It is a good idea to be familiar with these classic procedural names, such as the Royle, Camitz, or Huber transfers for thumb abduction or opposition in median nerve palsy[2,3,16,25] (Box 28.1); the Brand, Jones, and modified Boyes transfer for radial nerve palsy [2–3,4,25] (Box 28.2); or the Brand, Stiles-Bunnel, or Zancolli Lasso procedures used in the treatment of ulnar nerve palsy[2,3,15,25] (Box 28.3). There are many more names, procedures, and modifications described in the literature.[15] Make sure you confer with the surgeon to specify exactly which donor muscles were utilized (Fig. 28.11 through Fig. 28.13).

Not so common tendon transfer procedures are listed in Table 28.2.

Common Nerve Transfer Procedures

Select nerves have been identified as candidates for nerve transfers to help clients regain specific motor and/or sensory function (Table 28.3).[5-9]

BOX 28.2   Common Tendon Transfer for Radial Nerve Palsy[2,3,15,25]

Pronator teres to extensor carpi radialis brevis (ECRB) for wrist extension

Boyes: Flexor digitorum superficialis (FDS) (middle) to extensor digitorum communis (EDC) for metacarpophalangeal (MP) extension and FDS (ring) to extensor pollicis longus and extensor indicis proprius

Brand: Flexor carpi radialis (FCR) to EDC for MP extension and palmaris longus for thumb extension

Jones: Flexor carpi ulnaris to EDC for MP extension

In addition, FCR to abductor pollicis longus and extensor pollicis brevis for thumb radial abduction

---

BOX 28.3   Common Tendon Transfer Procedures for Ulnar Nerve Palsy[2–4,25]

Brand: Extensor carpi radialis brevis (ECRB) with a graft to the intrinsic muscles via the lateral bands

Burkhalter: Flexor digitorum superficialis (FDS) of the middle is inserted onto the proximal phalanx (P1), not the lateral band

Modified Stiles-Bunnel: FDS of the ring and middle is split into slips and inserted into the lateral band of each finger or the lateral part of the proximal phalanx (P1)

Zancolli Lasso: FDS is passed through the pulley and sutured back onto itself to improve metacarpophalangeal flexion

Additional procedures described to restore power pinch and thumb adduction:

Boyes: Brachioradialis is extended with a free graft and passed between the third and fourth metacarpals to insert on the adductor tubercle of the thumb

Smith-Hastings: ECRB is transferred to adductor pollicis at the first metacarpal for restoration of power pinch

---

?   Questions to Ask the Doctor

Whenever possible, ask to see the operative report. Make sure you and the surgeon share a realistic understanding of the expected outcomes. In addition, you should ask the surgeon the following questions:

- Which specific muscles or nerves were transferred to what insertion sites?
- Were pulleys created to alter the course of the pull?
- What was the quality of the transferred muscle tendon unit, or nerve?
- Were grafts needed (to increase the length)?
- What type of suturing technique was utilized?
- How long should the extremity be immobilized?
- How was the tension of the transferred muscles determined?

Postoperative Treatment: General Guidelines

Postoperative treatment can be divided into three phases for easy reference: early, intermediate, and late. General guidelines for therapeutic intervention are described first, followed by examples

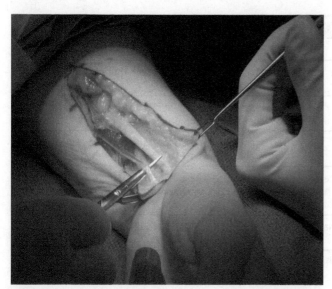

FIG. 28.11 Dissection of the palmaris longus tendon on the right and the flexor carpi radialis tendon on the left.

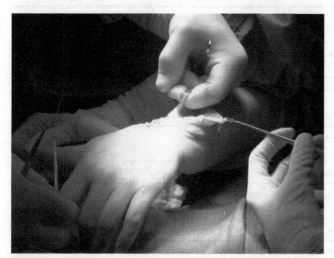

FIG. 28.12 Identifying the extensor pollicis longus tendon.

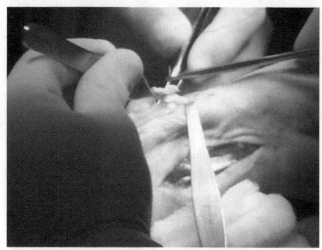

FIG. 28.13 Pulvertaft weave of tendons.

of different tendon transfers and specific therapeutic interventions. Several case studies that highlight these interventions are presented.[17,18]

Timing of the Rehabilitation Protocols

Tendon Transfers: The Early Phase (Weeks 1 to 4)

Postoperative treatment begins with positioning the involved extremity in a protective cast that prevents any tension on the transferred tissues. This allows healing to take place without overstretching or rupturing the transfers.[1-3] Nerve transfers are held in a protected position for a shorter period of time than tendon transfers in order to prevent adherence of the nerve to the surrounding tissue.[7-9] During this early phase of rehabilitation:

- Create an exercise program for the noninvolved digits and joints.
- Monitor your client's extremity for edema.
- Make sure the cast is secure and fits well.
- Educate your client on the time required for adequate healing.
- Begin desensitization techniques as needed
- Review the time frame and anticipated course of therapy.

The client may be anxious to see the results of the surgery and learn what the functional outcomes might be. Educate your client on the different phases of the rehabilitative course. Explain that all transferred structures require adequate time for healing. At each session, it may be beneficial to review the functional goals, the time frame, and the anticipated course of therapy.

◯ *What to Say to Clients*

"Move all of your uninvolved joints outside of the postoperative dressings while the tendon transfers heal. Perform regular active exercises of everything not in the cast. Periodically, elevate your arm to reduce swelling. You must inform the surgeon immediately if the cast seems loose."

If the cast becomes loose, offer to fabricate a thermoplastic orthosis as an alternative to a new cast, as this will be a bit more comfortable for your client.

Tendon Transfers: The Intermediate Phase (Weeks 4 to 6)

During the intermediate phase of postoperative rehabilitation, therapeutic intervention is much more involved and hands on. The postoperative cast can be removed. Replace it with a thermoplastic orthosis, maintaining the same protected positioning as the cast.[1,11] As you examine your client's extremity, note the placement of volar and dorsal incisions. The amount of scarring after tendon transfers can be quite extensive on both sides of the extremity because the surgery requires a great deal of exposure to locate and secure the donor tendons in their new insertion sites. You can now initiate scar management techniques. Be sure to include friction massage, desensitization, ultrasound, and perhaps elastomer and silicone gel products. Silicone gel products also work to hydrate the scar tissue as well as compress it[1,17] (Fig. 28.14).

Utilize therapeutic heat in the form of heat packs, whirlpool, and/or fluidotherapy to improve the elasticity of your client's tissue, as well as to reduce joint stiffness and increase the blood flow to the involved area.[1] Begin AROM to isolated joints. Perform

TABLE 28.2   Not So Common Tendon Transfer Procedures[11]

Condition	Indications	Procedure	Orthosis
Spinal cord injury	Lack of key pinch and pronation	Brachioradialis to FPL	Dorsal forearm-based orthosis with thumb adducted, wrist in neutral, and elbow free
Spinal cord injury	Lack of elbow extension	Biceps to triceps	Elbow extension orthosis at night Elbow flexion block during day
Spinal cord injury	Lack of palmar grasp	ECRL to FDP	Dorsal blocking orthosis with wrist in neutral, MP joints in flexion, and IP joints in extension
Brachial plexus birth palsy	Lack of shoulder external rotation/abduction	Latissimus dorsi and teres tendons to posterior shoulder cuff	Airplane orthosis with arm in 30 to 40 degrees of external rotation and 120 degrees of abduction
Brachial plexus birth palsy	Lack of elbow flexion	Steindler (Flexor-Pronator transfer)	Elbow flexion orthosis in 100 to 110 degrees of elbow flexion

ECRL, Extensor carpi radialis longus; *FDP,* flexor digitorum profundus; *FPL,* flexor pollicis longus; *IP,* interphalangeal; *MP,* metacarpophalangeal.

TABLE 28.3   Common Nerve Transfers[7,8]

Functional Loss	Donor Nerve	Recipient nerve(s)	Comments
Shoulder function and stability	1. Spinal accessory 2. Triceps or medial pectoral nerve	1. Suprascapular nerve 2. Axillary nerve	
Elbow flexion	Fascicles from intact median (to FCR, FDS, PL) and ulnar nerves (to FCU)	Biceps and brachialis branches of musculocutaneous nerve	
Wrist and finger extension	Dual nerve transfer from median nerve: 1. Nerve to FDS 2. Nerve to FCR	1. ECRB (for wrist extension) 2. PIN (for digital extension)	
Forearm pronation,	Branches of ulnar nerve to FCU or branches of radial nerve to ECRB	Nerve to PT	
Finger flexion	Musculocutaneous, radial and/or ulnar nerve	AIN	
Thumb opposition	Proximal branches of median nerve (AIN to PQ)	Recurrent branch of the median nerve	May require interposition graft
First web space sensation	Common digital nerve to third web space	Nerve to the first web space	

AIN, anterior interosseus nerve; *ECRB,* extensor carpi radialis brevis; *FCR,* flexor carpi radialis; *FCU,* flexor carpi ulnaris; *FDS,* flexor digitorum superficialis; *PIN,* posterior interosseus nerve; *PL,* palmaris longus; *PQ,* pronator quadratus; *PT,* pronator teres.

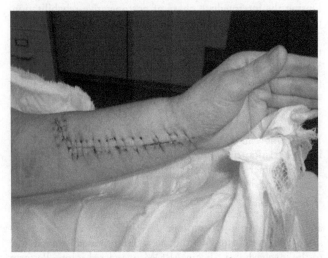

FIG. 28.14 Scarring after tendon transfer surgery.

gentle active and active-assisted motions for short sessions several times a day to reduce joint stiffness. For example, isolated joint motions might be thumb interphalangeal (IP) joint flexion and extension, or MP joint flexion and extension following tendon transfers for extensor pollicis longus (EPL) and extensor digitorum communis (EDC) (Fig. 28.15).

Precaution. *Remember to avoid composite motion and overstretching of the transferred tissues.*

When you observe good-quality muscle contractions, you can begin facilitation of the target muscle(s) in earnest. This is the core of the rehabilitation program.[1,9,18] The advantage of preoperative conditioning and education becomes apparent here. Clients who are able to recruit previously conditioned muscles learn to quickly activate these muscles with their new functions. Introduce **facilitation techniques** for those clients who show signs of difficulty initiating the desired motion. Facilitation techniques (Box 28.4) are specific strategies utilized to recruit the target muscle to function in its new capacity

(Fig. 28.16 through Fig. 28.18). Motor reeducation is critical to allow for cortical remapping and recruitment of muscles.[6-9,18] Normal movement patterns and muscle balance are emphasized through repetition, active exercises, and activities. Following nerve transfers, assess the muscles for evidence of reinnervation.[18] Initiate this movement with activation of the donor muscle. Motor retraining involves cocontraction of both the donor muscle and recipient muscle to enhance activation. Biofeedback units can provide visual and auditory feedback to help maximize the desired motions and also to minimize compensatory muscle activity.[18]

Sensory retraining and reeducation is another vital component of the therapeutic process, especially for clients who have received sensory nerve transfers. Clients may require additional education in this area to understand the (abstract) concepts of sensory relearning exercises and support to stay motivated to perform them regularly.[19]

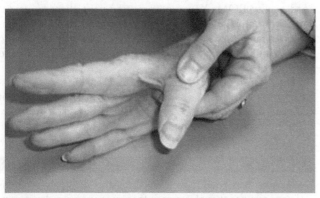

FIG. 28.15 Isolated motion at the thumb interphalangeal joint.

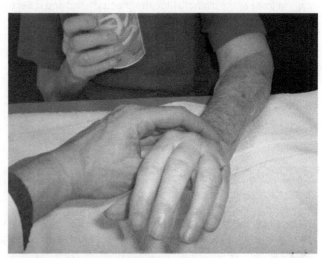

FIG. 28.16 Place and hold facilitation technique for wrist extension.

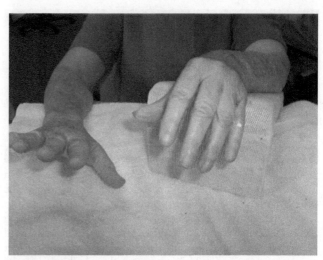

FIG. 28.17 Place and hold facilitation technique for both hands simultaneously.

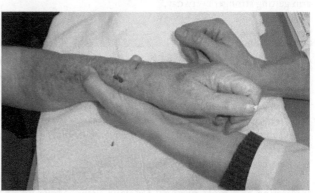

FIG. 28.18 Providing resistance to donor muscle.

| BOX 28.4 | Facilitation Techniques |

Place and hold: Place your client's wrist or finger in the desired position, and ask them to maintain this position. Count to 10. Educate your client to perform this on their own.

Using both hands simultaneously: Have your client perform the desired motion with both hands at the same time.

Using the donor muscle action: Have your client try to perform the donor muscle's original action, and monitor for the new muscle action to occur.

Resistance to the donor muscle: Offer gentle resistance to the donor muscle (its original action).

Verbal cues: Encourage the desired motion through words and description.

Tapping, vibration: Gently tap over the donor muscle, or use a small vibrator on this area to initiate stimulation of the donor muscle.

Visual and functional cues: Ask your client to imagine holding an object or performing a task with the involved hand. Look for small muscle activity in the desired motion.

Mirror training: Place the affected hand behind the mirror, and have your client perform the desired function with both hands. However, your client will be able to see only the noninvolved hand and its reflection in the mirror. Monitor the involved hand for motor activity.

Neuromuscular electrical stimulation (NMES): Use NMES to recruit the donor muscle activity. Place the smaller electrodes over the motor points for the donor muscles and place the larger dispersive pad over a noncontractile area.

Clinical Pearl

The use of mirrors in hand therapy is well established for reducing pain in amputees and for enhancing motor retraining in clients following stroke. This may also be a helpful technique to implement with tendon and nerve transfer clients.[20,21] To facilitate a donor or target muscle, place the mirror vertically in front of the client to hide the affected hand and reflect the noninjured hand. The client moves the noninjured hand in the desired motion and receives visual feedback that both hands are moving together. It is recommended that the client performs this activity twice a day in a quiet environment, and concentrate on the hand in the mirror while moving both hands at the same time.[20,21] Graded motor imagery, which stresses left-right recognition and imagined motions may also be a useful technique to try in therapy.[20-22]

Clinical Pearl

Encourage clients to perform slow and controlled repetitions to promote good patterns of use. Be aware that the target muscle may fatigue quickly. Thirty minutes or less may be all that is tolerated in a session. Do not overdo the exercise sessions!

Clinical Pearl

Dynamic orthoses that assist functional motions may also be helpful initially, in order to promote correct movement patterns. As the client gains muscular control, the orthosis can be modified to reduce its assistive force and let the muscles perform the motion.

What to Say to Clients

"As you begin to use your target muscles, make sure your motion is accurate and precise. Make sure your arm performs the specific desired motion. If you notice a slight change of direction, your arm is tired and you must take a break. Try 10 repetitions as a starting point. Do several short sessions throughout the day, and afterward put your orthosis on to rest. The orthosis helps to maintain the best position of your arm until it is strong enough to do this on its own. Do not be alarmed at how quickly your arm gets fatigued! It takes time for all structures to adjust to their new roles. You will see your arm getting stronger every day."

Precautions and Concerns

- *Do not perform passive motion or stretching in the direction against the transferred muscle's key function. For example, avoid passive wrist flexion following tendon transfers for wrist extension, as this places tension and stress on the sutured tendons.*
- *No resistance to the desired motion*
- *No composite motion that puts tension on the transferred muscle or nerve*
- *Do not overwork the target muscle*

Now is the time to make the therapeutic process more interesting and more personal for your client. Move beyond standard and rote exercises. Introduce functional activities into the rehabilitative program once the target muscle's activation is consistent and AROM is within functional limits. Do not forget to include functional activities that were outlined during preoperative goal setting. Provide many opportunities to practice activities that have personal meaning for your client.

Tendon Transfers: The Late Phase (Weeks 6 to 12)

At 6 to 8 weeks postsurgery (in most cases), you can begin to add strengthening exercises to your client's therapeutic sessions, including motion against gravity. The emphasis remains on good-quality ROM. You can encourage your client to gradually discontinue use of their orthosis, except when their extremity shows fatigue. Encourage the incorporation of the hand into your client's ADLs, including bathing, dressing, leisure, and work activities.

Do not rush to add PROM in the opposite direction of transferred muscles. These passive exercises are to be added only if necessary, as they continue to put strain and tension on the suture site of the transferred muscles.[1,11]

What to Say to Clients

"Now your transferred tissues have healed in their new positions and your arm has enough strength for you to use every day in your regular routines and actions. Try to use your hand normally for all of your activities of daily living. Try to eat and get dressed using both hands. Make sure your movements are correct and do not substitute with your other muscles. Do not overdo it! If your hand feels tired, rest it, and wear your orthosis."

Nerve Transfers: Early Phase

Kahn and Moore[23] propose a rehabilitation approach to nerve transfers focusing on donor activation strategies with an emphasis on patient education along with early and frequent training sessions. Their protocol also includes three phases of rehabilitation using manual muscle testing (MMT) as a guide to the type of exercises and motions to be highlighted. The early phase includes frequent exercise sessions to actively contract the donor muscles and to perform passive joint range of motion exercises to limit joint tightness and contractures. They label this high-repetition, low-resistance movement as "flooding" of the new neural pathway.

Nerve Transfers: The Middle Phase

MMT of the target muscle is assessed on regular visits. Resistance to the donor muscle can elicit a small contraction in the recipient muscle. This indicates a positive motor response. Exercises are then advanced to gravity eliminated movements of the target muscle and active assisted exercises. Flooding of the recipient muscle continues. Place and hold exercises against gravity can be initiated when the MMT is graded as a 2+ to 3/5.

Nerve Transfers: The Late Phase

When MMT indicates that the client can perform full range of motion against gravity, (3/5), resistive exercises can begin. Remember to pace the exercise sessions, as fatigue and frustration with slow progress can occur.

Kahn and Moore[23] suggest using metaphors to describe the transfer process so that clients have a better understanding of what is involved with their anatomy. They offer the example of a lamp and electrical cord to represent the nerve and the muscle. When the cord is cut or not plugged in, the lamp does not work. Another analogy is that of a highway and detours to suggest the need for alternate pathways to the muscle.

Diagnosis-Specific Information That Affects Clinical Reasoning

Operative Treatment: Restoration of Opposition/Opponensplasty

The most disabling functional loss after injury to the median nerve is the loss of thumb opposition. Opposition refers to the complex action of bringing the thumb up and out of the palm. Indications that this function may need restorative care are median nerve palsy, a congenital deformity (such as, thumb hypoplasia), trauma to tendons and nerves, and/or a disease process (such as, Charcot Marie Tooth syndrome). During the preoperative evaluation, look for tightness of the first web space. Begin with gentle stretching of this passively. You can also address a tight first web space by initiating activities that promote wide abduction. Fabricate a static progressive web spacer orthosis to maintain the stretch at night (Fig. 28.19).[16]

The primary muscles for opposition are the abductor pollicis brevis (APB), opponens pollicis (OP), and flexor pollicis brevis (FPB). A variety of procedures involve different donor muscles to restore the loss of these muscle's actions (see Box 28.1).

The therapist must know which muscle was used as the donor tendon, as this directly affects the choice of postoperative protective orthosis, the correct facilitation techniques, and activity selection.

Following the 3 to 4 weeks of immobilization in a postoperative cast, fabricate a long opponens orthosis for your client to protect the transferred tendon if it crosses the wrist. Make sure to place the thumb in wide abduction. Instruct your client to wear the orthosis day and night initially and to remove it only for exercises.

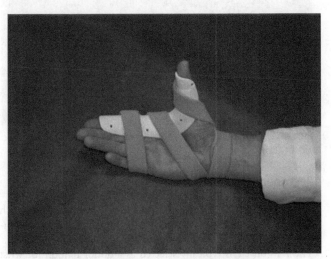

FIG. 28.19 Orthosis to stretch the first web space.

The easiest facilitation technique is the place and hold exercise. Using this technique, place the client's wrist or finger in the desired position (of the target muscle), and ask him or her to hold the wrist or finger in place against gravity. For example, if the flexor digitorum superficialis (FDS) to the ring has been used as a donor muscle to restore thumb abduction, place the client's thumb in abduction, and ask the client to hold it there while flexing the ring finger simultaneously. Count aloud as the client maintains the thumb position. Try to hold for 5 seconds, and increase gradually to 10 seconds. Do this for several repetitions. Do not be discouraged by the lack of full motion or the inability to sustain the position for more than a few seconds. This weakness and fatigue will gradually improve, and your client will start to see progress shortly. He or she will soon be able to recruit the target muscle more quickly and sustain the contraction for longer periods. As soon as your client can facilitate the action independently and without much effort, encourage the use of the thumb during ADLs. Facilitate wide thumb abduction and opposition by creating activities that incorporate the use of large diameter objects for grasp. Progress your client gradually to activities that require holding smaller diameter objects.

As you note improved control over the thumb's AROM, instruct your client to reduce orthotic wear during the day. Make sure your client is comfortable using the thumb in all ADLs. Do this gradually over time. Have your client continue to wear their orthosis during the night and for protection when around crowds and in unfamiliar settings until 12 weeks postsurgery.

Operative Treatment: Restoration of Wrist and Digital Extension

Serious injuries to the radial nerve cause loss of wrist extension from the functions of the ECRB, extensor carpi radialis longus (ECRL), and extensor carpi ulnaris; loss of finger extension from EDC, extensor indicis proprius (EIP), and extensor digiti minimi; and loss of thumb extension and abduction from EPL, extensor pollicis brevis, and abductor pollicis longus. This injury is often called "wrist drop deformity" due to the classic wrist flexion or dropped wrist posture (see Fig. 28.1).[15]

There may be a sensory deficit in the dorsal first web space if the level of injury occurs proximal to the branching of the radial nerve into its two terminal branches: the radial sensory nerve and the posterior interosseous nerve. Although this area has minimum functional impact, your client may still be susceptible to burns in this area without being aware of them.

Always educate your client regarding the potential for burns and injuries to insensate areas of skin (see Fig 28.10). Note the bandage over dorsal first web where the client burned herself removing items from a hot oven.

Preoperative Treatment

Preoperative treatment is always geared toward maintenance of function and prevention of, or correction of joint contractures. A loss of grip strength may be present due to the lack of wrist stabilizers. It is difficult for your client to extend their digits and release objects.[10] They may allow the wrist to drop into flexion

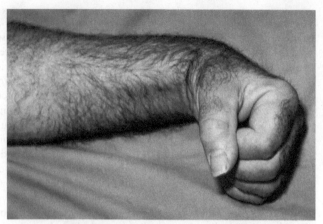

FIG. 28.20　Client with radial nerve palsy.

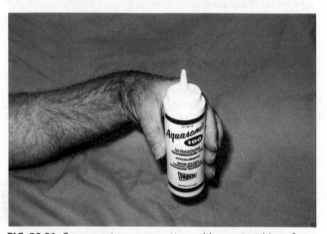

FIG. 28.21　Compensatory grasp pattern with overstretching of wrist extensors.

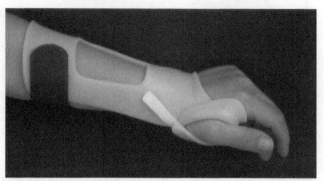

FIG. 28.22　Dorsal wrist cock up orthosis.

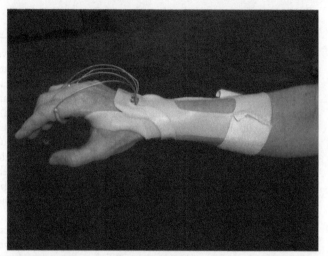

FIG. 28.23　Dynamic orthosis for radial nerve palsy with wires for metacarpophalangeal extension.

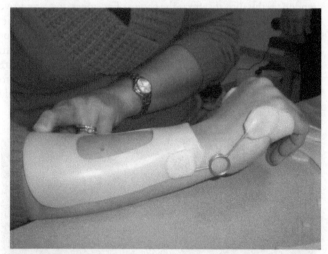

FIG. 28.24　Dynamic orthosis for radial nerve palsy with coils for wrist extension.

and pronation to achieve digital release (Figs. 28.20 and 28.21). Over time, this can cause overstretching of the paralyzed muscles and become a fixed deformity. Address contractures or joint tightness of the wrist by stretching and the use of static, static progressive, and/or functional orthoses.

Preoperative treatment addresses the lack of functional wrist and digital extension through creative orthotic fabrication. Clients who require a forceful grip may benefit most from a static wrist orthosis, either dorsal or volar based. Consider the benefits of a dorsal-based wrist orthosis that does not block the sensory input from the palm (Fig. 28.22).

Clients needing more wrist or finger mobility may prefer a dynamic wrist or finger orthosis (Figs. 28.23 and 28.24).[10]

> ### ⓘ Clinical Pearl
>
> There are many different orthotic designs and many different thermoplastic materials to choose from; each one provides a different functional solution. Remember to keep your design simple. Involve your client in the fabrication process. Make sure your completed orthosis is easy to don and doff and improves or enhances your client's function. Otherwise, it will not be utilized.

Postoperative Treatment

Tendon transfers following radial nerve palsy are performed with the combined goals of restoring wrist extension, finger extension at the MP joint level, and thumb extension and abduction.[2] The PT muscle is typically selected as a donor tendon for wrist extension (leaving the pronator quadratus available for active pronation), and additional donor muscles are included to power and restore digital and thumb extension. Typical donor muscles may include flexor carpi radialis (FCR) or FDS of the middle to EDC, and PL to EPL. However, there are many variations to these procedures.

> ### ◎ Clinical Pearl
>
> You must ask the surgeon specifically which donor muscles were utilized to power each deficit. Become familiar with the most commonly performed tendon transfers by your referring surgeons (Boxes 28.1, 28.2, and 28.3).

The indications for restoration of wrist extension may also include cases of cerebral palsy where there is unbalanced wrist posturing in flexion due to increased flexor tone.[24] This posture makes hand function difficult, as it places the wrist extensors in an overstretched position while causing shortening of the wrist and digital flexors. The donor muscle typically utilized in cases of cerebral palsy to enhance wrist extension is the flexor carpi ulnaris, which is surgically repositioned to assist the ECRL in active wrist extension.[24] Assessing the client for voluntary control of the digits with the wrist placed in extension is critical.[1,11] Do this by holding the wrist in extension, have the client make a fist with his or her digits, and then open them. If the client does not exhibit voluntary control of the digits in this position, he or she may use the tenodesis motion to allow his or her digits to open and release objects. Enhancing wrist extension hampers his ability to use his or her digits in this method and may not be beneficial.[11]

Early Phase

Following tendon transfer surgery for wrist extension, the upper extremity is typically placed in a long arm cast with the elbow positioned in 90 degrees of flexion (to protect the origin of the PT muscle). The forearm is positioned in pronation, the wrist is positioned in 30 to 40 degrees of wrist extension, and the MP joints are positioned in 0-degree extension. The IP joints can be left free.[1-3,11,24] Cast immobilization usually lasts 3 to 4 weeks.

> ### ◖ What to Say to Clients
>
> "Make sure you elevate your arm to mobilize your shoulder joint so that it does not get stiff. Do this also to reduce swelling in your digits. You need to actively bend and straighten your non-immobilized digits throughout the day to keep them from getting stiff as well."

At 4 weeks, the cast is replaced with a long arm thermoplastic orthosis fabricated to maintain the arm in the same position as previously described. Instruct your client to remove this orthosis during the day for AROM exercises. As your client gains ROM and demonstrates good control over the transferred tendons, orthotic wear is reduced to nighttime protection only—up and through 12 weeks.[1]

> ### ♡ Tips From the Field
>
> Some surgeons will allow the long arm orthosis to be modified to a wrist cock-up orthosis at 6 to 8 weeks postsurgery. This is much more comfortable for your client. Make sure to check with the surgeon regarding their choice of orthotic design.

Intermediate Phase

Introduce the facilitation techniques previously described to activate the transferred muscles (Box 28.4).

Begin activation of the donor tendon with a simple place and hold in wrist extension. Place your client's wrist in extension, and have your client try to hold the wrist in this position for 5 to 10 seconds initially. Gradually increase the length of this muscle contraction. Or try having your client extend their wrist actively with both hands simultaneously. If no response can be elicited, offer some resistance to the transferred muscle's original function. For example, if PT was used as a donor muscle for wrist extension, give some resistance to pronation while the client attempts to supinate the forearm. You should see some indication of active wrist extension with this maneuver. Do not expect full wrist ROM or even 50% of wrist ROM! The transferred tendon is very weak and still needs time to heal and strengthen. Approach these facilitation techniques very slowly and carefully.

If multiple tendon transfers have been performed in the same surgery, approach each one as a separate entity with facilitation strategies for each motion. For example, following the wrist extension exercises described earlier, you can attend to the digital and thumb transfers and facilitate these in a similar fashion with place and hold exercises for MP joints in extension and for the thumb in extension. If a muscle transfer was utilized that includes both of these functions together, such as the Boyes transfer[2,3] that incorporates the FDS (ring) to both the EPL and the EIP, you must work with these two motions as a single function (Box 28.2).

Make sure your client is able to demonstrate active wrist and finger extension and maintain an isometric contraction. Gradually introduce more activities into therapy sessions that require these motions.

Late Phase

At 8 to 12 weeks after surgery, your therapeutic intervention should focus on your client's ability to move through functional if not full ROM in all affected joints. You can add strengthening exercises to the routine. Sustained grip activities and progressive resistance exercises for wrist and finger extension are good choices. By now, your client should demonstrate using their involved extremity for all ADLs. Discuss any areas of concern or weakness. If it is not necessary for your client to regain full wrist flexion for functional activities, do not perform passive stretches into wrist flexion. You do not want to stretch out the tendon transfer.

Operative Treatment: Restoration of Thumb Extension With Tendon Transfers

Thumb extension may be lost either due to radial nerve injury or due to muscle and tendon trauma independent of other muscle involvement. Clients may experience a closed rupture of the EPL tendon after a distal radius fracture.[2] Tendon rupture is also common in clients with rheumatoid arthritis. The EIP is typically chosen as a donor muscle for the thumb extensor.[2] Following tendon transfer surgery, the wrist and thumb are placed in full extension, including the IP joint of the thumb. After 3 to 4 weeks of postoperative immobilization, fabricate a long opponens orthosis, including the IP joint of the thumb in full extension.

♡ Tips From the Field

Orthoses as Aids to Movement

To facilitate active thumb extension at the thumb MP joint, fabricate a small thumb IP extension orthosis. This allows the client to generate force specifically at the thumb MP joint and not involve the IP joint in the exercise (Fig. 28.25).

Similarly, to facilitate digital MP flexion and extension without IP flexion, fabricate a circular digital extension orthosis for all four digits that helps to generate force specifically at the MP joints and block the force going distally. Your client can practice active MP flexion and extension exercises wearing the orthosis and will later be able to recruit this motion without the orthosis (Figs. 28.26 and 28.27).

Operative Treatment: Restoration of the Intrinsic Muscles

Clients with injury to the ulnar nerve or with ulnar nerve palsy may present with weak wrist flexion, deficits in power grip, a flattened metacarpal arch, the loss of lumbrical function and MP flexion, and decreased pinch strength. High ulnar nerve injury is defined as proximal to the insertion of the flexor group, and low ulnar nerve injury is defined as distal to innervation of FDP. Low ulnar nerve injuries typically demonstrate clawing of the ulnar digits due to hyperextension of the MPs from unopposed extrinsic extensors

and strong over pull of the unopposed FDP.[2,3,25] In high-level ulnar nerve injuries, the FDP is also affected, and therefore there is no clawing deformity. Ulnar nerve palsy causes difficulty in grasping objects as the digits begin rolling into flexion starting with the IP joints followed by late MP joint flexion. The normal MP joint flexion pattern powered by the intrinsic muscles is lost, and it is extremely difficult to hold objects in the hand.[11] In fact, as your client attempts to grasp an object, you will note that his or her digital flexion begins at the fingertips that roll into flexion, closing up the hand before it actually encounters the object. The sensory deficit of ulnar nerve involvement also contributes to the functional loss.[4]

◎ Clinical Pearl

Two additional signs of ulnar nerve involvement are as follows[4,10]:
1. Wartenberg's sign: Eccentric abduction of the little finger due to unopposed extensor digiti minimi (EDM) and paralysis of palmar adductors (Fig. 28.28).
2. Froment's paper sign: Substitution of flexor pollicis longus for adductor pollicis (AP) and first dorsal interosseous; the sign is positive if the client flexes the IP joint with key pinch (Fig. 28.29).
   Be sure to look for these signs in your evaluation, and record your tests as positive if present.

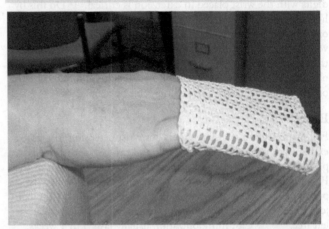

FIG. 28.27 Blocking orthosis to facilitate metacarpophalangeal extension.

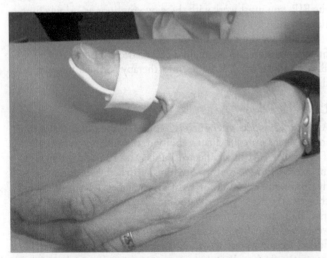

FIG. 28.25 Facilitation of thumb metacarpophalangeal extension.

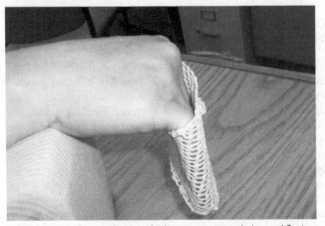

FIG. 28.26 Blocking orthosis to facilitate metacarpophalangeal flexion.

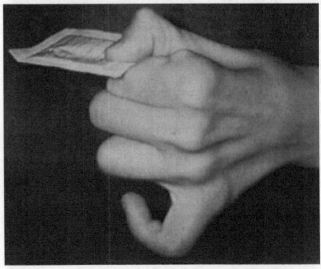

FIG. 28.28 Wartenberg's sign. (From Burke SL: *Hand and upper extremity rehabilitation: a practical guide.* ed 3, Philadelphia, 2005, Churchill Livingstone.)

Preoperative Treatment

Goals of preoperative treatment for ulnar nerve palsy include preventing contractures of the MP and proximal interphalangeal joints and maintaining the normal length of the extrinsic flexor muscles.[10] Provide your client with an anticlaw orthosis. This simple orthosis supports the metacarpal arch and holds the ulnar digits in flexion at the MP joint, preventing overstretching of the intrinsic muscles. It can be either a static or dynamic orthosis (see Figs. 28.5 and 28.6).

The surgeon may select from a variety of surgical procedures to correct the deformities associated with ulnar nerve paralysis[2,3,25] (Box 28.3).

Postoperative Treatment

Following surgery and the normal immobilization period of 3 to 4 weeks, fabricate an immobilization orthosis to maintain the MP joints in flexion. This can be either a forearm-based dorsal blocking orthosis or a volar wrist orthosis with MPs in flexion and IPs in extension. After 4 weeks of immobilization, instruct your client to begin gentle AROM exercises. Be sure to include isolated motions at the elbow, wrist, and MP joints.[1-3] It is important to mobilize one joint at a time to avoid increased tension on the transfer. Instruct the client to gently flex and extend the MP joints from their resting posture in full flexion.

Precautions and Concerns Following Tendon Transfers for Ulnar Nerve Function

- Avoid full metacarpophalangeal extension. (This may overstretch the transfer.)
- Avoid passive flexion and extension of the interphalangeal joints.

Initiate facilitation techniques to the transferred muscles. Use the facilitation techniques described earlier. As your client progresses to full control of digital motion, include functional activities of meaning into therapy. Encourage active use of the involved hand during all ADLs. Modify the original forearm-based orthosis to a hand-based orthosis. Tell your client to practice but not to overstress composite flexion of the digits.

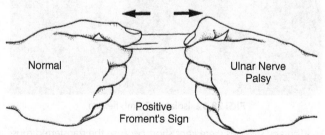

FIG. 28.29 Froment's paper sign. (From Burke SL: *Hand and Upper Extremity Rehabilitation: a Practical Guide.* 3rd ed. Philadelphia, PA: Churchill Livingstone; 2005.)

Avoid heavy resistance toward full extension, as this may cause overstretching of the transfer.[1-3] Begin gentle strengthening exercises at 8 weeks after surgery. Monitor your client for good quality motion. Full activity can be resumed by 12 to 14 weeks, depending on each individual. Gradually wean your client from orthotic wear.

Additional Tendon Transfer Protocols

The most commonly performed tendon transfer protocols have been described here. Preoperative and postoperative rehabilitation protocols for nerve transfers follow these same general guidelines. Always make sure to thoroughly investigate which tendons and nerves were involved in each procedure. Carefully evaluate the client for functional deficits, and create functional goals for the surgery. Protect the transferred muscles and/or nerves in a tension-free position as indicated. Begin activation of the target muscles. Utilize facilitation techniques, and motor and/or sensory reeducation therapies as needed to activate the transfers. Always incorporate meaningful functional activities into the treatment.

What's New in the Field?

Studies have compared immediate active mobilization of tendon transfers in clients to the conventional postoperative immobilization of 3 to 4 weeks, which is typically prescribed.[26] The benefits of a reduced course of rehabilitation are significant, with less time away from work being an important consideration. Early active motion was also compared with a dynamic orthosis protocol.[27] Early mobilization protocols appear to be safe and cost effective. Clients report less pain and regain function and motion more quickly. Additional studies indicate that the use of "wide awake" procedures in the absence of general anesthesia may also benefit tendon transfer clients. Adjustments for tension on the transferred muscle can be performed prior to skin closure. The client is also able to make an immediate association and perform the desired motion in the operating room.[28]

Tendon transfers and, more recently, nerve transfers have produced improved functional outcomes for clients with devastating nerve injuries and/or congenital deformities. Advances in surgical techniques and attention to detail in motor relearning and postoperative rehabilitation protocols have led to successful nerve transfer procedures for peripheral nerve injuries, with earlier reinnervation times and quicker return to function than traditional tendon transfers. The indications for and use of nerve transfers is increasing with newly described protocols for each specific nerve injury.

Strategies for Success

Tendon and or nerve transfer surgery can offer clients greatly improved functional outcomes. A team approach, including surgeon, client, and therapist along with other health care individuals if needed, benefits everyone involved. Careful preoperative evaluation, appropriate client selection, and thorough observation and planning must be done prior to surgery. Nerve transfers can benefit clients with limited sensory function as well.[5,7,8,9,18]

Defining the most critical functional goals of the client is imperative, as well as assessing the available muscles and nerves to achieve these goals. Client education regarding every aspect of the surgery and rehabilitation process enhances cooperation and outcomes. Judicious use of orthoses and activities of meaning will enhance your therapeutic interventions. Pay careful attention to the anatomy and the timetable of healing to create a successful rehabilitation process.

CASE STUDIES

CASE STUDY 28.1 ■ Radial Nerve Palsy and Restoration of Wrist, Finger, and Thumb Extension

SK is a 74-year-old, right hand dominant female living alone in an assisted living facility. She sustained a humeral fracture on her left side after a fall on the pavement. The arm was placed in a long arm cast for about 5 weeks. It was only after the cast was removed that she reported the inability to extend her wrist and her digits. A diagnosis of radial nerve palsy was made, and she was referred to hand therapy for ROM exercises and orthotic fabrication.

A dynamic MP extension orthosis was provided for the client to use during functional activities throughout the day. In addition, a wrist cock-up orthosis was provided for nighttime wear. After 3 to 4 months with no discernible nerve regeneration, the surgeon began plans to perform tendon transfer surgery.

The therapist performed a detailed client interview and determined that the client was having trouble with basic ADLs, including the ability to feed and dress herself unassisted. Her hobbies at the assisted living facility included playing cards, typing a community newsletter for the group, and participating in communal activities. She was unable to type or hold cards in her involved left hand, and therefore was no longer participating in any of the group activities at the home. The therapist performed a full preoperative evaluation, including manual muscle testing to determine which muscles could be used as possible donor muscles. SK demonstrated above fair muscle grades in all median nerve and ulnar nerve innervated muscles.

The surgeon performed the following tendon transfers:
- PT to ECRL
- FCR to EDC
- PL to EPL

After surgery, SK was placed in a long arm cast for 4 weeks with the elbow positioned in 90 degrees of flexion, the forearm in pronation, the wrist in 30 degrees of extension, and the MP joints in 0 degrees of extension (Figs. 28.30 and 28.31).

SK was instructed to mobilize her shoulder and digits throughout the period of immobilization. At 4 weeks postsurgery, the postoperative dressings were removed, and the therapist fabricated a long arm orthosis, maintaining this same positioning of the arm. Gentle isolated motions were initiated for wrist, digits, and thumb (Fig. 28.32 through Fig. 28.35).

At this time, facilitation techniques were initiated to activate the transferred muscles. Place and hold exercises were introduced for all of the transferred muscles, and resistance to supination was utilized to recruit the PT (donor muscle to the wrist extensors). These two facilitation techniques proved to be extremely successful and helped to activate the transferred muscles. Before long, SK could do these by herself (Fig. 28.36).

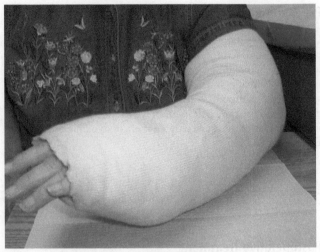
FIG. 28.30 Postoperative dressings.

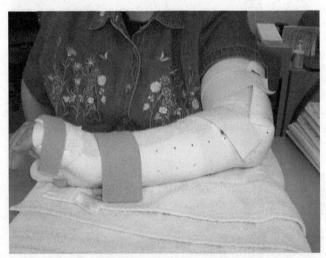
FIG. 28.31 Long arm orthosis.

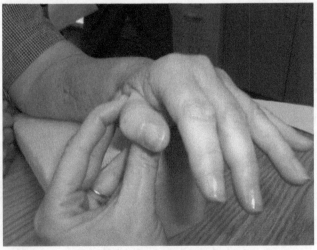
FIG. 28.32 Isolated thumb flexion.

Therapy sessions were kept short because the transferred muscles showed fatigue quickly. As the muscles gained strength, SK was able to sustain the contraction for longer periods of time and more frequently throughout the session. Along with the facilitation techniques, therapy sessions included activities of meaning to the client,

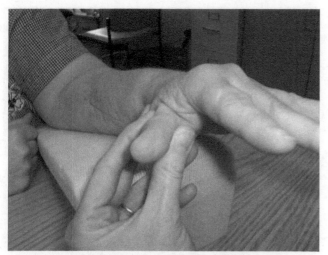

FIG. 28.33 Isolated thumb extension.

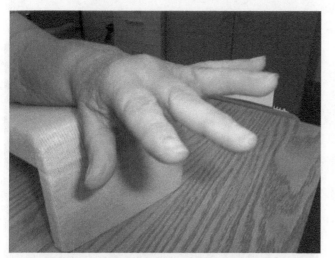

FIG. 28.34 Isolated metacarpophalangeal extension.

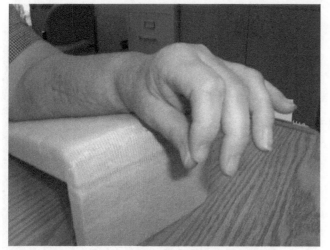

FIG. 28.35 Isolated metacarpophalangeal flexion.

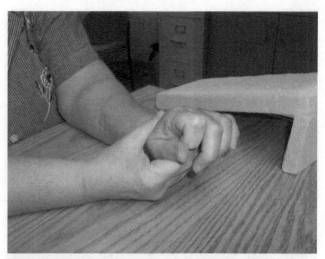

FIG. 28.36 Client performing place and hold independently to recruit wrist extension.

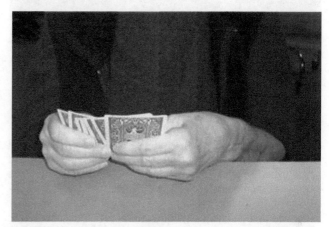

FIG. 28.37 Including activities of meaning into therapy sessions—holding cards.

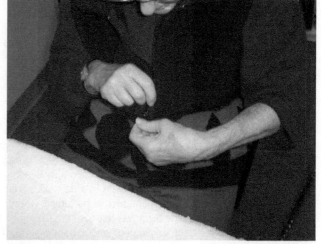

FIG. 28.38 Including activities of meaning into therapy sessions—self-dressing.

such as holding playing cards, simulated typing, and drinking with the involved hand (Fig. 28.37 through Fig. 28.39).

At 6 weeks postsurgery, the long arm orthosis was modified to a wrist cock up orthosis for nighttime use only. SK was encouraged to incorporate the left upper extremity in all ADLs. She progressed

through strengthening exercises for wrist extension and was discharged to a home program at 11 weeks postsurgery. It is important to note that while SK never achieved full wrist extension against gravity, she did realize adequate wrist extension for all ADLs.

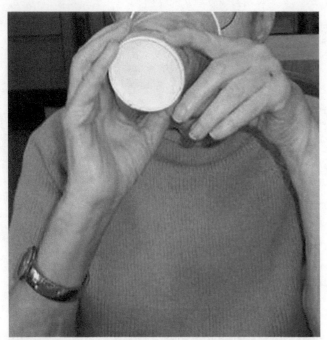

FIG. 28.39 Including activities of meaning into therapy sessions—self-feeding.

CASE STUDY 28.2 ▪ Median Nerve Palsy and Abductorplasty

CB is a 62-year-old, right-handed female with severe carpal tunnel syndrome, which has been progressively worsening over time, and has resulted in thenar muscle wasting and weak opposition. She reports pain, numbness, and difficulty manipulating objects. The surgeon performed carpal tunnel release surgery and, at the same time, performed an abductorplasty to restore thumb abduction. In this case, the FDS of the ring finger was selected as a donor muscle and inserted into the APB muscle. CB was referred to therapy at 2 weeks postsurgery for fabrication of a long opponens orthosis, protecting both the surgical site and maintaining wide thumb abduction. Initially, exercises were performed for the uninvolved digits, and shoulder and elbow ROM was encouraged to reduce swelling and prevent joint stiffness. Scar management of the volar forearm scars was also begun along with desensitization techniques. At 4 weeks postsurgery, the orthosis was taken off for daily active exercise sessions. The place and hold facilitation technique was initiated with the thumb placed in wide abduction, and the client was asked to maintain the position. In addition, she was asked to oppose the thumb to the ring finger. CB learned to actively recruit the motion of the FDS via some resistance to the ring finger in flexion.

Activities progressed from those incorporating a wide grasp, such as holding small balls, to those that demanded a smaller and stronger pinch, like placing Chinese checkers in a tray. ADLs were introduced to the therapeutic regiment, such as buttoning, writing, and computer typing. Slowly the client was able to return to her previous level of full independent functioning. Tendon transfer surgery paired with carpal tunnel release surgery was successful at eliminating the client's complaints of numbness and tingling in her median nerve innervated digits, as well as restoring stronger and more functional thumb motion (Fig. 28.40 through Fig. 28.42).

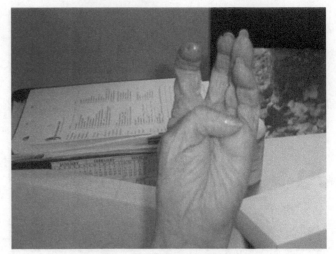

FIG. 28.40 Thumb abduction.

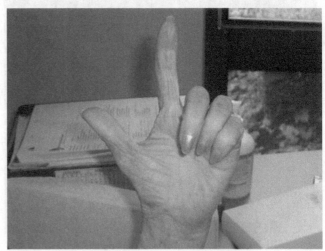

FIG. 28.41 Thumb extension.

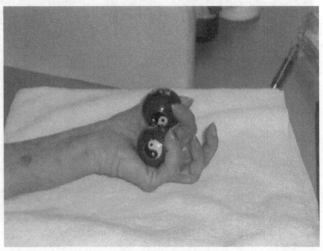

FIG. 28.42 Thumb activity holding and manipulating chime balls.

References

1. Duff SV, Humpl D: Therapist's management of tendon transfers. In Skirven TM, Osterman AL, Fedorczyk JF, et al.: *Rehabilitation of the hand and upper extremity*, ed 6, Philadelphia, 2011, Mosby, pp 781–791.
2. Seiler III JG, Desai MJ, Payne HS: Tendon transfers for radial, median, and ulnar nerve palsy, *J Am Acad Orthop Surg* 21(11):675–684, 2013.
3. Wilbur D, Hammert WC: Principles of tendon transfer, *Hand Clinics* 32(3):283–289, 2016.
4. Cook S, Gaston RG, Lourie GM: Ulnar nerve tendon transfers for pinch, *Hand Clinics* 32(3):369–376, 2016.
5. Korus L, Ross DC, Doherty CD, Miller TA: Nerve transfers and neurotization in peripheral nerve injury, from surgery to rehabilitation, *J Neurol Neurosurg Psychiatry* 87(2):188–197, 2016.
6. Rinker B: Nerve transfers in the upper extremity: a practical user's guide, *Ann Plast Surg* 74:S222–S228, 2015.
7. Tung TH, Mackinnon SE: Nerve transfers: indications, techniques, and outcomes, *J Hand Surg* 35(2):332–341, 2010.
8. Moore AM, Novak CB: Advances in nerve transfer surgery, *J Hand Ther* 27(2):96–105, 2014.
9. Tung TH: Nerve transfers. In Skirven TM, Osterman AL, Fedorczyk JF, et al.: *Rehabilitation of the hand and upper extremity*, ed 6, Philadelphia, 2011, Mosby.
10. Moscony AMB: Common peripheral nerve problems. In Cooper C, editor: *Fundamentals of hand therapy: clinical reasoning and treatment guidelines for common diagnoses of the upper extremity*, St Louis, 2007, Mosby Elsevier, pp 201–250.
11. Ashworth S, Kozin SH: Brachial plexus palsy reconstruction: tendon transfers, osteotomies, capsular release and arthrodesis. In Skirven TM, Osterman AL, Fedorczyk JF, et al.: *Rehabilitation of the hand and upper extremity*, ed 6, Philadelphia, 2011, Mosby, pp 792–812.
12. Uddin Z, MacDermid J, Packham T: The ten test for sensation, *J Physiother* 59(2):132, 2013.
13. Fess EE: Functional tests. In Skirven TM, Osterman AL, Fedorczyk JF, et al.: *Rehabilitation of the hand and upper extremity*, ed 6, Philadelphia, 2011, Mosby.
14. Von der Hyde R, Droege K: Assessment of functional outcomes. In Cooper C, editor: *Fundamentals of hand therapy: clinical reasoning and treatment guidelines for common diagnoses of the upper extremity*, St Louis, 2007, Mosby Elsevier, pp 115–127.
15. Cheah AEJ, Etcheson J, Yao J: Radial nerve tendon transfers, *Hand Clinics* 32(3):323–338, 2016.
16. Chadderdon RC, Gaston RG: Low median nerve transfers (opponensplasty), *Hand Clinics* 32(3):349–359, 2016.
17. Pettengill K: Therapist management of the complex injury. In Skirven TM, Osterman AL, Fedorczyk JF, et al.: *Rehabilitation of the hand and upper extremity*, ed 6, Philadelphia, 2011, Mosby, pp 1238–1251.
18. Novak CB: Rehabilitation following motor nerve transfers, *Hand Clinics* 24(4):417–423, 2008.
19. Vikström P, Carlsson I, Rosén B, Björkman A: Patients' views on early sensory relearning following nerve repair—a Q-methodology study, *J Hand Ther*, 2017. https://doi.org/10.1016/j.jht.2017.07.003.
20. McCabe C: Mirror visual feedback therapy. a practical approach, *J Hand Ther* 24(2):170–179, 2011.
21. Plumbe L, Peters S, Bennett S, Vicenzino B, Coppieters MW: Mirror therapy, graded motor imagery and virtual illusion for the management of chronic pain (Protocol), *Cochrane Database Syst Rev* (1), 2013. CD010329-1.
22. Dilek B, Ayhan C, Yagci G, Yakut Y: Effectiveness of the graded motor imagery to improve hand function in patients with distal radius fracture: a randomized controlled trial, *J Hand Ther*, 2017. https://doi.org/10.1016/j.jht.2017.09.004.
23. Kahn LC, Moore AM: Donor activation focused rehabilitation approach: maximizing outcomes after nerve transfers, *Hand Clinics* 32(2):263–277, 2016.
24. Koman LA, Li Z, Patterson Smith B, et al.: Upper extremity musculoskeletal surgery in the child with cerebral palsy: surgical options and rehabilitation. In Skirven TM, Osterman AL, Fedorczyk JF, et al.: *Rehabilitation of the hand and upper extremity*, ed 6, Philadelphia, 2011, Mosby, pp 1651–1658.
25. Ratner JA, Kozin SH: Tendon transfers for upper extremity peripheral nerve injuries. In Skirven TM, Osterman AL, Fedorczyk JF, et al.: *Rehabilitation of the hand and upper extremity*, ed 6, Philadelphia, 2011, Mosby, pp 771–780.
26. Rath S: A randomized clinical trial comparing immediate active motion with immobilization after tendon transfer for claw deformity, *J Hand Surg Am* 34:488–494, 2009.
27. Giessler GA, Przybilski M, Germann G, et al.: Early free active versus dynamic extension splinting after extensor indicis proprius tendon transfer to restore thumb extension: a prospective randomized study, *J Hand Surg Am* 33:864–868, 2008.
28. Lalonde DH, Kozin S: Tendon disorders of the hand, *Plast Reconstr Surg* 128(1):1e–14e, 2011.

29

Arthritis

Cynthia Clare Ivy

Arthritis is the leading cause of disability in the United States.[1] By the year 2040, at least 25.9% of all adults are expected to be diagnosed with arthritis and **arthritis attributable activity limitation** (AAAL).[2,3] Moreover, it is one of the most prevalent and disabling chronic conditions worldwide in older adults.[4,5] There are more than 100 types of arthritis,[6] with **osteoarthritis** (OA) being the most common joint disorder throughout the world.[7] OA is characterized by cartilage degradation, bone remodeling, osteophyte formation, joint inflammation, and loss of normal joint function.[8] **Rheumatoid arthritis** (RA), a multisystem condition marked by chronic destructive synovitis, is prevalent in 0.5% to 1% of people in developed countries and is the most common autoimmune inflammatory arthritis in adults.[9] Other types of rheumatic diseases include **juvenile arthritis** (children); **systemic lupus erythematosus** (SLE) (a systemic autoimmune disease characterized by inflammation and blood vessel abnormalities); **gout** (a disorder caused by uric acid or urate crystal deposition); **bursitis** (inflammation of the bursa); and **fibromyalgia** (diffuse widespread pain often with specific tender points).[9,10]

In the United States, 54.4 million adults have been told by a physician that they have some form of arthritis, and almost half of these individuals have AAAL.[11] In people over the age of 60, women experience hand OA more often than men. In people younger than 60, men experience this condition more often than women.[12] Women tend to develop OA in the distal interphalangeal (DIP) joints, proximal interphalangeal (PIP) joints, and at the base of the thumb in the carpometacarpal (CMC) joint. Men tend to develop OA in the wrist and metacarpophalangeal (MP) joints.[12] Furthermore, 50% of individuals with DIP involvement will also have PIP involvement.[13]

With this level of prevalence, many hand therapists find these clients on their caseload. The hand therapist must understand the disease process, potential deformities, and limiting factors affecting activities of daily living (ADLs), and know how to educate clients about their disease and treatment options. Arthritis and management of clients with arthritis is a very expansive topic. This chapter presents basic principles and common issues you will see in the hand clinic. However, it is not comprehensive, and I encourage the reader to seek additional information from other sources.

Osteoarthritis

Pathology

OA is often called the "wear-and-tear disease." However, this may be an oversimplification, as advancing research has determined that there are several types of OA, some more inflammatory in nature.[14-16] There is evidence that, in addition to mechanical factors, genetics and metabolic components also play a role in the pathogenesis of OA.[16,17] Chondrocytes, the only cells located in cartilage, do not behave the same in individuals with OA.[17,18] They produce pro-inflammatory cytokines and enzymes that degrade the cellular matrix.[19] This degradation corresponds to failure of the articular cartilage to act as a shock absorber, resulting in progression of the disease. Mechanical factors such as abnormal loading of the joint from trauma, heavy labor, joint instability, and obesity increase the risk of OA.[17]

Aging is also a risk factor, although OA is not inevitable as one ages.[20] As we grow older, cellular senescence results in joint surface fraying and softening—decreasing the ability of the chondrocytes to maintain or repair cartilage.[20] If a joint is then stressed, such as with a fracture in older age, the joint is more vulnerable to tissue degeneration because the cartilage cannot repair itself as well.[20] In addition to cartilage breakdown, new bone formation (**osteophytosis**) can occur in joints, resulting in pain and movement limitations. **Osteophytes**, or bone spurs, may occur at the MP, PIP, or DIP joints.

These may contribute to nodules called **Bouchard nodes** at the PIP joint and **Heberden nodes** at the DIP joint.[21] Deformities can develop such as **mallet finger** (inability to actively extend the DIP), and lateral deviation or flexion deformities at the PIP joint (**boutonniére**). Clients will often present with reduced ROM, pain, **crepitus** (grating or popping), and signs of inflammation.[22]

Timelines and Healing

There is no cure for OA at this time. Current scientific thought is that molecular abnormalities lead to illness, anatomical abnormalities, and physiological changes.[23] Treatment is based on the specific needs of each client and the stage of the disease. Staging is often done radiographically. Magnetic resonance imaging (MRI) has allowed experts to be more specific when staging the severity of the disease.[24] In the early stage, there is a reduction in the joint spaces and swelling of the periarticular tissues, sometimes without symptoms.[23] The moderate stage is marked by osteophytes, subchondral sclerosis, and cysts.[25] In the later stages, bone erosion, subluxation, and fibrotic ankylosis are observed.[24]

Postoperatively, wound healing timelines guide therapy intervention for clients with arthritis. Most postoperative treatment guidelines incorporate a balance between specific orthoses and gentle exercise during the proliferative stage (4 days to 3 weeks after surgery) when the fibroblasts lay beds of collagen. Therapy guidelines encourage scar management during the remodeling stage (which can last several years) when there is a gradual increase in the tensile strength of the collagen fibers.[26] Postoperative therapy should also include attention to edema management, ROM, and participation in ADLs during recovery.

Evaluation

Evaluation of the client with arthritis should include an assessment of function, pain, active range of motion (AROM), joint stability, and joint inflammation. The evaluation of function should include home, work, and leisure activities. Clients often seek help when their meaningful activities are threatened. Standardized tests, including the Canadian Occupational Performance Measure[27] and the Arthritis Impact Measurement Scales health status questionnaire[28] can be helpful in collaboratively determining the client's ADL limitations and goals. Pain can be measured at rest and with activities using a 10 cm visual analog scale, with 0 being no pain and 10 being severe pain, or any of 7 pain scales researched for use with arthritis.[29] **Precaution.** *Passive range of motion (PROM) measurements are generally not recommended, especially if there is a lack of joint stability. Do not apply passive stretch to a joint that lacks stability, as this can cause further damage in the presence of arthritis.*

Document areas of inflammation by specifying which joints are involved. If the joint is warm and red, it may be in an acute inflammatory stage. Evaluation of thumb base OA can be guided by the Eaton classification system, which is widely used to define severity as well as to guide treatment.[30] These stages are highlighted in Table 29.1. Treatment should be based on clinical findings as well as each client's unique values and priorities. Radiographic staging can be used as a marker by which to monitor progression of the disease process.

Evaluate thumb joint stability by having the client attempt a tip pinch. Ligament stability may be questioned if the thumb MP and interphalangeal (IP) joints are unable to maintain a

TABLE 29.1	Eaton Radiographic Classification for Staging Basal Joint Arthritis
Eaton Stage	**Radiograph**
Stage I	Normal appearance of articular surface and slight joint space widening.
Stage II	Minimal sclerotic changes of subchondral bone with osteophytes and loose bodies less than 2 mm.
Stage III	Trapeziometacarpal joint space markedly narrowed and cystic changes present. Subluxation of the metacarpal may have occurred. Osteophytes and loose bodies greater than 2 mm.
Stage IV	Presence of scaphotrapezial joint disease with narrowing.

From Eaton RG, Glickel SZ. Trapeziometacarpal osteoarthritis. Staging as a rationale for treatment. *Hand Clin.* 1987;3(4):455.

near-neutral position during pinch. Assessing lateral joint stability of the digits is important at the PIP and DIP joints. Test the involved joint(s) by stabilizing the proximal phalanx and gently moving the distal phalanx laterally in each direction. A greater degree of joint play is evident when joint stability is decreased. Lateral deviation of the IP joints at rest should also be noted. Document fixed deformities that cannot be corrected passively when *gently* positioned by the therapist. Fixed joint deformities in OA can include DIP joint flexion or angulation, thumb CMC joint adduction, and thumb MP joint extension or flexion. Pain with either the adduction stress test (in which the thumb is parallel to the index finger with forceful adduction) or the extension stress test (applied force of the thumb into the plane of the palm) appear to be the tests with the highest sensitivity and specificity in assessing CMC joint OA in the thumb.[31]

General Guidelines for Nonsurgical Treatment of Upper Extremity Osteoarthritis

OA has been the most commonly studied condition in the hand therapy literature over the past several years, and a large number of these studies address nonoperative approaches.[32] Nonoperative treatment begins with a thorough evaluation to determine the client's specific needs. Interventions may include joint protection education, pain relieving modalities, exercise, orthoses, and adaptive equipment.

Joint Protection

Joint protection principles are a group of suggestions for modifying activities using altered ergonomic positioning and adaptive techniques and tools to decrease stress and damage to the joints. With OA, special attention is focused on positioning and off-loading of the thumb CMC joint and the IP joints. Common joint protection principles for both OA and RA are categorized by themes in Fig. 29.1. Biomechanical studies have become more sophisticated and have allowed scientists to better understand both static and dynamic forces on joints during functional tasks.[33,34] The use of adaptive equipment may help normalize kinematics and decrease stresses in the small joints. Because excessive pinching during ADLs imparts large forces to the unstable thumb CMC joint, educating clients in techniques that decrease pressure and force applied to the thumb CMC joint is important.[35-37]

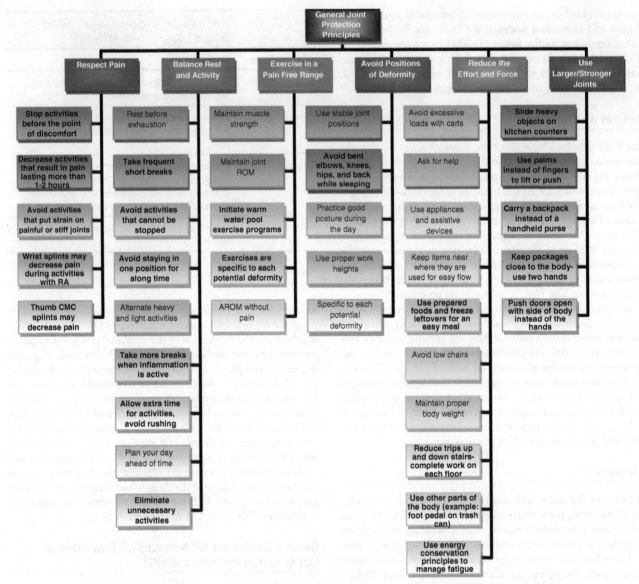

FIG. 29.1 Overview of joint protection principles. *AROM,* Active range of motion; *CMC,* carpometacarpal; *RA,* rheumatoid arthritis; *ROM,* range of motion. (Based on concepts by Cordery; Melvin;[156] Meenan, et al.;[28] and Hammond, et al.[143,145] Chart is used with permission from Beasley J. Osteoarthritis and rheumatoid arthritis. *J Hand Ther.* 2012;25(2):163-172.) Chart is used with permission from Beasley J: Osteoarthritis and rheumatoid arthritis, *J Hand Ther.* 25(2):163-172, 2012.

Several studies and reports support joint protection education and adaptive equipment for improving hand function and pain in clients with OA.[38-40] The European League Against Rheumatism (EULAR) published a systematic review recommending joint protection education combined with an exercise regimen for all clients with hand OA.[41] Adaptive equipment used in one study included enlarged writing grips, Dycem, an angled knife, a book holder, and other equipment that resulted in improvements in grip strength and global hand function.[42] Adaptive equipment that can help increase leverage and also distribute pressure in the hand includes larger-diameter pens, broad key holders, large plastic tabs on medicine bottles, and car door openers. As handle diameter increases, less digital force is needed to hold objects. In normal hands, the most comfortable handle is 19.7% of the user's hand length,[43] and the ideal tool handle design is a cylinder with

a 33 mm diameter.[44] To decrease the maximum push/pull force on a tool, a cylindrical handle should be parallel to the push/pull direction.[45,46] Handle designs that reduce wrist ulnar deviation require the least amount of grip force.[47]

Clients often place strong forces on their hands when lifting themselves from a seated position. In some cases, adaptive equipment such as a lift chair, a shower chair, or elevated toilet seat can compensate for lower extremity weakness by assisting with sit-to-stand movement, thereby reducing stress placed on the hands. Additional joint protection principles include pacing and planning (also called "energy conservation"), using adaptive equipment to reduce force requirements, avoiding prolonged grip, avoiding repetitive thumb movements, carrying objects closer to the body, and distributing weight over several joints.[40,41,48-50]

The hand therapist can help clients understand the benefits of incorporating basic joint protection principles in the presence of both OA and RA. Clients benefit from general education about arthritis, information about managing pain during activity, and tips on changing habits. Intervention should include assistance with goal setting and regular visits to the therapist.[51]

Physical Agent Modalities

Superficial heat often provides soothing relief from painful joints and can be incorporated into a self-management regimen.[52] Types of superficial heating agents include paraffin, Fluidotherapy, hot packs, microwave packs, hydrotherapy, and electric mitts. Deeper heating may be applied with continuous-wave ultrasound in the therapy clinic. Decreasing pain and maintaining or improving ROM is a primary goal when using these agents. It is interesting to note that studies examining the benefits of heat and ultrasound have found only weak to moderate evidence supporting the use of heat modalities in decreasing pain and improving grip strength in clients with OA.[39,53] More recent systematic reviews support these findings; however, they do recommend a combination of therapies, including therapeutic exercise, heat, and orthoses for the best results in reducing pain and improving function.[54-56] In practice, most clients report getting substantial relief with heat modalities. **Precaution.** *When clients benefit from superficial heat modalities and use them in their home exercise program (HEP), the therapist must instruct clients carefully to avoid the possibility of burns.*

Exercise

In determining an exercise program for individuals with OA, the initial evaluation becomes paramount. One must observe the current level of deformity, joint laxity, and changes in hand posture during activities. Exercise programs must be individualized. Specific exercises may be beneficial while a standard exercise set for all clients with OA could be detrimental.[57,58] A Cochrane systematic review concluded that there is low-quality evidence for small to moderate positive effects of exercise on hand pain, function, and finger joint stiffness.[59] Most of the studies about exercise and OA revolve around thumb CMC joint OA.[55,60-64] One systematic review found no evidence that resistance training has any significant effect on grip strength or hand function.[65] There appears to be growing support, however, for targeted strengthening of the opponens pollicis (OP) muscle and the first dorsal interosseous muscle in clients with thumb CMC joint OA. This seems to help because the two muscles provide a force coupling that results in slight distraction of the first metacarpal from the trapezium.[66-72] Strengthening these muscles also counterbalances the deforming forces that result in dorsal subluxation of the base of the first metacarpal and adduction of the thumb.[57,73]

General AROM exercises for the hand include wrist flexion and extension, gentle digital flexion and extension, and thumb opposition. Combining joint protection and pain-free home exercises is an effective intervention for improving hand function, as measured by grip strength and self-reported global functioning in individuals with hand OA. When orthosis use and exercise are added to a joint protection program there is greater improvement of pain, stiffness, grip strength, and ability to perform ADLs, than when using a joint protection program alone.[42] Exercise programs that utilize AROM as opposed to pinch strengthening are found to be more effective.[39,42] Even light putty-pinching exercise delivers large forces to an unstable CMC joint that can

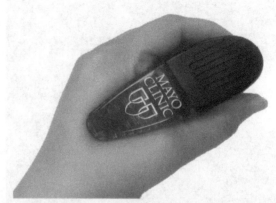

FIG. 29.2 A chip clip can be used to provide a trigger point release to the adductor pollicis muscle and stretch to the first web space. The clip should be covered with moleskin or a similar material to increase comfort for the client. Keep the clip in place 30 to 90 seconds until relief is felt.[87] (From Mayo Clinic patient education materials.)

aggravate a potential deformity.[35] Grip strengthening can also aggravate inflamed flexor tendons, thus exacerbating pain and symptoms in a digit that is triggering or locking. Stability must not be sacrificed for potential improvements in strength.[38]

A stable pain-free thumb provides a buttress for the fingers to grip and pinch effectively, and specific exercises should improve strength of muscles that help stabilize the thumb. One method of supporting the thumb in a stable position while simultaneously contracting the OP and the flexor digitorum indicis (FDI) is to have the client gently squeeze a tennis ball while lifting the index and long fingers off the ball as in making "bunny ears."[74] Stretching and massage,[63] as well as myofascial trigger point release of the first web space, may assist in relieving pain and first web space adduction.[75] Thumb web space stretching can be accomplished by having the client grasp a 1-inch (2.5 cm) wooden dowel as well as implementing techniques to relax the adductor pollicis (AP).[38] A chip bag clip with moleskin can also be used (Fig. 29.2). **Precaution.** *Therapy exercises should never create deforming forces or cause pain in the arthritic client.*

One systematic review exploring effects of resistance training on muscle strength, joint pain, and hand function in individuals with OA concluded that there is no evidence that resistance training has a significant effect on grip strength or hand function, and that the pain-relieving effect is small.[66] However, there may be merit in basic physical conditioning to help decrease pain and improve grip strength.[76,77] A study on low-impact general conditioning demonstrated increased aerobic capacity, decreased depression, and decreased anxiety in individuals with arthritis.[78]

Orthoses

Orthoses are the mostly widely studied and effective intervention for decreasing pain during hand use in people with OA.[55,60,62,79-81] Orthoses are used to protect joints and help reduce pain by statically holding the joint(s) in place. They decrease load by positioning the affected joint(s) during ADL hand use and by supporting the joint(s) to prevent distortion from deforming forces. Supportive orthoses are typically worn during the day during activity; however, some clients report pain reduction with nighttime use only. Systematic reviews and meta-analyses of randomized controlled trials have shown that orthosis use alone improves function and decreases pain.[60,62,79]

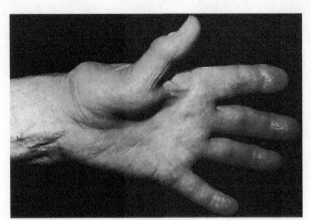

FIG. 29.3 The type III thumb deformity involves subluxation of the CMC joint, MP joint hyperextension, and IP joint flexion. (From Terrono AL, Nalebuff EA, Phillips CA. The rheumatoid thumb. In: Skirven TM, Osterman AL, Fedorczyk JM, et al., eds. *Rehabilitation of the Hand and Upper Extremity.* 6th ed. St Louis, MO: Elsevier; 2011, p. 1347.)

There are almost as many orthosis styles for thumb CMC joint OA as there are studies. However, most suggest a hand-based orthosis that allows the IP freedom of movement.[82] If the MP joint is included in the orthosis it is usually flexed at 10 to 20 degrees, and the thumb is positioned in a 3-point pinch positioning with the index and middle fingers. The choice of orthosis should be adapted to the type of activity the client partakes in and adapted to individual differences.[55] If the orthosis fits well, the client will report decreased pain with pinch activities, as it is stabilizing the CMC joint in the proper position. Radiographs during active pinch can verify if the orthosis is properly maintaining the metacarpal on the trapezium.[82]

Regarding orthotic intervention for the IP joints, I have had success in reducing pain and improving function with Silipos sleeves and custom gutter or circumferential orthoses that include only the involved joint. These are worn during activity to protect the joint from further trauma. In addition, a custom 3-point style orthosis can be used to correct lateral deviation at the PIP or the DIP, and help make hand use more comfortable.

Thumb Osteoarthritis

OA can affect all joints of the thumb, and **swan neck** is one of the most common deformities. It is characterized at the thumb CMC joint by metacarpal adduction and dorsal subluxation from the trapezium, MP joint hyperextension, and IP joint flexion (Fig. 29.3). Pinch is often painful because CMC subluxation becomes more pronounced during heavy pinch activities. The thumb IP joint sometimes assumes a flexed posture. When evaluating the thumb, determine the specific pattern of deformity so that treatment can be designed to oppose deforming forces with adaptive techniques, client-specific exercises, and orthoses.

? Questions to Ask the Doctor

- What joints of the thumb are involved (as seen on the radiographs)?
- Is there also joint involvement of the wrist?
- Is the client using any medications for this condition?

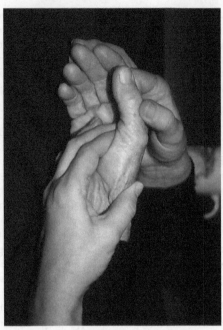

FIG. 29.4 When the thumb deformity is passively correctable, the placement of the therapist's hands often determines the forces that are needed to apply the orthosis correctly. (Concept courtesy Judy Leonard, OTR, CHT. From Beasley J. Soft orthoses: indications and techniques. In: Skirven TM, Osterman AL, Fedorczyk JM, et al., eds. *Rehabilitation of the Hand and Upper Extremity.* 6th ed. St Louis, MO: Elsevier; 2011, p. 1614.)

( ) What to Say to Clients

About the Condition

"Here is a picture (radiograph) of a thumb with osteoarthritis. The problem often starts at this joint (CMC). When cartilage wears down and joint ligaments weaken, this joint can slide out of place. Over time, the thumb has difficulty moving away from the palm of the hand. The next joint of the thumb (MP) then has to do extra work, and it often stretches out and hyperextends."

About Orthoses

"We are going to try a couple of orthoses, also referred to as splints, which may help give your thumb more stability. We have several options, but we need to see which works best for you. Some people prefer one type of orthosis for night wear and a less restrictive one for day wear."

About Exercise

"Heavy pinch activities and exercises put stress on this (CMC) joint and can decrease joint stability. It is important that you exercise your hand gently. Your exercises should not hurt. Some people like to exercise in a warm-water pool or heat their hand up with a heating pack prior to exercising."

Evaluation Tips

- Determine whether the thumb deformity is passively correctable. Gently stabilize the base of the metacarpal on the trapezium and then place the CMC joint in abduction and the MP joint in flexion (Fig. 29.4). This is the proper position for the orthosis.

- Determine how the disease process is affecting the client's function, and the client's goals for therapy. This allows you to design an individualized program that may increase the client's sense of self-efficacy. Collaborative treatment planning assists in developing rapport with your client and often leads to greater adherence to their program.[81]

> © **Clinical Pearl**
>
> If the thumb deformity is not passively correctable, the orthosis can help provide support but cannot change the deformity.

> ♡ **Tips from the Field**

The therapist has several choices when selecting an orthosis for the client with thumb OA. The orthosis can be custom fabricated of lightweight thermoplastic material (Fig. 29.5), or in some cases soft material (for example, neoprene) can be used if the strapping is applied properly to counteract deforming forces. There are also several prefabricated options available. Alternatives include the neoprene Comfort Cool Thumb CMC Restriction Splint (Fig. 29.6) (available from North Coast Medical Inc., Morgan Hill, CA) and the Push MetaGrip (available from HandLab). Custom hand-based orthoses that support the thumb in palmar abduction and the CMC and MP joints in slight flexion also give good results. Client acceptance of orthoses is likely due to decreased pain and improved joint stability during pinching activities. Clients often misinterpret this as an increase in strength.

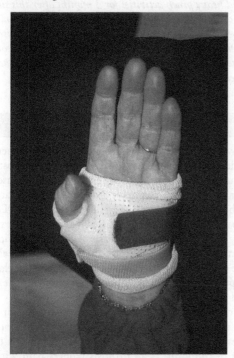

FIG. 29.5 The hand-based thumb spica orthosis for deformities that are passively correctable can help decrease pain. The orthosis places the metacarpal in gentle palmar abduction and the metacarpophalangeal joint in slight flexion. The wrist strap gives the splint additional stability to stabilize the carpometacarpal joint. (From Beasley J. Therapist's examination and conservative management of arthritis of the upper extremity. In: Skirven TM, Osterman AL, Fedorczyk JM, et al., eds. Rehabilitation of the Hand and Upper Extremity. 6th ed. St Louis, MO: Elsevier; 2011, p. 1339.)

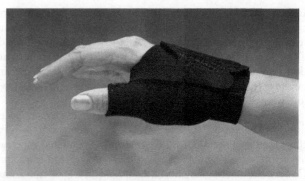

FIG. 29.6 Comfort Cool Thumb CMC Restriction Splint has an additional strap to support and gently compress the CMC joint. The splint also gently positions the metacarpal in abduction. (Photo and splint courtesy North Coast Medical, Inc., Morgan Hill, CA. From Beasley J. Soft orthoses: indications and techniques. In: Skirven TM, Osterman AL, Fedorczyk JM, et al., eds. Rehabilitation of the Hand and Upper Extremity. 6th ed. St Louis, MO: Elsevier; 2011, p. 1614.)

Sometimes clients have large thumb IP joints that make donning and doffing orthoses difficult. The orthosis must be large enough to fit over the IP, while still providing support to the proximal phalanx. One easy way to enlarge the thermoplastic orthosis thumbhole (when the material is still slightly warm) is to remove the orthosis from the client and then insert closed scissors into the thumb portion of the splint and gently open the scissors. Another technique is to pry open the seam that supports the proximal phalanx (after the orthosis has cooled) and secure the seam with a Velcro strap. The strap can be loosened and the unsecured seam expanded during orthotic application and removal. An additional solution is an orthosis that does not include the MP joint or has a dorsal proximal phalanx flap to help position the MP in flexion.[83] If the joints proximal to the trapezium are also affected by OA, such as the scaphoid and trapezoid (this is referred to as **pantrapezial arthritis**), consider an orthosis design that crosses the wrist and includes the thumb.

Clients usually respond favorably to orthoses if they are comfortable and fit correctly. Many clients wear a soft orthosis during the day and a more rigid orthosis at night.[82] Other clients feel that the rigid orthosis supports the thumb better during the day. In clients with bilateral involvement, fabricate one orthosis at a time to determine how the client responds before making one for the other hand.

> ▷ **Precautions and Concerns**
>
> - *After making an orthosis, check for pressure areas. The client should return for at least one follow-up visit to assess fit and make any necessary adjustments.*
> - *An orthosis that is clean is not being worn. Usually, a clean orthosis is one that is uncomfortable to wear and needs adjustment. Some clients hesitate to ask for adjustments for fear of offending their therapist.*

Surgical Treatment for Thumb Osteoarthtitis

Therapy After Carpometacarpal Interposition Arthroplasty

CMC interposition arthroplasty involves excision of the trapezium, which allows the metacarpal to return to an abducted position and eliminates the "bone-on-bone" pain of OA. There are now several surgical techniques to reconstruct the joint. Typically, a donor tendon is rolled up and interpositioned in the joint space. The ligaments are usually reconstructed and help provide CMC joint stability. This is referred to as **ligament reconstruction tendon interposition**.[84] Hyperextension of the MP joint can be corrected as well. In most cases the client is in a cast for 4 to 6 weeks, and then is referred to hand therapy.

The postoperative course varies from surgeon to surgeon. When the surgeon allows CMC joint AROM, it is important to help the client learn to move properly. These clients were often compensating before surgery by only moving their thumb IP and MP joints. One exercise to relearn thumb CMC movement is to flex the thumb IP and MP joints (and try to keep them flexed) while moving the CMC joint in gentle flexion and extension. Techniques to restore the thumb web space and strengthen the first dorsal interosseous muscle may also be helpful in the promotion of CMC stability.[85]

The postoperative orthosis will be worn for 6 to 12 weeks from the date of surgery, dependent on surgeon preference. Most clients gain AROM quickly and want to resume activities as soon as possible. Many ADLs require a strong pinch and must be delayed until approved by the surgeon. Decisions to return to work depend on the type of activities the job requires. **Precaution.** *Many surgeons recommend waiting at least 3 months from the date of surgery before performing any heavy pinching activities.*

? Questions to Ask the Doctor

- At the time of cast removal, should we apply a hand-based or forearm-based orthosis?
- At what point may we begin gentle AROM of the CMC joint?
- At what point may we discontinue the orthosis?
- How long should the client wait before doing heavy ADL pinching?

What to Say to Clients

About the Surgery

"The surgery helped correct your joint positioning. When it heals completely, you will have a pain-free and stable thumb joint! The donor tendon was rolled up and placed in the joint between the trimmed bones. That is sometimes called an anchovy."

About the Orthosis

"We need to make you an orthosis to protect your thumb while it heals. To get the best result, we need to maintain a good balance between mobility and stability. You will need to wear your orthosis between exercise sessions and at night until discontinued by the surgeon. It is important that your orthosis be comfortable and not cause any pressure areas."

About Exercise

"When it is approved by your surgeon, we will start gently exercising your new thumb joint. It is a joint that you have not moved in a long time, so I will need to show you some exercises to retrain your thumb to move correctly. Eventually we can work on gentle strengthening. We usually start with grip-strengthening exercises that do not involve the thumb because we do not want to put too much stress on the thumb before it is fully healed. The success of this surgery depends on the stability of your thumb. Doing pinch activities too soon can compromise the stability of your surgical repair."

Evaluation Tips

- Many clients who arrive for therapy are surprised at how long the recovery is for this surgical procedure.
- After being in a cast for several weeks, the skin will be very dry and the scars may be sensitive. The client will appreciate a gentle cleaning of the skin and an application of lotion. If the scars can tolerate it, initiate gentle scar massage. Instruct the client to do scar massage a couple of times each day as part of their HEP.
- Be aware and look for signs of complex regional pain syndrome with this population.

♡ Tips From the Field

Orthoses

The thumb orthoses tips previously outlined apply to the orthosis worn after surgery for CMC interposition arthroplasty. Special attention should be paid to avoid pressure from the orthosis at the incision site and at the base of the thumb near the superficial branch of the radial nerve. This area can be very sensitive. Some clients progress from a forearm-based to a hand-based orthosis. Some clients, after being cleared to return to work, prefer a soft neoprene orthosis (see Fig. 29.6) to help make the transition. This orthosis supplies gentle support while allowing some motion for hand use.

➤ Precautions and Concerns

- *Avoid heavy pinch activities for 3 months after this surgery.*
- *The orthosis should not force the thumb into position.*
- *If the superficial branch of the radial nerve is irritated after surgery, some clients report relief using a transcutaneous electrical nerve stimulation (TENS) unit. A silicone gel pad can also be helpful.*

Distal Interphalangeal Joint Osteoarthritis

Clients with OA at the DIP joints often have enlargements called "Heberden nodes."[12] These nodes appear because osteophytes (bony outgrowths) form near the extensor tendon insertion on the distal phalanx. When these nodes are present at the PIP joints, they are called "Bouchard nodes."[12] OA at the DIP joints can be painful initially, but pain usually decreases over time. Clients may get pain relief using a circumferential or resting trough style joint orthosis.[86,87] Joint protection education is also useful for these clients. In addition, wrapping the joint with elastic wrap or a Silipos sleeve may provide pain relief through light compression and protection from being bumped.

Clients sometimes come to therapy for an orthosis to help determine whether or not to have the DIP joint surgically fused. Clients wear the orthosis during ADLs to mimic a fusion of the joint. If an orthosis relieves pain without too much alteration in function, clients are likely to do well with DIP joint fusion.

? Questions to Ask the Doctor

- Is the client a candidate for DIP fusion? If so, would the physician like us to try immobilizing the joint with an orthosis to see if the client responds well to that?

About the Condition

"The end joints of the fingers (DIP) are one of the most common sites of osteoarthritis. These joints can be painful at first, but the pain gradually goes away."

About Orthoses

"If you are having pain, we can try taping, a Silipos sleeve protector, or immobilizing your joint(s) with an orthosis. If you are considering surgery to fuse your joint(s), wearing an orthosis during hand use may help you make a decision about this elective surgery."

About Exercise

"Many people with morning stiffness use heat prior to exercise to help increase mobility before starting their day. They usually apply the heat for 10–20 minutes. Also, during your daily activities, avoid holding objects tightly with the fingers for long periods of time. This position contributes to deformity and pain."

Determine each client's specific needs at the evaluation. For example, some clients do not wish to wear an orthosis, whereas others are there only for an orthosis.

Orthoses

Because of the presence of Heberden nodes and joint inflammation, orthoses for the DIP joints need to conform well and provide even pressure distribution. Thin or "light" orthotic materials are recommended, and the material should have excellent drape characteristics, such as Polyform or Orfit. Orthoses are usually made on the dorsal surface to allow for tactile input of the volar surface of the fingertip during activity (Fig. 29.7). To hold these splints in place, a non-adhesive wrap, such as Coban is recommended.

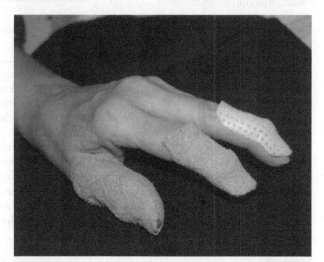

FIG. 29.7 Orthoses to the distal interphalangeal joints are usually only used with clients who are demonstrating a painful flare-up, with clients who are considering a surgical fusion, or with clients following surgical fusion.

During acute flare-ups, the skin is very sensitive on the dorsal DIP joint. Orthoses should conform well to prevent pressure and sliding on the digit, but should not be so snug as to feel constrictive. The DIP orthosis may need to be modified with changes in swelling.

Rheumatoid Arthritis

RA, the most common autoimmune inflammatory arthritis in adults,[9] decreases a person's ability to perform ADLs,[88] increases mortality,[88,89] and negatively impacts quality of life.[90] RA is characterized by synovial inflammation; autoantibody production; cartilage and bone destruction that leads to deformity; and systemic manifestations that include cardiovascular, pulmonary, psychological, and skeletal conditions.[91,92] RA causes intense joint pain and is chronic and progressive. Genetic and environmental factors have been linked to this disease.[92-95] Initially, the inflammatory process associated with RA manifests itself primarily in the synovial tissue[96]; joint destruction occurs when the synovial pannus expresses enzymes allowing cartilage penetration, cartilage damage, and joint erosion.[96,57]

The evaluation and treatment of clients with RA can be challenging for even the most experienced hand therapist. The disease affects the intricate balance of the hand when joints and soft-tissue structures become compromised. Treatment should be tailored to the client's occupational profile, deformity (or potential deformity), stage of disease, functional needs, and priorities. Education about the disease and treatment options is critical to newly diagnosed clients.

Pathology

RA typically affects the hand joints symmetrically, and commonly includes the MP, PIP, thumb, and wrist joints.[94,97] Early symptoms include prolonged morning stiffness, extreme fatigue, and swelling of the PIP joints.[97,98]

Flexor **tenosynovitis** can reduce digital motion and strength, and result in trigger fingers.[99] Interosseous tenosynovitis is present in 47.7% of people with RA.[100] Synovitis of the hand joints is the first sign of pathology in what is called the "pre-clinical phase" of RA, and this is the phase when medical management usually begins.[101,102] Onset of RA symptoms can be abrupt, but, more commonly, a slower progression occurs over several weeks.

A variety of deformities affect the hands of people with RA. The classic "zig-zag" deformity consists of carpal ulnar slide displacement with metacarpal radial deviation, followed by MP joint ulnar deviation.[103] **Rheumatoid nodules**, a common early extraarticular expression of RA, can occur over pressure areas at the elbows and digits, but are usually not painful.[104,105] Over the last two decades, disease-modifying biological pharmacology interventions have improved the management of RA and reduced joint damage and disability through early use of medications.[106,107]

Theories on the pathogenesis of RA include a relationship between genetics, environment, and chance.[108] One thought is that there is first an unknown environmental trigger that activates an innate immunity and that causes a signal to induce an immune response. The immune response leads to the production of autoantibodies that cause a joint-specific inflammatory reaction to occur. The inflammation becomes a chronic process leading to tissue destruction and remodeling.[109] Mechanical factors (such as the way people use their hands) can predispose sites to greater erosion. These are called "mechanically vulnerable" sites[110]; examples are the second and third MP joints. It is unclear why this is; however, articular bone erosion does not appear to repair in RA as it does in other inflammatory arthropathies.[108]

Recent classification criteria promotes treating RA with a strategic algorithm. However, a classic article published in the *Journal of the American Medical Association* in 1949 classifies the progression of RA into four stages.[110] These stages were developed prior to the widespread use of disease-modifying medications. Knowledge of these stages can be helpful when treating the many clients who are not taking RA medications for a variety of reasons.

The authors describe the acute phase, or stage I, with joint swelling and inflammation that is warm when palpated. Stage II is marked by a decrease in symptoms. Nodules may be evident in the joint **bursa** (a fluid-filled sac that decreases friction) or along tendons. Joint ROM is usually less painful and there are no obvious deformities, but deterioration of structures continues. In the destructive, "chronic active" stage III, the client often presents with less pain but has irreversible joint deformities. Stage IV is described as "chronic inactive" or "skeletal collapse and deformity." The joint deformities may include instability, dislocation, spontaneous fusion, and bony or fibrous **ankylosis** (stiffening of a joint).[110]

Understanding the pathogenesis of RA has led to the development of disease-modifying anti-rheumatic drugs (DMARDs), glucocorticoids, and biological DMARDs; and this has led to new recommendations for early medical management of RA.[111] There are 12 recommendations for the management of RA that have been updated by the EULAR. The recommendations involve using DMARD therapy as soon as the diagnosis of RA is made, with the aim of reaching a sustained remission or low disease activity in all patients.[111]

Timelines and Healing

The development of the recommendations from EULAR and widespread use of DMARDs is the closest there is to a cure at this time. Despite medical advances, it is important to appreciate that arthritis remains a chronic condition,[112] and medical advances do not necessarily permanently change the destructive behavior of the immune system.[113,114] Hand therapists can assist clients in managing symptoms through client education, physical agent modalities, orthoses, joint protection, and adaptive equipment. The therapist and client with RA frequently develop a lifelong relationship whereby the client may call with specific needs throughout the progression of the disease.

Evaluation

A thorough evaluation of the client includes an assessment of grip strength, ROM, occupational profile, current ADL status, joint deformities, stage of disease process, previous surgeries, expectations of therapy, and pain.

Occupational Profile

An occupational profile is "a summary of a client's occupational history and experiences, patterns of daily living, interests, values, and needs."[115] Completion of an occupational profile will help the hand therapist better understand the client's current priorities and assist in developing an individualized program.

Grip Strength

Taking periodic grip and pinch strength measurements can assist the therapist and client in measuring progress. Individuals with RA who have reduced grip strength demonstrate limitations in ADLs.[116,117] A study published in 2018 concluded that although grip strength improved over the course of 5 years after initial diagnosis and treatment, it remained much lower than expected.[118] Research has demonstrated improved grip strength after an extended occupational therapy information program,[119] and improvement after a tailored exercise program of hand strengthening and stretching.[120]

Range of Motion

Measurements of hand AROM vary depending on the time of day and whether or not the client is experiencing inflammation on the day of the visit. Goniometric measurement can be useful in determining progression of the disease, but deformities can make taking precise measurements difficult in the later stages. Measurements of composite digital flexion, active digital extension, and thumb opposition often provide functional information. Tracing a digit or hand on a sheet of paper can also help track changes in motion and deformity. The degree of ulnar deviation at the MP joints can provide helpful information for measuring progression of joint deformities; this measurement should be done with the digits in full active available extension.

> **◎ Clinical Pearl**
>
> Ulnar deviation often varies with metacarpophalangeal (MP) flexion and extension because of ligament laxity. Therefore the position of the MP joint should be reported in combination with ulnar drift measurements.

Tendon rupture can cause a loss of AROM resulting in loss of function. Rupture occurs as the tendon glides over roughened and irregular bones. The tendon, which may be weakened by inflamed synovium, can fray and eventually break. Although both flexor tendons and extensor tendons can rupture, the extensors are more vulnerable because of their proximity to the distal radius, ulna, and carpal bones.[121] The extensor tendons of the third, fourth, and fifth digits are particularly vulnerable. Rupture of the extensor pollicis longus at **Lister's tubercle** (a bony prominence) and extensor digitorum communis (EDC) at the distal end of the ulna frequently occur. The extensor digiti minimi and the EDC tendons to the ring and small fingers are the most common extensor tendon ruptures in RA.[122] Due to the poor integrity of these tendons, restoration is often through tendon transfers rather than tendon repair.[121]

Strength

Adams et al.[123] reported that hand grip strength acts as a reliable indicator of upper extremity functional ability. Because grip strength testing can be painful and stressful to arthritic joints, one trial versus three is adequate.[124,125] The B&L Engineering pinch gauge is considered the gold standard tool for measuring pinch strength.[126] Joint instability, rather than weakness, is usually more problematic during ADLs because even with adequate muscle strength, clients will be unable to maintain grip on objects if their joints collapse into deformity.

Activities of Daily Living

Evaluation of function begins when a client enters the clinic. Observing a client removing their coat and sitting at a table can be invaluable in understanding their ability to pinch, grasp, and complete functional activities. Joint deformities can be observed and may be accentuated with simple activities. The speed by which clients enter the clinic often provides qualitative information about pain levels and the involvement of lower extremities.

The therapist must gain an understanding of the client's home and support systems when planning the HEP and orthotic designs. For example, a client may need special strap adaptations or the assistance of a caregiver to don an orthosis. Identifying realistic goals with the client is very important. An activity diary can provide insight into the needs of clients and encourages them to be active participants in the treatment process.[127] A diary helps clients determine problem areas with ADLs, including which joints are involved and whether the difficulties are due to pain, power, or position.

Pain

Pain caused by acute inflammation is usually greatest in the early stages of the disease. Pain analog scales can be used to monitor the effectiveness of treatment, but clinical observation suggests that these clients, in the later stages, rate their pain much lower than anticipated by the therapist. Orthoses help decrease pain but should be balanced with the ADL requirements of each client. Rheumatoid nodules can be painful and should be noted in the evaluation because they may affect orthotic design or strap placement. Pain and/or numbness from nerve compression caused by **synovitis** may also be present. Compression of the median nerve (carpal tunnel syndrome) is one of the most commonly seen conditions at the wrist. The ulnar nerve can be compressed at **Guyon's canal** (wrist) and at the **cubital tunnel** (elbow).

Joint Deformities

Palpate joint deformities to help determine whether they are fixed or passively correctable, dislocated, or partially dislocated. Note this information in your evaluation. Include verbal descriptors as well as goniometric measurements. Common wrist and hand deformities are discussed in the following sections.

Swan Neck

A **swan neck deformity** is characterized by flexion of the DIP joint and hyperextension of the PIP joint. Synovitis of the flexor tendons can erode the **volar plate** (a thick fibrocartilaginous structure on the volar aspect of the PIP), which normally helps prevent PIP joint hyperextension. Flexor tendon synovitis also limits PIP joint flexion and causes the client to primarily use the MP joints for digital flexion.[128] This results in an **intrinsic plus position** (MP flexion with IP joints extended) during grasping activities, caused by an altered pull of the intrinsic muscles. This altered pull tends to facilitate dorsal subluxation of the lateral extensor tendons and PIP joint hyperextension. The DIP joint then flexes reciprocally. The action of the extensor mechanism is

concentrated at the PIP joint, resulting in PIP hyperextension if the volar plate is lax or disrupted.

I have observed improved function and client satisfaction with Oval-8 orthoses, which position the PIP joint in slight flexion. A study showed greater acceptance and tolerance of prefabricated orthoses as opposed to custom-made orthoses for swan neck deformities.[129] Another study reported that SilverRing Splints improved dexterity in select clients with RA.[130]

Boutonnière

The **boutonnière deformity** is characterized by PIP joint flexion and DIP joint hyperextension. Synovitis causes the central extensor tendon to become weakened, lengthened, or disrupted from the bony and capsular attachments, allowing the PIP joint to rest in flexion. The lateral bands then rest volar to the axis of the PIP joint, causing an altered mechanical pull that results in PIP joint flexion and DIP joint hyperextension.

Metacarpophalangeal Joint Ulnar Deviation and Palmar Subluxation

The MP joints, unlike the PIP hinge joints, have more planes of movement. They can flex, extend, abduct, adduct, pronate, and supinate. With this degree of mobility, the hand collapses into deformity if the restraining system of tendons, ligaments, or bony structures is disrupted by synovitis and joint erosion. Additional factors that can contribute to the development of MP ulnar deviation include asymmetry of the metacarpal heads; accumulation of fluid within joint spaces; and the line of pull of the flexor, extensor, and intrinsic muscles along with ulnar and volar forces applied during activity.[131] The flexor tendons exert strong ulnar and volar forces at the MP joint. Lateral pinch activities, gripping an object, writing, and even gravity, tend to place ulnar and volar deviating forces at the MP joints.

The deformity may also include radial deviation of the wrist (Fig. 29.8). With ligament instability, the carpal bones can shift into a variety of deformities. Ulnar displacement of the proximal carpal row results in radial deviation of the hand.[107] A forearm-based wrist orthosis can be used to stabilize the wrist during ADLs. Orthoses can decrease pain and improve grip strength but may decrease hand AROM.[132] Both soft and hard night resting orthoses help reduce pain.[133]

RA deformities can make orthotic fabrication and fitting challenging. When applying an orthosis to a hand with MP joint ulnar deviation and palmar subluxation, consider the position of the metacarpals, which are often in radial deviation. Aligning the MP joints into anti-ulnar deviation position may contribute to CMC joint radial deviation deformity. The orthosis should be designed to address all of the issues involved in the zigzag deformity.[133,134] The resting anti-deformity (and most comfortable position) is: wrist in 10 to15 degrees extension; metacarpals in neutral; no deviation at the wrist or the MP joints; PIPs and DIPs in 10 degrees flexion; and thumb in comfortable radial abduction with thumb MP and IP joints in 10 to 15 degrees flexion.[135]

Clinical Pearl

Ulnar deviation and palmer subluxation of the metacarpophalangeal joints is the most common deformity seen in rheumatoid arthritis.

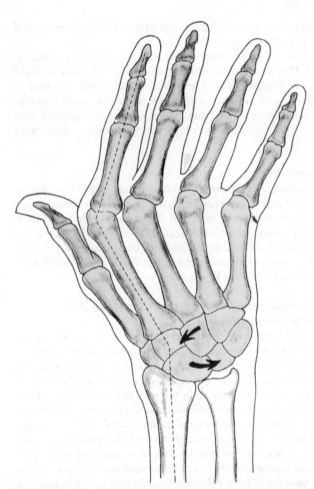

FIG. 29.8 The zigzag deformity with wrist radial deviation and metacarpophalangeal joint ulnar deviation. The dashed line indicates the position of the Rheumatoid hand and wrist at rest. Note radial deviation of wrist and ulnar deviation of MP joints. The arrows indicate the deforming forces of the carpus gliding ulnarly and tilting radially on the distal radius. (From Melvin JL. *Rheumatoid Disease: Occupational Therapy and Rehabilitation*. 3rd ed. Philadelphia, PA: FA Davis; 1989, p. 281. Redrawn with permission.)

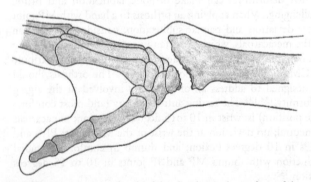

FIG. 29.9 The natural volar tilt of the distal articular surface of the radius and chronic synovitis can result in volar subluxation of the carpus on the radius. (From Melvin JL. *Rheumatoid Disease: Occupational Therapy and Rehabilitation*. 3rd ed. Philadelphia, PA: FA Davis; 1989, p. 280. Redrawn with permission.)

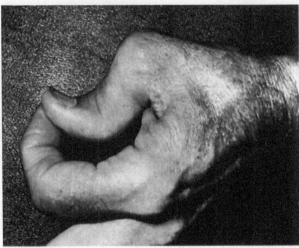

FIG. 29.10 The type I RA thumb deformity with metacarpophalangeal joint flexion and distal joint hyperextension. (From Terrono AL, Nalebuff EA, Phillips CA. The rheumatoid thumb. In: Skirven TM, Osterman AL, Fedorczyk JM, et al., eds. *Rehabilitation of the Hand and Upper Extremity*. 6th ed. St Louis, MO: Elsevier; 2011, p. 1345.)

Volar Subluxation of the Carpus on the Radius

Ligament laxity caused by chronic synovitis at the wrist and the natural volar tilt of the distal articular surface of the radius can result in volar subluxation of the carpus on the radius (Fig. 29.9). An orthosis for this condition usually includes a volar component to support the wrist.[136] The research on wrist orthoses is inconclusive at this time, although one systematic review found that clients who wore wrist and resting hand orthoses preferred using them.[137]

Distal Ulna Dorsal Subluxation

Instability of the distal ulna is common in RA. The distal ulna is normally less prominent in supination and more prominent in pronation. The RA disease process often weakens the ligamentous structures causing dorsal prominence of the distal ulna, pain, and crepitation with forearm rotation.[138] This instability and dorsal prominence of the ulna may lead to extensor tendon disruption at the wrist level. Orthoses to provide stability to the distal ulna can be helpful in decreasing pain with pronation and supination.[139]

Thumb Deformities

Common patterns of thumb deformity in the rheumatoid thumb are described in Table 29.2. Type I, with MP flexion and IP hyperextension, is common (Fig. 29.10). Type III, with CMC flexion, subluxation, adduction, MP hyperextension, and IP flexion is also common (see Fig. 29.3). With the Type III deformity, orthotic use is comparable to the previously described OA thumb deformity recommendations. The reader is referred to Terrono et al.[140] for further information on RA thumb deformities.

Crepitus

Crepitation during AROM sounds like crunching or popping. Volar inspection of the hand should include palpation of the first annular (A1) pulley (on the volar aspect of the MP joints) as the client flexes and extends the digits. A thickening of the flexor tendons, triggering, or periodic locking of the digit in flexion indicates flexor tenosynovitis.

Skin Condition

An evaluation of the skin should include color, temperature, and swelling. In the initial stage, the skin is often red and warm. In the later stages, the skin may be very thin and bruise easily, which may be due to long-term use of steroids and antiinflammatory medications. Fragile skin characteristics can affect postoperative healing and reduce tolerance to orthoses. **Precaution.** *Skin tears may occur with only minimal shearing, such as rubbing from dressings or at the edge of a table.*

General Guidelines for Nonsurgical Treatment of Upper Extremity Rheumatoid Arthritis

Joint Protection

The latest EULAR recommendations call for education of individuals with inflammatory arthritis.[141] Joint protection education includes providing information about avoiding potential deforming forces and positions that may overload vulnerable joints. Therapy intervention includes practice with and instruction in the use of both adaptive equipment as well as adaptive techniques (such as using an open palm to open a water bottle versus a lateral pinch). A systematic review published in 2017 describes strong evidence supporting the effectiveness of joint protection education in managing symptoms of RA and improving independence in ADLs.[142]

Common general joint protection principles for both OA and RA are categorized by themes in Table 29.3. For more complete information on specific principles and techniques as applied to specific deformities, the reader is referred to works by Cordery and Rocchi.[143,144] Educational-behavioral joint protection programs that involve skill practice, goal setting, and HEPs are more effective than short instruction and/or information booklets; as demonstrated by fewer deformities, less morning stiffness, improved ADL scores, and improved joint protection adherence.[145] Combining joint protection with adaptive device provision improves hand function and reduces pain.[39]

Joint protection principles for RA should address current and potential deformity. For example, joint protection for a client with a tendency to develop a swan neck deformity should avoid activities that place the PIP joints in full extension, such as holding a book. In contrast, if the client has a tendency toward a boutonnière deformity, PIP flexion activities (such as using a hook grasp to carry a purse) should be discouraged. Clients with MP joint ulnar deviation tendencies should be aware of activities that place ulnar deviating forces on the MP joints and use alternative grasping techniques (Table 29.3). With the thumb, joint protection principles focus on decreasing the amount of force used for pinching activities, such as use of levers and larger barrel tools.

Physical Agent Modalities

The use of heat in the form of continuous-wave ultrasound, warm water, paraffin, and heating pads;[146] the use of cold in the form of water and ice; and finally electrotherapy such as TENS have been used to treat the pain associated with RA. In addition to decreasing pain, these agents are also used as adjuncts to help maintain

TABLE 29.3	Joint Protection Principles for the Metacarpophalangeal Joints With Rheumatoid Arthritis
Activities that Aggravate Metacarpophalangeal Ulnar Deviation	**Joint Protection Techniques**
Closing a jar with the right hand	Use the heel of the hand to close the jar or use a jar opener with two hands.
Smoothing a sheet with shoulder adduction	Use shoulder abduction to smooth the sheet.
Stirring with a spoon using forearm pronation and lateral pinch on spoon	Stir with the forearm in neutral with the spoon head held on the ulnar side of the hand using a cylindrical grasp.
Resting the hand on the chin, with ulnar forces to the digits	Avoid resting the hand on the chin or place the chin in the palm.
Lifting a cup of coffee	Use two hands and a light-weight cup.
Cutting foods	Use a knife with a 90-degree handle, a pizza cutter, or electric knife.
Lateral pinch to turn the key in the car door or ignition	Use a built-up key turner.
Carrying a purse strap with a lateral pinch	Use a fanny pack, back pack, or shoulder bag.

Melvin JL, Ferrel KM, eds. *Adult rheumatic diseases.* Vol 2. Bethesda, MD: The American Occupational Therapy Association; 2000.

and improve range of motion. Paraffin wax,[146] ultrasound,[147] and low-level laser[148] have been found to decrease morning stiffness and improve range of motion. However, be aware that the literature reveals the efficacy of physical agent modalities is relatively low when compared to exercise, joint protection, and other forms of client education and orthosis use.[142,146-149] **Precaution.** *During the acute inflammatory phase when joint temperatures are elevated, heat is contraindicated because it can promote inflammation.*

Cryotherapy, which lowers joint temperatures, reduces pain, and decreases inflammation is more appropriate during the acute phase, but many clients cannot tolerate cooling treatments.

Exercise

Range of Motion

The guiding principle of exercise is to work within the client's comfortable AROM to prevent overstretching of joint structures that may be vulnerable due to inflammation. General exercises include AROM of the wrist, digit flexion and extension, and thumb opposition. Shoulder and elbow AROM in the supine position is also beneficial for preventing stiffness. Clients often obtain better shoulder motion in supine because the effects of gravity are reduced. Generalized conditioning for clients with RA has been found to improve stamina and muscle strength and is recommended as routine practice when working with clients who have RA.[150,151] Clinically, clients report the psychosocial benefits of *group* exercise in a warm pool, tai chi class, and other pain-free exercise programs.[134]

TABLE 29.2   Rheumatoid Arthritis Thumb Deformities

Type	Also Called	Carpometacarpal	Metacarpophalangeal	Interphalangeal
I	Boutonnière deformity	Not involved	Flexion	Hyperextension
II	(Uncommon)	Flexion and adduction	Flexion	Hyperextension
III	Swan neck deformity	Flexion, adduction, and subluxation	Hyperextension	Flexion
IV		Adduction and flexion as it progresses	Radially deviated and UCL unstable	Not involved
V		May or may not be involved	Unstable volar plate, hyperextension	Not involved
VI	Arthritis mutilans	Collapse resulting from bone loss at any level		

UCL, Ulnar collateral ligament.
Based on categories by Terrono AL, Nalebuff EA, Phillips CA. The rheumatoid thumb. In: Skirven TM, Osterman AL, Fedorczyk JM, et al., eds. *Rehabilitation of the Hand and Upper Extremity*. 6th ed. St Louis, MO: Elsevier; 2011, p.1345.

Strengthening

Stability must not be sacrificed for a potential improvement in strength. Grip strengthening can place the digits in increased ulnar deviation during flexion if unmonitored. However, with the careful eye of a therapist and an individually tailored and monitored home program, strengthening exercises that do not cause pain or undue loading through the hand can help improve strength,[120,152,153] hand function,[120,153,154] and pain in clients with RA. The literature supporting this reports very few adverse effects, but most of the research was performed on clients well-managed on medications.[154] **Precaution.** *Strengthening programs for the rheumatic hand should be used with caution to avoid aggravation of deformities. Avoid intrinsic plus positioning of the hand, ulnar deviation of the MPs, radial deviation of the wrist, and painful grip and pinch during exercise. Therapy exercises should never create deforming forces or cause pain.*

Orthoses

Client-specific orthoses are important in RA. An example of this would be a night resting orthosis for a client who sustains displacement of an old index MP joint arthroplasty which subsequently results in a PIP flexion contracture. By using a day orthosis to passively hold the PIP in greater extension, the client is able to use the finger in pinch and grasp activities. By positioning the index in extension and supporting all digits in more neutral alignment at the MP joints, the client is able to rest comfortably at night. For further reference on mechanical forces in the hand when designing specific orthoses for RA please refer to the works of Dr. Paul Brand[155] and Judy Melvin[156].

? Questions to Ask the Doctor

- Are there any tendon ruptures?
- Is surgery an option for this client in the future?
- What are your thoughts on an individually crafted hand-strengthening program?

() What to Say to Clients

About the Condition

"When you have rheumatoid arthritis, the lining of the joint becomes active and damages the structures around the joints, causing them to move."

About the Orthosis

"The orthosis is designed to keep your fingers and wrist in good alignment. It should be comfortable and can help decrease your pain. Some clients like to wear soft orthoses during the day for heavier activities. This supports your fingers while letting you do some activities."

About Exercise and Joint Protection

"Learning ways that you can protect your joints can be helpful. Adaptive equipment can also be helpful to decrease the stress on the joints as you do some activities. I can help you determine your best options. Exercise should be gentle, pain free, and avoid positions of deformity."

Evaluation Tips

Even with severe deformities, clients are somehow able to do a great deal with their hands. Be sure to find out if the client really wants, and will wear, an orthosis before fabrication. Adaptive equipment should also be used with the client's individual needs and expectations in mind.

♡ Tips From the Field

Orthoses

The goal of splinting is to gently position all involved joints. If the digits alone are aligned radially in the orthosis without supportive correction of the wrist, the wrist can be pulled into further radial deviation. A strap at the head of the metacarpals provides a necessary stop to counterbalance the long lever arm alignment pull of the digital straps or spacers. However, the hand/wrist should never be forced into position because we cannot correct a severe deformity with splinting.

Another method for applying ulnar pull to the wrist is to secure a double-sided Velcro loop strap to the inside of the orthosis at the head of the metacarpals. The gentle pull of this strap helps keep the wrist from its tendency to follow the digits and pull into radial positioning. The gentle pull of radial alignment straps help keep digits in proper position, counteracting the ulnar deviation forces. Some clients also wear soft neoprene digit alignment orthoses during the day to protect their hands during ADLs (Fig. 29.11).

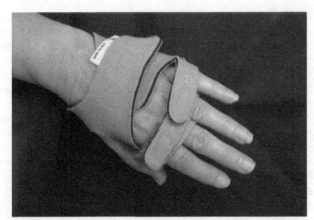

FIG. 29.11 A soft neoprene anti-ulnar deviation orthosis is often helpful for day wear when a client with rheumatoid arthritis demonstrates metacarpophalangeal ulnar deviation. (Rolyan Hand-Based In-Line Splint from Sammons Preston, Mississauga, ON.)

Small foam spacers provide a soft but forgiving alignment to the MP joints and yield to changes in digit size caused by edema or inflammation. Some clients prefer small thermoplastic spacers with moleskin covering.

Client Adherence to the Plan of Care

Clients will wear orthoses that fit well and are comfortable. Some clients return for new orthoses every year due to wear and tear. If a client returns with a clean orthosis, it is most likely not being worn. Most clients need orthoses for both hands, which can make nighttime trips to the bathroom difficult. Alternating an orthosis between the right hand and the left hand every other night can be helpful in managing this situation.

➤ Precautions and Concerns

The digits and wrist should never be forced into an aligned position. It is important to avoid the use of the long lever arm of the digit to extend the MP joint. If the proximal phalanx tilts rather than glides into position, it can wear away at the dorsal lip of the phalanx. This results in an orthosis that actually increases pain and absorption of the joint surface.[155] *Clients who are fitted with night orthoses should be made aware of proper application techniques to avoid this joint tilting, and the orthosis should be formed properly, allowing the joint to glide into position.*

Swan Neck Deformity

( ) *What to Say to Clients*

About the Condition

"Rheumatoid arthritis can loosen the stability of your joints, ligaments, and tendons. As you use your hand, the middle joints (PIPs) of your fingers tend to buckle backward and your end joints (DIPs) bend. This makes it difficult to grasp objects."

About Orthoses

"There are several styles of orthoses that can work for you. These orthoses allow your fingers to bend and prevent your middle joints (PIPs) from buckling backward."

About Exercise

"It is important that you maintain the bending ability of the middle joints (PIP flexion). This is done by taking your other hand and gently bending it toward the palm."

Evaluation Tips

Take care to measure both active and passive ROM of the PIP and DIP joints. If the joints are passively correctable, the client is usually a good candidate for a swan neck orthosis.

♡ *Tips From the Field*

Orthoses

Orthoses to correct a swan neck deformity (prevent PIP joint hyperextension, allow PIP flexion) are needed long term, and therefore should be durable. Dexterity can be improved using the orthosis.[130] There is research evidence of greater client acceptance and tolerance for prefabricated swan neck orthoses.[129] A good option is the plastic Oval-8 splint. It is available in many sizes and fitted in the clinic using a heat gun to adjust the orthosis (Fig. 29.12). A metal custom-sized splint called the SIRIS (or SilverRing) splint is another option. The therapist measures for this orthosis with a special tool that is available from the company. These splints allow hand use for most ADLs and do not need to be removed for hand washing.

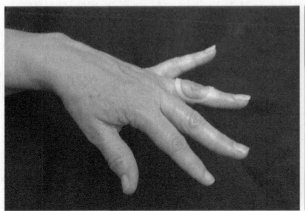
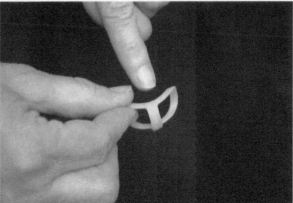

FIG. 29.12 The plastic Oval-8 splint is available in a variety of sizes and can be obtained from 3-Point Products, Inc. (Stevensville, MA).

> **Precautions and Concerns**

Take care to ensure that orthoses are not too tight or too loose. If they are too loose, clients often lose them; if they are too tight, they can cause pressure areas.

In the case of SilverRing splints, clients should have a good understanding of how to adjust the orthosis to account for changes in finger size from day to day. Some clients with sensitive skin may react to the metal; if needed, a special coating is available from the manufacturer.

Editor's note: Acknowledgement and thank you to Jeanine Beasley, who laid the foundation for this chapter in the first and second editions.

CASE STUDY

CASE STUDY 29.1 NONOPERATIVE TREATMENT OF RHEUMATOID ARTHRITIS ■

Bonita is a 53-year-old nurse with RA. She works 40 hours a week in the cardiac care unit of a local hospital and reports that her pain is largely under control with medication. She has two children in college and likes to play the organ at church. Bonita reports that with some activities, such as playing the organ, her right-hand PIP joints hyperextend at the index and ring fingers. This requires her to push even harder on the organ keys, which is sometimes painful. She would like some support that would give her index and ring finger (PIP) joints stability, yet allow her to do her activities.

Bonita was fitted with size 5 and 6 plastic Oval-8 splints (from 3-Point Products, Inc., Stevensville, MD) because there is evidence of greater acceptance and tolerance of prefabricated orthoses[129] than custom-made orthoses for this condition. She was shown the proper way to apply the orthoses to prevent PIP joint hyperextension, yet to allow full PIP joint flexion. She was instructed that the orthoses would be tighter when applied in the opposite direction and that this might be useful if her swelling were to decrease. Bonita was instructed in joint protection principles, including avoiding the intrinsic plus position, as she holds books or an electronic tablet. She was shown gentle PROM exercises for the PIP joints to help maintain PIP flexion.

Bonita returned to the clinic 1 week later with her husband. She reported increased finger stability while playing the organ. She felt the orthoses increased the stability of her PIP joints at work and during various other ADLs. Her husband had heard about the Silver-Ring splints and wanted to purchase a SilverRing (SIRIS) orthosis for Bonita's ring finger with her birthstone for their anniversary. The therapist was aware of a study that found SilverRing splints improved dexterity in selected patients with RA.[130]

Bonita was measured for the SilverRing splint using the EZ-Sizer. The correct size was determined, and the order form was completed. Her husband had purchased the birthstone previously, and this was included for placement on the ring splint with the order. The couple mailed in the order form and the stone.

The SilverRing orthosis arrived 8 days later and was fit to the client during her next hand therapy session. She was instructed in how to adjust the orthosis by bending the rings together (for a looser fit) or apart (for a tighter fit). This would help the ring splint fit appropriately when there were edema fluctuations. Bonita continued to wear her plastic Oval-8 orthosis on her index finger.

Bonita stopped by the clinic 2 weeks later. She had lost her Oval-8 splint. She reported decreased pain and increased stability with her orthosis and was wearing them day and night. They allowed full PIP joint flexion but prevented PIP hyperextension. She also felt she needed less pain medicine with the orthoses in place during activities. Her missing Oval-8 splint was replaced, and she was encouraged to contact the therapist if further assistance was needed.

References

1. Publication CDC: Prevalence of disabilities and associated health conditions among adults — United States, 1999, *Morb Mortal Weekly Rep* 50(7):120–125, 2001. http://www.jstor.org/stable/23312102.
2. Hootman JM, Helmick CG, Barbour KE, Theis KA, Boring MA: Updated projected prevalence of self-reported doctor-diagnosed arthritis and arthritis-attributable activity limitation among US adults, 2015–2040, *Arthritis Rheum* 68(7):1582–1587, 2016. https://doi.org/10.1002/art.39692. https://onlinelibrary.wiley.com/doi/abs/10.1002/art.39692.
3. Mchugh J: Epidemiology: arthritis more common than expected, *Nature Rev Rheum* 14(1):3, 2018. https://doi.org/10.1038/nrrheum.2017.203. https://search.proquest.com/docview/1978778814.
4. Australian Institute of Health and Welfare: *A snapshot of arthritis in australia 2010*, Canberra, 2010, Australian institute of Health and Welfare (AIHW).
5. Peeters G, Alshurafa M, Schaap L, de Vet HCW: Diagnostic accuracy of self-reported arthritis in the general adult population is acceptable, *J Clin Epidemiol* 68(4):452–459, 2015. http://www.sciencedirect.com.ezproxy 2.library.arizona.edu/science/article/pii/S0895435614003953. doi: //doi-org.ezproxy2.library.arizona.edu/10.1016/j.jclinepi.2014.09.019.
6. Centers for Disease Control and Prevention, (CDC). Arthritis in general. Accessed April 1, 2018.
7. Vos T, Flaxman AD, Naghavi M, et al.: Years lived with disability (YLDs) for 1160 sequelae of 289 diseases and injuries 1990–2010: a systematic analysis for the global burden of disease study 2010, *Lancet* 380(9859):2163–2196, 2012. https://doi.org/10.1016/S0140-6736(12)61729-2. https://www.clinicalkey.es/playcontent/1-s2.0-S0140673612617292.
8. Kraus VB, Blanco FJ, Englund M, Karsdal MA, Lohmander LS: Call for standardized definitions of osteoarthritis and risk stratification for clinical trials and clinical use, *Osteoarthr Cartil* 23(8):1233–1241, 2015. http://www.sciencedirect.com/science/article/pii/S1063458415008997. https://doi.org/10.1016/j.joca.2015.03.036.
9. Helmick CG, Felson DT, Lawrence RC, et al.: Estimates of the prevalence of arthritis and other rheumatic conditions in the United States. part I, *Arthritis Rheum* 58(1):15–25, 2008. https://doi.org/10.1002/art.23177. http://www.ncbi.nlm.nih.gov/pubmed/18163481.
10. Lawrence RC, Felson DT, Helmick CG, et al.: Estimates of the prevalence of arthritis and other rheumatic conditions in the United States. Part II, *Arthritis Rheum* 58(1):26–35, 2008. https://doi.org/10.1002/art.23176. http://www.ncbi.nlm.nih.gov/pubmed/18163497.
11. Haugen IK, Englund M, Aliabadi P, et al.: Prevalence, incidence and progression of hand osteoarthritis in the general population: the framingham osteoarthritis study, *Ann rheum Dis* 70(9):1581–1586. 2011. https://doi.org/10.1136/ard.2011.150078. http://www.ncbi.nlm.nih.gov/pubmed/21622766.
12. Kaufmann RA, Lögters TT, Verbruggen G, Windolf J, Goitz RJ: Osteoarthritis of the distal interphalangeal joint, *J Hand Surg* 35(12):2117–2125, 2010. https://doi.org/10.1016/j.jhsa.2010.09.003. https://www.clinicalkey.es/playcontent/1-s2.0-S0363502310010634.

13. Barbour KE, Helmick CG, Boring M, Brady TJ: Vital signs: prevalence of doctor-diagnosed arthritis and arthritis-attributable activity limitation—United States, 2013-2015. *MMWR, Morb Mortal Weekly Rep* 66(9):246, 2017. https://search.proquest.com/docview/1878088158.

14. Gazeley DJ, Yeturi S, Patel PJ, Rosenthal AK: Erosive osteoarthritis: a systematic analysis of definitions used in the literature, *Semin Arthritis Rheum* 46(4):395–403, 2017. https://doi.org/S0049-0172(16)30209-8 [pii].

15. Malfait AM: Osteoarthritis year in review 2015: Biology, *Osteoarthr Cartil* 24(1):21–26, 2015. https://doi.org/10.1016/j.joca.2015.09.010. https://www.clinicalkey.es/playcontent/1-s2.0-S1063458415013242.

16. Boesen M, Ellegaard K, Henriksen M, et al.: Osteoarthritis year in review 2016: imaging, *Osteoarthr Cartil* 25(2):216–226, 2016. https://doi.org/10.1016/j.joca.2016.12.009. https://www.clinicalkey.es/playcontent/1-s2.0-S1063458416304691.

17. Mobasheri A, Batt M: An update on the pathophysiology of osteoarthritis, *Ann Physical Rehabil Med* 59(5):333–339, 2016. http://www.sciencedirect.com/science/article/pii/S1877065716300847. //doi.org/10.1016/j.rehab.2016.07.004.

18. Goldring MB: Chondrogenesis, chondrocyte differentiation, and articular cartilage metabolism in health and osteoarthritis, *Therapeutic Advances Musculoskeletal* 4(4):269–285, 2012. https://doi.org/10.1177/1759720X12448454. doi: 10.1177/1759720X12448454.

19. Fernandes JC, Martel-Pelletier J, Pelletier J: The role of cytokines in osteoarthritis pathophysiology, *Biorheol* 39(1-2):237–246, 2002. https://www.scopus.com/inward/record.uri?eid=2-s2.0-0036286667&partnerID=40&md5=a0963228ac0c265db9885db3b7e1ce12. [Accessed 28 April 2018].

20. Martin J, Buckwalter J: Aging, articular cartilage chondrocyte senescence and osteoarthritis, *Biogerontol* 3(5):257–264, 2002. https://doi.org/S0049-0172(16)30209-8. http://www.ncbi.nlm.nih.gov/pubmed/12237562.

21. Gazeley DJ, Yeturi S, Patel PJ, Rosenthal AK: Erosive osteoarthritis: a systematic analysis of definitions used in the literature, *Seminars Arthritis Rheum*, 2016. https://doi.org/10.1016/j.semarthrit.2016.08.013. https://www.clinicalkey.es/playcontent/1-s2.0-S0049017216302098.

22. Punzi L, Frigato M, Frallonardo P, Ramonda R: Inflammatory osteoarthritis of the hand, *Best Pract Res Clin Rheum* 24(3):301–312, 2009. https://doi.org/10.1016/j.berh.2009.12.007. https://www.clinicalkey.es/playcontent/1-s2.0-S1521694209001521.

23. Kraus VB, Blanco FJ, Englund M, Karsdal MA, Lohmander LS: Call for standardized definitions of osteoarthritis and risk stratification for clinical trials and clinical use, *Osteoarthr Cartil* 23(8):1233–1241, 2015. http://www.sciencedirect.com/science/article/pii/S1063458415008997. https://doi.org/10.1016/j.joca.2015.03.036.

24. Haugen IK, Lillegraven S, Slatkowsky-Christensen B, et al.: Hand osteoarthritis and MRI: development and first validation step of the proposed Oslo hand osteoarthritis MRI score, *Ann Rheum Dis* 70(6):1033–1038, 2011. https://doi.org/10.1136/ard.2010.144527. http://www.ncbi.nlm.nih.gov/pubmed/21436160.

25. van der Kraan PM, van den Berg WB: Osteophytes: relevance and biology, *Osteoarthr Cartil* 15(3):237–244, 2007. http://www.sciencedirect.com/science/article/pii/S106345840600327X. doi: //doi.org/10.1016/j.joca.2006.11.006.

26. Cooper C: *Chapter 1 - fundamentals of clinical reasoning: hand therapy concepts and treatment techniques. Fundamentals of hand therapy*, Elsevier Inc, 2007, pp 3–21. https://doi.org/10.1016/B0-32-303386-5/50004-7.

27. Law M, Baptiste S, McColl M, Opzoomer A, Polatajko H, Pollock N: The Canadian occupational performance measure: an outcome measure for occupational therapy, *Canadian J Occupational Ther* 57(2):82–87, 1990. https://doi.org/10.1177/000841749005700207. http://journals.sagepub.com/doi/full/10.1177/000841749005700207.

28. Meenan RF, Mason JH, Anderson JJ, Guccione AA, Kazis LE: AIMS2. the content and properties of a revised and expanded arthritis impact measurement scales health status questionnaire, *Arthritis Rheum* 35(1):1–10, 1992. https://doi.org/10.1002/art.1780350102. http://www.ncbi.nlm.nih.gov/pubmed/1731806.

29. Hawker GA, Mian S, Kendzerska T, French M: Measures of adult pain: Visual analog scale for pain (VAS pain), numeric rating scale for pain (NRS pain), McGill pain questionnaire (MPQ), Short-Form McGill pain questionnaire (SF–MPQ), chronic pain grade scale (CPGS), short Form-36 bodily pain scale (SF–36 BPS), and measure of intermittent and constant osteoarthritis pain (ICOAP), *Arthritis Care Res* 63(S11):S252, 2011. https://doi.org/10.1002/acr.20543. https://onlinelibrary.wiley.com/doi/abs/10.1002/acr.20543.

30. Eaton RG, Glickel SZ: Trapeziometacarpal osteoarthritis: staging as a rationale for treatment, *Hand clinics* 3(4):455, 1987. http://www.ncbi.nlm.nih.gov/pubmed/3693416.

31. Gelberman RH, Boone S, Osei DA, Cherney S, Calfee RP: Trapeziometacarpal arthritis: a prospective clinical evaluation of the thumb adduction and extension provocative tests, *J Hand Surg* 40(7):1285–1291, 2015. https://doi.org/10.1016/j.jhsa.2015.04.012. https://www.clinicalkey.es/playcontent/1-s2.0-S0363502315004505.

32. Takata SC, Wade ET, Roll SC: Hand therapy interventions, outcomes, and diagnoses evaluated over the last 10 years: a mapping review linking research to practice, *J Hand Ther*, 2017. http://www.sciencedirect.com.libproxy.nau.edu/science/article/pii/S0894113016302770. //doi-org.libproxy.nau.edu/10.1016/j.jht.2017.05.018.

33. Luker K, Aguinaldo A, Kenney D, Cahill-Rowley K: Ladd A Functional task kinematics of the thumb carpometacarpal joint, *Clin Orthop Relat Res* 472(4):1123–1129. 2014, https://doi.org/10.1007/s11999-013-2964-0. http://www.ncbi.nlm.nih.gov/pubmed/23549712.

34. Halilaj E, Rainbow M, Got C, et al.: In vivo kinematics of the thumb carpometacarpal joint during three isometric functional tasks, *Clin Orthop Relat Res* 472(4):1114–1122, 2014. https://doi.org/10.1007/s11999-013-3063-y. http://www.ncbi.nlm.nih.gov/pubmed/23681597.

35. Cooney WP, Chao EY: Biomechanical analysis of static forces in the thumb during hand function, *J Bone Joint Surg* 59(1):27–36, 1977. https://doi.org/10.2106/00004623-197759010-00004. http://jbjs.org/article.aspx?articleid=16988.

36. Wu JZ, Sinsel EW, Zhao KD, An K, Buczek FL: Analysis of the constraint joint loading in the thumb during pipetting, *J Biomechanical Engineer* 137(8):7, 2015. https://doi.org/10.1115/1.4030311. https://doi.org/10.1115/1.4030311.

37. Bensghaier A, Romdhane L, Benouezdou F: Multi-objective optimization to predict muscle tensions in a pinch function using genetic algorithm, *Comptes rendus - Mécanique* 340(3):139–155, 2012. https://www.sciencedirect.com/science/article/pii/S1631072112000277. https://doi.org/10.1016/j.crme.2012.01.002.

38. Beasley J: Clinical relevance commentary in response to: effectiveness of a fine motor skills rehabilitation program on upper limb disability, manual dexterity, pinch strength, range of finger motion, performance in activities of daily living, functional independence, and general self-efficacy in hand osteoarthritis: a randomized clinical trial, *J Hand Ther* 30(3):274–275, 2017. https://doi.org/S0894-1130(17)30126-6 [pii].

39. 7 Valdes K, Marik T: A systematic review of conservative interventions for osteoarthritis of the hand, *J Hand Ther* 23(4):334–351, 2010. https://doi.org/10.1016/j.jht.2010.05.001. https://www.clinicalkey.es/playcontent/1-s2.0-S0894113010000505.

40. Dziedzic K, Nicholls E, Hill S, et al.: Self-management approaches for osteoarthritis in the hand: a 2×2 factorial randomised trial, *Ann Rheum Dis* 74(1):108–118, 2015. https://doi.org/10.1136/annrheumdis-2013-203938. http://www.ncbi.nlm.nih.gov/pubmed/24107979.

41. Zanghi HA, Ndosi M, Adams J, et al.: EULAR recommendations for patient education for people with inflammatory arthritis, *Ann Rheum Dis* 74(6):954–962, 2015. https://doi.org/10.1136/annrheumdis-2014-206807. http://www.narcis.nl/publication/RecordID/oai:cris.maastrichtuniversity.nl:publications%2F57311db7-678f-4cbc-aabf-913463598fdf.

42. Stamm TA, Machold KP, Smolen JS, et al.: Joint protection and home hand exercises improve hand function in patients with hand osteoarthritis: a randomized controlled trial, *Arthritis Rheum* 47(1):44–49, 2002. https://doi.org/10.1002/art1.10246. http://www.ncbi.nlm.nih.gov/pubmed/11932877.

43. Kong Y, Lowe BD: Optimal cylindrical handle diameter for grip force tasks, *Int J Ind Ergon* 35(6):495–507, 2005. https://doi.org/10.1016/j.

ergon.2004.11.003. https://www.sciencedirect.com/science/article/pii/S0169814104002148.

44. Sancho-Bru JL, Giurintano DJ, Pérez-González A, Vergara M: Optimum tool handle diameter for a cylinder grip, *J Hand Ther* 16(4):337–342, 2003. https://doi.org/10.1197/S0894-1130(03)00160-1. https://www.sciencedirect.com/science/article/pii/S0894113003001601.

45. Young JG, Woolley C, Armstrong TJ, Ashton-Miller JA: Hand-handhold coupling: Effect of handle shape, orientation, and friction on breakaway strength, *Human Factors: J Hum Factors Ergon Society* 51(5):705–717, 2009. https://doi.org/10.1177/0018720809355969. http://www.ingentaconnect.com/content/hfes/hf/2009/00000051/00000005/art00007.

46. Seo NJ, Armstrong TJ: Effect of elliptic handle shape on grasping strategies, grip force distribution, and twisting ability, *Ergonomics* 54(10):961–970, 2011. https://doi.org/10.1080/00140139.2011.606923. http://www.tandfonline.com/doi/abs/10.1080/00140139.2011.606923.

47. Hallbeck MS, Cochran DJ, Stonecipher BL, Riley MW, Bishu RR: Hand-handle orientation and maximum force, *Hum Factors Ergon Society Annual Meeting Proceedings* 34(10):800–804, 1990. https://doi.org/10.1177/154193129003401029. http://www.ingentaconnect.com/content/hfes/hfproc/1990/00000034/00000010/art00029.

48. Hochberg MC, Altman RD, April KT, et al.: American college of rheumatology 2012 recommendations for the use of nonpharmacologic and pharmacologic therapies in osteoarthritis of the hand, hip, and knee, *Arthritis Care Research* 64(4):465–474, 2012. https://doi.org/10.1002/acr.21596. https://onlinelibrary.wiley.com/doi/abs/10.1002/acr.21596.

49. Conaghan PG, Dickson J, Grant RL: Guidelines: care and management of osteoarthritis in adults: summary of NICE guidance, *BMJ* 336(7642):502–503, 2008. https://doi.org/10.1136/bmj.39490.608009. AD https://www.jstor.org/stable/20509118.

50. Beasley J: Osteoarthritis and rheumatoid arthritis: conservative therapeutic management, *J Hand Ther* 25(2):163–172, 2012. https://doi.org/10.1016/j.jht.2011.11.001. https://www.clinicalkey.es/playcontent/1-s2.0-S0894113011001529.

51. Hammond A, Bryan J, Hardy A: Effects of a modular behavioural arthritis education programme: a pragmatic parallel-group randomized controlled trial, *Rheumatology* 47(11):1712–1718, 2008. https://doi.org/10.1093/rheumatology/ken380. http://www.ncbi.nlm.nih.gov/pubmed/18815153.

52. Bjurehed L, Brodin N, Nordenskiold U, Bjork M: Improved hand function, self-rated health and decreased activity limitations - results after a two month hand osteoarthritis group intervention, *Arthritis Care Res (Hoboken)*, 2017. https://doi.org/10.1002/acr.23431 [doi].

53. Zhang W, Doherty M, Leeb BF, et al.: EULAR evidence based recommendations for the management of hand osteoarthritis: report of a task force of the EULAR standing committee for international clinical studies including therapeutics (ESCISIT), *Ann Rheum Dis* 66(3):377–388, 2007. http://www.ncbi.nlm.nih.gov/pubmed/17046965. https://doi:10.1136/ard.2006.062091.

54. Lue S, Koppikar S, Shaikh K, Mahendra D, Towheed TE: Systematic review of non-surgical therapies for osteoarthritis of the hand: an update, *Osteoarthr Cartil* 25(9):1379–1389, 2017. https://doi.org/S1063-4584(17)31028-2 [pii].

55. Aebischer B, Elsig S, Taeymans J: Effectiveness of physical and occupational therapy on pain, function and quality of life in patients with trapeziometacarpal osteoarthritis – a systematic review and meta-analysis, *Hand Ther* 21(1):5–15, 2016. https://doi.org/10.1177/1758998315614037. https://doi.org/10.1177/1758998315614037.

56. Ahern M, Skyllas J, Wajon A, Hush J: The effectiveness of physical therapies for patients with base of thumb osteoarthritis: systematic review and meta-analysis, *Musculoskelet Sci Pract* 35:46–54, 2018. https://doi.org/S2468-7812(18)30045-6 [pii].

57. Colditz JC: An exercise program for carpometacarpal osteoarthritis based on biomechanical principles, *J Hand Ther* 26(1):81–82, 2013. https://doi.org/10.1016/j.jht.2012.10.002. https://www.clinicalkey.es/playcontent/1-s2.0-S0894113012001573.

58. Valdes K, von der Heyde R: An exercise program for carpometacarpal osteoarthritis based on biomechanical principles, *J Hand Ther* 25(3):251–263, 2012. https://doi.org/10.1016/j.jht.2012.03.008. https://www.clinicalkey.es/playcontent/1-s2.0-S0894113012000427.

59. Osteras N, Kjeken I, Smedslund G, et al.: Exercise for hand osteoarthritis: A cochrane systematic review, *J Rheum* 44(12):1850–1858, 2017. https://doi.org/10.3899/jrheum.170424 [doi].

60. Ahern M, Skyllas J, Wajon A, Hush J: The effectiveness of physical therapies for patients with base of thumb osteoarthritis: systematic review and meta-analysis, *Musculoskelet Sci Pract* 35:46–54, 2018. https://doi.org/S2468-7812(18)30045-6 [pii].

61. Deveza LA, Hunter DJ, Wajon A, et al.: Efficacy of combined conservative therapies on clinical outcomes in patients with thumb base osteoarthritis: protocol for a randomised, controlled trial (COMBO), *BMJ Open* 7(1), 2017. https://doi.org/10.1136/bmjopen-2016-014498. https://search.proquest.com/docview/1858001906.

62. Lue S, Koppikar S, Shaikh K, Mahendra D, Towheed TE: Systematic review of non-surgical therapies for osteoarthritis of the hand: an update, *Osteoarthr Cartil* 25(9):1379–1389, 2017. http://www.sciencedirect.com.libproxy.nau.edu/science/article/pii/S1063458417310282. https://doi.org.libproxy.nau.edu/10.1016/j.joca.2017.05.016.

63. O'Brien VH, McGaha JL: Current practice patterns in conservative thumb CMC joint care: survey results, *J Hand Ther* 27(1):14–22, 2014. https://doi.org/10.1016/j.jht.2013.09.001. https://www.clinicalkey.es/playcontent/1-s2.0-S0894113013001270.

64. Spaans AJ, van Minnen PL, Kon M, Schuurman AH, Schreuders AR, Vermeulen GM: Conservative treatment of thumb base osteoarthritis: a systematic review, *J Hand Surg* 40(1):21.e6, 2015. https://doi.org/10.1016/j.jhsa.2014.08.047. https://www.clinicalkey.es/playcontent/1-s2.0-S0363502314014336.

65. Magni NE, McNair PJ, Rice DA: The effects of resistance training on muscle strength, joint pain, and hand function in individuals with hand osteoarthritis: a systematic review and meta-analysis, *Arthritis Res Ther* 19, 2017. https://search.proquest.com/docview/1916623472. https://doi.org/10.1186/s13075-017-1348-3.

66. Villafane JH, Valdes K, O'Brien V, Seves M, Cantero-Tellez R, Berjano P: Conservative management of thumb carpometacarpal osteoarthritis: an italian survey of current clinical practice, *J Bodyw Mov Ther* 22(1):37–39, 2018. https://doi.org/S1360-8592(17)30038-4 [pii].

67. Brand PW: Mechanics of individual muscles at individual joints. In *Clinical mechanics of the hand*, ed 3, p 131. United States. http://catalog.hathitrust.org/Record/004059512.

68. McGee C, Mathiowetz V: Evaluation of hand forces during a joint-protection strategy for women with hand osteoarthritis. *Am J Occup Ther* 71(1):7101190020p8, 2017. https://doi.org/10.5014/ajot.2017.022921 [doi].

69. McGee C, O'Brien V, Van Nortwick S, Adams J, Van Heest A: First dorsal interosseous muscle contraction results in radiographic reduction of healthy thumb carpometacarpal joint, *J Hand Ther* 28(4):375–381, 2015. https://doi.org/10.1016/j.jht.2015.06.002. https://www.clinicalkey.es/playcontent/1-s2.0-S0894113015000988.

70. O'Brien VH, Giveans MR: Effects of a dynamic stability approach in conservative intervention of the carpometacarpal joint of the thumb: a retrospective study, *J Hand Ther* 26(1):44–52, 2013. http://www.sciencedirect.com/science/article/pii/S0894113012001603. //doi.org/10.1016/j.jht.2012.10.005.

71. Ladd A, Crisco J, Hagert E, Rose J, Weiss A: The 2014 ABJS Nicolas Andry award: The puzzle of the thumb: Mobility, stability, and demands in opposition, *Clin Orthop Relat Res* 472(12):3605–3622, 2014. https://doi.org/10.1007/s11999-014-3901-6. http://www.ncbi.nlm.nih.gov/pubmed/25171934.

72. DeMott L: Novel isometric exercises for the dynamic stability programs for thumb carpal metacarpal joint instability, *J Hand Ther* 30(3):372, 2016. https://doi.org/10.1016/j.jht.2016.09.005. https://www.clinicalkey.es/playcontent/1-s2.0-S0894113016301740.

73. O'Brien VH, Giveans MR: Effects of a dynamic stability approach in conservative intervention of the carpometacarpal joint of the thumb: a retrospective study, *J Hand Ther* 26(1):44–52, 2013. https://doi.

org/10.1016/j.jht.2012.10.005. https://www.clinicalkey.es/playcontent/1-s2.0-S0894113012001603.

74. DeMott L: Novel isometric exercises for the dynamic stability programs for thumb carpal metacarpal joint instability, *J Hand Ther* 30(3):372, 2016. https://doi.org/10.1016/j.jht.2016.09.005. https://www.clinicalkey.es/playcontent/1-s2.0-S0894113016301740.

75. Villafañe JH, Cleland JA, Fernández-de-Las-Peñas C: The effectiveness of a manual therapy and exercise protocol in patients with thumb carpometacarpal osteoarthritis: a randomized controlled trial, *J Orthopaedic Sports Phy Ther* 43(4):204–213, 2013. https://doi.org/10.2519/jospt.2013.4524. http://www.ncbi.nlm.nih.gov/pubmed/23485660.

76. Rogers MW, Wilder FV: The effects of strength training among persons with hand osteoarthritis: a two-year follow-up study, *J Hand Ther* 20(3):244–250, 2007. http://www.sciencedirect.com/science/article/pii/S0894113007000324. //doi.org/10.1197/j.jht.2007.04.005.

77. Osteras N, Kjeken I, Smedslund G, et al.: Exercise for hand osteoarthritis: a cochrane systematic review, *J Rheumatol* 44(12):1850–1858, 2017. https://doi.org/10.3899/jrheum.170424 [doi].

78. Minor MA, Hewett JE, Webel RR, Anderson SK, Kay DR: Efficacy of physical conditioning exercise in patients with rheumatoid arthritis and osteoarthritis, *Arthritis Rheum* 32(11):1396–1405, 1989. https://doi.org/10.1002/anr.1780321108. http://www.ncbi.nlm.nih.gov/pubmed/2818656.

79. Roll SC, Hardison ME: Effectiveness of occupational therapy interventions for adults with musculoskeletal conditions of the forearm, wrist, and hand: a systematic review. *Am J Occup Ther* 71(1):7101180010p12, 2017. https://doi.org/10.5014/ajot.2017.023234 [doi].

80. Valdes K, Naughton N, Algar L: Linking ICF components to outcome measures for orthotic intervention for CMC OA: a systematic review, *J Hand Ther* 29(4):396–404, 2016. https://doi.org/S0894-1130(16)30076-X [pii].

81. Cole T, Robinson L, Romero L, O'Brien L: Effectiveness of interventions to improve therapy adherence in people with upper limb conditions: a systematic review, *J Hand Ther*, 2017. http://www.sciencedirect.com.libproxy.nau.edu/science/article/pii/S0894113017302818. //doi-org.libproxy.nau.edu/10.1016/j.jht.2017.11.040.

82. Beasley J: Therapist's examination and conservative management of arthritis of the upper extremity. In *Rehabilitation of the hand and upper extremity*, ed 6, p 1343.e2. https://doi.org/10.1016/B978-0-323-05602-1.00103-3. https://www.clinicalkey.es/playcontent/3-s2.0-B9780323056021001033.

83. Colditz JC: The biomechanics of a thumb carpometacarpal immobilization splint: design and fitting, *J Hand Ther* 13(3):228–235, 2000. https://doi.org/10.1016/S0894-1130(00)80006-X. https://www.sciencedirect.com/science/article/pii/S089411300080006X.

84. Johnson J, Goitz RJ: Ligament reconstruction and tendon interposition, *Operative Techniques Orthopaedics* 28(1):16–22, 2018. http://www.sciencedirect.com/science/article/pii/S104866661730112X. http://doi.org/10.1053/j.oto.2017.12.005.

85. O'Brien VH, Giveans MR: Effects of a dynamic stability approach in conservative intervention of the carpometacarpal joint of the thumb: a retrospective study, *J Hand Ther* 26(1):44–52, 2013. https://doi.org/10.1016/j.jht.2012.10.005. https://www.clinicalkey.es/playcontent/1-s2.0-S0894113012001603.

86. Ikeda M, Ishii T, Kobayashi Y, Mochida J, Saito I, Oka Y: Custom-made splint treatment for osteoarthritis of the distal interphalangeal joints, *J Hand Surg* 35(4):589–593, 2010. https://doi.org/10.1016/j.jhsa.2010.01.012. https://www.clinicalkey.es/playcontent/1-s2.0-S0363502310000687.

87. Kjeken I, Smedslund G, Moe RH, Slatkowsky–Christensen B, Uhlig T, Hagen KB: Systematic review of design and effects of splints and exercise programs in hand osteoarthritis, *Arthritis Care Res* 63(6):834–848, 2011. https://doi.org/10.1002/acr.20427. https://onlinelibrary.wiley.com/doi/abs/10.1002/acr.20427.

88. Pincus T, Callahan LF, Sale WG, Brooks AL, Payne LE, Vaughn WK: Severe functional declines, work disability, and increased mortality in seventy-five rheumatoid arthritis patients studied over nine years, *Arthritis Rheum* 27(8):864–872, 1984. https://doi.

org/10.1002/art.1780270805. http://www.ncbi.nlm.nih.gov/pubmed/6431998.

89. Solomon DH, Karlson EW, Rimm EB, et al.: Cardiovascular morbidity and mortality in women diagnosed with rheumatoid arthritis, *Circulation* 107(9):1303–1307, 2003. https://doi.org/10.1161/01.CIR.0000054612.26458.B2. http://circ.ahajournals.org/cgi/content/abstract/107/9/1303.

90. Chaigne B, Finckh A, Neto D, Alpizar Rodriguez D, Ribi C, Chizzolini C: SAT0393 health related quality of life in rheumatoid arthritis and systemic lupus erythematosus patients in switzerland: not the same impact, *Ann Rheum Dis* 74(Suppl 2):801, 2015. https://doi.org/10.1136/annrheumdis-2015-eular.4188. https://search.proquest.com/docview/1901787275.

91. Kourilovitch M, Galarza-Maldonado C, lOrtiz-Prado E: Diagnosis and classification of rheumatoid arthritis, *J Autoimmunity* 48:26–30, 2014. https://doi.org/10.1016/j.jaut.2014.01.027. https://www.clinicalkey.es/playcontent/1-s2.0-S0896841114000304.

92. Joshi VR: Rheumatology, past, present and future, *J Assoc Phys India* 60(1):21–24, 2012. https://www.scopus.com/inward/record.uri?eid=2-s2.0-84855526359&partnerID=40&md5=19f1d0ca11b98bb62fd01216c0b05f80. [Accessed 18 June 2018].

93. Gregersen PK, Jack S, Winchester RJ: The shared epitope hypothesis. an approach to understanding the molecular genetics of susceptibility to rheumatoid arthritis, *Arthritis Rheum* 30(11):1205–1213, 1987. https://doi.org/10.1002/art.1780301102. https://doi.org/10.1002/art.1780301102.

94. Liao K, Alfredsson L, Karlson E: Environmental influences on risk for rheumatoid arthritis, *Cur Opini Rheum* 21(3):279–283, 2009. https://doi.org/10.1097/BOR.0b013e32832a2e16. http://www.ncbi.nlm.nih.gov/pubmed/19318947.

95. Karlson EW, Chang S, Cui J, et al.: Gene-environment interaction between HLA-DRB1 shared epitope and heavy cigarette smoking in predicting incident rheumatoid arthritis, *Ann Rheum Dis* 69(1):54–60, 2010. https://doi.org/10.1136/ard.2008.102962. http://www.ncbi.nlm.nih.gov/pubmed/19151010.

96. Scott IC, Galloway JB, Scott DL: *Inflammatory arthritis in clinical practice*, ed 2, London [u.a.], 2015, Springer.

97. Aletaha D, Neogi T, Silman AJ, et al.: 2010 rheumatoid arthritis classification criteria: an American college of rheumatology/european league against rheumatism collaborative initiative, *Ann Rheum Dis* 69(9):1588, 2010. https://pure.amc.nl/portal/en/publications/2010-rheumatoid-arthritis-classification-criteria-an-american-college-of-rheumatologyeuropean-league -against-rheumatism-collaborative-initiative(9d2fbd1d-f75f-4859-9d7a-ef12d3f4be72).html.

98. Stephanie N, Christina B, Erik T, de Laar MA: Fatigue and factors related to fatigue in rheumatoid arthritis: a systematic review, *Arthritis Care Res* 65(7):1128–1146, 2013. https://doi.org/10.1002/acr.21949. https://doi.org/10.1002/acr.21949.

99. Horsten NCA, Ursum J, Roorda LD, Schaardenburg VD, Dekker J, Hoeksma AF: Prevalence of hand symptoms, impairments and activity limitations in rheumatoid arthritis in relation to disease duration, *J Rehabil Med* 42(10):916–921, 2010. https://doi.org/10.2340/16501977-0619. http://www.narcis.nl/publication/RecordID/vu2:oai:dare.ubvu.vu.nl:1871%2F20924.

100. Rowbotham E, Freeston J, Emery P, Grainger A: The prevalence of tenosynovitis of the interosseous tendons of the hand in patients with rheumatoid arthritis, *Eur Radiol* 26(2):444–450, 2016. https://doi.org/10.1007/s00330-015-3859-0. http://www.ncbi.nlm.nih.gov/pubmed/26045344.

101. Navalho M, Resende C, Rodrigues AM, et al.: Bilateral MR imaging of the hand and wrist in early and very early inflammatory arthritis: tenosynovitis is associated with progression to rheumatoid arthritis, *Radiology* 264(3):823–833, 2012. https://doi.org/10.1148/radiol.12112513. http://www.ncbi.nlm.nih.gov/pubmed/22723498.

102. Villeneuve E, Nam JL, Bell MJ, et al.: A systematic literature review of strategies promoting early referral and reducing delays in the diagnosis and management of inflammatory arthritis, *Ann Rheum Dis* 72(1):13–

22, 2013. https://doi.org/10.1136/annrheumdis-2011-201063. http://w ww.ncbi.nlm.nih.gov/pubmed/22532640.

103. Chung KC: Clinical management of the rheumatoid hand, wrist, and elbow. In: ed 1. 2016 ed. Cham: Springer International Publishing; 2016:184–285. http://lib.myilibrary.com?ID=907051. 10.1007/978-3-319-26660-2.

104. Nyhäll-Wåhlin B, Turesson C, Jacobsson L, et al.: The presence of rheumatoid nodules at early rheumatoid arthritis diagnosis is a sign of extraarticular disease and predicts radiographic progression of joint destruction over 5 years, *Scandinavian J Rheum* 40(2):81–87, 2011. https://doi.org/10.3109/03009742.2010.509103. http://www.ncbi.nlm.nih.gov/pu bmed/20919947.

105. Tilstra JS, Lienesch DW: Rheumatoid nodules, *Dermatologic Clinics* 33(3):361–371, 2015. https://doi.org/10.1016/j.det.2015.03.004. https: //www.clinicalkey.es/playcontent/1-s2.0-S0733863515000170.

106. van Dongen H, van Aken J, Lard L, et al.: Efficacy of methotrexate treatment in patients with probable rheumatoid arthritis: a double-blind, randomized, placebo-controlled trial, *Arthritis Rheum* 56(5):1424–1432, 2007. https://doi.org/10.1002/art.22525. http://www.ncbi.nlm.nih.gov/ pubmed/17469099.

107. Bukhari MAS, Wiles NJ, Lunt M, et al.: Influence of disease-modifying therapy on radiographic outcome in inflammatory polyarthritis at five years: results from a large observational inception study, *Arthritis Rheum* 48(1):46–53, 2003. https://doi.org/10.1002/art.10727. http://www.ncb i.nlm.nih.gov/pubmed/12528102.

108. McInnes IB, Schett G: Pathogenetic insights from the treatment of rheumatoid arthritis, *Lancet* 389(10086):2328–2337, 2017. http://www .sciencedirect.com/science/article/pii/S0140673617314721. //doi.org/1 0.1016/S0140-6736(17)31472-1.

109. Holmdahl R, Malmström V, Burkhardt H: Autoimmune priming, tissue attack and chronic inflammation — the three stages of rheumatoid arthritis, *Eur J Immunol* 44(6):1593–1599, 2014. https://doi.org/10.1002/ eji.201444486. https://onlinelibrary.wiley.com/doi/abs/10.1002/ eji.201444486.

110. Steinbroker O, Traeger CH, Batterman RC: Therapeutic criteria in rheumatoid arthritis, *J Am Med Association* 140(8):659–662, 1949. https://doi.org/10.1001/jama.1949.02900430001001. https://doi.org/ 10.1001/jama.1949.02900430001001.

111. Smolen JS, Landewé R, Bijlsma J, et al.: EULAR recommendations for the management of rheumatoid arthritis with synthetic and biological disease-modifying antirheumatic drugs: 2016 update, *Ann Rheum Dis* 76(6):960–977, 2017. https://doi.org/10.1136/annrheum-dis-2016-210715. https://doi.org/10.1136/annrheumdis-2016-210715.

112. Tuyl HD, Felson DT, Wells G, Smolen J, Zhang B, Boers M: Evidence for predictive validity of remission on long-term outcome in rheumatoid arthritis: a systematic review, *Research* 62(1):108–117, 2010. https://doi .org/10.1002/acr.20021. http://www.narcis.nl/publication/RecordID/vu 2:oai:dare.ubvu.vu.nl:1871%2F46200.

113. Catrina AI, Svensson CI, Malmström V, Schett G, Klareskog L: Mechanisms leading from systemic autoimmunity to joint-specific disease in rheumatoid arthritis, *Nature Rev Rheum* 13(2):79–86, 2017. https://doi.org/10.1038/nrrheum.2016.200. https://www.ncbi.nlm.nih .gov/pubmed/27974851.

114. Klareskog L, Catrina AI, Paget S: Rheumatoid arthritis, *Lancet* 373:659–672, 2009.

115. The American Occupational Therapy Association: AOTA occupational profile template, *Am J Occup Ther* 71(Suppl 2):S13, 2017. https://doi .org/10.5014/ajot.2017.716S12. https://www.ncbi.nlm.nih.gov/pub med/29309016.

116. Nordenskiöld U: *Daily activities in women with rheumatoid arthritis*, Scandinavian Univ. Press, 1997.

117. Hallert E, Björk M, Dahlström Ö, Skogh T, Thyberg I: Disease activity and disability in women and men with early rheumatoid arthritis (RA): an 8-year followup of a Swedish early RA project, *Arthritis Care Res* 64(8):1101–1107, 2012. https://doi.org/10.1002/acr.21662. https://onl inelibrary.wiley.com/doi/abs/10.1002/acr.21662.

118. Rydholm M, Book C, Wikström I, Jacobsson L, Turesson C: Course of grip force impairment in patients with early rheumatoid arthritis over the first five years after diagnosis, *Arthritis Care Res* 70(4):491–498, 2018. https://doi.org/10.1002/acr.23318. https://onlinelibrary.wiley.co m/doi/abs/10.1002/acr.23318.

119. Mathieux R, Marotte H, Battistini L, Sarrazin A, Berthier M, Miossec P: Early occupational therapy programme increases hand grip strength at 3 months: results from a randomised, blind, controlled study in early rheumatoid arthritis, *Ann Rheum Dis* 68(3):400–403, 2009. https://doi. org/10.1136/ard.2008.094532. http://www.ncbi.nlm.nih.gov/pub med/19015209.

120. Lamb SE, Williamson EM, Heine PJ, Adams J, Dosanjh S, Dritsaki M, et al.: Exercises to improve function of the rheumatoid hand (SARAH): a randomised controlled trial, *Lancet* 385(9966):421–429, 2015. https:// doi.org/10.1016/S0140-6736(14)60998-3. https://www.clinicalkey.es/p laycontent/1-s2.0-S0140673614609983.

121. O'Sullivan MB, Singh H, Wolf JM: Tendon transfers in the rheumatoid hand for reconstruction, *Hand Clinics* 32(3):407–416, 2016. https://doi. org/10.1016/j.hcl.2016.03.014. https://www.clinicalkey.es/playcontent/ 1-s2.0-S0749071216300269.

122. Moore JR, Weiland AJ, Valdata L: Tendon ruptures in the rheumatoid hand: Analysis of treatment and functional results in 60 patients, *J Hand Surg* 12(1):9–14, 1987. https://doi.org/10.1016/S0363-5023(87)80151-X. https://www.sciencedirect.com/science/article/pii/S036350238780151X.

123. Adams J, Burridge J, Mullee M, Hammond A, Cooper C: Correlation between upper limb functional ability and structural hand impairment in an early rheumatoid population, *Clin Rehabil* 18(4):405–413, 2004. https://doi.org/10.1191/0269215504cr732oa. http://journals.sagepub.c om/doi/full/10.1191/0269215504cr732oa.

124. Coldham F, Lewis J, Lee H: The reliability of one vs. three grip trials in symptomatic and asymptomatic subjects, *J Hand Ther* 19(3):318–327, 2006. https://doi.org/10.1197/j.jht.2006.04.002. https://www.sciencedi rect.com/science/article/pii/S0894113006000949.

125. Kennedy D: The reliability of one versus three trials of pain-free grip strength in subjects with rheumatoid arthritis, *J Hand Ther* 22(4):387–388, 2009. https://doi.org/10.1016/j.jht.2009.07.015. https://www.clin icalkey.es/playcontent/1-s2.0-S0894113009000908.

126. Mathiowetz V, Vizenor L, Melander D: Comparison of baseline instruments to the Jamar dynamometer and the B&L engineering pinch gauge, *OTJR: Occupation, Participation and Health* 20(3):147–162, 2000. https://doi.org/10.1177/153944920002000301. http://journals.s agepub.com/doi/full/10.1177/153944920002000301.

127. Devore GL: Preoperative assessment and postoperative therapy and splinting in rheumatoid arthritis. In Hunter JM, Schneider LH, Mackin EJ, et al.: *Rehabilitation of the hand: surgery and therapy*, ed 3, Philadelphia, 1990, Mosby, pp 942–952.

128. Rehim SA, Chung KC: Applying evidence in the care of patients with rheumatoid hand and wrist deformities, *Plast Reconstr Surg* 132(4): 885–897, 2013. https://doi.org/10.1097/PRS.0b013e31829fe5e1 [doi].

129. Knipping A, ter Schegget M: A study comparing use and effects of custom-made versus prefabricated splints for swan neck deformity in patients with rheumatoid arthritis, *Hand Ther* 5(4):101–107, 2000. https://doi.org/10.1177/175899830000500401. http://journals.sagepub .com/doi/full/10.1177/175899830000500401.

130. Spicka C, Macleod C, Adams J, Metcalf C: Effect of silver ring splints on hand dexterity and grip strength in patients with rheumatoid arthritis: an observational pilot study, *Hand Ther* 14(2):53–57, 2009. https:// doi.org/10.1258/ht.2009.009012. http://journals.sagepub.com/doi/full/ 10.1258/ht.2009.009012.

131. Flatt AE: *The care of the arthritic hand*, United States, 1995, Mosby, p 1. http://catalog.hathitrust.org/Record/003006265.

132. Steultjens EEMJ, Dekker JJ, Bouter LM, Schaardenburg DD, Kuyk MAMAH, Van den Ende ECHM: Occupational therapy for rheumatoid arthritis (review), *Cochrane Database Syst Rev* (1):CD003114, 2004. https://doi.org/10.1002/14651858.CD003114.pub2. http://

www.narcis.nl/publication/RecordID/oai:repository.ubn.ru.nl:2066%2F58846.

133. Callinan NJ, Mathiowetz V: Soft versus hard resting hand splints in rheumatoid arthritis: pain relief, preference, and compliance, *Am J Occup Ther* 50(5):347–353, 1996. https://doi.org/10.5014/ajot.50.5.347. https://www.ncbi.nlm.nih.gov/pubmed/8728664.

134. Biese J: Arthritis. In *Fundamentals of hand therapy: clinical reasoning and treatment guidelines for common diagnoses of the upper extremity*, ed 1, St. Louis, 2007, Elsevier Inc, pp 348–375.

135. Ivy CC, Dell RB: General principles of rehabilitation after surgical reconstruction of the rheumatoid hand, *Tech Hand Up Extrem Surg* 4(1):69–75, 2000. https://doi.org/10.1097/00130911-200003000-00010. https://www.ncbi.nlm.nih.gov/pubmed/16609414.

136. Colditz JC: Arthritis. In Malick MHKM, editor: *Manual on management of specific hand problems*, Pittsburgh, 1984, AREN, pp 112–136.

137. Egan M, Brosseau L, Farmer M, et al.: Splints and orthosis for treating rheumatoid arthritis, *Cochrane Database of Syst Rev* 4(4):112–136, 2001. https://doi.org/10.1002/14651858.CD004018.

138. Swanson AB: Pathomechanics of deformities in hand and wrist. In Hunter JM, Schneider LH, Mackin EJ, et al.: *Rehabilitation of the hand: surgery and therapy*, ed 3, Philedelphia, 1990, Mosby, pp 891–902.

139. Beasley J: Soft splints: indications and techniques. In ed 6, Skirven TM, Osterman AL, Fedorczyk JM, et al.: *Rehabilitation of the hand and upper extremity*, vol. 2. Philedelphia, 2011, Elsevier Inc, pp 1610–1619.

140. Terrono AL, Nalebuff EA, Philips CA: The rheumatoid thumb. In Skirven TM, Osterman AL, Fedorczyk JM, et al.: *Rehabilitation of the hand and upper extremity*, ed 6, Philedelphia, 2011, Elsevier Inc, pp 1344–1355.

141. Zanghi HA, Ndosi M, Adams J, et al.: EULAR recommendations for patient education for people with inflammatory arthritis, *Ann Rheum Dis* 74(6):954–962, 2015. https://doi.org/10.1136/annrheumdis-2014-206807. http://www.narcis.nl/publication/RecordID/oai:cris.maastrichtuniversity.nl:publications%2F57311db7-678f-4cbc-aabf-913463598fdf.

142. Siegel P, Tencza M, Apodaca B, Poole JL: Effectiveness of occupational therapy interventions for adults with rheumatoid arthritis: a systematic review, *Am J Occup Ther* 71(1):7101180050p1, 2017. https://doi.org/10.5014/ajot.2017.023176. https://www.ncbi.nlm.nih.gov/pubmed/28027042.

143. Cordery J, Rocchi M: Joint protection and fatigue management. In Melvin JJG, editor: *Rheumatologic rehabilitation: assessment and management*, vol. 1. Bethesda, MD, 1998, American Occupational Therapy Association, pp 279–322.

144. Cordery JC: Joint protection; a responsibility of the occupational therapist, *Am J Occup Ther* 19(5):285, 1965. https://www.ncbi.nlm.nih.gov/pubmed/5832168.

145. Hammond A, Freeman K: The long-term outcomes from a randomized controlled trial of an educational–behavioural joint protection programme for people with rheumatoid arthritis, *Clin Rehabil* 18(5):520–528, 2004. https://doi.org/10.1191/0269215504cr766oa. http://journals.sagepub.com/doi/full/10.1191/0269215504cr766oa.

146. Robinson V, Brosseau L, Casimiro L, et al.: Thermotherapy for treating rheumatoid arthritis, *Cochrane Database Syst Rev* (1):CD002826, 2002. https://www.ncbi.nlm.nih.gov/pubmed/11869637.

147. Casimiro L, Brosseau L, Robinson V, et al.: Therapeutic ultrasound for the treatment of rheumatoid arthritis, *Cochrane Database Syst Rev* (3):CD003787, 2002. https://www.ncbi.nlm.nih.gov/pubmed/12137714.

148. Brosseau L, Robinson V, Wells G, et al.: Low level laser therapy (classes I, II and III) for treating rheumatoid arthritis, *Cochrane Database Syst Rev* (4):CD002049, 2005. https://doi.org/10.1002/14651858.CD002049.pub2. https://www.ncbi.nlm.nih.gov/pubmed/16235295.

149. Vlieland Vliet, Theodora PM: New guidelines on nondrug treatment in RA, *Nature Re Rheum* 6(5):250, 2010, https://doi.org/10.1038/nrrheum.2010.59.

150. Hurkmans E, van der Giesen FJ, Vliet Vlieland TP, Schoones J, Van den Ende: ECHM: Dynamic exercise programs (aerobic capacity and/or muscle strength training) in patients with rheumatoid arthritis, *Cochrane Database Syst Rev* (4):CD006853, 2009. https://doi.org/10.1002/14651858.CD006853.pub2. https://www.ncbi.nlm.nih.gov/pubmed/19821388.

151. Minor MA, Hewett JE, Webel RR, Anderson SK, Kay DR: Efficacy of physical conditioning exercise in patients with rheumatoid arthritis and osteoarthritis, *Arthritis Rheum* 32(11):1396–1405, 1989. https://doi.org/10.1002/anr.1780321108. https://www.ncbi.nlm.nih.gov/pubmed/2818656.

152. O'Brien AV, Jones P, Mullis R, Mulherin D, Dziedzic K: Conservative hand therapy treatments in rheumatoid arthritis--a randomized controlled trial, *Rheum (Oxford, England)* 45(5):577–583, 2006. https://doi.org/10.1093/rheumatology/kei215. https://www.ncbi.nlm.nih.gov/pubmed/16319099.

153. Bergstra SA, Murgia A, Te Velde AF, Caljouw SR: A systematic review into the effectiveness of hand exercise therapy in the treatment of rheumatoid arthritis, *Clin Rheum* 33(11):1539–1548, 2014. https://doi.org/10.1007/s10067-014-2691-2 [doi].

154. Hammond A, Prior Y: The effectiveness of home hand exercise programmes in rheumatoid arthritis: a systematic review, *Br Med Bull* 119(1):49–62, 2016. https://doi.org/10.1093/bmb/ldw024 [doi].

155. Brand P, Hollister AM, Agee JM: Transmission. In Brand PWHA, editor: *Clinical mechanics of the hand*, vol. 3. St. Louis, 1999, Mosby, pp 61–99.

156. Melvin JL, Ferrel KM, editors: *Adult rheumatic diseases* (vol. 2). Bethesda, MD, 2000, The American Occupational Therapy Association.

30 Burns

Lisa Deshaies
Maura Ann Walsh

According to the American Burn Association, a burn of any depth to the hand is classified as a major injury that requires treatment at a specialized burn center. However, therapists may see clients with burns in a variety of clinical settings after acute management of the injuries. Burn injuries are caused by thermal, chemical, or electrical action. The causes are numerous and include house fires, motor vehicle accidents, and contact with an electrical current or hot objects or liquids at home or at work.[1,2]

> ◎ **Clinical Pearl**
>
> Dorsal hand burns are most often flame or explosion injuries; palmar burns occur more frequently from chemicals, friction, or high-voltage contact.[3]

Along with their effect on hand function, burns can have a significant impact on a person's social and psychological functioning as well as quality of life.[4,5,6] Scarring, perceived disfigurement, and loss of control over the body and the environment may lead to significant body image changes, social avoidance, anxiety about the future, and hopelessness.[7] Reduced income and reluctance to discuss emotions may also be contributing factors.[8] Other psychological symptoms that commonly develop after a burn injury are sleep disturbances, depression, anxiety disorders, feelings of guilt, shame, and blame, and posttraumatic stress.[7,9,10]

Related cognitive, emotional, and physiological problems (such as lack of concentration, apathy, pain, and low energy) can influence the client's recovery, making it difficult for the client to fully participate and follow through with treatment. Significant others are also affected and have concerns of their own.[11]

To plan the appropriate intervention, therapists who treat burn injuries must thoroughly understand the related anatomy and the wound healing and scar maturation processes. Emotional support for the client as well as significant others is crucial to a positive outcome.

Anatomy

The skin is the largest organ of the human body. Its essential functions include providing protection against bacterial invasion, preventing excessive loss of body fluids, regulating body temperature through perspiration, shielding deep structures from injury, absorbing certain substances (for example, vitamin D), and receiving sensory feedback from the environment.[12-14] Without the protection skin affords, exposed underlying tissues (for example, muscle and tendon) become desiccated, and nerve endings are exposed. An important nonphysiological function of the skin is to provide a cosmetic covering of the body that is unique to each individual.

Normal skin is composed of two basic layers, the epidermis and the dermis. The **epidermis** is the thin, avascular, outermost layer, which accounts for only about 5% of the skin's thickness. The **dermis,** which is much thicker, contains blood vessels, nerves, hair follicles, sweat and sebaceous glands, and the epithelial bed from which the skin regenerates. The thickness of the skin varies according to its location.

> ◎ **Clinical Pearl**
>
> On the hand, the dorsal skin is much thinner than the palmar skin.

> ◎ **Clinical Pearl**
>
> For the hand to function fully, the dorsal skin must be nonadherent and elastic, allowing hand closure, and the palmar skin must be thick enough to withstand forces arising from daily use.[3,15]

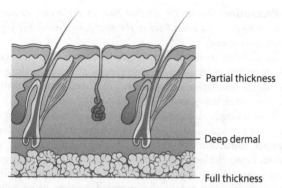

FIG. 30.1 Classification of burns by thickness. (From Leveridge JE. Burns. In: Prosser R, Conolly WB, eds. *Rehabilitation of the Hand and Upper Limb*. Edinburgh, UK: Butterworth Heinemann; 2003.)

The structure and function of the skin also vary. Dorsal hand skin contains hair follicles and sebaceous glands, whereas palmar skin does not. Palmar skin contains a greater number of sensory end organs.

The delicate balance of the intrinsic and extrinsic musculotendinous systems also can be affected by a burn injury.[3]

Diagnosis and Pathology

The temperature and duration of exposure to heat and the characteristics of the skin burned determine the amount of tissue destruction. Burn injuries are classified by both depth and extent. The larger and deeper the burn, the worse the prognosis.[12,16,17] Other factors include premorbid diseases and associated trauma.[16] Burn depth is assessed by visual examination to determine the extent of damage to or the destruction of anatomical structures. Depth can be described by degree (that is, first, second, third, or fourth) or by thickness (superficial partial thickness, deep partial thickness, full thickness, and full thickness burn with subdermal injury); thickness is the more descriptive and contemporary method (Fig. 30.1). Because skin thickness varies, a burn to the hand may involve tissues at different depths.

A **superficial partial-thickness burn** (which corresponds to first- and second-degree burns) involves the epidermis and possibly portions of the upper dermis. This type of burn is red or bright pink, blistered, soft, and wet. Sensation is intact, and the exposure of nerve endings results in pain and sensitivity to temperature, air, and light touch. Because the epithelial bed is intact, this type of burn can reepithelialize spontaneously in 2 weeks or earlier, therefore skin grafting is not necessary.

A **deep partial-thickness burn** (which corresponds to a deep second-degree burn) involves the epidermis and a deeper portion of the dermis. Hair follicles, sebaceous glands, and epithelial elements remain intact. This type of burn is mottled red or waxy white, soft, wet, and elastic. Sensation may or may not be present, depending on the extent to which nerve endings have been exposed or damaged. Reepithelialization can occur in approximately 3 to 6 weeks, but skin grafting may be done to expedite wound closure.

Precaution. *A deep partial-thickness burn may convert to a full-thickness burn.*

A **full-thickness burn** (which corresponds to a third-degree burn) involves the epidermis and the entire dermis, including hair follicles, nerve endings, and the epithelial bed. Sebaceous glands may be involved if the burn extends to the subcutaneous fat layer. Sensation is absent because nerve endings have been destroyed. This type of burn is white or tan, waxy, dry or leathery, and rigid. Spontaneous reepithelialization is impossible, and skin grafting is required.

A **full-thickness burn with subdermal injury** (which corresponds to a fourth-degree burn) involves deep tissue damage to fat, muscle, or possibly bone. Electrical burns often cause this type of injury. These burns require extensive debridement of necrotic tissue, followed by skin grafting. Amputation may be necessary if the damage is too extensive and severe.[13,17]

The extent of a burn is determined by estimating the percentage of the body surface burned. The two methods used for this are the rule of nines and the Lund-Browder chart. The extent of injury is described as the percentage of the **total body surface area (TBSA)** burned. A rough estimation is that the palm of the client's hand represents approximately 1% of the client's body surface. Each side of the hand is considered 1.5% of the body surface; therefore a person with circumferential burns to both hands would have a 6% TBSA burn.[17]

Timelines and Healing

The objective with any wound, including a burn, is to obtain quick healing to minimize scar formation and associated sequelae. The length of time required for wound closure is the most important determinant of scar development. Age, genetics, and burn depth and location are other variables.[18]

Wound healing is a dynamic cellular process that consists of three overlapping phases. Phase 1, the inflammatory (or exudative) phase, is characterized by inflammation and the presence of neutrophils and macrophages, which are responsible for clearing debris and preparing the wound for repair. This phase begins when the wound occurs and lasts 3 to 5 days. Phase 2, the fibroblastic (or proliferative or reparative) phase, lasts 2 to 6 weeks. It is characterized by the presence of fibroblasts, which lay down collagen and myofibroblasts, which cause **wound contraction.** The newly formed epithelium is very thin and fragile, and the tensile strength of the wound increases with collagen proliferation. Collagen is deposited in a random, disorganized fashion. Wound contraction continues even after epithelialization but to a lesser degree. Phase 3, the maturation (or remodeling) phase, may last for years. Collagen continues to cross-link, and tensile strength increases progressively.[19,20] Typically, 50% of normal tensile strength has been regained by 6 weeks, and the ultimate tensile strength is only about 80% of that of normal skin.[19,21] As scars mature, collagen deposition slows, and the breakdown of excessive collagen proceeds until scar maturity is reached.

Hypertrophic scars may develop after burns, with a reported prevalence rate of 32% to 72%.[9] Risk factors include dark skin, burns to the upper limb, burn severity, time to heal (longer than 3 weeks), and multiple surgical procedures. Hypertrophic scars are raised, thick, red, tight, and itchy. They also contract, often with deforming force. Scars that cross joints are the most problematic because **scar contraction** can lead to loss of functional joint mobility, with a reported prevalence of 38% to 54% in clients admitted to a burn center.[22] Scar hypertrophy and contraction are most active for the first 4 to 6 months.[23] Clients with full range of motion (ROM) early on may lose motion in the ensuing months; therefore long-term follow-up therapy is needed. Scars that soften over the first 6 to 12 months have an improved prognosis for full joint function.[17] As long as scars are active, they may be responsive to intervention with conservative therapy. Once scars have matured, surgical intervention is required to improve ROM or cosmetic appearance.

Phases of Burn Recovery

Four overlapping phases of recovery have been described for burn injuries: (1) emergent, (2) acute, (3) skin grafting, and (4) rehabilitation.[23] The emergent phase comprises the first 2 to 3 days after injury. The acute phase is considered to be the interval from day 2 or 3 to wound closure, which can occur by spontaneous healing or surgical intervention. The skin grafting phase is the period during which grafting is performed to cover wounds in the acute phase or as a component of reconstructive surgery in the rehabilitation phase. The rehabilitation phase lasts from wound closure to scar maturity.

◎ Clinical Pearl

Edema and poor positioning are the primary deforming forces in the emergent and acute phases. After the wound has been closed in the skin grafting and rehabilitation phases, scar contraction becomes the major deforming force.

Nonoperative Treatment

The course of treatment is influenced by the depth and extent of the burn injury, the client's medical status, the stage of wound healing, and the physician's plan of care. Nonsurgical management is an option for partial-thickness burns because they are able to regenerate epithelium.[3,13,23] Treatment is aimed at preventing infection, promoting healing, and minimizing complications.

Dressings

Dressings are used to protect the wound and provide an optimum environment for healing. Dressings may be the adherent or nonadherent type, and they can serve a number of purposes, including infection control, comfort, wound immobilization, fluid absorption, debridement, and early pressure.[16,19] Numerous dressing products and wound care/dressing change schedules are available. The selection of dressings and topical agents depends on the type and status of the wound; it also is often influenced by the physician's preference. Therapists must work closely with the physician so that they fully understand the dressing program and the rationale for it.

Positioning

Positioning is important in the early phases of burn recovery to minimize edema because edema can cause ischemia, intrinsic muscle tightness, deforming positions, loss of motion, adhesions, and fibrosis.[23] Edema is a natural component of the wound healing process, and burns create local and systemic responses.[24] Postburn edema develops rapidly within the first hour, peaks up to 36 hours after injury, and usually resolves within 7 to 10 days.[23] Edema still present in later stages is a matter of great concern.

Precaution. *To ensure arterial flow to the hand, elevate the hand no higher than heart level in the emergent phase while keeping the elbow extended.*[23]

In addition to elevation, use pressure techniques (for example, compression wraps, sleeves, or gloves) as needed, taking care to monitor circulation and skin integrity because fragile wounds and scars break down easily.

Positioning is also used to prevent loss of motion from soft-tissue shortening. The position of comfort typically is that of shoulder adduction and internal rotation, elbow flexion, wrist flexion, finger flexion, and thumb adduction. Loss of motion can occur in joints not even involved in the burn injury. Facilitate proper positioning out of the expected pattern using pillows, bulky dressings, foam wedges, or orthoses.

◎ Clinical Pearl

Remember a burn treatment adage: the position of comfort is the position of deformity.

Orthoses

Orthoses can be used to facilitate wound healing by immobilizing the wound and protecting key structures in the hand. It is important to note that not all hand burns require orthotic intervention. The decision to use or not to use an orthosis depends on the depth and extent of the burn and the client's ability to tolerate positioning, exercise, and function. Most superficial partial-thickness burns do not require an orthosis because healing is completed within 3 weeks. An orthosis should be considered if healing is compromised, tendons are exposed, or there is a significant limitation in active extension or flexion of hand joints.[23] In some cases an orthosis may be indicated for a client who is unable to actively move the hand or for a client who may move too aggressively. Orthoses are used more often with deeper burns. Despite static orthotic intervention in the early phases of wound healing to prevent burn scar contracture, the incidence of contracture has been reported as 5% to 40%, with weak evidence supporting their effectiveness.[25]

◎ Clinical Pearl

In the emergent and early acute phases, edema can lead to poor positioning and the classic burn deformity of wrist flexion, metacarpophalangeal hyperextension, interphalangeal flexion, thumb adduction, and a flattened palmar arch.

Unless otherwise indicated, immobilize the hand with the wrist in extension, the metacarpophalangeal (MP) joints in flexion, the interphalangeal (IP) joints in extension, and the thumb in abduction. Slight wrist extension encourages MP flexion by means of a tenodesic effect, and MP flexion in turn puts tension on the collateral ligaments to prevent shortening. Proximal interphalangeal (PIP) joint extension protects the vulnerable extensor mechanism, and thumb abduction maintains the first web space. Considerable variation in ideal joint angles can be found in the literature.[26] A consensus calls for wrist extension of 15 to 30 degrees, MP flexion of 50 to 80 degrees, full IP extension or slight flexion, thumb abduction midway between radial and palmar abduction, MP flexion of 10 degrees, and full thumb IP extension (Fig. 30.2).[13,18,23] For isolated burns to the palmar surface, position the wrist in neutral to slight extension, the fingers in full extension and abduction,

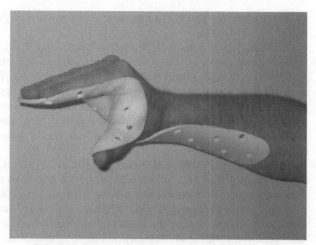

FIG. 30.2 Positioning orthosis for an acute hand burn.

and the thumb in radial abduction and extension.[23] *Never force joints into the ideal position.* Although prefabricated orthoses are available, custom orthoses made from perforated material are preferable because they allow a more precise fit and can be adjusted to accommodate changes in edema and joint mobility. Orthoses can be secured by gauze wraps, elastic bandages, or straps.

Precaution. *Carefully monitor and adjust how the orthosis is secured to ensure there is no vascular compromise.*[23]

For clients with significant involvement of the IP joints, the surgeon may opt to place Kirschner wires across the joints to obtain complete immobilization and protection of the extensor mechanism.[3]

Orthoses may also be used in the later phases of recovery to prevent or correct **scar contracture.** To prevent contracture, use static orthoses, placing joints in positions opposite the direction the scar will pull. Common burn scar contractures in the hand are wrist flexion from volar burns, wrist extension or flexion from dorsal burns, thumb adduction from a burn to the first web space, MP and IP extension from dorsal hand burns, and MP and IP flexion from volar hand burns. Have the client wear the static orthosis at night only, if possible, to avoid compromising functional hand use during the day. Use serial static orthoses, dynamic orthoses (also known as "elastic mobilization"), or static progressive orthoses (also known as "inelastic mobilization") to regain ROM with joint and/or scar contracture. Place scars under tension in an elongated position to promote new cell growth, collagen remodeling, and tissue lengthening.[14,27]

Circumferential burns may require alternating use of different orthoses to address all scars.[18]

Exercise

Exercise is important in the early phases of burn recovery to control edema, promote tendon gliding, and help maintain ROM and strength. Have the client perform active motion with the dressings removed while you carefully monitor the status of the wound. Muscle pumping exercises with a low number of repetitions can help with edema. Include lumbrical position exercises and abduction/adduction of the fingers to contract intrinsic muscles. If the client is unable to move effectively through full ROM, perform *gentle* active assistive or passive motion. It is important to stay within wound and pain tolerance; take care to put your hands on the most stable and least painful areas of the wound.

Precaution. *Aggressive motion at this stage is harmful to fragile tissue and results in more scarring.*[23] *To prevent tendon rupture, do not perform IP motion if extensor tendon involvement is known or suspected.*

In the later phases of recovery, emphasize exercises to achieve full active and passive wrist and hand motion. Include gentle passive exercises for individual joint tightness. Composite wrist and finger flexion or extension exercises may also be needed for scars that cross several joints (commonly seen with dorsal hand burns). Look for the scar to blanch, which indicates it is being effectively stressed.[23] Resistive exercises can help with regaining strength and muscle endurance. Stronger muscles are better able to move against tightening scars. Have the client perform resistive exercises in both directions to address scar and tendon adhesions. Use exercises and therapeutic activity to promote strength, dexterity, coordination, and hand function.

Joint mobilization for stiff joints can begin during the scar maturation phase once the scar has adequate tensile strength to tolerate the friction caused by mobilization techniques.

Continuous passive motion (CPM) has been reported to be an effective adjunct to therapy in the treatment of hand burns for clients who show little active motion because of pain, anxiety, or edema.[28]

Precaution. *Be very careful using CPM if extensor tendon injury is involved or suspected, as this technique might be too forceful for the delicate extensor mechanism.*

Functional Hand Use

Functional hand use in daily activities should be encouraged as much as possible throughout all phases of recovery. Assistive devices, such as built-up handles, can facilitate functional use if limitations exist. Using the hand has important physical and psychological benefits; it facilitates motion, strength, endurance, tendon glide, and edema reduction, and it gives the client a sense of self-control and sufficiency. However, keep in mind that improvement in pain, healing, motion, and strength does not always lead to spontaneous reintegration of the hand into tasks. Clients may be fearful of pain or of injuring fragile tissues. Acknowledge these concerns and provide support to help the client overcome them.

Scar Management

The goal of scar management is to modulate scars as much as possible to achieve a flat, smooth, supple, and cosmetically acceptable scar. Because scar formation is an unavoidable component of wound healing, the best we can hope to accomplish is to minimize scarring by altering its physical and mechanical properties through interventions, such as compression, silicone products, massage, and physical agent modalities. The exact mechanisms by which these interventions work are not well understood, and objective support of their efficacy is less than adequate, but they have produced positive clinical effects.[29-31]

Compression can be provided through a variety of means, including orthoses, compression wraps, and pressure garments. The processes of hypertrophic scarring and scar contraction begin shortly after injury; therefore early application of pressure is advised (that is, within 2 weeks of wound closure).[18,23,32] As a rule of thumb, use interim compression bandages and gloves until the hand is ready to be measured for a custom-fitted

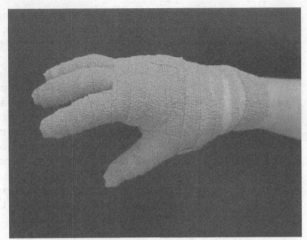

FIG. 30.3 Self-adherent compression wrap.

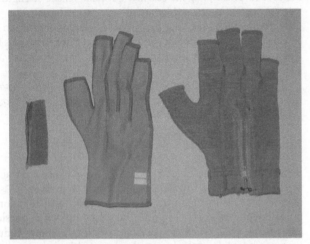

FIG. 30.4 Prefabricated digital sleeve, prefabricated glove, and custom pressure glove.

pressure garment. Pressure from self-adherent elastic wraps is effective in both edema and scar management, and these wraps can be used over light dressings as needed (Fig. 30.3).[18,32] Grade the amount of pressure to make sure it is tolerable. Prefabricated digital sleeves and gloves are an option once the scar is able to tolerate the shear forces created by putting them on, taking them off, and motion while wearing them. Measure for a custom glove only after edema has plateaued, wounds are smaller than a quarter, and the scar is ready to tolerate the heavier pressure and friction custom gloves impose (Fig. 30.4).[23] To be most effective, compression devices should be worn continually except during skin hygiene routines and exercise. It may take time for clients to tolerate full-time wear.

Silicone products are available in many forms, including sheets and putty. Some silicone gel sheets are self-adherent, whereas others must be held in place. Silicone can be used alone, but is often combined with pressure, although the effectiveness of using both together has been mixed.[33,34] Some manufacturers make pressure garments with a thin silicone lining, but these may be more difficult for a client to put on and remove because of increased friction from the silicone. The recommended wearing time for silicone is a minimum of 12 to 24 hours a day; close monitoring is required, since its occlusive nature may cause maceration.[18,23]

Precaution. *Do not apply silicone over open wounds or fragile skin.*

Massage, delivered manually or with a vibrator, may be helpful for freeing restrictive fibers, reducing itching, and relieving pain.[35,36] Begin with gentle massage of newly healed skin to avoid blister formation and skin breakdown. As tensile strength improves, progress to greater pressure causing scar blanching and massage with circular motions to work the scar in all directions. Lubricate the scar before massage to precondition the tissue. Massage should be performed at least twice a day.[18,23]

Physical agent modalities (for example, hot packs, paraffin, fluidotherapy, and ultrasound) have been used for burn scars to precondition tissues for exercise and activity.[18,23] Heat can reduce pain and improve elasticity of collagen fibers, making the scar easier to mobilize. Paraffin combines the benefits of heat and skin lubrication, both of which are useful before motion. Fluidotherapy can also help with desensitization of hypersensitive scars. Dense burn scars are best heated by ultrasound.

Precaution. *Care must be taken with heat modalities because scars may have diminished sensation and heat tolerance. Never use heat on open wounds or broken skin.*

Operative Treatment

Full-thickness burns require surgical intervention because reepithelialization is not possible. Deep partial-thickness burns that would require prolonged spontaneous healing (generally longer than 2 to 3 weeks) may be treated surgically to improve functional and cosmetic results.[3,17]

Early excision of nonviable burned skin (known as "escharotomy" or "fasciotomy") may be needed to establish a healthy wound bed and to maintain blood perfusion.[2,3,18] The wound then can be covered with tissue transfers, cultured epithelial skin, or skin substitutes. A **heterograft (xenograft)** is skin taken from another species, such as a pig. A **homograft (allograft)** is human skin, most often taken from a cadaver. Heterografts and homografts are used as a temporary wound covering until the client's own skin can be used. An **autograft** is the client's own skin, taken as a graft harvested from a **donor site** and placed on the recipient wound site.[15,37] It may be a **split-thickness skin graft (STSG)** or a **full-thickness skin graft (FTSG).** The thicker the graft, the more dermal appendages it will contain. Thinner STSGs typically are used to cover the dorsal hand. Thicker STSGs or FTSGs commonly are used for the palmar surface because they provide better sensibility and durability.[15] STSGs may be applied as is (known as a "sheet graft"), perforated to allow drainage of fluid (known as a "meshed graft"), or meshed and expanded to cover more surface area. A **flap**, which includes fascial and/or muscle layers, may be needed for deep wounds with exposed tendon or bone.[37,38] Grafts and flaps require time to heal and leave scars at both the recipient and donor sites.

Clinical Pearl

Scar contraction of grafts occurs; the thinner the graft, the more it will shrink.[37]

Grafts that are meshed and expanded tend to produce more scarring and contraction than sheet or unexpanded mesh grafts.[15,17] Cultured epithelial grafts are composed of sheets of epidermal cells grown in a laboratory. These very thin, fragile grafts are used for clients who do not have adequate donor sites; they afford poor coverage for hands.[15,23]

Postoperative therapy for burn wounds treated surgically is crucial for maximizing functional outcomes. Postoperative protocols vary according to the surgical procedure and the surgeon's preference. STSGs and FTSGs typically are immobilized for several days after surgery to allow establishment of vascularity and graft adherence. Cultured skin grafts are progressed more slowly than standard STSGs because of their fragile nature. Flaps usually are immobilized for slightly longer than grafts because they do not take as readily. Grafts and flaps are like any other healing wound in that time is required for collagen deposition and improvement of tensile strength. Initiate and cautiously progress positioning, orthotic intervention, exercise, and scar management as soon as graft or flap stability allows.

Precaution. *Healing tissues are very susceptible to injury in the first 3 weeks, especially from shearing forces.[3,15] Monitor carefully for signs of blistering or breakdown. Discuss with the surgeon whether therapy can proceed or should be discontinued temporarily.*

Surgery is an integral part of the rehabilitation phase for contracture release and reconstruction. Surgical intervention also may be used after the scar has reached maturity. In children, surgery may be needed periodically until growth is complete because of a discrepancy between the rapid rate of bony growth relative to the slower rate of scar tissue growth. Scar contracture release involves introducing more skin in areas where tight scarring has caused ROM limitations. Tissue transfers as described previously are common, as are local rotational and advancement flaps (for example, Z-plasties).[15,17,37] Postoperative treatment follows guidelines and timelines similar to those for wound coverage.

? Questions to Ask the Doctor

Nonoperative Clients

- What are the wound care and dressing guidelines?
- Will an orthosis be needed?
- Are there any known or suspected problems with tendon or joint integrity?
- Are any precautions necessary with regard to elevation, motion, or compression?

Operative Clients

- What surgery was performed? (Obtain a copy of the operative report if possible.)
- What type of graft or flap was used?
- What was the intraoperative ROM?
- How well had the graft or flap taken when postoperative dressings were removed?
- What are the wound care and dressing guidelines?
- Are there any problems with tendon or joint integrity?
- Will an orthosis be needed?
- Are any precautions required with regard to elevation, motion, or compression?
- What postoperative protocol would you like followed?

(·) What to Say to Clients

About the Injury

"A burn causes serious injury to the skin. Skin is important for preventing infection and for protecting deeper structures in our hands.

Here is a diagram showing the layers of the skin and key anatomical features, such as hair follicles, sweat glands, oil glands, and nerve endings. The burn you sustained injured your skin to this depth, and this is how your skin will be affected."

Customize your information according to the client's level of injury and the symptoms related to pain and sensation.

About Wound Care and Healing

"The primary concern is to help you heal as quickly as possible to prevent infection and to minimize scarring. This is the wound care and dressing program that has been designed for you. It is important that you understand it, feel comfortable with it, and follow it closely."

Clients may have less pain and anxiety if they perform or assist with their wound care. Educate and practice with the client and significant others as often as needed to increase their comfort level. If a tissue transfer will be or was used, explain the purpose of it and what the client can expect at the recipient and donor sites.

About Scar Management

"Wounds heal with a process of scar formation. It may take several months or years for your active scars to complete the process of becoming mature. Active scars are red and may become thick, raised, and firm. Active scars also tend to become tight and may get very itchy, especially in the first 2 or 3 months. As the scars mature, you'll see the redness fade to your more normal skin color, and the scars will be flatter, softer, and less itchy. Scars are more sensitive to sunlight; therefore you should use sunscreen or gloves to protect them. You should wash your hands with mild soap; don't use anything with a strong detergent, which can dry your skin. Dry scars crack or injure more easily, and they may itch more. Over time your scars will become more durable, but they will never be quite as resilient as your normal skin. Because the feeling in your scars may not be normal, you'll have to rely more closely on visually inspecting them for signs of injury. Scars also don't have the natural ability to stay moist; therefore you will need to lubricate your skin frequently throughout the day to keep it healthy. Avoid moisturizers with a high perfume or alcohol content, which can cause dryness. Although we can't prevent scarring, we can try to keep your scars as flat, soft, and mobile as possible using interventions such as massage, pressure, and silicone."

Educate the client and significant others so that they understand the scar management program, how to monitor for skin problems, and how to care for pressure and silicone devices properly.

About Orthoses

"Orthoses are used to help keep your active scars from becoming tight and causing loss of joint motion. They can also be used to regain motion you may have lost since your burn injury. It is important to follow the wearing schedule we set and to watch out for any problems with your skin that orthoses may cause."

Make sure that the client and significant others understand the purpose of each orthosis, the wearing schedule, and how to care for the orthosis.

About Exercise

"Exercise is important to keep your joints and scars mobile. The exercises designed for you include some for stretching your scars, some to help your tendons glide, and some to make your hand stronger. Always make sure to moisturize your scars well before you start your exercises so that they don't crack."

Educate the client and significant others about the purpose of each exercise and when and how each should be performed.

About Function

"One of the best ways to keep your hand moving is to use it as much as possible during all your normal daily activities. Although it may be a little awkward at first, using your hand will help your scars stay supple, your joints remain loose, and your muscles become strong. You may have to be a little more careful to protect your scars by monitoring for signs of pressure, blistering, or injury."

If assistive devices are used, explain, "These devices will help you use your hand better right now until it becomes easier for you to hold things or to do more with your hand."

Evaluation Tips

- Be careful and gentle when placing your hands or tools (for example, a goniometer) over healing wounds, fragile scars, and insensate or hypersensitive areas.
- Contractures may be caused by scar tightness, joint tightness, or both. Differentiate between a scar contracture and a joint contracture by watching for blanching and by palpating for tension of the scar.
- Scars that cross several joints need to be assessed closely. Assess individual joint active range of motion (AROM) and passive range of motion (PROM) with the scar in a relaxed position to measure the true joint motion. Tension on the scar may limit motion and make it appear that joint mobility is affected. For example, in a client with dorsal hand burns, place the wrist and MP in full extension while measuring PIP flexion. Once you have determined individual joint mobility, assess composite active and passive motion to determine if and how the scar is limiting motion.
- Use photographic images to help track wound healing and scar appearance. Quantify open wounds by measuring their size in centimeters and by describing their features (for example, color, integrity, drainage, and odor).[19] Quantify scars using scar assessment tools, such the Vancouver Burn Scar Scale, which rates pigmentation, vascularity, pliability, and height.[39,40] Assessing the client's subjective rating of the scars through visual analog scales is also beneficial, as the client's perception may not match yours. Despite the objective improvement you see, the client may not share your opinion that the scars are better.[41] Remember also to evaluate donor sites.
- Use hand tracings to evaluate and track changes in web spaces. You can obtain the most accurate representation by using a thin ballpoint refill without the pen body.
- Do not use volumetric measurement if open wounds are present without first obtaining the physician's permission. Always disinfect the volumeter after use.
- Watch for signs and patterns of peripheral nerve involvement. Nerve damage can be caused by direct injury, infection, or neurotoxicities. Localized compression caused by tight scars, poor positioning, or edema is also common.[23]
- Discuss how the burn is affecting the client's overall ability to function. Ascertain which activities are most important for the client to resume, and determine the factors that are most interfering with the client's ability to function.

> ## Clinical Pearl
> If the joint reaches maximum end-range and the scar blanches, scar tightness is contributing to the limitation. If the scar does not blanch at end-range, the limitation is caused by joint or other soft-tissue tightness.

Diagnosis-Specific Information That Affects Clinical Reasoning

Each client has unique clinical, functional, psychological, social, and cultural needs. Individualize treatment based on your evaluation results and an understanding and appreciation of each person. Empower the client and significant others to be involved throughout therapy through education and an open approach that fosters active participation. Provide the client with a sense of control by presenting choices whenever possible. Because the scar maturation process may take several years, make sure you give clients all the tools they need to manage their own care. Tailor information and teach clients how to perform interventions for themselves at every possible opportunity rather than doing the treatment for them; this facilitates better long-term outcomes.[42] Treatment needs also are dictated by the depth and location of the burn, the timing of injury and surgical procedures, the stage of wound healing, and the phase of burn recovery. Anticipate potential scar contractures and direct treatment at preventing or correcting them. The principles of hand burn treatment can be applied to burns on any area of the body.

Precaution. *Work closely with the physician on the plan of care and report any new problems promptly.*

Dorsal burns to the hand commonly result in a thumb web space contracture that limits functional positioning of the thumb and finger web space contractures that limit digital abduction and possibly MP flexion. Loss of MP, IP, and composite finger flexion is also typical. In some cases, the hand may have assumed an intrinsic minus position from poor early positioning, edema, or scar contraction (Fig. 30.5). A boutonnière deformity also may be present if the extensor mechanism was damaged. Palmar burns often cause limited thumb, finger, and composite extension.

Keep in mind that every scar is unique, and clients will have a variety of clinical problems; therefore perform a thorough

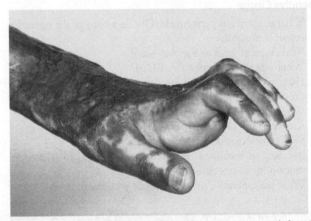

FIG. 30.5 Dorsal hand burn resulting in the intrinsic minus deformity position. (From Thornes N: Therapy for the burn patient. In: Prosser R, Conolly WB, eds. *Rehabilitation of the Hand and Upper Limb*. Edinburgh, UK: Butterworth Heinemann; 2003.)

evaluation to identify needs. The treatment of burn injuries is a dynamic process. Prioritize treatment based on the scars that are most active and the most functionally limiting. Reevaluate often and shift treatment in response to changing needs. Circumferential scars are especially challenging because they involve scars that pull in both directions, possibly limiting joint flexion and extension.

♡ Tips from the Field

Edema

If open wounds or fresh grafts are present, obtain the physician's permission before taking volumetric measurements. When elevating the hand, keep the elbow as straight as possible to aid flow. To provide more even pressure, use foam inserts placed in the palm, between the fingers, or on the dorsum of the hand under compressive wraps and prefabricated gloves.

Wound Care

When applying a dressing to the hand, make sure to wrap the digits individually and separately from the hand so as not to restrict motion unnecessarily and impede hand function (Fig. 30.6). If the thumb is involved in the dressing, pay attention to thumb positioning, and wrap it to facilitate functional palmar abduction. Wrap dressings over gauze pads in finger web spaces to provide early pressure. Keep the thickness of dressings consistent if an orthosis or interim garment is to be worn over them.

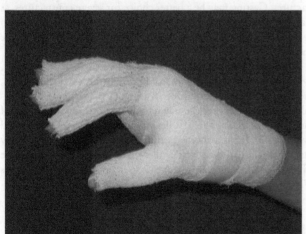

FIG. 30.6 Hand dressing that allows unimpeded motion.

Scar Management

Scar hypersensitivity is a common problem that often must be addressed before the client is able to tolerate other interventions, such as orthoses, pressure, or massage. Hypersensitive scars on the palmar surface can also significantly impede hand function. Use graded stimuli to lessen sensitivity, taking care to stay within the scar's pressure and shear force tolerances to avoid injury.

Use inserts under compression devices to augment pressure in difficult areas, such as the web spaces and the palmar arch. Inserts can be made from products such as thermoplastics, silicone or foam (Fig. 30.7).[18,23,32] Grade pressure to the tolerance of the scar. A graded sequence may be compressive wraps using self-adherent elastic materials, progressing to a prefabricated glove made from

soft material, progressing to a custom-fitted pressure glove. Order custom garments with the client's specific needs in mind. Zippers or Velcro closures make it easier for the client to put on and remove gloves with less trauma to fragile skin. Open tips allow for better finger sensation and hand function. Most manufacturers offer different grades of fabric from which the glove can be made. Select the material based on scar tolerance and functional demands. Very fragile scars may need a glove made of soft material; scars with good tolerance in a very active client may require a more durable material. Panels of soft material can be strategically placed in areas prone to discomfort or scar breakdown, such as bony prominences and the thumb web space (Fig. 30.8). Suede or other fabric patches and strips can be sewn onto the palmar surface to increase the glove's durability and prevent objects from slipping on slick fabric.[23]

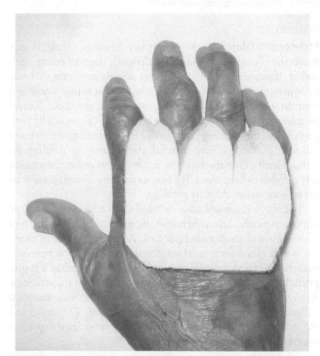

FIG. 30.7 Silicone gel sheet in the thumb web space and foam inserts in the finger web spaces to augment pressure under the glove.

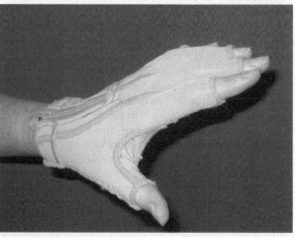

FIG. 30.8 Custom pressure glove with dorsal zipper, open tips, and a soft panel in the thumb web space.

Compression materials stretch as the client wears them throughout the day. Laundering the garments helps materials return to their original state. Provide the client with two sets of all garments so that each day a clean one can be put on that provides the appropriate amount of pressure. Custom garments generally last 2 to 4 months under normal wearing conditions. Some clients struggle to keep to the wearing schedule because these garments are tight, they can be uncomfortably hot to wear, and they may limit dexterity and functional sensation. To improve follow-through, provide clients with a choice of design and color, teach them the purpose of the garments, and frequently discuss their experience of wearing garments.[43]

Precaution. *Watch for allergic reactions, skin maceration or breakdown, and circulation or sensory impairments caused by compression garments, silicone, and inserts.*

Orthoses

Make sure to fabricate orthoses over any dressings, inserts, or garments the client will be wearing underneath them to ensure optimal fit. If you are molding an orthosis directly over scars that may be hypersensitive or heat sensitive, apply a thin cotton sleeve or a light dressing before placing warm material on the client. Relieve pressure over bony prominences or other areas of concern by temporarily placing padding over them before molding the orthosis; this will "bubble out" the material. Avoid lining or padding the orthosis itself unless absolutely necessary, as this makes the orthosis very difficult to keep clean. If lining or padding is used, place it on the orthotic material before molding.

Because wounds and scars are fragile, it is critical to smooth all edges completely. Select thermoplastic material based on the type of orthosis and its intended purpose. A material with full memory is well suited for a serial static orthosis that will be remolded numerous times. A material with excellent conformability is appropriate for an orthosis designed to apply pressure to uneven scars. A material with good rigidity is desirable for an orthosis that must withstand the force of a strongly contracting scar. The choice and placement of strapping also must be carefully considered to prevent the creation of pressure or shear forces.

To prevent unnecessary stiffness or disuse, design wearing schedules that leave the hand free for function and motion as much as possible.

Precaution. *With very active scars, just a few hours without an orthosis may result in significant loss of motion.*

As scars become more mature, wearing time can gradually be reduced, especially if the client's activity level or pressure devices are sufficient to control scar shortening.

Serial casts, serial static orthoses, dynamic orthoses, and static progressive orthoses all can be used to treat the wrist and hand. The type of orthosis used depends on the location of the scar, the direction of scar contraction, and the therapist's preference. Orthotic intervention to apply stress to burn scars often involves placing joints in positions not commonly used for other hand conditions, such as the wrist in flexion, the MP joints in extension, the thumb in radial abduction, or all joints in composite extension. Think creatively to design an orthosis that provides the most benefit. Leave uninvolved joints free whenever possible. Consider using a less restrictive orthosis during the day and a more restrictive orthosis at night. Orthoses may require frequent remolding or modification as edema diminishes, the shape of the scar changes, or scar tightness improves or worsens.

Thumb web space contractures respond well to serial static orthoses. An orthosis that conforms completely to the web space often is most effective. Position the thumb in the plane of abduction where you can achieve maximal stretch (as noted by scar blanching), and ensure stress is not placed on the MP ulnar collateral ligament. Strapping can be anchored around the wrist to apply pressure in the desired direction and to keep the orthosis firmly in place (Fig. 30.9).

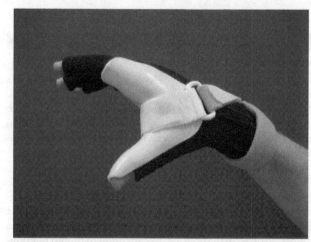

FIG. 30.9 Thumb abduction orthosis for scar contracture of the first web space.

Serial casts or gutter orthoses can be used for IP flexion contractures. Casting may be a better choice for severe contractures, as plaster conforms better than thermoplastics. Gutter orthoses can be secured with self-adherent compression wrap for a more secure and conforming fit.

MP extension contractures can be treated with serial static, dynamic, or static progressive MP flexion orthoses. In some cases, use of a simple wrist extension orthosis or a hand-based lumbrical bar orthosis during the day combined with functional use of the hand can encourage MP flexion. This can be complemented by use at night of a more restrictive orthosis designed to apply sustained stress to the scar. A full-contact palmar orthosis can be effective for flexion contractures caused by palmar hand burns (Fig. 30.10).

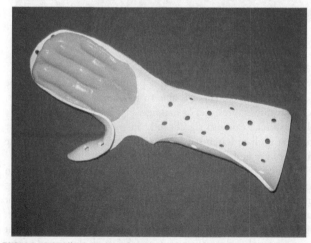

FIG. 30.10 Full-contact orthosis with silicone elastomer putty insert for palmar scar contracture.

Exercise

Include exercises for scar stretching, ROM, and tendon gliding as appropriate. Strengthening exercises are also useful because strong muscles are better able to pull against tight scars. Gripping and putty exercises are effective for encouraging composite flexion of the hand. Scars should be well lubricated before exercising. Exercises for nonburned areas may be needed to regain motion or strength lost through immobilization or disuse.

Promoting Function

Use assistive devices to help promote functional use through all phases of burn recovery. Build up handles on utensils or use universal cuffs to assist with grasp. Tight scars can limit dexterity and slow speed of performance. Improvement in skin integrity, pain, motion, and strength does not automatically equate with spontaneous return to functional hand use. Integrate therapeutic activities (for example, woodworking or leather crafts) and meaningful functional tasks into the therapy program to help clients see their functional potential and gain confidence in their hand use. Discuss self-care, home, community, leisure, or vocational demands with each client and address specific interfering factors. Reintegrating into social activities can be especially difficult for clients with scarring. Work with the client to figure out ways to return to activities as independently, safely, and comfortably as possible. Keep in mind that the ultimate goal is a return to the client's prior level of function.

Psychosocial Adjustment

Recovery from a burn injury goes beyond the healing of anatomical structures. Be aware of factors that may interfere with treatment and recovery, such as pain, anxiety, and depression. Take time to establish rapport and trust with your client. Provide encouragement, understanding, and emotional support throughout therapy. Facilitate client involvement and a sense of self-control during the therapeutic process to the fullest extent possible. Refer the client to other health care providers as appropriate to help address problems. Educate the client and significant others about resources for support. Many national and local organizations offer information, peer counseling, support groups, and recreational activities for burn survivors and their significant others. Find information through the American Burn Association and the Phoenix Society for Burn Survivors.

Reassessment

Reassess scar activity and ROM frequently because the scar's status can change quickly for the better or worse. Adjust the treatment program, goals, and priorities accordingly. Share the results with the client and significant others, to serve as positive reinforcement if improvements are noted or to motivate them to more closely follow therapy recommendations if no gains are seen or the scar's status has deteriorated. Collaborate closely to problem solve issues as soon as they arise.

Clinical Pearl

To be effective, compression must conform to the scar.

Precautions and Concerns

- *Facilitate wound healing and control edema to reduce the extent of scarring.*
- *Follow appropriate infection control procedures during wound care and dressing changes.*
- *When using orthoses on an edematous hand, never force joints into the ideal position. Instead, position the joints as close to the ideal as possible, and modify the orthosis gradually over time as edema diminishes.*
- *Be especially careful with PIP joints when extensor tendon injury is known or suspected; mobilize these joints only with permission from the physician.*
- *When orthoses and pressure devices are used, monitor closely for signs of skin breakdown.*
- *Be cautious with the use of thermal treatments over newly healed wounds or scars.*
- *Carefully assess the client's work environment. Clients with a large-percentage body burn have a decreased tolerance for hot temperatures. Chemicals also may pose an increased risk to scars.*

CASE STUDY

CASE STUDY 30.1

DL is a 24-year-old, right-hand dominant auto mechanic who sustained 4% TBSA circumferential burns to his right hand in a small explosion at work. The palmar wound was a mix of superficial and deep partial-thickness burns that crossed the wrist into the forearm; the dorsal injury involved deep partial-thickness burns. The client was admitted to a local burn unit, where he underwent early excision and grafting of the dorsal hand injury with STSGs from his right thigh. The palmar burn was treated with nonsurgical management. DL was referred to the outpatient hand clinic for therapy 3 weeks after surgery.

Treatment

DL arrived at the therapy clinic with his hand wrapped in a bulky dressing, even though he had no open wounds. He stated that it was "too painful" to leave his hand uncovered. He had mild edema, most notably on the dorsum of the hand. The following values were recorded for the right hand:

	AROM (degrees)	PROM (degrees)
Index finger MP	30/55	25/60
PIP	35/65	30/85
DIP	5/40	0/50
Middle finger MP	25/40	15/50
PIP	40/70	40/80
DIP	10/50	5/60
Ring finger MP	25-55	20–65
PIP	40/75	35/80
DIP	15/35	10/35
Small finger MP	10/30	10/40
PIP	55/70	35/75
DIP	20/55	10/60
Thumb MP	20/45	20/55
IP	0/5	0/15
Abduction	0–30	0–35

AROM, Active range of motion; *DIP,* distal interphalangeal; *IP,* interphalangeal; *MP,* metacarpophalangeal; *PIP,* proximal interphalangeal.

The scars were not hypertrophic but were very red, dry, and tight, as noted by blanching at end-ranges of motion. The hand did not appear to have been recently washed. Grip strength measured 15 lbs. All motor function was intact. Touch-pressure sensation was normal with monofilament testing, but hypersensitivity of the palmar surface was noted throughout the evaluation. DL lived with his girlfriend, who accompanied him to therapy. He was able to perform his basic activities of daily living using his left hand only.

The immediate treatment priorities were determined to be reducing hypersensitivity, resolving edema, and improving ROM for both hand opening and closing. Hypersensitivity and a fear of pain or damage to his skin were limiting DL's ability to care for his hand and to want to move it or use it. This issue initially was addressed by having him gently wash his hand and apply lotion to scars at the beginning of therapy sessions. DL was reluctant to do this for the first few sessions, and he needed a lot of encouragement to do a thorough job. After the third session, his hand consistently appeared clean upon his arrival for therapy. He also was able to tolerate having the therapist massage his scars after he performed massage for the first few minutes.

DL felt unable to leave his hand unbandaged, but he did agree to try a self-adherent compressive wrap to help manage edema and provide some light pressure to his scars. Foam inserts were placed in the palm and web spaces and on the dorsum of the hand. The wrap was applied with very light pressure at first, and DL was able to tolerate a little more pressure each time as hypersensitivity diminished and his trust of his therapist increased. Two weeks into therapy, the edema had almost resolved, and the hypersensitivity had improved enough that DL felt he could wear a soft, prefabricated pressure glove. This allowed him to move more freely and to remove the glove often for skin hygiene, massage, and progressive desensitization with textures. When the edema had resolved completely, DL began wearing a custom-fitted pressure glove.

Increasing ROM was addressed through a combination of orthoses, exercise, and functional use. DL lacked motion in both flexion and extension, and the therapist had to prioritize which joints and motions to focus on first. Gaining MP flexion and PIP extension were selected as priority concerns. Gutter orthoses were made for each finger and worn over the compression wrap. The aim was to serially gain IP extension ROM and transfer flexor forces to the MP joints to improve active MP flexion ROM. A volar wrist orthosis with the wrist in extension was also fabricated for use during the day to encourage MP flexion and prevent contraction of the volar forearm scar that crossed the wrist. Orthoses worn at night were geared toward improving composite extension ROM. A volar wrist-hand orthosis was fabricated with the wrist and fingers in maximum extension and the thumb in maximum abduction. Because each finger IP needed to be positioned at a different angle, the wrist-hand orthosis was fabricated over the existing gutter orthoses for a more precise fit. Once IP extension had improved, lacking only about 15 degrees to neutral, and active MP flexion also had improved (in

about 2 weeks), gutter orthoses were weaned off during the day to facilitate IP flexion and functional use of the hand. The daytime wrist orthosis was discontinued shortly thereafter.

Active and gentle passive exercises for all joints were initiated and had to be progressed slowly. As DL's hypersensitivity and edema improved, so did his ability to tolerate more vigorous exercises. Strengthening exercises were graded from squeezing a large, soft foam ball to putty. Later in the program, DL was able to perform weight well exercises with progressive resistance.

To help DL begin to integrate functional use of his hand at the beginning of therapy, soft, large-diameter tubing was used on his eating utensils and toothbrush. Because he was able to do tasks easily using his left hand, he was reluctant to consider trying with his right hand "until it got better." Once he understood the therapeutic value of active daily use for reducing the edema, hypersensitivity, and scar tightness, he was willing to integrate functional use as part of his home exercise program (HEP). When he saw that his hand looked and felt better after he began using it, he became eager to do more at home. DL shared with the therapist that he was a drummer who occasionally performed with a band made up of friends. The therapist was able to tap into this interest as a means to motivate DL by making drumming a focus of his HEP. He was asked to bring in a small drum and his drumsticks, and together DL and the therapist were able to devise modifications for his right drumstick. Soft padding was wrapped around the proximal end of the stick to a diameter large enough to allow him to hold it. As composite finger flexion improved, the diameter of the padding was reduced. Therapeutic activities were performed in the therapy clinic to improve fisting and strength. These included leather stamping and a woodworking project in which he fabricated a weight well for himself to use at home. The final activities involved tool use simulating work tasks. DL was concerned about being able to wear his pressure glove at work without getting it dirty. He brought in vinyl gloves that he typically wore on his hands at work and found that a larger size fit well over his pressure glove. He began doing some work on his car at home.

Result

Throughout the therapy program, DL was educated in all aspects of his injury and care. Building trust, fostering his sense of control over his care, providing him with choices, allowing him to see his progress by continually sharing reevaluation results, and tapping into motivating interests were keys to his successful rehabilitation. Upon discharge from therapy, DL had regained full AROM, and hypersensitivity had resolved. Grip strength was 75 lbs. He was wearing his pressure glove full time. He returned to using his right hand as dominant for all activities, which was enough to maintain full composite flexion without requiring orthoses. He continued to wear a night orthosis that positioned his wrist and hand in composite extension whenever he felt his volar scars were tightening. He felt confident about managing his scars long term and knew how to progress his hand-strengthening exercises at home. His physician cleared him to return to work shortly after therapy ended.

References

1. Wolf SE, Cancio LC, Pruitt BA: Epidemiological, demographic, and outcome characteristics of burns. In Herndon D, editor: *Total burn care*, ed 5, New York, 2018, Elsevier, pp 14–27.
2. Culnan DM, Capek KD, Huang T: Acute and reconstructive care of the burned hand. In Herndon D, editor: *Total burn care*, ed 5, New York, 2018, Elsevier, pp 589–608.
3. Germann G, Hrabowski M: Burned hand. In Wolf SW, Hotchkiss RN, Pederson WC, et al.: *Green's operative hand surgery*, ed 7, Philadelphia, 2017, Elsevier, pp 1926–1957.
4. Rosenberg L, Rosenberg M, Rimmer RB, et al.: Psychosocial recovery and reintegration of patients with burn injuries. In Herndon D, editor: *Total burn care*, ed 5, New York, 2018, Elsevier, pp 709–720.

5. McAleavy AA, Wyka K, Peskin M, et al.: Physical, functional, and psychological recovery from burn injury are related and their relationship changes over time: a burn model system study, *Burns* 44:793–799, 2018.

6. Knight A, Wasiak J, Salway J, et al.: Factors predicting health status and recovery of hand function after hand burns in the second year after hospital discharge, *Burns* 43:100–106, 2017.

7. Aili Low JF, Meyer WJ, Willebrand M, et al.: Psychiatric disorders associated with burn injury. In Herndon D, editor: *Total burn care*, ed 5, New York, 2018, Elsevier, pp 700–708.

8. Reeve J, Frances J, McNeill R, et al.: Functional and psychological outcomes following burn injury: reduced income and hidden emotions are predictors of greater distress, *J Burn Care Res* 32:468–474, 2011.

9. Lawrence JW, Mason ST, Schomer K, et al.: Epidemiology and impact of scarring after burn injury: a systematic review of the literature, *J Burn Care Res* 33:136–146, 2012.

10. Kornhaber R, Childs C, Cleary M: Experiences of guilt, shame and blame in those affected by burns: a qualitative systematic review, *Burns* 44:1026–1039, 2018.

11. Sundara DC: A review of issues and concerns of family members of adult burn survivors, *J Burn Care Res* 32:349–357, 2011.

12. Brownson EG, Gibran NS: Evaluation of the burn wound: management decisions. In Herndon D, editor: *Total burn care*, ed 5, New York, 2018, Elsevier, pp 87–92.

13. Malick MH, Carr JA: *Manual on management of the burn patient*, Pittsburgh, 1982, Harmarville Rehabilitation Center Educational Resource Division.

14. Richard RL, Staley MJ: Biophysical aspects of normal skin and burn scar. In Richard RL, Staley MJ, editors: *Burn care and rehabilitation: principles and practice*, Philadelphia, 1994, FA Davis, pp 49–69.

15. Pedersen WC: Nonmicrosurgical coverage of the upper extremity. In Wolf SW, Hotchkiss RN, Pederson WC, et al.: *Green's operative hand surgery*, ed 7, Philadelphia, 2017, Elsevier, pp 1528–1573.

16. Voigt CD, Celis M, Voigt DW: Care of outpatient burns. In Herndon D, editor: *Total burn care*, ed 5, New York, 2018, Elsevier, pp 50–57.

17. Simpson RL: Management of burns of the upper extremity. In Skirven TM, Osterman AL, Fedorczyk JM, et al.: *Rehabilitation of the hand and upper extremity*, ed 6, Philadelphia, 2011, Elsevier, pp 302–316.

18. Serghiou MA, Ott S, Cowan A, et al.: Burn rehabilitation along the continuum of care. In Herndon D, editor: *Total burn care*, ed 5, New York, 2018, Elsevier, pp 476–508.

19. von der Heyde RL, Evans RB: Wound classification and management. In Skirven TM, Osterman AL, Fedorczyk JM, et al.: *Rehabilitation of the hand and upper extremity*, ed 6, Philadelphia, 2011, Elsevier, pp 219–232.

20. Hawkins HK, Jay J, Finnerty CC: Pathophysiology of the burn scar. In Herndon D, editor: *Total burn care*, ed 5, New York, 2018, Elsevier, pp 466–475.

21. Peacock EE: *Wound repair*, ed 3, Philadelphia, 1984, WB Saunders.

22. Oosterwijk AM, Mouton LJ, Schouten H, et al.: Prevalence of scar contractures after burn: a systematic review, *Burns* 43:41–49, 2017.

23. Tufaro PA, Bondoc SL: Therapist's management of the burned hand. In Skirven TM, Osterman AL, Fedorczyk JM, et al.: *Rehabilitation of the hand and upper extremity*, ed 6, Philadelphia, 2011, Elsevier, pp 317–341.

24. Edgar DW, Fish J, Gomez M, et al.: Local and systemic treatments for acute edema after burn injury: a systematic review of the literature, *J Burn Care Res* 32:334–347, 2011.

25. Schouten HJ, Nieuwenhuis MK, van Zuiljen PPM: A review on static splinting therapy to prevent burn scar contracture: do clinical and experimental data warrant its clinical application? *Burns* 38:19–25, 2012.

26. Richard R, Staley M, Daugherty MB, et al.: The wide variety of designs for dorsal hand burn splints, *J Burn Care Rehabil* 15:275–280, 1994.

27. Brand PW, Hollister AM: *Clinical mechanics of the hand*, ed 3, St Louis, 1999, Mosby.

28. Covey MH, Dutcher K, Marvin JA, et al.: Efficacy of continuous passive motion devices with hand burns, *J Burn Care Rehabil* 9:397–400, 1988.

29. Ault A, Plaza P, Paratz J: Scar massage for hypertrophic burns scarring: a systematic review, *Burns* 44:24–38, 2018.

30. Nedelec B, Carter A, Forbes L, et al.: Practice guidelines for the application of nonsilicone or silicone gels and gel sheets after burn injury, *J Burn Care Rehabil* 36:345–374, 2015.

31. Ai J-W, Liu J-T, Pei S-D, et al.: The effectiveness of pressure therapy (15-25 mmHg) for hypertrophic burn scars: a systematic review and meta-analysis, *Sci Rep* 7:40185, 2017, https://doi.org/10.1038/srep40185.

32. Staley MJ, Richard RL: Scar management. In Richard RL, Staley MJ, editors: *Burn care and rehabilitation: principles and practice*, Philadelphia, 1994, FA Davis, pp 380–418.

33. Steinstraesser L, Flak E, Witte B, et al.: Pressure garment therapy alone and in combination with silicone for the prevention of hypertrophic scarring: randomized controlled trial with individual comparison, *Plast Reconstr Surg* 128:306e–313e, 2011.

34. Li-Tsang CWP, Zheng YP, Lau JCM: A randomized clinical trial to study the effect of silicone gel dressing and pressure therapy on posttraumatic hypertrophic scars, *J Burn Care Res* 31:448–457, 2010.

35. Bell PL, Gabriel V: Evidence based review for the treatment of post-burn pruritus, *J Burn Care Res* 30:55–61, 2009.

36. Field T, Peck M, Hernandez-Reif M, et al.: Postburn itching, pain, and psychological symptoms are reduced with massage therapy, *J Burn Care Rehabil* 21:189–193, 2000.

37. Levin LS: Management of skin grafts and flaps. In Skirven TM, Osterman AL, Fedorczyk JM, et al.: *Rehabilitation of the hand and upper extremity*, ed 6, Philadelphia, 2011, Elsevier, pp 244–254.

38. Jones NF, Lister GD: Free flaps to the hand and upper extremity. In Wolf SW, Hotchkiss RN, Pederson WC, et al.: *Green's operative hand surgery*, ed 7, Philadelphia, 2017, Elsevier, pp 1574–1611.

39. Sullivan T, Smith J, Kermode J, et al.: Rating the burn scar, *J Burn Care Rehabil* 11:256–260, 1990.

40. Tyack Z, Simons M, Spinks A, et al.: A systematic review of the quality of burn scar rating scales for clinical and research use, *Burns* 38:6–18, 2012.

41. Jones LL, Calvert M, Moiemen N, et al.: Outcomes important to burns patients during scar management and how they compare to the concepts captured in burn-specific patient reported outcome measures, *Burns* 43:1682–1692, 2017.

42. Szabo MM, Urich MA, Duncan CL, et al.: Patient adherence to burn care: a systematic review of the literature, *Burns* 42:484–491, 2016.

43. Coghlan N, Copley J, Aplin T, et al.: Patient experience of wearing compression garments post burn injury: a review of the literature, *J Burn Care Rehabil* 38:260–268, 2017.

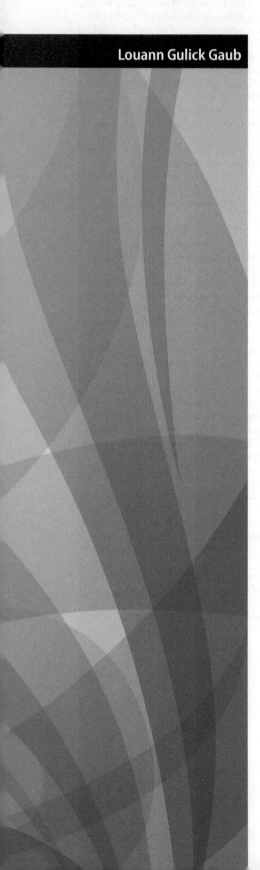

31

Infections

Louann Gulick Gaub

Hand therapists are often the first persons to identify early signs of inflammation or infection in their clients, such as redness (**rubor** or **erythema**), edema (**tumor**), heat (**calor**), and pain (**dolor**). By knowing the signs of infection, therapists can promptly communicate problems with the physician, leading to earlier diagnosis and treatment. Prompt attention could make the difference between a non-surgical solution and a surgical one. Delayed treatment can lead to greater adhesions, stiffness, joint contractures, amputation, or further disability.[1]

In a 2014 practice analysis by the Hand Therapy Certification Commission, most hand therapists who responded reported treating clients with infection. Wound management is considered a component of hand therapy used as an adjunct to upper extremity mobility and functional treatment techniques.[2] Therapists working in upper extremity rehabilitation must be able to identify signs of infection, document observations in the medical record, and communicate with the treating physician. Hand therapists play an integral role in treating and educating clients about infection.

The terms "inflammation" and "infection" are not synonymous. **Inflammation** is a protective response to injury "caused by a physical, chemical, or biologic agent."[3] The abnormal stimulation initiates a reaction in the body to destroy or remove the material, or to repair and heal the area.[3] An inflammatory response may occur when "infectious agents such as bacteria, viruses, and other pathogenic microorganisms" invade.[3] Therefore an infectious agent can cause inflammation. An **infection** is the "invasion and multiplication of microorganisms in body tissues."[4] There must be a susceptible host and a sufficiently virulent agent to destroy normal tissue. The body reacts by forming antibodies and with the physiological response of inflammation.[4]

Infection can lead to loss of tissue and even death. It can occur with a minor scratch or with a major trauma. Since the initial use of penicillin in 1942,[5,6] the incidence of hand infections and complications has greatly decreased. However, bacteria evolve and the sensitivity of bacteria to antibiotics can change over time. Many infected wounds contain more than one type of offending organism, and some bacteria have adapted to a point that available antibiotics may not affect them. One such resistant organism is **methicillin-resistant *Staphylococcus aureus* (MRSA)**. There has been an increased incidence of MRSA in hospitals and in the community. MRSA infections are reported to be responsible for 34% to 73% of all hand infections.[7]

Prevention

Since the passage of the Patient Protection and Affordable Care Act in the United Sates (2010), health care providers have had a heightened interest in preventing infection, as infection can lead to higher hospital readmission rates. High rates of unanticipated returns to the hospital are costly and may indicate problems with quality of care. Under the Affordable Care Act, hospitals can be penalized for high readmissions. Further, Medicare and Medicaid may move toward a payment system of "bundling" for each episode of care, which would include all care within the first 30 days of the incident.[8] Infections are costly, and a move to this type of payment system would further incentivize hospitals in the United States to prevent infections.

Hand hygiene is key in preventing cross-transmission of infection in health care facilities. The greater the staff's compliance with hand washing, the lower the rates of MRSA infections.[9,10] Washing with soap and warm water or using an alcohol-based rub are effective in achieving good hand hygiene.[9] The United States Centers for Disease Control and Prevention released guidelines for surgical site infection prevention in 2017, which include having patients shower with soap prior to surgery, using alcohol-based skin preparations in the operating room, avoiding use of topical antimicrobial agents on surgical incisions, and controlling blood glucose levels during surgery.[11]

Hand surgeries are increasingly being performed outside the traditional operating room. Greater than 70% of all Canadian carpal tunnel releases are performed under local anesthesia in field-sterile minor procedure rooms without increase in infection rates.[12] The "wide-awake" approach to hand surgery, such as in tendon repair, reduces costs and does not increase infection rates.[13]

General Principles

Infection occurs when certain criteria are met. A causative infectious microorganism must be present in sufficient number or strength, and there must be a susceptible host. In response to the organism's invasion, the body may form antibodies and undergo physiological inflammatory changes. The microorganisms will be fought off by the host or develop into an infection.[4] While heat, redness, swelling, pain, and loss of function may be outward signs of inflammation, the physiological changes inside the host are complex and deserve further study beyond this chapter. Generally, the physiological process includes: (1) an accelerated flow of blood (with dilation of the arterioles and opening of new capillaries in the area of injury), (2) increased capillary permeability (causing protein-rich fluid from the blood vessels to leak into extravascular areas), and (3) leukocytic exudation (cells fighting foreign substances or disease move outside the blood vessels and travel to the site of injury or invading microorganisms).[3]

The susceptibility of the host to infection depends on many factors, such as severity of the injury and whether or not multiple systems are involved. Certain conditions increase the susceptibility to infections, such as diabetes mellitus, acquired immune deficiency syndrome (AIDS), Raynaud disease, malnutrition, obesity, renal failure, burns, immunosuppression, alcoholism, and drug abuse.[7,14,15] Steroid use can predispose clients to infection. Certain systemic conditions, such as diabetes mellitus, can decrease tissue oxygenation due to impaired blood flow. Cell metabolism requires oxygen, and efficient tissue oxygenation is needed to prevent infection.[16] Ischemia from a microvascular disease, or trauma that affects normal blood flow, can prevent bacteria from leaving the infected area and makes it more difficult for antibiotics to take effect.[7]

Many types of microorganisms can cause infection in the hand but the most common is *Staphylococcus aureus*, which may comprise up to 60% of all hand infections.[7] The second most common pathogen found in hand infections is *β-hemolytic Streptococcus*. Many wounds are polymicrobial (contain more than one pathogen), such as bite injuries.[7] Infections may start out as **cellulitis**, a superficial infection of the skin and subcutaneous tissue that normally does not produce an **abscess** (a localized collection of pus). The involved area is tender, warm, and marked by erythema. An incision and drainage procedure is not routinely performed for cellulitis, but is done if an abscess develops.[1,7]

Untreated trivial injuries may lead to very serious hand infections that progress rapidly, leading to **lymphangitis.** Lymphangitis involves the superficial lymphatic vessels that arise from the skin, but can also lead to involvement of the deep lymphatic vessels following the course of the arterial system. Some signs of lymphangitis include fever, nausea, tachycardia, and red streaking up the hand and forearm. An abscess may form at the elbow or axilla if the infection is left untreated[6] (Fig. 31.1). Cellulitis and lymphangitis are considered superficial spreading infections.

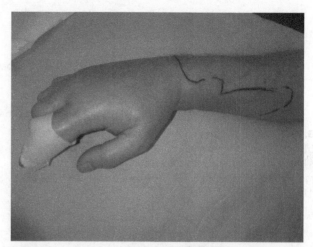

FIG. 31.1 Lymphangitis and purulent flexor tenosynovitis. Markings on forearm indicate progressing erythema and edema. (Courtesy Dr. James Nappi, Hand & Microsurgery Associates, Columbus, OH.)

There are other types of infections found in the hand such as subcutaneous abscesses, and synovial sheath and deep space infections. Subcutaneous abscesses include paronychias, felons, and subepidermal abscesses. With any infection of the hand, edema may be more present dorsally because of loosely organized connective tissue and the direction of flow of the lymphatic system over the back of the hand.[14]

Anatomy and Pathology

Perionychium

The **perionychium** comprises the whole nail structure consisting of the nail bed (germinal and sterile matrix), nail plate, nail fold, eponychium, hyponychium, and paronychium (Fig. 31.2). The nail fold is the proximal depression into which the proximal nail fits. The nail fold has a dorsal roof (eponychium).[17,18,19] The **lunula** is the white arc seen at the base of the nail just distal to the eponychium. The highly vascularized nail bed shows through the nail and is normally pink in color.[19] The **hyponychium**, between the nail bed and the distal nail, helps protect against fungal and bacterial contamination. The hyponychium contains leukocytes and lymphocytes that provide defense against invasion of the subungual area (under the nail). The **paronychium** is the lateral skin on the edge of the nail plate and bed.[17,18,19]

The fingernail is important aesthetically as well as functionally. The nail provides counter-pressure against the finger when pinching or holding an object, which improves sensitivity. The fingernail protects, regulates temperature, and promotes dexterity.[17,18,19] In a traumatic fingertip injury, a **subungual hematoma** (confined mass of blood under the nail) may develop from bleeding underneath the nail plate. Bleeding separates the nail bed from the nail plate and can cause throbbing pain due to pressure. A hematoma can be evacuated by creating a hole in the nail. This procedure is performed by the physician.[18]

Paronychia

Paronychia refers to an infection of the soft tissue around the nail or nail plate (Fig. 31.3). It is the most common infection in

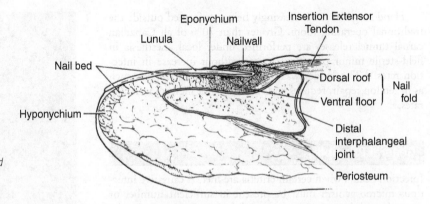

FIG. 31.2 Anatomy of the nail bed. (From Sommer NZ, Brown RE. The perionychium. In: Wolfe SW, Hotchkiss RN, Pederson WC, et al., eds. *Green's Operative Hand Surgery*. 6th ed. Philadelphia, PA: Churchill Livingstone; 2011.)

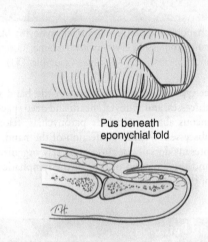

A

Pus beneath eponychial fold

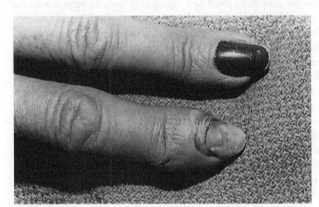

FIG. 31.4 Chronic paronychia. (From Mackin EJ, Callahan AD, Skirven TM, et al., eds. *Rehabilitation of the Hand and Upper Extremity*. 5th ed. St Louis, MO: Mosby; 2002.)

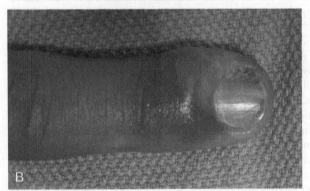

B

FIG. 31.3 Inflamed paronychium and eponychium with pus below the eponychial fold. A. Illustrated. B. Client presentation. (From Stevanovic MV, Sharpe F. Acute infections. In: Wolfe SW, Hotchkiss RN, Pederson WC, et al., eds. *Green's Operative Hand Surgery*. 6th ed. Philadelphia, PA: Churchill Livingstone; 2011.)

the hand.[1,20] It may be acute or chronic. Hangnails, nail biting, or manicures are often the cause.[1,7,20,21] In children, paronychia is associated with thumb or finger sucking. Erythema, swelling, and pain may occur at the lateral fold or base of the fingernail.[21] The most common causative organism of an acute paronychia is *Staphylococcus aureus*.[7,22]

Chronic paronychia is more common in people who immerse their hands in water or detergents frequently, such as dishwashers and office cleaners.[23] Finger suckers and individuals with diabetes are more susceptible to chronic paronychias.[20]

Normally, the hyponychium protects the subungual space from invading organisms. When the finger is repeatedly immersed in water and exposed to an alkaline environment, the protective barrier is violated and bacterial or fungal organisms enter more easily.[18] It was previously believed that *Candida albicans* caused most chronic paronychias; however, these are now classified more as dermatitis caused by environmental irritants. Even though *Candida albicans* may be found, the fungus disappears when the physiological barrier is improved. It is more of an eczematous condition that responds better to steroids than antifungals.[23] Individuals with chronic paronychias suffer with repeated erythema and drainage. A decrease in vascularity of the nail fold due to recalcitrant inflammation may lead to separation of the nail fold from the nail plate.[7] If the nail is not adequately treated, it may exhibit permanent deformity (Fig. 31.4).

Eponychia

When infection involves the tissue over the base of the nail in addition to one lateral fold beside the nail, it is more accurately called an **eponychia.** In an eponychia, pus develops near the lunula, the white arch visible at the base of some fingernails.[20] Due to inflammation at the base of the nail, a disruption of the seal between the nail fold and nail plate allows organisms to invade the tissue. An infection can begin on one side of the nail as a paronychia, then extend around the base to the opposite side of the nail, called a "run-around infection."[1,14]

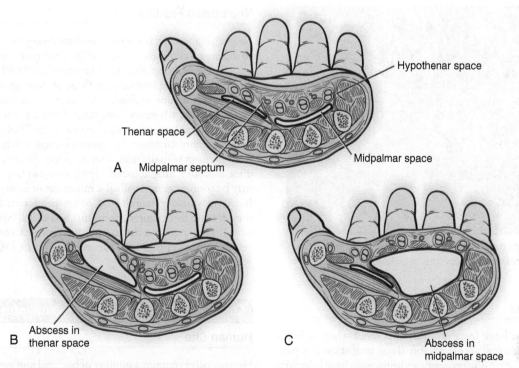

FIG. 31.5 Deep palmar spaces. (A) Potential spaces of the mid palm. (B) Thenar space abscess. (C) Midpalmar space abscess. (From Stevanovic MV, Sharpe F. Acute infections. In: Wolfe SW, Hotchkiss RN, Pederson WC, et al., eds. *Green's Operative Hand Surgery.* 6th ed. Philadelphia, PA: Elsevier Churchill Livingstone; 2011.)

Felon

An infection involving the distal finger pad is called a **felon**. The finger pad or pulp is divided into multiple compartments by fibrous septa. A subcutaneous abscess (pus) in these tiny compartments causes pressure, swelling, redness, and intense pain. A penetrating trauma, such as with splinters or finger-stick blood tests, can be the mechanism of injury.[21] If left untreated, the abscess from the felon can extend into the distal phalanx and lead to osteomyelitis (inflammation of bone and marrow) or **osteitis** (inflammation of bone). The tip of the finger holds the highest concentration of sensory receptors in the hand,[20] so when pressure develops in the finger pulp, pain is usually severe.

Flexor Tendon Sheath Infection

The flexor tendons in the hand move within synovial sheaths. These sheaths are poorly vascularized and tendons receive much of their nutrition via synovial fluid diffusion.[20] Synovial fluid is an enticing environment for bacterial growth. When infection occurs within the sheath, a **pyogenic flexor tenosynovitis** (or purulent flexor tenosynovitis) develops.[14,21] Increased pressure from bacterial proliferation within the sheath leads to even less blood supply and can cause tendon necrosis and rupture. Flexor sheath infections are most commonly caused by *Staphylococcus aureus* and *β-hemolytic Streptococcus.*[20,21,24]

Dr. Allen Kanavel, a pioneer in the treatment of hand infections in the early 20th century, described four signs (**Kanavel cardinal signs**) to identify pyogenic flexor tenosynovitis: (1) a semiflexed finger position, (2) uniform swelling of the finger, (3) tenderness along the tendon sheath, and (4) excruciating pain with passive extension of the finger.[7,14,20,21,24]

Even when treated early, pyogenic flexor tenosynovitis can lead to permanent tendon scarring, residual digit stiffness, and lack of function.[25] Tendon necrosis or the spread of infection to deep fascial spaces can occur. Although uncommon, radial and ulnar bursal infections may occur in association with flexor tendon sheath infections of the thumb or small fingers. There may be tenderness and swelling at the distal wrist crease and along the hypothenar or thenar eminence in addition to the cardinal signs of Kanavel in either the small finger or thumb.[20]

> ### Clinical Pearl
>
> Identify flexor tenosynovitis by the presence of four cardinal signs: (1) semiflexed finger position, (2) uniform swelling of the finger, (3) tenderness along the tendon sheath, and (4) excruciating pain with passive finger extension.[7,14,20,21,24]

Deep Space Infection

Infection can develop in a number of spaces in the upper extremity (Fig. 31.5). These include the (1) thenar, (2) hypothenar, (3) midpalmar spaces in the hand, and (4) Parona's space in the forearm (distal volar forearm deep to the flexor tendons). More superficial spaces are the (5) dorsal subcutaneous space, (6) dorsal subaponeurotic space, and (7) interdigital web spaces (collar-button abscesses occur here).[7,20] Infection may be caused by a penetrating injury or spread from an adjacent flexor tendon sheath infection.[7] Clients may present with tenderness and swelling over the palmar spaces. Dorsal hand swelling is usually present, since the palm consists of tight fascia that limits the accumulation of swelling volarly. The presence of infection in the fascial spaces is a medical emergency and usually requires surgical drainage.[7,14,20]

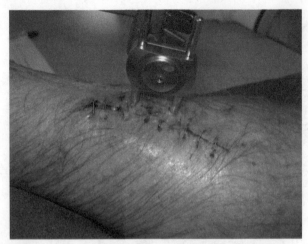

FIG. 31.6 Infection around the proximal screw site of an external fixator in the forearm. (Courtesy Louann Gulick Gaub.)

Osteomyelitis

Infection in the bone (**osteomyelitis**) can result when an infection is not eradicated in nearby soft tissue or if there is a penetrating trauma.[20,26] A felon, septic arthritis, soft-tissue infection, open fracture, or bite injury can lead to osteomyelitis. The most common pathogens are *Staphylococcus aureus* and *Streptococcus*, and immunocompromised clients are predisposed to these infections.[7] Intact bone cortex provides a good barrier to penetration by pathogens, but trauma to the bone allows a pathway for infection. If local inflammation causes necrosis of the bone, called a **sequestrum**, pathogens can more easily live there due to the deficient vascularity. Antibiotics are less effective in areas of necrotic bone.[26]

When hardware is required for fixation of a bone fracture, pathogens can enter the bone and an infection can develop around a pin or screw site (Fig. 31.6). Most pin tract infections are minor if treated with antibiotics and good wound care.[20] Incidence of pin tract infections is low, ranging from 0.5% to 21%.[20,26,27,28,29] External fixation has a higher rate of infection than internal fixation.[29] Most infections from pins and screws are minor and do not lead to significant osteomyelitis if treated early. However, these infections can necessitate the early removal of hardware and can result in necrosis of the bone if the infection is not controlled.[20,26]

Septic Arthritis

When infectious pathogens invade and colonize a joint, septic arthritis may occur. The presentation includes fusiform joint swelling (wider around the joint and tapered at both ends), erythema, and pain with movement of the joint. The most common pathogens are *β-hemolytic Streptococcus* and *Staphylococcus aureus*. Gout or other crystalline arthropathies have a similar clinical presentation, so cultures and crystal analysis can help with a more accurate diagnosis by the physician.[7] Septic arthritis usually occurs after a penetrating injury or spreads from another infected area such as a felon or pyogenic flexor tenosynovitis.[1] Surgical drainage and intravenous (IV) antibiotics are the optimal course of treatment, but some physicians may initiate treatment with oral antibiotics.[7,30]

Necrotizing Fasciitis

Necrotizing fasciitis is a serious medical emergency that requires emergent surgical debridement of necrotic tissue and IV antibiotics. Bacteria infect the fascia (connective tissue) and spreads quickly, destroying surrounding tissue. A delay in treatment can result in loss of limb or death. Most deaths stem from organ failure and sepsis. Mortality rates range from 23% to 76%.[7] This serious bacterial infection, also known as the "flesh-eating infection," is more common in immunocompromised individuals. Risk increases with diabetes, cancer, kidney disease, chronic liver disease, and IV drug abuse.[7,31] Symptoms can begin quickly but may be confusing, especially if a minor cut or injury is the cause. Individuals usually exhibit pain or erythema initially, and then they develop fever, fatigue, vomiting, and chills. Necrotizing fasciitis is fairly rare, but the Centers for Disease Control and Prevention estimates that there are at least 700 to 1100 cases each year in the United States.[31]

Common Mechanisms of Injury and Infection

Human Bite

Human saliva contains a number of bacterial and viral organisms. There are up to 50 species of bacteria in the human mouth.[7] The hand can become contaminated with saliva by several means: a fist striking a tooth, nail biting, a dental instrument, or a bite. A **fight bite** or **clenched-fist injury** results when a client strikes someone's mouth and their teeth lacerate skin over the dorsum of the hand. This thinly protected area is vulnerable to metacarpal and phalanx fractures, infections in the joint capsule, and laceration of extensor tendons.[1,7,14,21] Clients may not seek medical attention initially because the wound seems unimportant, but delay in treatment increases the chance of a severe infection and osteomyelitis.[14,21] After surgical drainage and antibiotics, the wound is usually left open to heal by **secondary intention** (gradually heals and closes on its own).

Animal Bite

The saliva of dogs and cats contains a number of disease-causing organisms, the most common offender being *Pasteurella multicida*.[14,32-34] Cuts and scratches can even become infected if an animal licks them.[33] Dog bites comprise 80% of animal bites and are more common than cat bites. Cat bites, however, are more likely to result in infection; 50% of cat bites will become infected.[7] Cat teeth are sharp and thin, causing puncture wounds. These wounds may introduce bacteria deep into the tissue, close quickly, and are difficult to clean. Dog teeth are bigger and more blunt, causing soft-tissue damage from crushing and tearing. If bitten by an animal, immediately wash with soap and warm water. Seek immediate medical attention, especially in the presence of a compromised immune system (such as diabetes, liver disease, human immunodeficiency virus [HIV]/AIDS).[33] Most animal bite wounds are left open to heal by secondary intention.

Intravenous Drug Abuse

IV drug abusers attempt venous access and commonly use dirty needles. They may inject chemicals into soft tissue, causing infection and necrosis. These infections usually begin as a subcutaneous abscess and progress to infections of the tendon sheaths, joints, or fascial spaces. Drug abusers may not seek prompt medical attention and may have poor adherence to the treatment regime. Additionally, IV drug abusers tend to have a deficient immune response and higher rates of malnutrition, hepatitis, and HIV/AIDS.[14,32] Forearm infections due to IV drug abuse may create swelling and pressure in the deep tissues, a condition known as compartment syndrome. This compression can lead to deoxygenation of the muscles, nerves, and blood vessels. Severe edema, pain in the forearm with finger flexion, and pain with passive finger extension may be an indication of **Volkmann contracture.** This is a serious emergency, as the muscles are dying. A fasciotomy (surgical opening of skin and fascia) may then be required to drain infection from the tissue and lower the tissue pressure.[32]

Mycobacteria

The most common mycobacterial infection in the hand is *Mycobacterium marinum*. It is often difficult to diagnose, since the symptoms can be diverse and may not occur for weeks or months after innoculation.[35] The infection often begins with a puncture wound or skin abrasion followed by contact with fish fins or fish tanks. People also get mycobacterial infections at beaches, lakes, and pools, as it is found in water and soil. The presentation includes skin lesions or nodules along lines of lymphatic drainage, or localized tenosynovitis of the flexors or extensors.[14] Since the infection may be prolonged and relatively painless, clients may not receive timely treatment. This delay can result in synovial structures being destroyed.[14,35]

Fungal Infections

Fungal infections occur in the hand but rarely require surgery. Contamination with soil, thorns, or splinters may cause an infection, such as **sporotrichosis.** These infections present with painless papules that can eventually spread along paths of lymphatic drainage.[35] Fungal infections can also attack the nail and lead to thickening and discoloration. *Candida*, one species of pathogen, can produce nail deformity. It is most frequently seen in those with peripheral vascular disease, Raynaud disease, or Cushing syndrome.[34] *Candida* infections can occur when individuals frequently expose their hands to wet or alkaline environments, as the hyponychium loses its ability to fend off infections.[18] Fungal organisms may be treated with systemic or topical antifungal medications.[18] However, new evidence classifies many fungal infections as more eczematous conditions, which respond better to steroids than antifungals.[23]

Viruses

The two most common viral infections of the hand are herpetic whitlow and periungual warts.[18] Periungual warts, caused by the human papillomavirus, are usually more of a cosmetic problem. There are various treatments, both surgical and nonsurgical, but most warts resolve within 2 years. However, eradication of warts is the optimal treatment, since surrounding tissue may be invaded during this time.[35]

Herpetic whitlow is caused by the herpes simplex virus and can be contracted through mucous membranes or broken skin. It can be spread by touching the fingers (with open skin) to herpes lesions in the mouth or genital areas.[21,35] Herpetic whitlow is often seen in health care workers who do not use standard precautions when exposed to secretions in the mouth. Fluid-filled vesicles on the finger, swelling, discomfort, or redness are characteristic of herpetic whitlow. It can be confused with a felon or paronychia, since some symptoms are similar.[7,21,34] The virus usually resolves on its own within 3 weeks. Incision is contraindicated because doing so may result in a secondary bacterial infection.[7,14,18,21,34] After vesicles resolve, the virus is latent and reoccurs with stressors in 20% of individuals.[7]

Timelines and Healing

Clients with infections who delay seeking medical treatment risk severe tissue damage. The longer the delay, the more the individual is at risk. Wound and infection resolution timelines depend on the location of infection, the client's medical status, extent of injury, and structures involved. Delayed treatment and complex cases may require incision and drainage, compartment release, reconstructive surgeries, or even amputation.

Nonoperative Treatment

Prompt wound care after injury can help prevent infection. When possible, immediately wash or flush out wounds with soap and warm water to help remove dirt, saliva, or foreign bodies that contain bacteria.[33] If the injury is more severe, prompt medical attention is important. Some injuries seem trivial, such as a small bite over the metacarpal during a fight, and individuals may not seek immediate medical attention. Remind your clients: *When in doubt, it is safest to consult a medical expert early on.*

> ### ◎ Clinical Pearl
>
> If infection and acute inflammation are present, the involved area should be immobilized to help prevent the spread of infection and to reduce pain and edema. The area should be immobilized in a position that prevents deformity or stiffness, such as the **safe position (intrinsic plus position)**; with the wrist in slight extension, the MP joints in flexion, and the IP joints in extension (unless not appropriate for injured structures).

Nonoperative treatment for the acute paronychia consists of oral antibiotics (usually anti-staphylococcal), warm soaks, and resting of the digit. Surgical drainage is performed if an abscess (pus) develops. Chronic paronychia may be more difficult to treat, especially if the client works in moist environments with substances that impair the hyponychium's natural barrier against fungi and bacteria. Chronic paronychia can be treated with antifungal or antimicrobial agents along with avoidance of prolonged immersion of hands in water and alkalines.[19] Some studies suggest that topical steroids are the drug of choice for chronic paronychias.

Felons, infections in the pulp of the finger, should be treated with appropriate oral antibiotics (usually antistaphylococcal) promptly. Otherwise, surgical drainage is inevitable to prevent further spread to other tissues and necrosis of the distal phalanx.[1,14] Pyogenic (or purulent) flexor tenosynovitis is also best treated immediately, certainly within 12 to 24 hours of onset. If treated very early, nonoperative treatment may include oral or IV antibiotics (usually fighting *Staphylococcus aureus* or *β-hemolytic Streptococcus*), immobilization in a splint, warm soaks, and elevation.[19,21]

Infection within the flexor tendon sheath can spread rapidly, impair function of the tendon, spread to other fascial spaces, and lead to necrosis of the tendon. These infections are closely monitored, since surgical intervention is often needed.[1,7,19,21,25]

It is important to understand that hand therapists do not diagnose any infection or condition described in this chapter. The therapist's role is to describe the clinical appearance of the hand to the physician if signs of infection are observed: erythema, an increase in drainage, purulent drainage, increase in pain, or increase in edema. The physician will make the diagnosis.

Operative Treatment

Postsurgical therapy may include wound care, edema control, splinting for rest and protection, and range-of-motion (ROM) exercises depending on the involved structures. Surgical intervention for acute paronychia involves evacuation of pus around the nail fold. The surgeon may remove part or all of the nail.[7,22] If nonoperative treatment has not been effective for the chronic paronychia, nail removal and a procedure called "eponychial marsupialization" may be required. This procedure removes the elliptical area of skin in the proximal nail fold to encourage improved drainage.[7,14,22,23,34]

Other infections, such as felons, animal or human bites, or pyogenic flexor tenosynovitis, may be treated surgically by incision and drainage if conservative treatment does not resolve the infection within 48 hours.[14,20-22] Hand therapists are more likely to treat these more complicated cases postoperatively. Treatment is individualized according to the structures involved and extent of injury.

Hand therapists often treat clients with internal or external hardware fixation of their fractures. Infection rates with Kirschner wire fixation are low. Superficial pin track infection occurs in about 3% to 8.3% of clients.[17,28,29] Pins placed in the metacarpals or phalanges have a higher incidence of infection than pins placed in the wrist and forearm (distal radius and ulna).[17] Exposed pins increase the incidence of infection compared to pins that are buried beneath the skin.[29,36]

? Questions to Ask the Doctor

- What structures were involved in the infection?
- What are the precautions or guidelines for active or passive range of motion (AROM, PROM)?
- What are the wound care guidelines (for example, soaking, frequency of dressing changes, dressing technique, packing an open wound)?
- Do you want the client to do home dressing changes?
- Is splinting desired? If so, what structures should be immobilized and in what position? Should the wrist be included in the orthosis?

() What to Say to Clients

If Infection Is Suspected

"Check your hand for an increase in redness, swelling, heat, and/or pain. Call your physician's office if you develop a fever, if you feel sick, or if you suspect your symptoms are worsening. Identifying early signs of infection can make a big difference in the speed of your recovery."

Postoperative Clients

"It is important to keep your hand elevated above your heart to minimize swelling. Swelling can lead to stiffness and pain.

Managing swelling early promotes better recovery of hand function. It is also important to adhere to the wound care instructions to decrease your risk for infection."

Evaluation Tips

- If you suspect infection, describe and measure the symptomatic area (for example, the area of erythema) so that you can later compare it with observations during subsequent visits.
- If you suspect infection, do not cause unnecessary pain by taking measurements of ROM or proceeding with therapeutic exercise. *Contact the physician's office right away to describe your observations while the client is in your clinic.* You may find that ROM or therapeutic activities are contraindicated.
- Find out if any treatment is contraindicated, such as PROM or resistive exercise.
- Check dressings to document amount of drainage, color, and odor.
- Watch for and document skin maceration (soft white-colored skin caused by prolonged exposure to moisture).
- Monitor and document appearance around pin or screw sites. Slight erythema may be present postoperatively but should be closely monitored for increased redness or other infection signs. Pin tract infections can lead to osteomyelitis.[20,27] Pin care should be done according to the physician's preference.

Diagnosis-Specific Information That Affects Clinical Reasoning

Prompt treatment is important when infection begins. If you observe signs of infection, call the physician while the client is present in your clinic. If you are not sure, try to determine the client's ability to monitor worsening symptoms while at home. Instruct the client in what signs to look for, and how to contact the physician's office if symptoms worsen. If the client feels uncomfortable with the decision making or is unable to accurately make that decision, recommend more frequent therapy visits so that you can monitor the situation more closely.

Precaution: *If infection is suspected, it is better to have it documented that the physician's office was contacted than to wish later that this had been done.*

Wound care guidelines are determined by the treating physician. If the status of the wound changes (for example, drainage volume increases and is soaking through the dressing, or wound color is changing), the dressing procedure might need to be changed. Therapists who work closely with hand surgeons can often make these decisions independently due to their close working relationship and training. Therapists who do not have this understanding and relationship with a particular referring physician should discuss any wound care changes before proceeding with treatment.

♡ Tips from the Field

Orthoses

Orthosis needs are determined based on the particular structures involved. It may be necessary to immobilize several hand joints in order to provide comfort or to protect healing tissues. Discuss orthotic options with the physician. The client with pyogenic flexor tenosynovitis, for example, may initially benefit from an orthosis that includes the wrist and positions the hand in intrinsic-plus position. Stiffness may develop as a result of their tenosynovitis and adhesions, so a proximal interphalangeal (PIP) extension orthosis or flexion mobilization orthosis may help in achieving optimal range of motion. For a felon or paronychia, a distal interphalangeal extension orthosis can be fabricated to rest and protect the fingertip.

Wound Care

Instruct clients in the signs of inflammation, such as redness, swelling, pain, and heat. Hand therapists should understand that some degree of these signs accompany the normal early inflammatory stage of a wound healing. Purulence does not always indicate infection.[36] It is best to have the physician assess the wound if infection is suspected. The wound may be left open to heal by secondary intention so that purulent material can easily drain. The physician may request that you and/or the client lightly pack the open wound with strip gauze to keep the superficial wound open and allow the deeper portion to heal first (Fig. 31.7). Wounds that are left open, such as fingertip amputations allowed to heal conservatively, do not necessarily have an increased risk for infection.[37]

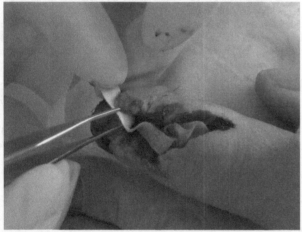

FIG. 31.7 Wound packing with strip gauze. Wound left open to heal by secondary intention. (Courtesy Louann Gulick Gaub.)

Wound care may also include debridement of slough (dead tissue that is moist and white-yellow in color) or eschar (dead tissue that is hard, dry, and black in color), since these nonviable tissues impede the normal cellular response. Eschar forms a mechanical block that does not allow the wound to close and can increase the growth of bacteria in the wound.[36] If you do not feel comfortable performing any wound care technique, you should discuss this with the referring physician.

Hand therapists have an important role in wound healing and infection control. Techniques that may prevent or control infection are protecting the wound with an appropriate dressing (barrier to the environment), cleaning the wound (mild soap and water or saline),[38] removing necrotic tissue, and managing excess drainage. Topical antiseptics may or may not be recommended by the physician, since they are cytotoxic and can destroy not only bacteria but also cell walls in healthy tissue.[33,36] With infection, warm water soaks two to four times per day may be effective in promoting drainage and cleansing the wound.[22,34,38]

Edema Control

Managing edema is important, as excessive edema can negatively affect the restoration of soft-tissue length and joint motion. After injury or surgery, all wounds have some edema. Edema is part of the normal inflammatory response to injury and is a result of excess fluid in the intercellular spaces.[37] However, excessive swelling can increase risk for infection, delay the healing process, and increase stiffness and scarring.[36,37] It is best to prevent excessive edema than to treat it after it becomes a problem. Managing edema may include elevation, compression with external wraps, gentle AROM if appropriate for the injury, and use of cold modalities if not contraindicated (for example, with clients who have circulatory compromise).[36-38]

Therapeutic Modalities

Using therapeutic modalities can be helpful for treating edema, pain, and stiffness. However, therapists should be cautious about using modalities when their client has an active infection. Some modalities may be contraindicated, such as ultrasound, contrast baths, intermittent pneumatic compression pumps, kinesiotaping, or iontophoresis.[38]

> **Precautions and Concerns**

- *Watch for redness, swelling, heat, pain, or fever. Instruct clients to check for these signs at home and to contact their physician immediately if infection is suspected.*
- *If the client is not adhering to restrictions or dressing guidelines, note this in your documentation.*

CASE STUDY

CASE STUDY 31.1

Gina, a 40-year-old woman, sustained a cat bite in her home. She washed her finger, applied a Band-Aid, and continued her daily routine without concern. About 12 hours later, significant pain, erythema, and edema developed rapidly. In the emergency department, the hand surgeon observed signs consistent with purulent flexor tenosynovitis of Gina's dominant index finger, and he opted for surgical incision and drainage. The flexor tendon sheath was incised, decompressed, and irrigated; serous fluid and purulence were drained. The first annular (A1) pulley was also released. Following surgery, Gina stayed overnight in the hospital for monitoring and IV antibiotics.

Two days postoperatively, Gina came to hand therapy. Her bulky surgical dressing was removed, her hand was soaked in warm water and liquid soap, and the wound packing was removed. The surgeon had left the wound open to heal by secondary intention. There were no visual signs of infection. The wound was loosely repacked with narrow strip packing gauze and a dry dressing was applied. The client and her husband were instructed in twice daily soaking and wound packing at home. Gina was able to perform tendon-gliding exercise with minimal difficulty. The therapist fabricated a custom PIP extension orthosis for night wear to correct a 20-degree PIP flexion contracture. Three weeks later, Gina's wound was almost fully closed and she had full ROM. Prompt and appropriate medical attention averted lasting tendon dysfunction.

Acknowledgment

The author would like to thank Cynthia Cooper who laid an excellent foundation for this chapter in the first edition.

References

1. Patel DB, Emmanuel NB, Stevanovic MV, et al.: Hand infections: anatomy, types and spread of infection, imaging findings, and treatment options, *Radiographics* 34(7):1968–1986, 2014.
2. Keller JL, Caro CM, Dimick MP, et al.: Thirty years of hand therapy: the 2014 practice analysis, *J Hand Ther* 29(3):222–234, 2016.
3. Inflammation (n.d.): *Farlex Partner Medical Dictionary*. Retrieved February 26 2018 from https://medical-dictionary.thefreedictionary.com/Inflammation, 2012.
4. Infection. (n.d.): *Medical Dictionary for the Health Professions and Nursing*. Retrieved February 26 2018 from https://medical-dictionary.thefreedictionary.com/Infection, 2012.
5. Arias CA, Murray BE: Antibiotic-resistant bugs in the 21st century—a clinical super-challenge, *N Engl J Med* 360:439–443, 2009.
6. Flynn JE: Severe infections of the hand: a historical perspective. In Jupiter JB, editor: *Flynn's hand surgery*, ed 4, Baltimore, 1991, Williams & Wilkins.
7. Osterman M, Draeger R, Stern P: Acute hand infections, *J Hand Ther* 39(8):1628–1635, 2014.
8. Curtin CM, Hernandez-Boussard T: Readmissions after treatment of distal radius fractures, *J Hand Ther* 39(10):1926–1932, 2014.
9. Mathur P: Hand hygiene: back to the basics of infection control, *Indian J Med Res* 134(5):611, 2011.
10. Nadimpalli G, Bhamare S, Rao NP, Ingole S: Incidence of methicillin-resistant Staphylococcus aureus (MRSA) infection among patients and hospital staff and impact of preventive measures in reduction of MRSA infection rate: a prospective observational study, *Int J Basic Clin Pharmacol* 5(6):2336–2340, 2018.
11. Berrios-Torres SI, Umscheid CA, Bratzler DW, et al.: Centers for Disease Control and Prevention guideline for the prevention of surgical site infection, 2017, *JAMA Surgery* 152(8):784–791, 2017.
12. LeBlanc MR, Lalonde DH, Thoma A, et al.: Is main operating room sterility really necessary in carpal tunnel surgery? A multicenter prospective study of minor procedure room field sterility surgery, *Hand* 6(0):60–63, 2011.
13. Lalonde D: How the wide-awake approach is changing hand surgery and hand therapy: inaugural AAHS sponsored lecture at the ASHT meeting, San Diego, 2012, *J Hand Ther* 26(2):175–178, 2013.
14. Taras JS, et al.: Common infections of the hand. In Skirven TM, Osterman AL, Fedorczyk JM, et al.: *Rehabilitation of the hand and upper extremity*, ed 6, Philadelphia, 2011, Elsevier Mosby.
15. Fitzgibbons PG: Hand manifestations of diabetes mellitus, *J Hand Surg Am* 33:771–775, 2008.
16. Guo SA, DiPietro LA: Factors affecting wound healing, *J Dent Res* 89(3):219–229, 2010.
17. Wilhelmi B, et al.: "Nail pathology, medscape reference", 2017.
18. Wegener EE: Identification of common nail and skin disorders, *J Hand Ther* 23:187–197, 2010.
19. Zook EG: Anatomy and physiology of the perionychium, *Hand Clin* 18:553–559, 2002.
20. Stevanovic MV, Sharpe F: Acute infections. In Wolfe SW, Hotchkiss RN, Pederson WC, et al.: *Green's operative hand surgery*, ed 6, Philadelphia, 2011, Elsevier Churchill Livingstone.
21. Clark DC: Common acute hand infections, *Am Fam Physician* 68(11):2167–2176, 2003.
22. Ritting AW, O'Malley MP, Rodner CM: Acute paronychia, *J Hand Surg Am* 37(5):1068–1070, 2012.
23. Relhan V, Goel K, Bansal S, Garg VK: Management of chronic paronychia, *Indian J Dermatol* 59(1):15, 2014.
24. Kennedy CD, Huang JI, Hanel DP: In brief: Kanavel's signs and pyogenic flexor tenosynovitis, *Clin Orthop Relat Res* 474(1):280–284, 2016.
25. Draeger RW, Bynum Jr DK: Flexor tendon sheath infections of the hand, *J Am Acad Orthop Surg* 20(6):373–382, 2012.
26. Honda H, McDonald JR: Current recommendations in the management of osteomyelitis of the hand and wrist, *J Hand Surg Am* 34:1135–1136, 2009.
27. Hsu LP, Schwartz EG, Kalainov DM, et al.: Complications of K-wire fixation in procedures involving the hand and wrist, *J Hand Surg Am* 36(4):610–616, 2011.
28. Rizvi M, Bille B, Holtom P, et al.: The role of prophylactic antibiotics in elective hand surgery, *J Hand Surg Am* 33(3):413–420, 2008.
29. Richard MJ, Wartinbee DA, Riboh J, et al.: Analysis of the complications of palmar plating versus external fixation for fractures of the distal radius, *J Hand Surg Am* 36(10):1614–1620, 2011.
30. Kowalski TJ, Thompson LA, Gundrum JD: Antimicrobial management of septic arthritis of the hand and wrist, *Infection* 42(2):379–384, 2014.
31. Centers for Disease Control and Prevention: Necrotizing Fasciitis, page last reviewed: July 3, 2017. https://CDC.gov.
32. Cahill JM: Special infections of the hand. In Jupiter JB, editor: *Flynn's hand surgery*, ed 4, Baltimore, 1991, Williams & Wilkins.
33. *LSU School of Veterinary Medicine: What you should know about animal bites, Official Web Page of Louisiana State University (website)*, http://www.vetmed.lsu.edu/animal_bites.htm, Accessed June 17, 2013.
34. Keyser JJ, Littler JW, Eaton RG: Surgical treatment of infections and lesions of the perionychium, *Hand Clin* 6(1):137–153, 1990.
35. Abzug JM, Cappel MA: Benign acquired superficial skin lesions of the hand, *J Hand Surg Am* 37:378–393, 2012.
36. Von Der Heyde R, Evans RB: Wound classification and management. In Skirven TM, Osterman AL, Fedorczyk JM, et al.: *Rehabilitation of the hand and upper extremity*, ed 6, Philadelphia, 2011, Elsevier Mosby.
37. Villeco JP: Edema: a silent but important factor, *J Hand Ther* 25:153–160, 2012.
38. Hartzell TL, Rubinstein R, Herman M: Therapeutic modalities—an updated review for the hand surgeon, *J Hand Surg Am* 37(3):597–621, 2012.

32

Dupuytren Contracture

Steven Kempton
Mojca Herman
Prosper Benhaim

Introduction

Dupuytren disease is a benign fibroproliferative disorder of the fascia of the hand and fingers, resulting in progressive thickening and shortening of the palmar fascia. As the disease progresses, cord formation at the palm and finger level can lead to flexion deformities of the digits and ultimately loss of functional finger extension.[1] Joint contractures often form in the flexed fingers, especially at the level of the proximal interphalangeal (PIP) joint, and must be recognized as an additional contributor to the deformity.

Dupuytren contracture is both common and incurable, but several treatment options are available. The aim of current intervention involves the preservation and improvement of hand function by either surgical or chemical division (fasciotomy) or surgical removal (fasciectomy) of the diseased tissue. Correctional treatment for Dupuytren contracture includes surgical intervention and nonoperative options, such as needle aponeurotomy and collagenase *Clostridium histolyticum* (Xiaflex and Xiapex) injections. Adjunctive treatment options, such as dynamic external fixation for severely affected joints, skin-grafting procedures, fat injections, steroid injections, and radiation therapy have a role in specific subsets of patients. Unfortunately, recurrence of Dupuytren contracture is common following all treatment options and should be discussed with the patient.

Hand therapy is important in the postoperative care of patients with Dupuytren disease. Hand therapists communicate closely with the hand surgeon, while guiding rehabilitation to gain maximal finger extension and improved hand function. Common therapy interventions include orthoses, wound/scar management, edema control, motion exercises, strengthening, and patient education for safe activity reintegration. The aim of this chapter is to discuss the management of Dupuytren disease, with particular attention paid to therapy implications. This chapter is written by a team of physicians and a hand therapist; as such, we use the terms "patient" and "client" interchangeably.

Diagnosis

Dupuytren contracture is a genetically inherited disease. The overall prevalence is 0.2% to 56%, depending on the particular population studied. The prevalence is higher in those of Northern European descent and is more commonly seen in males and those over the age of 60 years.[2] The disease is commonly associated with diabetes mellitus, alcohol abuse, hand trauma, human immunodeficiency virus infection, and medications used to treat epilepsy. Recognizing Dupuytren disease involves knowledge of normal hand anatomy and a practitioner skilled in detailed hand examination.[3] The diagnosis of Dupuytren contracture is often made by primary care physicians and hand surgeons. Hand therapists routinely see Dupuytren nodules and skin pitting in the course of treating other hand conditions, and are sometimes the first health care practitioner to identify the condition for clients.

Early diagnosis of Dupuytren contracture is important for client education and timing of early intervention. The disease predictably progresses through histological proliferative, involutional, and residual phases.[4,5] Nodule formation and skin pitting around the distal palmar crease are the earliest signs representing the proliferative phase and precede cord formation. These nodules are not usually tender but may be so in 5% to 10% of cases.[5] Cord formation and metacarpophalangeal (MP) and PIP joint contracture correspond to the involutional phase. The ring finger is the most commonly affected, followed by the small, middle, thumb, and index in order of decreasing frequency.[6] The diagnosis is made clinically, without need for radiographic imaging or other specific testing.

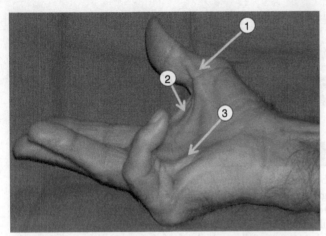

FIG. 32.1 Dupuytren cords affecting the hand. *(1)* Pretendinous cord over the first metacarpal resulting in thumb metacarpophalangeal (MP) contracture. *(2)* Commissural cord causing first web space contracture. *(3)* Pretendinous cord of the fourth metacarpal causing ring finger MP contracture with radial collateral cord extending into small finger causing MP and proximal interphalangeal joint contracture.

Dupuytren diathesis represents a more aggressive form of the disease and is characterized by male predominance, with earlier occurrence before the age of 50 years, positive family history, and bilateral hand involvement. Patients often present with knuckle pads and other ectopic sites of disease, including the plantar surface of the feet (Ledderhose disease) and the penis (Peyronie disease).[7]

Pathoanatomy

The palmar aponeurosis of the hand functions to stabilize the palmar skin to the underlying skeleton and is the primary target for Dupuytren pathology. The palmar aponeurosis fascial sheet consists of superficial longitudinal fibers and deep transverse fibers. These fibers stabilize structures in the palm by connecting the skin to the underlying skeleton while maintaining gliding of the flexor tendons. This fascial layer has been organized into identifiable bands and ligaments that represent normal anatomy.[4,5] Dupuytren cord formation represents pathological transformation of normal bands and can result in contracture of the digits. The pretendinous cord is the most commonly encountered, and is mostly responsible for MP joint contracture (Fig. 32.1).[4]

Indications for Intervention

The decision to intervene surgically on Dupuytren disease should be made with the thoughtful consideration that invasive procedures on the hand carry the risk of hastening disease progression elsewhere in the hand.[8] Therefore, indications for treatment factor in objective joint contracture severity in combination with subjective concerns including pain, cosmetic appearance, and functional limitations. Conventional treatment indications include MP joint contracture of greater than 30 degrees, PIP joint contracture of at least 15 degrees, and loss of functional capacity in the hand.[6]

Nonoperative Treatment

While surgery remains the gold standard treatment of Dupuytren contracture, nonsurgical options are available for patients who are either not surgical candidates or hesitant to proceed with an operation. Hand therapy as an alternative to correctional procedures has been investigated. These reports represent small case series that suggest utilizing a static night extension orthosis combined with stretching and massage may improve digital extension. However, these case studies indicate that this type of therapy is more effective in early proliferative disease and requires strict compliance.[9,10]

While the evidence to support hand therapy alone as a treatment consideration remains insufficient to direct management options, it may be a reasonable option for some patients hoping to avoid surgery and to maintain their current level of function. It should be noted, however, that therapy will not stop the progression of the disease. For patients presenting with painful Dupuytren nodules, corticosteroid injection may help to soften and flatten the nodules.[11]

◎ Clinical Pearl

When hand therapy clients present for treatment of Dupuytren-related digital flexion contractures (usually referred by their primary care physician), ask the client if they have ever consulted with a hand surgeon about treatment options. If not, consider facilitating a referral (either directly with the client or through the referring physician). These clients need to be aware of all their treatment options, which can only be determined after examination by a hand surgeon.

Minimally Invasive Options

Nonsurgical physician-administered interventions have been developed to correct flexion contractures. These include needle aponeurotomy and injection of collagenase—both followed by manual manipulation—to break up Dupuytren cords. These procedures avoid large incisions on the palm, but still result in patient discomfort and may demonstrate earlier recurrence rates when compared to surgery.

Needle Aponeurotomy

Percutaneous needle fasciotomy or needle aponeurotomy (NA) is a minimally invasive technique that uses a small hypodermic needle as a percutaneous scalpel blade to weaken the affected cords to the point where finger manipulation can result in cord rupture and improve finger extension. It should be performed with particular caution in PIP joint contractures when there is a large nodule or cord between the PIP joint flexion crease and the proximal digital crease.[12] NA is strongly discouraged in infiltrative disease, Dupuytren diathesis, or constitutionally treatment-resistant Dupuytren disease, since this will likely result in rapid recurrence.[13] Young age is also a relative contraindication for NA, due to the high likelihood of recurrence.

For precise surface anesthesia, superficial intradermal injections are infiltrated at multiple focal positions along the entire length of the cords targeted for release. Care is taken to avoid partial or complete digital nerve block to allow for

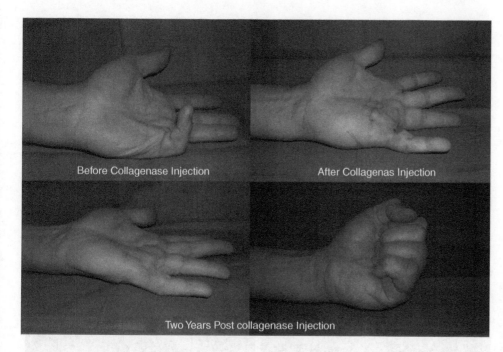

Before Collagenase Injection

After Collagenas Injection

Two Years Post collagenase Injection

FIG. 32.2 Small finger Dupuytren's contracture before and after collagenase injection, and 2 years after collagenase injection.

sensory preservation during the procedure. The needle aponeurotomy is performed with a hypodermic needle, with different surgeons preferring different sized needles. Smaller needles will typically be employed using a combination of perforation and sweeping maneuvers designed to weaken the cords. Larger needles are more typically utilized in a windshield wiper back and forth fashion with the goal of creating a transverse percutaneous fasciotomy. Needle aponeurotomy may either be performed in the surgeon's office or the operating room. With needle aponeurotomy, the recurrence rates are 10% to 20% per year.[14]

The definition of recurrence following Dupuytren release is challenging because of the variable techniques employed. Surgery can completely remove the diseased fascia, while NA and collagenase disrupt cords, leaving disease behind. Van Rijssen et al. redefined recurrence, indirectly, as an increase of the total passive extension deficit of 30 degrees or more in a ray.[12] This measure is reproducible and clinically more relevant when comparing surgical and nonsurgical interventions.

Collagenase

In 2010, the United States Food and Drug Administration approved the clinical use of injectable collagenase produced by the *Clostridium histolyticum* species (Xiaflex) to treat Dupuytren contracture. The same injectable, under the name Xiapex, was approved for use in 2011 in the European Union. Health Canada approved Xiaflex in 2012; and the Australian Therapeutic Goods Administration approved Xiaflex in 2013.

Clinical efficacy and safety of Dupuytren treatment with collagenase was established in two double-blind, placebo-controlled studies.[15,16] In a recent retrospective review comparing NA to collagenase, Nydick et al. showed that short-term (3 months) clinical outcomes and patient satisfaction were equal. Both clinical success (defined as reduction of contracture to within 0–5 degrees of normal) and mean reduction in contracture were similar between groups.[17]

The number of required or recommended collagenase injections is not known and is currently being investigated. The optimum timing of postinjection manipulation after collagenase injection remains unanswered and is typically between 24 and 72 hours postinjection, although a number of physicians have manipulated the treated fingers as long as 1 to 2 weeks after the initial collagenase injection. Following collagenase injection, 5-year recurrence rate was found to be 47%, which is comparable to surgical treatments.[18]

Final Manipulation

Once the cords have been weakened/divided at multiple sites with needle aponeurotomy or collagenase injection, the patient is tested to confirm that all flexor tendons and all digital nerves remain intact. Once this is verified, the treated sites are injected with local anesthetic to achieve combined palmar and digital blocks that will allow forceful manipulation of the fingers without significant pain. The fingers are passively stretched to achieve complete rupture of the cords and to break any residual tethering (Fig. 32.2). The wrist is flexed as each finger is being extended to minimize risk of tendon rupture.

After manipulation following both NA and collagenase injection, any open skin tears are dressed with antibiotic ointment and nonadherent gauze, and an extension orthosis is fabricated. Patients are instructed to wash their hands daily with soap and water and to reapply antibiotic ointment and nonadherent gauze until the wounds are healed. Patients are usually sent to hand therapy within 1 to 3 days of manipulation.

Operative Treatment

Surgery for Dupuytren contracture remains the gold standard treatment option. It offers the most complete release of flexion contracture, the option for excision of diseased fascia, and the lowest overall recurrence rate (5%–10% per year). A variety of

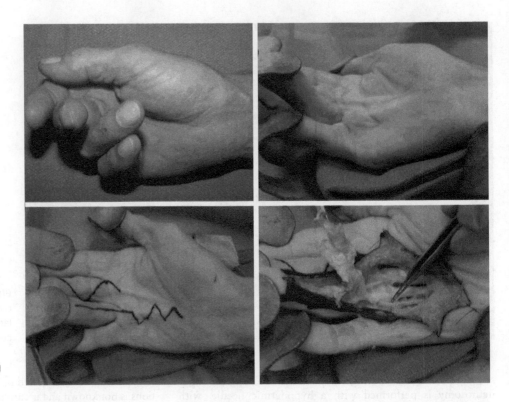

FIG. 32.3 Palmar fasciectomy for Dupuytren's contracture to the ring and middle fingers.

surgical options are available. Despite technique, the goal of surgery is either to divide or excise diseased palmar fascia.[4] In the case of skin deficiency at the time of surgical closure, wounds may be left open to heal or, alternatively, full-thickness skin grafts may be used.

Fasciotomy

Fasciotomy is reserved for those patients too ill to undergo surgery. The fascia is incised to release the contracture. This procedure is associated with a higher recurrence rate compared to fasciectomy.[19]

Regional Fasciectomy

Regional fasciectomy is the most commonly performed procedure for the treatment of Dupuytren disease. All of the diseased fascia is removed, leaving behind normal fascia. It is unlikely that the disease will recur in the excised areas. New disease, however, may occur in adjacent areas (Fig. 32.3).

Dermatofasciectomy

Dermatofasciectomy refers to the removal of the skin in conjunction with the underlying diseased fascia. This procedure may be considered for patients with aggressive disease due to Dupuytren diathesis or those who have recurrent contractures. The skin is replaced with full-thickness skin grafts from either the medial arm or groin.

Total Fasciectomy

Total fasciectomy refers to the removal of all diseased and normal fascia. This should be considered only for patients with Dupuytren diathesis involving a large portion of the hand. With this type

of extensive disease, both Dupuytren cords and PIP joint volar capsular contracture may be present. Single-stage fasciectomy may result in the need for skin grafting due to skin deficiency, and may result in digital ischemia through vascular spasm.[20] In such cases, success has been achieved with the use of a dynamic external fixation device to straighten the PIP joint slowly, over weeks, followed by PIP joint capsulotomy and fasciectomy in a second stage.[21,22]

The wide-awake approach to Dupuytren surgical intervention is a developing trend in hand surgery and involves fasciectomy under local anesthetic with epinephrine but without a tourniquet. Epinephrine is a vasoconstrictor and controls the bleeding. Studies have shown results equivalent to cases done under general anesthesia with the advantage of avoiding general anesthesia risks and allowing for decreased costs.[23,24]

The mainstay of care following surgical fasciectomy involves a bulky dressing with a volar orthosis holding the MP and PIP joints in extension. The initial postoperative dressings remain in place for several days to minimize risk of palmar hematoma; furthermore, nonabsorbable sutures are left in place for at least 14 days.

Hand therapy is a critical component of postoperative care and patients should be instructed by the surgeon that therapy is key to regaining and maintaining finger extension. Therapy also focuses on wound care, edema control, restoring good finger flexion, and improving overall hand function. Therapy should be in the form of a no-tension protocol as described by Evans et al., consisting of gentle active and passive range of motion until the inflammatory phase subsides.[25] A no-tension protocol maximizes tissue oxygenation and nutrition while avoiding complications with unnecessary inflammation, edema, or delayed healing that can occur with aggressive therapy.[25] The no-tension approach also involves orthosis fabrication in a position where there is no wound tension for up to 3 weeks. Too much tension causes inflammation and myofibroblast stimulation, whereas continuous limited tension remodels and softens collagen.[26]

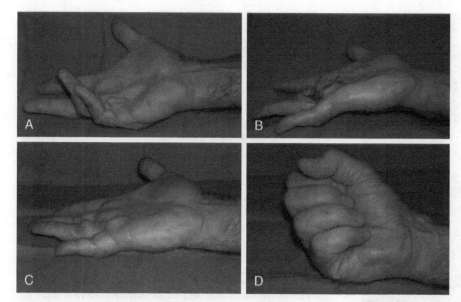

FIG. 32.4 (A) Dupuytren contracture limiting extension of ring and small fingers.
(B) Dupuytren cords are ruptured by forceful manipulation of fingers after collagenase injection. This sometimes results in skin tears, which then heal by secondary intention.
(C) Functional finger extension is restored, along with preservation of
(D) finger flexion.

Complications

The most common complications following fasciectomy for Dupuytren contracture are hematoma (2%–15%), infection (1%–3%), and skin flap necrosis (1%–3%).[27] Patients may also experience numbness in the operative fingers, which is often transient but may represent nerve injury requiring repair. Arterial injury can also occur and is typically repaired intraoperatively. *Therapists should monitor patients closely following vascular repair and use compression with caution.*

Arterial spasm is common and can be caused by arterial stretch with finger extension. If the finger turns white during therapy, the therapist should return the finger to a flexed position and warm the hand. If there is no improvement in perfusion, the hand surgeon should be notified as soon as possible for suture removal and possible reexploration.[4]

Dupuytren flare response sometimes occurs 2 to 3 weeks postoperatively, presenting as stiffness, edema, and pain out of proportion to exam. Flare tends to be more common in females.[28]

Complex regional pain syndrome (CRPS) may present in a similar fashion to Dupuytren flare. It usually occurs later, approximately 4 to 6 weeks postsurgery. If CRPS is suspected, the hand therapist should refer the patient back to the surgeon for appropriate medical management and potential secondary referral to a pain management specialist. In cases where there is more edema than anticipated, or suspected early CRPS, the physician may elect to prescribe a rapidly tapering steroid dosing regimen (for example, a Medrol dosepak) to minimize edema, inflammation, and pain.

⊙ *Clinical Pearl*

Monitor hand therapy clients carefully for infection, excessive edema, and significant pain following any procedure or surgery to release Dupuytren contracture. Do not hesitate to *immediately* refer clients back to the surgeon for evaluation and medical management of these issues. Even if you are not sure there is a problem, it is better to have the surgeon assess the situation. *Early* identification of infection, flare, and beginning CRPS can divert significant postoperative complications.

Complications following NA are generally less than with open techniques. Skin tearing is the most common complication with a reported incidence of 3%.[14] The most commonly reported complications following collagenase injection are localized pain, swelling, bruising, itching, transient regional lymph node pain and enlargement, as well as skin tears (Fig. 32.4). Less common complications include tendon rupture, neurapraxia, and CRPS.[15]

Therapy Guidelines Following Dupuytren Contracture Release

This section offers general guidelines for therapists treating clients who have undergone Dupuytren contracture release. The length of time skilled intervention is required can range from a few visits to a few months. Clients who undergo nonsurgical manipulations (NA and collagenase injections) typically do not require skilled intervention for longer than a month. Clients who undergo fasciectomy surgery can require skilled therapy for 2 to 3 months postsurgery.

Progression of the rehabilitation timeline is determined on a case-by-case basis. It is dependent on the severity of open wounds, rate of tissue healing, tissue response to therapy, and the client's goals for rehabilitation. The timeline will be progressed more slowly for postsurgical clients with large open wounds. The therapist should collaborate with the surgeon prior to the first therapy session to determine accurate timelines for all of the therapy components.

First Therapy Visit

The client's first visit to the hand therapy clinic usually occurs 1 to 2 days after nonsurgical manipulation, and about a week after surgical fasciectomy.

- Remove the bulky dressing and perform the initial evaluation. Assess wound/s, edema, range of motion (ROM), pain, sensation, and functional hand use.
- Educate the client on wound care and monitoring for infection and maceration (the softening of skin resulting from prolonged exposure to moisture).
- Educate the client on edema management techniques.
- Educate the client on monitoring sensation and functional impact.

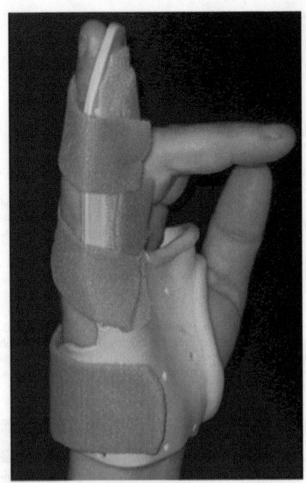

FIG. 32.5 A custom hand-based night extension orthosis is fabricated for the affected/neighboring fingers.

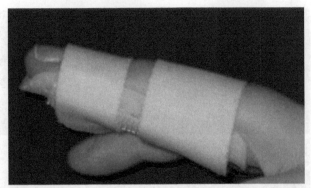

FIG. 32.6 A finger-based proximal interphalangeal (PIP) joint extension orthosis is fabricated if indicated for intermittent daytime wear, especially for clients who have a significant baseline PIP joint contracture.

- Carefully reassess wounds, edema, pain, sensation, ROM, functional hand use, and fit of orthoses. Review the home exercise program and, based on the information obtained during reassessment, update the program. Reiterate to the client that open wounds are not a contraindication to performing ROM exercises.
- Review the orthoses wear schedule(s). If needed, remold orthoses to progress toward the goal of full finger extension. Studies show that orthoses can improve finger extension following post-collagenase or post-needle aponeurotomy manipulation.[30] Orthoses may also require trimming due to edema reduction or the minimization of dressings as wounds heal.
- Review progress toward short-term goals for improved digital flexion and extension, wound closure, decreased edema and pain, and increased light functional hand use.
- Reinforce the timeline for resuming more strenuous activities and confirm that the client is not currently over using their hand.

The number and frequency of subsequent visits is based on clinical presentation and specific skilled needs.

Two to Three Weeks After Manipulation/Surgery

- Carefully monitor finger ROM. If the client is struggling to regain composite flexion, consider introducing composite taping or a dynamic PIP/DIP (distal interphalangeal) flexion orthoses. Confirm that clients are performing intrinsic stretching exercises.
  Evaluate and adjust orthoses at every visit to achieve maximal potential extension.
- Once the wounds have closed, educate the client to incorporate scar-remodeling techniques.
- Continually review the timeline for resuming more strenuous activities. It is not uncommon for clients to want to resume more demanding activities in advance of tissue readiness once all wounds have closed. Educate clients that if they overuse their hand, tissues may respond with increased swelling, pain, stiffness, and possible loss of ROM; this can delay progress.
- Watch for a "flare" reaction between 2 and 4 weeks postprocedure. Flares are not common; however, complaints will include increased edema, joint stiffness, pain, and a loss of ROM. If a client experiences a flare, refer them back to the

- Instruct the client to perform frequent, light-force active and passive ROM exercises with attention focused on digital extension and intrinsic stretching. Educate the client that sutures and/or open wounds are not a contraindication to performing exercises; rather, the exercises are critical to ensuring the best possible outcome.
- Fabricate a custom hand-based night extension orthosis for the affected/neighboring fingers. Also fabricate a finger-based PIP joint extension orthosis (if needed) for intermittent daytime wear; this is especially important for clients who have a significant baseline PIP joint contracture. Ask clients to bring their orthoses to every therapy session for reevaluation of fit (Figs. 32. 5 and 32.6).
- Instruct the client to immediately resume light functional activities using the affected (sometimes bandaged) hand, and to avoid strenuous activity for 4 to 6 weeks. If surgery was extensive, recommend they avoid strenuous activity for 8 to 10 weeks.

Second Therapy Visit: One Day to One Week Later

The timeline for the second visit is dependent on the client's clinical presentation at initial evaluation, the client's understanding of the home program, and the skilled interventions that are required. It can occur as early as 1 day after the first therapy visit but is often a few days to a week later.

physician for medical treatment, which might include a short course of oral steroids or even steroid injections. Do not be over zealous with passive ROM exercises during this time.

Three to Four Weeks After Manipulation/Surgery

- Full motion potential should be achieved by 4 weeks postmanipulation. This can take longer following fasciectomy.
- Monitor clients who may have developed a "flare" between 2 and 4 week postprocedure.
- As appropriate to the client's pain and inflammation levels, initiate graded progressive strengthening exercises. Transition clients to a home strengthening program in 1 to 2 weeks.

Four to Six Weeks After Manipulation/Surgery

- Perform a final reassessment, finalize the home program (including exercise and orthoses needs), and discharge the client to a well-established home program.
- Remember, some clients will progress more slowly through this timeline.

( ) What to Say to Clients

Client education is tailored to individual needs and clinical presentation during the course of hand therapy. The following sections summarize general information and education that should be provided.

Wound Care and Scar Management

Dupuytren release results in varying degrees of open wounds. It is important that clients become comfortable looking at their wounds and performing their own dressing changes (sometimes with the assistance of friends or family members). It is essential to educate clients how to monitor for infection. Tell them to be alert to the following signs and symptoms of infection: increased pain, periwound redness, excessive drainage, foul-smelling discharge, fever, chills, and red streaking up the arm. Instruct clients to immediately contact their surgeon (or seek emergency medical attention) and avoid waiting until the next therapy session for verification of possible infection. Remind clients to follow all medication instructions given by the physician. Tell clients that it is important to complete the entire course of antibiotic(s), regardless of how they feel or think the wound is progressing.

Referring physicians often have their own preferences regarding the cleaning regimen, dressings, ointments, and frequency of dressing changes. Open wounds may benefit from an over-the-counter topical antibiotic ointment (such as Neosporin, Polysporin, or Bacitracin) to facilitate moist wound healing. Laws vary with regard to therapists providing and/or administering medication (even over-the-counter medications and ointments). Check the laws that govern your practice before applying/administering any medication. Instruct clients to cover the wound with ointment, then to place a single layer of nonadherent gauze (such as Xeroform or Adaptic) over the wound, and then wrap everything with light gauze.

Clients should change the gauze dressing two to three times per day to prevent it from drying up and sticking to the wound. Pulling off an adherent dressing disturbs healing tissue. *It is critical to avoid desiccation (drying out) of the wound, especially if there are exposed tendons.*

Clients often make the mistake of trying to protect the wound with an abundance of antibiotic ointment and too many layers of gauze. This can cause skin maceration and eventual skin breakdown. Instruct clients to use ointments and dressings sparingly, and to monitor the periwound area for white and wrinkly skin (a sign of maceration). If maceration is detected, clients should allow the skin to air out and then reduce the amount of ointment utilized. The goal is a moist wound, not a wet wound. When the wound stops draining, transition from a gauze dressing to a Band-Aid until the wound is completely healed.

Educate the client on the physician-directed timelines for when it is acceptable to get wounds "clean wet" as well as "dirty wet." Allowing the hand to get clean wet means using the hand for activities such as showering, shampooing, and washing the hands with soap and water. This is usually allowed at postprocedure day 5 to 7 (or day 10–14 if tendon is exposed). Allowing the hand to get dirty wet means using the hand for activities such as washing dishes, swimming in pools/lakes/oceans, soaking in the Jacuzzi, and gardening. These activities are almost always restricted until wounds are fully healed.

Initiate scar management once wounds are fully healed. Scar management techniques modulate external scar formation to achieve flatter, smoother, suppler, and more cosmetically appealing scars. Initiate compression within 2 weeks of wound closure; use compression products such as silicone gel sheets, scar conformers (such as tape and compression garments), and elastomer (such as Otoform Kc) until aesthetic goals are achieved.

Scar massage is another scar management technique that clients should perform several times each day for a few minutes at a time. Educate the client to massage gently and to use lotion or oil to avoid blister formation and skin breakdown. Clients should also monitor for a tissue inflammatory response, which can encourage excessive scar tissue growth.

Although there is limited high-level evidence supporting the efficacy of scar massage and use of compression products for scar management, these techniques and products are widely used in hand therapy because of their anecdotal benefits.

Edema Management

It is common for the hand to swell following Dupuytren contracture release. There are many techniques therapists use to manage swelling: elevation; gentle retrograde massage; compressive dressings/gloves/stockinettes (such as Coban for digits and Tubigrip for wrists); active motion; and cold therapy. See Chapter 8 for detailed information on edema control techniques.

Range of Motion Exercises

Clients must be instructed to begin ROM exercises immediately upon starting hand therapy. Clients are often afraid to move because of bleeding and open wounds. *Educate clients that they must begin moving regardless of swelling, stitches, or open wounds.* Prioritize digital extension and intrinsic stretching.

ROM exercises typically encompass both active and gentle passive ROM (flexion and extension) movements at every finger joint, especially the MP and PIP joints. Exercises should be performed frequently to allow the tissue to accommodate to the new stresses. Tissue responds better to frequent sessions of light-force

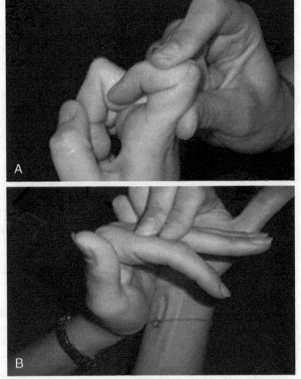

FIG. 32.7 (A) Demonstration of intrinsic stretching. Metacarpophalangeal (MP) extension with proximal interphalangeal (PIP) flexion. (B) Demonstration of reverse blocking by passively holding the MP joint in flexion and actively extending the PIP joint.

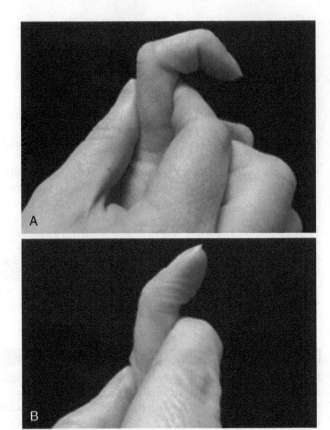

FIG. 32.8 Individual joint blocking of the (A) proximal interphalangeal and (B) distal interphalangeal joints for maximal differential excursion of the (A) flexor digitorum superficialis and (B) flexor digitorum profundus, respectively.

exercise than to infrequent sessions of high-force exercise. Many therapists suggest that gentle, controlled exercises be performed 5 to 10 repetitions, 4 to 6 times per day.

Clients often report that it is difficult to maintain ROM at the 2 to 3 weeks postprocedure time frame. This is because of the proliferative nature of soft-tissue healing. The therapist and client should monitor ROM closely and continue frequent gentle motion exercises. Educate clients to expect this natural occurrence to avoid frustration and unnecessary setbacks resulting from over-aggressive exercise sessions during this time frame.

Passive Finger Motion

Passive ROM should include individual flexion/extension of the MP, PIP, and DIP joints; composite finger flexion/extension; and intrinsic stretching (Fig. 32.7A).

Active Finger Motion

Active ROM should include tendon gliding exercises, composite fisting, finger abduction/adduction, and individual blocking of the PIP and DIP joints for maximal differential excursion of the flexor digitorum superficialis and flexor digitorum profundus tendons (Fig. 32.8). Regaining active digital flexion is usually not difficult for clients. This is partially because the hand was postured in flexion prior to the contracture release, and partially because clients naturally want to work on making a fist. Hand therapists should take proactive steps to prevent clients from developing intrinsic tightness, which may negatively affect active digital motion.

Focus on digital extension exercises, particularly active extension at the MP and PIP joints. Instruct the client in the following exercises for the MP joint: (1) isolated extensor digitorum communis exercises (active MP joint extension with PIPs/DIPs positioned in flexion); (2) finger lifts (palm flat on the table while actively extending the MP joint), both individually and together; (3) active MP joint flexion/extension with PIP/DIP joints held in extension; and (4) active finger abduction/adduction with fingers in full extension (Fig. 32.9A and B).

For the PIP joint, instruct the client in reverse blocking exercises (see Fig. 32.7B). Reverse blocking requires the client to flex the MP joint, place dorsal support against the proximal phalanx, and actively extend the PIP/DIP joints. Doing this allows the extensor digitorum to exert more leverage across the PIP joints and provides a better position for the lumbrical muscles to extend the PIP/DIP joints, thus isolating PIP extension. In some cases, clients require instruction in wrist, forearm, elbow, and shoulder ROM if there was prolonged immobilization or fear of movement.

Strength

Assess grip and pinch strength, and perform manual muscle testing of the wrist and forearm. Assess proximal strength if appropriate to the client's goals. Instruct the client in a graded, progressive strengthening program designed to help them achieve their functional goals. Limit formal strengthening in the clinic to purposeful sessions requiring skilled need and skilled monitoring. Transition clients to a home strengthening program within 1 to 2 weeks.

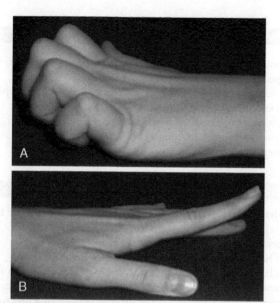

FIG. 32.9 (A) Demonstration of isolated extensor digitorum communis exercises (active MP joint extension with PIPs/DIPs positioned in flexion). (B) Demonstration of individual finger lift. Palm flat on the table while emphasizing active extension at the MP joint.

Sensation

Digital nerves are commonly disturbed or stretched during contracture release procedures. This usually presents in the form of a temporary neurapraxia. Educate clients to monitor an insensate hand during functional use. Clients must be aware of sharp or hot items encountered in daily life activities; this is crucial to avoid unnecessary injury. If sensation fails to improve, instruct clients to discuss concerns directly with the physician.

Orthoses

A custom volar extension orthosis is typically fabricated after Dupuytren release to take advantage of the newly extended tissue. Some studies refute the routine use of orthotics following fasciectomy.[26,31,32] However, there are simply not enough quality studies that accurately measure client adherence to orthotic use to determine its effectiveness and clinical significance.[29]

Following collagenase injections, a hand-based extension orthosis for the affected digits is usually recommended for 8 weeks of nighttime wear.[15] Some physicians will recommend 12 to 16 weeks of nighttime extension orthosis use. The length of time clients should continue nighttime extension orthotic use is based on each client's ability to maintain active and passive digital extension. The orthosis is fabricated at the first therapy visit (over dressings, if necessary) and requires remolding/adjusting as the dressings are modified, as swelling subsides, and as increased extension is gained. The orthosis is gradually remolded into more extension as tissues allow. *The orthosis should be comfortable, not cause any pressure areas, and avoid aggressive positioning that causes flare or compromises vascular structures.*

Additionally, if a finger had a significant PIP joint contracture released, with extensor tendon attenuation, consider fabricating a custom finger-based extension orthosis to be worn intermittently during the day for several weeks. It is postulated that holding the PIP joint in full passive extension with a finger orthosis, and limiting full active and passive PIP joint flexion for several weeks, may contribute to improved extension.[33] This will also

allow the lateral bands that may have migrated volar to the axis of the PIP joint to realign, and may allow for relative tightening of an attenuated central slip.

As active PIP joint flexion is initiated, monitor for extensor lag. Active flexion is advanced as long as active extension is maintained. Consider using a relative motion flexion orthosis in cases of significant PIP joint extensor lag.[34] Relative motion orthoses have been shown to improve active PIP joint extension. *However, use caution to ensure that the relative MP joint flexion in these orthoses does not cause a secondary MP joint flexion contracture.* In most cases, use a relative motion orthosis during the day and the extension orthosis at night.

> ### ◎ Clinical Pearl
>
> Clients often worry that wearing the night extension orthosis will hamper rehabilitation of the hand because the hand feels very stiff when the orthosis is removed in the morning. These clients will sometimes just stop wearing the night orthosis. Educate clients that it is normal to experience stiffness when they first take the orthosis off in the morning. After a few repetitions making a gentle fist, the significant stiffness should resolve. Educate the client that continuing the night extension orthosis for several weeks is important for a good outcome.
>
> Conversely, it is important to educate clients that wearing the orthosis for prolonged periods of time will not prevent recurrence of the disease.

Modalities

There are numerous modalities that can be utilized during hand therapy following Dupuytren contracture release. There is data that suggests low-level laser therapy alters cellular function and induces biological healing, and is therefore beneficial for open wound closure.[35] For edema and pain modulation, interferential current and transcutaneous electrical nerve stimulation have high client satisfaction ratings and are widely used despite the lack of rigorous supportive scientific data.[36] Cold therapy is also recommended as an adjunct to other therapeutic interventions.

Once the wounds are closed, superficial thermal agents such as paraffin and moist heat are beneficial for increasing collagen extensibility, improving blood flow, and offering some pain relief while decreasing joint stiffness. Thermal (continuous wave) ultrasound can also be used on scar tissue to increase the temperature of isolated deep and superficial tissue to promote intracellular activity and tissue exensibility.[36]

See Chapter 9 for more information on using physical agent modalities in the hand clinic.

Resuming Functional Activities

Light functional activities using the affected hand (such as eating, grooming, dressing, and light meal preparation) are immediately encouraged. More strenuous activities (such as golf, tennis, gardening, and use of screwdrivers and hammers) should be avoided for at least 4 to 6 weeks postprocedure. If surgery was extensive, strenuous activity should be restricted for 8 to 10 weeks.

> ### ♡ Tips From the Field
>
> Take time at the onset of therapy to explain to clients the diagnosis, clinical presentation, and expectations for therapy. Even though physicians try to prepare clients for bruising and skin tears, as well

as for the duration of postprocedure hand therapy, clients often have different expectations of the rehabilitation process. Strive to impart to clients a good understanding of the process, commitment, and personal responsibility required for successful hand rehabilitation.

Clients must be capable of monitoring their own wound, and this means the client must be able to look at the wound. If a client reports that looking at open skin tears, blood, or large incisions might be difficult at the first postoperative visit, the dressing can be removed with the client in supine. This minimizes the risk for a vasovagal reaction (a sudden drop in heart rate and blood pressure that can cause the client to faint). It is, however, critical to coach the client to look at the wound daily to monitor for infection.

The presence of open wounds often interferes with taking accurate joint ROM measurements. A gross description of available movement, such as the distance from the fingertip to the distal palmar crease, can be utilized during this time.

It is imperative to recognize and manage secondary deficits resulting from long-standing contractures. Long-standing PIP joint flexion contractures can contribute to central slip extensor tendon attenuation at the PIP joint, lateral band migration resulting in a boutonnière deformity, or volar plate and collateral ligament shortening. Long-standing MP joint flexion contractures can result in limited PIP joint motion due to intrinsic muscle tightness.

Reinforce to clients that they must perform ROM exercises despite sutures or open wounds. Tell them to expect some bleeding during range of motion exercises, but they should exercise anyway.

As the wounds heal and tissues begin to contract, carefully monitor finger extension. Do not allow skin or scar tightening to affect ROM.

Screen for ROM deficits in the entire upper extremity, and address any issues in the home exercise program.

Monitor the client's pain response at every session because Dupuytren flare and/or CRPS are potential complications.

> **Precautions and Concerns**

Communicate with the referring physician to determine if there are any specific restrictions or precautions to be aware of.
- *Closely monitor for signs of infection and refer back to the physician immediately if infection is suspected.*
- *Watch for signs of Dupuytren flare and/or CRPS.*
- *When making the orthosis, take special care not to create excessive tension on the tissue.*

? Questions to Ask the Doctor

Ask the referring physician any questions you have that are not answered by information included with the therapy referral. Do this prior to the client's first therapy visit.
- What postprocedure day can hand therapy be initiated?
- What type(s) of orthoses does the client require? Which fingers should be included in the orthotic(s)? What is the recommended wear schedule? If the surgeon performed a first web-space contracture release, is a C-bar orthosis necessary to prevent first web-space contracture?
- If the surgeon placed a Penrose drain during the fasciectomy, when can the drain be removed?
- Are there any restrictions or precautions?
- Are there any specific instructions for dressings and/or wound care management?
- When can the wound get wet? (Clarify "clean wet" versus "dirty wet.")
- Is the client cleared for both active and passive ROM? If not, what is the timeline to initiate these motions? When can light strengthening be initiated?
- When can the client resume strenuous activity?

References

1. Shih B, Bayat A: Scientific understanding and clinical management of Dupuytren disease, *Nat Rev Rheumatol* 6:715–726, 2010.
2. DiBenedetti DB, Nguyen D, Zografos L, et al.: Prevalence, incidence, and treatments of Dupuytren's disease in the United States: results from a population-based study, *Hand* 6(2):149–158, 2011.
3. Hindocha S, McGrouther DA, Ardeshir Bayat: Epidemiological evaluation of Dupuytren's disease incidence and prevalence rates in relation to etiology, *Hand* 4(3):256–269, 2009.
4. Khashan M, Smitham PJ, Khan WS, Goddard NJ: Dupuytren's disease: review of the current literature, *Open Orthop J* 5:283–288, 2011.
5. Ketchum LD: The rational for treating the nodule in Dupuytren's disease, *Plast Reconstr Surg Glob Open* 2(12):e278, 2014.
6. Rayan GM: Dupuytren disease: anatomy, pathology, presentation, and treatment, *JBJS* 89A:190–198, 2007.
7. Hindocha S, Stanley JK, Watson S, Bayat A: Dupuytren's diathesis revisited: evaluation of prognostic indicators for risk of disease recurrence, *J Hand Surg Am* 31(10):1626–1634, 2006.
8. Elliot D: The early history of contracture of the palmar fascia, *J Hand Surg* 13B:246–253, 1988.
9. Ball C, Nanchahal J: The use of splinting as a non-surgical treatment for dupuytren's disease: a pilot study, *Br J Hand Ther* 7(3):76–78, 2002.
10. Larocerie-Salgado J, Davidson J: Nonoperative treatment of PIPJ flexion contractures associated with Dupuytren's disease, *J Hand Surg Eru* 37(8):722–727, 2012.
11. Sood A, Therattil PJ, Kim HJ, Lee ES: Corticosteroid injection in the management of Dupuytren nodules: a review of the literature, *Eplasty* 15:e42, 2015.
12. Van Rijssen AL, Gerbrandy FSJ, Linden HT, Klip H, Werker PMN: A comparison of the direct outcomes of percutaneous needle fasciotomy and limited fasciectomy for Dupuytren's disease: a 6-week follow-up study, *J Hand Surg* 31A:717–725, 2006.
13. Degreeef I, De Smet L: Risk factors in Dupuytren's diathesis: is recurrence after surgery predictable? In Degreef I, editor: *Therapy resisting Dupuytren's disease. New perspectives in adjuvant treatment*, Leuven, 2009, KatholickeUniversiteit, pp 50–55.
14. Morhart M: Pearls and pitfalls of needle aponeurotomy in Dupuytren's disease, *Plast Reconst Surg* 135(3):817–825, 2015.
15. Hurst LC, Badalamente MA, Hentz VR, et al.: Injectable collagenase clostridium histolyticum for Dupuytren's contracture, *NEJM* 361(3):968–979, 2009.
16. Gilpin D, Coleman S, Hall S, Houston A, Karrasch J, Jones N: Injectable collagenase clostridium histolyticum: a new nonsurgical treatment for Dupuytren's disease, *J Hand Surg Am* 35(12):2027–2038, 2010.
17. Nydick JA, Olliff BW, Garcia MJ, Hess AV, Stone JD: A comparison of percutaneous needle fasciotomy and collagenase injection for Dupuytren disease, *J Hand Surg Am* 38(12):2377–2380, 2013.
18. Peimer CA, Blazar P, Coleman S, Kaplan FT, Smith T, Lindau T: Dupuytren contracture recurrence following treatment with collagenase clostridium histolytium (CORDLESS [collagenase option for reduction of Dupuytren's long-term evaluation of safety study]): 5-year data, *J Hand Surg Am* 40(6):1597–1605, 2015.
19. Rodrigo JJ, Niebauer JJ, Brown JL, Doyle JR: Treatment of Dupuytren's contracture: long-term results after fasciotomy and fascial excision, *J Bone Joint Surg* 58A380–387, 1976.

20. Lawson GA, Smith AA: Dynamic external fixation in the treatment of Dupuytren's contracture. In *Dupuytren's disease and related hyperproliferative disorders*, 2012, pp 297–303.

21. Rives K, Gelberman R, Smith B, et al.: Severe contractures of the proximal interphalangeal joint in Dupuytren's disease: result of a prospective trial of operative correction and dynamic extension splint, *J Hand Surg Am* 17:1153–1159, 1992.

22. Houshian S, Gynning B, Schroder H: Chronic flexion contracture of proximal interphalangeal joint treated with the compass hinge external fixator. A consecutive series of 27 cases, *J hand Surg Br* 27(4):356–358, 2002.

23. Nelson R, Higgings A, Conrad J, Bell M, Lalonde D: The wide-awake approach to Dupuytren's disease: fasciectomy under local anesthetic with epinephrine, *Hand* 5(2):117–124, 2010.

24. Bismil QMK, Bismil MSK, Bismil A, et al.: The development of one-stop wide awake Dupuytren's fasciectomy service: a retrospective review, *JRSM Short Rep* 3(7):48, 2012.

25. Evans RB, Dell PC, Fiolkowski P: A clinical report of the effect of mechanical stress on functional results after fasciectomy for Dupuytren's contracture, *J Hand Ther* 15:331–339, 2002.

26. Kemler MA, Houpt P, van der Horst CM: A pilot study assessing the effectiveness of postoperative splinting after limited fasciectomy for Dupuytren's disease, *J Hand Surg Br* 37(8):733–737, 2012.

27. Krefter C, Marks M, Hensler S, Herren DB, Calcagni M: Complications after treating Dupuytren's disease. a systematic literature review, *Hand Surg Rehabil* 36(5):322–329, 2017.

28. Zemel NP: Dupuytren's contracture in women, *Hand Clin* 7(4):707–711, 1991.

29. Sweet S, Blackmore S: Surgical and therapy update on the management of Dupuytren's disease, *J Hand Ther* 27(2):77–84, 2014.

30. Skirven TM, Bachoura A, Jacoby SM, Culp RW, Osterman AL: The effect of a therapy protocol for increasing correction of severely contracted proximal interphalangeal joints caused by Dupuytren disease and treated with collagenase injection, *J Hand Surg Am* 38(4):684–689, 2013.

31. Jerosch-Herold C, Shepstone L, Chojnowski AJ, Larson D, Barrett E: Night-time splinting after fasciectomy or dermofasciectomy for Dupuytren's contracture: a pragmatic, multi-center, randomised controlled trial, *BMC Musculoskelet Disord* 12:136–145, 2011.

32. Larson D, Jerosch-Herold C: Clinical effectiveness of post-operative splinting after surgical release of Dupuytren's contracture; a systematic review, *BMC Musculoskelet Disord* 9:104–110, 2008.

33. Skirven TM, Bachoura A, Jacoby SM, Culp RW, Osterman AL: The effect of a therapy protocol for increasing correction of severely contracted proximal interphalangeal joints caused by Dupuytren disease and treated with collagenase injection, *J. Hand Surg* 38(4):684–689, 2013.

34. Hirth MJ, Howell JW, O'Brien L: Relative motion orthoses in the management of various hand conditions a scoping review, *J Hand Ther* 29(4):405–432, 2016.

35. De Abreu Chaves ME, De Araujo AR, Cruz Piancastelli AC, Pinotti M: Effects of low-power light therapy on wound healing: LASER xLED, *An Bras Dermatol* 89(4):616–623, 2014.

36. Hartzell TL, Rubinstein R, Herman M: Therapeutic modalities—an updated review for the hand surgeon, *J Hand Surg* 37A:597–621, 2012.

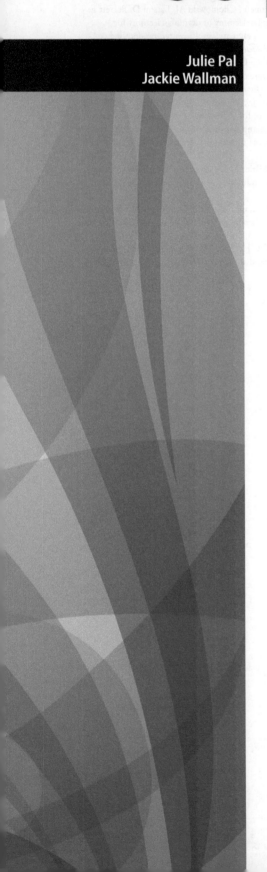

33

Ganglions and Tumors of the Hand and Wrist

Julie Pal
Jackie Wallman

Tumors of the forearm and hand can arise from any tissue in the upper extremity, including synovium, fat, skin, lymphatics, nerves, blood vessels, or bone. Tumors are classified into three categories: (1) tumor-mimicking lesions; (2) benign tumors; and (3) malignant tumors.[1] A hand therapist is likely to see these clients on their caseload because of the prevalence with which these clients come to our referring physicians. For this reason, it is important to understand the common sequence of diagnosis and treatment, the tissues involved, and how to manage both the physical care and psychological implications of an upper extremity tumor.

Ganglion Cysts

Ganglion cysts are the most common tumors, accounting for 15% to 60% of all cases of the hand and wrist.[1] The presentation and diagnosis can be confusing, and treatment is variable. A thorough medical history is vital for providing appropriate client care. Both the physician and the hand therapist should be aware of related trauma or repetitive use of the extremity, any period of rapid change in ganglion cyst growth, and/or pain. Although malignancy is unlikely, significant changes in growth, size, and appearance warrant prompt referral to a hand surgeon.

Diagnosis and Epidemiology

A ganglion is a mucin-filled soft-tissue cyst, formed from the synovial lining of a joint or tendon sheath.[2] Theories on formation of ganglions include mucoid degeneration, synovial herniation, and trauma to the joint capsule or ligaments.[2] Ganglions are generally painless. They tend to fluctuate in size with time and activity, and they may or may not resolve without intervention. Ganglions can appear gradually over time or suddenly. They usually occur singly and in very specific locations, but they have been reported in almost every joint of the wrist and hand.[2] If enlarged, the ganglion can produce pain secondary to pressure on nearby tissues. Clients tend to report pain in positions of extreme wrist flexion, extension, or with weight-bearing activities through the wrist.[1] The posterior interosseous nerve (PIN) in the dorsal wrist capsule, the median nerve as it passes through the carpal tunnel, and the ulnar nerve within Guyon's canal at the wrist have all been known to be symptomatic when there is a ganglion near these structures.[2] Usually, ganglion cysts arise from the scapholunate joint and ligament in the wrist. The main cyst is connected by a mucin-filled cleft interconnecting the cyst to the underlying joint (Fig. 33.1).[2]

Demographics

Ganglions can occur at any age in either gender, and they can resolve spontaneously or require therapeutic or surgical intervention. Ganglions occur more frequently in women between the teenage years through middle adulthood. They are found more often in clients with ligamentous laxity. A recent history of trauma or injury is present in 10% of cases, or there may be a history of repetitive use of the hand or extremity.[2] Ganglions have been diagnosed in children, and spontaneous healing almost always occurs within 2 years of diagnosis in a child. A pediatric client is seldom a surgical candidate for ganglion excision.[1]

Anatomical Sites

Dorsal wrist ganglions are the most common type of ganglion cyst, comprising 60% to 70% of all hand and wrist ganglions.[2] They are seen over the dorsum of the wrist, usually between the extensor pollicus longus and extensor digitorum communis, at the level of the scapholunate ligament. **Volar wrist ganglions** are the second most common type,

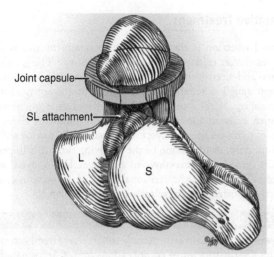

FIG. 33.1 The ganglion and scapholunate *(SL)* attachments are shown with connection to the joint via mucin clefts through capsule. *L*, Lunate; *S*, scaphoid. *(From Athanasian EA. Bone and soft tissue tumors. In: Wolfe SW, Hotchkiss RN, Pederson WC, et al. eds. Green's Operative Hand Surgery. 6th ed. Philadelphia, PA: Churchill Livingstone; 2011.)*

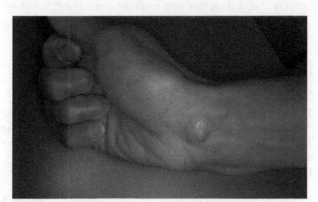

FIG. 33.2 Volar wrist ganglion.

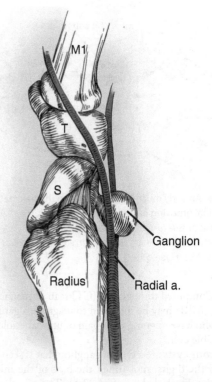

FIG. 33.3 The usual relationship of the ganglion to the radial artery and the volar capsule. *M1*, First metacarpal; *S*, scaphoid; *T*, trapezium. *(From Athanasian EA. Bone and soft tissue tumors. In: Wolfe SW, Hotchkiss RN, Pederson WC, et al. eds. Green's Operative Hand Surgery. 6th ed. Philadelphia, PA: Churchill Livingstone; 2011.)*

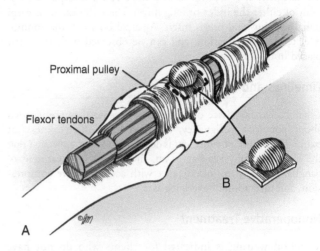

FIG. 33.4 (A) Volar retinacular ganglion in situ on the proximal annular ligament (A1 pulley) of the flexor tendon sheath. **B,** Excised specimen with a surrounding margin of tendon sheath. *(From Athanasian EA. Bone and soft tissue tumors. In: Wolfe SW, Hotchkiss RN, Pederson WC, et al. eds. Green's Operative Hand Surgery. 6th ed. Philadelphia, PA: Churchill Livingstone; 2011.)*

comprising 15% to 20% of cases. They are usually associated with the underlying scapholunate ligament and less often with the scaphotrapezial joint. A volar wrist ganglion is commonly seen on the radial aspect of the wrist (over the flexor carpi radialis tendon) (Fig. 33.2). When evaluating a volar wrist ganglion, the therapist should palpate the cyst and perform an **Allen's vascular test**. A mass that is pulsatile in nature or obstructs blood flow to the hand is indicative of a vascular tumor, but it can easily be misidentified as a volar wrist ganglion because of the proximity to the radial artery and the scapholunate joint (Fig. 33.3).

Retinacular cysts are a type of ganglion that develops from a tendon sheath rather than a joint. A **volar retinacular ganglion** is palpable and symptomatic near the proximal interphalangeal (PIP) joint or the metacarpophalangeal (MP) joint. An **extensor retinacular ganglion** is uncommon but, if detected, usually involves the first dorsal compartment (abductor pollicis longus and extensor pollicis brevis) and can be associated with **deQuervain tenosynovitis** (inflammation of the synovial lining surrounding the extensors within the first dorsal compartment). Retinacular cysts form on the tendon sheath itself, not on the tendon within (Fig. 33.4).

Hidden or **occult ganglions** can be a source of unexplained wrist pain and disproportionate tenderness.[2] Due to the deep

location in the wrist, this type of ganglion is a common source of pressure on the PIN within the dorsal capsule, causing dorsal wrist pain.[2] The ganglion may be detected by placing the client's wrist in marked volar flexion.[2] An **intraosseus ganglion** is rare and usually is detected with involvement of the scaphoid or

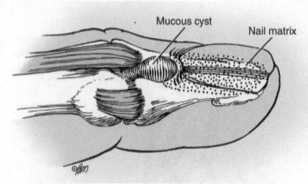

FIG. 33.5 An early mucous cyst resting on the nail matrix may cause longitudinal grooving of the nail in some cases. (*From Athanasian EA. Bone and soft tissue tumors. In: Wolfe SW, Hotchkiss RN, Pederson WC, et al. eds. Green's Operative Hand Surgery. 7th ed. Philadelphia, PA: Elsevier; 2017, page 2005, Figure 59.29.*)

lunate. Computed tomography (CT) scan or magnetic resonance imaging (MRI) may be indicated to diagnose a ganglion in these clients who have ongoing wrist pain of unclear etiology and without a visible cyst.

Mucous cysts are a type of ganglion that is seen on the dorsal joints of the digits, most often the base of the middle phalanx and/or the distal phalanx (Fig. 33.5). There is close association between mucous cysts and osteoarthritis of the distal interphalangeal (DIP) and PIP joints.[2] The mucous cyst typically forms on the DIP joint over an osteophyte known as a **Heberden node.** Longitudinal grooving of the nail secondary to pressure on the nail matrix may be seen with this.[2] A **carpal boss** is an osteoarthritic spur that forms over the carpometacarpal (CMC) joint of either the index or long finger where the extensor carpi radialis longus and brevis insert. A carpal boss is firm, nonmobile, tender to palpation, and can be observed with the wrist placed in flexion.

Timelines and Healing

Clients seek the advice of a physician because they are worried about potential malignancy, impaired function, weakness, or pain.[2] The course of treatment is dependent on the approach that the client and physician agree on. Indications for treatment of ganglia include pain, interference with activity, nerve compression, and ulceration of overlying skin.[3]

Nonoperative Treatment

Watchful waiting is indicated for clients who do not have persistent pain or functional limitation.[2] The surgeon may also choose to aspirate the cyst with or without a corticosteroid. Studies have shown 60% recurrence of ganglions with this approach, although resolution can occur with repeated aspiration.[1]

> ### ◎ *Clinical Pearl*
>
> Aspiration and/or corticosteroid injection is not commonly performed for volar wrist ganglions because of proximity to the radial artery and potential for complications.[1] Surgery is best reserved for clients with persistently symptomatic ganglions.

Operative Treatment

Surgical resection is the most effective treatment and is classically used after exhausting nonsurgical options.[4] The ganglion is excised and a portion of the attached joint capsule is removed to prevent ganglion recurrence while protecting ligaments for carpal stability. If the tumor is solid or diagnosis is questionable, an open excision allows for biopsy of the tumor. A client who chooses to have a mucous cyst excised usually does so for aesthetic reasons, pain, or ulceration of the overlying skin. It is important for the underlying osteophyte to also be excised to avoid recurrence.[1] Occasionally, the excisional aspect of the mucous cyst and underlying osteophyte requires a skin graft or flap.[5]

> ### ◎ *Clinical Pearl*
>
> Newer techniques in arthroscopic surgery have been shown to minimize postoperative complications from scar formation in dorsal wrist ganglions. The procedure is most suitable if the ganglion is on the dorsal aspect of the wrist in association with the scapholunate ligament. These procedures can be performed with minimal tissue trauma and better evaluation of the radioscaphoid and midcarpal joints of the wrist. This helps ensure that a ganglion with multiple clefts is excised in its entirety.[5]

Timeline for Therapy

Nonoperative

Therapeutic timelines vary considerably depending on whether the client has joint stiffness, functional impairment, and/or pain. Therapeutic approaches aim to preserve and improve function while decreasing pain. Intervention should include:

1. Symptom management: Providing tissue support with the use of a resting orthosis
2. Gentle home exercise programs (HEPs): Aimed at maintaining or improving range of motion (ROM) and/or function
3. Instruction in pain management: Using heat and cold modalities (as well as instruction in contraindications and precautions for both). For example, the client should not use heat if pain and edema have increased; in this case, a cold pack would be appropriate for acute symptoms.

Postoperative

If the client has an open tumor excision, a bulky dressing will be in place for approximately 5 days. ROM is usually initiated within the first 2 weeks postoperatively. Initially, it is best to avoid heat modalities, passive range of motion (PROM), or aggressive active range of motion (AROM). The client should be instructed in gentle AROM exercises to reduce scar formation, decrease stiffness, and reduce edema in the wrist and digits. These activities may be painful initially; clients are instructed to perform exercises slowly. With dorsal wrist ganglion excision, volar wrist flexion *must* be emphasized.

If a skin graft or local flap is used for coverage following a DIP joint mucous cyst excision, the DIP joint will be immobilized and the graft will be protected for approximately 2 weeks prior to beginning motion. Another reason to immobilize following a mucous cyst excision would be if the extensor tendon had to be detached and reattached to excise the cyst.

Precaution. *Following mucous cyst excisions, be cautious when considering passive joint stretching to avoid exacerbation of the underlying osteoarthritic joint changes.*

- What structures were involved?
- If the ganglion was at the wrist, is wrist stability a concern?
- What are the expectations for recovery of ROM?
- When is AROM to be initiated?
- Should PROM be avoided?
- Are there any precautions?
- Is an orthosis indicated? If so, in what position? Should it be used for stability or for symptom management?[6]

( ) **What to Say to Clients**

Nonoperative Approach

"You may notice a fluctuation in the size of your ganglion from time to time. You may also notice a fluctuation in size when you change the position of your hand and wrist. With heavy or repetitive use, pain and symptoms may increase but usually subside with tissue rest. Wearing a wrist orthosis may be helpful."

Operative Approach

"You might experience stiffness and pain with the use of your hand following surgery. Allow yourself time to heal. It is important to use your wrist, but your symptoms will increase with heavy use or activity. The goal is to have decreased pain. To achieve this, avoid the 'no pain, no gain' approach to rehabilitation."

Evaluation Tips

- Postoperative stiffness is best avoided with early and gentle wrist and digit ROM.
- Begin with AROM, especially volar wrist flexion. Avoid aggressive active motion or passive stretching initially.
- Pinch and grip strength testing should not be performed as part of the initial evaluation if the client has been referred to hand therapy following a surgical excision. Strength testing is too stressful to the early recovering tissues.
- History of acute trauma, activity with resultant wrist pain, or onset of a ganglion may be indicative of an underlying scapholunate sprain or other ligament sprain. Avoid aggressive ROM and strengthening if the ganglion is a result of trauma. If pain and functional limitations persist, the client should be reevaluated by a hand surgeon.
- Dorsal wrist ganglions can be easily confused with extensor tendon synovitis or a CMC boss. If the client has diffuse dorsal wrist edema and/or pain with wrist and/or digit extension, the client most likely has extensor tenosynovitis. A CMC boss can be distinguished by a bony landmark at the base of the second or third metacarpal.

Diagnosis-Specific Information That Affects Clinical Reasoning

Addressing the client's initial concerns when they are diagnosed with a ganglion is important. Typically, improved use of their

hand without pain or improved cosmesis is the client's primary goal. "Perfect" ROM and strength should not take precedence over pain reduction and stability of the wrist.

♡ **Tips From the Field**

Orthoses

A forearm-based wrist orthosis can help support tissue and joints of the wrist in clients who are being managed conservatively (no surgery). The orthosis should be functional so that the client is able to perform activity with minimal pain. The client uses the orthosis as needed for symptom relief.

On occasion, a DIP protection orthosis may be indicated for a client who has had a mucous cyst excision.

Client Expectations

Communication is vital between therapist and client for a successful outcome. The hand therapist must be clear about realistic goals for therapy and the importance of controlled progression of exercise and activity. Likewise, the therapist should pay close attention to the client's goals and concerns in order to tailor a treatment plan that achieves these objectives.

Flare-Ups

It is inevitable that clients will aggravate their symptoms from time to time. A flare of pain or edema is best treated with rest, orthosis use, heat or cold, and activity modification. Symptoms will resolve as long as the tissues are not continually aggravated.

Scar Maturation

A client who has had a ganglion cyst excised should be taught scar management techniques as soon as the sutures are removed and the skin is healed enough to tolerate this type of friction and pressure. The client should be instructed in scar massage with gentle pressure and skin mobilization in order to limit excessive scar formation and adhesions to underlying structures. Silicone gel sheeting or paper tape can be used by the client on healed incision sites to assist with controlled scar formation.

Complications

The most common postoperative complication is early ganglion recurrence following surgical excision. If a ganglion has not been excised completely, there is a high likelihood that it will return. Repeat excision can be performed; however, scar formation and adherence to underlying structures are of utmost concern with repeat surgical excision in the same area. **Neuroma** formation can also be a complication following a surgical procedure if there is damage to a branch of a nearby sensory nerve.

Stiffness of the wrist or digits can be expected following a ganglion excision and exacerbated by prolonged orthosis use. If volar wrist flexion limitations persist following dorsal wrist ganglion excision, a very gentle static progressive wrist flexion orthosis is indicated. Treatment techniques such as "heat and stretch" with the wrist placed in flexion to tolerance during heat application can also be helpful. If the client has underlying osteoarthritis of the digits or wrist, care should be taken when initiating gentle passive stretches to avoid a flare reaction and increased pain.

> **Precautions and Concerns**

- *With an excised dorsal wrist ganglion, the therapist should address and closely monitor wrist flexion because this motion is very difficult for the client to regain.*
- *Monitor postoperative wound healing. Exercise that puts excessive stress on a wound or incision with sutures delays healing and increases scar formation.*
- *If a skin graft or flap is required for a mucous cyst excision, avoid tension on the graft. Heat and cold modalities and DIP joint motion are contraindicated until approved by the surgeon. The client may require a protective DIP orthosis.*
- *AROM of the fingers and thumb are important postoperatively to avoid digital stiffness, to prevent and improve edema in the hand, and to maintain soft tissue mobility. Provide a HEP for gentle digital AROM early in therapy.*

Other Tumors of the Hand and Wrist

Most of the soft-tissue masses that occur in the forearm and hand are benign. Of those that are benign, many can be diagnosed clinically, require no treatment, and are asymptomatic.[2] Most of the soft-tissue tumors in the forearm and hand are not painful. The exceptions are glomus tumors, which are known to be very painful, or tumors that cause compression of a nerve. A small percentage of the tumors are malignant and may require aggressive medical treatment.

Diagnosis and Epidemiology

Diagnosis of a tumor relies on a thorough history and physical examination by a physician. Plain radiographs are often indicated to look for involvement of bone or presence of calcification within soft tissues. If malignancy is a possibility, MRI may be indicated, as it is currently the test of choice to further delineate the anatomy of tumors.[1] Ultrasound, bone scans, and CT scans may also be used to further study the tumor. If malignancy is suspected, a **biopsy** (a sample taken surgically from the tumor) with possible excision is often performed to definitively diagnose the tumor and determine the best course of action.

Types of Tumors

Giant-cell tumors are the second most common soft-tissue tumors seen in the upper extremity. Other names for this benign tumor are **fibrous xanthoma, localized nodular tenosynovitis,** and **pigmented villonodular tenosynovitis.**[2] Although their various names indicate otherwise, the tumor does not uniformly contain giant cells and is not typically associated with the tendon sheath.[2] Giant-cell tumors can be located on the volar or dorsal surface of the hand or finger. The most common location is on the volar surface of the proximal phalanx.[1]

Lipomas are common soft-tissue tumors comprised of mature fat cells and characterized by their soft consistency. Typically, these tumors are not painful unless their slow growth causes compression of a nerve. Their size and location can vary widely in the upper extremity. The most common location within the hand is the deep palmar space.[1]

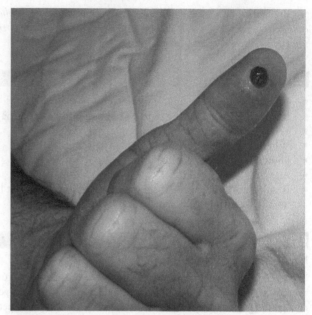

FIG. 33.6 Pyogenic granuloma of the tip of the thumb. (*From Haase SC, Chug KC. Skin tumors. In: Wolfe SW, Hotchkiss RN, Pederson WC, et al. eds.* Green's Operative Hand Surgery. *6th ed. Philadelphia, PA: Churchill Livingstone; 2011.*)

Vascular tumors in the forearm and hand can be either congenital or acquired. These tumors are typically a blue, red, or purple lesion. They may or may not be painful or **pulsatile** (pulse is palpable).[1] Failure of congenital differentiation results in **hemangiomas** (benign tumors of dilated blood vessels), **congenital arteriovenous malformations** (abnormal connection between arteries and veins), and **lymphangiomas** (tumors of lymphatic vessels).[1] Common acquired vascular tumors are pyogenic granulomas and glomus tumors. A **pyogenic granuloma** presents as a red mass that bleeds easily (Fig. 33.6). It is generally accepted that this tumor is caused by trauma and subsequent infection. **Glomus tumors** are benign tumors comprised of all tissues contained in a glomus body. A glomus body is a normal structure comprised of an arteriovenous anastomosis within the retinacular layer of the skin that functions as a thermoregulator. Glomus tumors are most commonly seen in the subungual region of the finger (under the fingernail).[7] The triad of symptoms that often accompany these tumors are cold hypersensitivity, paroxysmal pain, and pinpoint pain.[7] Occasionally, these tumors will invade bone space and erode bone tissue.[7]

An **epidermal inclusion cyst** develops following a penetrating injury in which a fragment of keratinizing epithelium is pushed into the subcutaneous tissue. This tissue proliferates and forms keratin that, over the course of several years, produces a tumor. These cysts most commonly occur in males who are 30 to 40 years of age; and the most common location is the left long finger or thumb.[2]

The two most common types of nerve tumors are **neurilemomas (schwannomas)** and **neurofibromas**. These benign tumors are rare and account for only 1% of tumors of the hand.[1] Neurilemomas are slow-growing tumors that arise from Schwann cells. They are most commonly located in the flexor surface of the forearm or hand. These tumors present in clients who are 40 to 60 years of age and can be misdiagnosed as ganglion cysts.[2] Neurofibromas also arise from Schwann cells but also involve the nerve tissue, which may cause neurological symptoms.[1]

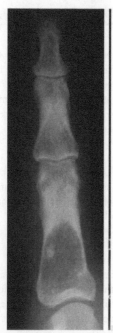

FIG. 33.7 Enchondroma. Magnetic resonance imaging confirming the intraosseous nature of the lesion. (*From Athanasian EA. Bone and soft tissue tumors. In: Wolfe SW, Hotchkiss RN, Pederson WC, et al. eds. Green's Operative Hand Surgery. 7th ed. Philadelphia, PA: Elsevier; 2017, page 2020, Figure 59.49 A.*)

Benign tumors of the epithelium include the common wart, or **verruca vulgaris,** caused by infection with the human papillomavirus. These tumors may involve any part of the hand and are commonly found at sites of trauma. **Dermatofibroma**, also known as **cutaneous fibrous histiocytoma**, and **keratoacanthoma** are benign epithelial tumors. These lesions are significant because they can be confused with malignant epithelial lesions on the forearm and hand due to their appearance and coloration.[1]

The most common primary bone tumor in the hand is an **enchondroma** (Fig. 33.7), accounting for 90% of hand bone tumors. Interestingly, approximately 35% of all enchondromas occur in the hand. These benign cartilaginous tumors are most commonly found in the proximal phalanx, followed by the metacarpal and middle phalanx.[2] These tumors are often diagnosed when a client presents with a fracture caused by a minor trauma or with an area of localized (usually painless) edema.[2] These lesions may also be an incidental finding on plain radiographs.[2]

There are three types of malignant epithelial tumors: **squamous cell carcinoma**, **melanoma**, and **basal cell carcinoma**. Squamous cell carcinoma is the most common type of skin cancer in the forearm and hand, and may spread to deeper tissues. Melanoma is almost as common and potentially life threatening due its tendency to rapidly spread to the lymph nodes. Basal cell carcinoma is the least common skin cancer in the forearm and hand, and tends to stay localized.[1] All of these tumors seem to have a direct link with sun exposure.

Soft-tissue sarcomas are malignant tumors that originate in muscle and connective tissues. They are rarely seen in the forearm and hand. They can be aggressive and metastasize; therefore they are often aggressively managed with amputation, chemotherapy, and radiation therapy.[1]

Timelines and Healing

Timelines and healing for tumors vary widely. The medical management and general health of a client who undergoes surgical excision of a tumor will determine the rate of wound closure. The type and extent of damage to tissues caused by the tumor and the course of treatment will certainly be a factor in functional outcome. A complex case involving a client with multiple comorbidities and treated with radiation therapy may have poor tissue quality and slower healing.

Nonoperative Treatment

- Since many tumors spontaneously resolve, delayed treatment is the conventional treatment for hemangiomas that appear soon after birth.
- Warts are treated nonsurgically (for example, cryotherapy or topical salicylate).
- Congenital arteriovenous malformations on the hand are initially treated with compression gloves, elevation, and medication.[1]

Operative Treatment

- Treatment for giant-cell tumors is surgical excision. Recurrence rates for these tumors are high—up to 50%.[8]
- Large lipomas can be difficult to excise. Recurrence rates are low.[1]
- If surgery is deemed necessary for hemangiomas, it can be complex due to separating normal and abnormal tissues and risk of vascular compromise. Feeder vessels are ligated and the tumor is excised.[1] Surgery for a lymphangioma is equally as challenging but poses less risk to distal vascularity.
- Excision of congenital arteriovenous malformations is reserved for painful lesions or those that have failed conservative management.[1]
- Surgical excision is the commonly accepted treatment of pyogenic granulomas; however, the use of electrocautery, silver nitrate, and laser have been attempted with some success.[1]
- The treatment of symptomatic glomus tumors includes excision of the tumor after first removing the nail plate and is followed by repair of the nail bed.[1]
- Inclusion cysts are excised with the goal of removing the entire wall of the cyst, as well as its contents, in order to minimize risk for recurrence.[1]
- Neurilemomas can typically be excised without damage to the nerve fibers. Postoperative neurological deficits following excision of neurofibromas are not uncommon due to the involvement of underlying nerve tissue. Ten percent of clients have multiple neurofibromas, which is known as von Recklinghausen disease or neurofibromatosis.[1]
- Usually, dermatofibromas are excised for differential diagnosis and to rule out malignancy.
- Medical management of malignant tumors depends on the clinical findings. Extensive surgery and reconstruction may be required to restore function. Chemotherapy and radiation therapy may also be utilized.

? Questions to Ask the Doctor

- What structures were involved?
- What are the guidelines for wound care?
- What are the precautions and guidelines for AROM?
- What type of orthosis, if any, is needed?
- What is the long-term prognosis?
- If reconstruction for aesthetics or function is warranted, what other surgeries are planned?

( ) What to Say to Clients

"It will take time to heal from the surgery to remove your tumor. The surgery will leave a scar on your skin and below the surface. It will be important for you to perform the exercises that I give you, but you also need to give your hand time to rest between exercise sessions. Our main goals for therapy are to manage your scar tissue and swelling and regain the motion in your hand in order to help you return to everyday activities without pain. It is possible that the tumor you had removed may reoccur and require additional treatment in the future."

To prepare for discussions with clients, gather information from the physician and surgical reports. Be prepared to answer questions about anatomy that is involved with the tumor. Anatomy books are often helpful. Set timelines and realistic expectations to regain functional use of the client's hand. Clients will often ask if you have seen similar cases before; answer honestly.

Evaluation Tips

- First and most importantly, listen to your clients. You may be the first person they have been able to confide in about their concerns. Be gentle and supportive. They are most likely worrying about malignancy of their tumor and may be dealing with the impact of serious medical findings.
- Prioritize wound healing.
- Screen or assess sensory perception so that the client can be instructed in protective safety precautions as needed.
- Try to avoid any aspects of evaluation that cause pain.

◎ Clinical Pearl

Be aware that dressing changes, especially during the initial visit, may bother some clients more than others. Reactions can vary widely, so be prepared to assist clients with symptoms of nausea or being "light headed." This may be especially true for clients who are concurrently undergoing radiation or chemotherapy treatment with hand therapy.

Diagnosis-Specific Information That Affects Clinical Reasoning

The hand therapist must communicate with the physician in order to have a clear picture of the medical diagnosis and treatment plan for each client. As discussed, there is variability in each type of tumor in presentation, location, functional implications, and medical management. This can make treating these clients challenging but rewarding.

♡ Tips From the Field

Orthoses

When an orthosis is needed, keep in mind the purpose of the orthosis, the anatomy that is involved, and the functional demands of the client. Tissues may be fragile and care should be taken to assure that the orthosis is comfortable. It is important to support the tissues adequately while preventing future deformities, especially if a nerve has been compromised.

Client Expectations

Be positive and reassure clients about their functional use and hand appearance. Help them set realistic expectations and see gains they have made with review of measurements and/or documentation of return to activities of daily living (ADLs).

Activities of Daily Living

Assisting the client in recovering functional use of their upper extremity is an important part of the hand therapist's role. Find out what ADLs are important to the client and incorporate these into treatment and goal setting. Also, consider use of adaptive equipment or task modification to assist the client in participating in home or work activities.

⊳ Precautions and Concerns

- *Be aware that some physical agent modalities are contraindicated for a client who has had a malignant tumor excised.*
- *Instruct the client in ROM exercises of uninvolved joints to prevent stiffness and reduce edema.*

CASE STUDIES

CASE STUDY 33.1 ■ Mucous Cyst

A 66-year-old, retired, right-hand dominant female came to therapy 8 days following a right carpal tunnel release and right thumb interphalangeal (IP) joint mucous cyst excision. She stated that the majority of her trouble before surgery was numbness in her fingers due to carpal tunnel syndrome. She elected to have the mucous cyst excised, since "the doctor was already going to be operating on my right hand anyway." During the initial evaluation the client stated that her finger numbness was already improving and she was independent with all home exercises related to the carpal tunnel release. She admitted that the majority of her pain and discomfort following surgery was with her thumb, and it bothered her that she was not able to bend her thumb well for functional activity and opposition. Her thumb IP motion was significantly limited and painful compared to the opposite hand, and her ADL function was limited due to inability to use her thumb. At 12 days postsurgery, the client was given gentle thumb AROM exercises, instructed in scar massage techniques, and fitted with a thumb compressive sleeve to provide support and to help decrease edema.

After 6 weeks of therapy the client confided that all symptoms of carpal tunnel syndrome had resolved, but she continued to have residual pain and stiffness in her thumb IP joint. However, she was now able to use her right thumb for most activities and was instructed in a long-term HEP for maintenance of thumb function. The home program included AROM, use of heating agents for comfort, and a resting static IP extension orthosis to help support and rest the joint and to avoid an IP extensor lag. The client was pleased with the improvements through hand therapy following her surgery. When the client was discharged, she was comfortable with self-managing her symptoms and participating in the home program.

CASE STUDY 33.2 ▪ Ganglion

A 37-year-old, right-hand dominant female came to therapy following an office visit with the hand surgeon. She explained to the therapist that she detected a volar wrist ganglion years ago that resolved spontaneously. However, with the recent birth of her third child, the ganglion reappeared and became painful with most activities. After electing to see a physician, she was referred to therapy for fabrication of a forearm-based wrist orthosis to assist with symptom management and to rest the surrounding tissues. The client explained that she was not interested in surgery; and she stated that the physician had explained that she was not a candidate for an injection or aspiration of the cyst due to the proximity of the ganglion to the radial artery and potential for injury to the artery with those procedures.

The therapist fabricated a forearm-based wrist orthosis in a neutral wrist position and educated the client in wrist and digital ROM to avoid stiffness. The therapist also explained to the client that she would need to wear the orthosis more often at first to help alleviate her acute symptoms, but that orthosis wear could be reduced as pain resolved. The client planned to use the orthosis during homemaking tasks and cooking, but to leave it off while caring for her infant. She assured the therapist that she agreed with the therapeutic plan and was motivated to carry out her treatment independently. The client planned to call and schedule a follow-up appointment only if pain and limitations of function persisted. The client called 1 month later and stated that her symptoms had nearly resolved and that the ganglion was not even visible most days. She had no further questions and was discharged from therapy.

References

1. Sweet S, Kroonen L, Weiss L: Soft tissue tumors of the forearm and hand. In Skirven TM, Osterman AL, Fedorczyk JM, et al.: *Rehabilitation of the hand and upper extremity*, ed 6, St Louis, MO, 2011, Mosby, pp 289–301.
2. Athanasian EA: Bone and soft tissue tumors. In Wolfe SW, Hotchkiss RN, Pederson WC, et al.: *Green's operative hand surgery*, ed 6, Philadelphia, PA, 2011, Churchill Livingstone, pp 2141–2195.
3. Teh J, Vlychou M: Ultrasound guided interventional procedures of the wrist and hand, *Eur Radiol* 19:1002–1010, 2009.
4. Gallego S, Mathoulin C: Arthroscopic resection of dorsal wrist ganglia: 114 cases with minimum follow-up of 2 years, *Arthroscopy* 26:1675–1682, 2010.
5. Edwards SG, Johansen JA: Prospective outcomes and associations of wrist ganglion cysts resected arthroscopically, *J Hand Surg Am* 34:395–400, 2009.
6. Cooper C: Ganglion cysts and other common tumors of the hand and wrist. In Cooper C, editor: *Fundamentals of hand therapy*, St Louis, MO, 2007, Mosby, pp 412–420.
7. Koman LA, Paterson Smith B, Smith TL, et al.: Vascular disorders. In Wolfe SW, Hotchkiss RN, Pederson WC, et al.: *Green's operative hand surgery*, ed 6, Philadelphia, PA, 2011, Churchill Livingstone, pp 2197–2240.
8. Plate AM, Lee SJ, Steiner G, et al.: Tumorlike lesions and benign tumors of the hand and wrist, *J Am Acad Orthop Surg* 11:129–141, 2003.

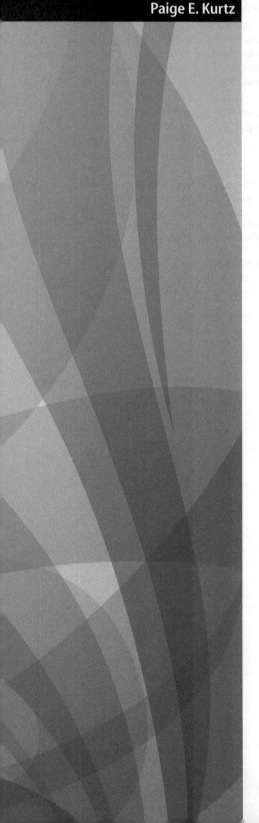

34

Traumatic Hand Injury Involving Multiple Structures

Paige E. Kurtz

Traumatic hand injuries can be both daunting and rewarding for the treating therapist. It can be intimidating deciding where to start with a new client because so many hand structures and systems need to be protected and treated at once. However, once therapy is underway, and throughout the rehabilitation process, the experience of participating in a client's recovery from initial evaluation to final status with good function can be remarkably rewarding.

The systems approach is the easiest way to evaluate, prioritize, and treat complex hand injuries. The therapist should evaluate each involved system individually; then, for each system, determine the stage of the injury and how it can best be treated within the constraints of necessary precautions. This approach makes it much easier to choose the correct interventions for each system according to its stage. Systems that must be considered include the skin (wound/graft), tendons (flexors, extensors, or both), nerves, blood vessels (veins and arteries), and bones (fractures, fusions, and joint surfaces). Pain and edema are additional considerations.

Plan ahead throughout the course of therapy. If future surgery is expected, incorporate that fact into treatment planning and goal setting. For example, if tenolysis or tendon grafting is likely, maximize passive range of motion (PROM); if tendon transfer is expected, maximize the strength of potential donor muscles. Continually educate your clients about where they are in the process, what may be coming next, and how adherence to the current plan of care will benefit them in the long run. Prepare these clients for a long course of therapy—possibly a year or longer—that may include several surgeries.[1]

Most traumatic hand injuries involve many different structures and systems. The most extreme and complex injuries require a **replant**; that is, an amputated finger, hand, or arm is reattached surgically to reestablish viability and function. Not all traumatic hand injuries involve a replant or **revascularization** (a surgical procedure to repair severed arteries or veins to restore blood supply to a limb). However, the precautions, decision making, and treatment processes are similar across the spectrum of these injuries.

Clinical Pearl

Keep in mind that the goal of rehabilitation following a traumatic hand injury is not to regain a completely normal hand. The goal is to regain maximal function with minimal pain.

As soon as possible, determine the reasonable functional outcome given the extent and location of the injury. Keep in mind that a client can be functional with less than "normal" range of motion (ROM). Work with your client to establish reasonable goals and expectations. Often, one of the most important parts of hand therapy is managing expectations and providing psychosocial support. Clients' satisfaction with their outcome is related to their expectations, as explained by the surgeon before surgery and reinforced by the therapist after surgery.[2] **Precaution.** *Achieving a pain-free hand with functional prehension, grasp, and grip is better than pushing to gain a few more degrees of ROM while jeopardizing stability. Usually, it is not worth risking the possibility of increasing pain and edema and reducing the chance of long-term success.*

Anatomy

Traumatic multisystem injuries can involve many different structures from the surface of the skin to the bone. Complex injuries, including replants and revascularizations, may occur at any level of the extremity, from the upper arm to the fingertips. To treat these injuries successfully, hand therapists must have a thorough working knowledge of the anatomy involved. Therapists must know the stages of wound healing; the anatomy and healing processes of veins and arteries, tendons, ligaments, and bone; and the biomechanics and interrelationships of these tissues and structures during functional movement.

Therapists must first understand the mechanics of a "normal" (uninjured) hand because this provides the basis for maximizing hand function after surgery. If you understand the implications of the injury and the surgery, you will be better able to set realistic goals and formulate a good treatment plan. Decision making is related to healing times and sequences and may depend on the surgery performed. Some structures may need to be protected while others must be mobilized early in therapy; this can be difficult to manage. Treatment of the traumatic hand injury can become a balancing act, requiring the hand therapist to determine which joints to move and which structures to protect, and to establish when stability is more important than mobility. Some stress on healing structures is good because it stimulates healing, but too much stress can cause a loss of stability. How aggressively to push a client in therapy depends on the skills and knowledge of the hand therapist, as well as the ultimate goals and expectations.

The therapist must know what tissues were disrupted and to what extent, the effect of different types of injuries on different tissues, and what surgical procedures were performed to repair those tissues. The position of the hand at the time of injury may affect which structures were injured and at which level (that is, the anatomical location of injury). The therapist must consider the effect of the injury on surrounding uninjured structures and attend to those uninjured structures throughout the extremity (for example, the shoulder or elbow) to prevent additional loss of function.

Consider the functional implications of the anatomy and the injury. Moran and Berger[3] have described seven maneuvers that constitute basic hand function; these include three types of pinch and four types of grasp. These maneuvers can be further categorized into two primary functional uses of the hand: pinch between the thumb and finger (or fingers) and grip. Pinch is affected by a radial-side hand injury, which influences prehension and fine motor coordination. Grip is more affected by an ulnar-side hand injury, which diminishes composite grip strength and stability. Keep these functional movements in mind when planning treatment and devising exercises and activities.[4]

Diagnosis and Pathology

Traumatic hand injuries can be caused by many types of force, from sharp lacerations to crush injuries. The mechanism of injury (for example, tearing, crushing, cutting, or twisting forces) and the cleanliness of the wound are important pathological factors. A closed crush injury may show little visible damage but may involve fractures or **ischemia** (deficient supply of blood) as a result of extensive damage to internal structures.

Primary treatment is typically performed in the emergency department, ideally with immediate referral to a hand specialist and/or replant team. The hand surgeon evaluates the injury with regard to what can and cannot be salvaged and restored to good function. Many systems and algorithms are available to aid problem solving and prioritization in the emergency department and operating room. Generally, the thumb, if salvageable, is always a priority for replantation. With multiple-digit amputations, the surgeon tries to replant as many as practical. Replants are nearly always attempted at any level in children. Incomplete amputations are also treated with maximum aggressiveness.[4] Box 34.1 lists surgical procedures often used to treat complex hand injuries.

Timelines and Healing

Operative Treatment

Initially, most or all involved structures are repaired surgically, depending on the timing of surgery and the extent of injury. The hand surgeon evaluates which structures can be repaired and which cannot be salvaged and therefore must be amputated

---

BOX 34.1 Surgical Procedures Used to Treat Complex Hand Injuries

Skin
- Skin may be sutured in primary repair.
- Graft or flap may be placed for wound coverage.
- Skin may be left open for secondary closure to allow further debridement and to prevent constriction over vascular structures.

Tendons
- Flexors and extensors are repaired.
- Tendon grafts or transfers or tendon removal may be performed in preparation for a future graft, often with insertion of a temporary spacer.

Nerves
- Nerves are repaired with or without grafting.

Blood vessels
- Veins and arteries are repaired with or without grafting.

Bone fixation
- Bone fixation is performed using bone grafts, fixators, wires, pins, plates, screws, or other devices.
- Joint arthroplasty implant may be inserted where joint surfaces cannot be repaired.
- Joint fusion may be performed.

◎ Clinical Pearl

- Finger flexors offer more function than extensors. However, during activities of daily living, wrist extension is generally more useful than wrist flexion. It is imperative to aim for a strong, stable wrist; without it, finger function and grip strength will be impaired.
- The importance of the thumb's contribution to overall hand function cannot be ignored; thus maintaining a good web space and opposition is critical.
- Keep in mind that regaining functional use of the hand is very difficult without functional sensibility.

or considered for later surgical interventions.[5,6] Irrigation and debridement are performed prior to repair to remove contaminants and nonviable tissue.

The order of repair generally begins with stabilization of the injury. Blood flow and fracture stabilization are the most critical and guide the surgeon's planning. Typically, bony injuries are fixed first, using techniques that are expedient but that also allow early ROM. Bone shortening may be utilized to allow for easier end-to-end repair of other structures. This can ultimately affect biomechanics of the surrounding structures, possibly resulting in compromised ROM and strength.

Tendon repairs are often performed next, unless vascular status is severely compromised. When both flexors and extensors are involved, the surgeon tries to restore balance between the two, giving priority to functional flexion. Generally, vascular and nerve repairs are performed next, and then skin coverage is addressed.

The initial goal of the surgeon is to restore the framework that allows the client and therapist to work toward a good functional outcome. The surgeon attempts to provide a reasonably strong structure, optimal skeletal alignment and joint mobility, good vascular flow, and the potential for functional tendon balance and glide. If the injury is extremely complex, scar, tendon and nerve grafts, joint contractures, and other deficits can be addressed by additional surgeries.

Involved systems may be in different stages of healing after surgery. For example, a finger fracture may have good stability because of internal fixation, but an overlying skin graft or infection may delay wound healing. The systems approach can be very helpful for treatment planning in such cases.

Prioritize the systems during the hand therapy evaluation. There is no firm hierarchy of systems; however, without healing in some systems, no further healing occurs in any of the others. The general order of importance is as follows:

1. Surgical repairs of arteries and veins (blood flow is critical for providing nutrients for healing and survival of the repaired structures)
2. Bone injury, ligament injury, and fracture fixation (ROM exercises require a stable support structure)
3. Prioritize flexor tendons over extensor tendons (functional use favors flexors, although balance should be maintained as much as possible)
4. Nerves and sensibility (nerve recovery is a slow process; nerve injuries tend to be protected when nearby blood vessels and tendons are protected)
5. Wound, scar, and soft tissue (promote healing while preventing and minimizing contractures)

Edema and pain must be managed throughout the entire process. Edema must be controlled and minimized because it contributes to stiffness and fibrosis. If pain is not managed, clients have a very difficult time participating in therapy (exercises, wound care, etc.).

The goals and priorities early in therapy (0–3 weeks after surgery, the acute phase) are to manage and protect repairs, prevent joint stiffness in all uninvolved joints, control edema, manage the wound, manage pain, educate the client, and provide psychosocial support. As the client progresses into the intermediate phase (3–6 weeks after surgery), therapy focuses more on increasing ROM of involved structures, managing scarring, continuing wound care and protection, and initiating functional use of the involved extremity. Later phases focus on building and maximizing ROM, endurance, strength, and function.

Whenever possible, obtain a copy of the operative report. Make sure you and the physician have the same understanding of treatment goals and expectations. Do not hesitate to ask for clarification when needed. Box 34.2 lists some appropriate questions to consider asking the physician.

Therapists spend considerable time developing rapport with clients, which results in therapists being more likely than the physician to hear about problems and concerns. Also, therapists see clients more regularly than the physician and are more likely to notice subtle changes that indicate potential problems.

◎ Clinical Pearl

Do not be afraid to confer with the referring physician in a timely manner on *any* information that appears to be important regarding the client's status, complaints, or problems.

() What to Say to Clients

About the Injury

Try to give clients perspective about their injury and rehabilitation goals. Teach clients that a good outcome is about getting enough movement in the hand to regain independence. Being able to use the hand for everyday tasks does not necessarily require normal ROM: "I am not going to worry about getting your hand back to normal. We are going to focus on you being able to use your hand for as many normal things as possible." Work to develop a partnership: "I'm the coach, but you have to practice every day. We will work together to get you the best use of your hand. If you do not do your exercises consistently at home, there is nothing we can do a few times a week here in therapy that will make up for it."

Discuss the ramifications of not adhering to contraindications and precautions: "If you are not careful about doing the exercises as I show you or you do not wear your orthosis, it could mean your hand will not heal as it should. If something goes wrong, it could even mean you'll need another surgery."

Clients come to rely on their therapists for information and they often ask questions they are afraid to ask the physician. Do not hesitate to refer the client to the physician for questions you cannot answer.

Clients adhere to the plan of care better and achieve better outcomes when the underlying anatomy and healing process are explained to them in common terms. Try to explain what they are attempting to achieve with specific exercises, using terms the client can understand. Provide basic information on how the flexors and extensors work and explain that many of the muscles that move the fingers originate near the elbow. Use models, pictures, or drawings to show specific anatomical features. Explain how the normal anatomy was affected by the injury and what outcome the client should expect. If future surgery is likely, make sure the client understands that and incorporate it into the goals of therapy.

About Orthoses

The orthosis is a critical component of protection and stability with traumatic injuries of the hand. Clients must understand that the orthosis may serve both protective and corrective functions; therefore it is essential that they wear it as directed by the therapist.

Help clients understand the importance of the orthosis and why the hand is positioned a certain way: "This orthosis is important for protecting the injured structures in your hand so that they can heal correctly. If you take it off and move your hand the wrong way, some of the repairs may not be able to handle the stress."

About Exercises

Most clients are afraid to move any part of the hand immediately after surgery, especially if they feel pain, have swelling or open wounds, or if they can see pins sticking out of the hand. The therapist must stress the importance of movement despite these issues: "You will not hurt your hand if you do the exercises just as I showed you. If you do not do the exercises, getting good movement back will be very difficult. We cannot wait for the swelling to go away, the pins to come out, or the wound to heal before we start moving. By that time, your fingers will be really stiff, and it will hurt more to move them." Make sure the client understands that "more" exercise is not necessarily better and that they should follow your direction on how often to exercise and how many repetitions to perform.

◎ *Clinical Pearl*

It may be helpful to use a client's cell phone to record a video of them performing the home program exercises. Video provides a good take-home record of how the exercises look when they are performed correctly. Many people do better when following along to a video than when reenacting exercises from a written paper.

BOX 34.2   Information Needed From the Physician

Therapists should make sure they obtain the following information from the client's physician or surgeon:
1. What do I need to protect, and what can I move?
2. What was injured, at what (anatomical) level, and what was repaired?
3. What type of injury was this (crush, tear, blade/laceration, type of blade, clean or dirty injury)?
4. What are your expected outcomes and goals?

With Surgical Repairs
1. What structures were repaired and how?
2. What is the quality of the repairs?
3. What is the strength of the repairs?
4. Is there tension on any repairs?
5. What is the most appropriate orthotic position to protect the repairs?[7]
6. What is the tendon quality; what is the relationship of the repair site to the pulleys?
7. How strong is any fracture fixation? Is anything fused? How is joint mobility? Was bone shortening performed?
8. Are any skin graft or flap precautions required?
9. Are any tissues or ROM to be protected?
10. Are there any tissues with questionable viability that should be watched closely?
11. What limits and restrictions were created by the surgical procedures?
12. What are your anticipated time frames for progression?
13. Were any structures not repaired? What is the plan for them?

Evaluation Tips

- Before seeing the client, gather all available information on the type of injury and the treatment to this point, especially the operative reports.
- The initial evaluation may be mostly "hands off" because of the client's pain and fear. This is a good time to establish trust and rapport. The initial evaluation is a time to do an overview assessment of the status of various systems and to perform the most basic but necessary aspects of early therapy (for example, wound care and orthosis fabrication).
- When you begin an evaluation, consider comorbidities and overall health status. Ask whether the client is a smoker or diabetic, or has any other health problems. These can delay healing in all systems and have a correlation to replant failure.
- Make sure to ask about support systems, including friends and family. Monitor clients' behavior toward the injured hand. Are they able to look at the hand? Do they treat the hand as if it belonged to someone else or as if they would like to get rid of it? To achieve a good outcome, the client must develop "ownership" of the injured hand and take some responsibility for recovery.
  Visually inspect the following:
- Vascular status (check skin color)
- Wound status (use wound color system: black, yellow, red)
- Finger stiffness (at the initial evaluation, measure full active range of motion [AROM] and PROM as appropriate, given precautions, and only if essential)
- Edema (minimal, moderate, or severe)
- Check ROM at uninvolved joints (for example, shoulder and elbow)

◎ *Clinical Pearl*

At the initial evaluation, obtaining specific measurements is not as important as making a global assessment of the client's status and establishing a baseline for treatment planning.

Diagnosis-Specific Information That Affects Clinical Reasoning

The following sections present a general discussion of the critical areas to evaluate for each system, precautions and contraindications, and healing guidelines and timelines. For more detailed information on specific systems, please refer to the relevant chapters elsewhere in this textbook.

Bone Injury: Fracture

With a complex injury, all surrounding unaffected joints should be moved immediately, if possible, depending on the type and location of fracture and the type of fixation. Beginning ROM exercises as soon as the physician permits helps enhance fracture healing. During the evaluation, consider precautions, the type of fixation, and the expected stability of structures. The surgeon may have elected to shorten bony structures at the time of fixation. This may allow for a cleaner more stable fixation and it facilitates end-to-end repair of tendons, nerves, and blood vessels in the area; however, it also may alter the mechanics of musculotendinous units in the arm and hand.

Surgical fixation may be achieved with pins/Kirschner wires, joint implants, plates and screws, interosseous wiring, or even joint fusion (Fig. 34.1). An important goal of surgery is to achieve as much stability as possible, creating the framework for movement in rehabilitation.[7,8] If the surgeon has established sufficient fracture fixation, ROM around a fracture site may be initiated immediately, starting from the midrange and progressing to full ROM as appropriate, observing precautions for tendons, nerves, and vascular structures.[9] **Precaution.** *Avoid excess stress at fracture/ fusion/pin sites and watch for signs of infection.*

If revascularizations were done in conjunction with fracture fixation, the chance of delayed healing or nonunion is greater because a decrease in blood flow decreases the delivery of nutrients to the area.

Revascularization: Arteries and Veins

Revascularizations and replants are often categorized together as the most complex injuries because injury to an artery or vein (or both) with revascularization affects peripheral blood flow, which in turn affects the potential for survival of every other structure in the hand. In complicated cases, surgeons may not repair both arteries into a digit; the digit therefore has decreased vascularity because of the repair and because it has only one functioning artery.[8,10]

After surgery, these clients are placed in a "hot" (75–80°F/24–27°C) room in the hospital to help increase peripheral circulation. Keep in mind that decreased circulation after arterial repair affects healing rates of wounds, tendons, and fractures in an extremity because of the decrease in peripheral circulation and delivery of nutrients to the area. Ideally, therapy should be performed in a comfortable warm room away from air conditioner vents. If possible, have the client exercise with the dressing off so that you can observe vascular status. While working with the client, monitor the color, capillary refill, and temperature in the injured hand. **Precaution.** *A dusky (grayish) finger or hand indicates severely diminished vascularity caused by arterial compromise; a purple color suggests venous congestion. Alert the referring physician if you note either a dusky or purple appearance. Either of these could signify distress, which could lead to failure of the replant.*[11]

A major precaution with revascularizations is to avoid anything that challenges the weakened peripheral vascular system. The client must not eat or drink anything vasoconstrictive, such as caffeine and chocolate. Smoking is prohibited because it causes

severe vasoconstriction, reduces peripheral circulation, and affects the blood's ability to carry oxygen.[12] Compressive bandages (for example, elastic stockinette, tape, or gloves) should not be used for 3 to 8 weeks, until the vascular status has stabilized. Monitor for compression caused by orthotic material and straps. Constantly check the color of the fingers with regard to capillary refill.

Another precaution is to avoid using cold treatments in the acute phase (3 to 6 weeks or longer after surgery). If the injury occurs during the winter, advise the client to keep the hand warm with a mitten, an oven mitt, or a scarf for both comfort and safety. Many experts recommend avoiding the use of whirlpool because it puts the hand in a dependent position; if a whirlpool is used, it must be run at neutral temperature.[13,14] Contrast baths should also be avoided because they may cause vasospasm followed by vasoconstriction.

Mild heat may be used at 4 to 8 weeks after surgery, once vascularity has stabilized. However, keep in mind that the insensate hand does not have a warning system to let the client know when a substance is too hot; it also cannot dissipate heat as well (that is, the tissue burns more easily). Although elevation is a good way to reduce edema, excessive elevation challenges the vascular system. After revascularization, the hand should not be held significantly above the level of the heart because this puts stress on the newly repaired arteries and can cause failure.[13]

Because neurovascular bundles are generally volarly located, artery and vein repairs often require positional protection similar to that of repaired flexor tendons (that is, a dorsally placed orthosis with the wrist and fingers flexed). If the bone was not shortened, the physician may need to use vein grafts to ensure adequate circulation without putting tension on the system. If tension is unavoidable, precautions must be observed, such as more flexed positioning in the orthosis and in therapy. If no other injuries or complications are involved, vascular structures can be moved soon after surgery. If tendon injuries or fractures occur in the same digit, follow the highest level of precautions to protect these structures appropriately.

Nerve Injury: Laceration and Repair

Like vascular injuries, nerve injuries often occur with flexor tendon injuries. In such cases, treat according to the appropriate flexor tendon repair protocol. Tension on the nerve guides decision making. As with tendon injuries, establishing early gliding is essential.

A nerve injury leaves part of the hand insensate. This may not be a significant problem in the early phase of therapy while the client is continually wearing the orthosis; however, it becomes a concern when the client begins to perform activities of daily living (ADLs) out of the orthosis. **Precaution.** *Teach the client to take care with ADLs (heat, sharp objects). The eyes must compensate for lack of sensation in the hand. The therapist must be cautious when using orthoses (particularly dynamic or static progressive orthoses), compression, as well as heat and ice. When the hand is insensate, there isn't a sensory warning system for ischemia. A client with decreased sensation may be unable to tell whether the temperature of an item is excessively hot or cold.*

A full sensibility evaluation is not necessary immediately after a traumatic hand injury. A cursory assessment may be performed initially to detect areas of sensory deficit. Because it takes some time for repaired nerves to reinnervate an area, a full sensibility evaluation is rarely worthwhile earlier than 1 month after surgery.

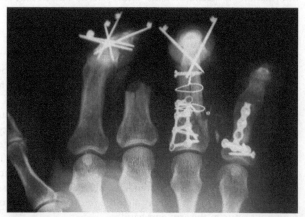

FIG. 34.1 X-ray film showing amputation and internal fixation.

Follow-up sensory assessments should be performed approximately once a month thereafter because nerves regrow slowly from the injury site to the distal fingertips.

After the client has regained protective sensation, begin sensory reeducation to teach the brain to recognize signals from the peripheral nerves.[13] Start with constant pressure and moving touch. Begin with the client's eyes open and progress to eyes closed; and alternate between the involved and uninvolved side or area. Mirror therapy may be a useful adjunct to facilitate sensory reeducation after nerve repairs.[15] Desensitization exercises should be performed for hypersensitivity.

> **◎ Clinical Pearl**
>
> Remember that sensitivity to cold and cold intolerance are possible for two or more years after a nerve injury.[12,16]

Flexor and Extensor Tendons: Tendon Repair

Most hand therapists treat flexor tendon repairs and extensor tendon repairs on a regular basis. However, flexor and extensor tendon injuries do not frequently occur together. Prioritizing becomes more difficult when both types of repairs must be treated at the same time. With a replant, or if both flexors and extensors have been lacerated/repaired, priority is almost always given to the flexors over the extensors because flexion is more important for function. However, the ideal is to maintain a normal balance between the two systems. A replanted hand or finger is usually immobilized in the position used for flexor tendon repair because this position is relatively balanced, slightly favoring the flexors and neurovascular bundles over the extensors. Gliding of involved structures should be implemented as soon as possible to increase the delivery of nutrients, enhance healing, reduce edema, and reduce the potential for adhesions.

Treatment rules are largely the same as those for typical hand therapy protocols with regard to healing phases. Therapy after replantation should follow a version of the referring physician's preferred flexor tendon repair protocol, modified to protect the extensors. Generally, begin wrist and metacarpophalangeal (MP) joint ROM, along with limited ROM of the proximal interphalangeal (PIP) and distal interphalangeal (DIP) joints. Limiting PIP and DIP flexion will help prevent extensor lag, while movement of the wrist and MPs will start to increase ROM and gliding via **synergistic movement**. Major precautions are similar to those for flexor and extensor tendon repair protocols: protect against a full active fist or full extension of the fingers and avoid resistance until the structures have healed. If bone shortening was performed, the normal biomechanics of both the flexors and extensors will have been modified; therefore completely normal ROM is not a practical expectation.

Edema

Edema causes increased resistance with AROM. This is a very important consideration in the introduction of early ROM for a complex traumatic hand injury. Long-standing edema leads to increased fibrosis and scar formation. Edema can be evaluated by means of circumferential or figure-of-eight measurement, volumetric measurement (after wound closure), or (quick but not objective) visual assessment of the edema as minimal, moderate, or severe.

Treatment for edema begins with elevation of the hand above heart level *but not significantly higher if vascular procedures were part of the surgical repair.* Excessive elevation challenges the damaged and repaired arterial system in the hand or arm.[14,17] It is important to avoid compression after revascularization until a strong stable vascular flow has been reestablished; this can take 6 to 8 weeks. AROM exercises can be performed, as appropriate in the treatment protocol, to create a pumping mechanism. Long-standing edema and the fibrosis that often occurs after a traumatic hand injury usually results in larger digits, and the client will probably have to have their rings resized. To determine the most stable size, the client should wait 6 to 12 months after the last surgery.

Compression may be used after the vascular system has stabilized. Available devices and techniques include elastic bandages, compressive gloves, elastic stockinette, manual edema mobilization, and retrograde massage.

Wound Healing and Scar Management

The presence of an open wound can change treatment priorities. Complex wounds often accompany complex injuries. Wound evaluation should include assessment and documentation of location, size, color (red/yellow/black), and drainage (type, color, and amount). Watch for signs of infection, which include redness that extends beyond the area of the wound, warmth, increased edema, increased pain, excessive drainage, and unusual colors and odors.

Skin grafts must be treated with special care until they have stabilized. The precautions are similar to those for a typical wound; however, special attention should be paid to avoiding friction and excessive compression over the graft site. Treat all wounds with care to avoid shear or mechanical stress from dressings and to prevent maceration of periwound areas while maintaining a moist wound bed. Good nutrition is critical for wound healing, including an adequate intake of protein and vitamins. Encourage the client to discuss nutrition questions with their physician or other experts.

Precaution. *Do not use cytotoxic chemicals, such as peroxide and povidone-iodine, on granulating wound tissue. Although these agents are helpful for reducing contaminants in a wound, they can also affect the viability of new tissues.*

In the early stages, wound care focuses on promoting healing and wound closure, preventing infection, and protecting healing structures.[14] In later stages, wound management involves efforts to modify and manage scarring through the use of scar massage, silicone gel sheets, Otoform elastomer, and paper or elastic tape. Therapy attempts to manage and control scarring while preventing future problems, such as the formation of adhesions and contractures. Keep in mind that scar heals all injured structures. Scar is essential for healing but it must be managed to minimize adhesions (which limit tendon glide) and scar contractures (which can pull hand structures into abnormal positions). It is important to control these two side effects of scarring because they limit ROM and affect hand function.

Scar tissue is different from normal skin tissue. It has less tensile strength and therefore may be more susceptible to abrasions and tearing. Scar tissue also sunburns easily and should be protected from sun exposure for approximately 6 months or until the scar is pale, soft, and supple.

> ### ◎ *Clinical Pearl*
>
> An easy way to protect scars on the hand is to cover them with a lip balm that has a high sun protection factor. The heavy waxy balm stays on the scar and the tube is portable and inexpensive.

Pain

Pain affects a client's ability to deal with the injury and to follow a home exercise program (HEP). Pain is normal with a complex injury. However, there is a higher incidence of complex regional pain syndrome with crush and complex injuries. When the pain is out of proportion to the injury for some time, a mental health consultation may be beneficial.[18]

Orthoses

Appropriate orthotic use and fabrication are important for supporting the injured hand, maintaining a position of balance, protecting the injured and repaired structures, and preventing future deformity. The orthosis typically used for a replant is similar to that for flexor tendon repairs: a forearm-based dorsal block orthosis with the MP joints in flexion and the interphalangeal (IP) joints in extension. The exact wrist position depends on the structures involved and the surgeon's preference.

> ### ◎ *Clinical Pearl*
>
> When fabricating an orthosis consider the locations of pins, the vascular supply with regard to strapping and pressure areas, and tension on nerve or tendon repairs. Avoid placing straps directly over repair sites. Use wide straps to distribute pressure.

> ### ◎ *Clinical Pearl*
>
> Prioritize the problems and orthosis design to support and protect the most significant concerns while maintaining a balance between the flexors and extensors.

Protocols for Mobilization

No true protocols exist for mobilization because injuries vary so widely. However, general guidelines are based on two approaches: delayed mobilization and early mobilization.

Delayed Mobilization

In some cases, delaying mobilization is appropriate because it allows the initial inflammatory response to decline while structures heal in a balanced position. As a result, fewer precautions are necessary after the immobilization period. Delayed mobilization may be used for young children or for any client who may not be fully cooperative.

If the physician prescribes this protocol without specific positioning parameters, immobilize the hand in protected position (flexed wrist and fingers, similar to the position used in a dorsal protective flexor-tendon repair orthosis) and keep it wrapped in a bulky compressive dressing for 3 weeks. At 3 weeks after surgery,

fit the client with a removable dorsal block orthosis (wrist flexion of 15 degrees, MPs flexed 50 to 70 degrees, and PIP/DIP joints fully extended to 0 degrees, unless different positioning is prescribed by the surgeon). Then begin gentle AROM exercise of the replanted digit or digits, along with full AROM and PROM of uninvolved digits. Initiate light manipulation activities as soon as practical to enhance ROM exercises.

At 4 weeks after surgery, add neuromuscular electrical stimulation (NMES) to assist with tendon glide. With medical clearance, initiate PROM in the replanted digit 6 weeks after surgery. If the fracture is clinically healed, add a dynamic or static progressive orthosis as needed. Have the client begin using their hand outside the orthosis for light ADLs after 6 weeks, making sure precautions for the insensate parts of the hand are observed. Start with using the hand for eating meals and slowly incorporate more ADLs. Add strengthening exercises at 8 to 10 weeks after surgery after verifying solid fracture healing (Table 34.1).[19]

Early Mobilization

Early protective motion (EPM) is a suggested replant treatment guideline that has been described in the hand therapy literature.[13,19,20] EPM allows for differential tendon glide and early movement while maintaining a balance between the flexors and extensors and minimizing tension on repaired structures by means of synergistic movement (in therapy this refers to mobilization of one or more joints by using the tendinous connections that run past those joints and the relationship between flexors and extensors).[21] Synergistic movement is seen with the natural flexion of the fingers that occurs when the wrist is extended and the natural extension of the fingers that occurs when the wrist is flexed. This protocol can be used for digital or hand replants characterized by stable fixation and a clean injury.

Early Protective Motion Phase I

The first treatment phase is EPM I. This phase begins 4 to 10 days after surgery (or 24 hours after discontinuation of anticoagulants), once viability of the replanted part has been established. Fit the client in a dorsal block orthosis with the wrist in neutral to slight flexion and the fingers in maximum practical MP flexion and IP extension. The orthosis may be refitted as tolerated to increase MP flexion and IP extension later in the program. Initiate in-clinic and home exercises at this time.

TABLE 34.1	**Delayed Mobilization Protocol for Replants**
Postoperative Timeline	**Exercise or Intervention**
0–3 weeks	No ROM
3 weeks	AROM of involved structures; PROM of uninvolved structures
4 weeks	NMES
6 weeks	Dynamic orthosis; PROM of involved structures; Initiate use of hand for ADLs
8–10 weeks	Strengthening exercises

ADLs, Activities of daily living; *AROM,* active range of motion; *NMES,* neuromuscular electrical stimulation; *PROM,* passive range of motion; *ROM,* range of motion.

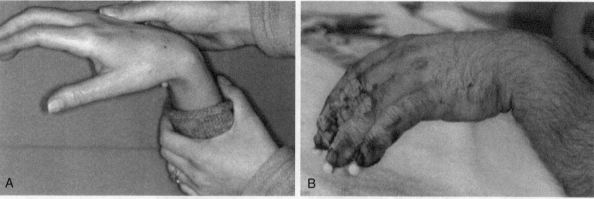

FIG. 34.2 (A) and (B) Early protective motion phase I wrist flexion and metacarpophalangeal/ interphalangeal extension.

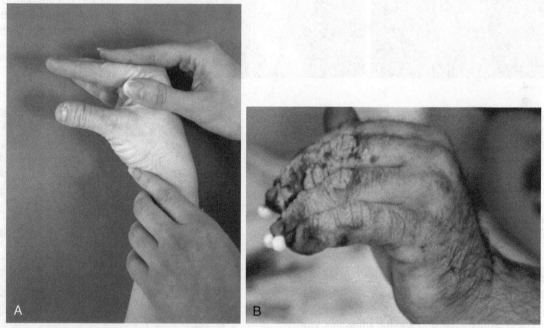

FIG. 34.3 (A) and (B) Early protective motion phase I wrist extension with metacarpophalangeal flexion.

Focus on using a gentle passive synergistic movement to proportionally move the MPs, IPs, and wrist. Help the client passively extend the MP and IP joints (naturally and with gentle assist) while the wrist is gently flexed (actively, if appropriate) (Fig. 34.2). Then help the client actively extend the wrist to neutral (with passive assist as needed) while you and gravity assist the fingers into MP flexion (Fig. 34.3). Ideally, PIP and DIP extension are increased at the same time through viscoelastic forces in the hand. This movement must be proportional and balanced between flexors and extensors. The goal of EPM I is to establish gliding of the intrinsic and extrinsic flexors and extensors, and movement of the wrist and MP joints, to minimize stiffness while protecting involved structures. **Precaution.** *EPM I should be modified if the MPs are tight or severely limited by edema or joint stiffness, if bony fixation is not stable enough to tolerate ROM in nearby joints, or if related structures were repaired under tension.*

AROM should be performed regularly for all uninvolved and proximal joints throughout the day. Exercises may be used to strengthen proximal musculature if the client is careful to avoid stressing the repaired distal structures. Contralateral strengthening by means of motor neuron retraining may be used to minimize loss of strength.

Early Protective Motion Phase II

The EPM protocol is advanced to *passive* EPM II at 7 to 14 days postsurgery, after a few days of EPM I movement. The goals of this phase are to reduce tendon adhesions, prevent/minimize PIP joint stiffness, provide differential tendon gliding, and improve tendon tensile strength. The client should continue EPM I while adding intrinsic plus ("tabletop" position) and intrinsic minus ("hook" position) exercises to enhance differential gliding and gentle contraction of the long flexors and extensors and the intrinsics. The wrist remains neutral throughout the hook position. To create the hook position, passively extend the MP joints and gently assist the PIP and DIP joints into slight flexion (Fig. 34.4). **Precaution.** *Limit PIP flexion to less than 60 degrees until 4 to 6 weeks after surgery to protect the central slip. If resistance is felt, do not progress ROM further.*

From the hook position, move to the tabletop position using gravity to assist flexion of the MP joints while assisting extension

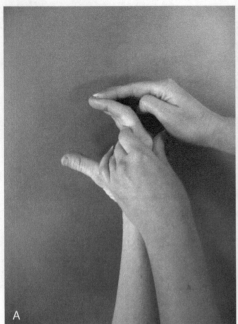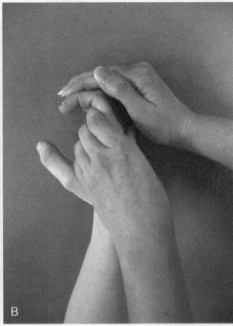

FIG. 34.4 Early protective motion phase II hook position. To create the hook position, keep the wrist in neutral and passively extend the MP joints. Then, gently assist the PIP and DIP joints from extension (A) into slight flexion (B).

of the PIP and DIP joints (Fig. 34.5). Interestingly, in the intrinsic plus (tabletop) position, the flexor digitorum superficialis (FDS) and flexor digitorum profundus (FDP) tendons are virtually inactive because MP flexion and PIP extension in this position are primarily achieved with contraction of the interossei and lumbrical muscles. Therefore a strong contraction in this position should not overly stress the repairs to the long flexors or extensors.

Significant edema or extensor tendon damage limits PIP joint ROM in this protocol and should be an indication to progress slowly.

◎ *Clinical Pearl*

Slow gentle movement helps reduce edema. Gentle stress on healing tissues can help stimulate healing. Some gliding of the extensors can reduce extension-limiting adhesions. With this in mind,[19,20] the "hook to tabletop" movement is the safest and most effective movement that allows ROM at all three joints of the fingers, along with gliding of both long flexors (the FDS and the FDP) and all components of the dorsal mechanism and the extrinsic extensor (extensor digitorum communis).[19,20]

Active EPM II is initiated 14 to 21 days after surgery. Progress to "place and hold" exercises by assisting the hand into the intrinsic minus hook position. Ask the client to hold the position with a gentle active contraction, then move the hand to the intrinsic plus (tabletop) position and ask for an active contraction. At this point, as appropriate and tolerated, add active gliding and isolated FDS gliding exercises and strengthen the interossei in the intrinsic plus position. This upgrade allows initiation of active gliding in noncomposite range while continuing to use synergistic movement and relying on balance to move the intrinsic and extrinsic flexors and extensors without overstressing any system. Initiate use of functional therapeutic activities as soon as possible. These may include picking up large beads and putting them into a container using modified prehension (Fig. 34.6). Returning to

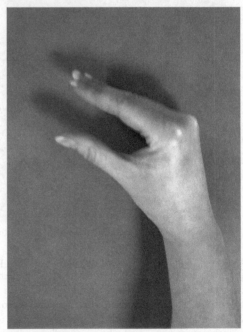

FIG. 34.5 Early protective motion phase II tabletop position.

"normal" activities as soon as possible helps the client regain a more functional and positive connection between the brain and the hand.

At 4 weeks after surgery, the client may begin gradually increasing wrist extension past neutral with the digits loosely flexed, increasing overall synergistic movement-related ROM. The client should also slowly progress toward full composite active flexion and extension at this time (depending on tightness). Continue to reassess the orthosis to ensure correct fit and positioning.

Six weeks or later after surgery, add gentle passive stretching, NMES as indicated for adhesions, more aggressive blocking

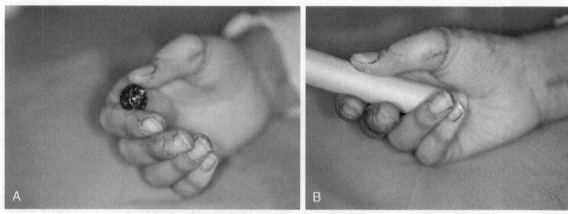

FIG. 34.6 (A) Functional prehension exercises. (B) Functional grasp exercise.

exercises, and upgrade functional activities. Continue to progress with caution given the likelihood that replanted or revascularized structures will heal more slowly than expected because of their diminished vascular and nutritional status. Introduce use of a dynamic or static progressive orthosis as needed for stiffness, but keep in mind that circulation will not be normal. Spread out pressure across as wide an area as possible with wide straps and cuffs and good orthosis contour and by keeping traction light. A serial static extension orthosis worn at night can provide gentle stretch over many hours and does not interfere with functional use during the daytime.

If the physician has assessed and verified fracture consolidation, add pinch and grip strengthening as early as 8 weeks after surgery. Continue to upgrade the program emphasizing reconditioning of the entire upper extremity. Table 34.2 presents highlights of the timelines and interventions for EPM. (See Silverman and colleagues[19,20] and Chan and LaStayo[13] for a more specific description of this protocol.)

Amputation

The hand surgeon generally makes every effort to salvage viable tissues in the hand. However, amputation is preferable to spending time and energy trying to save a finger that would ultimately remain stiff, insensate, and nonfunctional. This is especially true if the stiff finger would interfere with the functioning of the remaining digits.[9]

From a therapy standpoint, amputations are simple to treat because relatively few precautions are required. The primary focus is on promoting uncomplicated wound healing and desensitizing sensitive tissues. Neuroma formation is a possibility and this may be addressed through desensitization and use of a variety of gel sheeting products.

The most serious problem with amputations may be the psychological effect on the client. Although any traumatic injury may result in a malformed hand, the loss of a digit often causes the greatest stress and concern to the client. By emphasizing the positive effects of amputation on overall functional recovery, the therapist can aid the client in coping with this loss. Functional or cosmetic prostheses may be helpful later; showing the client pictures of these early can also be helpful. If the client continues to greatly mourn the loss, referral to a mental health professional may be appropriate.[22]

TABLE 34.2	Highlights of Early Protective Motion Protocol
Postoperative Timeline	**Exercise or Intervention**
4–10 days	**EPM I:** MP extension with wrist flexion MP flexion with wrist extension
7–14 days	**EPM II passive:** Continue EPM I Passively move client's fingers between "table" MP flexion with IP extension (intrinsic plus) and "hook" MP extension with IP flexion (< 60 degrees) (intrinsic minus)
14–21 days	**EPM II active:** Continue EPM I and EPM II passive Place and hold hook and table positions Progress to active hook and table Isolated FDS tendon exercises Interossei strengthening (intrinsic plus) Light functional activities
28 days	Increase wrist extension to full with flexed fingers Progress to full AROM and finger PROM Begin gentle blocking exercises
6 weeks	NMES Passive stretching of involved structures Full nonresistive use for ADLs (precautions for insensate hand) Dynamic orthosis use
8 weeks	Light strengthening exercises

ADL, Activity of daily living; *AROM,* active range of motion; *EPM,* early protective motion; *FDS,* flexor digitorum superficialis; *IP,* interphalangeal; *MP,* metacarpophalangeal; *NMES,* neuromuscular electrical stimulation; *PROM,* passive range of motion; *ROM,* range of motion.

Secondary Surgical Procedures

Despite the hard work of both the client and the therapist, secondary surgical procedures are common after a clinical plateau is reached. During the last phase of therapy, as you head toward discharge, consider the remaining issues that might be addressed with a secondary surgery. Assess for and address tightness of the joint capsule, intrinsic and extrinsic tightness, tendon and scar adhesions, and scar contracture. Plan ahead for future surgeries, which may include tenolysis, capsulectomy, joint contracture release, web-space revision, tendon grafting, and tendon transfers.[23] Maximizing PROM and strength is important before tenolysis and many other follow-up procedures. Communicate with the physician so that you understand the surgical procedures and objectives in advance, and then explain the next surgery to the client, in addition to the probable course of therapy, so that you can help them develop reasonable time and commitment expectations before undertaking another procedure.

Summary

Treating clients with traumatic hand injury requires simultaneous evaluation and management of many different types of structural defects and repairs. An organized logical systems approach allows you to assess each system individually and then prioritize the systems for treatment. Taking care to follow precautions is the guiding principle for treatment.

These injuries allow the hand therapist to facilitate significant improvements in appearance and function while working with a client over many months from initial evaluation to discharge. For this reason, treating these clients can be a very rewarding experience for a hand therapist.

Summary Thoughts on Diagnosis-Specific Information

- Determine which systems are involved, and then prioritize them.
- Determine the stage of each system, and decide how to treat this stage appropriately.
- Fracture fixation affects the appropriateness of early AROM and PROM.
- Healing varies with age, health, nutritional status, and smoking status. Vascular repairs can delay healing.
- Edema affects tendon glide and ROM by increasing resistance to movement, creating adhesions and fibrosis, and increasing pain.
- There is a fine line between being as aggressive as possible to improve the condition and being too aggressive. Some stress on healing systems encourages healing, but being too aggressive can lead to fracture nonunion, tendon rupture, or other problems. The ideal is to move everything as early as possible without compromising the surgical repair. **Precaution.** *Respect pain, monitor tissue responses, and adjust the therapeutic regimen accordingly if a flare reaction occurs.*
- Incorporate functional activities into therapy as soon as possible. Clients who are medically cleared to perform AROM can work on picking up, holding, and turning light objects in their hands or passing items from hand to hand.

Clinical Pearl

Clients tend to respond better to short, frequent exercise sessions of fewer repetitions performed more often, than to lengthy sessions performed infrequently.

- Work within a reasonable pain tolerance; ask clients to get to their end-range and then hold.
- Make therapy interesting, creative, functional, and purposeful.
- Consider functional outcomes and goals—strength needs versus endurance needs for work and ADLs.
- Strengthen every joint through the maximum available range. If you notice the client is "cheating" or cannot move a weight through full ROM, consider reducing the resistance.
- Strengthen proximal joints and the contralateral side as soon as possible after therapy. Use bilateral exercises and activities to demonstrate and "retrain" the involved hand.

➤ Precautions and Concerns

Revascularizations (Arterial and Venous Flow)

- *Decreased circulation after arterial repair affects the rate of healing for wounds, tendons, and fractures because of the decrease in peripheral circulation and delivery of nutrients to the area. Typical protocol timelines generally must be extended by a few weeks.*
- *Keep the hand warm and avoid exposure to cold or sudden/extreme temperature changes by using a mitten, an oven mitt, or a scarf.*
- *In the early phase of healing, be very gentle when changing dressings; avoid changing them in cold, drafty areas (for example, under an air conditioning vent).*
- *Emphasize to clients that they must not eat or drink anything vasoconstrictive, such as caffeine or chocolate. Smoking is prohibited. Appropriate hydration and nutrition are imperative for healing.*
- *Do not use compressive bandages (elastic tape, gloves, sleeves) until vascular status has stabilized.*
- *Prevent compression from orthosis material and straps.*
- *Constantly monitor the color of the fingers with regard to capillary refill.*
- *Do not use cold treatments in the acute phase.*
- *Do not use a whirlpool because it puts the hand in a dependent position.*
- *Do not use contrast baths because they may cause vasospasm followed by vasoconstriction.*
- *Mild heat may be used once vascularity has stabilized. However, the insensate hand does not have a warning system to let the client know when a substance is too hot; also, it cannot dissipate heat as well (that is, it burns more easily).*
- *Although elevation is a good way to reduce edema, excessive elevation challenges the vascular system; the hand should not be held significantly above the level of the heart if revascularization was a part of the surgery.*

Tendon Repairs

- *Protect against a full active fist or full extension of the fingers.*
- *Avoid resistance from excessive cocontraction in early stages.*
- *Edema increases resistance during early ROM exercises; modify your approach if you encounter resistance.*

Fractures

- *Avoid excess stress at fracture, fusion, or pin sites while mobilizing a complex injury.*
- *If revascularization has been done in conjunction with fracture fixation, expect delayed healing or nonunion as a result of a decrease in the delivery of nutrients to the area.*

Nerve Injury and Repair

- *Nerve injuries leave part of the hand insensate. Teach the client to use caution with ADLs (that is, avoid injury from exposure to heat or use of sharp objects).*
- *Use caution with use of dynamic or static progressive orthoses and any other external compression because of the lack of a warning system for ischemia.*
- *Also use heat and ice treatments cautiously.*
- *Remind the client that cold intolerance and pain after a nerve injury is common for two or more years.[24]*

Incisions, Wounds, and Grafts

- *Make sure that dressings do not exert shear or mechanical stress on healing wounds.*
- *Prevent maceration of periwound areas while maintaining a moist wound bed.*
- *Avoid using cytotoxic chemicals (for example, peroxide, povidone-iodine) on granulating wound tissue.*

CASE STUDIES

CASE STUDY 34.1

Michael a 15-year-old, right hand dominant, high school student sustained a complex laceration of his right hand while cutting a piece of wood with a saw blade during shop class. Because he was cutting wood, the wound was relatively clean. However, because the saw blade was an old one, it created a moderate amount of tearing damage. The following injuries were noted:

- Thumb: Amputation at the MP joint
- Index finger: Laceration of FDS and FDP, radial and ulnar neurovascular bundles
- Middle finger: FDS and FDP laceration, open fracture of the metacarpal neck, lacerations of the radial and ulnar digital arteries and veins in the digit (radial digital nerve [RDN], ulnar digital nerve [UDN], radial digital artery [RDA], and ulnar digital artery [UDA])
- Ring finger: Laceration of FDS and FDP, RDN, UDN, UDA
- Small finger: Extensor tendon laceration

The following procedures were performed:

- Thumb: Replant with MP arthrodesis, vein graft, flexor pollicis longus tendon repair, extensor repair, nerve repair, artery repair
- Index finger: Revascularization, repair of common digital artery to UDA, FDS/FDP repair in zone II, repair of RDN/UDN
- Middle finger: Debridement of metacarpal head and neck (intraarticular fracture), volar plate repair, repair of common digital artery to UDA, FDS/FDP repair in zone II, nerve repair
- Ring finger: RDN/UDN repair, FDS repair in zone II, excision of FDP, insertion of Hunter rod
- Small finger: Debridement, repair of 50% extensor laceration just proximal to PIP joint

Michael had his first outpatient appointment with the hand surgeon 6 days after surgery. The physician changed his dressing, and he was referred for an orthosis and hand therapy. The orthotic order stated: "Orthoplast to tips, thumb spica, wrist 10 degrees flexion, MPs at 90 degrees." The therapy referral requested "modified Duran protocol, no movement of thumb, ignore extensor in small finger (only partial injury)."

At his first hand therapy visit, Michael's hand was rebandaged with the lightest possible dressing, and he was fitted with a dorsal protective orthosis with slight wrist flexion and maximum reasonable MP flexion. The thumb was positioned in mid-abduction for protection in a safe position and to minimize the potential for webspace contracture (Fig. 34.7).

Although this had the elements of a complex injury, problem solving using the systems approach highlighted some exceptions worth considering in the treatment planning:

- The replant injury occurred in the thumb. Because of the importance of this digit, the surgeon opted for a delayed mobilization protocol to protect the revascularization and fusion. Also, because the thumb is relatively independent, it could be considered and treated separately from the other digits. While the thumb was primarily immobilized, synergistic movement exercises to the fingers would have some effect on gliding of some of the structures in and near the thumb.
- Most of the tendon injuries occurred in the flexors; therefore they could be treated as simple tendon lacerations with revascularization and nerve repair. According to the surgeon's orders, the small finger extensor tendon injury was not treated as a precaution, and this led to implementation of a modified version of the Duran flexor tendon repair protocol.
- Precautions for revascularization were followed throughout therapy for the vascular repairs.
- The fracture at the thumb MP joint was fused and was treated therapeutically as a fusion. The fracture at the middle finger MP joint did not significantly affect any protocols.

Initial Evaluation

At the initial evaluation, the following findings were noted:

- Pain: 3 to 5 on a scale of 1 to 10 (3–5/10)
- Edema: Moderate in digits and palm
- Sensibility: Not tested, anticipated loss secondary to nerve injuries
- Wounds: Slight serosanguineous drainage
- ROM: Passive flexion to within 1 inch of palm; extension of middle finger, ring finger, small finger to orthosis; index finger has 30-degree flexion contracture at PIP; ROM to thumb and wrist not attempted

The therapist kept the initial evaluation brief and cursory to get a good overview of the situation.

Therapy Goals

Short-Term Goals

1. Protect injury and surgical repair through use of the protective orthosis and education.
2. Increase passive flexion to the palm to enhance tendon glide, joint mobility, and prepare for AROM.
3. Promote wound healing and closure.
4. Initiate scar management program to minimize scarring and adhesions to maximize potential ROM.

Long-Term Goals

1. Increase PROM of fingers to within normal limits (WNL) for potential AROM and function.
2. Increase AROM of index finger, middle finger, and small finger to greater than 60% of normal limits for grasp/release of a 1-inch-diameter object.

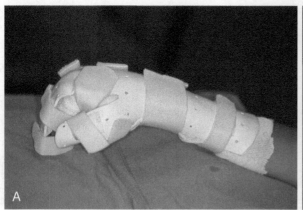
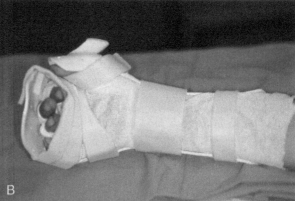

FIG. 34.7 (A) and (B) Dorsal protective orthosis with slight wrist flexion and maximum reasonable MP flexion. The thumb is positioned in mid-abduction.

3. Client to use hand in more than 50% of ADLs.
4. In cases in which the therapist does not know specifically what to expect in terms of outcome, the best course is to predict a basic level of function and ROM. PROM must be maximized if there is to be any hope of regaining full AROM and to obtain the best results after secondary surgery.

Home Exercise Program

Both the client and his mother were educated extensively about the surgical procedures performed, the expectations of surgery, and the necessity of a second surgery for replacement of the Silastic rod with an active tendon graft. They also were taught how to perform wound care, dressing changes, and ROM exercises. They were given the following initial HEP:

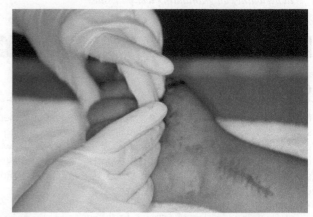

FIG. 34.8 Early passive range of motion at second postoperative visit.

Home Exercise Program to Be Done Every Other Hour

- Push the big knuckles down all together, hold 5 seconds (passive MP flexion).
- Push the big knuckle down, push the fingertip in, on each finger, one at a time; hold 5 seconds; do 3 to 5 times per finger (passive composite flexion) (Fig. 34.8).
- Push the big knuckles in as far as able, straighten fingers (one at a time), relax, repeat five times (passive MP flexion with active IP extension; enhances long flexor glide and intrinsic action).
Note that the HEP was written in common terms that the client and his mother would understand.
At the client's second visit for therapy, synergistic movement was added. The client was taught to combine wrist extension with a passive fist and then to flex the wrist and allow the fingers to extend naturally. The therapist was hopeful that some minimal gliding would occur in the thumb tendons without disrupting the healing and fusion there.

Three to Four Weeks After Surgery

At approximately 3 weeks after surgery, the physician gave approval to begin performance of a "place and hold" fist to try to mitigate the heavy scarring that was forming. Heavy scarring that limits ROM suggests that the client is forming good scar to heal the wounds and that the protocol may be progressed more rapidly. Transcutaneous electrical nerve stimulation was tried for pain management but was not helpful. About 4 weeks after surgery, active

finger flexion, extension exercises, and blocked finger flexion exercises were added.

The physician was consulted about beginning thumb AROM. He approved initiation of IP blocking exercises with the still-healing MP fusion protected, as well as abduction/adduction exercises. Because active finger and thumb ROM were now safe and acceptable, Michael began to use his hand for light prehension exercises in the clinic and at home. He was not yet allowed to use the hand for ADLs at home because of the concern that he might overdo it, especially with the thumb. He began functional prehension, picking up beads and grasping a foam tube (see Fig. 34.6). Because scarring was becoming more of a problem, scar massage was increased at the volar MP scars. Michael was an exception to the typical delays in healing after a replant or revascularization because he was young and still growing. His body was able to produce new tissue, especially scar tissue, faster than most adults. His program therefore could be speeded up when it became apparent that scar formation was becoming an issue.

Five to Six Weeks After Surgery

Five weeks after surgery, Michael's ROM evaluation showed that active MP flexion was WNL, PIP flexion averaged about 60 degrees, and DIP flexion was about 20 degrees. MP extension lag averaged 15 degrees, but the PIPs of the index, middle, and ring fingers were very limited in extension, at about −45 degrees. The client had full passive flexion of all fingers. The thumb web space showed tightness in both radial abduction (35 degrees) and palmar abduction

(25 degrees), and he had only 10 degrees of thumb IP flexion. He had very good wrist ROM with wrist extension at 55 degrees and flexion to 75 degrees. Sensibility was functional with diminished protective sensation; the Semmes-Weinstein evaluation showed the thumb, index finger, middle finger, and ring finger at 4.31 and the small finger at 3.61.

A note was sent to the physician at this time stating that Michael's tissue was "adherent, but gaining ROM" and that the web scar/contracture was a concern. The physician was asked when thumb PROM would be permitted, whether ultrasound treatment could be used for the scars, and whether the tolerable stretch for full passive extension of the fingers could be increased. The physician approved discontinuation of the protective orthosis, recommended the orthosis be modified to try to increase the thumb web space, and approved ultrasound treatment for the scars. He allowed use of a passive extension orthosis "as per normal protocol." He told the therapist, "I doubt he'll get much thumb IP motion, but it's okay to begin PROM." Discontinuing the protective orthosis at 5 weeks after surgery is a bit unusual, but this young client apparently was forming a significant amount of scar and healing more rapidly than a full-grown adult with the same injury. Sensibility, although diminished, was sufficient to protect him from additional injury and to allow use of the hand functionally in light ADLs.

Changes in therapy included conversion of the dorsal block orthosis to a volar design with Otoform elastomer to scar for PIP extension. A thumb web stretch also was built into the orthosis (Fig. 34.9). Michael began writing practice using a foam pen grip; he also practiced picking up marbles and in-hand manipulation skills. Moist heat was added at 6 weeks after surgery, and ultrasound treatment with extension stretch to the volar scars was added to increase passive extension of the fingers.

Seven Weeks After Surgery

At 7 weeks after surgery, the HEP consisted of the following:

- Web spacer orthosis with Otoform elastomer, 4 hours a day and at night
- AROM and PROM exercises, including blocking, opposition, place and hold, and wrist ROM, 10 repetitions, 4 to 6 times a day
- Scar massage
- Light to moderate use of the hand for ADLs, including writing and eating (Fig. 34.10)

In the clinic, Michael continued with moist heat, ultrasound treatment of scars, and one-on-one ROM exercises with emphasis on blocking. Mildly resistive activities were initiated, including use of a gripper with light tension (Fig. 34.11). The client used it in the normal position, gripping with the fingers, and also reversed it in his hand to pull down with the thumb. Putty rolling was done to stretch the fingers and elicit cocontraction of the finger and wrist flexors and extensors. The client also continued to practice writing and picking up pegs and marbles.

Eight Weeks After Surgery

At 8 weeks after surgery, a baseline grip evaluation was performed. The right grip strength average was 10 lbs and the left was 45 lbs. The physician approved gentle strengthening, including the addition of putty exercises to the HEP, gripping, pinching, and rolling. One of Michael's goals was to be able to carry a bucket of water or feed so that he could return to his summer job working on a farm. He therefore began a graded program of picking up and carrying weights in the clinic and at home, with the goal of working up to 20 lbs. A Baltimore Therapeutic Equipment work simulator program was

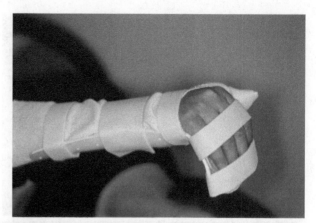

FIG. 34.9 At 6 weeks after surgery, the dorsal block orthosis was converted to a volar design with a thumb web stretch.

added to clinic sessions to help improve strength and endurance. By 12 weeks after surgery, the client primarily was performing a HEP with upgrades for strengthening.

Four to Six Months After Surgery

Michael's final evaluation was done approximately 4 months after surgery. Referring to his injured right hand, he said, "I can do anything with it," and he demonstrated lifting a 20-lb weight. Grip strength in the right hand had increased to 40 lbs. The findings at this evaluation are shown as follows:

Strength Measurements at Four Months after Surgery					
RANGE OF MOTION					
	Thumb	Index Finger	Middle Finger	Ring Finger	Small Finger
MP		0/90	0/100	0/105	0/95
PIP		−40/95	0/80	0/80	0/95
DIP		0/20	0/15	0/0	0/80
Semmes-Weinstein monofilament test	3.22	3.22	3.22	2.83	2.83

DIP, distal interphalangeal; *MP,* metacarpophalangeal; *PIP,* proximal interphalangeal.

	Right Hand	Left Hand
Grip strength	40 lbs	60 lbs
Lateral pinch	15 lbs	15 lbs
Three-jaw pinch	15 lbs	20 lbs

lbs, pounds.

Michael returned to the surgeon 6 months after surgery. He had decided that he did not want a tendon graft to the FDP of the ring finger; he felt that he was functional, and he did not want to go through rehabilitation again. At this time, several other surgical procedures were performed. These included release of

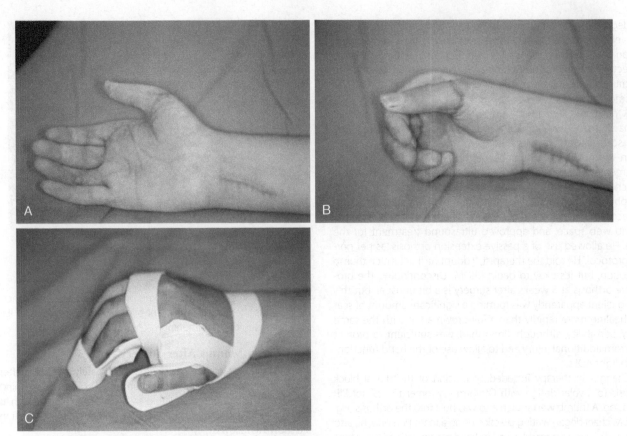

FIG. 34.10 (A) and (B) At 7 weeks after surgery, the client's home exercise program consisted of range of motion exercises. He also started using a web-spacer orthosis (C).

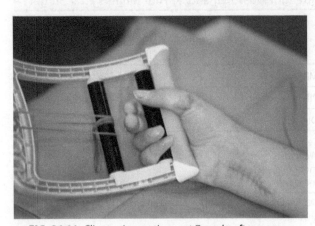

FIG. 34.11 Client using a gripper at 7 weeks after surgery.

a thumb web-space contracture (by Z-plasty); release of a volar skin contracture on the index finger (Z-plasty); and removal of the Hunter rod in the ring finger, which left the client with a superficialis finger (that is, he had no flexion force at the DIP, which meant he could end up with a boutonnière deformity).

Michael returned to therapy 9 days after surgery, and an orthosis was fabricated to maintain the web space and hold the index finger in full extension. He had minimal pain (0–2/10) and edema. Index finger extension was –30 degrees, thumb radial abduction was 65 degrees, and thumb palmar abduction was 60 degrees. The client was instructed in wound care and in full ROM exercises with emphasis on index finger PIP extension blocking and web-space stretching.

Because he was already familiar with therapy, he was seen only once a week for program and orthotic modifications and upgrades, which included the addition of strengthening exercises and a gel sheet.

Michael was seen for the last time in therapy 6 weeks after surgery. He reported full functional use of the hand in all ADLs and was prepared to return to his summer job soon thereafter. The final outcome measurements for this client are shown here:

Final Measurements				
RANGE OF MOTION				
	Index Finger	Middle Finger	Ring Finger	Small Finger
MP	0/90	0/100	0/95	0/90
PIP	–20/95	0/85	0/90	0/95
DIP	0/25	0/20	0/0	0/80

DIP, distal interphalangeal; *MP*, metacarpophalangeal; *PIP*, proximal interphalangeal.

STRENGTH MEASUREMENTS	
Right hand:	45 lbs
Left hand:	60 lbs
Thumb radial abduction:	60 degrees
Thumb palmar abduction:	60 degrees

References

1. Sturm SM, Oxley SB, Van Zant RS: Rehabilitation of a patient following hand replantation after near-complete distal forearm amputation, *J Hand Ther* 27:217–224, 2014.
2. Wilhelmi BJ, Lee WP, Pagensteert GI, et al.: Replantation in the mutilated hand, *Hand Clin* 19:89–120, 2003.
3. Moran SL, Berger RA: Biomechanics and hand trauma: what you need, *Hand Clin* 19:17–31, 2003.
4. Morrison WA, McCombe D: Digital replantation, *Hand Clin* 23:1–12, 2007.
5. Ng ZY, Askari M, Chim HL: Approach to complex upper extremity injury: an algorithm, *Semin Plast Surg* 29:5–9, 2015.
6. Win TS, Henderson J: Management of traumatic amputations of the upper limb, *BMJ* 348, 2014.
7. Huish SB, Hartigan BJ, Stern PJ: Combined injuries of the hand. In Mackin EJ, Callahan AD, Skirven TM, et al.: *Rehabilitation of the hand and upper extremity*, ed 5, St Louis, 2002, Mosby.
8. Rizzo M: Complex injuries of the hand. In Skirven TM, Osterman AL, Fedorczyk J, et al.: *Rehabilitation of the hand and upper extremity*, ed 6, Philadelphia, 2011, Mosby, pp 1227–1238.
9. Freeland AE, Lineaweaver WC, Lindley SG: Fracture fixation in the mutilated hand, *Hand Clin* 19:51–61, 2003.
10. Walsh JM, Chee N: Replantation. In Saunders RJ, Astifidis RP, Burke SL, et al.: *Hand and upper extremity rehabilitation: a practical guide*, ed 4, St. Louis, 2016, Elsevier.
11. Maricevich A, Carlsen B, Mardini S, et al.: Upper extremity and digital replantation, *Hand* 6:356–363, 2011.
12. Jones NF, Chang J, Kashani P: The surgical and rehabilitative aspects of replantation and revascularization of the hand. In Skirven TM, Osterman AL, Fedorczyk J, et al.: *Rehabilitation of the hand and upper extremity*, ed 6, Philadelphia, 2011, Mosby, pp 1252–1272.
13. Chan SW, LaStayo P: Hand therapy management following mutilating hand injuries, *Hand Clin* 19:133–148, 2003.
14. Pettengill KM: Therapist's management of the complex injury. In Skirven TM, Osterman AL, Fedorczyk J, et al.: *Rehabilitation of the hand and upper extremity*, ed 6, Philadelphia, 2011, Mosby, pp 1238–1252.
15. Rosen B, Lundborg G: Training with a mirror in rehabilitation of the hand, *Scand J Plast Reconstr Surg Hand Surg* 39:104, 2005.
16. Gustafson M, Hagberg L, Holmefur M: Ten years follow-up of health and disability in people with acute traumatic hand injury: pain and cold sensitivity are long-standing problems, *J Hand Surg Eur* 36(7):590–598, 2011.
17. Beris AE, Lykissas MG, Korompilias AV, et al.: Digit and hand replantation, *Arch Orthop Trauma Surg* 130:1141–1147, 2010.
18. Savas S, Inal EE, Yavuz DD, et al.: Risk factors for complex regional pain syndrome in patients with surgically treated traumatic injuries attending hand therapy, *J Hand Ther* 31:250, 2018.
19. Silverman PM, Willette-Green V, Petrilli J: Early protective motion in digital revascularization and replantation, *J Hand Ther* 2:84–101, 1989.
20. Silverman PM, Gordon L: Early motion after replantation, *Hand Clin* 12:97–107, 1996.
21. Novak CB, von der Hyde RL: Rehabilitation of the upper extremity following nerve and tendon reconstruction: when and how, *Semin Plast Surg* 29:73–80, 2015.
22. Grob M, Papadopulos NA, Zimmerman A, et al.: The psychological impact of severe hand injury, *J Hand Surg Eur* 33(3):358–362, 2008.
23. Neumeister MW, Brown RE: Mutilating hand injuries: principles and management, *Hand Clin* 19:1–15, 2003.
24. Cannon NM: *Diagnosis and treatment manual for physicians and therapists*, ed 4, Indianapolis, 2001, Hand Rehabilitation Center of Indiana, 196–200.

35

The Stiff Hand

Susan Weiss

We should regard the hand as a mobile organ and never
let it stiffen. It must move to thrive.

—Sterling Bunnell, 1947

The interesting thing about hand stiffness is that it is encountered in every clinical practice. Hand stiffness is a complication that is incurred from an array of frequent, as well as not-so-frequent, issues. Occasionally, a client comes to us with a stiff hand—years after an initial injury—and we are challenged to restore functional pain-free motion. Additionally, many of the disorders we treat can yield the sequela of stiffness. This chapter addresses how to prevent, evaluate, and treat stiffness. We will examine common treatment regimens that can be utilized to assist our clients with what they want most, which is to return to full function.

Diagnosis

Broadly speaking, the term *stiffness* implies that there is a mechanical resistance to deformation. This resistance results in limited joint mobility, and there are many sources that contribute to it: muscle tightness, tendon adhesions, scars, skin and subcutaneous tissue loss, joint capsule tightness, articular problems, or a combination of these and/or other factors. Stiffness can also be psychosomatic or result from nonuse. Nonuse of the affected hand may occur due to pain, denervation, or immobilization, and this triggers a cascade of problems that further perpetuate stiffness. Nonuse results in muscle atrophy (and further weakness), edema, muscle collagen fiber cross-linkage, and abnormal motor programs (Fig. 35.1). Even brief periods of immobilization can result in reduced somatosensory representation on the brain and the development of abnormal movement patterns. This results in both mechanical and cerebral challenges to regaining motion in the stiff hand. This cycle must be altered in order to "undo stiffness."

Timelines and Healing

Hand stiffness can begin at any stage of the healing process. When soft tissue is wounded, our bodies move into the **inflammatory phase** of healing. The response is a local infiltration of white blood cells that clean up debris and help fight off infection. Although some inflammation is normal and necessary for healing, edema should be treated early and aggressively. Edema contributes to pain, adhesions, and disuse throughout the healing process—all leading to eventual stiffness. Generally speaking, edema in this phase is controlled with elevation, gentle active range of motion (AROM) if allowed, compression, possibly cold modalities, and positional orthoses.

The **proliferative phase** (fibroblastic stage) of healing begins once the injured area is clean and free from damaged tissue, foreign matter, and bacteria. This phase is characterized by random collagen formation designed to fill the wound and bridge the gap. This can take up to a few weeks to complete. It is important to get the injured hand moving as early as is safely possible (which depends on the nature of the injuries). If there is prolonged immobilization, collagen disorganization persists—resulting in weakening and additional stiffness.[1] Active joint motion in this phase has the capacity to promote healthy collagen formation, which is compatible with function.[1] During this phase, disuse leads to weakness of muscles, which contributes to stiffness. Stiffness early in this phase typically has a soft end-feel, and edema is often pitting during this time (Fig. 35.2). If the application of appropriate stress is applied in this phase, chronic stiffness can perhaps be avoided.

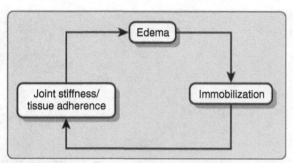

FIG. 35.1 Cycle of nonuse. (From Skirven TM, Osterman AL, Fedorczyk JM, et al. eds. *Rehabilitation of the Hand and Upper Extremity.* 6th ed. Philadelphia, PA: Mosby; 2011, p. 896.)

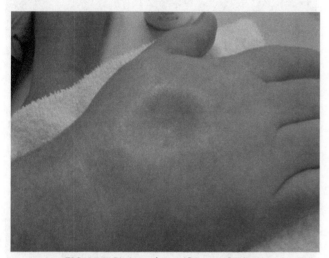

FIG. 35.2 Pitting edema. (Courtesy S. Weiss.)

During the **maturation phase** of healing, the process of laying down collagen normalizes and strong cross-linkages between collagen fibers form. The length of the maturation phase varies based on many factors but can continue for up to two years.[2] After the maturation stage, the therapist's options for treating stiffness become fewer with regard to intervention opportunities. Casting motion to mobilize stiffness (CMMS) is discussed as an intervention later in the chapter and can be an effective treatment strategy for the chronically stiff hand.

> **◎ Clinical Pearl**
>
> Edema and pain perpetuate nonuse → which perpetuates weakness and alterations in motor programs → which leads to stiffness → which causes further pain and edema → which perpetuates further nonuse → etc.
>
> This cycle *must* be broken to allow clients to regain motion and function.

Evaluation

The first steps in evaluating a client with a stiff hand involve seeking background information on: (1) the client's medical condition, (2) date of onset of the medical condition or surgery, (3) specific physician orders, and (4) precautions (movements and activities to avoid). This is accomplished via a medical record review, communication with referral sources, and an interview of the client. The data will guide the therapist's clinical reasoning through the evaluation and treatment planning processes. Therapists often observe how clients use their hands while engaging in manual occupations. This helps the therapist obtain a functional assessment. Observing how a client uses the entire upper extremity can provide beneficial insights into a client's movement patterns, movement quality, and substitution patterns. Photography and videography are extremely useful for this.

Visual inspection of the affected extremity will include looking for atrophy, redness, bruises, wounds, scars, skin creases, trophic changes, deformities, and the arches of the hand. Our palpation and hands-on examination helps detect issues with any nodules, tender points, scar and skin limitations, bony protrusions, and capillary refill. The interview establishes the client's chief complaints, daily routines/functional limitations, and therapy goals.

Goniometry

Range of motion (ROM) assessment helps determine the nature and extent of stiffness in a given joint, and is the most commonly used assessment for joint mobility.[3] To determine whether weakness or soft-tissue/bony restrictions are sources of limited joint mobility, we take both active and passive measurements. Generally speaking, a goniometric measurement of the hand is subject to a 5 degree measurement error;[4] and because of this, goniometric measurements need to have a discrepancy of greater than 5 degrees for there to be a "real difference."[5] Of interest, the iPhone goniometer was studied to assess accuracy of wrist ROM and was shown to have less than a 2 degree difference compared to a universal goniometer.[6] This technology could be helpful for engaging clients as partners in their own hand rehabilitation.

Strength

Often, strength evaluations cannot be performed in the early stages of healing, but both grip and pinch strength should be performed and documented once allowed.

Sensation

If our clients have impaired sensation, it will interfere with normal hand functioning. Baseline sensory testing is useful because we need to be aware of this limitation. We test sensation with assessments such as the Semmes-Weinstein (monofilaments), two-point discrimination, or the Moberg pick-up test.

Edema

We must assess edema in any client who has stiffness as a result of trauma, an inflammatory condition, dependent posturing, weakness, or nonuse.[7] If you think of edema as glue, you will understand why we do everything possible to avoid it; and if it is unavoidable, we do our best to mitigate it as quickly as possible. Edema fluctuates with diet, exercise, activity, temperature, and time of day. It is important to try to test at the same time of day and to document both hands.[7] Use the volumetric *difference* between the two hands as your indicator of change from week to week.

> **◎ Clinical Pearl**
>
> When clients insist they are swollen but objective measurements indicate zero swelling, know that they are not fabricating this. Swollen interstitial fluids can have up to a 30% overload before edema is detected by the naked eye or with any measuring tools.[7]

Neurological Tone Assessment

Clients with spasticity or flaccidity may experience stiffness. In nearly all cases, therapists should prevent prolonged client posturing that encourages contracture development.

Intrinsic Tightness Testing

These tests are used when proximal interphalangeal (PIP) joint passive flexion is limited and the therapist wants to determine if extrinsic finger extensors, intrinsics (lumbricals), or joint capsule tightness are responsible. If placing the metacarpophalangeal (MP) joint in flexion lessens available passive PIP flexion, there is extrinsic extensor tightness (Fig. 35.3). When a position of MP extension lessens passive PIP flexion, there is intrinsic (lumbrical) tightness (Fig. 35.4).[8] If the posture of the MP joint does not at all influence passive PIP joint flexion, yet passive PIP motion is still limited, a contracted joint capsule is likely the problem.[8]

Intrinsic tightness is common in clients who have sustained hand crush injuries, metacarpal fractures, and in those with rheumatoid arthritis. In addition to the reduced grasp associated with intrinsic tightness, there is evidence to support that this tightness may, at times, be partially responsible for the development of carpal tunnel syndrome.[9]

Distal Interphalangeal Joint Assessment

Lack of distal interphalangeal (DIP) flexion is typically hindered by either a contracted joint capsule or oblique retinacular ligament (ORL) tightness (Fig. 35.5). An ORL tightness test (Fig. 35.6) determines the source of limited passive DIP joint flexion. If you place the PIP in extension and your client's passive DIP flexion measurements become more limited than when in flexion, then ORL tightness is present. If changing the posture of the PIP joint does not alter your DIP flexion measurements, then the joint capsule is likely contracted. A tight ORL often accompanies a boutonnière deformity and, along with the management of a PIP flexion contracture, requires therapeutic attention (Fig. 35.7).

Hand Therapy Interventions

Early intervention and prevention are key factors to focus on when clients present with the potential for hand stiffness. If prevention is not implemented or is unsuccessful, stiffness is one of the most precarious problems to treat. Indulge in every opportunity you have for prevention. If you are able to persuade local physicians to refer clients early, you will have far less catastrophic cases of hand stiffness. Early regimes can be simple and only require one or two visits. Clients can be issued a home program consisting of breathing techniques, relaxation, elevation, edema control, and positional orthotics. You can also instruct clients in appropriate early motion of uninvolved joints, as well as encourage allowable functional activities.

Many clients are simply afraid to use the injured extremity and go into protection mode, which facilitates the cycle depicted in Fig. 35.1. A therapy visit or two provides clients the confidence they need to begin early motion exercises. This limits edema and leads to less joint stiffness and/or tissue adherence. You can also teach clients what to watch out for—that the MP joints will want to posture into extension and the PIP and DIP joints will migrate toward

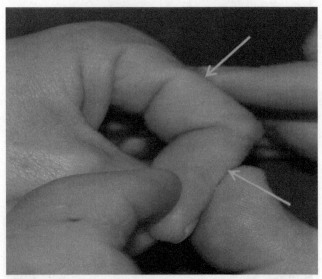

FIG. 35.3 Test for extrinsic extensor tightness. Position: Place metacarpophalangeal (MP) joint in maximal flexion. Test: Passively flex the proximal interphalangeal (PIP) joint, as indicated by the arrows. Rule out PIP joint contracture by repeating with the MP joint extended. Interpret: Extrinsic extensor muscle tightness is present if PIP joint motion is greater when MP is extended than when is flexed. PIP joint contracture is present if position of MP does not influence PIP flexion.

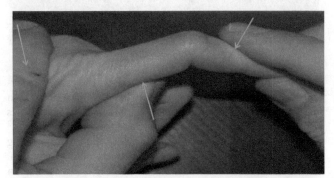

FIG. 35.4 Test for intrinsic tightness. Position: As indicated by the arrows, place metacarpophalangeal (MP) joint in full extension. Test: Passively flex the proximal interphalangeal (PIP) joint. Rule out PIP joint contracture by repeating with the MP joint flexed. Interpret: Intrinsic muscle tightness is present if PIP joint motion is greater when MP is flexed than when is extended. PIP joint contracture is present if position of MP does not influence PIP flexion.

flexion. These early therapy sessions give the therapist a chance to develop an open line of communication with clients, as well as with referring physicians. This allows clients to interact more easily with you when concerns arise. An educated client can detect early signs of problems and contact you or the physician to implement early intervention and avoid potential disasters.

Orthoses Application

One of most unique opportunities we have as therapists is the ability to utilize orthoses when treating clients with hand stiffness. There is consistent evidence in the literature—although

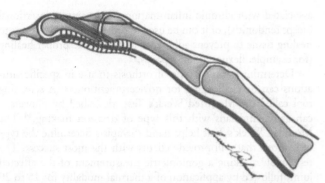

FIG. 35.5 Anatomy of oblique retinacular ligament (ORL). The ORL originates from the volar surface of the A2/C1 pulleys of the proximal phalanx and travels "obliquely" toward the dorsum of the distal phalanx where it inserts into the extensor mechanism. (From Skirven TM, Osterman AL, Fedorczyk JM, et al. eds. *Rehabilitation of the Hand and Upper Extremity.* 6th ed. Philadelphia, PA: Mosby; 2011.)

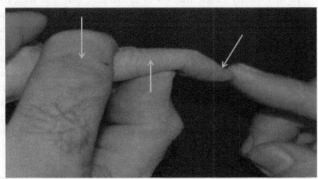

FIG. 35.6 Test for oblique retinacular ligament (ORL) tightness. Position: As indicated by the arrows, place the proximal interphalangeal (PIP) joint in full extension. Test: Passively flex the distal interphalangeal (DIP) joint. Rule out PIP joint contracture by repeating with the PIP joint flexed. Interpret: ORL tightness is present if DIP joint motion is greater when PIP is flexed than when extended. DIP joint contracture is present if position of PIP does not influence DIP flexion.

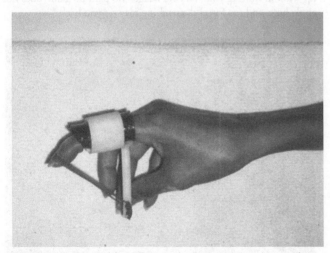

FIG. 35.7 Dynamic oblique retinacular ligament stretching orthosis to increase distal interphalangeal joint passive flexion. (Courtesy S. Weiss.)

mostly case studies—to suggest that the use of orthoses will improve joint motion in the stiff hand.[10] With our knowledge and skill set, we can provide our clients a range of orthotic interventions. We can fabricate a safe and comfortable orthosis when they need to be in a protected position (Fig. 35.8), or we can provide a more complex static progressive orthosis to improve joint range (Fig. 35.9).

This brings us to some important concepts that all hand therapists must understand when using orthoses. The concepts involve how much time clients should wear their orthoses and how much pull to provide. To safely elongate soft tissue, tissue stress must occur in the elastic range. If soft tissue elongates beyond this point then elongation will result in microtears, inflammation, and fibrosis. The literature indicates that 200 grams or a half-pound of force is adequate stress to elongate soft tissue.[11] However, in practice, force measurements of dynamic

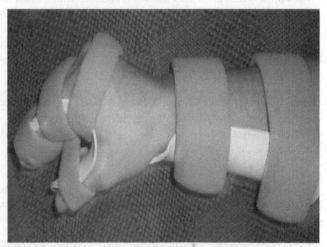

FIG. 35.8 Volar forearm-based "safe position" hand orthosis. (Courtesy C. McGee.)

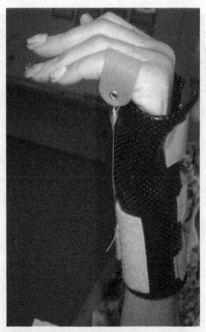

FIG. 35.9 Circumferential forearm-based static progressive metacarpophalangeal joint flexion mobilizing orthosis. (Courtesy S. Weiss.)

orthosis components are rarely used; we rely on our clients' subjective report of perceived tension in the orthosis. Ideally, the client should report a sensation of stretching but have no pain while using any mobilization orthosis.[12]

Although the amount of tissue stress is critical, so is the *duration* of applied stress. The longer the "total end-range time"—duration of time a contracted joint is placed at its maximal length—the better the results.[13] Studies have shown that **low-load prolonged stress** and **total end-range time (TERT)** are key factors in resolving soft-tissue contractures and regaining passive motion in stiff joints.[13,14]

The goal of applying stress to tight and shortened tissue is to achieve permanent elongation of the tissue and to encourage remodeling and realignment of collagen fibers, which will then facilitate improvements in joint motion. Permanent elongation of soft tissue can be achieved by either **creep loading** or by **stress relaxation loading**.[11] Creep loading is obtained with a constant force and varying displacement, which is provided by the application of a dynamic orthosis (Fig. 35.10).[11] In contrast, stress relaxation loading is achieved with incremental changes in force and a constant displacement—provided by the application of a static progressive orthosis (Fig. 35.11).[11]

> ### ◎ Clinical Pearl
>
> It is important to consider that mobilization using orthotic intervention is most effective when implemented within 2 months of the onset of stiffness.[14]

The application of stress to soft tissue can contribute to change in the periarticular structures and surrounding musculature, which will yield increased ROM and function. When stiffness is present, the goals of orthotic interventions are to remodel collagen fibers, remediate tendinous adhesions, and lengthen tight tissues.[10,14] However, an orthotic intervention may also be indicated to rest inflamed tissue to allow healing and prevent sclerosis

associated with chronic inflammation (for example, insertional biceps tendonitis); or it can be used to provide controlled stress to healing tissue to prevent adherence and promote proper healing (for example, flexor tendon repairs).[15]

Determining which type of orthosis to use in specific situations can be challenging for novice practitioners. A screening tool called the **Modified Week's Test**, described by Flowers,[16] can assist clinicians with this type of decision making.[14] The Modified Week's Test helps hand therapists determine the type of orthosis that will provide clients with the most success. The test involves taking a goniometric measurement of the affected joint, followed by application of a thermal modality for 15 to 20 minutes, followed by manual therapies (joint mobilization and therapeutic stretching) to the stiff joint. Redo the measurement. If the joint motion improves by 10 to 20 degrees, fit the client with a serial-static or dynamic orthosis. If the gain is less than 10 degrees, a static progressive orthosis will be most effective.

Practitioners also inquire as to how long they should have clients use a mobilization orthosis. This ultimately depends on the type of mobility deficit (flexion vs extension), and how long the stiffness has been present. For example, Glascom, Flemming, and Tooth[17] report that PIP extension contractures maximally respond to a dynamic orthotic intervention within 12 weeks; however, PIP flexion contractures will not maximally respond until 17 weeks or more. Similarly, these authors describe that extension contractures respond well to 6 hours of daily TERT, whereas flexion contractures may respond best after 11 hours of TERT. Lastly, regardless of the type of mobility deficit, when stiffness has been present for 8 weeks or less, it responds better to an orthotic intervention than stiffness that has been present for 3 months or longer.[17]

> ### ( ) What to Say to Clients
>
> To maximize client adherence to the plan of care, and to help your client understand why you are using a mobilization orthosis, it is helpful to tell them something along the lines of "Much of the soft tissue in your arm is like a rubber band. Rubber bands break when stretched too far and too quickly, and just like a rubber band, your muscles and tendons are stretchy but will also tear when stretched too hard or too fast. This is why a gentle but long stretch is necessary to loosen things up without hurting you. The old adage, 'no pain no gain,' does not apply here, and too forceful stretching may set you back."

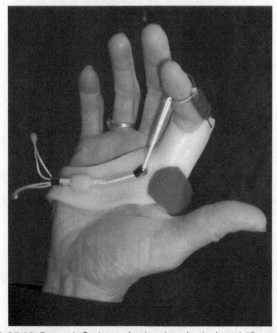

FIG. 35.10 Dynamic flexion orthosis using elastic thread. (Courtesy S. Weiss.)

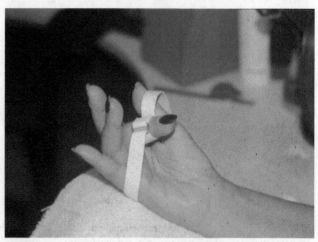

FIG. 35.11 Static-progressive flexion orthosis using a cinch strap. (Courtesy S. Weiss.)

Casting Motion to Mobilize Stiffness (CMMS)

Colditz describes a casting technique utilized to facilitate more normal movement patterns when treating the chronically stiff hand (Fig. 35.12A).[18] The casting motion to mobilize stiffness technique selectively places proximal joints in specific positions so that distal joints can move in a specified range (Fig. 35.12B). These specified positions are designed to create new movement patterns to allow for revival of normal motion (Fig. 35.12C). This is an active motion program facilitated by casting of proximal joints.[18] Cast position is not arbitrary and is determined based on the patterns of motion that are impaired, and ones you are attempting to facilitate. Colditz proposes a minimum of 2 to 4 weeks of casting. However, an extremely stiff hand will often require 8 or more weeks of casting. Some practitioners have replaced what was discussed earlier in the chapter regarding static progressive and dynamic orthosis application with CMMS, as it addresses movement patterns through active range of motion. The somatosensory cortex is not influenced by passive motion as it is with active motion. The cast provides a safe haven to facilitate normal movement patterns with cognitive involvement. Clients stay in the cast until they spontaneously demonstrate the desired movement pattern for two weeks and then they begin the process of weaning from the cast.[18]

Massage

Hand therapists have long recognized that edema control is essential to preventing stiffness, and we have utilized retrograde massage to combat edema. Retrograde massage has traditionally been performed in a firm, proximal-to-distal manner. This "milking" action can be too aggressive for the delicate lymphatic system.[19] Evidence suggests massage should be much lighter and only provide minimal traction to the skin.[19] It should start and end proximally to clear the lymph channels and allow fluid to move. This technique is called **manual edema mobilization**.[19] Manual edema mobilization can be beneficial for all kinds of swelling following upper extremity trauma and surgery.

Taping

Kinesiotape (also called K-tape) can be considered when treating the stiff swollen hand, as it is designed to mimic the elastic properties of our skin. The tape lifts the skin, which allows greater interstitial space and can encourage edema reduction.[20] Further research is warranted on the benefits of kinesiotaping to reduce edema and prevent stiffness in the hand.

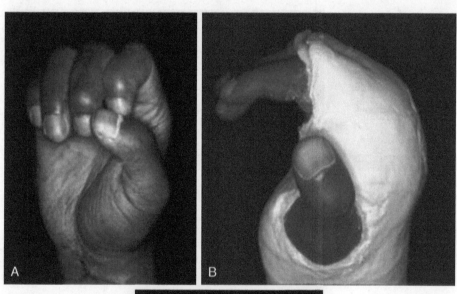

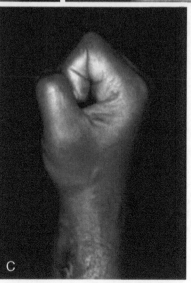

FIG. 35.12 Casting motion to mobilize stiffness.[4] A. Chronic stiff hand. B. Cast applied. C. Normal motion. (From Skirven TM, Osterman AL, Fedorczyk JM, et al. eds. *Rehabilitation of the Hand and Upper Extremity.* 6th ed. Philadelphia, PA: Mosby; 2011.)

Early Active Mobilization

Early active motion will likely dismantle the edema-disuse-stiffness cycle, when not contraindicated. If motion is restricted at a specific joint, active mobilization of the joints distal and proximal to the immobilized segment(s) should be instituted to avoid undue edema, capsular-ligamentous shortening, and adhesion formation. This is where an early visit to a hand therapist can be beneficial. When physicians instruct their patients to wiggle their fingers daily, the patients do just that; they gently wiggle, and they DO NOT (really) MOVE (much)! By the time these clients get to hand therapy, they are already getting stiff. If referred to therapy early (before this happens), the hand therapist can instruct clients in an active motion program that prevents adaptive shortening of the tissues. Active motion exercises combined with elevation are extremely effective and act as a pump to assist with edema reduction.

Active motion orthoses are also valuable tools in your therapy toolbox. Exercise orthoses can be customized to facilitate tendon gliding and to improve active glide of the commonly shortened intrinsic muscles. Fig. 35.13 is an example of a custom orthosis designed to facilitate active intrinsic function. These are easy to fabricate from scrap material and clients can use them in the clinic and at home.

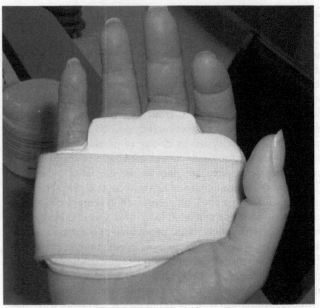
FIG. 35.13 Exercise orthosis. (Courtesy S. Weiss.)

Physical Agents

Physical agent modalities can be coupled with your treatment regime and may be useful in modulating pain and edema. This reduction in pain allows the hand therapist to perform activities and therapeutic interventions with the client to increase ROM. Physical agents can also be combined with stretch techniques (Fig. 35.14).

> ### ◎ Clinical Pearl
>
> Neuromuscular electrical stimulation (NMES) and biofeedback can be useful tools to help reestablish "lost" motor programs that result from immobilization and disuse. When limited joint mobility appears to be related to your client's difficulty with recruiting primary and secondary movers, try helping your clients refresh their "motor memories" using these modalities.

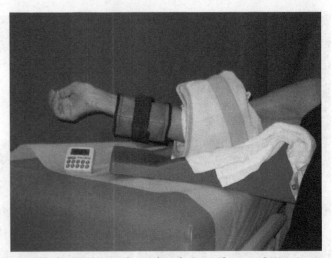
FIG. 35.14 Heat and stretch technique. (Courtesy S. Weiss.)

> ### ◎ Clinical Pearl
>
> When surface scarring appears to be restricting the glide of superficial tendons, you may notice that this scarring moves in concert with the tendons. Ultrasound applied to this scar tissue, massage, and, lastly, a small piece of Dycem or Theraband to stabilize the surface scar during "tendon gliding"–type exercises may facilitate a nonsurgical "lysis of adhesions."

> ### ◎ Clinical Pearl
>
> Simple techniques, such as diaphragmatic breathing, can assist clients with relaxing and reducing guarding of the injured extremity.

Holistic Care

Complementary health approaches within the scope of occupational/physical therapy practice have a positive correlation with facilitating good outcomes in hand therapy. Meditation, mindfulness, acupressure, and yoga are viable considerations to incorporate into your upper extremity clinical practice or your clients' home programs.

Home Program

Hand therapy intervention requires consistent follow through by the client/family/caregiver(s). This can be challenging, especially when relatively complex exercises and orthoses are used as part of the home program. I recommend the following to help foster learning and carry over of home exercises and activities:

- Use video on the client's cell phone to record the performance of therapeutic activity or exercise, or orthosis application. Digital photography can also be beneficial.

- Verbal instructions should always be accompanied by written and/or video instructions.
- Be certain that client educational materials are being written at the sixth-grade reading level. Consider using readability scorecards[21] to assess the readability of your materials.
- Consider designing your handouts for older adults to improve legibility. Use large fonts (12-point), clear fonts (Arial or Helvetica), and good contrast between foreground and background colors (white paper with black print works well).
- Consider having non-English handouts available in the language(s) commonly spoken by your clients. Alternately, design handouts with more pictures and fewer words.
- Always have the client/family/caregiver(s) demonstrate their exercises and how to apply orthoses after you have instructed them. You may need to do this several times until you are confident they "get" it.

Stretching, Manual Treatments, and Strengthening

ROM and strengthening regimes are carefully prescribed after you determine the safety measures for your client. As with many of our therapeutic interventions, dosage, force, and speed have little definitive data to support them. We must use our clinical expertise and intuition as to how much, how often, and how long each client should perform each and every exercise. Chapter 10 of this textbook offers some guidance with this.

Respecting tissues is a key component of successful outcomes. Active motion is often superior to passive motion, as it will stimulate the lymphatic system and help reduce edema. Manual therapy with joint mobilization is a useful strategy when clients have capsular tightness and limited inflammation. On the other hand, overzealous mobilization will land your client right back to the cycle displayed in Fig. 35.1. There is moderate support in the literature for the use of manual joint mobilization to reduce stiffness.[10]

Here are a few examples of creative activities for the clinic or your clients' home programs:
Differential tendon gliding (Fig. 35.15)
Stretching tight extrinsic long flexor muscles with the use of putty (Fig. 35.16)
Interossei strengthening activity (Fig. 35.17)
Intrinsic tightness stretching: the client can place their hand over the MPs to provide overpressure (Fig. 35.18)
Figs. 35.19 A and B demonstrate active engagement of the intrinsic muscles by having the client roll the cylinder up from the palm of the hand to the hook fist position. Fig. 35.19A portrays the use of a larger dowel when intrinsic function is more limited. Fig. 35.19B shows a more advanced capability of end-range when the intrinsic muscles have become more functional.

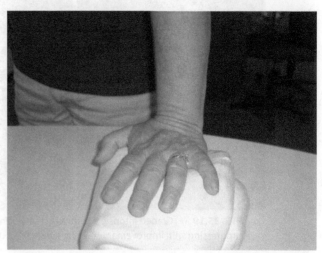
FIG. 35.16 Extrinsic flexor tightness stretch. (Courtesy S. Weiss.)

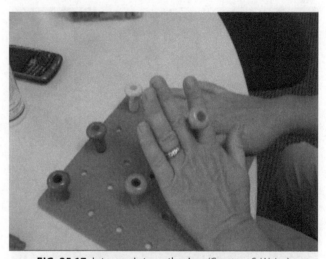
FIG. 35.17 Interossei strengthening. (Courtesy S. Weiss.)

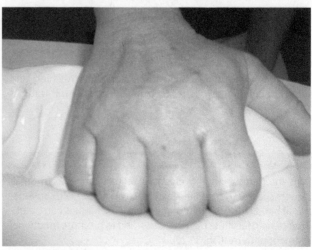
FIG. 35.18 Intrinsic tightness stretch. (Courtesy S. Weiss.)

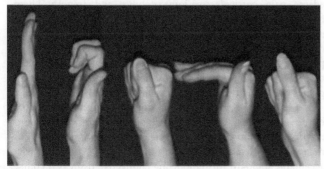
FIG. 35.15 Differential flexor tendon gliding exercises. (From Skirven TM, Osterman AL, Fedorczyk JM, et al. eds. *Rehabilitation of the Hand and Upper Extremity*. 6th ed. Philadelphia, PA: Mosby; 2011.)

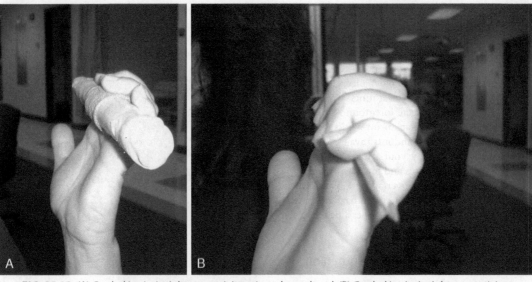

FIG. 35.19 (A) Graded intrinsic tightness activity using a large dowel. (B) Graded intrinsic tightness activity progressing with improvement to using a pencil. (Courtesy S. Weiss.)

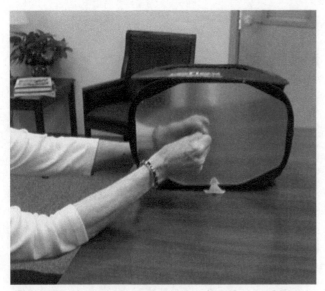

FIG. 35.20 Motor imagery using a mirror box. (Courtesy S. Weiss.)

◎ Clinical Pearl

It is imperative to teach clients to perform stretching and strengthening activities *gently*. Forceful motion will traumatize tissue.

◎ Clinical Pearl

Pain interferes with movement. This can range from small muscle spasms to complete avoidance of motion with no functional hand use. Graded motor imagery techniques can be utilized to help facilitate pain reduction and to promote functional moment patterns (Fig. 35.20).

♡ Tips from the Field

Table 35.1 provides a quick-tip descriptive recipe for intervention planning specific to many joint restrictions experienced across the three phases of healing. It is not designed to illustrate the clinical reasoning that either justifies or precludes utilization of these activities.

Assessing Therapy Outcomes

A client-centered hand therapist frequently revisits satisfaction, participation, and progress toward the client's goal attainment. The literature does not clearly describe how frequently to reassess; however, the recommended dosage or duration of an intervention can assist therapists in planning reassessment. For example, serial casting is most effective when applied for a period of 6 days.[13] For this reason, a reassessment of joint motion is often performed once a week following cast removal. Generally speaking, the frequency of reassessment and choice of tools depends on your intervention frequency/duration, third-party payer constraints, and institutional policy.

Most interventions for the stiff hand are intended to impact edema, pain, passive/active joint mobility, and strength. Therefore reassessment should be performed frequently (ideally by the same therapist, in the same standardized fashion, and at the same relative time of day) to determine responsiveness to your therapeutic interventions. New assessments may be introduced along the way, given that some may be contraindicated during early phases of healing (for example, strength testing).

Videography is useful for recording mechanical and cerebral improvements, and most hand therapists perform weekly goniometric assessments of the targeted areas. Cummings and Tillman[22] report that a 3-degree gain in joint ROM per week is an acceptable standard for remodeling connective tissue. Of course, given that hand goniometry is subject to a 5-degree measurement error, a difference of more than 5 degrees is the most convincing evidence that your interventions are impacting change.

What to Do If Progress Slows

There will be times when your interventions will not be successful. When joint mobility does not progress after exhaustive treatment, it may be necessary to reevaluate the intervention plan. First, check with your client to determine if their habits, roles, and routines are barriers to performing their home program. You may need to help your client identify how to best incorporate therapeutic activities, exercises, and orthotic interventions into their lifestyle. Sometimes, lack of progress means that you haven't yet found the right approach for a particular client, or that the intervention approach you have chosen needs refinement. Turn to the literature to learn more about best practices, as these are constantly changing. Be creative yet scientific when trying new things. Lastly, although it is not in our nature to give up on clients, a referral back to the physician may be necessary. If this is necessary, know that you are not failing your client. Rather, you are advocating on their behalf to expedite progress and keep costs down.

Operative Interventions

Surgical interventions or medical procedures may be required when hand therapy has plateaued in remediating or preventing stiffness. Hand rehabilitation clients occasionally undergo the following surgeries if therapeutic interventions fail to achieve their goals. These are some of the procedures that our surgical colleagues may suggest:

- Open capsulectomy: For capsular contracture that does not respond to conservative measures. After surgery, early hand therapy and mobilization is recommended.
- Tenotomy: Releases long-standing musculotendinous tightness by "lengthening" a tendon through the surgical division of the tendon.
- Tenolysis: The surgical removal of scar tissue impacting gliding of tendon. Preoperative hand therapy is important for maximizing PROM. Early postoperative hand therapy is recommended after this procedure to keep the tendon moving and to minimize new adhesions.
- Surgical decompression of tendon sheaths or pulleys: Utilized when stenosing tenosynovitis is the culprit in movement restriction.
- Surgical release and skin grafting: Performed when cutaneous scarring is impeding movement.
- Palmar fasciotomy or palmar needle aponeurotomy: This may be used when diseased palmar fascia is restricting digital extension.

TABLE 35.1   Intervention Highlights across Phases of Healing and Physiological Barriers

Healing Phase	Physiological Barriers	Therapist Interventions	Orthotic Ideas
Inflammatory	Edema	<ul><li>Elevation</li><li>PAMs<ul><li>Cryotherapy in most cases</li><li>High-volt electrical stimulation</li><li>Pulsed ultrasound</li></ul></li><li>Proximal lymphatic decongestion</li><li>Pumping/proximal motion</li><li>Light compression</li></ul>	Static orthosis may help immobilize inflamed structures to reduce inflammation
	Pain/anxiety	<ul><li>Elevation</li><li>PAMs<ul><li>Cryotherapy in most cases</li><li>High-volt electrical stimulation</li><li>Pulsed ultrasound</li><li>TENS</li></ul></li><li>Early controlled use of permitted digits/segments</li><li>Guided imagery/relaxation</li></ul>	Static orthosis may help immobilize inflamed structures to control pain
	Nonuse of affected extremity	<ul><li>Early controlled use of permitted digits/segments</li><li>Imagery/mirror therapy</li><li>AROM to permitted joints distal and proximal to injury (ideally within 2 days) every 2 hours 5–10 repetitions for 5 seconds</li></ul>	Use of orthoses that are as "least restrictive" when medically indicated. Be certain to avoid unwarranted restriction of adjacent joints.
	Decreased knowledge	<ul><li>Education<ul><li>Protection</li><li>Home program</li></ul></li></ul>	Education on orthosis care and wear schedule
Proliferative	Edema	<ul><li>See inflammatory phase</li><li>Controlled active use of affected extremity during occupations<ul><li>Must find balance between activity and elevation</li><li>Elevate when not engaged in activity</li><li>Schedule breaks for elevation</li></ul></li></ul>	

TABLE 35.1	Intervention Highlights across Phases of Healing and Physiological Barriers—cont'd			
Healing Phase	**Physiological Barriers**		**Therapist Interventions**	**Orthotic Ideas**
	Pain/anxiety		• See inflammatory phase • Monitor for CRPS	Static/protective orthosis may control pain and support use during aggravating occupations
	Forearm tightness (radioulnar joints)	Pronation	• AROM • Gentle passive motion	Supination/pronation orthosis
		Supination	• AROM • Gentle passive motion	Supination/pronation orthosis
	Wrist tightness (radiocarpal and ulnocarpal joints)	Extrinsic (due to muscular or skin tightness)	• Moist heat to extensor and flexor wads • AROM to wrist with tenodesis and also in composite manners (wrist flexion/finger flexion and wrist extension/finger extension) • Gentle passive motion (wrist flexion/finger flexion and wrist extension/finger extension)	If immobilization is indicated (unless contraindicated), wrist should be positioned in 15 degrees of extension to prevent flexion contracture. With volar wrist scarring, wrist should also be positioned in slight wrist extension. With dorsal wrist scarring, a more neutral wrist is preferred to prevent extensor contracture.
	MP/PIP tightness	Intrinsic	• Active "intrinsic minus" stretches	Hand-based "intrinsic minus" orthosis with MPs extended to facilitate active stretches. A dynamic outrigger can be added in mid-proliferative phase.
		Extrinsic (due to muscular or skin tightness, or adhesions)	• Moist heat to flexor/extensor wads • PIP blocking exercises • Controlled active movement • Gentle passive movement • Controlled active use in daily occupations • Differential tendon glides	Static or serial static orthosis at night and during times of rest. Intrinsic plus position is best for extensor tightness and a modified resting pan orthosis is best for flexor tightness. In mid-proliferative phase, dynamic orthosis can be used.
	DIP tightness	ORL	• DIP blocking exercises with PIP held in extension	PIP flexion blocking orthosis to isolate DIP flexion
		FDP (due to muscular or volar skin tightness, or adhesions)	• Differential tendon glides • AROM to wrist and also in composite manners (wrist extension/finger extension) • Gentle passive motion (wrist extension/finger extension)	Static or serial static modified resting pan orthosis
	Nonuse of affected extremity/weakness		• Biofeedback to assist with recruitment/cortical remapping • NMES to difficult-to-recruit muscles • Early controlled use in daily occupations • Early isolative active motion specific to commonly "forgotten" muscle groups (e.g., ECRB, FDS, etc.) • Active assistive exercises when antigravity strength is limited	Blocking orthosis to assist with isolation of difficult-to-recruit muscles

	Decreased knowledge		• Education
			  • Controlled active use/restrictions
			  • Home program
			  • Orthosis wear schedule
				Education on orthosis care and wear schedule

Maturation	Edema		• Manual edema mobilization • Chip bags if fibrotic • Active movement • Compression • Elastic taping techniques	
	Pain		• See inflammatory phase • Imagery and mirror therapy	

Continued

TABLE 35.1	Intervention Highlights across Phases of Healing and Physiological Barriers—cont'd			
Healing Phase	**Physiological Barriers**		**Therapist Interventions**	**Orthotic Ideas**
	Forearm tightness (radioulnar joints)	Pronation	If no change from thermal modalities and manual therapy, unlikely to respond to passive or active stretching because collagen cross-linking is so pervasive. In this case, an orthotic intervention is required.	Pronation/supination static progressive orthosis
		Supination	If no change from thermal modalities and manual therapy, unlikely to respond to passive or active stretching because collagen cross-linking is so pervasive. In this case, an orthotic intervention is required.	Pronation/supination static progressive orthosis
	Wrist tightness (radiocarpal and ulnocarpal joints)	Extrinsic (due to muscular or skin tightness)	• Moist heat and lotion to skin scarring • Scar massage	• Serial casting • Static progressive orthosis
		Capsular	• Heated ultrasound	• Serial casting • Static progressive orthosis
	MP/PIP tightness	Intrinsic		• Hand-based intrinsic minus orthosis with static progressive outrigger • Casting motion to mobilize stiffness
		Extrinsic (due to muscular or skin tightness, or adhesions)	• Heated ultrasound to site of adhesion • Moist heat and lotion/massage to skin scarring	• Forearm-based static progressive orthoses • Serial casting • Casting motion to mobilize stiffness[15]
		Capsular	• Heated ultrasound	• Hand or finger-based static progressive orthosis • Serial casting • Casting motion to mobilize stiffness
	DIP tightness	ORL	• Heated ultrasound	• PIP flexion blocking orthosis with static progressive DIP flexion mobilizing outrigger
		FDP (due to muscular or volar skin tightness, or adhesions)	• Heated ultrasound to site of adhesion	• Static progressive orthosis
		Capsular		• DIP static progressive extension mobilizing outrigger
	Nonuse of affected extremity/weakness		• Biofeedback to assist with recruitment/cortical remapping • NMES to difficult-to-recruit muscles • Early controlled use in daily occupations • Early isolative active motion specific to commonly "forgotten" muscle groups (e.g., ECRB, FDS, etc.) • Active assistive exercises when antigravity strength is limited	• Blocking orthoses to assist with isolation of difficult-to-recruit muscles

	Decreased knowledge		• Education
			  • Controlled active use/restrictions
			  • Home program
			  • Orthosis wear schedule
				• Education on orthosis care and wear schedule

AROM, Active range of motion; *CRPS,* complex regional pain syndrome; *DIP,* distal interphalangeal; *ECRB,* extensor carpi radialis brevis; *FDP,* flexor digitorum profundus; *FDS,* flexor digitorum superficialis; *MP,* metacarpophalangeal; *NMES,* neuromuscular electrical stimulation; *ORL,* oblique retinacular ligament; *PAMs,* physical agent modalities; *PIP,* proximal interphalangeal; *TENS,* transcutaneous electrical nerve stimulation.

? Questions to Ask the Doctor

Unless standing protocols are already in place, seeking clarification on postoperative orders is important prior to starting therapy with your client. Ask the physician questions such as:

- Is it okay for me to begin active motion, blocking exercises, passive motion, or resistance activities/exercises?
- What is the client's activity status? When can they begin using the hand for light resistive activities such as oral care or self-feeding?
- If you have concerns about protocol, would you like to progress your client or try a different approach?

Communicate your clinical reasoning and be diplomatic when approaching the referring physician. For example, say, "I have a 17-year-old client who is an instrumentalist and she is exceptionally responsible. Could we attempt an early passive motion program rather than cast immobilization?" When necessary, convey evidence-based reasoning and present scientific literature to support your requests. Develop good working relationships with referring physicians, as this is pivotal to your learning and your clients' successful outcomes.

Summary

Our clients' return to functional hand use is the ultimate outcome measure of our interventions. Table 35.2 is a guide to generalized ROM goals for functional upper extremity use. Clients should be capable of engaging in most daily activities if these active goniometric measures are achieved. Therapeutic intervention and open communication will impact clients' ability to participate in

TABLE 35.2 Functional Goniometric Measures of the Distal Upper Extremity

	Joint	Joint Active Motion (Degrees)
Hand[23]	Second to fifth MP flexion	61
	Second to fifth PIP flexion	60
	Second to fifth DIP flexion	39
	First MP flexion	21
	First IP flexion	18
Wrist[24]	Flexion	54
	Extension	0
	Ulnar deviation	40
	Radial deviation	17
Forearm[25]	Supination	60
	Pronation	40
Elbow[26]	Flexion	130
	Extension	−30

DIP, Distal interphalangeal; *IP*, interphalangeal; *MP*, metacarpophalangeal; *PIP*, proximal interphalangeal.

meaningful play, work, and leisure activities. Our goal as hand therapy practitioners is to maximize function and quality of life for clients despite their upper extremity disorders. Treating clients with our unique expertise facilitates these intentions.

References

1. Madden JW: Wound healing: the biological basis of hand surgery, *Clin Plast Surg* 3(1):3–11, 1976.
2. Cyr LM, Ross RG: How controlled stress affects healing tissues, *J Hand Ther* 11(2):125–130, 1998.
3. Flinn NA, Jackson J, McLaughlin Gray J, et al.: Optimizing abilities and capacities: range of motion, strength, and endurance. In Radomski M, Latham CA, editors: *Occupational therapy for physical dysfunction*, ed 6, Philadelphia, 2008, Wolters Kluwer/Lippincott Williams & Wilkins, pp 81–185.
4. Long C: Intrinsic-extrinsic muscle control of the fingers: electromyographic studies, *J Bone Joint Sur* 50(5):973–984, 1968.
5. Groth GN, VanDeven KM, Phillips EC, et al.: Goniometry of the proximal and distal interphalangeal joints, Part II: placement preferences, interrater reliability, and concurrent validity, *J Hand Ther* 14(1):23–29, 2001.
6. Modest J, Clair B, DeMasi R, et al.: Self-measured wrist range of motion by wrist-injured and wrist-healthy study participants using a built-in iPhone feature as compared with a universal goniometer, *J Hand Ther*, July 2018. In Press.
7. Villeco JP: Edema: therapist's management. In Skirven TM, Osterman AL, Fedorczyk JM, Amadio PC, editors: *Rehabilitation of the hand and upper extremity*, ed 6, Philadelphia, PA, 2011, Mosby, pp 845–857.
8. Bunell S: *Surgery of the hand*, ed 2, Philadelphia, 1948, JB Lippencott.
9. Cobb TK, An KN, Cooney WP: Effect of lumbrical muscle incursion within the carpal tunnel on carpal tunnel pressure: a cadaveric study, *J Hand Sur Am* 20(2):186–192, 1995.
10. Michlovitz SL, Harris BA, Watkins MP: Therapy interventions for improving joint range of motion: a systematic review, *J Hand Ther* 17(2):118–131, 2004.
11. Brand PW, Hollister A: *Clinical mechanics of the hand*, ed 3, St Louis, 1999, Mosby.
12. Colditz JC: Therapist's management of the stiff hand. In Skirven TM, Osterman AL, Fedorczyk JM, et al.: *Rehabilitation of the hand and upper extremity*, ed 6, Philadelphia, 2011, Elsevier Mosby, pp 894–921.
13. Flowers KR, LaStayo P: Effect of total end range time on improving passive range of motion, *J Hand Ther* 7(3):150–157, 1994.
14. Glascow C, Tooth L, Fleming J, et al.: Dynamic splinting for the stiff hand after trauma: predictors of contracture resolution, *J Hand Ther* 24:195–206, 2011.
15. Klein L: Early active motion flexor tendon protocol using one splint, *J Hand Ther* 16(3):199–206, 2003.
16. Flowers KA: Proposed hierarchy for splinting the stiff joint, with emphasis on force application parameters, *J Hand Ther* 15(2):158–162, 2002.
17. Glascow C, Fleming J, Tooth L: The long-term relationship between duration of treatment and contracture resolution using dynamic orthotic devices for the stiff proximal interphalangeal joint: a prospective cohort study, *J Hand Ther* 25:38–47, 2012.
18. Colditz JC: Plaster of Paris: the forgotten splinting material, *J Hand Ther* 15:144–157, 2002.
19. Miller LK, Jerosch-Herold C, Shepstone L: Effectiveness of edema management techniques for subacute hand edema: a systematic review, *J Hand Ther* 30:432–446, 2017.

20. Morris D, Jones D, Ryan H, Ryan CG: The clinical effects of Kinesio Tex taping: a systematic review, *Physiother Theory Pract* 29(4):259–270, 2013.

21. Seubert D: *Design readability scorecard*. 2010, *Health communications* (website) www.healthcommunications.org: Accessed October, 20, 2012.

22. Cummings GS, Tillman LI: Remodeling of dense connective tissue in normal adult tissues. In Currier DP, Nelson RM, editors: *Dynamics of human biologic tissues*, Philadelphia, 1992, FA Davis, p 45.

23. Hume MC, Gellman H, McKellop H, et al.: Functional range of motion of the joints of the hand, *J Hand Surg* 15(2):240–243, 1990.

24. Ryu JY, Cooney WP, Askew LJ, et al.: Functional ranges of motion of the wrist joint, *J Hand Surg* 16(3):409–419, 1991.

25. Safaee-Rad R, Shwedyk E, Quanbury AO, et al.: Normal functional range of motion of upper limb joints during performance of three feeding activities, *Arch Phys Med Rehabil* 71(7):505–509, 1990.

26. Morrey BF, Askew LJ, Chao EY: A biomechanical study of normal functional elbow motion, *J Bone Joint Surg Am* 63(6):872–877, 1981.

27. Carswell A, McColl MA, Baptiste S: The Canadian Occupational Performance Measure: a research and clinical literature review, *Can J Occup Ther* 71(4):210–222, 2004.

36
The Neurological Hand

Gillian Porter
Lara Taggart

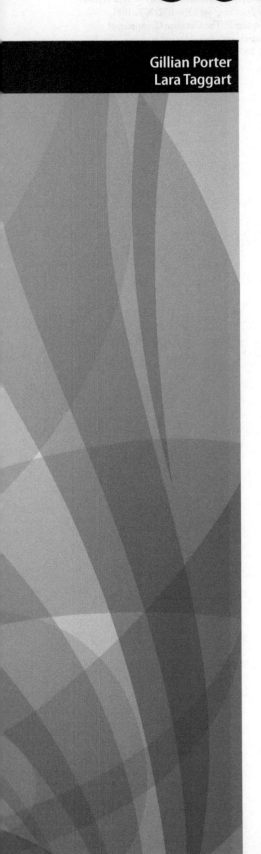

The neurological hand can be complex. Motor and sensory impairments, **spasticity/hypertonicity**, **learned disuse/nonuse**, and perceptual issues make rehabilitation of this type of hand a challenge. And since not every neurological injury or impairment has the same symptoms among clients,[1] predicting outcomes in a neurological client's hand progress can be difficult. However, when clients with neurological conditions make progress with hand skills or experience increases in functional use of the hand, the reward is significant. This chapter is designed to assist clinicians in the assessment and treatment of the neurological hand and to offer suggestions for orthotic options to promote optimal positioning at rest and in function.

Common Diagnoses Associated With the Neurological Hand

The range of diagnoses associated with neurological hand conditions include but are not limited to the following: multiple sclerosis (MS), cerebral palsy (CP), spinal cord injury (SCI), cerebrovascular accident (CVA), traumatic brain injury (TBI), Parkinson disease (PD), and **dystonia**.

Acquired Brain Injury: Cerebrovascular Accident and Traumatic Brain Injury

Brain injury can lead to a broad spectrum of symptoms and disabilities. Persons with acquired brain injury from CVA and TBI can exhibit motor disorders in which the upper extremities often show clinical symptoms such as spasticity, decreased muscle strength, incoordination, impaired sensation, and inability to bear weight symmetrically.[2]

Functional recovery following a stroke is nonlinear, with the most rapid recovery occurring during the first 3 months. Therapists used to be taught that brain recovery was nearly complete within 3 to 6 months following stroke. However, more current scientific investigation has dispelled this belief. Research shows that although muscle strength in the paretic upper extremity (UE) shows its greatest recovery in the initial 6 months post stroke, some individuals achieve motor recovery many years after CVA. There are studies of eventual complete or near-complete brain recovery in rats following lab-induced CVA. Neuroscientists have discovered that the brain continues to repair itself even when motor changes or functional improvements may not be evident. There is no research to show that recovery from stroke stops at 6 months.

It has been estimated that 3 months after a stroke, only 20% of clients attain full recovery of UE function, and 30% to 66% of these individuals are unable to use their affected UE for meaningful activity.[3] Intervention to increase hand skills is very individualized, and the level of functional return varies between individuals. Therefore, as therapists, it is important to assess both the current functional hand status as well as the client's priorities for hand use.

There is poor consistency between researchers and clinicians in the use of terminology to describe changes in motor ability after stroke. Recovery is a dynamic process that cannot be encapsulated at one point in time. However, use of a descriptive UE functional guideline to assist with goal writing and intervention planning is helpful. This is further addressed later in the chapter.

Using neuroimaging techniques to diagnose acute capsular stroke, Wenzelburger and colleagues[4] found that lesions in the posterior regions of the internal capsule were associated with chronic dexterity deficits in the affected UE. At baseline assessment, muscle strength was the only predictor significantly associated with dextrous hand function at 6 months poststroke. Duncan and colleagues[5] reported that motor and sensory scores on the Fugl-Meyer Assessment (FMA) at day 5 after stroke accounted for 74% of the variance in the composite scores at 6 months post stroke. However, it is not possible to delineate the contribution of UE sensation to the recovery of discrete dextrous hand function from such composite scoring of the sensorimotor functions in the UEs.[5]

Multiple Sclerosis

MS is the most common autoimmune, inflammatory, demyelinating disease of the central nervous system (CNS). MS is characterized by a combination of damage to both gray matter and white matter, with an ensuing loss of tissue leading to cortical atrophy. The neurological symptoms with respect to the hand include sensory disturbances, motor impairment, intention tremor, ataxia, and impaired motor coordination.[6] The clinical symptoms of MS are highly variable depending on the site and extent of CNS involvement. However, difficulty with object manipulation caused by deterioration of hand dexterity is a common and important clinical feature with even mildly involved clients living with MS.[7] Additionally, UE dysfunction seems to be related to a decrease or loss of light-touch pressure and two-point discrimination sensations in the hand, as well as decreased elbow flexion strength. UE strengthening and sensory retraining of the hand may contribute to improved UE function in clients with MS. Testing of both static and dynamic manipulation tasks may be needed for a more complete assessment of hand function in various populations. However, an explicit overview of arm-hand training programs is lacking for the MS population.

Cerebral Palsy

Hemiparetic CP is a common neurological disorder that affects sensorimotor function and development in children. Functional motor developmental delay or deconditioning of the affected limb is known to contribute to compensatory use of the intact limb rather than attempted use of the affected limb. Subsequently, the affected limb undergoes reduction in muscle size or atrophy and associated muscle weakness. Neurofacilitation approaches are now integrating weight-bearing and muscle-strengthening exercise with neuromuscular electrical stimulation (NMES), **biofeedback**, **forced use**, repetitive training, and **bilateral arm training**. These approaches are based on contemporary motor learning and control theories to maximize motor recovery in individuals with neurological impairments.

Spinal Cord Injury

Cervical spinal cord injury (cSCI) can lead to devastating impairments and yet, to date, there is no reliable medical treatment to reverse the condition. In humans, cSCI, including complete and incomplete **tetraplegia**, represents about 62% of all spinal cord injuries.[8] This type of injury can cause severe impairments affecting the use of the UEs. Regaining partial or full arm and hand function can make significant improvements in clients' quality of life and is considered to be a priority for clients with cSCI.[9] It is very important for therapists to have sensitive and reliable methods to evaluate forelimb motor functions. Donnelly et al.[10] identified functional limitations in the cSCI population associated with several broad areas. The study surveyed 41 clients with cSCI in the early stage of recovery for their perceived level of satisfaction and performance in these areas. The top five identified areas of concern were: functional mobility, including transfers and wheelchair use (19%); dressing (13%); grooming (11%); feeding (8%); and bathing (7%).

> ### ⊚ Clinical Pearl
>
> Clients recently diagnosed with a neurological condition benefit from having both a physiatrist (a physician who specializes in physical medicine and rehabilitation) and a neurologist (a physician who treats the nervous system) throughout their recovery.[11] Many clients will have a neurologist assigned at the acute stage of their injury and may need to seek a different physician or neurologist to continue managing their care in the later stages of recovery. A neurologist typically oversees needs such as routine tests to monitor any changes in recovery. Both neurologists and physiatrists may manage medication specific to a client's neurological injury, such as to address seizures, spasticity, and **neurogenic** pain. Having consistent follow-up with a physician is essential, especially if a client is experiencing some of the most common challenges to progression of the neurological hand—spasticity, pain, and edema.

Common Challenges of the Neurological Hand

Neurological conditions typically present with one or more of the following UE challenges: hemiplegia/hemiparesis, edema, spasticity/hypertonicity, decreased coordination, tremor, sensory disturbances, muscle atrophy, weakness, pain, and/or joint stiffness/decreased range of motion (ROM).

Spasticity

One of the most common challenges for the neurological hand is spasticity. In a survey of over 500 stroke survivors, 58% experienced spasticity, and only 51% of those with spasticity had received treatment.[12] Spasticity can be difficult to manage and has the potential to sabotage recovery.

First, it is important to determine if a client's spasticity is being medically managed by a medication (muscle relaxer or antispasmodic) such as oral Baclofen, Zanaflex, Flexeril, Valium, or Dantrium,[13,14] Botox injections, or an intrathecal baclofen pump (ITB).[14] Second, it is important to understand the client's oral medication routine, Botox injection cycle, and/or ITB program. In a perfect world, a client has a consistent relationship with the physician managing the spasticity and monitoring the effectiveness of interventions. However, it is not uncommon for the therapist to encourage a client to seek medication for spasticity management, or suggest to a client's physician a more comprehensive tone management program that includes medication.

Spasticity is known to develop and change over weeks, months, and years after brain injury,[15] which when left undiagnosed or undermanaged can lead to debilitating UE changes. Unmanaged spasticity interferes with successful function of the affected UE,[15] increasing the odds of developing patterns of learned nonuse that may become extremely difficult to overcome.

When a client's spasticity is being managed pharmacologically, it is worthwhile to discover the client's dosage and routine for oral medication or ITB therapy, when the last series of Botox injections occurred, and/or when the next series of Botox injections will occur. Understanding a client's routine with antispasticity medication promotes better treatment planning in therapy. Botox injections, for example, are usually received every 3 to 4 months, with the first noticeable effects typically occurring within the first 2 weeks of injections.[16] If a client is seeking therapy toward the end of the injection cycle, intervention may not be as successful.

An oral medication or ITB dose schedule is important to understand because the best results are often achieved soon after receiving a dose. Some ITB dose schedules can be programmed to correlate with a client's therapy schedule and/or times of the day when the client is most likely to incorporate the affected UE in functional activities. Therapy following a dose of oral medication may offer positive results in reducing spasticity to benefit intervention; however, these muscle relaxers may also have the negative side effect of decreasing a client's ability to remain alert and attentive to therapy.

It is good practice for therapists to collaborate with a client's physician on the client's degree and location of spasticity and its impact on function. Therapists commonly utilize measures, such as the Ashworth Scale, Modified Ashworth Scale (MAS), or Tardieu Scale, to assess levels of spasticity in specific UE muscles and then provide the physician with these findings. Such communication should include remarks about the impact of spasticity on function, particularly during grasp and release demands in various reaching patterns. This collaboration will provide a comprehensive picture of the client's ability to utilize the affected UE while under the influence of spasticity. It is also important to communicate to physicians the degree to which a client uses the affected hand in functional activities and/or exercise following Botox injections. This information is important to the physician because the physician will want to avoid delivering too strong a Botox dose that renders grasp too weak to carry objects or complete repetitive grasp-release training.

Severe cases of spasticity may cause soft-tissue shortening and decreased joint ROM. In these cases, Botox can be administered prior to orthotic positioning or serial casting to promote the most optimal conditions for increasing soft-tissue length and joint ROM.

If clients are not progressing because of spasticity, it may be worthwhile to place their therapy visits on hold with plans to resume after more comprehensive spasticity management is achieved. This way, a client has the opportunity to receive the maximal benefit of therapeutic intervention.

It is important to encourage clients to ask their physician questions about the options available to manage spasticity, as well as their potential risks and side effects.

Pain

Pain is an obvious challenge to a client's ability to effectively incorporate the affected hand into meaningful tasks. Referring a client to a neurologist, physiatrist, or pain specialist is critical to managing pain, particularly if the pain is neurogenic. Clients may benefit from asking their physicians the possible side effects of pharmacological intervention and discussing a dosage regime that will lead to minimal interference with daily activities and rehabilitation. Clients may also wish to inquire about holistic interventions for pain management.

Edema

Edema reduces ROM, coordination, and effectiveness of grasp and pinch. Edema can result from trauma, dependent positioning of the affected UE, a comorbid medical condition, poor positioning habits while seated or lying down, and medications.

For persistent cases of edema that do not respond to basic edema management techniques or are suspected to be the result of medication, it is important to refer clients to the appropriate physician (neurologist, physiatrist, or cardiologist) to discuss options for decreasing the edema. When a client has severe edema, referring to a lymphedema specialist may be necessary, not only to address the problem but also to ensure the movement of fluid does not overwhelm a client's cardiovascular status.

> **Clinical Pearl**
>
> Therapists working with neurological clients often benefit from asking questions and providing feedback to physicians regarding issues such as blood pressure, oxygen saturation rate, or any other medical issue that could interfere with a client's ability to participate in therapy.

> **Clinical Pearl**
>
> Therapists working with neurological patients' UEs often request prescriptions from physicians regarding equipment that may benefit neuro-reeducation and positioning of the affected hand: orthoses, transcutaneous electrical stimulation (TENS)/NMES units, and compression garments.

> **What to Say to Clients**
>
> Clients often ask, "Will I ever regain 100% function in my (affected) hand?" This is a difficult question to answer, particularly since no two clients with the same neurological condition are the same.[1] Recovery varies based on many factors, starting with the type of diagnosis. Conditions such as CVA and TBI depend on location and extent of injury, the number and extent of challenges present (that is, spasticity, edema, pain, cognition, visual-perceptual issues, and so on), compensatory patterns of movement, orthopedic issues, patterns of learned nonuse, and other issues. Understanding the difference in how a neurological hand clinically presents in the various stages of recovery is also important. For example, the answer to this question for someone with a paralyzed UE within the acute phase of a CVA will be different than the answer for someone who possesses a chronic neurological hand several years post injury. More degenerative conditions, such as MS and PD, require a different approach. Maintenance, prevention, and adaptation, especially in the chronic stages of these conditions, can be a more appropriate focus than recovery of lost function.[1] The following sections give some suggested comments and considerations for treating clients with hemiplegic/hemiparetic hands and for clients with progressive conditions.

Hemiplegia/Hemiparesis

Weakness (hemiparesis) or paralysis (hemiplegia) in one of the UEs is one of the most common challenges when treating clients who have survived a CVA or TBI. Recovery of the hemiparetic/hemiplegic UE is often categorized in stages: the acute stage, the postacute stage, and the chronic stage.

Acute Stage

The acute stage starts at the time of initial injury and continues to the time of discharge from hospital/inpatient rehabilitation. This is a difficult stage because many clients have concomitant concerns (that is, problems with mobility, activities of daily living [ADLs], speech, vision, cognition, and so on) complicating the recovery of the hemiplegic hand. Areas of focus in therapy at this stage tend to be, but are not limited to, ADL performance, bed mobility, transfers, community mobility, positioning, and UE orthosis needs.

The affected hand's available ROM, fine motor coordination, sensation, and the presence of other challenges such as a client's visual-perceptual and cognitive capacity impact a therapist's approach to involving the hand in self-care. A paralyzed, edematous hand requires a therapist to teach the client and family positioning, self-passive range-of-motion (PROM) exercises, and edema management techniques. An affected hand with emerging movement and beginning spasticity will require self-active range of motion (AROM) exercises, an orthosis, and client/family education regarding functional return. Concomitant visual perceptual and/or cognitive deficits such as a **visual field hemianopsia/neglect**, decreased cognitive attention, and sensory deficits require the additional challenge of increasing clients' attention to the affected UE. Increasing awareness to the affected UE is important for sensory reeducation and decreasing the risk of injury during transfers and functional mobility.

Since a primary focus of acute rehabilitation following brain injury is ADL training, including the affected hand in these activities is dependent on how well the hand contributes to functional performance. How to involve the affected UE as an assist in self-care is addressed later in this chapter. The challenge at this stage is balancing the focus of increasing a client's independence in self-care and addressing the recovery of the affected UE. If paralyzed, inclusion of the affected hand in self-care is limited. Therefore training a client to dress, shower, and complete toilet hygiene will often rely on unilateral techniques. If a neurological hand's deficits are limited to decreased fine motor skills, encouraging a client to continue utilizing the affected hand as either the dominant hand or an equal assist during fine motor activities is important. Humans are inclined to find the most efficient and effective method of completing a task to conserve energy.[17] If the less affected hand can complete a task faster with better quality, or if a client has not experienced adequate success in utilizing the affected hand, a pattern of learned nonuse may result. Learned nonuse of the affected UE in the beginning stages of recovery presents significant challenges in restoring hand function.

Points to consider and comments for clients and family at the acute stage:

1. Encourage functional use and inclusion of the affected UE in daily activities. Neuroscientists have discovered a "use it or lose it" phenomenon in brain cells during development and in adult brains following stroke, Alzheimer's disease, and other motor neuron diseases.[18]

Clinical Pearl

Brain cells that are not stimulated by activity will self-destruct. Encouraging the affected UE to participate in meaningful daily tasks (such as hair brushing) can stimulate better quality of movement as well as increase the relevancy of a task for the client.[13] Increasing engagement of the affected UE in purposeful activities at this stage helps maintain neuronal connections for activities that are deeply embedded within the brain from years of repetition.

2. Develop the mantra: "Repetition, repetition, repetition, *with variety.*" Research on motor learning has revealed that repetition in random practice format (that is, repetition of specific tasks with variability in sequence) is better than a blocked practice format (that is, repetition of the same task) within a treatment session.[13] Otherwise known as *motor variability* or *repetition without repetition,*[19] this concept suggests the movements required for a specific task (such as tying shoes) need high repetition in a variety of contexts in order to promote more successful completion of the actual task. In other words, clients need lots of practice to learn/relearn how to use their affected hand in functional tasks.

3. A client's emerging movement will often look different than the client's movement before the injury. As movement returns, clients may have a difficult time figuring out how to use their affected hand,[13] or are deterred from using their affected hand because the emerging movement does not appear familiar. For example, clients knew how to tie shoes prior to their injury, and likely did so without thinking of the hand movements required to complete the task. As they attempt familiar tasks (such as tying shoes) after the injury, the affected hand may not be able to contribute as expected. Assist clients in recognizing what they see now is only a beginning. Clients need to know, although their movements may not look the same, different movement patterns can be used to successfully complete a task and will evolve throughout recovery.

Clinical Pearl

It has been proposed that synergistic movement patterns can be used as part of a strategy to allow for variance in motor performance.[20] These movement patterns have the potential to represent the beginning of "normal" movement or result in compensatory movement strategies. Although there are treatment approaches that suggest it is best to avoid abnormal patterns of movement,[1] discouraging such variance may deter movement in the affected hand altogether and lead to learned nonuse.

4. Be cautious when discussing recovery expectations. Clients have reported hearing comments from health care professionals that there is no hope for recovery. Pessimistic comments leave a lasting impression that can deter clients from working on their recovery and contribute to a negative attitude about their hands. We have seen clients who started out with a nonfunctional hand in the acute stage and went on to be discharged from outpatient therapy writing and typing with their affected hand!

5. Dispel the theory that recovery plateaus within the first 6 months of brain injury.

Clinical Pearl

Neuroplasticity is recognized as the injured brain's ability to anatomically and functionally change as a result of: (1) activation of parallel pathways to maintain function within a damaged area, (2) activation of silent pathways, and (3) synaptogenesis, or the formation of new connections.[21]

One study involving brain imaging of stroke survivors revealed improvement in function correlated with increased activity in multiple areas of the brain.[22] Studies such as this support the idea that plasticity occurs even in the later stages of recovery. Furthermore, a client's ability to capitalize on returning movement may not occur for a long time post injury. For instance, having the ability to plan and realize variance in movement, such as how to incorporate a lateral pinch in daily activities where a tip-to-tip pinch was formally used, can take time for the client to discover and the brain to problem solve.

6. ROM, positioning, and orthotic needs can be addressed at this stage with client/family/health care worker education.[13] Clients, families, and caregivers need to know how to don/doff the orthosis, how to care for the orthosis, and the signs of improper fit. Posting signs with instructions and pictures to assist health care staff with adhering to a positioning and/or orthotic routine may be necessary.
7. Educate clients and families on spasticity (if applicable) and encourage consistent contact with a physician to manage tone.
8. Reinforce bilateral UE involvement in self-care.

◎ Clinical Pearl

Research has shown improvement in affected UE functional performance as a result of bilateral training.[23]

One study involving transcranial magnetic stimulation noted subjects experienced increased speed and functional ability to complete tasks with the affected UE after bilateral training.[24] This was accompanied by a significant increase in corticomotor representation of the involved limb within the affected hemisphere. For more details on bilateral training, see the "Tips from the Field" section later in this chapter.

Post-Acute Stage

This stage starts when the client is released from hospital/inpatient rehabilitation and continues up to 12 months post injury. In many cases, emerging motor and sensory return occurs in this stage. Although there may still be lingering associated concerns to address, a more intent focus on hand rehabilitation can begin. Ideally, a client arrives with an assigned neurologist and/or physiatrist, in possession of a resting hand orthosis, and with any spasticity well managed. If not, these areas need to be addressed in addition to functional return of the hand. Clients may arrive to outpatient therapy making statements such as, "I want my hand back," or "When I get my hand back, I will…." Family members may also press for therapy to "fix [the client's] hand." Providing realistic feedback is a balance between keeping clients motivated while also preparing them for the likelihood they may not achieve 100% recovery. Of course, recovery varies depending on the severity of injury and the individual.[25] Regardless, it is important to stress that the neurological hand has the potential to continually improve.

As clients start noticing other clients and the difference between hand presentations, it may be meaningful for them to appreciate that every presentation is unique. As a therapist, comparing clients can be both a benefit and a hazard. It can be beneficial as one prepares for the hand's progression, or hazardous if it limits a therapist's approach to treating the neurological hand. Clients may also wonder why their affected lower extremities (LE) are making greater progress than their hands. It may be beneficial to educate them on the location of their stroke, the

motor homunculus, and how the UE is typically more involved than the LE following a brain injury, such as a CVA.[26]

At this stage, relearning once-automatic tasks with a hand that is now difficult to control often leads to frustration and can result in a pattern of learned nonuse. Concurrent cognitive and motor planning issues have the potential to confound recovery and increase client frustration.

Additional points to consider and comments for clients and family at the acute stage:
1. No two neurological conditions are alike. This is important to realize because individuals may compare themselves to other clients.
2. Recovery of function takes time, practice, and commitment. Remind clients that they did not originally learn to tie their shoes from one attempt. Consider timing them to provide realistic feedback of their efforts, because clients will often feel as though a task took "forever" when, in fact, it may have only taken a couple of minutes.
3. Promote an environment that encourages clients to self-learn and explore the unexpected. When a client figures out how to accomplish a difficult task independently, there is greater potential for carryover outside of therapy.
4. Clients need to be successful. Plan activities for that "just right challenge" and grade accordingly in order to promote success. Whichever direction is required to grade an activity for successful results, client engagement is essential in realizing the hand's potential.
5. Encourage realistic short-term goals. When faced with goals such as, "I want to play my classical guitar again," stated by a client with trace digit movement 4 months after a stroke, it is important to avoid dismissing the goal. Instead, return with a comment such as, "That is a good long-term goal. Here is where your hand is now, and in order to achieve your long-term goal, we will need to achieve this short-term goal first."
6. Be positive and supportive when a client incorporates the affected hand in daily activities. Clients can be their own worst critic because the functional return of their affected hand may not appear the same as at prior level of function. Providing positive feedback may assist in increasing their confidence to utilize the affected hand with greater consistency.
7. Identify patterns of learned nonuse and tenaciously seek ways to include the affected hand as a functional assist to break these patterns. The earlier learned nonuse habits can be broken, the better. Consider reviewing a constraint protocol if appropriate, or introducing a tool such as the motor activity log (MAL) to help clients identify functional activities in which to incorporate the affected UE.
8. Respect the former role of the affected hand. Asking clients to complete activities with their affected nondominant hand that would otherwise be performed by their dominant less affected hand is not likely to be well received by the client.

Chronic Stage

This stage begins at 12 months post injury and can continue for months or years. Clients at this stage may be seeking an update to their home exercise program, have experienced a change in status with their hand, or are interested in exploring additional ways in which to incorporate their affected hand in daily activities. Some clients in the chronic stage had very little treatment during the acute and post-acute stages and may want therapy to address their affected hand for the first time. Clients in the chronic stage of recovery often arrive with an assigned neurologist and/or physiatrist, in possession of a resting hand orthosis, and with their spasticity managed (if applicable). If not, these areas need to be addressed during therapy. Clients may require an updated orthosis to accommodate orthopedic changes to their hand and/or changes in their spasticity.

Additional points to consider and comments for clients and family at the chronic stage:

1. It is important to reiterate that clients can regain function several years post brain injury.
2. Since learned nonuse patterns have the potential to be well ingrained in chronic survivors, it may be beneficial to focus on bilateral UE tasks because this may encourage more automatic use of the affected hand during functional tasks.
3. In cases of learned nonuse, encourage the client to identify a specific number of tasks the affected hand can complete on a regular basis as a starting point for automatic use in functional activities. For example, have the client agree to use the affected hand to carry objects during mobility or to stabilize objects as an assist to the less-affected UE.

Progressive Conditions

For clients diagnosed with progressive conditions such as Parkinson disease (PD), MS, or other conditions that contribute to declining fine motor skills or grip and pinch effectiveness, the focus of therapy can differ. This depends on the severity of fine motor deficits; length of time from initial diagnosis or appearance of first symptoms; and comorbid issues such as arthritis, decreased sensation, fatigue, and decreased cognitive skills. The length of time from initial diagnosis or appearance of first symptoms is not necessarily a predictor of fine motor performance or response to techniques involving recovery of function, because these conditions often have variability in presentations. Therefore it is important to evaluate and treat each client with a progressive condition on an individual basis and focus on the fine motor skills with respect to function (that is, buttoning, writing, typing, meal preparation, feeding, grooming, and so on).

One study indicated a positive response to modified Constraint Induced Therapy (mCIT) on behalf of clients with PD in Hoehn and Yahr stages II to III as demonstrated by improvement in action research arm test (ARAT), FMA, and box and block test (BBT) scores.[27] Of particular interest is the finding that **bradykinesia** may be reduced through mCIT activities. However, a significant limitation in this study is the fact the researchers did not assess functional performance in daily activities. Therefore they could not infer that their results led to increased or more effective use of the affected hand in daily activities requiring fine motor skills. In both MS and PD, research has shown that the more chronic and severe the symptoms, the more difficulty a client will have with dexterity.[28,29] This results in clients requiring more assistance and modification to tasks involving dexterity.[28]

Challenges to completing tasks that involve fine motor coordination for individuals with PD include, but are not limited to, tremors, decreased initiation of movement ("freezing"), weakness in pinch and grasp, medication "off-time," and decreased attention to tasks (particularly when tasks are out of their visual field).[1] People with PD respond well to completing movement with high amplitude and high effort.[30] Though anecdotal, clients report increased ease in fine motor activities (such as handwriting or buttoning) when, prior to initiating these tasks, they sit with increased trunk extension and "activate" their hands by completing high-amplitude "finger flicks."

Challenges for individuals with MS include, but are not limited to, fatigue, weakness in pinch and grasp, decreased sensation, and decreased attention.[1] Research is limited on individuals with MS recovering lost function. Therapy should focus on preserving existing skills through fine motor exercises and consistent use of the hand in meaningful activities while educating clients to avoid fatigue.

Points to consider and comments for clients and family with progressive conditions:

1. Time of day may impact effectiveness of dexterity because medication regimes, level of alertness, or degree of fatigue may correlate with performance. Try to organize tasks with high dexterity demands with the times of day performance has its best potential.
2. Though recovery of lost function may not be attainable for clients with more chronic and severe symptoms, modification and adaptation can assist in increasing a client's participation in both basic and instrumental activities of daily living tasks that require dexterity, while decreasing dependence on caregiver support.
3. Encourage upright posture and "finger flicks" prior to engaging in (and throughout as needed) fine motor tasks with individuals who have PD.
4. Promote tasks that accentuate existing fine motor skills in order to preserve the current level of functional ability. This may decelerate disease progression and reduce caregiver burden over the long term.
5. Respect the client's dexterity skill level within the context of the client's overall presentation and promote realistic functional goals for the client and family. For example, a client with PD who also possesses concomitant cognitive, fine motor control, and motor planning deficits can preserve independence in feeding if more finger foods are available at mealtimes. In severe cases involving cognitive and motor-planning deficits, utensil management can often be frustrating, and training these clients to use adaptive equipment (AE) may not be successful.

Tips for Evaluating the Neurological Hand

Commonly used assessments for evaluating hand function in the neurological setting are as follows:
- Box and block test (BBT)
- Nine hole peg test (NHPT)
- Action research arm test (ARAT)
- Fugl-Meyer Assessment (FMA)
- Motor activity log (MAL)
- Stroke impact scale (SIS)
- Functional independence measure (FIM)
- Wolf-Motor Function Test (WMFT)
- Functional test for the hemiplegic/paretic upper extremity (FTHUE)
- Jebsen-Taylor Hand Function Test
- Grip and pinch dynamometer testing

Improving motor impairment, increasing daily function, and enhancing quality of life are the primary goals of stroke rehabilitation. The assessments listed above represent some of the tools used to evaluate the neurological hand. When choosing an appropriate evaluation tool, it is important to use your clinical observations. Some assessments are more appropriate for a higher-functioning hand, whereas other assessments are better for a lower-functioning hand.

The BBT assesses gross manual dexterity by counting the number of blocks that can be transported individually from one compartment of a box to another within 1 minute. Higher scores are indicative of better manual dexterity. The reliability, validity, and responsiveness of the BBT have been established in clients with stroke. The NHPT is a timed test of fine manual dexterity. Participants place nine pegs in nine holes and then remove them as quickly as possible. The time needed to complete the task is measured in seconds, and a lower score indicates better dexterity. The NHPT has been demonstrated to have high reliability, validity, and responsiveness in clients with stroke. The ARAT assesses the ability to handle objects based on 19 items that are divided into 4 subscales of grasp, grip, pinch, and gross movement scored by a 4-level ordinal scale ranging from 0 (no movement) to 3 (normal movement). A total scale score maximum of 57 indicates normal performance. The ARAT has established reliability, validity, and responsiveness in clients with stroke.

Three other well-developed outcome measures are widely used to assess UE motor impairment for persons with spasticity and hemiplegia.[31] The FMA assesses motor impairment and is reported to be highly correlated with FTHUE scores,[13] the MAL evaluates daily function, and the SIS determines quality of life. All have adequate reliability and validity. Both the MAL and SIS rely on self-report data.

Adequate validity has been established for the BBT in clients with acute stroke, MS, and TBI, and in elderly clients with UE impairment. The ARAT has good construct validity in measuring UE motor function for clients with chronic stroke. BBT and ARAT had better concurrent validity than the NHPT in clients with chronic stroke at pre- and posttreatment with better correlations to the FMA and MAL. These findings attest to the relationship between motor impairment and daily functions.

The FIM is part of the uniform data system for rehabilitation in the acute phase. The FIM is one of the most widely used methods of assessing functional status in persons with a disability.[32] The FIM includes 18 items, each with a maximum score of 7 and a minimum score of 1. Total possible FIM scores range from 18 to 126. The areas examined by the FIM include self-care, sphincter control, transfers, locomotion, communication, and social cognition. These areas are further divided into motor and cognitive domains.[33] The FIM is intended to serve as a basic indicator of the severity of disability.

The WMFT was designed to assess functional motor ability of clients with moderate to severe UE motor deficits. It has been found to be useful for characterizing the motor status of higher-functioning chronic clients who have experienced a stroke or TBI. The intertest and interrater reliability is high for both performance time and functional ability rating scales. However, the test has limited usefulness for lower-functioning chronic clients. The problem is that such clients are only able to complete less than half of the items on the WMFT, which lends to a sparse sampling of their motor ability. A graded version of the test was developed to address this problem.

The FTHUE is an UE assessment that tests the client's ability to complete ADLs in order of increasing complexity. It consists of 7 levels requiring clients to complete 17 tasks based on Brunnstrom's hierarchy of motor return.[34] Task complexity ranges from evidence of an **associated reaction** during resisted elbow flexion of the less affected UE to the fine motor skills required to remove a rubber band placed on the outside of a client's affected UE digits without using the less affected UE. Activities are timed and graded based on a quality of movement scale. This test was found to be reliable under test–retest conditions.

Lastly, the Jebsen-Taylor Hand Function Test looks at seven subtests to assess hand function. The seven timed subtests include handwriting; turning over cards; grasping and releasing small objects (for example, pennies, paper clips); stacking checkers; picking up and releasing beans with a spoon; and grasping and releasing large empty, and then weighted, cans. This test has good test–retest reliability and good concurrent validity compared to other tests of upper limb dexterity.

Choosing an appropriate evaluation tool is one step in assessing a client's involvement of the affected hand in daily tasks. It is also important to obtain additional information, such as the following:
- Chief complaint/reason for referral
- History of present illness; onset of injury
- Past medical history
- History and present use of orthoses
- Prior therapy: Ask about other therapy services the client has received, as well as type (inpatient or outpatient), when, and duration
- Social history
- Living situation; support systems
- Mobility; use of assistive devices, if any
- Driving status
- Employment: Inquire if a client is considering return to gainful employment or volunteer work. It is important to assess the extent to which the affected hand will be incorporated in activities such as carrying, stabilizing, writing, typing, using tools, and so on.
- Communication; use of assistive technologies, if applicable
- ADLs; use of durable medical equipment (DME) and AE; level of independence
- PROM/AROM: Assess presence and cause of limitations, such as pain, edema, soft-tissue restriction, **joint contractures**, spasticity
- Edema
- Spasticity: Assess using Ashworth Scale, MAS, or Tardieu Scale, and ask about past and present methods of tone management
- Sensation: Light touch, two-point discrimination, sharp/dull
- **Kinesthesia**
- Pain/temperature
- **Stereognosis**
- Cerebellar testing: **Dysdiadochokinesia, dysmetria**
- Cognitive testing
- Visual perception testing: There are many aspects of vision related to hand function, as vision often guides UE engagement. Visual deficits that could interfere with a client's ability to engage the hand in activities include, but are not limited to, visual field neglect/inattention, visual field hemianopsia, and difficulty with tracking/pursuits, **diplopia**, and fixation.
- Identify the client's goals

Diagnostic-Specific Information That Affects Clinical Reasoning

Functional Progression of the Neurological Hand

After assessing a client and the affected hand using the aforementioned objective measures, it is important to evaluate how a client uses the affected hand during daily activities. Assessing hand performance with measurements such as the WMFT and the Jebsen-Taylor Hand Function Test reveals only a portion of movement potential. A therapist needs to understand what a client does with the hand throughout the course of his or her day. Assessing a client's ability to achieve a perfect tip-to-tip pinch between the thumb and index finger to grasp a paperclip in the WMFT may be irrelevant if the client's most effective and commonly used pinch during daily activities is a lateral pinch. A client might also achieve test scores that would indicate normal, or near-normal, ability to complete functional tasks using the affected hand but fail to incorporate the hand due to learned nonuse. Learned nonuse can occur regardless of whether the affected hand was a client's dominant or nondominant hand prior to injury.

The influence of hand dominance on stroke recovery has limited research. One study concluded greater reliance on the ipsilateral UE to the lesion when the lesion is in the right hemisphere, demonstrating a strong right hand preference among right-hand dominant survivors.[35] This means if a right-hand dominant individual has a right hemisphere injury, there is a greater preference to utilize the right hand during daily tasks. Conversely, left-hand dominant survivors did not demonstrate increased hand preference when their injury was in the left hemisphere, and instead demonstrated more bilateral UE involvement in tasks.[35]

Understanding the developmental progression of grasp can be helpful for identifying needs in ROM and motor control to achieve basic grasps and progress to more complex grasp skills. Examining the hand in this manner also allows the therapist to set realistic goals in grasp skills because it would be logical, per developmental progression, for the neurological hand to master a gross grasp prior to a refined pinch. However, the neurological hand may not follow developmental milestones in the recovery of hand skills. Challenges (such as spasticity, difficulty with motor planning, joint deformities, lack of coordination, and decreased sensation) can interfere with the developmental progression of the neurological hand. Instead of using these parameters to set goals for hand function, it may be beneficial to recognize the type of grasp most likely to be achieved by a client, and its potential effect on daily activities. Goals can then be established according to functional potential. The following list is extracted in its entirety from its source and is offered as a reference from which to derive functional goals.

Functional Levels of the Hemiplegic Upper Extremity[36]

I. Classification of Function—Seven Levels
   Level 1—No voluntary motion, no functional use
   Level 2—Beginning active motion, no functional use
   Level 3—Dependent Stabilizer: Minimal voluntary motion, able to do the following types of activities:
   1. Move arm away from side while putting shirt into pants on affected side.
   2. Move arm away from side while adjusting side or back of shirt with less affected UE.
   3. Stabilize shirt at bottom for buttoning in front.
   4. Stabilize wet cloth at lap level while less affected UE applies soap.
   5. Weigh down paper while less affected UE is writing.
   Level 4—Independent Stabilizer: Moderate mass flexion pattern, including some shoulder motion against gravity, and moderate gross grasp are capable of performing the following types of activities:
   1. Hold up trousers while transferring to/from toilet.
   2. Hold toothbrush while less affected UE applies toothpaste.
   3. Hold handle and help open a drawer or refrigerator.
   4. Stabilize a mixing bowl at table level while the less affected UE mixes/stirs.
   5. Stabilize a bottle with a cap while the less affected UE twists the cap open.
   Level 5—Gross Motor Assist: Strong mass flexion pattern, some elbow extension control, moderate gross grasp (some release is helpful but not necessary), and some lateral pinch should be able to perform the following types of activities:
   1. Assist less affected UE in pulling donning/doffing socks/nylons.
   2. Reach and wash less affected UE and armpit.
   3. Hold dish while washing/wiping with less affected UE.
   4. Hold and assist in manipulating a broom for sweeping.
   5. Assist less affected UE in wringing a rag or sponge.
   Level 6—Functional Assist: Ability to combine components of strong mass flexion and extension patterns, including fair plus shoulder control, strong grasp/release, and strong pinch/release are able to perform the following types of activities:
   1. Assist in tying bows.
   2. Assist in fastening a zipper.
   3. Hold a utensil and stabilize food item while less affected UE cuts.
   4. Hold/stabilize pot lid while less affected UE pours out liquid.
   5. Hold pencil and begin to write legibly.
   Level 7—Refined Functional Assist: Fair plus to good isolated control in shoulder, elbow, and wrist, strong grasp/release, lateral and palmar prehension, and ability to manipulate individual digits are able to perform the following types of activities:
   1. Lace shoes
   2. Thread needle
   3. Manage safety pin to secure material
   4. Screw nut onto bolt
   5. Pick up coins
II. Classification of Function—Four Levels
   Level 1—Placement of Arm
   1. No prehension
   2. Move then fix in space (stabilize paper, bear weight)
   Level 2—Use in Relationship to an Object
   1. Shoulder adduction to clamp object under arm
   2. Forearm hook to carry objects
   3. Finger hook to carry objects
   4. Fixed hand to push and pull as weight to stabilize object
   Level 3—Use of Prehension
   1. Supportive—holds handrail
   2. Transports—moves objects
   3. Use of tool—use of object to accomplish a task
   Level 4—Skilled Independent Finger Motion
   1. Typing
   2. Playing piano
   Examples of goals:
1. Client will consistently demonstrate UE wrist/digit control to maintain cylindrical grasp of water bottle to work toward inclusion as a gross assist in daily activities.
2. Client will use the right UE as a functional assist by demonstrating pinch/release skills during 25% or more of dressing both upper and lower body.
3. Client will incorporate the UE as an equal refined functional assist during meal preparation demands (that is, cutting, chopping, dicing, mixing, stirring, and so on).

Assessments to Consider Based on Functional Level of the Hemiplegic Upper Extremity

Level 1—Test measurements not likely appropriate

Level 2—FTHUE

Level 3—FTHUE, WMFT (simple tasks), FMA, grip and pinch dynamometer, SIS, MAL

Level 4—FTHUE, WMFT (simple tasks), FMA, grip and pinch dynamometer, SIS, MAL

Level 5—FTHUE, WMFT (simple and complex tasks), FMA, grip and pinch dynamometer, SIS, MAL

Levels 6 and 7—FTHUE, WMFT (simple and complex tasks), FMA, grip and pinch dynamometer, SIS, ARAT, BBT, NHPT, Jebsen-Taylor Hand Function Test, MAL

Common Presentations/Physiological Changes That Interfere With Functional Grasp and Release

1. Intrinsic minus position or "claw hand" (interphalangeal [PIP/DIP] joints in flexion with metacarpophalangeal [MP] joints in neutral)
2. Flexor synergistic pattern placing wrist/digits/thumb in a rigid flexed position insufficient for grasp/release
3. Indwelling or cortical thumb involving a thumb-in-palm posture
4. Spasticity/hypertonicity pattern, including digital MP flexion with PIP/DIP joints in extension and wrist in extension (lumbrical grip with wrist in extension)
5. Spasticity/hypertonicity in thenar eminence (thumb adducted and/or opposed at carpometacarpal and MP to insufficient position for grasp)
6. Flexor tendon shortening (active insufficiency) with extensor tendon lengthening (passive insufficiency)
7. Ataxic/dystonic movement leading to difficulty with coordination
8. Decreased sensation
9. Reaching pattern with forearm in supination rendering an ineffective hand position for grasp and release
10. Decreased arch control limiting grasp capability (that is, client only able to complete span grasp secondary to decreased intrinsic control to form arches necessary for cylindrical or lumbrical grasp)
11. Digit-initiated wrist movement limiting position of hand for grasp
12. Composite digit movement or lack of ability to manipulate individual digits making pinch control difficult or nonexistent
13. Joint instability/deformities: Subluxations, collateral ligament laxity, shifting volar plate, boutonnière, swan neck
14. Contractures

♡ **Tips from the Field**

The following tips are adapted from approaches developed by clinicians using evidence-based practice.

Tip 1: Addressing Spasticity

For the purpose of this chapter, moderate to severe UE spasticity refers to neurological clients who lack volitional control over wrist and digit flexion or extension due to increased spasticity. One would think removing spasticity immediately and in its entirely would be advantageous. However, some clients have learned to use spasticity to their advantage. Therefore therapists should be sensitive to the fact the client may have adopted movement patterns that depend on spasticity/hypertonicity. For example, clients with spastic hemiplegia may have learned to use the increased muscle tone in their weak LE to support functional transfers and gait. Removing this increased tone by treating the spasticity might unmask the underlying weakness and prevent these functions. Spasticity in the hand may assist a client to achieve a functional grasp and if reduced/removed, the client's grasp may be too weak to continue its role in functional tasks. It is important to educate clients that spasticity and muscle strength are not synonymous, and with the reduction of spasticity comes opportunity to develop the strength and motor control for improved volitional involvement in functional activities. Conversely, a client's spasticity can be so severe that it prevents any degree of functional involvement. Regardless of function, spasticity has the potential to lead to other challenges, such as deformities, pain, and inadequate hygiene.

Clients with spasticity experience difficulty inhibiting unwanted tone and facilitating volitional muscle control. Therefore it is important to educate clients on facilitation and **inhibition techniques.**

Facilitation and Inhibition Techniques

Facilitatory Techniques/Suggestions

- Quick stretch
- Vibration
- Kinesiotape
- NMES
- Overflow or associated reaction
- Tapping the muscle belly
- Stroking the muscle belly
- Working in synergistic patterns

Inhibitory Techniques/Suggestions

- Weight bearing
- Fatiguing antagonists of desired movement
- E-stim (quick successive contractions to relax flexors in order to exercise/strengthen extensors), or use of Bioness H200 Hand Rehabilitation System "Fast 3" program
- Kinesiotape
- Mental imagery
- Vibration (stimulation applied to the antagonist of the spastic muscle in order to decrease spasticity)
- Stretching program
- Orthoses
- Serial casting
- Referral for medical management of spasticity

Tip 2: Sensory Reeducation

Somatosensory dysfunction is common following stroke and can be present with other neurological diseases. The literature in this area highlights a broad range of interventions to address sensory deficits. However, the evidence is conflicting because one protocol is not distinctly identified as being superior over another.[37] Anecdotally, significant variability exists in both client sensory presentation and response to intervention, requiring an individualized approach in managing deficits. Variability in presentations and response to intervention is often associated with concurrent motor and/or cognitive deficits. The most notable findings indicate electrical somatosensory stimulation improves hand motor function.[38]

Somatosensory training can include:
- Contrast bathing
- Thermal stimulation
- Intermittent pneumatic compression
- Sensory training using robotics
- Brushing
- Weight bearing
- TENS/NMES with electrode placement protocols specific to sensory reeducation or use of a conduction glove.
- Stereognosis
- Vibration
- Tactile input

Tip 3: Edema

Three different treatment approaches to aid in the reduction of hand edema following stroke have been studied, including passive motion exercises, neuromuscular stimulation, and intermittent pneumatic compression.[39] Findings indicate that continuous passive motion and electrical stimulation are potentially more effective treatments for hand edema than intermittent pneumatic compression. Volumetric assessments of the hand appear to provide the best estimation of changes in edema (a change of 12 mL or more is considered clinically significant). However, measurement comparisons of the circumference of the hand at mid-finger, proximal to the MP joints, and wrist can also be used to document changes in the edematous hand.[40]

Treatment approaches to address edema may include:
- Medifit glove (compression glove)
- Kinesiotaping
- Contrast bathing
- Soft-tissue mobilization
- Positioning
- Fist pumps above the heart
- Caregiver education

Tip 4: Increase Attention to the Affected Upper Extremity
- Proprioceptive feedback
- Blend of active assist range of motion and resistance
- Resistance
- Vibration
- Perturbations
- Visual regard
- Mirror box therapy

Tip 5: Hand Dominance

Research studies on hand dominance and neurological conditions are limited. As presented earlier in this chapter, right-hand dominant individuals with a right brain injury prefer to use their right UE, whereas left-hand dominant individuals with a left brain injury prefer more bilateral UE involvement.[35] There is emerging research linking deficits in hand function to specific hemispheric damage. For example, evidence of hemispheric specialization in the control of automatic reach-to-grasp actions reveals left hemispheric specialization in visual-motor transformation of grasp pre-shaping and right hemispheric specialization in transport-grasp coordination.[41]

Tip 6: Weight Bearing

The incorporation of UE weight-bearing activities is an important and common practice for normalizing muscle tone in clients following brain injury. Repetitive UE weight bearing inhibits hypertonicity and facilitates activation of both agonist and antagonist muscle groups. While there is limited information regarding both objective evaluation and intervention for unilateral and bilateral training, one study concluded a strong correlation between UE weight-bearing measures and FIM motor scores. Bilateral UE weight-bearing conditions yielded the highest significant correlation. Based on these findings, therapists should consider utilizing bilateral motor training to improve weight bearing in an affected UE.[42]

One study examined external and internal factors that can affect weight bearing. External factors, according to Serrien et al.,[43] arise from information provided by the environment in which the movement is produced. Therefore the unilateral or bilateral condition itself is an external factor modifying the UE weight-bearing pressure. Internal factors, on the other hand, refer to the individual's related conditions from the CNS. For example, a client's attention can affect movement and symmetrical weight bearing of the extremity.[43]

In the clinic, it is not uncommon to incorporate the use of a static hand-shaped paddle to support digital MP and interphalangeal (IP) joints in a neutral position as the wrist is positioned into extension for weight bearing throughout the entire UE. Consideration should be given to accommodate changes in digit position, pressure, and comfort level as the wrist is moved into extension, as the degree of spasticity and flexor tendon shortening may impact the effectiveness and comfort of a hand paddle.

Tip 7: Constraint Induced Therapy and Modified Constraint Induced Therapy

Constraint induced therapy (CIT) protocols (that is, forced use) have been proven effective at improving UE function in CVA clients with benefits lasting longer than 1 year.[44] CIT and modified CIT protocols have specific inclusion and exclusion criteria, protocols for practice, and yield the best outcomes when supported by dedicated therapists/caregivers and a motivated client. If not supervised properly, poor adherence to the protocol can result, yielding less than desirable outcomes.[45]

Tip 8: Bilateral Training

Research involving imaging has shown improvement in affected UE functional performance following bilateral training.[23] The most effective protocol establishing whether bilateral UEs should move concurrently, with or without synchronicity, and with use of rhythmic cuing or visual feedback (such as mirror imaging) has yet to be identified. Further research is needed to identify how well the movement(s) learned in bilateral training can be translated to other tasks. Theoretically, the use of the less affected limb helps promote functional recovery of the affected limb through facilitative coupling effects between the upper limbs.[46]

One study noted the importance of intention for simultaneous movement as more significant than simultaneous movement alone.[47,48] Reports of anecdotal experience by clinicians indicate bilateral training has been effective in assisting clients to initiate movement in the affected UE, as well as to problem-solve movement patterns clients are otherwise unable to complete using their affected UE alone.

Tip 9: Electrical Stimulation

Neuromuscular Electrical Stimulation (NMES)/Functional Electrical Stimulation (FES)

NMES/FES is often used with the neurological hand. Functional electrical stimulation refers to the application of NMES to help achieve a functional task. FES is a technique that uses bursts of short electrical pulses to generate muscle contraction by stimulating motor neurons or reflex pathways.

Three forms of NMES are available:

1. Cyclic NMES, which contracts paretic muscles on a preset schedule and does not require participation on the part of the client
2. Electromyogram (EMG) triggered NMES, which may be used for clients who are able to partially activate a muscle and may have a greater therapeutic effect
3. Neuro prosthetic applications of NMES, which can ultimately improve or restore the grasp and manipulation functions required for typical ADLs.[49]

However, there are certain factors to consider with use of NMES. One factor is tendon shortening due to spasticity.

> **Clinical Pearl**
>
> If an individual has moderate to severe tone with tendon shortening, using electrical stimulation can elicit hyperextension of finger joints, which can threaten joint integrity. If this occurs, it is important to reduce the stimulation intensity to allow better positioning of the wrist and hand. This will protect the joints and promote the most optimal tendon excursion.

Evaluate stimulation intensity by how much extension or flexion of digits can be elicited before hyperextension is noted. Alter position to decrease stretch on shortened tendons or consider blocking proximal digit joints in neutral or slight flexion to allow better tendon excursion distally.

Several reviews and metaanalyses examining the benefit of NMES have been conducted. A metaanalysis of four studies concluded that FES enhanced strength.[50] However, conclusions are limited by the methodology of the trials (small sample size, inadequate blinding), and the difficulty in correlating improved strength with improved function. A systematic review by de Kroon et al.[51] assessed the effect of therapeutic electrical stimulation of the affected UE in improving motor control and functional abilities after stroke. The authors included six randomized controlled trials in their review and concluded that there is a positive effect of electrical stimulation on motor control. However, conclusions could not be drawn regarding its effect on functional abilities.

Transcutaneous Electrical Nerve Stimulation (TENS)

TENS capitalizes on the use of afferent stimulation to increase inflow of sensory signals to enhance plasticity, which, in turn, yields better outcomes in rehabilitation.[52] Several trials have examined the use of TENS treatment in the restoration of motor function following stroke. Many of the trials presented assessed motor function, pain, spasticity, and a variety of other outcomes in both the upper and lower extremities.[51] Evidence regarding the efficacy of using TENS to improve motor recovery, spasticity, and ADLs is conflicting.

Electromyogram With Neuromuscular Electrical Stimulation

Some devices combine EMG and electrical stimulation, requiring volitional muscle contraction of a desired movement. One disadvantage with electrical stimulation is the tendency for clients to passively allow the machine to do the work. However, with the addition of EMG capability, the electrical stimulation will not be evoked until there is an EMG reading reflecting trace AROM of the desired movement. EMG biofeedback uses instrumentation applied to the client's muscle(s) with external electrodes to capture motor unit electrical potentials. As the instrumentation converts the potentials into visual or audio information, the client has access to visual pictures and/or auditory indications of the degree to which they are activating the muscle.

Tip 10: Hand/Palmar Shaping

Grasping deficits have been described in terms of altered hand orientation as the hand approaches an object, which may correlate with compensatory movement strategies of the arm and trunk.[53] Compensatory movement in the proximal UE and trunk can occur as a result of deficits in hand configuration or aperture during grasp. Therefore, it is important to consider positioning and shape of the hand when assessing and treating reach-to-grasp movement.

Rehabilitation interventions for clients with grasp deficits should stress anticipatory hand pre-shaping required for objects of varying size and shape. It is important not only to know where there is a deficit (such as the difference in grip aperture), but it is also necessary to understand its cause (for example, weakness in the thenar or hypothenar muscles causing decreased arch control or uncoordinated grip). In order to address hand shaping, consider the following:

- Open/closed kinetic chain exercises
- Positioning to support distal movement (that is, decreasing proximal excursion to allow increased focus on distal control)
- Grading force of movement
- Closing the sensory loop
- Working in/out of synergistic patterns

Tip 11: Adaptive Movements

As the client attempts to use the affected hand, observe the patterns of muscle weakness, the degree of interjoint coordination, and the lack of joint and muscle flexibility due to decreased soft-tissue length or spasticity/hypertonicity. Notable adaptive movements include:

- Pre-grasp: No terminal extension of the digits, disproportionate opening of the hand to compensate for muscle imbalance, and/or decreased wrist control for optimal position of the hand for grasp.
- Grasping: If the client has the ability to extend digits, excessive force can be observed due to difficulty gauging the amount of force need to grasp. At times, clients will use the same force to grasp an empty plastic cup as they would to grasp a gallon of milk. Also, decreased palmar thumb abduction with thumb IP in extension can impede the ability to effectively achieve a pad-to-pad pinch.
- Releasing objects: Clients may attempt to utilize grasp driven by tenodesis. Though active wrist motion may be limited, wrist flexion may be accomplished through relaxation of hypertonicity instead of AROM in order to allow the digital tendons to lengthen (passively or actively) for release. The disadvantage of this technique causes limitations in ability to grasp and release larger objects, particularly in cases with limited active digit extension.

Tip 12: Mirror Box Therapy

Mirror box therapy can assist in reducing unilateral neglect because it brings attention to the affected UE.[54] While mirror box therapy can be an effective modality, it is not for everyone. Subjectively, it requires considerable skill in being able to maintain sustained attention. Clients observe their less affected UE complete motor tasks in the reflection of a mirror as a way to simulate the same movement in their affected UE.[55] Research involving transcranial magnetic stimulation and brain imaging has shown primary motor cortex excitability exists in the ipsilateral hemisphere of unilateral hand movement as subjects watch the mirror image of their less affected UE complete motor tasks.[56] This activity was completed without any active movement in the affected UE, which was occluded from view.

Tip 13: SaeboFlex and SaeboReach Orthoses

The use of neuro rehabilitation orthoses has gained recent popularity. Saebo's Functional neurological dynamic orthoses, the Saebo-Flex and SaeboReach, are devices used to treat clients with limited hand and arm function. For the purpose of this chapter, the most distal orthosis, the SaeboFlex, will be the primary focus. The SaeboFlex allows clients with moderate to severe UE hemiparesis to participate in the latest treatment advances by incorporating their affected hand in highly repetitive task-specific training. The concept behind this orthosis challenges the traditional neuro rehabilitative concept of "proximal to distal" recovery by introducing "distal to proximal" recovery. The SaeboFlex is a dynamic custom-fabricated wrist, hand, finger orthosis designed to strengthen grip and assist in release as needed.

Tip 14: Bioness H200 Hand Rehabilitation System

The Bioness H200 Hand Rehabilitation System (or Ness H200) is an advanced FES system intended to provide clients with a mechanism to regain function and movement of their affected UE. The device allows for the precise delivery of patterned FES to selected muscles in the forearm and hand to facilitate various grasp and release patterns.

Tip 15: TheraTogs

TheraTogs are an elasticized orthosis garment and strapping system that can be used to position the hand and wrist for grasp and release. TheraTogs promote the functional alignment of the UE, both proximally and distally, to include the wrist and thumb.

Tip 16: Robotics/Virtual Reality/Telerehabilitation

Robotics

Robotic devices can be used to assist a client in a number of circumstances. Robotic devices can aid with PROM to help maintain ROM and flexibility, temporarily reduce hypertonia, or resist passive movement. Robotic devices can also assist ROM when a client cannot achieve AROM independently. Robotics may be most appropriate for clients with dense hemiplegia, although robotics can benefit higher-level clients by increasing strength through resisted movement.[57]

The Hand Mentor by Kinetic Muscles, Inc., is an exercise therapy robotic device based on motor learning principles to engage the user, provide meaningful feedback during the performance of repetitive activities, and utilize a massed practice training schedule. The consistent, repetitive, and progressive nature of the Hand Mentor may increase the quantity and quality of sensorimotor information provided to the patient, which has been shown to modulate motor cortex function and excitability and promote motor learning. The Hand Mentor requires clients to utilize wrist and digit flexors and extensors, ideally actively, but can assist passively if needed during computerized audiovisual tasks that provide feedback of movement.

Virtual Reality

Virtual reality training is an innovative new treatment approach that may enhance cortical reorganization following stroke. To date, only a few randomized control trials have been conducted. One study involved two trials using popular gaming systems—the PlayStation EyeToy and the Nintendo Wii.[58] The authors hypothesized improvement in UE function following stroke could be attributed to the avoidance of learned nonuse behavior or by repeated task practice.

Telerehabilitation

Few examples of formal client testing involving telerehabilitation approaches are available. One study highlighted the feasibility of remote retraining of arm movement in stroke patients through Java Therapy software.[59] A participant trained at home using a computer mouse and keyboard as input devices while interacting with a web-based library of games and progress charts. The programs automatically recorded participant performance and the information was transmitted to a central database for analysis. The study concluded movement parameters of the participant improved over several training sessions.

Tip 17: Complementary Medicine

Complementary medicine tends to focus on noninvasive and stress-reducing techniques and can supplement or be used in conjunction with more conventional treatment methods. Certain Asian countries, such as China and Korea, have utilized acupuncture in treating stroke. However, scientific study in this area is controversial. Effectiveness of acupuncture in aiding stroke recovery indicates mixed results with questionable research design methods. For instance, several studies did not use a control group and for those including control groups, the participants were not clearly randomized. Yet, some studies indicate when acupuncture is used in conjunction with other therapy, the technique can be effective in improving specific motor function of extremities following stroke. The greatest benefit from this technique results from early intervention post stroke.[60]

Orthoses

Therapists make important decisions about whether or not to issue UE orthoses and at what stage in recovery to issue orthoses.[13] Therapists must also determine the most appropriate type of orthosis to issue. There are many variables to consider when assessing a client for an orthotic. Design options include: static/immobilization, dynamic/mobilization, static progressive, hand- or forearm-based, positioned on the volar or dorsum surface, and prefabricated/fabricated. Material properties to consider consist of, but are not limited to: conformability, resistance to stretch, memory, rigidity, bonding, working time, thickness, perforated or nonperforated, and neoprene.[61] Prefabricated options include products offered by: SaeboStretch, Softpro, Dynasplint Systems, and FREEDOM Omni Progressive, to name a few.

The neurological hand will often change throughout the course of recovery. Therefore choosing the type of orthosis and deciding when to introduce it to the client and caregiver requires thoughtful consideration. For example, a static, forearm-based resting hand orthosis fabricated for a client in inpatient rehabilitation may need to be adjusted, replaced, or discontinued months later due to changes in the hand. And if an orthosis is introduced without comprehensive education (how to don/doff, how to progress the wearing schedule, how to identify signs of possible harm), wearing the orthosis may actually lead to complications. Deformities, pain, injury, and edema can occur as a result of improper orthotic application and use, or changes in the hand that result in the orthosis no longer performing its original purpose.

The aims of an orthosis for a neurological client include reduction in spasticity and/or pain, lengthening of soft tissue, maintenance of joint alignment, improvement in functional outcome, and prevention of contracture/deformities and edema. Evidence regarding use of orthoses for the spastic UE is controversial.[61] There is some evidence that using orthoses in CVA does not reduce spasticity in the long term nor decrease a client's impairment/disability.[62] However, there is also support in the literature for using orthoses that provide low-load prolonged stretch at end-range to reduce spasticity/hypertonicity and contractures.[13] Therapists and clients alike have long provided anecdotal reports of increased relaxation and reduced tone in the digits and wrist during and after orthotic wear. Additionally, the evidence supports using orthoses to increase flexor tendon length, decrease the potential for passive insufficiency from extensor tendon lengthening, and promote neutral positioning of wrist and digit joints and tendons.[63]

Research suggesting superiority of a particular orthotic design over another with respect to the CVA hand is limited.[13] Historically, two different approaches to splinting the CVA hand have been debated: (1) the biomechanical approach, which emphasizes support of joint alignment, soft-tissue length, and prevention of contractures; and (2) the neurophysiological approach, which considers reflexive response, facilitation/inhibition through sensory input and positioning, and the neurological basis of spasticity.[13] It is important for therapists to consider a client's biomechanical needs for an orthosis as well as the potential for a neurological response to an orthosis. For example, clients may experience an increase in spasticity/hypertonicity from physical contact with an orthosis or the positioning of their wrist and digits in the orthosis. The former can be addressed by considering different material or location of input (volar or dorsal base of support or the addition of proximal joint support to decrease the stretch on a distal joint), and the latter by modifying the angles of the wrist and digits. This typically means decreasing the amount of stretch to the hypertonic muscles, such as modifying the orthosis to allow for increased digit and wrist flexion, thereby reducing the amount of stretch to the spastic/hypertonic flexors.[61] It is also important to evaluate the impact of an orthosis on a client's daily routine, as some orthoses may be too complicated to manage independently or may overwhelm an already strained caregiver. Either situation has the potential to lead to complications, inappropriate orthotic use, or no use of the orthosis at all.

In addition to these considerations, the following are evaluation tips and management strategies to consider when assessing a client's hand for an orthosis.[13,61]

Presentations Indicating the Need for an Orthosis

1. Soft-tissue restrictions to digit flexion or extension (both intrinsic and extrinsic), limited thumb–index finger web space, and lack of functional digit excursion with wrist movement (that is, increased digital flexion during neutral to extended wrist position)
2. Joint contractures
3. Decreased joint ROM, muscle weakness, tendon laxity, and decreased coordination causing difficulty with functional grasp
4. Hygiene issues due to moderate-severe spasticity or joint contracture
5. Resting hand posture in any position other than neutral

Points to Consider When Issuing an Orthosis

1. Client/caregiver ability to don/doff and manage an orthotic wearing schedule
2. Sensory deficits compromising an accurate reflection of the orthosis fit leading to potential injury
3. Impact on functional use, as orthoses have the potential to block functional movement. Orthotics that impede movement should ideally be worn when the client is least likely going to use the hand for grasp and release.
4. The presence of edema
5. Potential for pressure that could lead to possible injury
6. Instruction in orthotic use, maintenance, and follow-up care that is realistic for the client and caregiver. Consider developing an orthotic wearing schedule for the client and caregiver. Follow-up on their ability to progress the wearing schedule. Consider providing sequential photographs of the donning process and end result reflecting the correct positioning of the orthotic. Ensure clients and caregivers can demonstrate the donning/doffing process to promote successful and consistent use at home.

Common Orthoses Used to Address Neurological Hand Issues

1. Static or dynamic forearm-based resting hand orthoses: Prefabricated options are available from companies, such as SaeboStretch, Softpro, Dynasplint Systems, and FREEDOM Omni Progressive. Custom fabricated immobilization orthoses with or without finger separation and increased thumb abduction can be used to promote reflex inhibition.[61] These orthoses are typically worn overnight in a supported position because they have the tendency to restrict participation in grasp and release and cause an unwanted load on proximal joints.
2. Static progressive orthoses with adjustable dial or ratcheting components: Examples include orthoses from Joint Active Systems, Inc. and Dynasplint Systems. These are worn to provide prolonged, progressive stretch over specific period(s) of time throughout the day. After

wearing a static progressive orthosis clients should continue to wear the Dynasplint on a lower load stretch, or don a static or dynamic forearm-based resting hand orthosis, to enforce a low-load prolonged stretch. This assists in maintaining any gains made in tissue length from the static progressive orthosis. Caveats in maintaining these types of orthoses include the need for consistent follow-up by a therapist; clients/caregivers must be vigilant in managing a wearing schedule and observing/acting on concerns; and major adjustments and repairs typically require a company representative or orthotist.

3. Wrist cock-up orthoses: Prefabricated options include various over-the-counter brands that can be purchased at drug stores, and brands offered through DME providers. Commercial orthoses are offered with volar, dorsal, or circumferential support. Custom immobilization or mobilization orthoses can also be fabricated by the therapist. Wrist orthoses are worn to support the wrist in a position to promote optimal positioning of digits for grasp and pinch demands. This may involve a neutral or slightly flexed wrist position to promote tenodesis grasp. Wrist orthoses may also protect the wrist during transfers, particularly those transfers involving clients with visual neglect/hemianopsia. The best wrist orthosis is one that least interferes with grasp and pinch.

4. Orthoses to promote neuro-reeducation: One style of reeducation orthosis positions the second, third, fourth, and fifth digit MP joints in neutral and leaves the IP joints free to move. This allows the client to isolate PIP flexion/extension in these digits without MP joint interference. Other styles functionally position the hand and digits for grasp and release (MP blocking splint, intrinsic minus splint, hand-based anticlaw splint, Oval 8 or Silver Ring splints, thumb spica splint, digit IP and thumb abduction immobilization splints, digit mobilization splints, and so on). Caveats of these orthoses include frequent donning/doffing of the orthotic; consistent monitoring for skin redness and swelling; and client vigilance in using the orthosis appropriately and managing an often-complicated wearing schedule. Additionally, the static nature of these orthoses does not bode well in accommodating changes to spasticity during functional use.

5. Fabric-based orthoses: Examples include neoprene strapping, Comfort Cool Thumb Adductor Strap, Benik thumb strap or hand-based thumb or thumb-index finger support, TheraTogs, and digit buddy straps. These orthoses promote functional positioning of digits via dynamic blocking or facilitation. Caveats of these orthoses include frequent donning/doffing with the donning process being potentially complex, and the risk of spasticity/hypertonicity overcoming the orthotic support.

6. Serial casts: Serial casting can be used to treat contractures and has been proven effective in promoting elongation of tissue length.[61] Progressive casting over a period of days or weeks provides an excellent opportunity to apply a low-load prolonged stretch to spastic/hypertonic or contracted joints and soft tissue. Another benefit includes the reduction of spasticity secondary to the neutral warmth provided by the casting materials.[61] Casts are typically applied to promote a prolonged stretch just below maximal range and/or prior to activating spasticity.[61] Casts are left on for 3 to 5 days before checking skin integrity and response to treatment, and can be applied weekly for up to 3 to 5 weeks.[61] A successful result per cast is noted by a gain in ROM of 10 to 20 degrees.[64] Exclusion criteria can include edema, digit or wrist subluxation, fracture, heterotrophic ossification, open wounds, or client intolerance. Impaired sensation can also be a concern. Caveats to casting include decreased functional use of the casted UE, issues with skin integrity and pressure, poor tolerance or client agitation, increased edema, circulatory changes, and itching.[13,61] Subjectively, clients have benefited from the use of batting material alone wrapped around the digits to provide a prolonged stretch in extension without the addition of casting material. This technique provides a less aggressive therapeutic stretch and has the potential to decrease tone via neutral warmth. The soft batting material also allows the therapist easier access to the digits in order to assess a client's response to prolonged stretch.

Common Challenges With Treating the Neurological Hand

Spasticity UE weakness (proximal and/or distal)	Poor motor planning (apraxia)
Decreased coordination (ataxia, dysmetria)	Edema
Visual-perceptual deficits	Pain
Cognitive deficits	Soft-tissue limitations
Sensory impairments	Joint contractures
Decreased caregiver support	Depression
Poor case management	Learned nonuse/disuse
Socioeconomic issues lending to decreased access to resources	Behavioral issues
	Aphasia

References

1. Pedretti L, Early MB: *Occupational therapy: practice skills for physical dysfunction*, ed 5, St Louis, 2001, Mosby.
2. Rosenstein L, Ridgel AL, Thota A, et al.: Effects of combined robotic therapy and repetitive-task practice on upper-extremity function in a patient with chronic stroke, *Am J Occup Ther* 62(1):28–35, 2008.
3. van der Lee JH, Beckerman H, Lankhorst GJ: The responsiveness of the Action Research Arm test and the Fugl-Meyer Assessment scale in chronic stroke patients, *J Rehabil Med* 33(3):110–113, 2001.
4. Wenzelburger R, Kopper F, Frenzel A, et al.: Hand coordination following capsular stroke, *Brain* 128(1):64–74, 2005.
5. Duncan P, Reker D, Kwon S, et al.: Measuring stroke impact with the stroke impact scale: telephone versus mail administration in veterans with stroke, *Med Care* 43(5):507–515, 2005.
6. Reddy H, Narayanan S, Woolrich M, et al.: Functional brain reorganization for hand movement in patients with multiple sclerosis: defining distinct effects of injury and disability, *Brain* 125(12):2646–2657, 2002.
7. Verheyden G, Nuyens G, Nieuwboer A, et al.: Reliability and validity of trunk assessment for people with multiple sclerosis, *Phys Ther* 86(1):66–76, 2006.
8. UAB School of Medicine Department of Physical Medicine and Rehabilitation: *The UAB-SCIMS information network*, Spinal Cord Injury Model System Information Network (website) http://www.spinalcord.uab.edu/show.asp?durki=21819: Accessed August 20, 2012.
9. Augutis M, Anderson CJ: Coping strategies recalled by young adults who sustained a spinal cord injury during adolescence, *Spinal Cord* 50(3):213–219, 2012.
10. Donnelly C, Eng JJ, Hall J, et al.: Client-centered assessment and the identification of meaningful treatment goals for individuals with a spinal cord injury, *Spinal Cord* 42(5):302–307, 2004.
11. Health library: *Rehabilitation for stroke*, John Hopkins Medicine (website) http://www.hopkinsmedicine.org/healthlibrary/conditions/adult/cardiovascular_diseases/rehabilitation_for_stroke_85, P00805/: Accessed August 19, 2012.
12. National Stroke Association: *New survey emphasizes need for more, better care after stroke*, The National Stroke Association (website) http://www.stroke.org/site/DocServer/NSA_Stroke_Perceptions_Survey_Press_Release__final_.pdf?docID=1943: Accessed August 21, 2012.
13. Gillen G, Burkhardt A: *Stroke rehabilitation: a function-based approach*, ed 2, St Louis, 2004, Mosby.
14. Corey Witenko, Robin Moorman-Li, Carol Motycka: *Spasticity skeletal muscle relaxers*, eMedExpert (website) www.emedexpert.com/classes/skeletal-muscle-relaxers.shtml: Accessed July 4, 2013.
15. Gallichio JE: *Pharmacologic management of spasticity following stroke*, Physical Journal (website) http://ptjournal.apta.org/content/84/10/973: Accessed July 4, 2013.
16. Eric Chang, Nilasha Ghosh, Daniel Yanni: *Spasticity management*, Stroke Survivors Association of Ottawa (website) http://www.strokesurvivors.ca/new/SpasticityManagement.php: Accessed August 21, 2012.
17. Herzfeld R, Kramer H: *Re-wiring the brain, re-shaping the mind: an integral approach to transformation*, Integral New York's Ken Wilber Meetup (website) http://www.meetup.com/kenwilber-58/events/61658802/: Accessed August 20, 2012.
18. Queensland Brain Institute (QBI): *More brain research suggests "use it or lose it,"*, Science Daily (website) http://www.sciencedaily.com/releases/2008/02/080207091859.htm: Accessed August 21, 2012.
19. Bernstein NA: *The co-ordination and regulation of movements*, Oxford, 1967, Pergamon Press.
20. Latash L, Scholz JP, Schoener G: Motor control strategies revealed in the structure of motor variability, *Exerc Sport Sci Rev* 30(1):26–31, 2002.
21. Font MA, Arboix A, Krupinski J: Angiogenesis, neurogenesis and neuroplasticity in ischemic stroke, *Curr Cardiol Rev* 6(3):238–244, 2010.
22. Zorowitz R, Brainin M: Advances in brain recovery and rehabilitation 2010, *Stroke* 42:294–297, 2011.
23. Cauraugh J, Summers J: Neural plasticity and bilateral movements: a rehabilitation approach for chronic stroke, *Prog Neurobiol* 75(5):309–320, 2005.
24. Summers J, Kagerer F, Garry M, et al.: Bilateral and unilateral movement training on upper limb function in chronic stroke patients: a TMS study, *J Neurol Sci* 252(1):76–82, 2007.
25. *Mayo Clinic staff: Stroke rehabilitation: what to expect as you recover*, Mayo Clinic (website) http://www.mayoclinic.com/health/stroke-rehabilitation/BN00057: Accessed August 21, 2012.
26. Twitchell TE: The restoration of motor function following hemiplegia in man, *Brain* 74(4):443–480, 1951.
27. Lee K-S, Lee W-H, Hwang S: Modified constraint-induced movement therapy improves fine and gross motor performance of the upper limb in Parkinson disease, *Am J Phys Med Rehabil* 90:380–386, 2011.
28. Poole J, Nakamoto T, Skipper B, et al.: Dexterity, visual perception, and activities of daily living in persons with multiple sclerosis, *Occupational Therapy In Health Care* 24(2):159–170, 2010.
29. Pradhan S: Use of sensitive devices to assess the effects of medication on attentional demands of precision and power grips in individuals with Parkinson disease, *Med Biol Eng Comput* 49(10):1195–1199, 2011.
30. Farley BG, Fox CM, Ramig LO, et al.: Intensive amplitude-specific therapeutic approaches for Parkinson's disease: toward a neuroplasticity-principled rehabilitation mode, *Top Geriatr Rehabil* 24(2):99–114, 2008.
31. Fugl-Meyer AR, Jääskö L, Leyman I, et al.: The post-stroke hemiplegic patient. 1. A method for evaluation of physical performance, *Scand J Rehabil Med* 7(1):13–31, 1975.
32. Berglund K, Fugl-Meyer A: Upper extremity function in hemiplegia, *Scand J Rehabil Med* 18:155–157, 1986.
33. Stineman MG, Shea JA, Jette A, et al.: The functional independence measure: tests of scaling assumptions, structure, and reliability across 20 diverse impairment categories, *Arch Phys Med Rehabil* 77:1101–1108, 1996.
34. Winstein CJ, Rose DK, Tan SM, et al.: A randomized controlled comparison of upper-extremity rehabilitation strategies in acute stroke: a pilot study of immediate and long-term outcomes, *Arch Phys Med Rehabil* 85:620–628, 2004.
35. Rinehard JK, Singleton RD, Adair JC, et al.: Arm use after left or right hemiparesis is influenced by hand preference, *Stroke* 40(2):545–550, 2009.
36. *Occupational therapy: functional levels of the hemiplegic upper extremity*, Terapia-Ocupacional.Com (website) http://www.terapia-ocupacional.com/articulos/LevelsoftheHemiplegic.shtml: Accessed August 8, 2012.
37. Doyle S, Bennett S, Fasoli SE, et al.: Interventions for sensory impairment in the upper limb after stroke, *Cochrane Database Syst Rev* (6):CD006331, 2010.
38. Schabrun SM, Hillier S: Evidence for the retraining of sensation after stroke: a systematic review, *Clin Rehabil* 23:27–39, 2009.
39. Leibovitz A, Baumoehl Y, Roginsky Y, et al.: Edema of the paretic hand in elderly poststroke nursing patients, *Arch Gerontol Geriatr* 44:37–42, 2007.
40. Post MW, Visser- Meily JM, Boomkamp-Koppen HG, et al.: Assessment of edema in stroke patients: comparison of visual inspection by therapists and volumetric assessment, *Disabil Rehabil* 25:1265–1270, 2003.
41. McCombe-Waller S, Whitall J: Hand dominance and side of stroke affect rehabilitation in chronic stroke, *Clin Rehabil* 19:544–551, 2005.
42. Reistetter T, Abreu BC, Bear-Lehman J, et al.: UE weight-bearing after brain injuries, *Occup Ther Int* 16(3-4):218–231, 2009.
43. Serrien DJ: Interactions between new and pre-existing dynamics in bimanual movement control, *Exp Brain Res* 197(3):269–278, 2009.
44. Wolf SL, Winstein CJ, Miller J, et al.: Effect of constraint-induced movement therapy on upper extremity function 3 to 9 months after stroke: the EXCITE randomized clinical trial, *JAMA* 296(17):2095–2104, 2006.
45. Ploughman M, Shears J, Hutchings L, et al.: Constraint-induced movement therapy for severe upper-extremity impairment after stroke in an outpatient rehabilitation setting: a case report, *Physiother Can* 60(2):161–170, 2008.

46. Latimer CP, Keeling J, Lin B, et al.: The impact of bilateral therapy on upper limb function after chronic stroke: a systematic review, *Disabil Rehabil* 32:1221–1231, 2010.

47. McCombe-Walle S, Whitall J: Bilateral arm training: why and who benefits? *NeuroRehabilitation* 23:29–41, 2008.

48. Mudie MH, Matyas TA: Can simultaneous bilateral movement involve the undamaged hemisphere in reconstruction of neural networks damaged by stroke? *Disabil Rehabil* 22:23–37, 2000.

49. Popovic DB, Popovic MB, Sinkjaer T, et al.: Therapy of paretic arm in hemiplegic subjects augmented with a neural prosthesis: a cross-over study, *Can J Physiol Pharmacol* 82:749–756, 2004.

50. Glanz M, Klawansky S, Stason W, et al.: Functional electrostimulation in poststroke rehabilitation: a meta-analysis of the randomized controlled trials, *Arch Phys Med Rehabil* 77(6):549–553, 1996.

51. de Kroon JR, van der Lee JH, IJzerman MJ, et al.: Therapeutic electrical stimulation to improve motor control and functional abilities of the upper extremity after stroke: a systematic review, *Clin Rehabil* 16(4):350–360, 2002.

52. Sonde L, Kalimo H, Fernaeus SE, et al.: Low TENS treatment on post-stroke paretic arm: a three-year follow-up, *Clin Rehabil* 14(1):14–19, 2000.

53. Sangole AP, Levin MF: Palmar arch modulation in patients with hemiparesis after a stroke, *Exp Brain Res* 199:59–70, 2009.

54. Altschuler EL, Wisdom SB, Stone L, et al.: Rehabilitation of hemiparesis after stroke with a mirror, *Lancet* 353(9169):2035–2036, 1999.

55. *Mirror box therapy/mirror visual feedback*, Research and Hope (website) http://researchandhope.com/stroke/mirror-box-therapy: Accessed August 21, 2012.

56. Garry MI, Loftus A, Summers JJ: Mirror, mirror on the wall: viewing a mirror reflection of unilateral hand movements facilitates ipsilateral M1 excitability, *Exp Brain Res* 163:118–122, 2005.

57. Burgar CG, Lum PS, Shor PC, et al.: Development of robots for rehabilitation therapy: the Palo Alto VA/Stanford experience, *J Rehabil Res Dev* 37:663–673, 2000.

58. Fischer HC, Stubblefield K, Kline T, et al.: Hand rehabilitation following stroke: a pilot study of assisted finger extension training in a virtual environment, *Top Stroke Rehabil* 14:1–12, 2007.

59. Piron L, Tonin P, Trivello E, et al.: Motor tele-rehabilitation in post-stroke patients, *Med Inform Internet Med* 29(2):119–125, 2004.

60. Laures JS, Shisler RJ: Complementary and alternative medical approaches to treating adult neurogenic communication disorders: a review, *Disabil Rehabil* 26(6):315–325, 2004.

61. Jacobs ML, Austin N: *Splinting the hand and upper extremity: principles and process*, Baltimore, 2003, Lippincott Williams & Wilkins.

62. Lannin NA, Herbert RD: Is hand splinting effective for adults following stroke? A systematic review and methodologic critique of published research, *Clin Rehabil* 17(8):807–816, 2003.

63. Tyson SF, Kent RM: The effect of upper limb orthotics after stroke: a systematic review, *NeuroRehabilitation* 28(1):29–36, 2011.

64. Hill J: Management of abnormal tone through casting and orthotics. In Kovich KM, Bermann DE, editors: *Head injury: a guide to functional outcomes in occupational therapy*, Gaithersburg, MD, 1988, Aspen, pp 107–124.

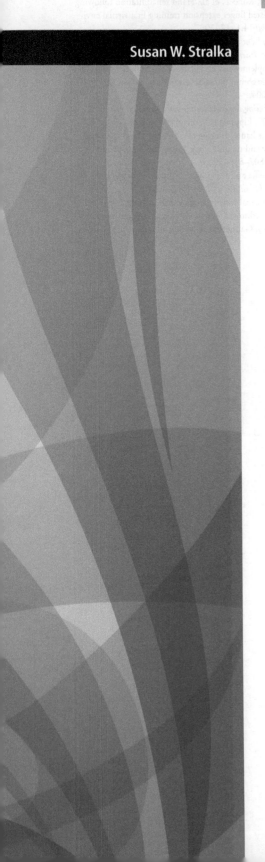

37 Complex Regional Pain Syndrome

Susan W. Stralka

Complex regional pain syndrome (CRPS) is a challenging problem that can potentially derail the best efforts of a well-intentioned therapist. CRPS usually occurs after injury or surgery and presents with clinical symptoms such as disproportionate continued burning pain that cannot be explained by the initial injury. One of the older terms for CRPS was reflex sympathetic dystrophy (RSD). This name originated at a time when the condition was believed to be driven by only the sympathetic nervous system; however, as we learned more about this disorder, the term "RSD" was abandoned. Recent research on the pathogenesis of CRPS has led to a better understanding of the disorder and its multiple mechanisms involving both the peripheral and central nervous symptoms as well as an aberrant inflammatory response.[1] Initially the pathophysiology of CRPS is dominated by a posttraumatic inflammatory reaction with involvement of the immune system. Most often, without early identification and adequate treatment, central sensitization develops because of continuous nociceptive input. Even though the exact etiology is still unknown, there is now a better understanding of the mechanisms that contribute to development, progression, and maintenance of this condition.[2]

The pain associated with CRPS usually starts in an injured limb, such as the hand or foot, and sometimes spreads to other body parts. The CRPS experience is not proportional to the magnitude of injury or surgery because it can occur even after very minor (or no) injury. Spontaneous CRPS (the occurrence of CRPS without a causative event) does occur and requires further differential diagnostic workup for rheumatic, inflammatory, or neuropathic diseases. Pain, sensory, motor, and trophic symptoms typically change throughout the course of CRPS as a result of the varying pathophysiology.[1,3,4]

Treatment of CRPS is challenging in part because evidence is relatively sparse in this realm. Unfortunately, therapeutic intervention is often aimed at treating only the peripheral symptoms while ignoring the central symptoms. Since CRPS symptoms change throughout its course, clinical signs and symptoms reflecting the *underlying* pathophysiological mechanisms must be addressed. The earlier CRPS is recognized and treated, the less likely it is to continue as a chronic pain disorder.[5]

Diagnostic Criteria

A good history and physical examination are essential for identifying CRPS, as diagnosis is primarily based on clinical presentation. The first diagnostic criteria for CRPS was proposed in 1994 by the International Association for the Study of Pain.[6] In 2007, an international group of experts met in Budapest to develop more accurate and valid criteria. The updated criteria have come to be known as the "Budapest Criteria."[6] The Budapest Criteria is now widely accepted as having a high rate of accuracy in identifying CRPS (Box 37.1).

Tests such as X-ray, magnetic resonance imaging (MRI), functional MRI (fMRI), three-phase bone scan, skin biopsy, sympathetic nerve tests, and electromyography do not rule in CRPS but may be used for differential diagnosis (identifying other diagnoses that present with signs and symptoms similar to CRPS). However, brain imaging studies, such as fMRI, have demonstrated alterations in central-motor processing in individuals with CRPS, and these recent findings could have implications for rehabilitation.[7,8]

Incidence and Factors for Developing Complex Regional Pain Syndrome

The exact incidence of CRPS is not known, but it has been estimated that there are between 20,000 to 80,000 new cases of CRPS diagnosed every year in the United

---

BOX 37.1 **Symptoms and Signs of Complex Regional Pain Syndrome**

The Budapest Criteria differentiates between "symptoms," which are reported by the client, and "signs," which are seen or felt by the person carrying out the examination.

Under the Budapest Criteria for a diagnosis of CRPS, a client must have at least one symptom in three of the following four categories:

1. Sensory: hyperaesthesia (an abnormal increase in sensitivity) and/or allodynia (pain caused by usually nonpainful stimuli)
2. Vasomotor: skin color changes or temperature and/or skin color changes between the limbs
3. Sudomotor/edema: edema (swelling) and/or sweating changes and/or sweating differences between the limbs
4. Motor/trophic: decreased range of motion and/or motor dysfunction (weakness, tremor, muscular spasm, dystonia) and/or trophic changes (changes to the hair and/or nail and/or skin on the limb)

At the time of clinical examination, at least one sign must be present in two or more of the following categories:

1. Sensory: hyperalgesia (to pinprick) and/or allodynia (to light touch and/or deep somatic [physical] pressure and/or joint movement)
2. Vasomotor: temperature differences between the limb and/or skin color changes and/or skin color changes between the limb
3. Sudomotor/edema: edema and/or sweating changes and/or sweating differences between the limbs
4. Motor/trophic: decreased range of motion and/or motor dysfunction (i.e., weakness, tremor, or muscle spasm) and/or trophic changes (hair and/or nail and/or skin changes).

Finally, it is important that no other diagnosis can explain the signs and symptoms.

Adapted from Harden RN, Bruehl S, Stanton-Hicks M, Wilson PR. Proposed new diagnostic criteria for complex regional pain syndrome. *Pain Med.* 2007;8:326-331.

States.[1] Women are three to four times more likely than men to develop this disorder.[9] CRPS is a complication in 3.8% of all wrist fractures. One study reported a CRPS rate of 25% in distal radius fractures.[10] Women with complicated fractures who have intense pain 1 week after trauma may be more prone to developing CRPS, as are those with a rheumatological disease. Other risk factors include baseline pain, high-energy injuries, and immobilization.[11,12]

A study published in the *Journal of Hand Therapy* in 2018 evaluated risk factors for the development of CRPS after hand surgery for treatment of traumatic injuries. These researchers found that individuals with crush injuries had a higher risk of developing CRPS.[13] This same study supported earlier research findings that significant pain in the first few days following surgery—in this study a pain score greater than 5 out of 10 in the first three days following surgery—increased patients' risk for developing CRPS.

Clinical Presentation

CRPS is divided into two subgroups: **CRPS type 1** and **CRPS type 2**. Type 1 occurs in individuals with no definitive evidence of a major nerve injury and can occur spontaneously. Type 2 occurs in individuals who have a known nerve injury. It is important to identify if there is a nerve issue that may warrant further investigation, but the presentation and management of both types are similar. Both types of CRPS present with signs that are characteristic of neuropathic pain: spontaneous burning pain; **allodynia** (when a stimulus that is not normally painful is perceived as painful); **hyperalgesia** (increased sensitivity to a painful stimuli with symptoms spreading beyond the nerve or tissue innervation); motor disturbances such as tremors, muscle spasms, dystonia, and decrease in speed of movement; changes in vascular tone; fluctuating skin temperature; skin and nail color changes; edema; and hypo- or hyperhidrosis (sweating changes).[14] Distal edema occurs in 80% of cases and is a result of vasomotor instability as well as lack of motion.

Central pain or **central sensitization** is a CRPS mechanism caused by dysfunction of the central nervous system (CNS), and this may explain why the symptoms sometimes spread around the body.[15] With central sensitization, there is cortical reorganization, body perception disturbances, and movement disorders such as dystonia. Perceptual disturbances or a dysfunctional representation

of the affected limb in the brain map causes finger misperception, impaired laterality recognition, abnormal body schema, astereognosis, as well as a feeling of the limb being foreign.[14] In some instances, these manifestations of CRPS are so severe that individuals have reported a desire to amputate the limb(s). Clearly, these disturbances must be targeted for treatment.

When allodynia is present along with motor symptoms, there is a poor prognosis for recovery unless treatment is aimed at targeting the burning or other unusual pain sensations. A primary strategy for pain reduction with or without allodynia must be implemented immediately before any improvement in motion can be achieved. Persistent allodynia without intervention can prevent the client from tolerating or participating in rehabilitation for CRPS.[14]

Additionally, somatosensory perceptual disturbances must be addressed. Traditional therapies often do not address these symptoms, but with CRPS, treating only the peripheral symptoms may result in limited improvement with the client failing to achieve their potential for function. Understanding the pathogenesis and mechanisms of CRPS allows the hand therapist to design appropriate interventions that include treatment of both the peripheral (bottom-up) and central (top-down) symptoms. This understanding enables the therapist to develop a mechanism-specific rehabilitation program.[16] (See treatment section below for top-down treatment approaches for allodynia and somatosensory perceptual disturbances.)

Peripheral mechanisms include inflammation, peripheral sensitization, and symptom-afferent coupling. Central mechanisms include neuroplastic changes such as cortical reorganization, afferent-efferent feedback conflicts, and central autonomic dysregulation.[2,14] There is great variability in presentation of signs and symptoms. Signs such as denial of the involved extremity (neglect-like phenomena) and loss of body schema indicate that mechanisms are changing from the peripheral to the CNS (cortical disorganization).[16] In 2014, Gierthmuhlen et al.[2] proposed eight mechanisms for the clinical signs and symptoms of CRPS. (Box 37.2)

Pathophysiology

The pathophysiological mechanisms of CRPS are not fully understood, but current research implicates multiple mechanism contributions from a maladaptive proinflammatory response and

BOX 37.2   **Eight Key Mechanisms for signs and symptoms of Complex Regional Pain Syndrome**

1. Inflammatory response
2. Neurogenic inflammation
3. Increased catecholamine circulation
4. Peripheral sensation
5. Sympatho-afferent coupling
6. Central sensitization
7. Maladaptive plasticity
8. Psychological symptoms.
Only the last three mechanisms were listed as having the potential to be treated by multidisciplinary rehabilitation.

Adapted from Gierthmuhlen J, Binder A, Baron R. Mechanism based treatment in complex regional pain syndromes. *Nat Rev Neurology.* 2014;10:518-528.

disturbances in sympathetic-mediated vasomotor control with maladaptive peripheral and central neuronal plasticity.[16] The initial peripheral injury triggers the release of proinflammatory cytokines leading to exaggerated inflammation at the injury site as well as in the dorsal horn, causing continuous CRPS symptoms. This continuous nociceptive input maintains central sensitization. The result is an increased responsiveness in the CNS intensifying both peripheral neurogenic inflammation and mechanical pressure sensitivity such as allodynia and temperature intolerance. As stated earlier, both the peripheral changes and central changes must be addressed. It is important to get these individuals to a physician specializing in pain management immediately, so that they can start receiving treatment for the systemic inflammation.

Biopsychosocial Model of Pain

Hand therapists must move from the biomedical model to a biopsychosocial approach when treating CRPS. This approach addresses the potential influence of pain that occurs in the biological, psychological, and social domains. Scientific evidence demonstrates that pain is a multidimensional experience. In addition to restoring sensory and motor function in the upper extremity, the therapist must address the affective and motivational aspects of individuals with CRPS. Numerous psychological components such as the client's beliefs, cognitive functioning, and emotional state can impact outcomes.

Louw and associates[17] present compelling evidence that educating clients about the neurobiology and neurophysiology components of CRPS has a positive effect on modifying pain, disability, anxiety, and stress. Emotional experience can impact outcomes as well. A biopsychosocial approach starts with educating the client about the neuroscientific etiology of CRPS. Both the client and therapist must understand the mechanisms causing maladaptive symptoms and be willing to change their thinking about traditional treatment methods. It is also important that the client understand that pain or movement does not mean tissue damage. It is the brain protecting the body. For the best results, the following should occur: (1) early identification of CRPS, and (2) immediate treatment starting with client education.

Biopsychosocial Model of Treatment

Unfortunately, there are few high quality randomized and controlled multicenter studies that address rehabilitation of individuals with CRPS. This condition is notoriously difficult to manage. The manifestations of CRPS impact our clients' ability to work and participate in social activities, resulting in substantial deterioration in quality of life along with high rates of depression.[18] A multidisciplinary approach should be established and led by a physician who specializes in treating neuropathic pain and CRPS. Intervention with nonnarcotic medication, regional and local blocks, physical therapy, occupational therapy, and psychological support must be accepted by the entire team.

Effective treatment starts with early identification, immediate intervention, and client education. After educating your client about CRPS, focus on symptom reduction. Because symptoms can vary among clients, it can be challenging to individualize treatments. Specific peripheral and central symptoms must be identified at the initial assessment so that an individualized plan of care can be developed. Establish a strategy for pain reduction and for decreasing allodynia or hyperalgesia. The neuropathic symptoms indicating a hypersensitive nervous system must not be ignored. Your client will make little progress until some amount of pain control has been achieved.

Along with education on CRPS, calming the nervous system should be an integral part of early treatment. Interventions to quiet the nervous system include cognitive-behavioral techniques, mindfulness, relaxation, and diaphragmatic breathing. These techniques reduce feelings of helplessness and increase the client's sense of control, as they provide the client something to do rather than just focusing on their symptoms. These strategies should be a part of the client's home program.

Clinical Pearl

McManus and associates[19] developed active self-management strategies to address CNS arousal: mindfulness, relaxation, cognitive-behavioral training, graded motor imagery, and sleep management. Ongoing stress reactions only strengthen the memory of pain. Incorporate these strategies into your treatment program to help modify dysfunctional neuroplasticity changes.

Continued assessment of tissue irritability helps the hand therapist manage and treat peripheral symptoms. Packman et al.[15] stated that mechanism-guided management continues to be promising in helping therapists select treatments most likely to be effective for their clients' signs and symptoms.

Since CRPS is an ongoing vasomotor instability, we must not exacerbate the symptoms. CRPS clients often develop fear of moving because of having experienced painful passive exercise. This can cause the client to fear active movement, which can be very debilitating. *The general rule for therapists is do not aggravate the symptoms or increase pain.* Also, remember to calm the CNS. It is imperative that traditional treatments, if used, should not magnify symptoms, but rather they should improve motion, decrease tissue irritability, and reduce pain. The client should never be pushed into intolerable pain. Exercises should focus on counting repetition or time, as opposed to being told, "Stop when your symptoms increase." Reassurance should continue throughout treatment, and the client must understand that moving with pain does not cause harm. Gentle yoga is helpful for individuals with CRPS because it is a cost-effective form of movement that helps with rehabilitating the body–mind relationship.

Treatment for Somatosensory Cortex Reorganization

In individuals with CRPS, the CNS undergoes functional and structural changes. Continued nociceptive input maintains central sensitization. It has been estimated that 70% to 75% of clients with CRPS have allodynia, which is a central mechanism. Somatosensory rehabilitation treatment should start as early as possible in the treatment of CRPS. Persistent neuropathic pain not only decreases function but also continues to cause *maladaptive* neuroplasticity in the CNS.

On the other hand, the same neuroplasticity (which is the brain's ability to remodel) is what allows sensory reeducation and sensory relearning to happen. Rosen and associates state that following nerve repair in the hand, "the hand speaks a new language to the brain."[20] The purpose of sensory reeducation is to enhance recovery of sensory function so that both the hand and brain, "speak the same language." Dr. Rosen and others have stated that sensory reeducation should start immediately following nerve repair and with CRPS. Functional improvement using sensory reeducation is based on normalization of the distorted brain map or homunculus. The goal is to restore the cortical hand representation by treating changes that are disorganized in the brain. By changing the disorganization in the brain, many clients report that symptoms improve.

The target of somatosensory rehabilitation is the skin, which has a network of cutaneous endings as the entry point to the nervous system. Both desensitization and somatosensory rehab have been used to treat allodynia. Desensitization starts outside the painful area using textures, vibration, pressure, or percussion, and slowly progresses into the painful area. Desensitization efforts should not be allowed to exacerbate symptoms. The idea behind this method is to flood the area of altered sensation with intense sensory stimuli and to allow for sensory accommodation. Unfortunately, there are times when this increases allodynia, so hand therapists should be constantly alert for symptom increases.

Mirror therapy along with cortical audio-tactile interaction has been shown on MRI to improve cortical organization.[20] Anecdotally, individuals with allodynia report improvements using mirror therapy. The noninvolved hand is placed in front of the mirror, and the involved hand behind the mirror in the same position, if possible. Touching the healthy, noninvolved hand gives the illusion in the mirror that the involved hand is being touched. Often the client gets a perception of tactile stimuli felt on the injured hand, which is still behind the mirror, and this may activate the cortical hand area due to visuo-tactile interaction.

Spicher[21] describes a somatosensory rehabilitation method for pain control that may contribute to regulating both peripheral and central sensitization. Spicher states that neuropathic pain such as CRPS results from CNS damage and is the cause of allodynia. His research was based on identifying specific nerve branch injuries and then using comfortable somatosensory stimulation over an area related to the same nerve but away from the injury. It was his belief that a comfortable stimuli would be felt over the painful sensation area. His method is called the somatosensory rehab model (SRM) and may cause the correct neurotransmitter to generate from the comfortable stimulation to reduce the aberrant signaling. Packman et al.[15] published a 2018 article in the *Journal of Hand Therapy* that presents in-depth information on the SRM.

> ### ◎ Clinical Pearl
>
> Nijs and colleagues[22] describe central sensitivity with widespread hypersensitivity to bright light, touch, noise, mechanical pressures, and high and low temperatures. These things need to be avoided when treating clients with CRPS (to not continue to increase the CNS sensitivity). Choosing the correct treatment area is important so that the CNS starts to calm down.

> ### ◎ Clinical Pearl
>
> Graded motor imagery and mirror therapy might be useful for reducing pain and disability.[23] These techniques assist in correcting the brain's cortical body maps by reducing the incongruence between motor commands and sensory feedback.[24] Graded motor imagery is a brain-based treatment (top down), which targets the activation of different brain regions in a graded manner.[25] Treatment consists of three different components: rehabilitation of left/right discrimination, motor imagery rehearsal, and mirror therapy.

Addressing Psychosocial Factors

Treatment should start with neuroscience education. This should be followed closely with addressing cognitive-behavioral components and sensory/motor strategies that will allow the client to move without increasing the level of symptoms. At the same time, we must remember that psychosocial factors are present and frequently become intertwined with physical factors. Often, clients with high pain levels feel helpless. Educating the client and providing specific strategies to address symptoms of CRPS can help the client feel they have some control.

With central sensitization, the clinical approach should be aimed at dealing with both the mind and body. Treatment should start immediately using a biopsychosocial approach. Education can have a positive effect on pain and disability, catastrophizing, and physical performance.[17] Neuroscience education can lessen the cognitive-affective contributions by reducing facilitation and turning on descending inhibitory pain pathways. It is imperative that clients understand that pain is complex and the brain responds to protect the individual. This neuroscience education component must be easily understood by the client and reinforced by the hand therapist.

Clients with CRPS need a support system, and there are times when, as hand therapists, we are that support. Clients may need psychological counselling before, during, and after treatment for CRPS. This is especially true for clients with and history of abuse and/or concomitant mental health issues, such as posttraumatic stress disorder or major depression. Mind and body must both be addressed for successful treatment.

Summary

There is much research showing that cognitive-behavioral education, early identification of both peripheral and central mechanisms, and approaches to correct abnormalities in the sensory map can change abnormal cortical disorganization.[19] For best results, treatment goals should be the restoration of function and self-management of symptoms, as opposed to total pain relief. Each case offers a unique opportunity to identify the symptoms and mechanisms and to determine ways to measure progress. A multidisciplinary team that addresses all mechanisms of CRPS, including mind and body aspects, usually produces the best results.[26]

References

1. Marinus J, Moseley L, Birklein F, et al.: Clinical features and pathophysiology of complex regional pain syndrome, *The Lancet Neurology* 10(7):637–648, 2011.
2. Gierthmuhlen J, Binder A, Baron R: Mechanism based treatment in complex regional pain syndromes, *Nat Rev Neurology* 10:518–528, 2014.
3. Birklein F, Oneil D, Schereth T: Complex regional pain syndrome: an optimistic perspective, *Neurology* 84(1):89–96, 2015.
4. Zyluk A, Puchalski P: Complex regional pain syndrome of the upper limb. A review, *Neurol Neuro Chir Pol* 48:200–2005, 2014.
5. Hamasaki T, Pelletier R, Bourbonnais D, et al.: Pain-related psychological issues in hand therapy, *J Hand Therapy* vol. 31(2):215–228, 2018.
6. Harden RN, Bruehl S, Stanton-Hicks M, Wilson PR: Proposed new diagnostic criteria for complex regional pain syndrome, *Pain Med* 8:326–331, 2007.
7. Lebel A, Becerra L, Wallin D, et al.: fMRI reveals distinct CNS processing during symptomatic and recovered complex regional pain syndrome in children, *Brain* 131:1854–1879, 2008.
8. Kuttikat A, Noreika V, Chennu S, et al.: Neurocognitive and neuroplastic mechanisms of novel clinical signs in CRPS, *Front Hum euroscience* 2016.
9. Shipton E: Complex regional pain syndrome-mechanisms, diagnosis and management, *Curr Anaesth Crit Care* vol. 20(issue 5):209–214, 2009.
10. Cowell F, Gillespie S, Cheung G, Brown D: Complex Regional Pain Syndrome: how to implement changes to reduce incidence and facilitate early management, *J Hand Therapy* vol. 3(2):201–205, 2018.
11. Royal College of Physicians: *Complex regional pain syndrome in adults in uk, guidelines for diagnosis, referral and management in primary and secondary care*, World Press, 2012.
12. Moseley L, Herbert R, Parsons T, et al.: Intense pain soon after wrist fractures strongly predicts who will develop Complex Regional Pain Syndrome, *J Pain* 15:16–23, 2014.
13. Savas S, Inai E, Yavuz, et al.: Risk factors for complex regional pain syndrome with surgically treated traumatic injuries attending hand therapy, *J Hand Therapy* vol. 31: number 2:250–254, 2018.
14. Bruehl S, Harden R, Galer B, et al.: Complex Regional Pain Syndrome: are there distinct subtypes and sequential stages of the syndrome? *Pain* 95(1-2):119–124, 2002.
15. Packman T, Holly J: Mechanism-specific rehabilitation, management of complex regional pain syndrome, proposed recommendations from evidence synthesis, *J Hand Therapy* vol. 31(2):238–249, 2018.
16. Cohen H, McCabe C, Harris N, et al.: Clinical evidence of parietal cortex dysfunction in correlation with extent of allodynia in CRPS, *Eur J Pain* 17(4):527–538, 2013.
17. Louw A, Diener I, Butler D, Puentedura E: The effect of neuroscience education on pain, disability, anxiety and stress in chronic musculoskeletal pain, *Arch Phys Med Rehab* 92(12):2041–2056, 2011.
18. Walsh M: *Therapist management of complex regional pain syndrome, in rehabilitation of the hand and upper extremity*, ed 6, 2011. Philadelphia.
19. McManus C: Mindfulness and physical therapy practice, *APTA PT in Motion* 9(1):24–32, 2017.
20. Rosen B: *Sensory reeducation in rehabilitation of the hand and upper extremity*, ed 6, 2011. Philadelphia.
21. Spicher C, Fehlmann P, Maihofner C, et al.: Management algorithm of spontaneous neuropathic pain and/or touch-evoked neuropathic pain illustrated by prospective observation in clinical practice of 66 chronic neuropathic pain patients, *E-news Somatosensitive Rehabilitation*(1) 4–28, 2016.
22. Nijs J, Ickman K: Chronic whiplash-associated disorders: to exercise or not, *The Lancet* 384(9938):109–111, 2014.
23. Smart K, Ward B, O'Connell N: Physiotherapy for pain and disability in adults with complex regional pain syndrome type 1 and 2, *Cochrane Library* 24, 2016.
24. Flor H: New developments in the understanding and management of persistent pain, *Current Opinion Psychiatry* 25(2):109–113, 2012.
25. Butler D, Moseley L: *Explain pain supercharged*, Noigroup, 2017.
26. Stralka S: Hand therapy treatment for pain in hand clinics-pain management by eds. Curtin,C and Chung K. vol. 32(1):63–69, 2016.

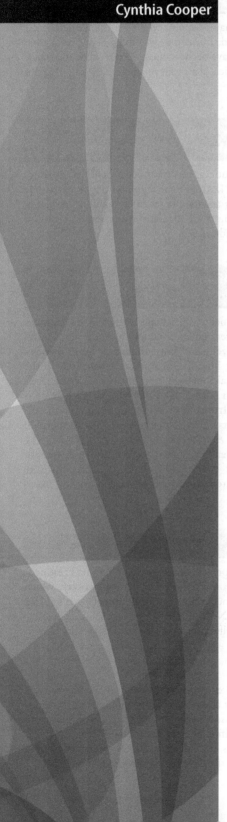

38 Chemotherapy-Induced Peripheral Neuropathy

Cynthia Cooper

Many people who have been treated with chemotherapy complain of upper extremity (UE) neuropathy that interferes with their performance of activities of daily living (ADLs) and work tasks. Those affected by UE neuropathy report that it negatively impacts their overall quality of life. Certain chemotherapy agents are known to cause this problem but are necessary for best medical management. However, medical guidelines sometimes require that patients' chemotherapy regimens be reduced or discontinued because of neuropathy.[1] This difficult choice may result in shortening their life spans.

In the oncology literature, there are no descriptions or acknowledgments of the value of hand therapy for individuals with chemotherapy-induced UE neuropathy. Articles in oncology journals refer to rehabilitation but appear to define rehabilitation as medication only and do not mention the potential value of hand therapy. Likewise, hand therapy literature has not identified this population as a diagnostic group that could benefit from our services. To make matters more challenging, oncologists are not typically in the habit of referring their patients with neuropathy to hand therapy. To encourage referrals from oncologists, we must spark their interest and their availability to learn about our services as hand therapists.

Definition of Chemotherapy-Induced Peripheral Neuropathy

Chemotherapy-induced peripheral neuropathy (CIPN) is defined as somatic or autonomic signs or symptoms resulting from damage to the peripheral nervous system (PNS) or autonomic nervous system (ANS) caused by chemotherapeutic agents.[2] CIPN tends to be worse in individuals with preexisting nerve entrapments or neuropathies.[3] Authorities acknowledge that reports of 30% to 40% incidence of CIPN are an underestimate. As more aggressive pharmacological agents are developed and survival rates increase in the future, this number is projected to grow.

Quality of life is adversely affected by CIPN. Also, symptoms can interfere with treatment, resulting in a reduction of dosage or even discontinuation of life-sustaining medications.[4,5] This is called a **dose-limiting factor**. Currently there are no proven methods to treat CIPN.

Anatomy and Physiology Related to Chemotherapy-Induced Peripheral Neuropathy

Peripheral nerves are comprised of nerve fibers with varied myelination, morphology, functions, and chemical features. These differing fibers vary in their resistance to and response to the toxicity of chemotherapy drugs. Most nutritional, metabolic, and toxic neuropathies are **axonopathies**, meaning the pathology is axonal. Chemotherapy toxicity can affect various components of the nervous system from the sensory cell bodies in the dorsal root ganglion to the distal axon.[1]

⊚ Clinical Pearl

The vulnerability of a nerve to chemotherapy is influenced by its length. Longer nerves are more vulnerable than shorter nerves. In general, sensory fibers tend to be at higher risk for anticancer drug toxic effects than motor fibers.

Anticancer drugs can injure any portion of the PNS or the central nervous system (CNS), or even muscle. Symmetrical distal polyneuropathy is the most common pattern of symptoms. Other patterns of peripheral nerve disease in CIPN are radiculopathy, plexopathy, polyradiculoneuropathy, mononeuropathy, and multiple mononeuropathy (also known as mononeuritis multiplex).

Symptoms

◎ Clinical Pearl

While the deficits of CIPN can be sensory, motor, or autonomic, most polyneuropathies are purely sensory.[6]

Paresthesias reportedly occur distally and symmetrically in a glove and stocking distribution and are worst on volar surfaces of the hands and plantar surfaces of the feet. It is my observation, having treated many clients with CIPN, that hand sensory symptoms are not always symmetrical and do not always present in a glove and stocking distribution. I base this observation on findings from use of the TEN test on these clients (see below).

In CIPN, **allodynia** (experiencing pain with stimuli that is not typically painful) is common and frequently occurs in response to hot or cold. Motor impairment occurs less frequently and usually has a later onset. Purely autonomic symptoms are uncommon, but some autonomic involvement combined with PNS involvement is common.

Impaired fine motor skills affect activities such as buttoning, donning earrings, manipulating clasps, and handling small objects. **Sensory ataxia**, an impairment in motor coordination caused by loss of sensory input, is more severe when the eyes are closed or the lighting is low. Proprioceptive sensory disturbances also occur, as demonstrated by a positive **Romberg sign**, which is a loss of balance that occurs when the individual stands with the eyes closed. Motor neuropathy presents with signs of weakness, cramps, atrophy, and fasciculation. Like sensory symptoms, the onset is typically distal. Findings of proximal weakness may be indicative of another condition, so be sure to mention this finding to the referring provider.

Nociceptive pain is defined as pain that is caused by structural dysfunction, such as the somatic pain of a fracture or the visceral pain of irritable bowel syndrome. **Neuropathic pain**—also known as nerve pain—is pain that results from injury to the somatosensory nervous system. This type of pain is difficult for clients to describe, but words such as sharp, cold, prickling, stinging, or burning are often used.

◎ Clinical Pearl

Neuropathic pain has been associated with depression more often than somatic pain. In my clinical experience, many hand therapy clients, not just those with CIPN, experience neuropathic pain. Hand therapists should be addressing this in their clinical reasoning and treatment plans.

Small Fiber Neuropathy

Most CIPNs are described as **mixed fiber neuropathies** because there is involvement of both large and small nerve fibers. Small fiber neuropathy is a result of damage to A-delta and C fibers, which are the smallest unmyelinated fibers. These fibers carry sensations of temperature and dull pain. Clients with small fiber neuropathy have intense neuropathic pain that is worse than those with large fiber neuropathy. They also demonstrate autonomic symptoms because autonomic fibers are small nonmyelinated fibers. It is harder to clinically diagnose small fiber neuropathy than large fiber neuropathy, in part because nerve conduction studies examine only large fibers that are myelinated and fast conducting.

Chemotherapy-Induced Peripheral Neuropathy Symptom Timeline

Symptoms of CIPN may disappear when the chemotherapeutic agents are discontinued, but some symptoms may persist even after the medications have been stopped. This is called the **coasting phenomenon**, which is a result of slow physiopathology or slow drug clearance.

Chemotherapeutic Agents Involved in Chemotherapy-Induced Peripheral Neuropathy

Certain chemotherapeutic agents have been identified as drugs that contribute to CIPN. At the time of this writing, they include microtubule-stabilizing agents, platinum compounds, cisplatin, oxaliplatin, carboplatin, vinca alkaloids, proteasome inhibitors, thalidomide, and lenalidomide.[7]

Diagnosis of Chemotherapy-Induced Peripheral Neuropathy

Simple clinical assessments are usually sufficient to diagnose CIPN. As noted earlier, nerve conduction studies are useful in identifying large myelinated fast conduction nerve involvement, but they do not identify small fiber dysfunction. In the oncology literature, scales of symptom severity describe levels of impact on function including ADLs.[8,9] One such scale is the National Cancer Institute Grading: Common Terminology Criteria for Adverse Events that scores neuropathic pain with grades 1 to 4.[10] Another scale is the Total Neuropathy Score, which reflects sensory, motor, autonomic, and strength symptoms with grades 1 to 4.[2] The National Cancer Institute Common Toxicity Criteria scores motor and sensory symptoms with grades 1 to 5.[11]

Neuroplasticity

Hand therapists are experts in sensory rehabilitation. Treatment programs are based on the concept of **neuroplasticity**, which refers to the fact that our brains can be neuronally reorganized in response to stimuli. Neuroplasticity involves learning, habituation, memory, and cellular recovery.[12,13] Key concepts of neuroplasticity are:

- Sensory perception is experienced by the CNS and is a dynamic process.
- Hand use affects receptor morphology. In other words, use it or lose it. Disuse of a hand leads to deteriorative and regressive changes in sensory receptors, whereas promoting hand use is thought to stimulate new receptors.[14]
- One single stimulus can excite multiple receptors because of the overlap of receptive fields of certain nerve fibers.

"Our perception of sensation is very complex and is affected by many variables, including posture, swelling, movement, and sensory stimulation, such as touching different materials. It has been shown that avoiding use of the hand worsens the sensory symptoms, and light use, visual imagery, and tactile stimulation can help it improve."

Evaluation and Treatment of Clients With Chemotherapy-Induced Peripheral Neuropathy

My work treating clients with CIPN has been based on extrapolation of hand therapy's traditional sensory interventions with modifications in order to target the unique characteristics of the CIPN population. I encourage readers to add to this program with additional interventions based on their clinical reasoning and their clients' presentation. The program that I currently use is described in the following section.

Evaluation

Begin with conversation and rapport building. Ask about the client's medical history, medications, surgeries, and past medical history, including prior injuries or nerve entrapments of the upper extremities. Learn about the lymphatic status including whether any nodes have been removed. Inquire about the client's social support system. Assess the impact of symptoms on ADLs. Consider using the Canadian Occupational Performance Measure, so that your treatment goals and plan are personalized and relevant to the client.

Ask about the client's pain. Discern whether it is neuropathic or nociceptive or both. Is it constant or intermittent? If it is intermittent, what are the provokers, if any? Is fatigue a factor influencing their sensory problem or pain?

If there are sensory symptoms, is the presentation one of sensory pain (burning or sharp shooting pain) or sensory impairment (numbness or tingling) or both? Map the areas of sensory complaints. Are there paresthesias? If so, are they positional? I have not found pressure threshold testing or moving or static two-point discrimination testing to be very meaningful clinically with this population, and in my experience, these tests are often too painful to justify using. The sensory test that has been most informing and meaningful to me with this population is called the TEN test.[15] In fact, I have found the TEN test to be a very useful sensory test with all my hand therapy clients, not just those with CIPN.

Observe the client's posture. Individuals who have had surgery have often developed postural accommodations for pain relief, and these accommodations may contribute to nerve entrapment or vulnerability. Measure the client's edema. Look for extrinsic or intrinsic tightness and excursion of flexor digitorum profundus (FDP) and flexor digitorum superficialis (FDS). Perform appropriate gentle provocative maneuvers using your clinical judgment, but be sure to avoid creating pain. These may include, but are not limited to, cervical screening, elevated arm stress test, palpation of epicondyles, middle finger test, elbow flexion test, Phalen's test, tests for Tinel's sign at the volar wrist and the cubital tunnel, thumb carpometacarpal grind test, and Finkelstein's test. Be careful performing upper limb tension testing because this may be provoking.

Treatment

I have found that a combination of three categories of hand therapy intervention is most effective in treating clients with CIPN: (1) manual therapy, (2) active range of motion (AROM) and nerve and tendon glides, and (3) desensitization/sensory reeducation. Each client will respond uniquely, so explore and determine which of these categories seem to be the most effective. Begin with client education regarding neuroplasticity. Welcome the client's significant other(s) to participate.

Significant others often feel helpless and want to be able to assist the client with CIPN in the therapy and home exercise program. Include them as much as possible so that they can be involved in providing symptom relief to their loved one.

Manual Therapy

Emphasize edema control. Try light, nonadherent compressive wraps, but be sure that these are not applied tightly. Do not perform manual edema mobilization or retrograde massage if the client has had any nodes removed. If the lymphatic system has been disrupted by surgery, refer the client to a trained lymphedema therapist and instead perform other interventions described later.

Instruct the client in breathing, as appropriate, particularly if the client is breathing shallowly from the chest. Gentle manual therapy can be very effective with sensory symptoms. Try a comfortable carpal tunnel stretch while the client actively extends and abducts the digits, and ask whether this is helpful for sensory pain and/or sensory normalization. Consider teaching the client's significant other how to do a gentle carpal tunnel stretch on them. Perform gentle palmar fascial stretches and gentle mobilizations, such as intermetacarpal sweeps. If the interphalangeal joints are painful, lightly stroke up the sides along the ulnar collateral ligaments and radial collateral ligaments, moving volar to dorsal. Myofascial techniques can also be very normalizing, especially over the volar and dorsal forearms. Be gentle with all manual techniques.

Active Range of Motion/Nerve and Tendon Gliding

Explain and emphasize the relevance of proximal motion for distal sensory symptomatology. Instruct in AROM in pain-free ranges, including trunk motion and scapular stabilization, as well as shoulder circles, as appropriate, and AROM for shoulder, elbow, wrist, and hand. Perform tendon gliding exercises and nerve glides/slides bilaterally and very gently, as appropriate. Include FDP and FDS tendon glides. Try soft isometric contractions of wrist flexors and extensors in neutral positions.

Desensitization/Sensory Reeducation

Explain that disuse due to sensory pain or impairment contributes to and reinforces the sensory symptoms. Explore strategies to maximize well-tolerated use of the hand. If sensory pain is reported, try applying paper tape over the areas of sensory pain (Fig. 38.1). I have found this to be surprisingly effective on sensory pain. Some clients report painful fingernails. If this is the case, try paper tape over the nails (Fig. 38.2). I have seen this simple strategy help clients use the computer again without pain.

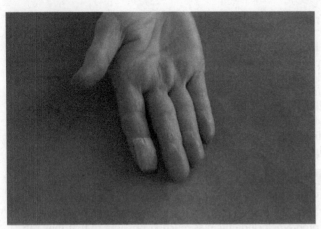

FIG. 38.1 Paper tape applied over areas of sensory pain. (Photo by Cynthia Cooper. Used with permission.)

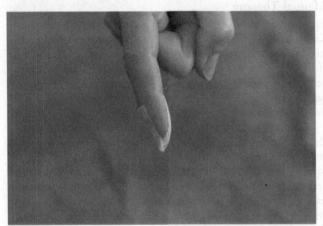

FIG. 38.2 Paper tape applied over painful fingernail. (Photo by Cynthia Cooper. Used with permission.)

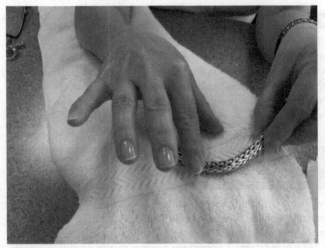

FIG. 38.3 Client performing sensory reeducation using a bracelet that she loved. (Photo by Cynthia Cooper. Used with permission.)

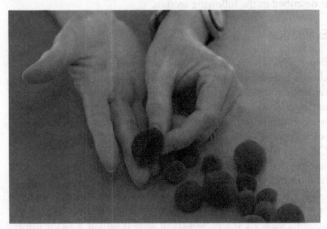

FIG. 38.4 Many clients enjoy using soft pom-poms for soothing and pleasant sensory stimulation. (Photo by Cynthia Cooper. Used with permission.)

Depending on the client's needs, perform desensitization and sensory reeducation based on hand therapy's traditional body of knowledge in these areas. Perform these interventions proximal to distal. Include the noninvolved areas peripheral to the involved areas and treat bilaterally. Instruct the client to think about where the sensation feels normal and where the demarcation is for sensory loss. Find desensitization materials that are meaningful to the client (Figs. 38.3 and 38.4). Most of my clients with CIPN seem to really like vibration for sensory stimulation.

Use laterality, graded motor imagery, and mirror box interventions (Fig. 38.5).[16,17] Try intentional confounding, such as having the client wear an exam glove to perform dexterity tasks, then removing the glove and performing the same tasks again (Fig. 38.6). This form of sensory training seems to help the client perceive or appreciate the available (albeit impaired) sensation, thereby promoting a sense of improved function; and it is based on exciting research by experts on the peripheral nervous system.[18]

Diagnosis-Specific Information That Affects Clinical Reasoning

Clients with CIPN are different clinically from our traditional hand therapy clients with peripheral nerve trauma or repair. CIPN clients tend to present with sensory symptoms that do not follow the distribution of a particular peripheral nerve. This is because the pathology of chemotherapy toxicity is different from that of a peripheral nerve injury or repair.

The fatigue factor for clients with CIPN may necessitate shorter therapy sessions. Monitor their tolerances to the visit, and be prepared for them to need to shorten or cancel the visit, possibly without notice if they are not feeling well enough to participate that day.

? Questions to Ask the Doctor

- Has the client had surgical disruption of the lymphatic system?
- What is the projected timeline of drug administration?

♡ Tips From the Field

- Light manual therapy can be very powerful for this population. Be prepared for the possibility of a moving emotional response from the client or a family member.

- Use your training in joint protection, work simplification, and energy conservation to maximize the function of clients with CIPN.
- Focus on ADLs. Something as simple as an assistive device that improves clients' function will be well appreciated by the client and their family.

Marketing Dilemmas/Strategies

Individuals with CIPN tell me that when they have complained to their doctors' offices about their neuropathy symptoms,

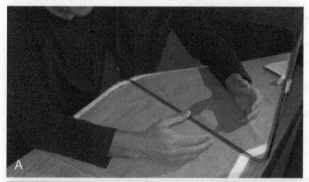
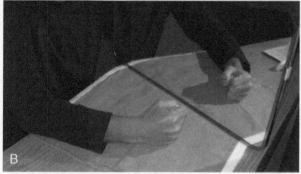

FIG. 38.5 Mirror box therapy. (From Skirven T, Osterman AL, Fedorczyk JM, et al. *Rehabilitation of the Hand and Upper Extremity.* 6th ed. Philadelphia, PA: Mosby; 2011.)

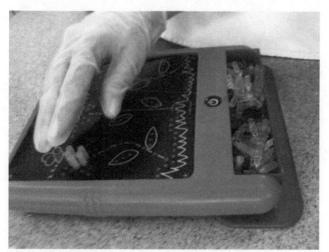

FIG. 38.6 Client performing pinch task with exam glove on, then patient will perform the same task with the glove off. (Photo by Cynthia Cooper. Used with permission.)

they have been told there is no nonmedicinal rehabilitation for this problem. My efforts to get referrals to hand therapy from oncologists over the past 10 years have been frustrating. One reason for this is the physician's office's perception that these patients are already overloaded with medical appointments and do not really have time or interest in yet another appointment. My personal experience with these clients indicates otherwise. Many have asked me why they were not referred earlier. Some have cried when they experienced relief at their first therapy visit. It seems to me that there is a profound and as yet unarticulated importance of sensory function to these individuals. Hand therapists are in a perfect position to explore this new territory. See Box 38.1 for a sample marketing letter to oncologists. See Box 38.2 for a sample screening tool that referrers might find useful.

BOX 38.1   Sample Marketing Letter

To Whom It May Concern:

I am an occupational therapist/ physical therapist/certified hand therapist at _____. I have a passion for working with oncology patients with upper extremity neuropathy. Although hand therapists routinely treat patients with other neuropathies, the oncology patients seem to have been overlooked by my profession, and this concerns me. I feel that patients with any subjective complaints of sensory changes or any signs of hand weakness/atrophy are good candidates for hand therapy. So far, I have found that gentle soft-tissue work, nerve gliding, and sensory reeducation techniques appear to be helpful, in addition to desensitization and other compensatory strategies, including adapted implements that maximize function. Most patients do not need more than a few therapy visits.

I would be very interested in communicating with you further regarding opportunities to treat your patients. If you would be available for a phone call or a meeting in person, I would welcome that.

Sincerely,

BOX 38.2   Sample Screening Tool

Hand Therapy Referral Screening Questions
- Do you have any numbness or tingling in your hands or fingers?
- Do you experience weakness in your arms or hands?

Referral Process
- Write a prescription for the patient to have hand therapy with _____ (name of therapist) _____.
- Patient calls _____ (phone number) _____ to schedule an appointment as a new client.

Documentation
You will receive reports regarding the patient's clinical status and progress.

Conclusion

Hand therapists who are interested in sensory problems have much to offer this population of potential clients who have not been identified in the hand therapy or oncology literature.

Recognizing this population and providing hand therapy services to these individuals can improve their quality of life, assist in their medical management, and provide hand therapists with personally rewarding work and new program growth and development.

References

1. Park SB, Goldstein D, Krishnan AV, et al.: Chemotherapy-induced peripheral neurotoxicity: a critical analysis, *CA Cancer J Clin* 63(6):419–437, 2013.
2. Gutiérrez-Gutiérrez G, Sereno M, Miralles A, et al.: Chemotherapy-induced peripheral neuropathy: clinical features, diagnosis, prevention and treatment strategies, *Clin Transl Oncol* 12(2):81–91, 2010.
3. Sioka C, Kyritsis A: Central and peripheral nervous system toxicity of common chemotherapeutic agents, *Cancer Chemother Pharmacol* 63(5):761–767, 2009.
4. Wolf S, Barton D, Kottschade L, et al.: Chemotherapy-induced peripheral neuropathy: prevention and treatment strategies, *Eur J Cancer* 44(11):1507–1515, 2008.
5. Majithia N, Temkin SM, Ruddy KJ, et al.: National cancer institute-supported chemotherapy-induced peripheral neuropathy trials: outcomes and lessons, *Support Care Cancer* 24(3):1439–1447, 2016.
6. Kaley TJ, DeAngelis LM: Therapy of chemotherapy-induced peripheral neuropathy, *Br J Haematol* 145(3):14, 2009.
7. Kajih RN, Moore CD: Management of chemotherapy-induced peripheral neuropathy, *US Pharm* 40(1):HS5–HS10, 2015.
8. Kaplow R, Iyere K: Grading chemotherapy-induced peripheral neuropathy in adults, *Nursing* 47(2):67–68, 2017.
9. Brewer JR, Morrison G, Dolan ME, et al.: Chemotherapy-induced peripheral neuropathy: current status and progress, *Gynecol Oncol* 140(1):176–218, 2016.
10. Barbour SY: Caring for the treatment-experienced breast cancer patient: the pharmacist's role, *Am J Health Syst Pharm* 65(10 Suppl 3):S16–S22, 2008.
11. Windebank AJ, Grisold W: Chemotherapy-induced neuropathy, *J Peripher Nerv Syst* 13:27–46, 2008.
12. Calford MB: Mechanisms for acute changes in sensory maps, *Adv Exp Med Biol* 508:451–460, 2002.
13. Malaviya GN: Sensory perception in leprosy-neurophysiological correlates, *Int J Lepr Other Mycobact Dis* 71(2):119–124, 2003.
14. Rosen B, Balkenius C, Lundborg G: Sensory re-education today and tomorrow: a review of evolving concepts, *Br J Hand Ther* 8(2):48–56, 2003.
15. Strauch B, Lang A, Ferder M, et al.: The TEN test, *Plast Reconstr Surg* 99(4):1074–1078, 1997.
16. Rosen B, Lundborg G: Training with a mirror in rehabilitation of the hand, *Scand J Plast Reconstr Surg Hand Surg* 39(2):104–108, 2005.
17. Rosen B, Lundborg G: Sensory reeducation. In Skirven TM, Osterman AL, Fedorczyk JM, et al.: *Rehabilitation of the hand and upper extremity*, ed 6, Philadelphia, 2011, Mosby, pp 634–645.
18. Rosén B, Bjorkman A, Lundborg G: Improved sensory relearning after nerve repair induced by selective temporary anaesthesia—a new concept in hand rehabilitation, *J Hand Surg Br* 31(2):126–132, 2006.

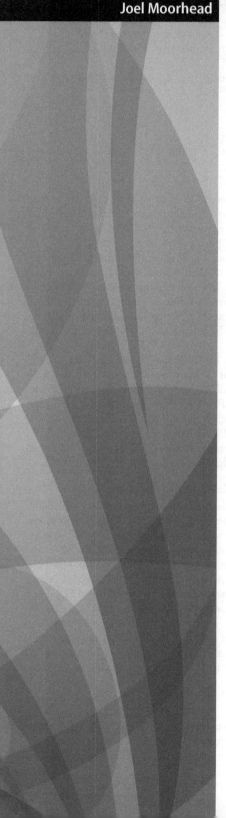

39

Clients With Functional Somatic Syndromes or Challenging Behavior

Joel Moorhead

Functional Somatic Syndromes

A functional somatic syndrome (FSS) is defined as a physical illness that cannot be explained by an organic disease and that involves no demonstrable structural lesion or established biochemical change.[1] The distinction between *disease* and *illness* is particularly important. A **disease** is an anatomical or physiological impairment of function in a structure or biochemical process. An **illness** is the client's personal experience of poor health. Clients frequently have illnesses that are not fully explained by available medical evidence of disease.

Hand therapists commonly see clients with complex biopsychosocial conditions that improve most rapidly with attention to both disease and illness. The relatively few clients with FSSs may benefit from early recognition and individualized treatment planning. FSSs can be classified as undifferentiated somatoform disorders, somatization disorders, factitious disorders, or malingering, depending on whether the client's actions are intentional or unintentional and whether motivation is conscious or subconscious.

Giving clients satisfying and health-promoting rehabilitative care is particularly challenging for therapists treating clients with FSSs. When the client's distress is disproportionate to the medical evidence of impairment, reducing the degree of impairment may not reduce the client's distress. The goal of this chapter is to help therapists become familiar with the types of FSSs seen in clinical practice so that they can build a therapeutic relationship with even the most challenging client.

Undifferentiated Somatoform Disorders

Clients with symptoms that are out of proportion to impairments most often manifest one of the somatoform disorders in which symptom magnification is subconscious and unintentional.

Clients with **hypochondriasis**, also known as illness anxiety disorder, show excessive concern about minor health disturbances or intense worry over the possibility of future ill health. Clients with **body dysmorphic disorder** become preoccupied with imagined or innocent variations in appearance. Clients with **conversion disorder** have a bodily event (for example, paralysis or seizure) that is psychological in origin. Clients with psychogenic pain and unspecified psychophysiological dysfunction have persistent symptoms without apparent organic origin and without other distinctive classifying features. Clients with medically unexplained pain may have other diagnostic features as well, which could lead to a diagnosis of one of the somatization disorders below.

Somatization Disorders

More controversial are the **somatization disorders**, in which clients experience persistent or recurrent symptoms without objective or measurable medical evidence of impairment. Although these disorders occur frequently, general agreement is lacking on the cause and the treatment, and even on the status of some of them as legitimate diagnoses. However, questioning the validity of the diagnosis does little to help the client become more functional and may do irreparable harm to the therapeutic relationship. This chapter makes no judgment on the diagnostic legitimacy of the somatization disorders, but it recognizes the high level of distress in many clients diagnosed with these conditions.

TABLE 39.1　Diagnostic Classification of Functional Somatic Syndromes

Diagnosis	ICD-10 Code[23] - All ICD-10-CM Code Assignments are Based on Physician Documentation. Consider Query to Physician to Clarify Documentation if Needed
Undifferentiated somatoform disorders	F45.1
Hypochondriasis	F45.21
Body dysmorphic disorder	F45.22
Conversion disorder	F44.4-F44.7
Psychogenic pain	F45.4
Unspecified psychophysiological malfunction	F59
Somatization disorders	F45.0
Fibromyalgia	M79.7
Chronic fatigue syndrome	R53.82
Idiopathic environmental intolerance	Possibly T78.40; may need physician query to clarify
Psychogenic tremor	F44.4
Factitious disorders	F68.1

ICD, International Classification of Diseases; *ICD-10-CM*, International Classification of Diseases, 10th revision, Clinical Modification

Fibromyalgia

Fibromyalgia is perhaps the most common somatization disorder. Established in 1990 by the American College of Rheumatology, the criteria for a diagnosis of fibromyalgia include pain on both sides of the body, above and below the waist, accompanied by tenderness at 11 or more of 18 specific tender point sites.[2] Fibromyalgia affects approximately 2% of the population, although clients with fibromyalgia may account for 10% to 20% of visits to rheumatology clinics. The prevalence is inversely related to income and level of education, and females are affected more frequently than males at a ratio of up to 6:1. Fifty-nine percent of clients with a diagnosis of fibromyalgia rate their health as fair or poor.[3] Clients with this diagnosis commonly have other, associated symptoms, including nonrestorative sleep, fatigue, headaches, diarrhea or constipation, numbness, tingling, stiffness, a sensation of swelling, anxiety, and depression. Clients with rheumatoid arthritis and osteoarthritis report similar levels of distress, according to one measurement tool, the Rheumatology Distress Index[4]; however, clients with fibromyalgia report higher levels of distress in the areas of anxiety, depression, sleep disturbance, global severity, and fatigue.[4] Fatigue is also prominent in another disorder in this classification, chronic fatigue syndrome.

Chronic Fatigue Syndrome

The case definition of **chronic fatigue syndrome (CFS),** or **chronic fatigue and immune dysfunction syndrome (CFIDS),** includes several important criteria: (1) the fatigue cannot be

BOX 39.1　Criteria for Chronic Fatigue Syndrome

Major Criteria
- Fatigue is unexplained by other diagnoses.
- Fatigue has been present longer than 6 months.
- Fatigue has a definite time of onset.
- Fatigue has resulted in decreased activity level not due to ongoing exertion.
- Fatigue is not substantially relieved by rest.

Minor Criteria
Four or more of the following symptoms are present:
- Impaired short-term memory or concentration
- Sore throat
- Tender lymph nodes
- Myalgias
- Arthralgias
- Headaches
- Nonrestorative sleep
- Postexertional malaise (lasting longer than 24 hours)

explained by other diagnoses; (2) it must persist for longer than 6 months; (3) it must have a definite time of onset; (4) it must result in a decreased activity level but cannot be the result of ongoing exertion; and (5) it must not be substantially relieved by rest.[5] This case definition, like that for fibromyalgia, was established primarily to identify subjects for clinical research. Salit[6] notes that these criteria "are not suitable for the determination of the presence and severity of illness, either in general medical settings or for medicolegal or insurance purposes" and that "clinical management should be based on an assessment of the client" (Box 39.1).

The case definitions for fibromyalgia and CFS overlap substantially. About 70% of clients with CFS meet the case definition for fibromyalgia, and 70% of clients with fibromyalgia meet the case definition for CFS.[7] Both disorders result in a high prevalence of work disability. Bombardier and Buchwald[8] found that 37% of clients with a diagnosis of CFS were unemployed. The prevalence of unemployment rose to 52% for clients diagnosed with CFS and fibromyalgia.[8]

Multiple Chemical Sensitivity Syndrome

A third somatization disorder that can affect perceived ability to work is **multiple chemical sensitivity (MCS) syndrome.** Clients with multiple chemical sensitivities, or **idiopathic environmental intolerance (IEI),** experience medically unexplained symptoms in response to low-level, identifiable environmental exposures.[9] Among the postulated mechanisms for MCS syndrome are **time-dependent sensitization (TDS)** and the development of **conditioned responses.** In TDS, repeated stressful episodes make an individual increasingly sensitive to low-level environmental stimuli.[10] With conditioned responses, cardiovascular, respiratory, gastrointestinal, or immunological responses are triggered by heightened perception of environmental stimuli.[11]

Psychogenic Tremors

As with MCS syndrome, stress can be a factor in the development of **psychogenic tremors.** Psychogenic tremors of the hands and arms can manifest in unusual ways and have variable clinical characteristics. The severity of the tremor may be task specific, with the tremor often improving when the client is distracted.[12] Shaking of the limbs or body can appear exaggerated, whereas finger tremors often are absent. A twisting or ballistic component to the tremor can create the appearance of chorea.[13] Psychogenic tremor as a somatization disorder appears unintentionally, and without conscious client awareness of motivation.

Factitious Disorders

Factitious disorders result from intentional client action but without conscious client awareness of motivation. They more often arise from a psychological need to be sick than from a conscious effort for material gain.[14] Clients with factitious disorders knowingly cause their own disease but are unaware of the underlying reason or reasons for their behavior. Several factitious disorders can affect clients' hands.

Munchausen's syndrome derives its name from Baron Karl Friedrich Hieronymous von Munchausen, an eighteenth-century nobleman known for telling vivid but untrue stories. Clients with Munchausen's syndrome may cut, bruise, bite, or inject their hands and then give an untruthful history to the medical professionals who care for the resulting injuries.[15]

Clients with **clenched fist syndrome** have stiff, tightly curled fingers that resist extension.[15] The thumb and index fingers often are spared, enabling the client to maintain a level of function with the involved hand. Nerve block of the affected upper extremity or examination under anesthesia produces some relaxation of the hand, but often not full extension of the involved fingers. Some edema of the hand may be present, but it is not as great as in a hand that is repeatedly traumatized. (See Case Study 39.1.)

Clients who repeatedly strike their hands on a wall or other hard surface eventually develop chronic dorsal hand edema, a condition that has been called "secretan's syndrome."[15] The fibrotic changes that develop in a repeatedly traumatized hand eventually create an appearance similar to the brawny edema that develops in the lower legs of clients with chronic vascular insufficiency.

Malingering

Malingering can be defined as the intentional presentation of false or misleading health information for personal gain. This personal gain is described as secondary gain, distinct from the primary gain of recovery from illness. Some malingering clients are seeking financial gain, whereas others are consciously seeking social or interpersonal benefits.[16] Although malingering generally is recognized as an uncommon condition (prevalence 5% or less), Mittenberg and colleagues[17] estimate that 29% of personal injury cases, 30% of disability cases, 19% of criminal cases, and 8% of medical cases probably involve malingering and symptom exaggeration.[17]

> ### Evaluation Tips: Findings Suggestive of Simulated or Exaggerated Upper Extremity Deficits

Inconsistent Force Generation

Manual muscle testing provides information to the examiner in several ways. First, normal strength through a joint's functional range of motion (ROM) reassures the examiner that no

abnormalities have been identified on this screening test. Second, examination of a client with organic weakness, such as that caused by neuropathy or myopathy, will disclose a smooth, consistent inability to resist the examiner's opposition. For example, the examiner will be able to flex the client's extended wrist smoothly despite the client's full effort to maintain wrist extension. An experienced examiner takes into account the client's age, muscle mass, and overall medical condition when assessing the significance of such a finding. Third, a client with disease or injury may be unable to maintain consistent force generation because of pain or structural instability. This results in a sudden release of resistance to the examiner's opposition. The client can be expected to describe the reason for this release of resistance clearly, providing information that is helpful for diagnosis and management. Fourth, the client may release resistance inconsistently, without other organic signs of impairment and without reporting incapacitating pain or instability. This "cogwheel," or "give-way," "weakness" is one of the physical signs reported by Waddell and colleagues[18] as suggestive of nonorganic pain.[18]

Nonphysiological Pain and Movement Patterns

Clients with simulated or exaggerated upper extremity deficits may exhibit additional **Waddell's signs**, including extreme reaction to light touch (overreaction), tenderness that does not conform to established myotomal or segmental patterns, and sensory disturbances that do not conform to established dermatomal or segmental patterns.[18] Other similar and easily observed tests include Mannkopf's test and O'Donoghue's maneuver.

Mannkopf's test relies on the observation that the pulse rate rises when a client experiences acute pain. The absence of a rise in heart rate of at least 5% on palpation of a reportedly painful area suggests symptom magnification. **O'Donoghue's maneuver** relies on the observation that passive range of motion (PROM), generally, is greater than active range of motion (AROM) when structures in and around a joint are painful. The possibility of symptom magnification is raised when AROM is greater than PROM.[19]

Associated Movements and Vicarious (Trick) Movements

Taking possibly simulated wrist extensor weakness as an example, several techniques can be used to assess the veracity of a client's complaints. A client simulating wrist extensor weakness may use the wrist normally when unaware that he or she is being observed. A client with a simulated wrist drop can be asked to make a fist while the examiner observes the actions of the wrist extensors. The wrist normally extends when a person makes a fist; only if the wrist extensors are truly paralyzed, as in a complete radial nerve injury, can the client make a strong fist without associated wrist extension.[16]

Even if the wrist extensors are truly paralyzed by radial nerve injury, a client with intact median nerve innervation will be able to extend the interphalangeal joint of the thumb. This vicarious, or trick, movement is mediated by the abductor pollicis brevis and flexor pollicis brevis muscles, both of which insert onto the extensor expansion of the thumb.[20] Absence of this movement may be an indicator of symptom magnification.

Correct diagnosis of symptom magnification or an FSS is important for several reasons. First, an accurate anatomical or physiological diagnosis for the client's complaints is an important step in determining what additional diagnostic tests, if any, are indicated. Second, the clinician becomes aware of the complexity of managing such a client and can plan to spend the needed additional time and mental energy to achieve a therapeutic alliance and a favorable outcome. Third, correct diagnosis is essential to designing a successful treatment plan.

♡ Tips From the Field

Treatment of Clients With Functional Somatic Syndromes
As mentioned previously, the distinction between disease and illness is very important in the treatment of clients with FSS. To recap, disease is a demonstrable alteration in anatomy or physiology with unfavorable consequences for the client; illness is the client's perception and experience of poor health. Both disease and illness are valid and important concerns for clients and the health care professionals who treat them.

◎ Clinical Pearl

Disease should be treated only when present; illness should always be treated.

Clients with a conversion disorder are unaware that their physical symptoms have a psychological origin. Clients with somatization disorders feel unwell and can become truly convinced that they have a life-threatening or incapacitating disease or injury; this phenomenon has been called **dissimulation**.[16] Clients with factitious disorders have diseases or injuries that require treatment; in addition, to prevent future disease or injury, attention must be paid to the factors that caused these clients to harm themselves. As Hippocrates observed, "It is more important to know the person who has the disease, than the disease the person has."[21]

Somatic Symptoms and Treatment Goals

Major diagnostic classifications now separately recognize the importance of somatic symptoms. The *Diagnostic and Statistical Manual of Mental Disorders* (DSM-5) recognizes somatic symptom disorder.[22] The 2018 ICD-10-CM Manual[23] includes specific codes for many FSSs (Table 39.1). Somatic symptom burden is increasingly recognized as a separate domain of health-related quality of life.[24]

The Somatic Symptom Scale-8 (SSS-8)[24] uses an 8-symptom survey asking respondents to indicate how much they have been "bothered by" each symptom in the past week, with options ranging from 0 (not at all) to 4 (very much). Somatic symptom burden is indicated by the sum of responses, with a possible range of 0 to 32. Most respondents are expected to report a minimal or low symptom burden (summary score 0–7). Scores of 8 to 32 indicate medium, high, or very high symptom burden. Summary scores predicted the incidence of healthcare visits in the past 12 months.

Each 1-point increase in the SSS-8 summary score was associated with a 12% increase in the number of health care visits in the past month.[24] If therapy can reduce the client's symptom burden, two favorable outcomes may result: (1) the client's health-related quality of life could increase, and (2) the client's utilization of health care services could decrease. These findings suggest that symptoms may be important "in and of

themselves,"[25] independent of any and all comorbid conditions. Given the "high prevalence and functional impairment associated with somatic symptoms,"[24] including a functional goal of symptom reduction in hand therapy treatment plans for clients with FSSs could result in greater independence and health-related quality of life.

Clients With Challenging Behaviors

Reaching Agreement on a Treatment Plan at Every Stage of Treatment

Treatment of clients with FSS requires attention to the biological, psychological, and social factors that influence a client's illness (that is, a biopsychosocial approach).[26] Kleinman[27] observes that clinicians tend to evaluate treatment success by improvement in signs of disease, whereas clients view success as healing of illness. The five-step strategy recommended by Kleinman recognizes the importance of the clinician and client finding enough common ground to reach agreement on a treatment plan (Box 39.2).

Not every client requires or wants the type of negotiated understanding produced by this five-step process. This is fortunate for the busy clinician, as the discussion can take a bit longer than the 10 to 15 minutes estimated by Kleinman. This is especially true when the client's and the clinician's models for explaining illness have little in common. The therapist often has the luxury of being able to work through these five steps gradually over two or three therapy visits, taking advantage of the natural rhythm and growing trust that develop between client and therapist over time. The experienced clinician is alert for opportune moments to explore psychological or social factors that may contribute to a client's illness.

Windows of Opportunity

In their study on client interaction with five experienced physicians, Branch and Malik[28] described "windows of opportunity" as unique moments in which clients briefly discuss personal, family, or emotional issues with clinicians. Based on the findings from their study, they suggested the following four ways clinicians can explore important issues efficiently:
- Listen attentively.
- Ask open-ended questions, such as, "Is there anything else I can do for you today?"

BOX 39.2   Five-Step Strategy for Reaching Agreement on a Treatment Plan

Step 1: The clinician develops an understanding of the client's explanatory model of his or her illness and the meaning of the illness to the client.
Step 2: The clinician presents his or her explanatory model for the client's illness in nontechnical terms.
Step 3: Clinician and client compare models.
Step 4: Clinician and client discuss illness problems.
Step 5: Clinician and client develop and agree on specific interventions and elements of a plan for treating the client's illness.

- Listen for and recognize changes in the client's emotions, appearance, posture, or voice. These windows of opportunity often occur in the middle of the visit. Ask a second question in a softer, gentler tone. Use silence, nods, and small comments to encourage the client to talk while you listen.
- Know when to end the conversation. Summarize the discussion and convey understanding and empathy.

Other authors have offered additional suggestions for establishing therapeutic relationships with challenging clients; these are presented in Box 39.3.

The health care professionals most likely to be sued are those whose clients feel that they were rushed, that they were not given enough information, and that their complaints were ignored.[29] Physician traits associated with malpractice suits include aloofness, lack of good communication with the patient, and too great a desire to accommodate or please the patient even if the request is not rational. It is very important to document when the client does not participate in his or her care. It also is important not to overly accommodate inappropriate requests (see Case Study 39.4).[30]

Participatory Decision Making

Clients who have been encouraged to participate in decision making demonstrate better follow-through on their decisions than those who have not been encouraged to participate. Clients with the best health outcomes are those who express their opinions, who indicate their preferences about their treatment during appointments, and who ask questions. Physicians who regularly include their patients in treatment decisions are those who offer opinions and talk about the advantages and disadvantages of the options, who ask for input about patient preferences, and who pursue mutual agreement about treatment plans. These physicians demonstrate a *participatory* style. They elicit greater patient cooperation and better health outcomes than physicians who have more controlling styles of decision making.[31] This probably is also true for hand therapists.

Participatory decision making can be defined as the practice of offering clients choices among several treatment options and of giving them a sense of control and responsibility for their care.[31] Kaplan and colleagues[31] studied physicians' practice habits to determine the characteristics that promote participatory decision-making styles. They found that physicians who demonstrate participatory decision making are willing to spend extra time with patients and have lower-volume practices.

Participatory physicians reported greater satisfaction with the autonomy they experienced in their personal lives. Short office visits in busier practices have demonstrated poorer outcomes. Medical office visits shorter than 18 minutes are associated with poor quality of information. Patients who had more time with their physicians rated the physicians more favorably. Physicians whose communication styles are less dominant receive higher satisfaction ratings than physicians who communicate in a more dominant manner.[31] In current practice, unfortunately, fiscal demands and business issues may challenge the ability of some physicians and hand therapists to provide participatory care.

Partnerships in Client Care

Quill[32] makes the following observations and recommendations:
- The relationship between the therapist and client is consensual, not obligatory. The therapist may speak with authority but should

> **BOX 39.3 Establishing Therapeutic Relationships With Challenging Clients**
>
> - Build trust. Positive client–therapist interactions require trust. Actions foster trust as much as words do. For example, return the client's phone calls and provide materials as promised.
> - Provide good instructions. Focus on the client's agenda whenever possible. Clear instructions that fit with the client's agenda result in better client satisfaction and improved outcomes.
> - Let the client talk without interruption at the beginning of the appointment. Identify which problems can be covered in the time available and which problems can be addressed at subsequent visits.
> - Stay attuned to your sense of frustration, as this may be a sign that you find the client to be "difficult" (see Case Study 39.2).
> - Be client centered. Use simple explanatory models that are easily understood. Avoid blaming the client; the therapeutic relationship can be harmed by the client's perception that he or she is being blamed (see Case Study 39.3).
> - If a consensus cannot be reached with a challenging client despite compassionate listening, it may be best to refer the client elsewhere. Barriers to reaching a consensus include unexpected resistance from the client and communication mismatch. Nonadherence to the plan of care or the expression of opposition from a client is exemplified by denial of disease, conscious or unconscious sabotaging of the treatment, or a need to control every detail (see Case Study 39.4).
> - Try to develop and convey unconditional positive regard for the client, family, and caregiver. Respect the client's autonomy and individuality and be willing to learn from clients' various backgrounds.
> - Give your undivided attention to complaining clients. Dissatisfied clients tell 20 people, and satisfied clients tell 3.
> - Avoid dealing with difficult clients when you are too tired or busy.
> - Don't downplay the client's perception of the seriousness of the complaints. Give each client time to describe his or her illness in its entirety. Listen responsively, but avoid interrupting.
> - Make a statement that is empathetic. Work to establish a good rapport with the client, and do not be defensive. Convey that you are working with, not against, the client.
> - Ask additional questions and take control of the situation. Ask what clients would like to be done or how they believe the problem can be solved. Create an action plan, and describe that plan in positive terms.
> - Explain changes in treatment ahead of time. Fewer problems arise when there are fewer surprises.
> - Follow up in a timely fashion and document the situation.

not be authoritarian. The client may ask questions, present alternatives, seek other opinions, or choose a different caregiver.
- The two parties must respect and trust each other.
- The client gets healed, cured, and/or relieved of pain. The provider derives enjoyment from being able to help, experi-

ences personal or intellectual satisfaction from solving a problem, and receives financial compensation.

- The client's request may be incompatible with what the health care professional feels is in the client's best interest, or it may conflict with the professional's personal beliefs. The caregiver should not compromise ethical, medical, or personal standards because of a client's request.
- Not all clients participate equally in their care. Caregivers may need to encourage clients to participate. It may be helpful, when appropriate, to request that clients participate more actively in their own treatment.

CASE STUDIES

CASE STUDY 39.1 ■

A 58-year-old woman had tightly clenched long, ring, and small fingers on her nondominant left hand. This posture had persisted for 2 years and had been refractory to treatment by medications for dystonia and muscle relaxation. The client was able to use the thumb and index fingers to some degree. A diagnosis of clenched fist syndrome was made. Further discussion revealed that the condition began at the time of a stressful change at her workplace.

Treatment Approach

Make sure the client understands that she has a condition that requires treatment and that the likelihood of improvement with treatment is excellent. Perform an examination under regional anesthetic block, and fit the client for a custom wrist-hand orthosis while the arm is still under the effects of anesthesia. See the client daily for at least 2 weeks to reinforce wearing of the wrist-hand orthosis to preserve the ROM gained by the procedure. Perform and teach assertive passive, active-assisted, and active ROM exercises with the goal of restoring full ROM. Consider a custom dynamic wrist-hand orthosis to speed restoration of full ROM. Consider the timing of recommending mental health counseling. Often the time to suggest counseling is when the client reports feeling sad or anxious, as many clients naturally will do as they become more comfortable with the therapist. Work closely with the referring physician to achieve the best outcome from a mental health referral.

CASE STUDY 39.2 ■

A female executive was seen after excision of a recurrent glomus tumor of the nondominant left small finger. She experienced a Code Blue that was narcotics induced. She stated at her next visit that her hand therapist had caused the code by upsetting her with a discussion of her therapy authorization status.

Treatment Approach

Validate the client's concerns. Tell her that you recognize that discussions about therapy authorization can be upsetting and that you are sorry she was upset. Ask how she would like to be kept informed about authorization status in the future. Recommend that the client discuss the factors that led up to the Code Blue with her physician. Call the physician so that he or she is prepared to discuss the Code

Blue with the client. Coordinate all care as a medical team and document the situation carefully.

CASE STUDY 39.3 ■

A 60-year-old, right dominant retired male executive suffered a radial collateral ligament injury to the small finger of his right hand while bicycling. He was shocked to learn that it would take longer than 2 weeks to recover from this injury. He could not accept this and demanded that he recover normal ROM and resolution of edema in 2 weeks' time.

Treatment Approach

Supervise the client's home program closely. Provide good explanations of the typical recovery timeline at every visit and include the physician in this explanation. Offer encouragement and enthusiasm for the client's progress, and explore ways he can pass the recovery time meaningfully.

CASE STUDY 39.4 ■

An operating room nurse was treated nonoperatively for a boutonnière deformity of the dominant long finger. She refused to make appointments and frequently arrived at hand therapy unscheduled. She was unwilling to wait to be seen, even though she had no scheduled appointment. She called and interrupted the department director to complain, wrote letters of complaint, and also complained to the hand surgeon about being told she needed to make appointments to be seen in hand therapy.

Treatment Approach

Provide a nonemotional, factual explanation to the department director and the physician, and be consistent in requiring all clients to have appointments for therapy. Offer the client the option of seeking care elsewhere if she prefers to do that.

Summary

Ideally, the hand therapy client and the hand therapist will have similar goals. Also ideally, the client will attend therapy as scheduled, describe his or her illness honestly and accurately, make clinically appropriate requests, participate actively in treatment, and follow the treatment plan. When the therapist–client relationship does not benefit from these positive attributes, the relationship can deteriorate.

Through their recognition of the various patterns of FSS and the characteristics of challenging clients, hand therapists can more effectively shape rewarding therapeutic relationships. These positive relationships can favorably affect the clinical outcome for even the most challenging clients. Challenging client situations are opportunities for professional growth and can bring out the best care we have to offer.

Acknowledgement

The author acknowledges Cynthia Cooper for her collaboration on this chapter in the first and second editions of this textbook.

References

1. Manu P: *Functional somatic syndromes*, Cambridge, 1998, Cambridge University Press.
2. Wolfe F, Smythe HA, Yunus MB, et al.: The American College of Rheumatology 1990 criteria for the classification of fibromyalgia: report of the Multicenter Criteria Committee, *Arthritis Rheumatism* 33:1863–1864, 1990.
3. Wolfe F, Anderson J, Harkness D, et al.: Health status and disease severity in fibromyalgia: results of a six-center longitudinal study, *Arthritis Rheumatism* 40:1571–1579, 1997.
4. Wolfe F, Skevington SM: Measuring the epidemiology of distress: the rheumatology distress index, *J Rheumatol* 27:2000–2009, 2000.
5. Fukuda K, Straus SE, Hickie I, et al.: The chronic fatigue syndrome: a comprehensive approach to its definition and study, *Ann Intern Med* 121:953–959, 1994.
6. Salit IE: The chronic fatigue syndrome: a position paper, *J Rheumatol* 23:540–544, 1996.
7. Aaron LA, Buchwald D: A review of the evidence for overlap among unexplained clinical conditions, *Ann Intern Med* 134(9 pt 2):868–881, 2001.
8. Bombardier CH, Buchwald D: Chronic fatigue, chronic fatigue syndrome, and fibromyalgia: disability and health-care use, *Med Care* 34:924–930, 1996.
9. Cullen MR: The worker with multiple chemical sensitivities: an overview, *Occup Med* 2:655–661, 1987.
10. Sorg BA, Prasad BM: Potential role of stress and sensitization in the development and expression of multiple chemical sensitivity, *Environ Health Perspect* 105(Suppl 2):467–471, 1997.
11. MacPhail RC: Evolving concepts of chemical sensitivity, *Environ Health Perspect* 105(Suppl 2):455–456, 1997.
12. Koller W, Lang A, Vetere-Overfield B, et al.: Psychogenic tremors, *Neurology* 39:1094–1099, 1989.
13. Deuschl G, Koster B, Lucking CH, et al.: Diagnostic and pathophysiological aspects of psychogenic tremors, *Mov Disord* 13:294–302, 1998.
14. Iverson GL, Binder LM: Detecting exaggeration and malingering in neuropsychological assessment, *J Head Trauma Rehabil* 15(2):829–858, 2000.
15. Kasdan ML, Stutts JT: Factitious disorders of the upper extremity, *J Hand Surg Am* 20(3 Pt 2):S57–S60, 1994.
16. Green LN: Malingering, dissimulation, and conversion-hysteria, *Trauma* 6:3–21, 2002.
17. Mittenberg W, Patton C, Canyock EM, et al.: Base rates of malingering and symptom exaggeration, *J Clin Exper Neuropsychol* 24(8):1094–1102, 2002.
18. Waddell G, McCulloch JA, Kummel E, et al.: Nonorganic physical signs in low back pain, *Spine* 5:117–125, 1980.
19. Kiester PD, Duke AD: Is it malingering or is it real? Eight signs that point to nonorganic back pain, *Postgrad Med* 106:77–84, 1999.
20. Parry CBW: Trick movements, *Proc Royal Soc Med* 63:674–676, 1970.
21. Novack DM, Epstein RM, Paulsen RH: Toward creating physician-healers: fostering medical students' self-awareness, personal growth, and well-being, *Acad Med* 74(5):516–520, 1999.
22. American Psychiatric Association: *Diagnostic and statistical manual of mental disorders*, ed 5, Arlington, VA, 2013, American Psychiatric Publishing.
23. International Statistical Classification of Diseases and Related Health Problems, 10th Revision, Clinical Modification. National Center for Health Statistics: 2018.
24. Glerk B, Kohlmann S, Kroenke K, et al.: The somatic symptoms scale - 8, *JAMA Intern Med* 174(3):399–407, 2014.
25. Barsky AJ: Assessing somatic symptoms in clinical practice (Invited Commentary), *JAMA Intern Med* 174(3):407–408, 2014.
26. Goldberg RJ, Novack DH, Gask L: The recognition and management of somatization: what is needed in primary care training, *Psychosomatics* 33:55–61, 1992.
27. Kleinman A: Clinical relevance of anthropological and cross-cultural research: concepts and strategies, *Am J Psychiatry* 135:427–431, 1978.
28. Branch WT, Malik TK: Using "windows of opportunity" in brief interviews to understand patients' concerns, *JAMA* 269:1667–1668, 1993.
29. Eisenberg L: Medicine: molecular, monetary, or more than both? *JAMA* 274:331–334, 1995.
30. Lerner AM, Luby ED: Error of accommodation in the care of the difficult patient, *J Psychiatry Law* 20:191–206, 1992.
31. Kaplan SH, Greenfield S, Gandek B, et al.: Characteristics of physicians with participatory decision-making styles, *Ann Intern Med* 124:497–504, 1996.
32. Quill TE: Partnerships in patient care: a contractual approach, *Ann Intern Med* 124:228–234, 1983.

Glossary

A1 pulley Located at the volar aspect of the metacarpophalangeal joints, it is where the flexor tendons often are constricted, as in trigger finger or stenosing tenosynovitis.

abscess Localized collection of pus.

accessory collateral ligament (ACL) of the proximal interphalangeal (PIP) joint The fibers insert more volarly on the volar plate.

adhesion Attachment of scar to surrounding tissue, such as tendon, ligament, fascia, or joint capsule.

agonist The muscle most directly involved in bringing about a movement. Also known as *prime mover*.

allodynia Experiencing pain with stimuli that is not typically painful.

allograft See *homograft*.

anatomic snuffbox The dorsal surface area that lies just distal to the radial styloid process. The tendons bordering it become more prominent when the thumb is extended.

angiofibroblastic hyperplasia Pathologic alterations seen in the tissue of clients with the diagnosis of tendinosis. A change in the gross appearance of the tissue is visible.

angiofibroblastic tendinosis Another term for *angiofibroblastic hyperplasia* or for *tendinosis*.

angiogenesis The process of creating new vessels in the tissue of a healing open wound.

ankylosis The stiffening of a joint by disease, injury, or surgery.

annulus fibrosis Multilayered ligamentous exterior of the disc.

antagonist Muscle that assists in joint stabilization, protecting ligaments and cartilaginous surfaces from sustaining potentially destructive forces. The antagonist opposes the agonist. It can slow down or stop the movement.

anterior interosseous syndrome An entrapment neuropathy of the motor branch of the median nerve.

anterior ulnar nerve transposition Release and repositioning of the ulnar nerve to an anterior position at the elbow.

antideformity (intrinsic-plus) position Wrist is extended or neutral, metacarpophalangeals (MPs) are flexed, inter-phalangeals (IPs) are extended, and thumb is abducted with opposition.

ape hand deformity The classic posture that results from loss of median nerve integrity. It is characterized by loss of thumb opposition and palmar abduction.

aphasia A language disorder that impacts the ability to communicate.

apraxia Impaired skilled movements independent of weakness, sensory loss, language comprehension deficits, or general intellectual deterioration.

arteriole The smallest artery in the body; often supplies the capillaries and becomes part of the capillary.

arteriole hydrostatic pressure The pressure of the blood fluid within the arteriole that is exerted against its walls.

arthrodesis Fusion of a joint to stabilize it and place it in a more functional position.

arthrokinematics The movement of articular surfaces and movement around a mechanical axis; this is the movement that takes place within the joint.

arthroscopic capsular plication Suturing folds into the glenohumeral (GH) capsule.

arthrosis Degenerative condition of a joint.

articular cartilage The hyaline cartilage that lines the ends of articulating bones. Hyaline or articular cartilage has no nerve supply and no blood supply; therefore it is dependent upon joint motion (which bathes it with the rich nutritious synovial fluid found in the joint capsule) to maintain health.

associated reaction Effortful activities of other parts of the body may generate inappropriate muscle activity causing involuntary movements in the paretic limbs (for example, elbow flexion in the paretic limb during walking that, in turn, may impact balance).

ataxia (ataxic) A lack of muscle coordination during voluntary movements, such as walking or picking up objects.

attenuating Weakening, stretching.

authenticity Operating from a core of sincerity and honesty regarding oneself. Being true to oneself and honoring one's own values and unique individuality. Knowing how one's personal attributes can contribute positively to the care of the client.

autograft Permanent skin graft using client's own skin.

autolytic debridement The ability of the body to break down its own necrotic tissue in a wound.

autonomic instability Sympathetic nervous system irritation.

avascular necrosis (AVN) The death of a bone resulting from decrease or loss of blood supply to that bone.

axial skeleton Skeletal components consisting of the skull, rib cage, spine, and pelvis.

axis of reference The plumb line envisioned as perfect balance within a specific plane; determines symmetry in the sagittal plane and anterior or posterior deviations in the coronal plane.

axon A process that emerges from the soma of the neuron (at the axon hillock) and that extends to target cells. It transmits action potentials or nerve signals. Typically information travels away from the cell body by way of the axon. Axons can be myelinated or unmyelinated.

axonopathies Disorders that disrupt the normal functioning of axons.

axonotmesis A compression lesion to a nerve where the axons distal to the lesion degenerate. The endoneurial tubes remain, however, so there is typically complete recovery of function. Also known as *Sunderland type 2 nerve injury*.

axoplasmic flow The flow of axoplasm (or cytoplasm) within the peripheral nerve's axon. There are three main flows: fast antegrade flow, slow antegrade flow, and retrograde flow. The role of the axoplasm in nerve homeostasis includes transport of neurotransmitters and transmitter vesicles for use in transmission of impulses at the synapse and carrying recycled transmitter vesicles from the nerve terminal to the soma.

Ballentine sign The collapse of the distal IP joints of the thumb and index and long digits when attempting to pinch; it may indicate a neuropathy of the forearm motor branch of the median nerve.

Bankart lesion Damage to the anterior glenohumeral (GH) capsule glenoid labrum.

basal cell carcinoma A malignant epithelial tumor.

base The proximal end of the metacarpal or phalangeal bone.

Bennett fracture dislocation Intra-articular, unstable, two-fragment fractures of the base of the thumb metacarpal that result in dislocation or subluxation of the carpometacarpal (CMC) joint of the thumb.

Berger test A provocative maneuver test used to identify possible lumbrical contribution to carpal tunnel syndrome (CTS). The patient holds a full fist position with the wrist in neutral for 30 to 40 seconds. The test is positive if pain and paresthesias occur.

bicondylar Having two condyles.

bilateral arm training A rehabilitation intervention that uses both limbs to complete a task; both arms are coupled symmetrically.

bilateral hand use Using two hands together in order to accomplish an activity. Follows unilateral hand use developmentally.

bimanual hand use Each hand performs differently in order to accomplish an activity. Examples are tying shoelaces or cutting with scissors.

biofeedback A complementary and alternative medicine technique in which a person learns to control bodily functions (such as their heart rate) using their mind.

biopsy A sample taken surgically from a tumor.

blocking exercises Exercises in which proximal support is provided to promote isolated motion at a particular site. Blocking exercises exert more force than non-blocked active range of motion (AROM).

body conformation The structure or outline of the body determined by the arrangement of its segments.

body dysmorphic disorder Preoccupation with imagined or innocent variations in appearance.

bony mallet finger injury A fracture of the terminal phalanx of the digit with accompanying terminal extensor tendon injury.

Bouchard node Bony outgrowth at the proximal interphalangeal (PIP) joints commonly seen in osteoarthritis (OA).

boutonnière deformity Finger posture with proximal interphalangeal (PIP) joint flexion and distal interphalangeal (DIP) joint hyperextension. This pathologic condition occurs with disruption of the central slip and volar displacement of the lateral bands.

bowstringing The result of a tendon that is not supported firmly in place by the pulley system. The tendon pulls away from the joint and strains against the skin when it is pulled proximally, creating the effect of bowstringing.

boxer's fracture Extra-articular fracture of the neck of the metacarpal of the hand; they occur most often at the fourth and fifth metacarpals.

bradykinesia Decrease in spontaneity and movement; it is one of the features of extrapyramidal disorders, such as Parkinson disease. The slowness of movement is most clear when initiating and executing actions or activities that require several successive steps.

brawny edema Firm, thick edema that does not move or become depressed with pressure.

bursa A fluid-filled sac that decreases friction between structures.

bursitis Inflammation of the bursa.

calor A term meaning "heat."

capitellum Eminence on the lateral aspect of the distal end of the humerus that articulates with the radial head; also known as *capitulum.*

capsule tightness A pattern of joint passive range of motion (PROM) tightness that is unaffected by the position of joints proximal or distal to the given joint.

caring moment The occasion when the therapist and client come together with their unique life histories and enter into the human-to-human transaction in a given focal point in space and time.

caritas Derived from the Greek word meaning to cherish, appreciate, and give special attention, if not loving attention, to; it connotes something that is very fine, that indeed is precious.

carpal boss See *carpometacarpal boss.*

carpal instability Dislocation or loss of contact between bones of the distal carpal row over the proximal carpal row in relation to the radioulnar joint.

carpal tunnel release A surgical procedure to decompress the median nerve in the carpal tunnel by cutting the transverse carpal ligament.

carpal tunnel syndrome (CTS) Median nerve compression at the carpal tunnel of the wrist.

carpometacarpal boss An osteoarthritic spur at the base of the second or third carpometacarpal (CMC) joint. The boss is more evident as a prominent, firm, bony, tender mass when the wrist is flexed.

carpometacarpal interposition arthroplasty Positioning of a donor tendon or implant in the carpometacarpal (CMC) joint space usually to stabilize and align the joint. This can be a treatment for osteoarthritis (OA) at the thumb CMC joint.

carpus A term used to describe the eight carpal bones of the wrist.

carry Transporting an object in the hand to another place.

carrying angle The normal valgus presentation of the elbow as the hand deviates away from the body when the upper extremity is observed in anatomic position.

catch-up clunk The lateral fluoroscopic view in palmar mid-carpal instability (MCI) often demonstrates a sudden dramatic shift of the position of the proximal carpal row when the wrist moves from radial to ulnar deviation. This is often associated with a clunk. This clunk occurs because the proximal carpal row is not moving synchronously from palmar flexion to dorsal flexion while moving from radial to ulnar deviation. The proximal carpal row gets behind and catches up, which leads to a dramatic clunk back into place.

cellulitis A superficial infection involving the skin and subcutaneous tissue usually without any localized abscess or pus.

central extensor tendon A part of the proximal interphalangeal (PIP) joint dorsal tendon; attaches to the middle phalanx at the dorsal tubercle.

central sensitization Loss of brain-orchestrated pain inhibitory mechanisms and hyperactivation of ascending pain pathways.

cervicobrachial pain Shoulder and arm pain originating from the cervical region.

chip bags Bags containing small pieces of foam of various densities that are placed inside pressure garments or low-stretch bandages or orthoses to reduce edema and soften indurated areas.

chondroblasts Cells that form cartilage; immature chondrocytes.

chondrocytes Cartilage cells; the functional unit of cartilage.

chronic fatigue and immune dysfunction syndrome (CFIDS) Fatigue that is unexplained by other diagnoses, persists for more than 6 months, has a definite time of onset, results in decreased activity level but may not be due to ongoing exertion, and is not substantially relieved by rest. At least four minor criteria also must be present.

chronic fatigue syndrome (CFS) See *chronic fatigue and immune dysfunction syndrome (CFIDS)*.

claw hand deformity Indicative of an ulnar nerve palsy. The fourth and fifth digits (in particular) posture into hyper extension at metacarpophalangeal (MP) joints and flexion at the interphalangeal (IP) joints. This indicates an intrinsic muscle paresis.

clenched-fist injury A wound occurring from a fist to the mouth.

clenched-fist syndrome Clients present with tightly curled fingers that are stiff and resist extension. The thumb and index fingers often are spared, enabling the client to maintain a level of function with the involved hand.

client self-report outcome measures Client questionnaires that measure health-related outcomes.

closed chain exercises Working against resistance with the extremity working against a stationary or mobile but motion-constrained object or surface.

close-packed position Joint position in which the capsule and ligaments are under the most tension with maximal contact between joint surfaces.

co-activation exercise Contraction of agonist and antagonist muscles that cross the joint simultaneously.

coasting phenomenon Worsening of symptoms after treatment has been ceased.

co-contraction Simultaneous contraction of agonist and antagonist muscles around a joint.

collagen The most abundant protein in the human body. It is the fundamental component of connective tissue, including fascia, fibrous cartilage, tendon, ligaments, bone, joint capsules, blood vessels, adipose tissue, and dermis.

collagenase enzymatic fasciotomy Injection of enzymes into the diseased cord followed by manipulation the next day.

collateral ligaments The main restraints to lateral and medial deviation forces. At the proximal interphalangeal (PIP) joint, they are 2 to 3 mm thick. They are very important to the joint's medial-lateral stability. There are two components: the proper collateral ligament (PCL) and the accessory collateral ligament (ACL), which are differentiated by their areas of insertion. The former inserts into bone, the latter into volar plate.

collector lymphatic A three-celled lymphatic vessel having bicuspid shaped valves every 6 to 8 mm that conduct lymph proximally in the body.

Colles fracture A complete fracture of the distal radius with dorsal displacement of the distal fragment and radius shortening. It is usually extra-articular, minimally displaced, and stable.

colloquial names Like street jargon, these names reflect regional geographic locales. They often make little sense to outsiders but within regional groups they carry distinct meaning.

comminuted fracture A bone fracture with multiple fragments.

compensatory movement patterns Patterns of movement that are utilized subconsciously to make up for the lack of normally functioning muscles.

complex elbow dislocation Joint displacement with associated fracture or fractures.

complex regional pain syndrome (CRPS) A compilation of symptoms, most notably increased sympathetic activity and vasomotor instability. Pain, discoloration, and a shiny, wax-like characteristic of the skin, temperature difference in the injured extremity as compared with the uninjured extremity, brawny edema, and persistent, unrelenting stiffness are often seen. Formerly referred to as *reflex sympathetic dystrophy*.

complex rotation Turning or rolling an object 180° to 360° in the finger pads. Turning a pencil in order to use the eraser end is an example.

composite motions Combined motions of the wrist, metacarpophalangeals (MPs), and interphalangeals (IPs).

concentric Muscle contraction resulting in approximation of the origin and insertion.

conditioned responses Cardiovascular, respiratory, gastrointestinal, or immunologic responses that are triggered by heightened perception of environmental stimuli.

congenital arteriovenous malformations Abnormal connection between arteries and veins.

construct validity Comparison between a new measure and an associated measure.

content validity Accurate measurement of a specific domain.

conversion disorder A bodily event (such as a seizure or paralysis) that is psychological in origin.

cord Ropelike collagen growth that shortens, causing flexion contracture.

coronal plane A vertical plane that divides the body into anterior and posterior halves.

coronoid Anterior portion of the trochlear notch of the proximal ulna.

coronoid fossa Depression on the anterior humerus proximal to the trochlea.

covalent bonds Strong chemical bonds formed by the sharing of a pair of electrons. Mature collagen is stronger than immature collagen because of its covalent bonds.

Cozen test The examiner's thumb stabilizes the client's elbow at the lateral epicondyle. With the forearm pronated, the client makes a fist and actively extends the wrist and radially deviates it with the examiner resisting the motion. Severe and sudden pain at the lateral epicondyle area indicates a positive test.

crepitus Grating or popping as the digit flexes and extends.

criterion validity Compares a new measure with a gold standard.

cross-bridges In the sarcomere of a muscle cell, the portion of the myosin filaments that pulls the actin filaments toward the center of the sarcomere during muscle contraction.

cubital tunnel The groove between the medial epicondyle and the olecranon of the ulna at the elbow.

cubital tunnel syndrome Compression of the ulnar nerve between the medial epicondyle and the olecranon.

cutaneous fibrous histiocytoma See *dermatofibroma*.

cyanosis Blue tinge to the skin because of a decrease in oxygen.

cylindrical grasp Flattening of the transverse arch facilitates holding of the fingers against the object. Having the hand around a jar is an example.

cytotoxic Anything that has the ability to kill cells.

debridement The removal of dead tissue from a wound so that healthy tissue is exposed in the wound bed.

decompression Procedure to decrease compressive forces or pressure on a nerve.

deep partial-thickness burn Burn involving the epidermis and deep portion of the dermis.

degrees of freedom Direction or type of motion at a joint.

delayed (or secondary) nerve repair A surgical repair of a severed nerve performed more than a week after the injury.

demyelination A pathological response to peripheral nerve axonal injury resulting in a transient state of disrupted nerve conduction along the injured segment.

dendrite A process that extends from the soma of the neuron and that conducts information toward the cell body. They are the input units of the nerve cell. Dendrites are typically tree-shaped processes that receive messages from adjacent neuron(s).

denuded skin Skin in which the epidermal layer has been broken down.

de Quervain disease Disease evident by pain over the radial styloid process that can radiate proximally or distally. Pain also occurs with resisted thumb extension or abduction, and Finklestein's test frequently is positive. Also known as *stenosing tenovaginitis* or *stenosing tenosynovitis*.

dermatofibroma An epithelial tumor composed of fibroblastic cells and some scattered histiocytes.

dermis Thicker layer of skin containing blood vessels, nerves, hair follicles, sweat and sebaceous glands, and the epithelial bed.

desensitization The systematic process of applying nonnoxious stimuli to peripheral tissues to reeducate and retrain the nervous system.

diaphragmatic breathing A form of breathing where air is brought in through the nose with a closed mouth, filling primarily the lower thoracic area. This engages the diaphragm in exhalation and inhalation. The movement of the diaphragm causes thoracic pressure changes in the lower thoracic duct and conducts lymph more proximal within the duct.

diaphysis The central shaft of the bone composed of cortical or dense bone.

differential tendon gliding exercise The relative freedom of movement between the flexor digitorum superficialis (FDS) and flexor digitorum profundus (FDP) tendons. This relative glide can be negatively impacted by inter-tendon adherence and can significantly restrict the ability to fully grasp. These exercises are a mainstay of conservative management of carpal tunnel syndrome (CTS).

digital stenosing tenosynovitis Also called trigger finger. A discrepancy exists between the volume of the flexor tendon and the size of the pulley lumen. The site of the problem typically is the first annular pulley (A1 pulley), which lies volar to the metacarpophalangeal (MP) joint in the area of the distal palmar crease.

DIP extensor lag See *distal interphalangeal (DIP) extensor lag*.

DIP flexion contracture See *distal interphalangeal (DIP) flexion contracture*.

diplopia The condition in which a single object is perceived as two objects.

directional preference Direction of motion that reduces or centralizes radiating pain of spinal origin.

disc herniation Damage to the annular wall of the disc resulting in disc deformity as the nucleus displaces into the lesion.

disease A physiologic or anatomic impairment in the function of a structure or biochemical process.

disease-specific measures Instruments intended to be highly responsive for individual diagnoses.

disk grasp Metacarpophalangeal (MP) hyperextension and finger abduction adjusted according to the object's size. Opening a lid of a jar is an example.

dissimulation A phenomenon in which clients with somatization disorder become convinced that they have a life-threatening or incapacitating disease or injury.

distal interphalangeal (DIP) extensor lag A finger posture in which the DIP joint droops; the patient is not able to actively extend the DIP, but this joint can be passively extended.

distal interphalangeal (DIP) flexion contracture A finger posture in which the DIP joint droops and cannot be passively extended to neutral.

distal radioulnar joint (DRUJ) The articulation between the distal radius and the distal ulna.

distal transverse arch of the hand The more distal of the two bony transverse arches of the hand. These mobile arches contribute to the normal resting posture (palmar concavity) of the hand and to normal hand function. The distal transverse arch is located at the heads of the metacarpals.

dolor Pain.

donor site Site from where skin graft or flap is harvested.

dorsal wrist ganglion Dorsal wrist ganglions are found in the dorsal aspect of the wrist, or dorsal to the scapholunate joint.

dose-limiting factor Side effects that are severe enough to prevent further increase in dosage of treatment or prevent continuation of the treatment at any dosage level.

double crush syndrome An irritation to a nerve in more than one place. Minor serial impingements along a nerve have been proposed to have an additive effect that can cause a nerve entrapment lesion distal to the initial lesion site.

Dupuytren diathesis Features in patients with a higher disease risk, severity, and recurrence.

Dupuytren disease Disease process resulting in thickening and contracture of the palmar fascia.

dynamic orthoses Orthoses that use moving parts (such as rubber bands or spring wires) to apply a gentle force.

dynamic posture A series of positions that constantly change during movement and function; they have components of stability and mobility.

dyscoordinate co-contraction Poor quality of movement that can result from co-contraction of antagonistic muscles.

dysdiadochokinesia Impairment of the ability to perform rapidly alternating movements.

dysmetria A condition in which there is improper judgment of distance during reaching/grasping tasks that results in overshooting or undershooting the intended target.

dystonia A movement disorder that causes involuntary contractions of muscles resulting in twisting and repetitive movements.

eccentric contraction Muscle contraction to stabilize movement resulting in increased distance between the origin and insertion.

eccentric strengthening Exercises designed to increase strength by applying load while physically lengthening the activated muscle.

eccentrically Muscle contraction to stabilize movement resulting in increased distance between the origin and insertion.

edema/ edematous Swelling/swollen.

ego self Oneself.

elastic mobilization orthoses See dynamic orthoses.

elasticity The property of a muscle to return to its normal length after being stretched or shortened.

elbow flexion contracture Loss of full passive elbow extension.

elbow flexion test A provocative maneuver designed to reproduce symptoms of ulnar nerve compression. The elbow is fully flexed for 5 minutes; a positive test is symptom reproduction.

elbow joint A complex structure comprising the ulnohumeral, radiohumeral and proximal radioulnar joints.

elevated arm stress test (EAST) Special test used to detect the presence of neurovascular compromise in the thoracic outlet. Also known as *Roos test*.

empathy Trying to put oneself in the client's place and identifying with a client's situation in a caring way without condescension or pitying of the client.

enchondral ossification The process by which the interpositional callus bone (that forms during the second repair stage of bone healing following fracture) is gradually converted to bone tissue by a process of mineralization.

enchondroma The most common primary bone tumors of hand bones; benign cartilaginous lesions. They compose 90% of bone tumors.

endoneurial tube A distensible elastic structure made up of closely packed collagen tissue. This tube provides an optimum environment for nerve fibers, electrically insulating individual nerve fibers from each other.

endoneurium The basement membrane that surrounds peripheral nerve fibers. It is closely packed together, and serves to electrically insulate axons from each other.

endoscopic release A technique for decompressing a peripheral nerve using an endoscope. Instead of surgically opening up the restricting tunnel, small portals are used to visualize and release the compressing tissue.

endosteum The lining of the medullary cavity of cortical bone; it consists of osteoclasts (bone destroying cells) and osteoblasts (bone forming cells).

enzymatic debridement The application of topical enzymes to break down necrotic tissue in a wound.

epidermal inclusion cyst Cyst that occurs following injury in which a segment of keratinizing epithelium is forced into subcutaneous tissue, where it produces keratin and becomes a tumor. It occurs most often in men who are between 30 and 40 years of age with the most common site being the distal phalanx of the left thumb and long finger.

epidermis Thin, avascular, outermost layer that accounts for only about 5% of the skin's thickness.

epineurium The external protective connective tissue covering that surrounds the nerve trunk. It is the outermost covering that functions to surround and cushion nerve fascicles.

epiphysis The end of a long bone. This part of the bone is composed primarily of cancellous or spongy bone tissue.

epithelialization The act of epithelial cells migrating across granulation tissue to completely cover a healing wound.

eponychia An infection that entails the entire eponychium along with one lateral fold. The pus collection usually occurs near the lunula.

equanimity The quality of being calm and even-tempered with patience or firmness of mind under stress.

erythema Reddening of the skin.

eschar A thick layer of necrotic collagen over a wound, usually black or dark brown.

Essex-Lopresti lesion Fracture of the radial head with rupture of the interosseous membrane.

excitability The properties of a muscle to respond to a stimulus and to maintain chemical potentials across its cell membranes.

excursion The length of tendon needed to move a joint through its full range of motion (ROM). The available excursion is limited by the surrounding connective tissue.

expendable donor muscles Muscles that perform a certain function of the extremity, but there are alternate muscles also performing that function. The transfer of the expendable muscle does not in itself cause another deficit of motor function.

extensibility The property of a muscle to be stretched, repeatedly and considerably, as needed, without being damaged.

extension outrigger orthoses An orthosis fabricated to support the finger(s) in extension and allow a controlled amount of flexion to allow tendon gliding. Slings with elastic attachments support the fingers in extension. An outrigger, or attachment to the sling, is used to direct the angle of pull of the slings.

extensor habitus Habitual posturing in digital extension. Especially common at the index finger, this posturing can lead to stiffness and functional limitations.

extensor retinacular ganglion Uncommon but, if detected, usually involves the first extensor compartment (abductor pollicis longus [APL] and extensor pollicis brevis [EPB]) and can be associated with de Quervain's tenosynovitis.

extensor tendon adhesion Restrictive attachments of surrounding scar tissue to the extensor tendon, preventing or limiting gliding of the extensor tendon.

external fixator A manufactured device for maintaining fracture alignment. It consists of pins, wires, or screws, and it attaches the appropriately aligned and stabilized injured bone to its external low-profile scaffold.

extra-articular fracture A fracture of the bone that does not cross into the joint space and does not interrupt the cartilage at the end of the bone.

extracellular matrix The network of fibrous and fluid material that is excreted by, surrounds, and supports living cells. It is critical to cellular growth and maintenance.

extrinsic extensor tightness Passive proximal interphalangeal (PIP)/ distal interphalangeal (DIP) flexion is limited when the metacarpophalangeal (MP) joint is passively flexed.

extrinsic muscles Muscles that originate proximal to the wrist.

extrinsic tendon tightness Condition that prevents a normal amount of finger motion, most notably when the wrist is moved. The extrinsic tendons are those that originate proximal to the wrist and insert within the hand. Because the extrinsic tendons cross the wrist, when the wrist moves, it creates tightness or slack in the tendons at the wrist.

exudate Drainage from a wound that is characterized by a creamy or yellow coloration because of sloughed cells, increased phagocytic activity, and higher protein level.

exudate edema Edema that is filled with plasma protein molecules.

facet joints These joints of the cervical spine are paired synovial joints with fibrous capsules.

facilitation To stimulate or maintain control of a muscle group by external inputs, such as vibration, muscle belly tapping, and so on.

facilitation techniques Specific strategies utilized to recruit the donor tendon to function in its new capacity after tendon transfer.

factitious disorders Disorders that arise out of a psychological need to be sick rather than a conscious effort for material gain. Clients with factitious disorders knowingly cause their own disease but are unaware of the underlying reasons for their behavior.

fall on an outstretched hand (FOOSH) Mode of injury; distal forearm or wrist fractures usually result from impact to the outstretched hand and wrist during falls.

fasciculus A bundle of pathway axons within the central nervous system (CNS).

fasciectomy Removal of diseased fascia through one or more incisions.

fasciotomy Local division of the diseased cord without its removal.

febricity The condition of having a fever.

felon A deep infection of the finger pad involving the tiny compartments of the pulp. Felons are very painful.

fibroblastic phase The reparative phase of healing during which time new tissue is laid down in the wound. The phase begins on about day 4 following injury and lasts for 2 to 6 weeks. Fibroblasts synthesize scar tissue with gradual increase of tensile strength. Also known as the *fibroplasia stage* or the *fibroplasia phase or stage*.

fibroblastic stage See *fibroblastic phase*.

fibroblasts Cells that respond to mechanical stimulus by producing type I collagen fibers that are found in tendons, ligaments, and joint capsules. They also produce glycosaminoglycans.

fibromyalgia A pain syndrome affecting the entire musculoskeletal system. Symptoms include chronic widespread musculoskeletal pain, sleep disturbances, morning stiffness, fatigue, anxiety, and depressive symptoms. The syndrome is often difficult to diagnose.

fibrosis Condition of increased or degenerated fibrous tissue.

fibrous xanthoma Another name for a giant-cell tumor.

fight bite injury See *clenched-fist injury*.

filariasis Found primarily in the southern hemisphere from infected mosquitoes injecting larvae into the bloodstream. The larvae can grow into filarial worms 20 cm long and destroy lymph nodes and vessels when they die, resulting in severe lymphedema.

finger-to-palm translation Grasping an object with the thumb and finger pads, and then moving the object into the palm.

firm end feel A stop-to-passive movement produced by a gradually increased tension.

first annular (A1) pulley See *A1 pulley*.

flap Segment of skin including muscle and/or fascial layers.

flexor synergistic pattern Voluntary contractions of a group of limb muscles producing a stereotypical pattern of limb movement. Flexor synergy is usually seen in the upper extremities with shoulder, elbow, wrist, and finger flexion.

flexor tendon adhesion Restrictive attachments of surrounding scar tissue to the flexor tendon, preventing or limiting gliding of the flexor tendon.

FOOSH See *fall on an outstretched hand (FOOSH)*.

force couple Two resultant forces of equal magnitude in opposite directions that produce rotation of a structure.

forced use Immobilization of the unaffected arm combined with intensive training of the affected arm.

forward elevation The motion involved in reaching forward and above the head as in getting objects from the cupboard; combination of shoulder and scapula motions.

foul purulent exudate Thick, pus-like wound drainage with a bad odor; ranges in color from yellow to green and is a sign of infection.

fracture An impairment of the skeleton's mechanical integrity that typically leads to functional deficits and pain.

fracture consolidation Healing with solidification of a broken bone.

free muscle transfer The entire muscle-tendon unit is transferred with intact nerve and blood supply preserved.

Froment sign Indicative of an ulnar nerve lesion; one will see flexion of the interphalangeal (IP) joint of the thumb as the flexor pollicis longus (FPL) attempts to compensate for the paralyzed or weak adductor pollicis during lateral pinch.

full-thickness burn Burn involving the epidermis and the entire dermis.

full-thickness burn with subdermal injury Burn involving the epidermis, the entire dermis, and deep tissue damage to fat, muscle, and possibly bone.

full-thickness skin graft (FTSG) Graft of epidermis and entire dermis.

functional somatic syndrome (FSS) A physical illness that is not explained by an organic disease or structural lesion or biochemical change.

functional stability of the PIP joint This is tested actively and passively. If the patient demonstrates normal active range of motion (AROM) (that is, no subluxation at the proximal interphalangeal [PIP] joint), there is adequate functional stability of the joint. If, however, there is subluxation with AROM, this suggests that major ligament disruption has probably occurred.

fusiform swelling Having tapering at both ends.

gamekeeper's thumb Chronic ulnar collateral ligament (UCL) instability of the thumb metacarpophalangeal (MP) joint.

ganglion Mucinfilled soft tissue cyst, formed from the synovial lining of a joint or tendon sheath.

ganglion cyst A synovial cyst that arises from the synovial lining of a joint or tendon sheath.

Gate theory Proposed by Melzack and Wall in the mid-1960s. They hypothesized that stimulation of the large, myelinated non-nociceptive, A-beta sensory fibers would effectively flood the main pain pathway (the Spinothalamic tract) to higher centers of the brain, effectively gating off pain signals to the cortex and thereby diminishing the perception of pain. Later investigations demonstrated that some details of the original theory were incorrect. Current research indicates that the pain message appears to be "gated off" from the brain when activation of the A-beta fibers (for example, by mechanically stimulating a painful area by rubbing it) causes local interneurons in the dorsal horn of the spinal cord to release a neurotransmitter that binds with the excited nociceptors. This neurotransmitter (called *Enkephalin*) effectively dampens the transmission of nociceptive signals by inhibiting the release of its neurotransmitter, substance P, thereby decreasing the sensation of pain.

generic measures Instruments used to compare health conditions.

giant-cell tumor The most common solid tumor of the hand. The tumor is grayish-brown with yellow patches. Despite its name, the giant-cell tumor does not tend to be located at a tendon sheath and does not contain exclusively giant cells. Also known as *localized nodular tenosynovitis, localized pigmented villonodular synovitis,* and *xanthomas.*

ginglymus joint Hinge joint; the distal interphalangeal (DIP) joint of the finger is a ginglymus joint.

glomus tumor Tumor arising from the neuromyoarterial apparatus or the glomus body. It tends to occur subungually (beneath the nail) and in distal finger pads. It causes cold sensitivity, lancing pain, and tenderness. Over time, glomus tumors can lead to erosion of bone.

glycosaminoglycan Monomer proteoglycans produced by fibroblasts and occupying the interstitial space between collagen fibers to provide lubrication and nutrition to the collagen fibers.

Golgi tendon organ A spindle-shaped structure at the junction of a muscle and a tendon. The organ senses muscle tension through tendon stretch and inhibits muscular contraction of the agonists and facilitates contraction of the antagonists.

gout A disease resulting from monosodium urate crystal deposition in the tissues or uric acid in the extracellular fluids.

granulation tissue The tissue that forms in an open wound and is composed of new collagen and capillary growth, resulting in red coloration. Re-epithelialization occurs over granulation tissue in open wounds.

grasp Attaining an object with the hand.

grating Similar to crepitus and usually occurs at a joint.

grind test Assessment usually done at the thumb carpometacarpal (CMC) joint to determine damaged cartilage. The CMC joint is compressed, and the head of the metacarpal is pressed and gently rotated against the trapezium. Pain and crepitus are positive findings.

ground substance See *extracellular matrix.*

Guyon canal A superficial passageway between the pisiform and hamate bones of the carpus through which the ulnar nerve and artery pass as they enter the hand.

hard end-feel An abrupt stop to movement produced when two hard surfaces converge. There is an unyielding quality at passive joint end-range. This is a stiffer joint and is less favorable for potential to improve.

head The distal end of the metacarpal or phalangeal bone.

Heberden nodes The bony outgrowths at the distal interphalangeal (DIP) joints commonly seen in osteoarthritis (OA).

hemangioma A benign tumor of dilated blood vessels.

hemiarthroplasty Prosthetic replacement of one joint surface.

hemiparesis (hemiparetic) Slight paralysis or weakness affecting one side of the body.

hemiplegia (hemiplegic) Paralysis affecting only one side of the body.

heterograft Temporary skin graft taken from another species, such as a pig. Also known as *xenograft.*

heterotopic ossification Abnormal growth of bone in nonosseous tissues.

high radial nerve plasy Injury at the mid-humeral level; the radial nerve is particularly vulnerable at this level, because it traverses around the spiral groove of the humerus moving medially to laterally.

Hill-Sachs lesion An osseous defect of the posterolateral portion of the humeral head, caused during traumatic anterior dislocation.

hinged external fixator Articulated device applied to stabilize a joint while allowing controlled joint motion.

homeostasis Cells need relatively stable conditions to function effectively and contribute to the survival of the body as a whole. Homeostasis is the condition in which the body's internal environment remains within certain physiological limits. Disease is homeostatic imbalance.

homograft Temporary skin graft taken from another human, most often from a cadaver. Also known as *allograft.*

hook grasp Useful for sustaining a grip to carry objects.

hope A positive attitude or orientation toward the future.

hyperalgesia Hypersensitivity.

hyperemic An increase in the quantity of blood flow to a body part; engorgement.

hypergranulation tissue An abnormal overgrowth of granulation tissue in a wound.

hypermobility Joint movement that takes place around a physiologic axis but is more than normal.

hyperpathia Pain that is more intense than normally expected and/or lasts longer than normally expected.

hypersensitivity When one experiences pain in response to non-noxious stimuli.

hypertonicity Excessive muscle tone, tension, or activity. There are three major types of hypertonicity: rigidity, spasticity, and flexor spasms.

hypertrophic scars Scars that are raised and thick.

hypertrophy Excessive development of a structure.

hypochondriasis Excessive concern about minor health disturbances or worry over the possibility of future ill health.

hypomobility Joint movement that takes place around a physiologic axis but is less than normal.

hyponychium The area between the nail bed and the distal nail. It contains leukocytes and lymphocytes that provide defense against invasion under the nail by fungal and bacterial contamination.

idiopathic environmental intolerance (IEI) Having multiple chemical sensitivities and experiencing medically unexplained symptoms in response to low-level, identifiable environmental exposures.

illness A client's personal experience of his or her poor health.

imbibition Primary means of obtaining nutrition for avascular tissues.

immediate active motion protocol Following a tendon repair, exercises that incorporate an active component of the repaired musculotendinous unit; generally begun within 5 days after repair.

immediate passive motion protocol Following a tendon repair, exercises that incorporate passive motion in the direction of the tendon repair; generally begun within 5 days after repair.

impingement Compression of soft tissue between bony structures.

induration The hardening or thickening of tissue.

indwelling thumb Hand fisted with thumb adducted and flexed toward palm.

infection The invasion of the body by pathogenic micro organisms.

inflammation A localized protective reaction of tissue to irritation, injury, or infection. It is characterized by pain, redness, swelling, and sometimes loss of function.

inflammatory phase of bone healing The initial phase of bone healing following fracture. Hallmarks of this phase include cellular and vascular responses that serve to promote the formation of a hematoma, which provides some early fracture stabilization.

inflammatory stage The initial stage of wound healing composed of the immediate vascular and cellular response in an attempt to clear the wound of debris or necrotic tissue. The completion of the inflammatory stage of wound healing facilitates the repair phase of wound healing. Also known as the *inflammatory phase*.

in-hand manipulation Adjusting an object in the hand after grasping it.

in-hand manipulation with stabilization Performance of any in-hand manipulation skill while stabilizing other objects in the same hand.

inhibition techniques To quiet/relax/dampen overactive muscle groups by external inputs, such as weight bearing, neutral warmth, and so on.

initial lymphatic The smallest of all lymphatic vessels and most superficial in the dermis layer of tissue. It is one cell thick and lined with overlapping oak leaf shaped endothelial cells.

innervation density The number of nerve endings in an area.

instability When joint motion occurs around a nonphysiologic axis.

interactional synchrony The way in which two persons behave in pattern and synchrony during a given interaction. Behaviors in the interaction may be nonrandom and patterned after one another in timing and in pattern. For example, when one party leans forward, the other person then leans forward as well.

interosseous ligament Sheet of fibrous tissue lying obliquely between the shafts of the radius and ulna.

interosseous muscle tightness Passive proximal interphalangeal (PIP)/distal interphalangeal (DIP) flexion is limited when the metacarpophalangeal (MP) joint is passively extended or hyperextended.

interposition arthroplasty Procedure in which soft tissue is inserted between debrided joint surfaces.

interstitium On a capillary level, the space between the cells.

intervertebral foramen (IVF) Bony canal that contains the spinal nerve.

intra-articular fracture A fracture that crosses into the joint space, interrupting the articular cartilage.

intraneural Contained within the nerve.

intraosseus ganglion A ganglion cyst found within the carpal bone.

intrinsic minus position Metacarpophalangeal (MP) joint extension with interphalangeal (IP) joint flexion.

intrinsic muscles Muscles that originate distal to the wrist and in the hand.

intrinsic plus position Metacarpophalangeal (MP) joint flexion with interphalangeal (IP) joint extension. Also known as the *safe position*.

intrinsic tightness Tightness of the interossei and lumbrical muscles and tendons, which originate and insert within the hand. The tendons run volar to the axis of motion at the metacarpophalangeal (MP) joint and dorsal to the axis of motion at the interphalangeal (IP) joints. Tightness of these muscles and tendons limits the position that stretches them, that of MP joint extension and IP joint flexion.

ion channels Portals or openings along a nerve cell membrane that allow the flow of ions into the nerve cell (axon). This causes a change in the electrical charge on each side of the cell membrane. A rapid change in electrical potential results in information being transmitted along the length of an axon, and can elicit a release of chemical transmitters to other neurons or to the electrically excitable membrane of a muscle.

ischemia Low-oxygen state; a condition of decreased blood flow to an area. Long-term ischemia may lead to hypoxia and tissue death.

isokinetic exercise When the velocity of limb movement is held consistent by a rate-controlled device.

isometric exercises A type of strength training in which the joint angle and muscle length do not change during contraction.

isometric maximum (IM) The amount of force that can be maintained by an isometric contraction for 1 second (1 IM).

isotonic contractions Contraction with muscle shortening.

jersey finger A rupture of the flexor digitorum profundus (FDP) from its attachment on the distal phalanx of the finger, caused by forceful extension of the flexed fingertip.

joint contracture Passive limitation of joint motion.

joint tightness Confirmed when the passive range of motion (PROM) of a joint does not change despite repositioning of proximal or distal joints.

juncturae tendinum Slips of extensor tendon that attach the ring finger extensor tendon to the extensor tendons of the adjacent fingers and variably the middle finger tendon to the index finger tendon.

Kanavel cardinal signs Four signs indicating flexor tenosynovitis: (1) posture with slight digital flexion, (2) uniform volar swelling of the involved digit, (3) tenderness along the tendon sheath, and (4) pain with passive extension of the involved digit.

Keinböck disease Avascular necrosis (AVN) of the lunate carpal bone. Manifestations of AVN include bony sclerosis and osteopenia. AVN can occur spontaneously, be a result of overuse, or be secondary to local trauma or systemic disease.

keratinocytes Cells that produce keratin.

keratoacanthoma Another name for a dermatofibroma.

kinematic chain Several joints that unite successive segments; can be open or closed.

kinesthesia Awareness of the position of body parts in space provided to the central nervous system by proprioceptors, the sensory receptors in muscles, joints, and tendons that monitor length/tension of the musculotendinous complex. Also known as *kinesthetic awareness*.

knowing the client Connecting with the client in an intentional and meaningful way; this can take place even within a limited time frame. Understanding of the needs of the client and how the client's life as a whole is affected by the client's health condition and treatment.

knuckle pad Firm nodule located on the dorsal aspect of the proximal interphalangeal (PIP) or metacarpophalangeal (MP) joint.

lag When passive range of motion (PROM) exceeds active range of motion (AROM) at a joint.

landmark An important visual cue, prominence, or conspicuous body part that serves as a guide in mapping the body.

lateral bands Bands that originate volar to the metacarpophalangeal (MP) joint axis. They have intrinsic muscle contributions and join dorsal to the proximal interphalangeal (PIP) joint axis. They unite to form the terminal extensor tendon.

lateral collateral ligament complex Group of tough, fibrous bands of tissue supporting the outer aspect of the elbow.

lateral pinch Useful for manipulating or holding a small object. Turning a key in the door is an example of lateral pinch.

lateral ulnar collateral ligament (LUCL) A component of the lateral collateral ligament complex of the elbow.

L-Codes The foundation for othotic billing; developed in the late 1970s by orthotists in order to standardize billing for orthoses and prostheses.

learned disuse/nonuse The loss of function as a result of unsuccessful attempts at movement.

Ledderhose disease Plantar nodules.

length-tension The relationship between the length of the fiber and the force that the fiber produces at that length.

ligamentotaxis Continuous longitudinal force applied to a comminuted fracture in order to bring fracture fragments more congruent. By applying this distraction force, the soft tissues surrounding the fracture facilitate reduction by molding the bony fragments.

Likert scale A summative scale based on degree of agreement/disagreement.

lipoma A common tumor consisting of mature fat cells, characterized by its soft consistency when palpated. Lipomas can occur anywhere that fatty tissue exists, but they occur most commonly in the deep palmar space of the hand.

Lister tubercle A bony prominence located at the distal dorsal end of the radius. The extensor pollicis longus (EPL) tendon passes around the ulnar side of this tubercle.

localized nodular tenosynovitis *See* giant-cell tumor.

locking During active range of motion (AROM), locking of the digit in flexion as the tendon passes through a pulley and gets stuck there, unable to actively extend. The finger usually can be straightened passively.

longitudinal arch The longitudinally oriented bony arch of the hand that is composed of a fixed or rigid portion apparent at the carpometacarpal (CMC) joint of the middle finger.

low-load, long-duration (LLLD) approach An approach to mobilization orthotic interventions where mild stress that is within the elastic range of a given soft tissue is applied over a longer duration. In theory, this helps to affect the growth and remodeling of heavily cross-linked collagen fibers that are restricting joint movement.

lunula The white arch visible at the base of some fingernails.

lymph In the extremities, it is a clear yellowish fluid filled with water molecules plus large molecule substances, such as plasma proteins, fat cells, hormones, minerals, ions, bacteria, and tissue waste products.

lymph nodes Round, oval, or kidney-shaped structures ranging from a pin head to an olive in size. They are a part of the lymph system with a complex of internal sinuses that are responsible for immunologic functions and filtration of lymph.

lymphangioma A tumor of lymphatic vessels.

lymphangion The chamber, or space, between the valves in the collector lymphatic. As the chamber fills and stretches, the one cell of smooth muscle contracts and lymph is propelled proximally into the next lymphangion.

lymphangitis A serious hand infection that progresses rapidly. Red streaking up the hand and forearm occurs along the lymphatic pathways, and an abscess may form at the elbow or axilla if the problem is left untreated. The causative organism is typically *Streptococcus*.

lymphatic bundles Groupings of small lymphatic vessels (that is, initial lymphatics and collector lymphatics); generally does not include lymph nodes.

lymphatic capillary Same as initial lymphatic.

lymphatic streaking Red streaks visible below the skin that travel from the site of an infection toward the axilla or groin areas.

lymphedema A permanent loss, destruction, damage, or removal of lymphatic vessels (that is, lymph nodes) that results in some degree of permanent swelling or potential for swelling. In America, the term is commonly associated with lymphedema resulting from lymphadenectomy and or lymph node radiation, primary, or filariasis lymphedema.

lymphorrhea Weeping of tissue occurs with an extremely congested edematous hand or arm. Lymph, a clear, yellowish fluid, escapes from the interstitium to the outside of the skin.

lymphovenous anastomoses A "joining" of small lymphatic and venous vessels.

macerated skin Softened skin that is very fragile and caused by prolonged exposure to moisture. Often looks white.

macrophage Specific type of cell present in the inflammatory and early fibroplasia phases of wound healing that assists in cleaning the wound of necrotic tissue and debris.

malaise The state of feeling generally unwell.

malingering The intentional presentation of false or misleading health information for personal gain.

mallet finger A finger posture in which the distal interphalangeal (DIP) joint droops. May involve an avulsion fracture.

malunion A fracture that heals with aberrant biomechanical consequences. A malunion of the distal radius following a fracture infers that the fracture healed with greater than 10° of dorsal angulation of the distal radius, rather than its normal volar angulation.

Mannkopf test The absence of a rise in heart rate of at least 5% on palpation of a reportedly painful area that suggests symptom magnification.

manual edema mobilization (MEM) A method of lymphatic decongestion of subacute or chronic edema post extremity trauma, extremity surgery, or stroke where the lymphatic system is overwhelmed but intact. Through the use of specific light massage techniques, three types of exercise techniques, a home self-management program, rerouting around scar tissue, use of pump point stimulation, methods to soften indurated tissue, and possible use of low-stretch bandaging, persistent edema (or the possibility of persistent edema) is significantly and usually permanently reduced.

manual lymphatic drainage (MLD) The manual decongesting of lymph through activating the lymph uptake through massage, low-stretch bandaging programs, and so on.

manual lymphatic treatment (MLT) A generic term used to describe massage principles for lymphedema that are common to all schools of lymphatic drainage.

mapping Techniques used to determine postural faults.

mast cells Cells that secrete substances that initiate inflammation to help fight infection.

maturation (remodeling) phase Third phase of tissue healing. This phase can last months or years with changing tissue architecture and improved organization of collagen fibers contributing to increased tensile strength. Also called *maturation stage*.

maturation stage See *maturation phase*.

mechanical debridement The use of non-selective methods (such as whirlpool agitation or wet-to-dry dressings) to remove necrotic tissue from a wound.

mechanoreceptors Specialized nerve endings that transmit information regarding position and motion.

medial collateral ligament complex Group of tough, fibrous bands of tissue supporting the inner aspect of the elbow.

melanoma A type of malignant epithelial tumor that can potentially be life-threatening due to rapid spread to lymph nodes.

mesoneurium The loose areolar tissue that surrounds peripheral nerve trunks.

metabolites By-products of metabolism; any substance produced by metabolism.

methicillin-resistant *Staphylococcus aureus* (MRSA) A pathogen that is highly resistive to typically-used antibiotics.

midcarpal instability (MCI) Classified as a carpal instability nondissociative (CIND) pattern and refers to instability between the proximal and distal carpal rows.

midcarpal shift test Performed by placing the patient's wrist in neutral and the forearm in pronation. A palmar force is applied to the hand at the level of the distal capitate. The wrist is then simultaneously axially loaded and ulnarly deviated. This test is considered positive if a painful clunk occurs that reproduces the patient's symptoms.

Mills tennis elbow test Originally described as a manipulation maneuver, the technique can be used as a clinical test instead. The client's shoulder is in neutral. The examiner palpates the most tender area at or near the lateral epicondyle, pronates the client's forearm, and fully flexes the client's wrist while moving the elbow from flexion to extension. Pain at the lateral epicondyle is a positive finding.

mindfulness The act of paying attention in a particular, intentional way: on purpose, in the present moment, and nonjudgmentally.

minimal detectable change A valid change in score that is not due to chance.

minimally clinically important difference (MCID) Meaningful difference in client function.

mirror box therapy Originally developed to help people deal with phantom limb pain, this approach works by using the reflection of one's less involved hand or leg to fool the brain into thinking the involved hand or foot is moving. In stroke, this may stimulate movement in the weak or paralysed limb.

mixed fiber neuropathies Neuropathies involving both small and large fibers.

mobilization orthoses See *dynamic orthoses*.

Modified Allen Test The modified Allen's test assesses the status of the blood supply within the hand through the ulnar and radial arteries of the wrist.

Modified Weeks Test A screening tool used to determine whether and which orthotic intervention is necessary. Changes in joint passive measurements are recorded following thermal modalities and manual therapies; based on such changes, a given orthotic approach may or may not be indicated.

modulation Long-lasting changes in the electrical potential of a neurons's cell membrane. Learning and memory, for example, require long-lasting, persistent changes in the strength of synaptic connections.

mononeuropathy Damage to a single nerve.

Monteggia fracture Fracture of the ulna with associated radial head dislocation.

MRSA See *methicillin-resistant Staphylococcus aureus* (MRSA).

mucous cyst Cyst seen exclusively on a bone spur of a joint (namely the distal interphalangeal [DIP]) and communicated with the joint via mucin pedicle.

multiarticulate Crossing multiple joints.

multiple chemical sensitivity (MCS) syndrome Having medically unexplained symptoms in response to low-level, identifiable environmental exposures. Also known as *idiopathic environmental intolerance*.

multiple mononeuropathy Multifocal asymmetric damage to multiple nerves.

Munchausen syndrome A practice in which clients may cut, bruise, bite, or inject their hands and then give an untruthful history to the medical professionals who care for them.

muscle fiber length equilibrium The length the muscle will maintain when it is unaffected by outside forces.

musculotendinous tightness Tightness confirmed when the passive range of motion (PROM) of a joint changes with repositioning of adjacent joints that are crossed by that muscle–tendon unit.

myelinated nerve fiber A nerve fiber (axon) that is surrounded by a myelin sheath. Myelin provides physical support and insulation for conduction of electrical signals by neurons.

myofibroblasts Cells that have a key role in tissue reconstruction after injury. They are highly specialized forms of fibroblasts and contribute to wound contraction.

myoplasticity The principle that muscle tissue adapts structurally and functionally to changes in activity level and/or to prolonged positioning of the muscle.

neck The area of the metacarpal between the head and the shaft.

negative intracapsular pressure Air pressure inside the joint capsule lower than pressure outside the capsule.

negative ulnar variance A condition in which the ulna is shorter than it should be compared with the radius. This can cause the radius to impinge on the proximal carpal row during forearm rotation and often leads to dorsal and radial wrist pain and an increase in the likelihood of distal radioulnar joint arthrosis developing.

nerve A bundle of pathway axons in the peripheral nervous system (PNS).

nerve decompression Surgical intervention performed to free the nerve from entrapment or impingement.

nerve gliding The longitudinal gliding of a peripheral nerve and its associated connective tissues layers in relation to the adjacent tissues.

nerve grafting A type of surgical nerve repair performed when repair cannot otherwise be completed without undue tension on the nerve's cut ends. Nerve grafts serve as a temporary tunnel or tube through which the regenerating axon can grow. Grafting can be performed using a commercially available conduit, an autograft, or an allograft.

nerve sliding Involves encouraging gliding of the nerve within its tissue bed while decreasing the tension at the proximal or distal ends of the range.

neural mobility The ability of the neural structures to adjust to changes in the nerve bed length through a combination of gliding and elongation.

neural plasticity The changing of the structure, function, and organization of neurons in response to new experiences; the brain's ability to reorganize itself by forming new neural connections, allowing neurons to compensate for injury and disease in response to new situations or to changes in their environment.

neural sensitization Activation of the small-diameter pain fibers within the nerve itself.

neurilemoma A rare, slow-growing, benign nerve tumor that arises from the Schwann cells.

neuritis Inflammation of a nerve.

neurofibromas A rare, benign nerve tumor that arises from the Schwann cells but also involves the nerve tissue.

neurogenic Originating in the nerves or nervous tissue; caused or affected by the nerves or nervous system.

neurological re-education Therapeutic procedure that reeducates movement, balance, coordination, kinesthetic sense, posture, and/or proprioception for sitting and/or standing activities; retraining a body part to perform some task the body part was previously able to do.

neurolysis The surgical dissection and exposure of a damaged nerve with the goal of freeing that nerve from soft tissue restrictions and/or scar adhesions.

neuron The basic unit of the nervous system.

neuropathic pain Pain caused by some form of peripheral nerve dysfunction. It is typically a sensory pain that is difficult for patients to describe in words and may be burning or electrical. Providing sensory protection and minimizing peripheral nerve irritation reduces this type of pain.

neuropathy Peripheral nerve pathology.

neuroplasticity The ability of neurons to change their function, chemical profile, or structure; the ability of the brain to adapt and change neuronal connections based on a variety of stimuli; the nervous system's capacity for adaptation or regeneration after injury.

neuropraxia A local conduction block within a nerve trunk; typically from compression on the nerve. Prognosis is excellent for complete recovery.

neurotization The implantation of a donor motor nerve into denervated vascularized muscle.

neurotmesis A complete nerve transaction or a nerve injury with such serious internal disorganization that no recovery is expected without surgical intervention.

nociceptive Free nerve endings that are within the mechanoreceptors and that react to painful stimuli.

nociceptive pain Pain that is caused by structural dysfunction, such as a fracture or an arthritic wrist.

nociceptors Specialized nerve endings that transmit pain signals.

nodes of Ranvier Interruptions in the myelin sheath that leave small patches of axon unmyelinated. These unmyelinated patches contain a high density of voltage-gated sodium channels that contribute to the generation of action potentials.

nodules Thickened closed-packed collections of cells and the primary pathologic manifestation of Dupuytren's contracture. Also often seen in rheumatoid arthritis.

non-occlusive dressing In theory, a dressing that allows the free passage of water, water vapor, and bacteria through the material.

non-prehensile movements Using the fingers or the entire hand to lift or push an object.

non-union Failure of the bone to heal or fuse.

normal default state See *zero position.*

normal resting balance State where the agonist and antagonist are equally at rest.

normative data Average scores for large groups of clients with similar diagnoses and abilities.

nucleus pulposus Pulpy semiliquid center of the disk.

oblique retinacular ligament (ORL) Ligament that originates from the flexor sheath, progressing volar to the proximal interphalangeal (PIP) joint axis and inserting at the terminal extensor tendon dorsally. The ORL tightens when the PIP joint extends. It provides concomitant PIP joint and distal interphalangeal (DIP) joint extension and helps prevent hyperextension of the PIP joint.

oblique retinacular ligament (ORL) tightness With the proximal interphalangeal (PIP) joint extended, passive distal interphalangeal (DIP) joint flexion is limited.

occlusive dressing In theory, a dressing that will not allow any passage of water, water vapor, and bacteria through the material.

occult ganglion One that is not observable by surface anatomy visualization. Provocative positioning may produce the ganglion.

O'Donoghue maneuver A finding of active range of motion (AROM) that is greater than passive range of motion (PROM), which raises the possibility of symptom magnification.

olecranon Posterior portion of the trochlear notch of the proximal ulna.

olecranon fossa Depression on the posterior humerus proximal to the trochlea.

oncotic pressure The pressure in the interstitium caused by plasma proteins.

open chain Movement occurring from muscle origin to insertion with the terminal joint free.

open chain exercises Working against resistance where the extremity is free to move in space resulting in movement of the distal segment.

open inferior capsular shift Surgical detachment and superior advancement of the inferior glenohumeral (GH) ligament.

open-packed position Joint position in which the capsule and ligaments are most lax and separation of the joint surfaces is greatest.

open reduction internal fixation (ORIF) Surgical fracture reduction technique in which the fracture is stabilized with internal hardware (for example, plates, screws, pins) secured directly to the fractured bone.

opponensplasty Tendon transfers to restore thumb opposition.

osteitis Inflammation of the bone.

osteoarthritis (OA) A gradual loss of articular cartilage and change in underlying bone caused by degenerative joint disease and chemical factors.

osteoblasts The functional building blocks of bone. These cells synthesize the organic compounds that mineralize into bone. They are found at the surface of bone tissue.

osteoclasts Cells responsible for bone dissolution and absorption.

osteocytes Mature osteoblasts.

osteoid matrix The noncalcified matrix of young bone; a precursor to bone.

osteomyelitis Infection of the bone.

osteophyte Abnormal growths of bone that occur within joints or at other sites where there is degeneration of cartilage. Otherwise known as *bone spurs*.

osteophytosis New bone formation occurring as a result of joint erosion.

osteotomy Surgical transection of a bone.

outrigger The structure from which the forces of a static progressive or dynamic orthosis are directed. They can be high-profile or low-profile.

overflow Uncontrolled or unconscious movements that have no definite cause, are associated with intentional movements, and are generally not associated with a well-defined neurological condition. Also called *motor overflow, neurological overflow,* or *synkinesis*.

pad-to-pad pinch See *two-point pinch*.

pallor Whiter-than-normal coloration of the skin.

palmar grasp Categorized into standard, cylindrical, disk, and spherical grasps.

palm-to-finger translation Moving an object from the palm into the thumb and finger pads.

pannus The formation of synovial hyperplasia that is a result of rheumatoid arthritis.

pantrapezial arthritis A disease affecting the joints adjacent to the trapezium, such as the scaphoid and trapezoid.

paresthesias Abnormal sensations such as numbness, prickling, and tingling.

paronychia A bacterial infection of the nail fold or the nail plate. Paronychia is the most common hand infection. It can be acute or chronic.

pathway A chain of communicating neurons in the nervous system.

percutaneous needle aponeurotomy/fasciotomy A needle is used to cut the contracted cord at multiple levels.

perineural Between the nerve and the nerve bed.

perineurium The middle connective tissue covering that surrounds each nerve fascicle. It is a mechanically strong sheath that serves as a diffusion barrier, helping to preserve the specialized microenvironment inside the fascicles.

perionychium Comprises the whole nail structure of the finger consisting of the nail bed, nail plate, eponychium, hyponychium, and paronychium.

periosteum The outer lining, or sleeve, that envelopes bones. It plays an integral part in bone healing following injury.

periwound skin The skin around the wound margins.

Peyronie disease Penile fibromatosis.

phagocyte cell A type of cell that can surround and digest bacteria and other foreign organisms that would be harmful to the body. These cells are essential to the "cleanup" aspect in the inflammation phase of wound healing.

phagocytosis Removal of dead tissue and foreign bodies.

phasic muscles Muscles that are anaerobic and contract at higher speeds and with greater force than tonic muscles; they fatigue more quickly. They are better suited for short-duration, high-intensity activities.

pigmented villonodular tenosynovitis Another name for a giant-cell tumor.

pillar pain Pain experienced on either side of a carpal tunnel incision. The exact etiology is unknown; it may be secondary to ligamentous or muscle irritation following surgery or to an alteration in the carpal arch. It usually lessens in intensity within the first year after surgery.

pilomotor Changes affect the goosebump flesh appearance of skin; *pilus* is Latin for "hair."

pincer grasp See *two-point pinch*.

PIP contracture See *proximal interphalangeal (PIP) flexion contracture*.

pitting edema Soft edema that stays depressed after pressure placed on the edematous tissue has been removed. The depressed area is referred to as "pitting."

place and active hold Gentle application of passive motion followed by an attempt by the client to maintain that position after removing the passive assistance. Also called *place and hold exercises*.

place and hold exercises See *place and active hold*.

plane synovial joint Joint with a synovium-lined capsule and relatively flat surfaces.

plexuses Networks of nerves. There are four plexuses of nerves in the human body; the two largest are the brachial plexus and the lumbar plexus.

plyometrics Exercises that link strength and speed of movement to produce an explosive-reactive type of muscle response.

polyneuropathy Bilateral damage to more than one peripheral nerve. Peripheral polyneuropathy may involve the feet as well as the hands.

positive ulnar variance A condition in which the ulna is longer than it should be when compared to the radius. In this scenario, the ulna may impinge on the triangular fibrocartilage complex (TFCC), particularly during forearm rotation. This kinematic alteration can cause a "wear and tear" injury to the TFCC, thus compromising ulnar wrist stability.

posterior interosseus nerve (PIN) This motor nerve branch of the radial nerve courses deep beneath the supinator muscle, traveling through the radial tunnel of the forearm. This tunnel is about 3 to 4 fingerbreadths in length, lying along the anterior aspect of the proximal radius. An injury to this motor branch will spare the radial wrist extensors, which receive their innervation above the level of the elbow joint.

posterolateral rotatory instability Recurrent partial displacement of the ulnohumeral and radiohumeral joints related to external rotation of the ulna on the trochlea of the humerus

posterolateral rotatory subluxation Transient partial displacement of the ulnohumeral and radiohumeral joints related to external rotation of the ulna on the trochlea of the humerus.

post-test probability The probability of the condition being present compared to pretesting.

postural fault Deviations from the normal function and structure of the body; contributes to pain and disability.

power grasp Uses the whole hand with thumb flexion or abduction according to the control needed for the task.

precision grasp Uses opposition of the thumb to the fingertips.

prehensile movements Grasping an object. Can be subdivided into precision grasp and power grasp.

premorbid Prior to injury.

primary dressing A dressing that makes direct contact with the wound.

primary healing Following fracture, the use of an internal rigid device that permits direct regrowth of bone across the fracture line allows the fracture to bypass the formation of callus and heal directly with bone tissue. The internal rigid stability offered by a plate and/or screws serves as a substitute external callus, providing the motionless environment required for bone healing.

primary instability Often a combination of global capsular laxity and pathological imbalances of the rotator cuff and shoulder muscles.

primary intention When a wound is closed with sutures or staples, it is said to heal by primary intention.

primary nerve repair Surgical repair of a severed nerve performed within a week of the injury.

procollagen Precursor of collagen.

proliferative phase of wound healing The second phase of wound healing in which the body begins to fill in the open space created by the wound.

pronator syndrome A condition caused by compression of the median nerve in the proximal forearm, characterized by diffuse pain in the medial forearm.

proper collateral ligament (PCL) of the proximal interphalangeal (PIP) joint Originates on the lateral aspect of the condyles of the proximal phalanx. The fibers insert volarly and distally on the middle phalanx lateral tubercles.

proprioception Awareness of joint position.

proprioception exercises Activities to enhance position and movement sense/control

proteoglycans Molecules that are fundamental components of connective tissue. They are composed of sugars linked to polypeptides and are found in the tissues and organs of the body.

proximal interphalangeal (PIP) flexion contracture A condition in which the PIP joint of the finger is unable to be extended passively.

proximal radioulnar joint Articulation between the radial head and the radial notch of the proximal ulna.

proximal transverse arch of the hand The more proximal of the two bony transverse arches of the hand. These arches contribute to the normal resting posture (palmar concavity) of the hand and to normal hand function. The proximal transverse arch is located at the carpus, which has a deep palmar concavity created by the interlocking carpal bones.

pseudarthrosis A false joint that occurs at the site of a nonunion fracture if there is any shearing force present. Abnormal shearing force stimulates undifferentiated mesenchymal cells to produce cartilage at the fracture site.

pseudoboutonnière An injury to the proximal interphalangeal (PIP) volar plate, usually the result of a PIP hyperextension injury. The pathology occurs to the volar surface.

psychogenic tremors A somatization disorder that appears unintentionally and without conscious client awareness of motivation, with shaking of the limbs or body that can appear exaggerated, often improving when the client is distracted.

psychometric properties Validity, reliability, and responsiveness of an instrument.

pulsatile A description for a tumor in which a pulse is palpable.

pump point stimulation A method of simultaneously massaging two groups of nodes, bundles of lymphatic vessels, or watershed areas (anatomical drainage dividing areas), which theoretically speeds up the movement of lymph through the nodes.

purulence A viscous, yellowish-white colored pus that indicates infection.

purulent exudate Pus-like wound drainage. Can be thick or thin and ranges in color from tan to yellow.

purulent flexor tenosynovitis Flexor sheath infections. Another term for purulent flexor tenosynovitis is *pyogenic flexor tenosynovitis*.

pyogenic granuloma A type of acquired vascular tumor that presents as a red mass that bleeds easily; thought to be caused by a trauma.

quadriga effect Exemplified by the shared muscle belly of the flexor digitorum profundus (FDP). When trying to make a fist, if one digit is stiff, the ability to actively flex other digits is limited.

qualitative Subjective information; often consists of client narratives.

quantitative Variables that are measured in a standardized fashion and result in numeric data.

radial head Eminence on the proximal end of the radius.

radial notch Recess on the proximal ulna that articulates with the radial head.

radial tunnel syndrome (RTS) A condition caused by compression of the radial nerve in the proximal forearm and characterized by dull aching or burning pain along the lateral forearm.

radiocarpal joint The articulation between the distal radius and the scaphoid and lunate.

radiohumeral joint Articulation between the radial head and the capitellum of the distal humerus.

reach Moving and extending the arm for placing or grasping an object.

reduction The realigned position of a displaced fracture.

referred pain Pain that originates from an area other than where it presents.

reflex disturbance Abnormal action of the cell, tissue organ, or organism caused by overstimulation or understimulation.

regional measures Instruments designed to demonstrate changes at the systems level.

reliability The degree of consistency with which an instrument or rater measures a variable.

remodeling phase of bone healing The final phase of bone healing following fracture. Repaired bone tissue is replaced and reorganized over months to years to provide the bone with its preinjury strength and structure. Otherwise known as the *maturation phase*.

repair phase of bone healing The second phase of bone healing following fracture. During this phase, the damaged cells (including the hematoma) are removed and replaced with callus bone. This callus is gradually converted to bone tissue by a process of mineralization called *enchondral ossification*.

repetitive task-specific training Takes a typical task completed in daily life (such as drinking from a glass) and breaks the task into the smaller parts required to complete it successfully. The individual is then taught small components of the movement needed to do the task (such as straightening out their elbow over and over again).

replant An amputated finger, hand, or arm is reattached surgically to re-establish viability and function.

resistance maximal (RM) Maximum resistance that a group of muscles can overcome once (1 RM).

responsiveness The ability of a test to demonstrate change. It often is referred to as sensitivity to (clinical) change and is established if change in scores accurately represents change in clinical status.

revascularization A surgical procedure to repair severed arteries or veins to restore blood supply to a limb.

reverse blocking exercises Exercises that hold the metacarpophalangeal (MP) joint in flexion while the interphalangeal (IP) joints are extended actively to maximize the extension force to the IP joints.

reverse catch-up clunk Often demonstrated under fluoroscopy as the wrist moves from ulnar deviation back to neutral. This clunk pattern represents the wrist returning to its original subluxated position.

rheumatoid arthritis (RA) A chronic, systemic disease characterized by synovial inflammation.

rheumatoid nodules These nodules are made up of granulomatous and fibrous tissue and are seen in 50% of all clients with rheumatoid arthritis. They are often largest at the elbow joint.

Rolando fracture Comminuted, intra-articular fracture of the first metacarpal base. It consists of three distinct fragments in either a "Y" or a "T" shape.

Romberg sign Indicates a loss of position sense; the patient loses balance when standing erect with the feet together and the eyes closed. Also called *Romberg test*.

rotator interval The region between the superior edge of the subscapularis and anterior edge of the supraspinatus tendons.

rubor Redness.

safe position Wrist in slight extension, the metacarpophalangeal (MP) joints in flexion, and the interphalangeal (IP) joints in extension. Also known as the *intrinsic plus position*.

sagittal plane A vertical plane that divides the body into right and left halves.

SAM protocol See *short arc motion (SAM) protocol*.

sanguinous exudate Thin, bright red, bloody wound drainage.

Saturday night palsy A radial nerve injury at the humeral level that results from compression from some hard external source; a classic example of a neuropractic lesion.

scaphoid non-union advanced collapse (SNAC) wrist A complication resulting from a scaphoid fracture that does not heal.

scapholunate advanced collapse (SLAC) wrist: a degenerative wrist condition affecting the radiocarpal and midcarpal joints that presents as instability, arthritis, and deformity.

scapholunate joint A joint formed from the scaphoid and lunate, found in the proximal carpal row of the wrist.

scaption Elevation of the arm in the plane of the scapula.

scapular kinematics Scapular movement in sequence and proportion to humeral movement.

scapulo-thoracic rhythm The way the scapula moves on the thorax and the humerus works with the scapula to achieve full elevation of the arm.

scar contraction Process of scar becoming tighter during healing.

scar contracture Tight scar limiting mobility.

Schwann cell A glial cell found only in the peripheral nervous system (PNS) that provides the myelin that envelops the nerve's axon.

schwannomas Another name for a *neurilemoma*.

scientific nomenclature systems Systems that successfully and accurately sort items and often utilize organizational structures that progressively move from comprehensive to fine detail. The scientific classification that groups living biological entities into eight hierarchal taxonomic ranks (life, domain, kingdom, phylum, class, order, family, genus, and species) is an excellent example of this type of ranked classification system.

secondary dressing A dressing placed over a primary dressing to either hold the primary dressing in place or absorb any exudate that leaks out from under the primary dressing.

secondary healing The ordered process of bone tissue repair and reorganization orchestrated by a cascade of signaling factors. It involves an intermediate phase in which connective tissue or callus is formed first and then is replaced by bone. Also known as *callus healing*, *indirect healing*, or *enchondral ossification*.

secondary intention The process of healing an open wound that is not surgically repaired, whereby it closes itself over time.

secondary nerve repair See *delayed nerve repair*.

segments The line between two points (joints) represented by dotted lines on the bone.

semi-occlusive dressing A dressing that generally does not allow the passage of water or bacteria through the material but allows the passage of water vapor.

sensitivity Few, if any, clients with the disease will have negative test results—a negative test rules out the condition.

sensorimotor Of, relating to, or involving both sensory and motor activity.

sensory ataxia Loss of coordination caused by loss of sensory input into the control of movement.

sequestrum Necrosis of the bone.

serial casting The use of a series of progressive casts to increase muscle length using low-load prolonged stress to contracted tissues. The casts are replaced at intervals, allowing the tissue to respond to increasing lengthened positions.

serial static othoses Orthoses that position the tissue for lengthening. They are remolded periodically.

serosanguinous exudate Pink, thin, blood-tinged wound drainage.

serous exudate Clear, thin, watery wound drainage.

shaft The diaphysis of the bone.

sharp debridement The use of any sharp instrument to remove necrotic tissue.

shift Moving an object linearly on the finger surface on radial side of the hand in order to reposition it on the finger pads. Repositioning a pen after grasping it is an example.

short arc motion (SAM) protocol A protocol designed by Evans that allows a controlled amount of active motion of a repaired tendon to achieve tendon gliding.

simple elbow dislocation Joint displacement without associated fracture.

simple rotation Turning or rolling an object less than or equal to 90° in the finger pads. Opening a small bottle cap is an example.

skier's thumb Injury to the ulnar collateral ligament (UCL) of the thumb metacarpophalangeal (MP) joint. If it is chronic, it is called gamekeeper's thumb.

sliding filament theory The cross-bridges on the myosin filament attach to the active site on the actin filament. When all of the cross-bridges in a muscle shorten in a single cycle, the muscle shortens by approximately 1%. Muscles have the capacity to shorten up to 60% of their resting length; therefore the contraction cycle must be repeated multiple times.

slough Soft, yellow-white, moist dead tissue in a wound made of fibrin, bacteria, dead cells, and wound exudate.

Smith fracture A complete fracture of the distal radius with palmar displacement of the distal fragment. It is the second most commonly seen distal radius fracture, and it is frequently unstable.

SNAC wrist See *scaphoid non-union advanced collapse (SNAC) wrist*.

soft end feel Quality of a spongy feel at passive joint end-range. This is favorable for potential to improve.

soft tissue sarcoma A malignant tumor that originates in muscle and connective tissues. They are rarely seen in the forearm and hand.

soma The nerve cell body; the metabolic center of the cell.

somatization disorders Persistent or recurrent symptoms with no measurable or objective medical evidence of impairment.

spasticity Clinical spasticity is velocity dependent resistance to stretch, where a lack of inhibition results in excessive contraction of the muscles, ultimately leading to hyperflexia (overly flexed joints).

specificity All persons who do not have the disease have negative test results—a positive test rules in the condition.

spherical grasp Incorporates wrist extension, digital abduction, some metacarpophalangeal (MP) and interphalangeal (IP) flexion, such as in holding a tennis ball. Requires control and balance of the intrinsic and extrinsic muscles.

spinal nerve A peripheral nerve formed from the sensory and motor nerve roots of a spinal segment that join together just as the nerve fibers leave the intervertebral foramen of the spinal column.

spiritual The way in which persons understand their lives in view of their ultimate meaning and value was the definition of spirituality proposed by McLain, Rosenfeld, and Breitbart.

split-thickness skin graft (STSG) Graft of epidermis and partial layer of dermis.

squamous cell carcinoma A malignant epithelial tumor, which may spread to deeper tissues.

standard precautions Guidelines from the Centers for Disease Control and Prevention for reducing the risk of transmission of body fluid pathogens in health care settings.

Starling equilibrium A balanced movement of fluid out of the arteriole, into the interstitium, and back into the venule or lymphatic vessel functioning on a gradient system from high to low pressure.

static orthosis Used to immobilize tissues, prevent deformity, prevent contracture of soft tissue, and provide substitution for motor function.

static posture A stationary position held against gravity.

static progressive orthoses Orthoses that apply mobilizing force using non-moving parts, such as monofilament, Velcro, or screws.

steady-state respiratory rate When the level of intensity of exercise enables one to sustain equilibrium of the respiratory system that can be maintained over time.

Stener lesion Proximal displacement of the thumb meta-carpophalangeal (MP) ulnar collateral ligament (UCL) with interposition of the adductor aponeurosis. This injury requires surgical correction because the interposition prevents healing of the ligament.

stereognosis The faculty of perceiving and understanding the form and nature of objects by the sense of touch.

strain Result of stress and is expressed mathematically as the change in length of soft tissue ÷ original length × 100.

stress Amount of force per unit area (that is, pressure) applied to soft tissue.

stress relaxation A decrease in stress after a material is initially strained and then held under moderate tension for a long time.

stroke The sudden death of brain cells in a localized area due to inadequate blood flow.

subcutaneous ulnar nerve transposition A surgical procedure where the ulnar nerve is transferred anteriorly and positioned below the subcutaneous fascia of the anterior forearm, medial to the median nerve.

submuscular ulnar nerve transposition Surgical procedure that involves moving the ulnar nerve and placing it in a well-vascularized muscular bed in the volar forearm. It involves separating the flexor-pronator muscle origin, then reattaching it to its origin on the medial epicondyle.

subungual hematoma Hematoma beneath the nail that causes throbbing and pain.

sudomotor A term meaning "sweating."

superficial partial-thickness burn Burn involving the epidermis and possibly portions of the upper dermis.

Superior Labral tear Anterior to Posterior (SLAP) lesions Hypothesized to be a result of increased torsional force from the biceps tendon that "peels back" the biceps and posterior labrum from the glenoid rim. The SLAP lesion then enhances the dynamic and static instability of the already unstable shoulder.

supraclavicular scalenectomy Surgical removal of the anterior scalene.

swan neck deformity Finger posture with proximal interphalangeal (PIP) joint hyperextension and distal interphalangeal (DIP) joint flexion. The metacarpophalangeal (MP) joint tends to be flexed.

synovial Pertaining to the lubricating fluid of the joints.

synovial bursa Structure containing synovial fluid surrounding tendons as they cross under pulley systems. The synovial bursa allows smooth gliding of the tendons with less friction, and provides nutrition to the tendon.

synovitis Inflammation of the synovial tissues, which can result in pain.

systemic lupus erythematosus A systemic autoimmune disease characterized by diverse clinical symptoms caused by inflammation and blood vessel abnormalities.

tendinitis An acute inflammatory response to injury of a tendon that produces the classical signs of heat, swelling, and pain. Also known as *tendonitis*.

tendinopathy Pathological changes to a tendon.

tendinosis Another term for *angiofibroblastic hyperplasia* or *angiofibroblastic tendinosis*.

tendon gliding Distance that the tendon travels when the muscle contracts; the amount of excursion depending on the location of the tendon.

tendonitis Tendon injury with classical signs of heat, swelling, and pain. Involved structures are painful with resistance and with passive stretch. Also known as *tendinitis*.

tenodesis Automatic movement of a joint produced by a more proximal joint; for example, wrist extension and finger flexion. Surgery can enhance or create a tenodesis effect by rerouting the transected tendon across a more proximal joint and attaching it more proximally.

tenosynovitis Inflammation of the synovial lining of the tendon sheath, which can affect digit motion and strength.

tensile strength The amount of force required to break a tendon. The tensile strength of a tendon gradually increases following injury and repair.

terrible triad of the elbow Elbow dislocation with associated fractures of the radial head and coronoid.

TERT See *total end range time (TERT)*.

tertiary intention Occasionally, a surgeon will leave a wound open after the irrigation and debridement procedure with the plan to return the client to surgery for wound closure in a few days. This is known as *delayed primary wound closure,* and the wound is said to heal through tertiary intention.

tetraplegia Replaces the term *quadriplegia,* which involves injury to the spinal cord in the cervical region with associated loss of muscle strength in all four extremities.

thermal capsulorrhaphy Selective heating of portions of the joint capsule, resulting in capsular shrinkage.

thoracic duct The lymphatic system culminates in this duct, the largest lymphatic structure.

three-jaw chuck See *three-point pinch.*

three-point pinch Thumb opposes the index and middle finger pads simultaneously. This pinch provides better prehension stability than does two-point pinch. Also called *three-jaw chuck.*

time-dependent sensitization (TDS) Repeated stressful episodes make an individual increasingly sensitive to low-level environmental stimuli.

Tinel sign A temporary tingling sensation experienced with percussion over an injured and/or healing nerve. Also known as *Hoffman-Tinel's sign.*

tip pinch Opposition of the tips of the thumb and index finger with all joints of the thumb and index finger partially flexed, forming a circle.

tone Continuous and passive/partial contraction of the muscle; the muscle's resistance to passive stretch during the resting state.

tonic muscles The primary dynamic joint stabilizers. Their nutrition comes primarily from delivery of oxygen. They are predominantly type I or slow-twitch muscles and are responsible for sustaining joint arthrokinematics over time.

total body surface area (TBSA) Estimate of burn extent relative to client's entire body surface.

total elbow arthroplasty Replacement of the ulnohumeral joint with a prosthetic joint.

total end range time (TERT) Amount of time a joint is passively held at its end range. In theory, increased passive range of motion (PROM) of a stiff joint is directly proportional to the duration of the application of the mobilizing orthotic intervention.

tract A bundle of pathway axons located in the central nervous system.

transpersonal caring relationship The type of relationship that connotes the sharing of authentic self between individuals and within groups in a reflective frame. It conveys a concern for the inner world of another. All parties are changed within the relationship.

transpersonal self Being able to know one's source of strength and meaning and being able and willing to tap into that strength while never assuming the client shares in these values. This approach requires that the therapist be able to sustain healthy personal boundaries and put aside personal concerns in order to care for the client.

transudate edema An edema found in early stages of inflammation or tissue injury when high capillary permeability of vessels has not occurred. It consists mainly of dissolved electrolytes and water molecules.

transverse arch of the hand A transversely oriented bony arch of the hand composed of the proximal transverse arch and distal transverse arch. The proximal transverse arch is at the level of the carpometacarpal (CMC) joint with the keystone being the capitate. The distal transverse arch is at the level of the metacarpophalangeal (MP) joints with the keystone being the second and third metacarpals.

transverse retinacular ligament (TRL) Arises from the lateral band volar surface, envelops the collateral ligaments, and inserts into flexor tendon sheath at the proximal interphalangeal (PIP) joint, thereby preventing lateral band dorsal displacement.

triangular fibrocartilage complex (TFCC) A hammocklike structure composed of cartilage and ligaments. It suspends the ulnar carpus and acts as both a force distributor between the ulnar head and triquetrum and a primary stabilizer for the distal radioulnar joint (DRUJ).

trigger point Palpable taut muscle bands that refer pain when compressed.

triggering Limited digital range of motion (ROM) caused by dragging of the flexor tendon as it passes through a pulley. The tendon may click or lock during ROM.

trochlea Spool-shaped region on the medial aspect of the distal end of the humerus that articulates with the trochlear notch of the ulna.

trochlear notch Rounded articular surface formed by the coronoid and olecranon of the proximal ulna, also known as the *semilunar* or *greater sigmoid notch.*

trophic changes Changes in tissue characterized by abnormal hair growth, nail bed changes, cold intolerance, and soft tissue atrophy (most notably at the fingertip pulps).

tropocollagen The basic molecular unit of collagen fibrils composed of three polypeptide chains.

tuft The distal end of the terminal phalanx of the digit.

tumor Swelling.

tunneling Narrow channels of open space (tissue damage) extending off the main wound cavity into other tissues beneath intact skin.

two-point pinch Thumb opposes only the index finger. Also called *pad-to-pad pinch* or *pincer grasp.*

type III deformity Categorized by Nalebuff, the thumb deformity includes metacarpal adduction, metacarpophalangeal (MP) joint hyperextension, carpometacarpal (CMC) subluxation, and distal joint flexion. The CMC joint slides out of its place on the trapezium during pinch activities.

ulnar impingement syndrome Another name for *ulnocarpal abutment syndrome.*

ulnar nerve Nerve arising from the medial cord of the brachial plexus and innervating the majority of the intrinsic muscles of the hand, as well as providing cutaneous sensation to the medial border of the hand and to the fifth and medial half of the fourth digits.

ulnar tunnel syndrome Compression of the ulnar nerve at the wrist within Guyon's canal. Also called *entrapment at Guyon's canal.*

ulnocarpal abutment syndrome A syndrome that can develop when the ulna is longer in comparison to the radius and it impinges on the triangular fibrocartilage complex (TFCC) and ulnar carpus during wrist and forearm motion. One often sees the development of pain and traumatic arthritis of the ulnar wrist, restricted ulnar deviation of the wrist, and diminished grip strength associated with this syndrome.

ulnohumeral joint Articulation between the trochlear notch of the proximal ulna and the trochlea of the distal humerus.

uncinate processes Wing-like projections from the superior portion of the cervical vertebrae that articulate with the inferior portion of the vertebrae above.

undermining Open space (tissue damage) directly beneath the wound margins.

uniaxial pivot joint A type of synovial joint that allows 1° of motion. An example is the distal radioulnar joint that allows rotatory motion called *supination* and *pronation*.

unstable fractures Fractures that displace spontaneously or with motion; these require some type of fixation method to ensure that healing occurs without malunion, angulation, or rotation of the bone.

valgus Away from midline of the body, abduction.

valgus instability Recurrent, elbow valgus (abduction) related to medial collateral ligament insufficiency.

validity The degree to which an instrument measures what it is intended to measure.

varus Toward midline of the body, adduction.

varus instability Recurrent, elbow varus (adduction) related to lateral collateral ligament insufficiency.

vascular tumor A tumor that directly involves the blood vessels. This type of tumor can be classified as either congenital or acquired.

vasoconstriction The act of blood vessels narrowing to reduce the amount of blood passing through.

vasodilation The act of blood vessels opening to allow more blood to pass through.

vasomotor Changes in the diameter of blood vessels with noticeable changes in the color and/or temperature of the hand.

venule The smallest venous structure.

verruca vulgaris A benign tumor of the epithelium. Also known as the *common wart.*

vertebral end plate Cartilaginous interface between the vertebral disc and the vertebral body.

visual analog scale (VAS) A continuous scale used to measure level of agreement/disagreement.

visual field hemianopsia Loss of vision in one-half of the visual field of one or both eyes.

visual field neglect A neuropsychological condition in which, after damage to one hemisphere of the brain, a deficit in attention to and awareness of one side of the body/space is observed. It is defined by the inability of a person to process and perceive stimuli on one side of the body or environment that is not due to a lack of sensation. Also known as *visual inattention.*

volar plate A fibrocartilaginous structure found in the metacarpophalangeal (MP) and interphalangeal (IP) joints that reinforce the joint capsules, enhance joint stability, and limit hyperextension.

volar plate of the proximal interphalangeal (PIP) joint See *volar plate.*

volar retinacular ganglion Retinacular cysts are a type of ganglion that develops from a tendon sheath, rather than a joint. A volar retinacular ganglion is palpable and symptomatic near the proximal inter phalangeal (PIP) joint or the metacarpophalangeal (MP) joint.

volar wrist ganglion Volar wrist ganglions are found volar to the scapholunate joint, or on the volar aspect of the wrist.

Volkmann contracture High tissue pressure causing necrosis and deoxygenation of muscles, nerves, and blood vessels. Severe edema, pain in the forearm with finger flexion, and pain with passive extension are signs of this serious emergency.

voluntary release Intentionally letting go of an object in the hand at a specific place and time.

von Recklinghausen disease Neurofibromatosis.

Waddell signs Signs of simulated or exaggerated deficits including extreme reaction to light touch (overreaction), tenderness that does not conform to established myotomal or segmental patterns, and sensory disturbances that do not conform to established dermatomal or segmental patterns.

Wallerian degeneration The breakdown of the axon distal to the site of the axon's injury.

Wartenberg sign Indicative of an ulnar nerve lesion; the fifth digit is postured in abduction and adduction to the fourth is weak or not possible. This indicates interosseous muscle weakness.

watershed areas Drainage areas within the lymphotome that slightly direct the lymph in to a different area. They are not actual structures. An analogy would be the way water flows on either side of a Continental Divide.

Watson test A test for identifying a scapholunate ligament tear or instability. Also known as the *scaphoid shift test.*

work of flexion The amount of tension developed in a tendon during active motion to overcome resistive factors (swelling, stiffness, internal friction, bulk of repair, tight pulleys).

wound contraction The act of specialized cells in the wound bed pulling the edges of the wound together making the wound smaller.

wound debris Anything embedded in the wound bed that should not be there.

wound margins The edges of a wound cavity.

wrist The common term used to describe the multiple articulations that exist between the distal radius, ulna, and eight carpal bones.

wrist drop deformity The classic deformity associated with a high radial nerve lesion. When the forearm is pronated, the wrist and digits are unable to actively extend.

wrist tenodesis exercise Exercise designed to passively move the digits and glide the tendons as a result of wrist motion. Wrist extension results in passive finger flexion due to tensioning of the flexor tendons as the wrist extends. Wrist flexion results in passive finger extension due to tensioning of the finger extensors across the wrist as it flexes.

xenograft See *heterograft.*

zero position The normal resting standing balanced position where the upper extremities align themselves in space against gravity, movement ceases, and loads are removed. The anatomical position with the arms resting at the side of the body and the forearm position is midway between supination and pronation.

Index

Note: Page numbers followed by "f" indicate figures, "t" indicate tables, and "b" indicate boxes.

Dynamic scapholunate instability
  proprioceptive reeducation in, 281–282, 281f
  therapeutic management, guideline, 282t
Dyscoordinate cocontraction, 5
Dysdiadochokinesia, 480
Dysmetria, 480
Dystonia, 474

E
Early active mobilization, for stiff hand, 466, 466f
Early controlled protected motion
  following surgical repair, 283–287
Early protective motion phase I (EPM I), 450–451
  wrist extension, 451f
  wrist flexion, 451f
Early protective motion phase II (EPM II), 451–453, 452b
  active EMP II, initiation, 452
  hook position, 452f
  tabletop position, 452f
Early protective motion protocol, 453t
Eaton radiographic classification, 385t
Eccentric exercises, 277
Eccentric muscle contraction, 120
Eccentric strengthening, design, 277
Eccentrically actions, 170
ECRB. *see* Extensor carpi radialis brevis
Edema, 2, 3f
  biological mechanism, 100
  characteristics, 57
  formation, 131
  increase, 449
  management, 100–103, 100b, 431
  measurements, 101, 230
    circumferential finger tape, usage, 57f
    volumeters, usage, 56f
  neurological hand and, 476, 476b
  observation, 57
  palpation, 57
  related to wound healing, 100–101
  stiff hand, 461, 461b
  versus swelling, 100–102, 100b
  types, 101
Edema gloves, 102
Edematous hand, requirement, 477
Effective radiating area (ERA), 107
Elastic cartilage, 117
Elastic mobilization, 407
  orthoses, usage, 5–6
Elastic traction, usage, 356f
Elastic tubular stockinette, 102
Elasticity, 23
Elbow
  anatomy, 203–205, 203b
  biomechanics, 205, 205b
  blood vessels, 205, 205b
  carrying angle, 30
  case studies on, 216–217, 216b–217b
  clinical reasoning, diagnosis-specific
    information (impact), 207–208, 208b
  complex dislocation, 208
  contracture release, 213, 214b
  diagnoses, 203–218
  distal humeral fractures, 205–206
  evaluation of, 207–208
  extension, forearm pronation, 211f
  flexion, contracture, 205
  fractures, 205–207
    consolidation, 206
  function, 203, 203b
  hinged external fixator, 211
  hyperextension, 192f
  joint, 203
    anterior/posterior views, 204f

Elbow (*Continued*)
  lateral collateral ligament complexes, 204, 204f
  lateral epicondylosis (tennis elbow), 312–313
  ligaments, 204, 204b
  limited motion of, static progressive orthoses
    for, 94, 95f
  medial collateral ligament complexes, 204, 204f
  motion exercises, 208b
  muscles, 205
  nerves, 205, 205b
  nonoperative treatment, 206
  olecranon fractures, 205, 205b
  operative treatment, 206–207, 207b
  orthoses, 208b
  posterolateral rotatory instability, 210
  posterolateral rotatory subluxation, 208
  radial head fractures, 205, 205b
  repair, 235
  serial static elbow extension orthosis, 213,
    214b–215b
  simple dislocation, 208, 209b
  stability, 206
  stable fractures, 207b
  static progressive elbow extension orthosis,
    214b–215b
  static progressive elbow flexion orthosis,
    214b–215b
  stiff, 212–214, 213b
    clinical reasoning, diagnosis-specific
      information (impact), 214–216, 214b,
      216b
    cocontraction, 213
    end range positioning, thermal modalities
      (combination), 215b
    evaluation tips of, 214–216
    fibrosis, 213
    hypertrophy, 212–213
    interposition arthroplasty, 213–214
    nonoperative treatment of, 213
    operative treatment of, 213–214, 214b
    orthoses, 214b–215b
    osteophytes, 213
    timelines/healing of, 213
  terrible triad of, 210
  timelines and healing, 206
  valgus instability, 210
  varus instability, 210
Elbow dislocation, 208–209
  clinical reasoning, diagnosis-specific
    information (impact), 209–210, 210b
  evaluation tips of, 209–210
  nonoperative treatment of, 209
  operative treatment of, 209, 209b
  orthoses, 209b–210b
  timelines/healing of, 209, 209b
Elbow hemiarthroplasty, 206–207
Elbow instability, 210–211
  clinical reasoning, diagnosis-specific
    information (impact), 212, 212b
  evaluation tips of, 212
  non-operative treatment of, 210–211
  operative treatment of, 211, 211b
  orthoses, 212b
  timelines/healing of, 210, 210b
Elbow tendinopathies
  anatomy of, 311
  case study on, 318–319
  diagnosis of, 312
  general pathology of, 311, 311b
Electrical stimulation, 102–103, 109–110, 109b
  functional, 109–110, 111f
  for muscle reeducation, 109
  neuromuscular, 109–110, 111f
  for pain management, 110–112

Electrical stimulation (*Continued*)
  Russian current, 110
  for scar remodeling, 110
  usage, 109, 109f, 109b
  for wound healing, 110
Electromyogram, neuromuscular electrical
  stimulation with, 482b–485b
Elevated arm stress test (EAST), 180
  test position for, 183f
Elevation, 101
Emotional display, regulation, 144
Emotional labor, 144
  narrative example, 144
  therapist reflection, 144
Empathy, 134, 134b
Empty can test, 198f
Enchondral ossification, 254–255
Enchondroma, 441, 441f
End range positioning, thermal modalities
  (combination), 215b
Endoneurial tube, 222
Endoneurium, 221
Endoscopic release, 245
Endosteum, 254–255, 299–300
Endurance, term (usage), 120
Energy
  requirements, age (effects), 121f
  total daily energy requirements, 121f
Enzymatic debridement, 157
Epidermal inclusion cyst, 440
Epidermis, 154, 404
  skin component, 155f
Epineurium, 221
Epiphyses, 300
Epithelialization, 155
Epithelium, benign tumors of, 441
EPL tendinitis, 312
Eponychia, 418
  inflammation, 418f
"Eponychial marsupialization," 422
Erector spinae, 38–39
Erythema (rubor), 164, 416
Eschar, 49, 156
"Escharotomy," 408
Essex-Lopresti lesion, 205b
European League Against Rheumatism (EULAR),
  386
Evidence-based practice, 15–20
  differential diagnosis, 17–19
  steps to, 15–17
Evidence hierarchy, 16, 16t
Excitability, 23
Excursion, 366
Exercise
  client education, 126, 126b
  concentric aspects, 123
  concentric exercise, 126
  considerations, 116
  core/proximal stabilization exercises, 125
  dose, calculation (example), 122f
  dosing, 120–121, 120b
    calculation, 121
  eccentric aspects, 123
  functional qualities, 120
  hypomobilities, progressions, 123–124
  isometric exercise, 126
  length-tension, relationship/implications,
    122–123
  orthosis, usage, 6, 7f–8f
  osteoporosis, 120–126
  perceived exertion
    rate, 125
    scales, Borg Rate, 125t
  program